Delmar's Drug Reference for Health Care Professionals

Delmar's Drug Reference for Health Care Professionals

SYLVIA NOBLES, CMA, MSN, CRNP

Former Director, Medical Assisting
Trenholm State Technical College
Montgomery, AL

Consultant

DELMAR
THOMSON LEARNING™

Australia Canada Mexico Singapore Spain United Kingdom United States

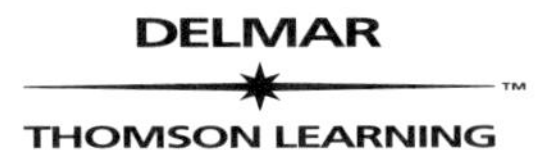

Health Care Publishing Director:
William Brottmiller

Executive Editor:
Cath L. Esperti

Acquisitions Editor:
Maureen Muncaster

Developmental Editor:
Marjorie A. Bruce

Editorial Assistant:
Jill Korznat

Executive Marketing Manager:
Dawn F. Gerrain

Database Program Manager:
Linda J. Helfrich

Project Editor:
Mary Ellen Cox

Production Editor:
James Zayicek

Art/Design Coordination:
Connie Lundberg-Watkins

Printed in the United States of America
3 4 5 XXX 05 04

For more information, contact Delmar,
3 Columbia Circle, PO Box 15015,
Albany, NY 12212-0515

Or you can visit our Internet site at
http://www.delmar.com

ISBN: 0-7668-2523-X

Notice to the Reader

The publisher and the authors do not warrant or guarantee any of the products described herein or perform any independent analysis in connection with any of the product information contained herein. The publisher and the authors do not assume and expressly disclaim any obligation to obtain and include information other than that provided by the manufacturer.

The reader is expressly warned to consider and adopt all safety precautions that might be indicated by the activities described herein and to avoid all potential hazards. By following the instructions contained herein, the reader willingly assumes all risks in connection with such instructions.

The publisher and the authors make no representations or warranties of any kind, including but not limited to the warranties of fitness for a particular purpose or merchantability nor are any such representations implied with respect to the material set forth herein, and the publisher and the authors take no responsibility with respect to such material. The publisher and the authors shall not be liable for any special, consequential, or exemplary damages resulting, in whole or in part, from the reader's use of, or reliance upon, this material.

The authors and publisher have made a conscientious effort to ensure that the drug information and recommended dosages in this book are accurate and in accord with accepted standards at the time of publication. However, pharmacology and therapeutics are rapidly changing sciences, so readers are advised, before administering any drug, to check the package insert provided by the manufacturer for the recommended dose, for any contraindications for administration, and for any added warnings and precautions. This recommendation is especially important for new, infrequently used, or highly toxic drugs.

Acknowledgments

This drug reference was developed from the database for ***Delmar's Nurse's Drug Handbook*** by George R. Spratto, PhD (Dean and Professor of Pharmacology, School of Pharmacy, West Virginia University, Morgantown, West Virginia) and Adrienne L. Woods, MSN, ARNP, FNP-C (Family Nurse Practitioner, Primary Care, at the Department of Veterans Affairs Medical and Regional Office Center, Wilmington, Delaware).

We would like to thank the Delmar team who kept us on schedule, taught us all sorts of computer skills, and gave invaluable guidance at all phases of the process. An extra special thanks goes to Marge Bruce for all of her patience, guidance, and support. Other Delmar team members include Maureen Muncaster, Mary Ellen Cox, James Zayicek, and Connie Lundberg-Watkins. Thank you one and all. Thanks are also extended to Datapage Technologies International, Inc. for their excellent work.

Sylvia Nobles extends appreciation to my colleagues and family members Alan K. Nobles, CRNA and Dawnita Granger, RN, BSN who both assisted in numerous areas of refinement of the project. Special appreciation is extended to Fayyaz A. Malik, M.D., Chief of Adult Medicine, Health Services, Inc. for his time in reviewing the drug listings for the book.

The author and Delmar team also want to thank J. A. Johnson, RPh for the many hours he devoted to reviewing, researching, and verifying content for the drug monographs.

Preface

Health care professionals encounter many challenges due to the information explosion of the 21st century. Perhaps the largest volume of information is to be found in the continually expanding area of medications. Not only are new medications introduced to the market at a more rapid pace, but information on new and revised uses and dosages, side effects, drug interactions, and new forms/administration procedures for current and older medications is also provided by drug manufacturers at an accelerated rate.

Delmar's Drug Reference for Health Care Professionals provides a concise yet thorough source of drug information for a wide variety of health care professionals, from medical assistants and medical transcriptionists to nurse practitioners and physician assistants.

The Drug Reference is organized for quick access to information on drug classifications in Chapter 2 and to A-Z drug monographs in Chapter 3. Drugs listed in Chapter 3 are identified by generic name. The Drug Reference was developed with the varied needs of health care professionals in mind.

Features of the Drug Reference include:

- Dosage forms and routes are clearly presented and are connected, when appropriate, with the target disease state.
- Boldface italics highlight life-threatening side effects of drug therapy.
- "Overdose Management" section for selected drugs provides a quick reference to symptoms and treatment of overdose.
- "Health Care Considerations" are presented in a problem-solving process format, with assessment, intervention, teaching, and evaluation guidelines all clearly identified. Specific criteria for evaluating the outcomes of drug therapy are provided in the "Outcomes/Evaluate" section.
- The section "Using the Drug Reference" outlines the content of each section of the drug monographs and provides a quick "how-to-use" overview.
- Numerous appendices provide useful, supplemental information for the health care professional.

QUICK GUIDE TO THE USE OF *DELMAR'S DRUG REFERENCE FOR HEALTH CARE PROFESSIONALS*

An understanding of the format of this drug reference will help you find information quickly.

- There are three chapters:
  1. Detailed information on how to use *Delmar's Drug Reference for Health Care Professionals*
  2. Alphabetical listing of many therapeutic/chemical drug classes with general information for the class, plus a listing of drugs in the class covered in Chapter 3
  3. Alphabetical listing of drugs by generic name

The individual entries follow a similar format. All items listed below may not appear in each drug entry but are represented where appropriate and when information is available.

General drug information (similar in format to Chapter 2) includes the following categories:

— COMBINATION DRUG HEADING indicates when two or more drugs are combined in the same product

— GENERIC NAME OF DRUG

— PHONETIC PRONUNCIATION of generic name

— FDA PREGNANCY CATEGORY to which drug is assigned; see Appendix 2 for the definition of these categories

— TRADE NAME(S) by which the drug is marketed; a maple leaf (🍁) indicates that the trade name is available only in Canada

— DRUG SCHEDULE If the drug is controlled by the U. S. Controlled Substances Act, the appropriate schedule is listed. See Appendix 1 for the definition of the five schedules as well as a listing of drugs with their schedules in both the United States and Canada

— Rx = prescription drug; OTC = nonprescription, over-the-counter drug

— See also reference to classification in Chapter 2, if applicable

— CLASSIFICATION is the chemical or pharmacologic class to which the drug has been assigned

— CONTENT (for combination drugs) is the generic name and amount of each drug in the combination product

— ACTION/KINETICS The action portion describes the mechanism(s) by which a drug achieves its therapeutic effect; not all mechanisms of action are known. The kinetics portion provides information about the rate of drug absorption, distribution, minimum effective serum or plasma level, biologic half-life, duration of action, metabolism and excretion.

The time it takes for half the drug to be excreted or removed from the blood, **t½**, is important in determining how often a drug is to be administered and how long to assess for side effects. Therapeutic serum or plasma levels indicate the desired concentration for the drug to exert its beneficial effect and is helpful in predicting the possible onset of side effects, as well as achievement of the desired drug effects.

— USES are the approved therapeutic applications for the drug. Investigational uses, when available, are also listed for selected drugs.

— CONTRAINDICATIONS notes disease states or conditions for which the drug should not be used. The safe use of many of the newer pharmacologic agents during pregnancy, lactation, or childhood has not been established and therefore should generally not be used.

— SPECIAL CONCERNS cover considerations for use with pediatric, geriatric, pregnant, or lactating clients. Situations and disease states when the drug should be used with caution are also listed.

— SIDE EFFECTS include potential drug-related undesired or bothersome effects, organized by body system or organ affected. Nearly all potential side effects are listed, unless otherwise noted. In any given clinical situation, a client may show no side effects, one or two side effects, or several side effects. Life-threatening side effects are identified by bold italic print.

— OVERDOSE MANAGEMENT lists the symptoms of drug overdose. The treatment portion of this category gives approaches and/or antidotes to treat the symptoms of the drug overdose. Designated by a special icon OD.

— DRUG INTERACTIONS lists the effects and, when known, the mechanism for drugs interacting with one another. Drug interactions may result from a number of different mechanisms (e.g., additive or inhibitory effects, interference with degradation of drug, increased rate of elimination, decreased absorption from the GI tract, receptor site competition or displacement from plasma protein binding sites). Potential lethal/adverse drug interactions are noted.

Any side effects that accompany the administration of a specific drug may be increased as a result of a drug interaction.

Drug interactions are often listed for classes of drugs. Therefore drug interactions are likely to occur for all drugs in the class.

— LABORATORY TEST CONSIDERATIONS indicates the effect of the drug on laboratory test values for the client. Some of the interferences are caused by the therapeutic or toxic effects of the drugs; others result from interference with the testing method itself. Interferences are described as increased (↑) or false positive (+) and as decreased (↓) or false negative (-).

— HOW SUPPLIED lists the various dosage form(s) available for the drug and amounts of the drug in each of the dosage forms.

— DOSAGE provides adult and pediatric doses as well as the dosage forms in which the drug is available. The dosage form or route of administration is clearly shown and is often followed by the disease state (in italics) for which the particular dosage is recommended. The listed dosage is to be considered as a general prescribing guideline; the exact amount of the drug to be given is determined by the provider. However, one should always question orders or prescriptions when dosages and routes of administration differ markedly from the accepted norm.

Health Care Considerations are guidelines to help the practitioner in applying the problem solving process to pharmacotherapeutics to ensure safe practice.

- Adminisration/Storage: Guidelines to the practitioner in preparing medications for administration, administering the medication, and proper storage and disposal of the medication; specific IV route delineated by a special icon **IV** .
- Assessment: Guidelines to assist the practitioner in what to obtain, identify, and assess before, during, and after drug therapy.
- Interventions: Guidelines for specific practitioner actions related to the drug being administered.
- Client/Family Teaching: Guidelines to promote education, active participation, understanding, precautions, and adherence to drug therapy by the client or family member.
- Outcomes/Evaluate: Identifies desired outcomes of drug therapy and client response.

— ADDITIONAL CONTRAINDICATIONS, ADDITIONAL SIDE EFFECTS, or ADDITIONAL HEALTH CARE CONSIDERATIONS provide information relevant to a specific drug but not necessarily to the class overall and serves to reinforce certain areas of importance. (Also refer to Chapter 2 which contains information for the class.)

— GENERAL INDEX is extensively cross-referenced (multiple trade names and the generic name for each drug are paired); information is coded as follows:

- **boldface** = generic drug name
- *italics* = therapeutic drug class
- regular type = trade name
- CAPITALS = combination drugs

Contents

Common Sound-Alike Drug Names

The following is a list of common sound-alike drug names; trade names are capitalized. In parentheses next to each drug name is the pharmacological classification/use for the drug.

Accupril (ACE inhibitor)	Accutane (antiacne drug)
acetazolamide (antiglaucoma drug)	acetohexamide (oral antidiabetic drug)
Aciphex (proton pump inhibitor)	Accupril (ACE inhibitor)
Adriamycin (antineoplastic)	Aredia (bone growth regulator)
albuterol (sympathomimetic)	atenolol (beta-blocker)
Aldomet (antihypertensive)	Aldoril (antihypertensive)
Alkeran (antineoplastic)	Leukeran (antineoplastic) Myleran (antineoplastic)
allopurinol (antigout drug)	Apresoline (antihypertensive)
alprazolam (anti-anxiety agent)	lorazepam (anti-anxiety agent)
Ambien (sedative-hypnotic)	Amen (progestin)
amiloride (diuretic)	amlodipine (calcium channel blocker)
amiodarone (antiarrhythmic)	amrinone (inotropic agent)
amitriptyline (antidepressant)	nortriptyline (antidepressant)
Apresazide (antihypertensive)	Apresoline (antihypertensive)
Arlidin (peripheral vasodilator)	Aralen (antimalarial)
Artane (cholinergic blocking agent)	Altace (ACE inhibitor)
asparaginase (antineoplastic agent)	pegaspargase (antineoplastic agent)
Atarax (antianxiety agent)	Ativan (antianxiety agent)
atenolol (beta-blocker)	timolol (beta-blocker)
Atrovent (cholinergic blocking agent)	Alupent (sympathomimetic)
Avandia (oral hypoglycemic)	Coumadin (anticoagulant)
Avandia (oral hypoglycemic)	Prandin (oral hypoglycemic)
bacitracin (antibacterial)	Bactroban (anti-infective, topical)
Benylin (expectorant)	Ventolin (sympathomimetic)
Brevital (barbiturate)	Brevibloc (beta-adrenergic blocker)
Bumex (diuretic)	Buprenex (narcotic analgesic)
Cafergot (analgesic)	Carafate (antiulcer drug)
calciferol (Vitamin D)	calcitriol (Vitamin D)
carboplatin (antineoplastic agent)	cisplatin (antineoplastic agent)
Cardene (calcium channel blocker)	Cardizem (calcium channel blocker)
Cataflam (NSAID)	Catapres (antihypertensive)
Catapres (antihypertensive)	Combipres (antihypertensive)
cefotaxime (cephalosporin)	cefoxitin (cephalosporin)
cefuroxime (cephalosporin)	deferoxamine (iron chelator)
Celebrex (NSAID)	Cerebyx (anticonvulsant)

Celebrex (NSAID)	Celera (antidepressant)
Cerebyx (anticonvulsant)	Celera (antidepressant)
chlorpromazine (antipsychotic)	chlorpropamide (oral antidiabetic)
chlorpromazine (antipsychotic)	prochlorperazine (antipsychotic)
chlorpromazine (antipsychotic)	promethazine (antihistamine)
Clinoril (NSAID)	Clozaril (antipsychotic)
clomipramine (antidepressant)	clomiphene (ovarian stimulant)
clonidine (antihypertensive)	Klonopin (anticonvulsant)
Cozaar (antihypertensive)	Zocor (antihyperlipidemic)
cyclobenzaprine (skeletal muscle relaxant)	cyproheptadine (antihistamine)
cyclophosphamide (antineoplastic)	cyclosporine (immunosuppressant)
cyclosporine (immunosuppressant)	cycloserine (antineoplastic)
Cytovene (antiviral drug)	Cytosar (antineoplastic)
Cytoxan (antineoplastic)	Cytotec (prostaglandin derivative)
Cytoxan (antineoplastic)	Cytosar (antineoplastic)
Dantrium (skeletal muscle relaxant)	danazol (gonadotropin inhibitor)
Darvocet-N (analgesic)	Darvon-N (analgesic)
daunorubicin (antineoplastic)	doxorubicin (antineoplastic)
desipramine (antidepressant)	diphenhydramine (antihistamine)
DiaBeta (oral hypoglycemic)	Zebeta (beta-adrenergic blocker)
digitoxin (cardiac glycoside)	digoxin (cardiac glycoside)
diphenhydramine (antihistamine)	dimenhydrinate (antihistamine)
dopamine (sympathomimetic)	dobutamine (sympathomimetic)
Edecrin (diuretic)	Eulexin (antineoplastic)
enalapril (ACE inhibitor)	Anafranil (antidepressant)
enalapril (ACE inhibitor)	Eldepryl (antiparkinson agent)
Eryc (erythromycin base)	Ery-Tab (erythromycin base)
etidronate (bone growth regulator)	etretinate (antipsoriatic)
etomidate (general anesthetic)	etidronate (bone growth regulator)
Fioricet (analgesic)	Fiorinal (analgesic)
flurbiprofen (NSAID)	fenoprofen (NSAID)
folinic acid (leucovorin calcium)	folic acid (vitamin B complex)
Gantrisin (sulfonamide)	Gantanol (sulfonamide)
glipizide (oral hypoglycemic)	glyburide (oral hypoglycemic)
glyburide (oral hypoglycemic)	Glucotrol (oral hypoglycemic)
Hycodan (cough preparation)	Hycomine (cough preparation)
hydralazine (antihypertensive)	hydroxyzine (antianxiety agent)
hydrocodone (narcotic analgesic)	hydrocortisone (corticosteroid)
hydromorphone (narcotic analgesic)	morphine (narcotic analgesic)
Hydropres (antihypertensive)	Diupres (antihypertensive)
Hytone (topical corticosteroid)	Vytone (topical corticosteroid)
imipramine (antidepressant)	Norpramin (antidepressant)
Inderal (beta-adrenergic blocker)	Inderide (antihypertensive)
Inderal (beta-adrenergic blocker)	Isordil (coronary vasodilator)
Indocin (NSAID)	Minocin (antibiotic)
Lamictal (anticonvulsant)	Lamisil (antifungal)
Lanoxin (cardiac glycoside)	Lasix (diuretic)
Lantus (insulin product)	Lente insulin (insulin product)

Lioresal (muscle relaxant)	lisinopril (ACE inhibitor)
Lithostat (lithium carbonate)	Lithobid (lithium carbonate)
Lithotabs (lithium carbonate)	Lithobid (lithium carbonate)
Lodine (NSAID)	codeine (narcotic analgesic)
Lopid (antihyperlipidemic)	Lorabid (beta-lactam antibiotic)
lovastatin (antihyperlipidemic)	Lotensin (ACE inhibitor)
metolazone (thiazide diuretic)	methotrexate (antineoplastic)
metolazone (thiazide diuretic)	metoclopramide (GI stimulant)
metoprolol (beta-adrenergic blocker)	misoprostol (prostaglandin derivative)
Monopril (ACE inhibitor)	minoxidil (antihypertensive)
nelfinavir (antiviral)	nevirapine (antiviral)
Norlutate (progestin)	Norlutin (progestin)
Norvasc (calcium channel blocker)	Navane (antipsychotic)
Ocufen (NSAID)	Ocuflox (fluoroquinolone antibiotic)
Orinase (oral hypoglycemic)	Ornade (upper respiratory product)
Percocet (narcotic analgesic)	Percodan (narcotic analgesic)
paroxetine (antidepressant)	paclitaxel (antineoplastic)
Paxil (antidepressant)	paclitaxel (antineoplastic)
Paxil (antidepressant)	Taxol (antineoplastic)
penicillamine (heavy metal antagonist)	penicillin (antibiotic)
pindolol (beta-adrenergic blocker)	Parlodel (inhibitor of prolactin secretion)
Platinol (antineoplastic)	Paraplatin (antineoplastic)
Pravachol (antihyperlipidemic)	Prevacid (GI drug)
Pravachol (antihyperlipidemic)	propranolol (beta-adrenergic blocker)
prednisolone (corticosteroid)	prednisone (corticosteroid)
Prilosec (inhibitor of gastric acid secretion)	Prozac (antidepressant)
Prinivil (ACE inhibitor)	Prilosec (GE drug)
Prinivil (ACE inhibitor)	Proventil (sympathomimetic)
Procanbid (antiarrhythmic)	Procan SR (antiarrhythmic)
propranolol (beta-adrenergic blocker)	Propulsid (GI drug)
Provera (progestin)	Premarin (estrogen)
Prozac (antidepressant)	Proscar (androgen hormone inhibitor)
quinidine (antiarrhythmic)	clonidine (antihypertensive)
quinidine (antiarrhythmic)	Quinamm (antimalarial)
quinine (antimalarial)	quinidine (antiarrhythmic)
Regroton (antihypertensive)	Hygroton (diuretic)
Rifamate (antituberculous drug)	rifampin (antituberculous drug)
Rimantadine (antiviral)	flutamide (antineoplastic)
Soriatane (antipsoriasis)	Loxitane (antipsychotic)
Stadol (narcotic analgesic)	Haldol (antipsychotic)
Tegretol (anticonvulsant)	Tequin (antibacterial)
terbinafine (antifungal agent)	terfenadine (antihistamine)
terbutaline (sympathomimetic)	tolbutamide (oral hypoglycemic)
tolazamide (oral hypoglycemic)	tolbutamide (oral hypoglycemic)
torsemide (loop diuretic)	furosemide (loop diuretic)

trifluoperazine (antipsychotic)	trihexyphenidyl (antiparkinson drug)
Trimox (amoxicillin product)	Diamox (carbonic anhydrase inhibitor)
Vancenase (corticosteroid)	Vanceril (corticosteroid)
Vasosulf (sulfonamide/decongestant)	Velosef (cephalosporin)
Versed (benzodiazepine sedative)	Vistaril (antianxiety agent)
Versed (benzodiazepine sedative)	VePesid (antineoplastic)
Xanax (antianxiety agent)	Zantac (H_2 histamine blocker)
Xenical (antiobesity)	Xeloda (antineoplastic)
Zebeta (beta-blocker)	DiaBeta (oral hypoglycemic)
Zinacef (cephalosporin)	Zithromax (macrolide antibiotic)
Zocor (antihyperlipidemic)	Zoloft (antidepressant)
Zofran (antiemetic)	Zantac (H_2 histamine blocker)
Zosyn (penicillin antibiotic)	Zofran (antiemetic)
Zovirax (antiviral)	Zyvox (antibiotic)
Zyvox (antibiotic)	Vioxx (COX-2 inhibitor)

Commonly Used Abbreviations and Symbols

aa, A	of each
ABG	arterial blood gas
a.c.	before meals
ACE	angiotensin-converting enzyme
ACLS	advanced cardiac life support
ACS	acute coronary syndrome
ACTH	adrenocorticotropic hormone
ad	to, up to
a.d.	right ear
ADA	adenosine deaminase
ADD	attention deficit disorder
ADH	antidiuretic hormone
ADL	activities of daily living
ad lib	as desired, at pleasure
ADP	adenosine diphosphate
AFB	acid fast bacillus
AHF	antihemophilic factor
AIDS	acquired immune deficiency syndrome
a.l.	left ear
ALL	acute lymphocytic leukemia
ALS	amyotrophic lateral sclerosis
ALT	alanine aminotransferase
a.m., A.M.	morning
AMI	acute myocardial infarction
AML	acute myelogenous leukemia
AMP	adenosine monophosphate
ANA	antinuclear antibody
ANC	absolute neutrophil count
ANS	autonomic nervous system
APTT	activated partial thromboplastin time
aq	water
aq dist.	distilled water
ARBS	angiotensin receptor blockade agents
ARC	AIDS-related complex
ARDS	adult respiratory distress syndrome
ASA	aspirin
ASAP	as soon as possible
ASHD	arteriosclerotic heart disease
AST	aspartate aminotransferase
ATC	around the clock
ATP	adenosine triphosphate
ATS/CDC	American Thoracic Society/Centers for Disease Prevention and Control
ATU	antithrombin unit
ATX	antibiotics
a.u.	each ear, both ears
AV	atrioventricular
AVB	abnormal vaginal bleeding
b.i.d.	two times per day

b.i.n.	two times per night
BMR	basal metabolic rate
BP	blood pressure
BPD	bronchopulmonary dysplasia
BPH	benign prostatic hypertrophy
bpm	beats per minute
BS	blood sugar, bowel sounds
BSA	body surface area
BSE	breast self-exam
BSP	Bromsulphalein
BUN	blood urea nitrogen
C	Celsius/Centigrade
CABG	coronary artery bypass graft
C&DB	cough and deep breathe
CAD	coronary artery disease
caps, Caps	capsule(s)
CBC	complete blood count
CCB	calcium channel blocker
C_{CR}	creatinine clearance
CD_4	helper T_4 lymphocyte cells
CDC	Centers for Disease Control and Prevention
C&DB	cough and deep breathe
CF	cystic fibrosis
CHF	congestive heart failure
CHO	carbohydrate
CLL	chronic lymphocytic leukemia
CLS	capillary leak syndrome
cm	centimeter
CML	chronic myelocytic leukemia
CMV	cytomegalovirus
CN	cranial nerve
CNS	central nervous system
CO	cardiac output
COMT	catechol-o-methyltransferase
COPD	chronic obstructive pulmonary disease
CP	cardiopulmonary
CPAP	continuous positive airway pressure
CPB	cardiopulmonary bypass
CPK	creatine phosphokinase
CPR	cardiopulmonary resuscitation
CRF	chronic renal failure
C&S	culture and sensitivity
CSF	cerebrospinal fluid
CSID	congenital sucrase-isomaltase deficiency
CT	computerized tomography
CTS	carpal tunnel syndrome
CTZ	chemoreceptor trigger zone
CV	cardiovascular
CVA	cerebrovascular accident
CVP	central venous pressure
CXR	chest X ray
dATP	deoxy ATP
DBP	diastolic BP
dc	discontinue
DEA	Drug Enforcement Agency
DI	diabetes insipidus
DIC	disseminated intravascular coagulation
dil.	dilute
dL	deciliter (one-tenth of a liter)
DM	diabetes mellitus
DNA	deoxyribonucleic acid

DOE	dyspnea on exertion
dr.	dram (0.0625 ounce)
DTR	deep tendon reflex
DVT	deep vein thrombosis
EC	enteric-coated
ECB	extracorporeal cardiopulmonary bypass
ECG, EKG	electrocardiogram, electrocardiograph
EDTA	ethylenediaminetetraacetic acid
EEG	electroencephalogram
EENT	eye, ear, nose, and throat
EF	ejection fraction
e.g.	for example
elix	elixir
emuls.	emulsion
ENL	erythema nodosum leprosum
ENT	ear, nose, throat
EPS	electrophysiologic studies, extrapyramidal symptoms
ER	extended release
ESR	erythrocyte sedimentation rate
ESRD	end-stage renal disease
ET	endotracheal
ETOH	alcohol
ext.	extract
F	Fahrenheit, fluoride
FBS	fasting blood sugar
FDA	Food and Drug Administration
FEV	forced expiratory volume
FFP	fresh frozen plasma
FOB	fecal occult blood
FS	finger stick
FSH	follicle-stimulating hormone
F/U	follow-up
FVC	forced vital capacity
g, gm	gram (1,000 mg)
GABA	gamma-aminobutyric acid
G-CSF	granulocyte colony-stimulating factor
GERD	gastroesophageal reflux disease
GFR	glomerular filtration rate
GGT, GGTP	gamma-glutamyl transferase: *syn.* gamma-glutamyl transpeptidase
GH	growth hormone
gi, GI	gastrointestinal
GnRH	gonadotropin-releasing hormone
GP	glycoprotein
G6PD	glucose-6-phosphate dehydrogenase
gr	grain
gtt	a drop, drops
GU	genitourinary
h, hr	hour
HA, HAL	hyperalimentation
HbAlc	hemoglobin A1c
HBV	hepatitis B virus
HCG	human chorionic gonadotropin
HCP	health-care provider
HCV	hepatitis C virus
HDL	high density lipoprotein
HFN	high flow nebulizer
H&H	hematocrit and hemoglobin
HIT	heparin-induced thrombocytopenia
HIV	human immunodeficiency virus
HMG-CoA	3-hydroxy-3-methyl-glutaryl-coenzyme A
HOB	head of bed

HPV	human papillomavirus
HR	heart rate
h.s.	at bedtime
HSE	herpes simplex encephalitis
HSV	herpes simplex virus
5-HT	5-hydroxytryptamine
HTN	hypertension
IA	intra-arterial
IBD	inflammatory bowel disease
IBS	irritable bowl syndrome
IBW	ideal body weight
ICP	intracranial pressure
ICU	intensive care unit
Ig	immunoglobulin
im, IM	intramuscular
IMV	intermittent mandatory ventilation
inh	inhalation
INR	international normalized ratio
I&O	intake and output
IOP	intraocular pressure
IP	intraperitoneal
IPPB	intermittent positive pressure breathing
ITP	idiopathic thrombocytopenia purpura
IU	international units
iv, IV	intravenous
IVPB	IV piggyback, a secondary IV line
JVD	jugular venous distention
kg	kilogram (2.2 lb)
KVO	keep vein open
l, L	liter (1,000 mL)
L	left
LDH	lactic dehydrogenase
LDL	low density lipoprotein
LFTs	liver function tests
LH	luteinizing hormone
LHRH	luteinizing hormone-releasing hormone
LOC	level of consciousness
LV	left ventricular
LVEF	left ventricular ejection fraction
LVFP	left ventricular function pressure
M	molar
m^2, M^2	square meter
m	meter
MAC	*Mycobacterium avium* complex
MAO	monoamine oxidase
MAP	mean arterial pressure
max	maximum
mcg	microgram
MCH	mean corpuscular hemoglobin
mCi	millicurie
MCV	mean corpuscular volume
MDI	metered-dose inhaler
mEq	milliequivalent
mg	milligram
MI	myocardial infarction
MIC	minimum inhibitory concentration
min	minute, minim
mist, mixt	mixture
mL	milliliter
mm^3	cubic millimeter

MRI	magnetic resonance imaging
MS	multiple sclerosis
MU	million units
MUGA	multigated radionuclide angiography
NaCl	sodium chloride
ng	nanogram
NG	nasogastric
NGT	nasogastric tube
NIDDM	non-insulin dependent diabetes mellitus
NKA	no known allergies
NKDA	no known drug allergies
noct	at night, during the night
non rep	do not repeat
NPN	nonprotein nitrogen
NPO	nothing by mouth
NR	do not refill (e.g., a prescription)
NSAID	nonsteroidal anti-inflammatory drug
NSR	normal sinus rhythm
NSS	normal saline solution
NYHA	New York Heart Association
N&V	nausea and vomiting
O_2	oxygen
OC	oral contraceptive
o.d.	once a day
O.D.	right eye
OH	orthostatic hypotension
OOB	out of bed
OR	operating room
os	mouth
O.S.	left eye
O_2 sat	oxygen saturation
OTC	over the counter
O.U.	each eye, both eyes
oz	ounce
PA	pulmonary artery
PABA	para-aminobenzoic acid
PAF	paroxysmal atrial fibrillation
PAWP	pulmonary artery wedge pressure
PBI	protein-bound iodine
p.c.	after meals
PCA	patient-controlled analgesia
PCI	percutaneous coronary intervention
PCN	penicillin
PCP	*Pneumocystis carinii* pneumonia
PDE	phosphodiesterase
PE	pulmonary embolus
PEEP	positive end expiratory pressure
PEF	peak expiratory flow
per	by, through
PFTs	pulmonary function tests
pH	hydrogen ion concentration
PID	pelvic inflammatory disease
p.m., P.M.	afternoon, evening
PMH	past medical history
PMI	point of maximal intensity
PMS	premenstrual syndrome
PND	paroxysmal nocturnal dyspnea
po, p.o., PO	by mouth
PPAR	peroxisome proliferator-activated receptor
PPD	purified protein derivative

PR	by rectum
p.r.n., PRN	when needed or necessary
PSA	prostatic specific antigen
PSP	phenolsulfonphthalein
PSVT	paroxysmal supraventricular tachycardia
PT	prothrombin time
PTCA	percutaneous transluminal coronary angioplasty
PTH	parathyroid hormone
PTSD	post traumatic stress disorder
PTT	partial thromboplastin time
PUD	peptic ulcer disease
PUVA	psoralen and ulraviolet A
PVC	premature ventricular contraction; polyvinyl chloride
PVD	peripheral vascular disease
q.d.	every day
q.h.	every hour
q2hr	every two hours
q3hr	every three hours
q4hr	every four hours
q6hr	every six hours
q8hr	every eight hours
q12hr	every 12 hours
qhs	every night
q.i.d.	four times a day
qmo	every month
q.o.d.	every other day
q.s.	as much as needed, quantity sufficient
RA	right atrium; rheumatoid arthritis
RBC	red blood cell
RDA	recommended daily allowance
RDS	respiratory distress syndrome
REM	rapid eye movement
Rept.	let it be repeated
RICE	rest, ice, compression and elevation
RNA	ribonucleic acid
R/O	rule out
ROM	range of motion
ROS	review of systems
RRMS	relapsing-remitting multiple sclerosis
R/T	related to
RV	right ventricular
RUQ	right upper quadrant
Rx	symbol for a prescription
SA	sinoatrial; sustained-action
SAH	subarachnoid hemorrhage
SBE	subacute bacterial endocarditis
SBP	systolic BP
sc, SC, SQ	subcutaneous
SCID	severe combined immunodeficiency disease
SGOT	serum glutamic-oxaloacetic transaminase
SGPT	serum glutamic-pyruvic transaminase
S., Sig.	mark on the label
SI	sacroiliac
SIADH	syndrome inappropriate antidiuretic hormone
SIMV	synchronized intermittent mandatory ventilation
SL	sublingual
SLE	systemic lupus erythematosus
SOB	shortness of breath
sol	solution
sp	spirits

SR	sustained-release
ss	one-half
SSRI	selective serotonin reuptake inhibitor
S&S	signs and symptoms
stat	immediately, first dose
STD	sexually transmitted disease
SV	stroke volume
SVT	supraventricular tachycardia
syr	syrup
t½	halflife
tab	tablet
TB	tuberculosis
TCA	tricyclic antidepressant
TENS	transcutaneous electric nerve stimulation
TIA	transient ischemic attack
TIBC	total iron binding capacity
t.i.d.	three times per day
t.i.n.	three times per night
TKR	total knee replacement
TNF	tumor necrosis factor
T.O.	telephone order
TPN	total parenteral nutrition
TSH	thyroid stimulating hormone
µ	micron
µCi	microcurie
µg	microgram
µm	micrometer
µM	micromolar
U	unit
U/A	urinalysis
UGI	upper gastrointestinal
ULN	upper limit of normal
ung	ointment
UO	urine output
URI, URTI	upper respiratory infection
US	ultrasound
USP	U. S. Pharmacopeia
ut dict	as directed
UTI	urinary tract infection
UV	ultraviolet
VAD	venous access device
VF	ventricular fibrillation
vin	wine
vit	vitamin
VLDL	very low density lipoprotein
VMA	vanillylmandelic acid
V.O.	verbal order
VS	vital signs
VT	ventricular tachycardia
WBC	white blood cell
XRT	radiation therapy
&	and
>	greater than
<	less than
↑	increased, higher
↓	decreased, lower
-	negative
/	per
%	percent
+	positive
x	times, frequency

CHAPTER ONE

How To Use HCDR-2002

Delmar's Drug Reference for Health Care Professionals is intended to be a quick reference to useful information on drugs. An important objective is also to provide information on the proper monitoring of drug therapy and to assist practitioners in teaching clients and family members about important aspects of drug therapy.

Chapter 2 includes general information on important therapeutic or chemical classes of drugs. The classes of drugs are listed alphabetically. Specific drugs in therapeutic or chemical classes are found in Chapter 3 (alphabetical listing of drugs). The information on each therapeutic or chemical class in Chapter 2 begins with a list of the drugs addressed in the drug class. Information on the specific drugs is provided under that drug in Chapter 3 as well as for many other drugs.

The format for information on individual drugs (and for drug classes when appropriate) is presented as follows:

Drug Names: The generic name for the drug is presented first; this is followed by the phonetic pronunciation of the generic name. The FDA pregnancy category A, B, C, D, or X (see Appendix 3 for definitions) to which the drug is assigned is also listed in this section. All trade names follow this; if the trade name is available only in Canada, the name is followed by a maple leaf (✱). If the drug is controlled by the U.S. Federal Controlled Substances Act, the schedule in which the drug is placed follows the trade name (e.g., C-II, C-III, C-IV or I, II, III, IV, V). See Appendix 1 for a listing of controlled substances in both the United States and Canada. A combination drug heading indicates that two or more drugs are combined in the same product.

Classification: This section defines the type of drug or the class under which the drug is listed. This information is most useful in learning to categorize drugs. To minimize the need to repeat general information, a cross reference to Chapter 2 is often made for drugs listed in Chapter 3. This information should also be reviewed by the reader.

General Statement: Information about the drug class and/or what might be specific or unusual about a particular group of drugs is presented. In addition, brief information may be presented about the disease(s) for which the drugs are indicated.

Action/Kinetics: The action portion describes the proposed mechanism(s) by which a drug achieves its therapeutic effect. Not all mechanisms of action are known, and some are self-evident, as when a hormone is administered as a replacement. The kinetics portion lists pertinent pharmacologic properties, if known, about rate of drug absorption, distribution, time for peak plasma levels or peak effect, minimum effective serum or plasma level, biologic half-life, duration of action, metabolism, and excretion. Metabolism and excretion routes may be important for clients with systemic liver disease, kidney disease, or both. Again, information is not available for all therapeutic agents.

The time it takes for half the drug to be excreted or removed from the blood, **t½** (half-life), is important in determining how often a drug is to be administered and how long to assess for side effects. **Therapeutic levels** indicate the desired concentration, in serum or plasma, for the drug to exert its beneficial effect and are helpful in predicting the onset of side effects or the lack of effect. Drug therapy is often monitored in this fashion (e.g., antibiotics, theophylline, phenytoin, amiodarone). An additional feature is a listing of commonly accepted therapeutic drug levels (see Appendix 7).

Uses: Approved therapeutic use(s) for the particular drug are presented. Some investigational uses are also listed for selected drugs.

Contraindications: Disease states or conditions in which the drug should not be used are noted. The safe use of many of the newer pharmacologic agents during pregnancy, lactation, or childhood has not been established. As a general rule, the use of drugs during pregnancy is contraindicated unless specified by the provider where the benefits of drug therapy far outweigh the potential risks.

Special Concerns: This section covers considerations for use with pediatric, geriatric, pregnant, or lactating clients. Situations and disease states when the drug should be used with caution are also listed.

Side Effects: Undesired or bothersome effects the client *may* experience while taking a particular agent are described. Side effects are listed by the body organ or system affected and are usually presented with the most common side effects in descending order of incidence. It is important to note that nearly all of the potential side effects are listed; in any given clinical situation, however, a client may show no side effects, or one or more side effects. If potentially life threatening, the side effect is indicated by boldface italic print.

Laboratory Test Considerations: The manner in which a drug may affect laboratory test values is presented. Some of these effects are caused by the therapeutic or toxic effects of the drugs; others result from interference with the testing method itself. The laboratory considerations are described as false positive (+), or increased (↑), values and as false negative (–), or decreased (↓), values.

OD Management of Overdose: When appropriate, this section provides a list of the symptoms observed following an overdose (*symptoms*) as well as treatment of the overdose (*treatment*).

Drug Interactions: This is an alphabetical listing of drugs that may interact with one another. The study of drug interactions is an important area of pharmacology and is changing constantly as a result of the influx of new drugs, clinical feedback, and increased client usage. The compilation of such interactions is far from complete; therefore, listings in this reference are to be considered *only* as general cautionary guidelines.

Drug interactions may result from a number of different mechanisms (e.g., additive or inhibitory effects, interference with degradation of drug, increased rate of elimination, decreased absorption from the GI tract, and competition for or displacement from receptor sites or plasma protein binding sites). Such interactions may manifest themselves in a variety of ways; however, an attempt has been made throughout the text to describe these interactions whenever possible as an increase (↑) or a decrease (↓) in the effect of the drug, and a reason for the change.

It is important to realize that any side effects that accompany the administration of a particular agent also may be increased as a result of a drug interaction.

The reader should be aware that drug interactions are often listed for classes of drugs. Thus, the drug interaction is likely to occur for all drugs in a particular class. Consult this information in Chapter 2.

How Supplied: The various dosage form(s) available for the drug and amounts of the drug in each of the dosage forms is presented. Such information is important as one dosage form may be more appropriate for a client than another. This information also allows the user to ensure the appropriate dosage form and strength is being administered.

Dosage: The dosage form and route of administration is followed by the disease state or condition (in italics) for which the dosage is recommended. This is followed by the adult and pediatric doses, when available. The listed dosage is to be considered as a general guideline; the exact amount of the drug to be given is determined by the provider. However, one should question orders when dosages differ markedly from the accepted norm.

Health Care Considerations: These guidelines were developed to assist in applying the problem solving process to pharmacotherapeutics. The Administration/Storage section assists the health care provider in preparing the medications for administration, administering the drug, and proper storage. All information relating to IV administration is listed under an IV icon for ready reference. Guidelines assessing the client before, during, and after prescribed drug therapy are identified, as are health care interventions appropriate for the prescribed drug therapy. Important client/family teaching issues related to the particular drug therapy are addressed. The client/family teaching section also includes instructions on how the drug is to be taken (e.g., with meals, at bedtime). Specific outcome criteria are listed to help evaluate the effectiveness of the prescribed drug therapy. Health care considerations that include assessments and interventions may contain specifics such as:

1. Gathering of physical data and client history.
2. Assessment of specific physiologic functions that may be affected by the drug.
3. Specific laboratory tests to monitor during drug therapy.
4. Identification of sensitivities/interactions and conditions that may preclude a particular drug therapy.
5. Recording specific indications for therapy and describing symptom characteristics related to this condition.
6. Physiologic, pharmacologic, and psychologic effects of the drug and how these may affect the client and impact on the health care process.
7. Adverse reactions that can arise as a result

of drug therapy and appropriate health care interventions.

8. Ensuring client safety when receiving drug therapy.

The practitioner must also assess the client for the *Side Effects* which must be recorded and reported to the provider. Severe side effects generally are cause for dosage modification or discontinuation of the drug.

Specific information for the client is provided for each drug. Client/family teaching emphasizes information to help the client/family recognize side effects, avoid potentially dangerous situations, and to alleviate anxiety that may result from taking a particular drug. Details on administration are included to enhance client understanding and adherence. Side effects that require medical intervention are included as well as specifics on how to minimize side effects for certain medications (i.e., take medication with food to decrease GI upset or take at bedtime to minimize daytime sedative effects).

The proper education of clients is one of the most challenging aspects of health care. The instructions must be tailored to the needs, awareness, and sophistication of each client. For example, clients who take medication to lower BP should assume responsibility for taking their own BP or having it taken and recorded. Clients should carry identification listing the drugs currently prescribed. They should know what they are taking and why, and develop a mechanism to remind themselves to take their medication as prescribed. Clients should carry this drug list with them whenever they go for a check-up or seek medical care. The drug list may also be shared with the pharmacist if there is a question concerning drugs prescribed, if the client is considering taking an over-the-counter medication, or if the client has to change pharmacies. The records, especially BP recordings, should be shared with the health care provider to ensure accurate evaluation of the response to the prescribed drug therapy. This may also alert the provider to any medication consumption by the client that they did not prescribe, were not aware of, or that may interfere with (i.e., potentiate, antagonize) the current pharmacologic regimen. The provider may also encourage the client to call with any questions or concerns about their therapy.

Finally, when taking the medical history, emphasis should be placed on the client's ability to read and to follow directions. Clients with language barriers should be identified, and appropriate written translations should be provided. In addition, client life-style, cultural factors, and income as well as the availability of health insurance and transportation are important factors that may affect adherence with therapy and followup care. The potential for a client being/becoming pregnant, and whether a mother is breast feeding her infant should be included in assessments. The age and orientation level, whether learned from personal observation or from discussion with close friends or family members, can be critical in determining potential relationships between drug therapy and/or drug interactions. Including these factors in the health assessment will assist all on the health care team to determine the type of therapy and drug delivery system best suited to a particular client and promotes the highest level of adherence.

An outcomes/evaluate section is included to assist in determining the effectiveness and positive therapeutic outcome of the prescribed drug therapy. Specific outcome criteria related to each drug are delineated.

The previous points are covered for all drugs or drug classes. When drugs are presented as a group (as in Chapter 2) rather than individually, the points may be covered only once for each group. In this case the practitioner should look for the appropriate entry in the drug class. For example, the *Contraindications, Side Effects, Drug Interactions,* and *Health Care Considerations* for all the insulins are so similar that they generally are listed only once in Chapter 2, under Insulins, in order to prevent lengthy duplication. However, the individual drug entries are cross-referenced to this general information.

Information that requires emphasis or is relevant to a particular drug is listed under appropriate headings, such as *Additional Contraindications, Additional Side Effects,* or *Additional Health Care Considerations.* These are *in addition to* and not *instead of* the regular entry, which is referenced and must also be consulted.

Additional information to assist in administering drugs and monitoring drug therapy is also included. For example, formulas for calculating IV flow rates and administration guidelines for some frequently administered IV antibiotics are included in Appendices 4 and 5, respectively. A list of sound-alike drug names is included in the front portion of the book to alert the provider to these similarities in an effort to prevent a potential lethal error. It is important to check drug names carefully to ensure that the prescribed drug is, indeed, the one that is being administered, as it is sometimes easy to confuse drugs that sound alike or are spelled similarly. Also helpful are the Elements of a Prescription (Appendix 2), Tables of Weights and Measures (Appendix 8), Commonly Used Abbreviations and Symbols (front portion of book), and the Guide to Drug Compatibility (in the back of the handbook).

The wound/dressing classification section (Appendix 6) identifies the therapeutic class of wound care products as well as the types of wounds appropriate for this therapy. Vitamins and vaccines are addressed as a group in Chapter 2. Finally, due to the rapidly changing area of pharmacotherapy, a monthly Internet and e-mail update service has been developed to ensure that you have all the tools necessary to practice currently and safely.

The Index is designed for maximum efficiency in finding a drug. Generic drug names are presented in boldface, trade names in regular type, therapeutic drug classes in italics, and combination drugs in all capital letters. In addition, each generic name is followed, in parentheses, by the most common trade name; and, each trade name is followed, in parentheses, by the generic name.

You are now ready to use Delmar's Drug Reference for Health Care Professionals. We hope that the text will be useful and assist you in your education, profession, and practice. The safe administration of drugs, assessment of potential interactions and adverse effects, as well as outcome evaluation are crucial parts of the health care process.

CHAPTER TWO

Therapeutic Drug Classifications

ALKYLATING AGENTS

See also the following individual entries:

Busulfan
Chlorambucil
Cisplatin
Cyclophosphamide
Dacarbazine
Lomustine

Action/Kinetics: Alkylating agents donate an alkyl group (carbonium ion) to biologically important macromolecules, such as DNA. The molecule is inactivated bringing *cell division* to a halt. This cytotoxic activity affects replication of cancerous cells and other cells, especially in rapidly proliferating tissues, such as the bone marrow, intestinal epithelium, and hair follicles. The toxic effects are usually cell-cycle nonspecific and become apparent when the cell enters the S phase and cell division is blocked at the G_2 phase (premitotic phase), resulting in cells having a double complement of DNA.

Resistance of cancer cells to alkylating agents usually develops slowly and gradually. Resistance seems to be the sum total of several minor adaptations, including decreased permeability of the cells, increased production of noncancer receptors (nucleophilic substances), and increased efficiency of the DNA repair system.

See *Health Care Considerations* for individual agents and *Health Care Considerations* for *Antineoplastic Agents*.

HEALTH CARE CONSIDERATIONS

Outcome/Evaluate: Clinical/radiographic evidence of tumor regression and disease stabilization.

ALPHA-1-ADRENERGIC BLOCKING AGENTS

See also the following individual entries:

Doxazosin mesylate
Prazosin hydrochloride
Tamsulosin hydrochloride
Terazosin

Action/Kinetics: Selectively block postsynaptic alpha-1-adrenergic receptors. Results in dilation of both arterioles and veins leading to a decrease in supine and standing BP. Diastolic BP is affected the most. Prazosin and terazosin do not produce reflex tachycardia. Terazosin also relaxes smooth muscle in the bladder neck and prostate, making it useful to treat BPH. Have many undesirable effects which, although not toxic, limit their use. Always start treatment at low doses and increase gradually.

See also *Beta-Adrenergic Blocking Agents*.

Uses: Alone or in combination with diuretics or beta-adrenergic blocking agents to treat hypertension. Doxazosin and terazosin are used to treat BPH. *Investigational:* Prazosin is used for refractory CHF, management of Raynaud's vasospasm, and to treat BPH. Doxazosin, along with digoxin and diuretics, is used to treat CHF.

Contraindications: Hypersensitivity to these drugs (i.e., quinazolines).

Special Concerns: The first few doses may cause postural hypotension and syncope with sudden loss of consciousness. Use with caution in lactation, with impaired hepatic function, or if receiving drugs known to influence hepatic metabolism. Safety and efficacy have not been established in children.

Side Effects: The following side effects are common to alpha-1-adrenergic blockers. See individual drugs as well. *CV:* Palpitations, postural hypotension, hypotension, tachycardia, chest pain, arrhythmia. *GI:* N&V, dry mouth, diarrhea, constipation, abdominal discomfort or pain, flatulence. *CNS:* Dizziness, depression, decreased libido, sexual dysfunction, nervousness, paresthesia, somnolence, anxiety, insomnia, asthenia, drowsiness. *Musculoskeletal:* Pain in the shoulder, neck, or back; gout, arthritis, joint pain, arthralgia. *Respiratory:* Dyspnea, nasal congestion, sinusitis, bronchitis, ***bronchospasm,*** cold symptoms, epistaxis, increased cough, flu symptoms, pharyngitis, rhinitis. *Ophthalmic:* Blurred vision, abnormal vision, reddened sclera, conjunctivitis. *GU:* Impotence, urinary frequency, incontinence. *Miscellaneous:* Tinnitus, vertigo, pruritus, sweating, alopecia, lichen planus, headache, edema, weight gain, facial edema, fever.

OD Management of Overdose: *Symptoms:* Extension of the side effects, especially on BP. *Treatment:* Keep supine to restore BP and normalize heart rate. Shock may be treated with volume expanders or vasopressors; support renal function.

Drug Interactions: Alpha-1 blockers ↓ the antihypertensive effect of clonidine.

Dosage

See individual agents.

Laboratory Test Considerations: ↑ Urinary VMA.Take the first dose of prazosin and terazosin at bedtime.

HEALTH CARE CONSIDERATIONS

Assessment

1. Note any history of PUD; drug should be used cautiously.
2. Record indications for therapy, type, onset, and characteristics of symptoms.
3. Monitor electrolytes, ECG, and VS. Base titration on standing BP due to postural effects.
4. Assess for heart or lung disease and note currently prescribed therapy. Some agents may cause vasospasm with Prinzmetal or vasospastic angina.
5. Use cautiously in older clients due to possibility of orthostatic hypotension. They may tolerate a slower, more gradual increase in dosage (i.e., terazosin 1 mg/day for 7 days followed by 2 mg/day for 7 days, etc., until desired response).

Client/Family Teaching

1. Take with milk or meals to minimize GI upset.
2. Take first dose at bedtime to minimize syncope and hypotensive effects. Use caution when performing activities that require mental alertness until drug effects realized.
3. Do not drive or undertake hazardous tasks for 12–24 hr after the first dose and after increasing dose or following an interruption of dosage.
4. Avoid symptoms of orthostatic hypotension by rising slowly from a sitting or lying position and waiting until symptoms subside.
5. Keep record of BP and weight. Report any weight gain or ankle edema; without a diuretic, one may experience retention of salt and water due to vasodilation.
6. Dizziness, lassitude, headache, and palpitations may occur as well as transient apprehension, fear, anxiety, and/or palpitations. Report if persistent so dosage may be adjusted.
7. Review life-style changes needed for BP control; i.e., dietary restrictions of fat and sodium; weight reduction; regular physical exercise; decreased use of alcohol; stress reduction; and smoking cessation.
8. Avoid excess caffeine and OTC agents (especially cold remedies).
9. Do not stop abruptly.

Outcome/Evaluate

- ↓ BP
- ↓ Nocturia, urgency/frequency

AMEBICIDES AND TRICHOMONACIDES

See also the following individual entries:

Atovaquone
Erythromycins
Metronidazole
Paromomycin sulfate
Tetracyclines

General Statement: Amebiasis is caused by the protozoan *Entamoeba histolytica. E. histolytica* has two forms: (1) an active motile form known as the trophozoite form and (2) a cystic form that is resistant to destruction and is responsible for the transmission of the disease. The obvious manifestations of amebiasis vary, including violent acute dysentery (characterized by sudden development of severe diarrhea, cramps, and passage of bloody, mucoid stools); others have few overt symptoms or are even completely asymptomatic.

Amoebae often migrate from the GI tract to other parts of the body (extraintestinal amebiasis). The spleen, lungs, or liver are frequently affected. The amoebae colonize in these organs and form abscesses that may rupture and thereby serve as infectious foci.

At present, no one drug can cure both intestinal and extraintestinal amebic infestations; thus, combination therapy is used. Often the more effective but toxic agents are used initially for a short period of time, while long-term eradication or prophylaxis is carried out with less toxic agents.

Infestation with the parasite *Trichomonas vaginalis* causes vaginitis. This is treated by various locally applied antitrichomonal agents—often effective amebicides—and also by the oral administration of metronidazole (usually prescribed for both sexual partners to prevent reinfection). Acid douches (vinegar or lactic acid) are a helpful adjunct to treatment.

The incidence of infections by the protozoan, *Giardia lamblia,* is transmitted in the feces. Symptoms include mucous diarrhea, abdominal pain, and weight loss. Drugs of choice are metronidazole and quinacrine.

See also *General Health Care Considerations for All Anti-Infectives.*

HEALTH CARE CONSIDERATIONS

AMEBICIDES

Assessment

1. Record onset and characteristics of symptoms; identify causative factors/conditions, any travel, and possible exposures.
2. Obtain CBC, electrolytes, nutrition profile, and cultures.
3. Assess for acute dysentery or extraintestinal amebiasis; agents are highly toxic.

Interventions

1. Clients are frequently on combination-drug therapy for amebiasis; observe for toxic reactions.
2. Provide supportive medical care with acute dysentery; assist to control diarrhea, maintain fluid and electrolyte balance, skin integrity, comfort, and to prevent complications caused by malnutrition. May have to curtail activity during acute disease phase.
3. Administer drugs only as ordered to allow for rest periods between courses of therapy.

Client/Family Teaching

1. Carriers must continue with drug therapy; review benefit to themselves, their families, and their co-workers.
2. Thorough hand washing is imperative, especially in factories, schools, and other institutions where disease is easily spread; disinfect toilets daily.
3. Food handlers must be particularly conscientious about washing hands after toileting; use soap, water, and clean towels.
4. Obtain regular periodic stool examinations to check for recurrence.
5. Client and carriers need to report for follow-up visits to ensure eradication of organisms. Do not self-medicate.

TRICHOMONACIDES

Client/Family Teaching

1. Review the prescribed method/frequency for administration.
2. Review methods for insufflation, suppositories, and douching; practice good feminine hygiene.
3. Wear a pad to prevent clothing or bed linen from becoming stained with vaginal suppositories, especially if they contain iodine (which does stain). Change pad frequently and immediately upon staining because it may serve as a growth medium for organisms.
4. Sexual partner may be an asymptomatic carrier and require therapy to prevent reinfection of female. Use condoms during sexual intercourse to prevent reinfections.

Outcome/Evaluate

- Negative cultures; resolution of infection
- Clinical/microscopic confirmation of eradication/prophylaxis of amebiasis and trichomoniasis

AMINOGLYCOSIDES

See also the following individual entries:

Gentamicin sulfate
Kanamycin sulfate
Neomycin sulfate
Paromomycin sulfate
Tobramycin sulfate

Action/Kinetics: Broad-spectrum antibiotics believed to inhibit protein synthesis by binding irreversibly to ribosomes (30S subunit), thereby interfering with an initiation complex between messenger RNA and the 30S subunit. This leads to production of nonfunctional proteins; polyribosomes are split apart and are unable to synthesize protein. Usually bactericidal due to disruption of the bacterial cytoplasmic membrane. Poorly absorbed from the GI tract; usually administered parenterally (exceptions: some enteric infections of the GI tract and prior to surgery). Also absorbed from the peritoneum, bronchial tree, wounds, denuded skin, and joints. Distributed in the extracellular fluid and cross the placental barrier, but not the blood-brain barrier. Penetration of the CSF is increased when the meninges are inflamed.

Rapidly absorbed after IM injection. **Peak plasma levels, after IM:** Usually ½–2 hr. Measurable levels persist for 8–12 hr after a single administration. **t½:** 2–3 hr (increases sharply in impaired kidney function). Ranges of t½ from 24 to 110 hr have been observed. Excreted mainly unchanged in urine. Resistance develops slowly.

See also *General Health Care Considerations for All Anti-Infectives.*

Uses: Are powerful antibiotics that induce serious side effects—**do not use for minor infections**. Gram-negative bacteria causing bone and joint infections, septicemia (including neonatal sepsis), skin and soft tissue infections (including those from burns), respiratory tract infections, postoperative infections, intra-abdominal infections (including peritonitis), UTIs. In combination with clindamycin for mixed aerobic-anaerobic infections. Also, see individual drugs.

Used for gram-positive bacteria only when other less toxic drugs are either ineffective or contraindicated. Use in CNS *Pseudomonas* infections such as meningitis or ventriculitis is questionable.

Contraindications: Hypersensitivity to aminoglycosides, long-term therapy (except streptomycin for tuberculosis).

Special Concerns: Use with extreme caution with impaired renal function or preexisting hearing impairment. Safe use in pregnancy and during lactation not established. Assess premature infants, neonates, and older clients closely; they are particularly sensitive to toxic effects. Considerable cross-allergenicity occurs among the aminoglycosides.

Side Effects: *Ototoxicity:* Both auditory and vestibular damage have been noted. The risk is increased with poor renal function and in the elderly. Auditory symptoms include tinnitus and hearing impairment, while vestibular symptoms include dizziness, nystagmus, vertigo, and ataxia.

Renal Impairment: May be characterized by cylindruria, oliguria, proteinuria, azotemia, hematuria, increase or decrease in frequency of urination; increased BUN, NPN, or creatinine; and increased thirst. *Neurotoxicity:* Neuromuscular blockade, headache, tremor, lethargy, paresthesia, peripheral neuritis (numbness, tingling, or burning of face/mouth), arachnoiditis, encephalopathy, acute organic brain syndrome. CNS depression, characterized by stupor, flaccidity, and rarely, ***coma, and respiratory depression in infants.*** Optic neuritis with blurred vision or loss of vision. *GI:* N&V, diarrhea, increased salivation, anorexia, weight loss. *Allergic:* Rash, urticaria, pruritus, burning, fever, stomatitis, eosinophilia. Rarely, ***agranulocytosis and anaphylaxis.*** Cross-allergy among aminoglycosides has been observed. *Miscellaneous:* Joint pain, ***laryngeal edema, pulmonary fibrosis,*** superinfection.

OD **Management of Overdose:** *Symptoms:* Extension of side effects. *Treatment:* Undertake hemodialysis (preferred) or peritoneal dialysis.

Drug Interactions

Bumetanide / ↑ Risk of ototoxicity
Capreomycin / ↑ Muscle relaxation
Cephalosporins / ↑ Risk of renal toxicity
Ciprofloxacin HCl / Additive antibacterial activity
Cisplatin / Additive renal toxicity
Colistimethate / ↑ Muscle relaxation
Digoxin / Possible ↑ or ↓ effect of digoxin
Ethacrynic acid / ↑ Risk of ototoxicity
Furosemide / ↑ Risk of ototoxicity
Methoxyflurane / ↑ Risk of renal toxicity
Penicillins / ↓ Effect of aminoglycosides
Polymyxins / ↑ Muscle relaxation
Skeletal muscle relaxants (surgical) / ↑ Muscle relaxation
Vancomycin / Additive ototoxicity and renal toxicity
Vitamin A / ↓ Effect of vitamin A due to ↓ absorption from GI tract

Laboratory Test Considerations: ↑ BUN, BSP retention, creatinine, AST, ALT, bilirubin. ↓ Cholesterol values.

1. Check expiration date.
2. Warn if drug being administered stings or causes a burning sensation.
3. During IM administration
• Inject deep into muscle mass to minimize transient pain.
• Use a Z track method for thin, elderly clients.
• Rotate/record injection sites.
4. With IV administration
• Dilute with compatible solution.
• Infuse at the rate ordered to prevent excessive serum concentrations.
5. Administer for only 7–10 days and avoid repeating course of therapy unless a serious infection is present that does not respond to other antibiotics.
6. Administer ATC to maintain therapeutic drug levels.

HEALTH CARE CONSIDERATIONS

Assessment

1. Assess for allergic reactions; note any knowledge/history of sensitivity to anti-infectives.
2. Weigh to ensure correct dosage.
3. Determine baseline liver, renal, auditory, and vestibular function; assess for nephrotoxicity.
4. Assess for presence and source(s) of infection. Record fever, culture/lab reports, and wound characteristics (i.e., color, odor, drainage).

Interventions

1. Monitor VS and I&O; increase fluids to prevent renal tubule irritation.
2. Monitor drug levels; (e.g., Amikacin levels > 30 mcg/mL are considered toxic.)
3. With vestibular dysfunction protect by supervising ambulation and providing side rails; assess and record (potential for) fall hazard.
4. Assess for ototoxicity; pretreatment audiograms may be helpful, as hearing loss is a dose-related side effect of drug therapy

most commonly associated with amikacin, kanamycin, neomycin, or paromomycin. Tinnitus, dizziness, and loss of balance are also signs of vestibular injury and more commonly seen with gentamicin and streptomycin. Deafness may occur several weeks after discontinuing drug.
5. Do not administer concurrently or sequentially with a topical or systemic nephrotoxic or ototoxic drug (e.g., potent diuretics such as ethacrynic acid or furosemide) unless provider designates benefits outweigh the risks.
6. Observe for neuromuscular blockade with muscular weakness leading to apnea, when administered with a muscle relaxant or after anesthesia. Have calcium gluconate or neostigmine available to reverse blockade.
7. Note cells or casts in the urine, oliguria, proteinuria, lowered specific gravity, or increasing BUN or creatinine, all of which indicate altered renal function.

Client/Family Teaching

1. Review goals of therapy and prescribed method of administration.
2. Take as prescribed, ATC, until prescription is finished.
3. Follow a well-balanced diet and consume at least 2–3 L/day of fluids.
4. Report symptoms of superinfection (black, furry tongue; loose, foul-smelling stools; vaginal itching).
5. Report alterations in hearing, vision, and/or ambulation.

Outcome/Evaluate

- Negative culture reports
- Resolution of infection with ↓ WBCs, ↓ fever, ↓ drainage; symptomatic improvement
- Therapeutic drug levels

AMPHETAMINES AND DERIVATIVES

See also the following individual entries:

Amphetamine sulfate
Dextroamphetamine sulfate
Mazindol
Methamphetamine hydrochloride
Phendimetrazine tartrate

Action/Kinetics: Thought to act on the cerebral cortex and reticular activating system (including the medullary, respiratory, and vasomotor centers) by releasing norepinephrine from central adrenergic neurons. High doses cause release of dopamine from the mesolimbic system. The stimulatory effect on the CNS causes an increase in motor activity and mental alertness, a mood-elevating effect, a slight euphoric effect, and an anorexigenic effect. The anorexigenic effect is thought to be produced by direct stimulation of the satiety center in the lateral hypothalamic feeding center of the brain. Peripheral effects are mediated by alpha- and beta-adrenergic receptors and include increases in both systolic and diastolic BP and respiratory stimulation. Readily absorbed from the GI tract and distributed throughout most tissues, with the highest concentrations in the brain and CSF. Duration of anorexia (PO): 3–6 hr. Metabolized in liver and excreted by kidneys. Excreted slowly (5–7 days); cumulative effects may occur with continued administration.

Psychic stimulation is often followed by a rebound effect manifested as fatigue. Tolerance will develop to all drugs of this class. There is a relatively wide margin of safety between the therapeutic and toxic doses of amphetamines. However, both acute and chronic toxicity can occur.

Uses: See individual drugs.

Contraindications: Hyperthyroidism, advanced arteriosclerosis, nephritis, diabetes mellitus, hypertension, narrow-angle glaucoma, angina pectoris, CV disease, and individuals with hypersensitivity to these drugs. Use in emotionally unstable persons susceptible to drug abuse and in agitated states. Psychotic children. Lactation. Appetite suppressants in children less than 12 years of age. Within 14 days of MAO inhibitors.

Special Concerns: Use with caution in clients suffering from hyperexcitability states; in elderly, debilitated, or asthenic clients; and in clients with psychopathic personality traits or a history of homicidal or suicidal tendencies.

Side Effects: *CNS:* Nervousness, dizziness, depression, headache, insomnia, euphoria, symptoms of excitation. Rarely, psychoses. In children, manifestation of vocal and motor tics and Tourette's syndrome. *GI:* N&V, cramps, diarrhea, dry mouth, constipation, metallic taste, anorexia. *CV:* Arrhythmias, palpitations, dyspnea, pulmonary hypertension, peripheral hyper- or hypotension, precordial pain, fainting. *Dermatologic:* Symptoms of allergy including rash, urticaria, erythema, burning. Pallor. *GU:* Urinary frequency, dysuria. *Ophthalmologic:* Blurred vision, mydriasis. *Hematologic:* ***Agranulocytosis,*** leukopenia. *Endocrine:* Menstrual irregularities, gynecomastia, impotence, and changes in libido. *Miscellaneous:* Alopecia, increased motor activity, fever, sweating, chills, muscle pain, chest pain.

Long-term use results in psychic dependence, as well as a high degree of tolerance.

OD **Management of Overdose:** *Symptoms of Acute Overdose (Toxicity):* Restlessness, irritability, insomnia, tremor, hyperreflexia, rhabdomyolysis, rapid respiration, ***hyperpyrexia,*** assaultiveness, hallucinations, panic states, sweating, mydriasis, flushing, hyperactivity, confusion, hypertension or hypotension, extrasystoles, tachypnea, fever, delirium, self-injury, arrhythmias, ***seizures, coma, circulatory collapse, death. Death usually results from CV collapse or convulsions.*** *Symptoms of Chronic Toxicity:* Chronic use/abuse is characterized by emotional lability, loss of appetite, severe dermatoses, hyperactivity, insomnia, irritability, somnolence, mental impairment, occupational deterioration, a tendency to withdraw from social contact, teeth grinding, continuous chewing, and ulcers of the tongue and lips. Prolonged use of high doses can elicit symptoms of paranoid schizophrenia, including auditory and visual hallucinations and paranoid ideation. *Treatment of Acute Toxicity (Overdosage):*

- Symptomatic treatment. After oral ingestion, induce emesis or perform gastric lavage, followed by use of activated charcoal. Acidification of the urine increases the rate of excretion. Give fluids until urine flow is 3–6 mL/kg/hr; furosemide or mannitol may be beneficial.
- Maintain adequate circulation and respiration.
- Treat CNS stimulation with chlorpromazine and psychotic symptoms with haloperidol. Treat hyperactivity with diazepam or a barbiturate. Reduce stimuli and maintain in a quiet, dim environment. Treat clients who have ingested an overdose of long-acting products for toxicity until all symptoms of overdosage have disappeared.
- IV phentolamine may be used for hypertension, whereas hypotension may be reversed by IV fluids and possibly vasopressors (used with caution).

Drug Interactions

Acetazolamide / ↑ Effect of amphetamine by ↑ renal tubular reabsorption
Ammonium chloride / ↓ Effect of amphetamine by ↓ renal tubular reabsorption
Anesthetics, general / ↑ Risk of cardiac arrhythmias
Antihypertensives / Amphetamines ↓ effect of antihypertensives
Ascorbic acid / ↓ Effect of amphetamine by ↓ renal tubular reabsorption
Furazolidone / ↑ Toxicity of anorexiants due to MAO activity of furazolidone
Guanethidine / ↓ Effect of guanethidine by displacement from its site of action
Haloperidol / ↓ Effect of amphetamine by ↓ uptake of drug at its site of action
Insulin / Amphetamines alter insulin requirements
MAO inhibitors / All peripheral, metabolic, cardiac, and central effects of amphetamine are potentiated for up to 2 weeks after termination of MAO inhibitor therapy (symptoms include hypertensive crisis with possible intracranial hemorrhage, hyperthermia, convulsions, coma); death may occur. ↓ Effect of amphetamine by ↓ uptake of drug into its site of action
Methyldopa / ↓ Hypotensive effect of methyldopa by ↑ sympathomimetic activity
Phenothiazines / ↓ Effect of amphetamine by ↓ uptake of drug at its site of action
Sodium bicarbonate / ↑ Effect of amphetamine by ↑ renal tubular reabsorption
Thiazide diuretics / ↑ Effect of amphetamine by ↑ renal tubular reabsorption
Tricyclic antidepressants / ↓ Effect of amphetamines

Dosage

See individual drugs. Many compounds are timed-release preparations.

Laboratory Test Considerations: ↑ Urinary catecholamines, ↑ plasma corticosteroid levels.

1. If prescribed to suppress appetite, administer 30 min before anticipated meal time.
2. Use a small initial dose; then increase gradually as necessary.
3. Unless otherwise ordered, give the last dose of the day at least 6 hr before bedtime.

HEALTH CARE CONSIDERATIONS

Assessment

1. Identify meds currently taking, indications, and effectiveness.
2. Record physical conditions that would preclude using drugs in this category i.e. ASHD, hyperthyroidism, DM, glaucoma.
3. Record age and if debilitated.
4. Monitor electrolytes, ECG, weight, VS, and CBC.
5. Under the Controlled Substances Act; follow appropriate policy for dispensing/handling to restrict availability and discourage abuse.

Interventions

1. If agitated or complains of sleeplessness, reduce dosage of drug.
2. If receiving MAO inhibitors or received them 7–14 days before amphetamine therapy, assess for hypertensive crisis. Monitor and report fever, marked sweating, excitation,

delirium, tremors, or twitching; pad side rails and have suction available.
3. Monitor VS. Assess for arrhythmias, tachycardia, or hypertension. CV changes with psychotic syndrome may indicate toxicity.
4. If somnolent or appears mentally or physically impaired, stop the drug. Observe for signs of psychologic dependence and drug tolerance.
5. Monitor height to assess for growth inhibition.

Client/Family Teaching

1. When anorexiants are used for weight reduction, their effect lasts only 4–6 weeks; use is short term. Follow an established dietary and exercise regimen to maintain weight loss and attend a behavioral modification weight control program.
2. Take only as prescribed, 1 hr before meals and last dose 6 hr before bedtime to ensure adequate rest. Abrupt withdrawal may cause symptoms.
3. Diets high in fiber, fruit, and fluids assist to reduce drugs' constipating effects. See dietitian to discuss weight control and/or reducing diets and to assist with food selections and meal planning when weight loss is the goal.
4. Record food intake and weight daily the first week and then at least once a week. May become anorexic; report any persistent, severe weight loss so therapy can be adjusted.
5. Report any changes in attention span and ability to concentrate.
6. Take only as directed; do not share meds. Report S&S of tolerance.
7. May cause a false sense of euphoria and well being and mask extreme fatigue. These may impair judgment and ability to perform potentially hazardous tasks, such as operating a machine or an automobile. Using amphetamines to treat fatigue is inappropriate because rebound effects may be severe.
8. Seek medical assistance if experiencing extreme fatigue and depression once drug is discontinued. Periodic "drug holidays" may be ordered to assess progress and prevent dependence.
9. Avoid OTC medications and ingesting large amounts of caffeine in any form. Read labels for the detection of caffeine since this contributes to CV side effects.
10. Manage dry mouth by frequent rinsing, chewing sugarless gum, or sucking sugarless hard candies.
11. Store safely out of child's reach.

Outcome/Evaluate

- ↑ Attention span/concentration
- Weight reduction
- ↓ Episodes of narcolepsy

ANGIOTENSIN-CONVERTING ENZYME (ACE) INHIBITORS

See also the following individual entries:

Benazepril hydrochloride
Captopril
Enalapril maleate
Fosinopril sodium
Lisinopril
Moexipril hydrochloride
Quinapril hydrochloride
Ramipril
Trandolapril

Action/Kinetics: Believed to act by suppressing the renin-angiotensin-aldosterone system. Renin, synthesized by the kidneys, produces angiotensin I, an inactive decapeptide derived from plasma globulin substrate. Angiotensin I is converted to angiotensin II by ACE. Angiotensin II is a potent vasoconstrictor that also stimulates secretion of aldosterone from the adrenal cortex, resulting in sodium and fluid retention. The ACE inhibitors prevent the conversion of angiotensin I to angiotensin II. This results in a decrease in plasma angiotensin II and subsequently a decrease in peripheral resistance and decreased aldosterone secretion (leading to fluid loss) and therefore a decrease in BP. There may be either no change or an increase in CO. Several weeks of therapy may be required to achieve the maximum effect to reduce BP. Standing and supine BPs are lowered to about the same extent. Are also antihypertensive in low renin hypertensive clients. ACE inhibitors are additive with thiazide diuretics in lowering blood pressure; however, β-blockers and captopril have less than additive effects when used with ACE inhibitors.

Uses: Alone or in combination with other antihypertensive agents (especially thiazide diuretics) for the treatment of hypertension. Some are effective in CHF as adjunctive therapy or to treat LV dysfunction. See also individual drug entries.

Contraindications: History of angioedema due to previous treatment with an ACE inhibitor. Use of fosinopril, ramipril, or trandolapril in lactation.

Special Concerns: Use during the second and third trimesters of pregnancy can result in injury and even death to the developing fetus. May cause a profound drop in BP following the first dose; start therapy under close medical supervision. Use with caution in renal disease (especially renal artery stenosis) as increases in BUN and serum creatinine have occurred. Use with caution in clients with aortic stenosis due to possible decreased coronary perfusion following vasodilator use. Most are used with caution during lactation. Geriatric clients may show a greater sensitivity to the hypotensive effects of ACE inhibitors although these drugs may preserve or improve renal function and reverse LV hypertrophy. For most ACE inhibitors, safety and effectiveness have not been determined in children.

Side Effects: See individual entries. Side effects common to most ACE inhibitors include the following. *GI:* Abdominal pain, N&V, diarrhea, constipation, dry mouth. *CNS:* Sleep disturbances, insomnia, headache, dizziness, fatigue, nervousness, paresthesias. *CV:* Hypotension (especially following the first dose), palpitations, angina pectoris, ***MI,*** orthostatic hypotension, chest pain. *Hepatic:* Rarely, cholestatic jaundice progressing to ***hepatic necrosis and death.*** *Miscellaneous:* Chronic cough, dyspnea, increased sweating, diaphoresis, pruritus, rash, impotence, syncope, asthenia, arthralgia, myalgia. ***Angioedema*** of the face, lips, tongue, glottis, larynx, extremities, and mucous membranes. ***Anaphylaxis.***

OD **Management of Overdose:** *Symptoms:* Hypotension is the most common. *Treatment:* Supportive measures. The treatment of choice to restore BP is volume expansion with an IV infusion of NSS. Certain of the ACE inhibitors (captopril, enalaprilat, lisinopril) may be removed by hemodialysis.

Drug Interactions

Allopurinol / ↑ Risk of hypersensitivity reactions
Anesthetics / ↑ Risk of hypotension if used with anesthetics that also cause hypotension
Antacids / Possible ↓ bioavailability of ACE inhibitors
Capsaicin / Capsaicin may cause or worsen cough associated with ACE inhibitor use
Digoxin / ↑ Plasma digoxin levels
Indomethacin / ↓ Hypotensive effects of ACE inhibitors, especially in low renin or volume-dependent hypertensive clients
Lithium / ↑ Serum lithium levels → ↑ risk of toxicity
Phenothiazines / ↑ Effect of ACE inhibitors
Potassium-sparing diuretics / ↑ Serum potassium levels
Potassium supplements / ↑ Serum potassium levels
Thiazide diuretics / Additive effect to ↓ BP

Dosage

See individual drugs.

Laboratory Test Considerations: ↑ BUN and creatinine (both are transient and reversible). ↑ Liver enzymes, serum bilirubin, uric acid, blood glucose. Small ↑ in serum potassium.Do not interrupt or discontinue ACE inhibitor therapy without consulting provider.

HEALTH CARE CONSIDERATIONS

Assessment

1. Note any previous therapy with ACE inhibitors or antihypertensive agents and the results.
2. Monitor VS (BP—both arms while lying, standing, and sitting), electrolytes, CBC, and renal function studies; check urine for protein (microalbuminuria).
3. Record hereditary angioedema (especially if caused by a deficiency of C1 esterase inhibitor).
4. Assess understanding of hypertension (or CHF) and prescribed therapy.
5. Record weight, risk factors, and medical problems. Identify life-style changes needed to achieve and maintain lowered BP. Assess motivation and ensure that a trial of "good behavior" with dietary modifications and regular exercise for 3–6 months has been done unless BP stage 2 or 3.

Interventions

1. Assess for neutropenia (esp. with captopril); precludes drug therapy.
2. Report any evidence of angioedema (swelling of face, lips, extremities, tongue, mucous membranes, glottis, or larynx) esp. after first dose (but may also be delayed response). Relieve S&S with antihistamines. If involves laryngeal edema, observe for airway obstruction. *Stop* drug; use epinephrine (1:1000 SC).
3. Monitor VS, I&O, weight, serum potassium, and renal function studies. Those hypovolemic due to diuretics, GI fluid loss, or salt restriction may exhibit severe hypotension after initial doses; supervise ambulation until drug response evident.
4. If undergoing surgery or general anesthesia with drugs that cause hypotension, ACE inhibitors will block angiotensin II formation; correct hypotension by volume expansion.

Client/Family Teaching

1. Take 1 hr before meals and only as directed.
2. Review prescribed dietary guidelines; do not use salt substitutes containing potassium.

3. Medication controls but does not cure hypertension; take as prescribed despite feeling better and do not stop abruptly.
4. Take BP readings at various times during the day and record to prevent treating "white collar" readings.
5. Do not perform activities that require mental alertness until drug effects realized; initially may cause dizziness, fainting, or lightheadedness.
6. Rise slowly from a lying position and dangle feet before standing; avoid sudden position changes to minimize postural effects.
7. Practice birth control; report if pregnancy suspected.
8. Report adverse side effects:
• Nonproductive, persistent, chronic cough
• Sore throat, fever, swelling of hands or feet, irregular heartbeat, chest pains, difficulty breathing, or hoarseness
• Excessive perspiration, dehydration, vomiting, and diarrhea
• Itching, joint pain, fever, or skin rash
9. Report edema and weight gain of more than 3 lb/day or 5 lb/week.
10. With diabetes (with or without hypertension), ACE inhibitors have been shown to reduce proteinuria and to slow the progression of renal disease.
11. Avoid any OTC medications, especially cold remedies, without approval.
12. NSAIDs and aspirin may impair the hypotensive effects of ACE inhibitors while antacids may decrease bioavailability.
13. Avoid excessive amounts of caffeine (e.g., tea, coffee, cola).
14. Regular exercise, proper diet, weight loss, stress management, and adequate rest in conjunction with medications are needed in the overall management of hypertension. Additional interventions such as reducing alcohol use, discontinuing tobacco products, and reducing salt intake may also assist in BP control.

Outcome/Evaluate

• ↓ BP
• Improvement in S&S of CHF
• ↓ Proteinuria/renal damage
• ↓ Morbidity post-AMI

ANTACIDS

See also the following individual entries:

Sodium bicarbonate

Action/Kinetics: Antacids act by neutralizing or reducing gastric acidity, thus increasing the pH of the stomach and relieving hyperacidity. If the pH is increased to 4, the activity of pepsin is inhibited. The ability of a specific antacid to neutralize acid is termed *acid-neutralizing capacity,* and antacids are selected on this basis. Acid-neutralizing capacity (ANC) is expressed as milliequivalents per milliliter and is defined by the HCl required to maintain an antacid suspension at pH 3.5 for 10 min in vitro. An antacid should neutralize at least 5 mEq/dose; also, to be considered an antacid, the compound should contribute to at least 25% of the ANC of a product.

Ideally, antacids should not be absorbed systemically, although substances such as sodium bicarbonate or calcium carbonate may produce significant systemic effects. The most effective dosage form for antacids is suspensions. Antacids also promote healing of peptic ulcers.

Antacids containing magnesium have a laxative effect, whereas those containing aluminum or calcium have a constipating effect. This is why clients are often given alternating doses of laxative and constipating antacids. Antacids containing aluminum bind with phosphate ions in the intestine forming the insoluble aluminum phosphate, which is excreted in the feces. This is of value in treating hyperphosphatemia of chronic renal failure. **Onset:** Depends on ability of the antacid to solubilize in the stomach and react with hydrochloric acid. The poorly soluble antacids (e.g., magnesium trisilicate) react slower with hydrochloric acid than do the more soluble compounds. **Duration of antacids:** 30 min if fasting; up to 3 hr if taken after meals.

General Statement: Hydrochloric acid maintains the stomach at a pH (1–2) necessary for optimum activity of the digestive enzyme pepsin and for stimulating the release of secretin when the acid contents of the stomach pass into the duodenum. Under certain circumstances, however, people suffer adverse reactions due to gastric acidity ranging from heartburn to life-threatening peptic or duodenal ulcers. Although production of acid has an important role in the development of gastric and duodenal ulcers, other factors are also involved. These include endogenous histamine (which can stimulate gastric acid secretion), antigen-antibody reactions, and the psychologic makeup of the client. Acute and chronic GI disturbances are among the most common medical conditions requiring treatment. Various drugs and dietary measures are used for the treatment of hyperacidity states and ulcers, and the use of antacids is an important part of such regimens.

Uses: Treatment of hyperacidity (heartburn, acid indigestion, sour stomach), gastric ulcer, duodenal ulcer, gastroesophageal reflux. Adjunct (with histamine H_2-receptor antagonists) in the treatment of hypersecretory conditions (e.g., Zollinger-Ellison syndrome), systemic mastocytosis, and multiple endocrine adenoma. Treatment of hypocalcemia, hypophosphatemia. Prophylaxis of renal calculi.

Contraindications: Sodium-containing products are contraindicated in CHF, hypertension, or conditions requiring a low-sodium diet. Pregnant or lactating women should not use antacids without physician approval. Children less than 6 years of age.

Special Concerns: Chronic use of aluminum-containing antacids may aggravate metabolic bone disease seen in geriatric clients; also, chronic use of aluminum-containing antacids may contribute to development of Alzheimer's disease. Taking too much of an antacid may result in an increased secretion of stomach acid. Antacids may mask the warning signs associated with ulcers and GI bleeding caused by NSAIDs.

Side Effects: *Aluminum-containing antacids:* Constipation, intestinal obstruction, aluminum intoxication, hypophosphatemia, osteomalacia. *Calcium carbonate, aluminum-magnesium hydroxide, magnesium oxide, soluble bismuth salts, sodium bicarbonate:* Milk-alkali syndrome (acute: headache, nausea, irritability, weakness; chronic: alkalosis, hypercalcemia, renal impairment). Rebound hyperacidity. *Magnesium-containing antacids:* Diarrhea, hypermagnesemia in clients with renal failure.

Drug Interactions

1. *Aluminum-containing antacids:* ↑ Effect of benzodiazepines. ↓ Effect of allopurinol, chloroquine, corticosteroids, diflunisal, digoxin, ethambutol, histamine H_2 antagonists, iron products, isoniazid, penicillamine, phenothiazines, tetracyclines, thyroid hormones, and ticlopidine by ↓ absorption from GI tract.
2. *Aluminum- and magnesium-containing antacids:* ↑ Effect of levodopa, quinidine, sulfonylureas, and valproic acid probably by ↓ excretion. ↓ Effect of benzodiazepines, captopril, corticosteroids, fluoroquinolones, histamine H_2 antagonists, hydantoins, iron products, ketoconazole, penicillamine, phenothiazines, salicylates, tetracyclines, and ticlopidine either by ↓ absorption from GI tract or ↑ excretion.
3. *Calcium-containing antacids:* ↑ Effect of quinidine by ↓ excretion. ↓ Effect of fluoroquinolones, hydantoins, iron products, salicylates, and tetracyclines either by ↓ absorption from GI tract or ↑ excretion.
4. *Magnesium-containing antacids:* ↑ Effect of dicumarol, quinidine, and sulfonylureas probably by ↓ excretion. ↓ Effect of benzodiazepines, corticosteroids, digoxin, histamine H_2 antagonists, hydantoins, iron products, nitrofurantoin, penicillamine, phenothiazines, tetracyclines, and ticlopidine either by ↓ absorption from GI tract or ↑ excretion.
5. *Sodium bicarbonate:* ↑ Effect of amphetamines, flecainide, quinidine, and sympathomimetics probably by ↑ excretion. ↓ Effect of benzodiazepines, hydantoins, ketoconazole, lithium, methenamine, methotrexate, salicylates, sulfonylureas, and tetracyclines either by ↓ absorption from GI tract or ↑ excretion.

Dosage

See individual drugs.

1. Clients who have an active peptic ulcer should take antacids every hour during waking hours for the first 2 weeks.
2. For PUD, it is recommended that most antacids be taken 1 hr and 3 hr after meals and at bedtime.
3. Tablets should be thoroughly chewed before swallowing and followed by a glass of milk or water. Effervescent tablets should completely dissolve in water before ingestion.
4. Liquid preparations have a more rapid action time and greater activity than tablets. Refrigerate to improve palatability.
5. Shake liquid suspensions thoroughly before pouring the medication. After administering, follow with water to ensure passage to the stomach. When administering via feeding tube, flush tube with water.
6. The absorption rate of many drugs may be affected by antacids. Enteric-coated tablets may dissolve prematurely. Therefore, if other oral drugs are to be taken, it should be done at least 2 hr after ingestion of the antacid.
7. Administer laxative or cathartic dose at bedtime, as medication takes about 8 hr to be effective and the effect should not interfere with the client's rest.

HEALTH CARE CONSIDERATIONS

Assessment

1. Document indications for therapy and type and onset of symptoms.
2. Note subjective reports of heartburn, indigestion, or epigastric pain. Document any precipitating factors such as foods as well as location, character, and duration of discomfort.

3. List other drugs taking to ensure none interact unfavorably.
4. Note if the client has problems with diarrhea. Antacids containing magnesium may have a laxative effect, worsening this problem; use aluminum-based product instead.
5. Determine if the client has a history of cardiac disease or hypertension. These clients often are on low-sodium diets, so prescribed antacids should also be low in sodium.
6. Note any radiologic studies or endoscopic findings; document H. pilorior urease or slant test results.

Interventions

1. Clients taking antacid preparations containing calcium or aluminum are prone to constipation. Encourage fluid intake of 2–3 L/day unless contraindicated and also increased consumption of foods high in bulk and fiber.
2. If the client has renal failure, increasing fluid intake to avoid constipation is not an option. Stool softeners may be necessary. Also, absorption of Na, Mg, Al, or Ca may precipitate alkalosis.
3. If constipation persists, determine if changing the antacid or using laxatives and/or enemas may be of some benefit.
4. Clients taking antacids that contain magnesium may report diarrhea. Document and report as a change in antacid or alternating a magnesium-based antacid with an aluminum- or calcium-based antacid may be indicated. Magnesium salts have a cathartic effect.

Client/Family Teaching

1. Take the tablets with water. The liquid acts as a vehicle, transporting the medication to the stomach, where the desired drug action occurs.
2. Take the drug at the prescribed times. Some may need to be taken on an empty stomach, whereas others, such as those used to bind phosphate, may need to be taken with meals.
3. Advise that refrigeration may improve taste.
4. Report any persistent constipation or diarrhea.
5. Advise that consumption of large amounts of TUMS can cause acid rebound.
6. Avoid taking OTC preparations unless specifically ordered.
7. Do not smoke or use alcoholic beverages as these alter drug effects.
8. Report any evidence of GI bleeding (dark black or tarry stools, coffee ground emesis).
9. Discuss the importance of following the specific dietary regime established as well as adhering to the medication protocol. Explain that antacids should be taken for 4–6 weeks after symptoms have disappeared as healing of the ulcer is not correlated with the disappearance of symptoms.
10. Instruct client to report if the symptoms for which they are being treated show little or no improvement after 2 weeks of therapy.

Outcome/Evaluate

- Improvement in or resolution of pretreatment symptoms
- Reports of ↓ gastric pain and irritation
- Evacuation of a soft, formed stool
- ↑ Gastric pH
- Promotion of duodenal ulcer healing
- Prophylaxis of renal calculi

ANTHELMINTICS

See also the following individual entries:

Albendazole
Ivermectin
Mebendazole
Praziquantel
Pyrantel pamoate
Thiabendazole

General Statement: Helminths (worms) may infect the intestinal lumen or the worm also may migrate to a particular tissue. Treatment of helminth infections is complicated by the fact that a worm may have one or more morphologic stages. Thus, it is important to ensure that therapy rids the body of eggs and larvae, as well as worms. Also, a client may be infected by more than one type of worm. Factors such as availability and cost of the drug, toxicity, ease of administration, and how long it takes to complete therapy also have a significant impact on successful treatment of helminths. Accurate diagnosis is extremely important before treatment is started because its success depends on selecting the drug best suited for the eradication of a specific infestation. Parasites that infest only the intestinal tract can be eradicated by locally acting drugs. Other parasites enter tissues and must be treated by drugs that are absorbed from the GI tract.

Since many parasitic infestations are transmitted by persons sharing bathroom facilities, the provider may wish to examine all members of the household for parasitic infestation. Treatment is often accompanied or followed by repeated laboratory examinations to determine whether the parasite has been eradicated.

Helminths can be divided into three groups: cestodes (flatworms, tapeworms), nematodes (roundworms), and trematodes (flukes). The following is a brief description of the more common helminths and the drug of choice to treat infections by that particular helminth.

CESTODES (FLATWORMS, TAPEWORMS): The more common tapeworms are the beef tapeworm (*Taenia saginata*), pork tapeworm (*T. solium*), dwarf tapeworm (*Hymenolepis nana*), and fish tapeworm (*Diphyllobothrium latum*). Tapeworm infestations are difficult to eradicate. **Drug treatment:** Praziquantel.

NEMATODES: **1. Filaria (filariasis).** Infections due to *Wuchereria bancrofti, Brugia malayi,* and *B. timori* are transmitted by mosquitoes. Mosquito control is the best means of combating this infestation. Other filarial infections include *Loa loa,* transmitted by the bite of a horsefly, and *Onchocerca volvulus* (onchocerciasis, river blindness), which is transmitted by the bite of a blackfly. **Drug treatment:** Diethylcarbamazine. Suramin sodium (available from Centers for Disease Control) is used to treat onchocerciasis.

2. Hookworm (uncinariasis). Intestinal infection caused by *Ancylostoma duodenale* or *Necator americanus.* **Drug treatment:** Mebendazole or pyrantel pamoate.

3. Pinworm (enterobiasis). Caused by *Enterobius vermicularis.* **Drug treatment:** Mebendazole, pyrantel pamoate, thiabendazole.

4. Roundworm (ascariasis). Caused by *Ascaris lumbricoides.* **Drug treatment:** Mebendazole, pyrantel pamoate.

5. Trichinosis. Caused by *Trichinella spiralis,* these parasites are transmitted by the consumption of raw or inadequately cooked pork. **Drug treatment:** Corticosteroids to control the inflammation caused by systemic infestation; mebendazole, thiabendazole.

6. Threadworm (strongyloidiasis). This parasite (*Strongyloides stercoralis*) infests the upper GI tract. **Drug treatment:** Thiabendazole.

7. Whipworm (trichuriasis). This threadlike parasite (*Trichuris trichiura*) lodges in the mucosa of the cecum. **Drug treatment:** Mebendazole.

TREMATODES: Schistosomiasis (blood flukes or bilharziasis) can be transmitted by *Schistosoma mansoni, S. japonicum, S. haematobium,* and *S. mekongi.* The infection is difficult to eradicate. **Drug treatment:** Praziquantel, oxamniquine (*S. mansoni* only).

See also *General Health Care Considerations for All Anti-Infectives.*

Side Effects: N&V, cramps, and diarrhea are common to most.

HEALTH CARE CONSIDERATIONS

Assessment

1. Record type, onset and characteristics of symptoms, any causative factors, and exposure(s).
2. Obtain specimens for microscopic exam.
3. Determine if pregnant; note ulcer presence.

Client/Family Teaching

1. Review instructions regarding diet, cathartics, enemas, meds, and follow-up tests.
2. *Good hygienic practices reduce the incidence of helminthiasis.*
3. Notify school that child is undergoing therapy; identify close contacts that should also be treated.
4. Specific practices are as follows:

PINWORMS

1. Therapy consists of a single dose with meals and is repeated in 2 weeks.
2. Prevent infestation with pinworms by:
   - Washing hands with soap and water before and after contact with infected person and when changing their clothes or bed linens
   - Washing hands frequently during the day, always after toileting, and before meals
   - Keeping nails short
   - Washing ova from anal area bid to prevent itching
   - Applying ointment to anal area to reduce scratching, which transfers pinworms. Scratching causes pinworms to attach to the fingers, which when placed in the mouth causes reinfection
   - Changing clothes daily and checking for evidence of eggs or worms
   - Wearing tight underpants
   - Wearing gloves to prepare food
   - Washing linens in hot water
   - Not sharing washcloths and towels and changing/laundering regularly
   - Disinfecting toilet daily; double flush after BM
   - For several days after therapy, wet mop or vacuum bedroom floor; do not sweep, as this spreads eggs
   - Wash bed linens and night clothes after therapy and do not shake
3. Eggs are not visible but contaminate everything they come in contact with (i.e., food, hands, clothes, linens, rugs). Eggs floating in the air can be swallowed and cause infestation; is very contagious and easily transmissable and all family members need to be checked.
4. After treatment, swab the perianal area each morning with transparent tape and re-

turn to provider. A cure is considered when no further eggs are found on microscopic exam for 7 consecutive days.

ROUNDWORMS, HOOKWORMS, WHIPWORMS:

1. Two to 3 weeks after therapy, stools should be microscopically examined for fecal egg count.
2. Record stool color and consistency; examine for expulsed worm.
3. Examine results of the enema for the head of the worm.
4. Advise that:

• Stools must go to the lab warm and be examined daily until no further roundworm ova are found

• Wash hands with soap and water frequently during the day, always after toileting, and before eating

• Wash all fruits and vegetables before eating; cook meats and vegetables thoroughly

• Wear shoes, do not defecate outside, use a bathroom, and double flush to ensure proper excretion disposal

TREMATODES:

1. Dizziness, drowsiness, N&V, headache, diarrhea, and pruritis may occur 3 hr after dosing and last for several hours.
2. Report any low-grade fever, discoloration of urine, or seizure activity.
3. If prior seizure disorder, hospitalize for treatment due to change in seizure threshold.

Outcome/Evaluate

• Knowledge of illness, prevention of transmission, and eradication/expulsion of organism

• Causes for repeated infestation; need for further treatment

ANTIANEMIC DRUGS

See also the following individual entries:

Ferrous fumarate
Ferrous gluconate
Ferrous sulfate
Ferrous sulfate, dried

Action/Kinetics: The normal daily iron intake for males is 12–20 mg and for females is 8–15 mg, although only about 10% (1–2 mg) of this iron is absorbed. Iron is absorbed from the duodenum and upper jejunum by an active mechanism through the mucosal cells where it combines with the protein transferrin. Iron is stored in the body as hemosiderin or aggregated ferritin which is found in reticuloendothelial cells of the liver, spleen, and bone marrow. About two-thirds of total body iron is in the circulating RBCs in hemoglobin. Absorption of the ferrous salt is three times greater than the ferric salt. Absorption is enhanced when stored iron is depleted or when erythropoesis occurs at an increased rate. Food decreases iron absorption by up to two-thirds. The daily loss of iron thorugh urine, sweat, and sloughing of intestinal mucosal cells is 0.5–1mg in healthy men; in menstruating women, 1–2 mg is the normal daily loss.

General Statement: Anemia is a deficiency in the number of RBCs or in the hemoglobin level in RBCs. The two main types of anemia are (1) iron-deficiency anemias, resulting from greater than normal loss or destruction of blood cells, and (2) megaloblastic anemias, resulting from deficient production of blood cells. Iron deficiency can affect muscle metabolism, heat production, and catecholamine metabolism and can cause behavioral or learning problems in children. The cause of the iron deficiency must be determined before therapy is started.

Uses: Prophylaxis and treatment of iron deficiency and iron-deficiency anemias. Dietary supplement for iron. Optimum therapeutic responses are usually noted within 2–4 weeks. *Investigational:* Clients receiving epoetin therapy (failure to give iron supplements either IV or PO can impair the hematologic response to epoetin).

Contraindications: Hemosiderosis, hemochromatosis, peptic ulcer, regional enteritis, and ulcerative colitis. Hemolytic anemia, pyridoxine-responsive anemia, and cirrhosis of the liver. Use in those with normal iron balance.

Special Concerns: Allergic reactions may result due to certain products containing tartrazine and some products containing sulfites.

Side Effects: *GI:* Constipation, gastric irritation, nausea, abdominal cramps, anorexia, vomiting, diarrhea, dark-colored stools. These effects may be minimized by administering preparations as a coated tablet. Soluble iron preparations may stain the teeth.

OD **Management of Overdose:** *Symptoms:* Symptoms occur in four stages—(1) Lethargy, N&V, abdominal pain, weak and rapid pulse, tarry stools, dehydration, acidosis, hypotension, and ***coma*** within 1–6 hr. (2) If client survives, symptoms subside for about 24 hr. (3) Within 24–48 hr symptoms return with ***diffuse vascular congestion, shock, pulmonary edema, acidosis, seizures, anuria, hyperthermia, and death.*** (4) If client survives, pyloric or antral stenosis, hepatic cirrhosis, and CNS damage are seen within 2–6 weeks. Toxic reactions are more likely to occur after parenteral administration. *Treatment (Iron Toxicity):*

- General supportive measures.
- Maintain a patent airway, respiration, and circulation.
- Induce vomiting with syrup of ipecac followed by gastric lavage using tepid water or 1%–5% sodium bicarbonate (to convert from ferrous sulfate to ferrous carbonate, which is poorly absorbed and less irritating). Saline cathartics can also be used.
- Deferoxamine is indicated for clients with serum iron levels greater than 300 mg/dL. Deferoxamine is usually given IM, but in severe cases of poisoning it may be given IV. Hydration should be maintained.
- It may be necessary to treat for shock, acidosis, renal failure, and seizures.

Drug Interactions

Antacids, oral / ↓ Absorption of iron from GI tract
Ascorbic acid / Doses of ascorbic acid of 200 mg or more ↑ absorption if iron
Chloramphenicol / ↑ Serum iron levels
Cholestyramine / ↓ Absoprtion of iron from GI tract
Cimetidine / ↓ Absorption of iron from GI tract
Fluoroquinolones / ↓ Absorption of fluoroquinolones from GI tract due to formation of a ferric ion-quinolone complex
Levodopa / ↓ Absorption of levodopa due to formation of chelates with iron salts
Levothyroxine / ↓ Efficacy of levothyroxine
Methyldopa / ↓ Absorption of methyldopa from GI tract
Pancreatic extracts / ↓ Absorption of iron from GI tract
Penicillamine / ↓ Absorption of penicillamine from GI tract due to chelation
Tetracyclines / ↓ Absorption of both tetracyclines and iron from GI tract
Vitamin E / Vitamin E ↓ response to iron therapy

Dosage

See individual drugs. Duration of therapy: 2–4 months longer than the time needed to reverse anemia, usually 6 or more months.

Laboratory Test Considerations: Iron-containing drugs may affect electrolyte balance determinations.

1. For infants and young children, administer liquid preparation with a dropper. Deposit liquid well back against the cheek.
2. Eggs and milk or coffee and tea consumed with a meal or 1 hr after may significantly inhibit absorption of dietary iron.
3. Ingestion of calcium and iron supplements with food can decrease iron absorption by one-third; iron absorption is not decreased if calcium carbonate is used and taken between meals.
4. Do not crush or chew sustained-release products.

HEALTH CARE CONSIDERATIONS

Assessment

1. Take a drug history, including:
   - Antacid use; any other drugs that may interact
   - OTC drugs, i.e., iron compounds or vitamin E use
   - Recent abdominal surgery; all currently prescribed drugs
   - Allergy to sulfites or tartrazines (may be present in some products)
2. Note any GI bleeding; tarry stools or bright blood in stool or vomitus.
3. Assess for thalassemia; obtain hemoglobin electrophoresis, as iron administration could be lethal.
4. Note any complaints of fatigue, pallor, poor skin turgor, or change in mental status, especially in the elderly.
5. Assess nutritional status and diet history through questioning and intake if possible.
6. Review pregnancies and menstruation history; note frequency, amounts, and heavy or abnormal bleeding. Pregnancy is an indication for preventive administration of iron.
7. Monitor VS, CBC, chemistry profile, stool for occult blood, reticulocytes, serum transferrin, and iron panel results. Discontinue if 500 mg of iron daily does not cause a 1 g-rise of hemoglobin in 1 mo. Note cause (i.e., iron-deficient or megaloblastic anemia) or if further workup is needed.

Client/Family Teaching

1. Adhere to prescribed regimen; report any problems immediately. Coated tablets may diminish GI effects such as nausea, constipation or diarrhea, gastric irritation, and abdominal cramps.
2. Review the form of iron prescribed (bi- or trivalent) and frequency of administration.
3. Take with meals to reduce gastric irritation. Milk products, eggs, and antacids inhibit absorption so avoid unless taking ferrous lactate. Coffee and tea consumed within 1 hr of meals may inhibit absorption of dietary iron.
4. Taking with citrus juices enhances iron absorption.
5. May cause indigestion, change in stool color (black and tarry or dark green), abdominal cramps, diarrhea, or constipation; may be relieved by changing the med, dosage, or time of administration.

6. Increase intake of fruit, fiber, and fluids to minimize constipating effects. Eat a well-balanced diet with foods high in iron (i.e., meat proteins, dried fruits) and affordable foods (i.e., raisins, dark green leafy vegetables, and liver versus apricots or prunes).
7. Will reduce tetracycline absorption. If to receive both, allow at least 2 hr to elapse between doses.
8. Store out of reach of children as an overdosage can be fatal.
9. Dilute liquid preparations well with water or fruit juice and use a straw to minimize teeth staining.
10. Pregnant women need an iron-rich diet. The American Academy of Pediatrics recommends an iron supplement for infants during their first year of life.
11. Follow administration guidelines for each product to minimize side effects. Do not self-medicate with vitamin, mineral, and iron supplements.

Outcome/Evaluate

- Resolution of anemia; If hemoglobin has not increased 1 g in 4 weeks, then reconfirm diagnosis
- Improvement in exercise tolerance and level of fatigue
- Improvement in skin pallor, color of nail beds, Hb and iron levels

ANTIANGINAL DRUGS—NITRATES/NITRITES

See also Beta-Adrenergic Blocking Agents, Calcium Channel Blocking Drugs, and the following individual entries:

Amyl nitrite
Isosorbide dinitrate
Isosorbide mononitrate, oral
Nitroglycerin sublingual
Nitroglycerin sustained release
Nitroglycerin topical ointment
Nitroglycerin transdermal system
Nitroglycerin translingual spray

Action/Kinetics: Nitrates relax vascular smooth muscle by stimulating production of intracellular cyclic guanosine monophosphate. Dilation of postcapillary vessels decreases venous return to the heart due to pooling of blood; thus, LV end-diastolic pressure (preload) is reduced. Relaxation of arterioles results in a decreased systemic vascular resistance and arterial pressure (afterload). The oxygen requirements of the myocardium are reduced and there is more efficient redistribution of blood flow through collateral channels in myocardial tissue. Diastolic, systolic, and mean BP are decreased. Also, elevated central venous and pulmonary capillary wedge pressures, pulmonary vascular resistance, and systemic vascular resistance are reduced. Reflex tachycardia may occur due to the overall decrease in BP. Cardiac index may increase, decrease, or remain the same; those with elevated left ventricular filling pressure and systemic vascular resistance values with a depressed cardiac index are likely to see improvement of the cardiac index. The onset and duration depend on the product and route of administration (sublingual, topical, transdermal, parenteral, oral, and buccal). **Onset:** Less than 1 min for amyl nitrite to 1 to 3 min for IV, sublingual, translingual, and transmucosal nitroglycerin or sublingual isosorbide dinitrate; 20 to 60 min for sustained-release, topical, and transdermal nitroglycerin or oral isosorbide dinitrate or mononitrate; and up to 4 hr for sustained-release isosorbide dinitrate. **Duration of action:** 3 to 5 min for amyl nitrite and IV nitroglycerin; 30 to 60 min for sublingual or translingual nitroglycerin; several hours for transmucosal, sustained-release, or topical nitroglycerin and all isosorbide dinitrate products; and up to 24 hr for transdermal nitroglycerin.

Uses: Treatment and prophylaxis of acute angina pectoris (use sublingual, transmucosal, or translingual nitroglycerin; amyl nitrite). Nitrates are first-line therapy for unstable angina. Prophylaxis of chronic angina pectoris (topical, transdermal, translingual, transmucosal, or oral sustained-release nitroglycerin; isosorbide dinitrate and mononitrate; erythrityl tetranitrate; pentaerythritol tetranitrate). IV nitroglycerin is used to decrease BP in surgical procedures resulting in hypertension, as well as an adjunct in treating hypertension or CHF associated with MI. *Investigational:* Nitroglycerin ointment has been used as an adjunct in treating Raynaud's disease. Also, isosorbide dinitrate with prostaglandin E_1 for peripheral vascular disease. Sublingual and topical nitroglycerin and oral nitrates have been used to decrease cardiac workload in clients with acute MI and in CHF.

Contraindications: Sensitivity to nitrites, which may result in severe hypotensive reactions, MI, or tolerance to nitrites. Severe anemia, cerebral hemorrhage, recent head trauma, postural hypotension, closed angle glaucoma, impaired hepatic function, hypertrophic cardiomyopathy, hypotension, recent MI. PO dosage forms should not be used in clients with GI hypermotility or with

malabsorption syndrome. IV nitroglycerin should not be used in clients with hypotension, uncorrected hypovolemia, inadequate cerebral circulation, constrictive pericarditis, increased ICP, or pericardial tamponade.
Special Concerns: Use with caution during lactation and in glaucoma. Tolerance to the antianginal and vascular effects may occur. Safety and efficacy have not been determined during lactation and in children.
Side Effects: *CNS:* Headaches (most common) which may be severe and persistent, restlessness, dizziness, weakness, apprehension, vertigo, anxiety, insomnia, confusion, nightmares, hypoesthesia, hypokinesia, dyscoordination. *CV:* Postural hypotension (common) with or without paradoxical bradycardia and increased angina, tachycardia, palpitations, syncope, rebound hypertension, crescendo angina, retrosternal discomfort, ***CV collapse,*** atrial fibrillation, PVCs, ***arrhythmias.*** *GI:* N&V, dyspepsia, diarrhea, dry mouth, abdominal pain, involuntary passing of feces and urine, tenesmus, tooth disorder. *Dermatologic:* Crusty skin lesions, pruritus, rash, exfoliative dermatitis, cutaneous vasodilation with flushing. *GU:* Urinary frequency, impotence, dysuria. *Respiratory:* URTI, bronchitis, pneumonia. *Allergic:* Itching, wheezing, tracheobronchitis. *Miscellaneous:* Perspiration, muscle twitching, methemoglobinemia, cold sweating, blurred vision, diplopia, ***hemolytic anemia,*** arthralgia, edema, malaise, neck stiffness, increased appetite, rigors. **Topical use:** Peripheral edema, contact dermatitis.

Tolerance can occur following chronic use. Nitrites convert hemoglobin to methemoglobin, which impairs the oxygen-carrying capacity of the blood, resulting in ***anemic hypoxia.*** This interaction is dangerous in clients with preexisting anemia.

OD **Management of Overdose:** *Symptoms (Toxicity):* Severe toxicity is rarely encountered with therapeutic use. Symptoms include hypotension, flushing, tachycardia, headache, palpitations, vertigo, perspiring skin followed by cold and cyanotic skin, visual disturbances, syncope, nausea, dizziness, diaphoresis, initial hyperpnea, dyspnea and slow breathing, slow pulse, ***heart block,*** vomiting with the possibility of bloody diarrhea and colic, anorexia, and increased ICP with symptoms of confusion, moderate fever, and paralysis. Tissue hypoxia (due to methemoglobinemia) may result in ***cyanosis, metabolic acidosis, coma, seizures, and death due to CV collapse.*** *Treatment (Toxicity):*

• Induction of emesis or gastric lavage followed by activated charcoal (nitrates are usually rapidly absorbed from the stomach). Gastric lavage may be used if the drug has been recently ingested.
• Maintain in a recumbent shock position and keep warm. Give oxygen and artificial respiration if required.
• Monitor methemoglobin levels.
• Elevate legs and administer IV fluids to treat severe hypotension and reflex tachycardia. Phenylephrine or methoxamine may also be helpful.
• Do not use epinephrine and similar drugs as they are ineffective in reversing severe hypotension.

Drug Interactions
Acetylcholine / Effects ↓ when used with nitrates
Alcohol, ethyl / Hypotension and CV collapse due to vasodilator effect of both agents
Antihypertensive drugs / Additive hypotension
Aspirin / ↑ Serum levels and effects of nitrates
Beta-adrenergic blocking drugs / Additive hypotension
Calcium channel blocking drugs / Additive hypotension, including significant orthostatic hypotension
Dihydroergotamine / ↑ Effect of dihydroergotamine due to increased bioavailability or antagonism resulting in ↓ antianginal effects
Heparin / Possible ↓ effect of heparin
Narcotics / Additive hypotensive effect
Phenothiazines / Additive hypotension
Sympathomimetics / ↓ Effect of nitrates; also, nitrates may ↓ effect of sympathomimetics resulting in hypotension

Dosage

See individual agents.
Laboratory Test Considerations: ↑ Urinary catecholamines. False negative ↓ in serum cholesterol.Store tablets and capsules tightly closed in their original container. Avoid exposure to air, heat, and moisture.

HEALTH CARE CONSIDERATIONS

Assessment

1. Note any sensitivity to nitrites.
2. Record location, intensity, duration, extension, and any precipitating factors (i.e., activity, stress) surrounding anginal pain. Use a pain-rating scale to rate pain.
3. If history of anemia, administer with extreme caution.
4. Nitrates are contraindicated with elevated intracranial pressure.
5. Note any changes in ECG or elevated cardiac panel. Document results of echocardiogram, stress test, and/or catheterization.

Interventions

1. Determine experience with self-administered medications; note if SL tablets ordered for the bedside.
2. While hospitalized, note drug required to keep angina under control. Record:
- How frequently given
- Intensity of pain (use a pain-rating scale; rate pain initially and 5 min after administration)
- Duration of attacks
- Whether relief is partial or complete
- Time it takes for relief to occur
- Any side effects
3. Report when consumed so effectiveness can be determined and usage monitored.
4. Monitor VS. Assess for sensitivity to hypotensive effects of nitrites (N&V, pallor, restlessness, and CV collapse).
5. Monitor for hypotension when receiving additional drugs; adjustment may be necessary. Supervise activities/ ambulation until drug effects realized.
6. Assess for signs of tolerance, which occur following chronic use but may begin several days after starting treatment; manifested by absence of response to the usual dose. (Nitrites may be discontinued temporarily until tolerance is lost, and then reinstituted. During interim, other vasodilators may be used.)
7. Observe for N&V, drowsiness, headache, or visual disturbances with long-term therapy (prolonged effects which require a change in drug).
8. Note change in activity and response to drug therapy. Determine if less discomfort experienced when performing regular activity.

Client/Family Teaching

1. Take oral nitrates on an empty stomach with a glass of water. The drug decreases myocardial oxygen demand and reduces workload of the heart.
2. To prevent postural hypotension, use inhalation products or take SL tabs while sitting or lying down. Make position changes slowly and rise only after dangling feet for several minutes.
3. Elderly clients should sit or lie down when taking nitroglycerin as they are more prone to hypotensive effects and may become dizzy and fall.
4. Do not change from one brand to another due to differences in effectiveness between products manufactured by different companies.
5. Always carry SL tablets for use in aborting an attack. Check expiration date; replace when needed or every 6 mo. A burning sensation under the tongue attests to drug potency.
6. Carry SL tablets in a *glass* bottle, tightly capped. Keep in original container as heat, moisture, and air cause deterioration. Do not use plastic containers; drug deteriorates in plastic; avoid child-proof caps as client must get to the tablets quickly.
7. If pain is not relieved in 5 min by first SL tablet, take up to 2 more tablets at 5-min intervals. If pain has not subsided 5 min after third tablet, client should be taken to the emergency room; *do not* drive; call 911.
8. Take SL tabs 5–15 min prior to any situation likely to cause pain (e.g., climbing stairs, sexual intercourse, exposure to cold weather).
9. Record attacks; report any increase in the frequency/intensity of attacks and loss of effectiveness.
10. Schedule frequent rest periods, pace activities, and avoid stressful situations. Use Tylenol for drug-induced headaches.
11. Follow instructions on how to apply topical nitroglycerin. Remove at bedtime and apply upon arising; some studies support a nitrate-free period of at least 8 hr may reduce or prevent nitrate tolerance.
12. Avoid alcohol; nitrite syncope, a severe shock-like state, may occur.
13. Inhalation products are flammable; do not use under situations where they might ignite.
14. Do not smoke. Review risks and lifestyle changes necessary to prevent further CAD (i.e., weight control, dietary changes, ↓ salt intake, modified regular exercise program, no alcohol/tobacco, and stress reduction).
15. Have family or significant other learn CPR; survival rate is greatly increased when CPR is initiated immediately.
16. Carry ID and list of prescribed drugs. Know what you are taking and why.

Outcome/Evaluate

- ↓ Myocardial oxygen requirements; ↑ activity tolerance
- Improved myocardial perfusion
- Relief of coronary artery spasm

ANTIARRHYTHMIC DRUGS

See also the following individual entries:

Calcium Channel Blocking Drugs
Digitoxin
Digoxin
Diltiazem hydrochloride
Disopyramide phosphate
Flecainide acetate

Moricizine hydrochloride
Phenytoin
Phenytoin sodium
Procainamide hydrochloride
Propafenone hydrochloride
Propranolol hydrochloride
Quinidine gluconate
Quinidine sulfate
Tocainide hydrochloride
Verapamil

Action/Kinetics: Examples of cardiac arrhythmias are *premature ventricular beats, ventricular tachycardia, atrial flutter, atrial fibrillation, ventricular fibrillation,* and *atrioventricular heart block.* The various antiarrhythmic drugs are classified according to both their mechanism of action and their effects on the action potential of cardiac cells. Importantly, one drug in a particular class may be more effective and safer in an individual client. The antiarrhythmic drugs are classified as follows:

1. Group I. Decrease the rate of entry of sodium during cardiac membrane depolarization, decrease the rate of rise of phase O of the cardiac membrane action potential, prolong the effective refractory period of fast-response fibers, and require that a more negative membrane potential be reached before the membrane becomes excitable (and thus can propagate to other membranes). Group I drugs are further listed in subgroups (according to their effects on action potential duration) as follows:

• Group IA: Depress phase O and prolong the duration of the action potential. Examples: Disopyramide, procainamide, and quinidine.
• Group IB: Slightly depress phase O and are thought to shorten the action potential. Examples: Lidocaine, phenytoin, and tocainide.
• Group IC: Slight effect on repolarization but marked depression of phase O of the action potential. Significant slowing of conduction. Examples: Flecainide, indecainide, and propafenone.

NOTE: Moricizine is classified as a group I agent but it has characteristics of agents in groups IA, B, and C.

2. Group II. Competitively block beta-adrenergic receptors and depress phase 4 depolarization. Examples: Acebutolol, esmolol, and propranolol.
3. Group III. Prolong the duration of the membrane action potential (relative refractory period) without changing the phase of depolarization or the resting membrane potential. Examples: Amiodarone, bretylium, and sotalol.
4. Group IV. Verapamil, a calcium channel blocker that slows conduction velocity and increases the refractoriness of the AV node.

Adenosine and digoxin are also used to treat arrhythmias. Adenosine slows conduction time through the AV node and can interrupt the reentry pathways through the AV node. Digoxin causes a decrease in maximal diastolic potential and duration of the action potential; it also increases the slope of phase 4 depolarization.

Special Concerns: Monitor serum levels of antiarrhythmic drugs since some drugs can cause toxic side effects which can be confused with the purpose for which the drug is used. For example, toxicity from quinidine can result in cardiac arrhythmias. Antiarrhythmic drugs may cause new or worsening of arrhythmias, ranging from an increase in frequency of PVCs to severe ventricular tachycardia, ventricular fibrillation, or tachycardia that is more sustained and rapid. Such situations (called proarrhythmic effect) may make it difficult to distinguish the proarrhythmic effect from the underlying rhythm disorder.

HEALTH CARE CONSIDERATIONS

Assessment

1. Note drug sensitivity and any previous experiences with these drugs.
2. Assess extent of palpitations, fluttering sensations, chest pains, fainting episodes, or missed beats; obtain ECG with arrhythmia documentation.
3. Assess heart sounds and VS.
4. Monitor BS, electrolytes, liver and renal function studies. Ensure that serum pH, electrolytes, pO_2 and/or O_2 saturations are WNL.
5. Assess life-style related to cigarettes and caffeine use, alcohol consumption, and lack of regular exercise. Certain foods, emotional stress, and other environmental factors may also trigger arrhythmias; identify and eliminate before instituting drugs.

Interventions

1. Use a cardiac monitor if administering drugs by IV route. Monitor for rhythm changes; report and document rhythm strips.
2. Monitor BP and pulse. A HR < 50 bpm or > 120 should be avoided. Review written parameters for BP and pulse ranges.
3. Monitor serum electrolyte and drug levels.

Client/Family Teaching

1. Drugs work by controlling the irregular heart beats so the heart can pump more efficiently.
2. Take drugs as ordered; If a dose is missed, do not double up on the next dose.

3. Record BP and pulse for review at next visit.
4. Avoid OTC products. Eliminate caffeine, cigarettes, and alcohol, as these alter drug absorption and may precipitate arrhythmias.
5. Keep follow-up visits so that therapy can be adjusted and evaluated.
6. Report concerns/fears or problems R/T sexual activity.
7. Always carry list of currently prescribed meds and condition being treated.
8. Family/significant other should learn CPR; survival rates are greatly increased when initiated immediately.

Outcome/Evaluate

- ECG evidence of arrhythmia control; restoration of stable cardiac rhythm
- Laboratory confirmation that serum drug concentrations are within therapeutic range

ANTICOAGULANTS

See also the following:

Warfarin sodium

Action/Kinetics: Drugs that affect blood coagulation can be divided into three classes: (1) *anticoagulants,* or drugs that prevent or slow blood coagulation; (2) *thrombolytic agents,* which increase the rate at which an existing blood clot dissolves; and (3) *hemostatics,* which prevent or stop internal bleeding. Carefully monitor the dosage of all agents since overdosage can have serious consequences. The major anticoagulants are warfarin, heparin, and low molecular weight heparin derivatives. The following considerations are pertinent to all types. Anticoagulants do not dissolve previously formed clots, but they do forestall their enlargement and prevent new clots from forming.

See also *Health Care Considerations* for individual agents.

Uses: Venous thrombosis, pulmonary embolism, acute coronary occlusions with MIs, and strokes caused by emboli or cerebral thrombi. Prophylactically for rheumatic heart disease, atrial fibrillation, traumatic injuries of blood vessels, vascular surgery, major abdominal, thoracic, and pelvic surgery, prevention of strokes in clients with transient attacks of cerebral ischemia, or other signs of impending stroke.

Heparin is often used concurrently during the therapeutic initiation period. *Investigational (Warfarin):* Reduce risk of postconversion emboli; prophylaxis of recurrent, cerebral thromboembolism; prophylaxis of myocardial reinfarction; treatment of transient ischemic attacks; reduce the risk of thromboembolic complications in clients with certain types of prosthetic heart valves; reduced risk of thrombosis and/or occlusion following coronary bypass surgery.

Contraindications: Hemorrhagic tendencies (including hemophilia), clients with frail or weakened blood vessels, blood dyscrasias, ulcerative lesions of the GI tract (including peptic ulcer), diverticulitis, colitis, SBE, threatened abortion, recent operations on the eye, brain, or spinal cord, regional anesthesia and lumbar block, vitamin K deficiency, leukemia with bleeding tendencies, thrombocytopenic purpura, open wounds or ulcerations, acute nephritis, impaired hepatic or renal function, or severe hypertension. Hepatic and renal dysfunction. In the presence of drainage tubes in any orifice. Alcoholism.

Special Concerns: Use with caution in menstruation, in pregnant women (because they may cause hypoprothrombinemia in the infant), during lactation, during the postpartum period, and following cerebrovascular accidents. Geriatric clients may be more susceptible to the effects of anticoagulants.

Side Effects: See individual drugs.

Dosage

See individual drugs.

Special Considerations

1. The elderly are more prone to developing bleeding complications.
2. Unusual hair loss and itching are common with the elderly; report immediately.
3. Many elderly use multiple pharmacies and shop for value; make sure they carry the name and dosage of all drugs prescribed.

HEALTH CARE CONSIDERATIONS

Assessment

1. Review history and drug profile to ensure none interact unfavorably.
2. Assess for defects in clotting mechanism or any capillary fragility.
3. Note indications for therapy, time frame (i.e., DVT (initial) 6 months; valve replacement—lifetime), and desired INR, PT/PTT and record.
4. Review PMH for conditions that may preclude therapy: PUD, chronic GI tract ulcerations, severe renal or liver dysfunction, infections of the endocardium.
5. Assess for alcoholism as anticoagulants are contraindicated.
6. Monitor CBC, PT/INR or PTT.

Interventions

1. Post/advise client receiving anticoagulant therapy.
2. Monitor PT/INR or PTT levels closely; adjust oral anticoagulant weekly, esp. if receiving one of the many drugs known to interact or compete.
3. Question about bleeding (gums, urine, stools, vomit, bruises). If urine discolored, determine cause, i.e., from drug therapy or hematuria. Indanedione-type anticoagulants turn alkaline urine a red-orange color; acidify urine or test for occult blood.
4. Sudden lumbar pain may indicate retroperitoneal hemorrhage.
5. GI dysfunction may indicate intestinal hemorrhage. Test for blood in urine and feces; check H&H to assess for abnormal bleeding.
6. Have vitamin K, FFP, or factor IX concentrate for warfarin overdoses and protamine sulfate for heparin overdose (generally for every 100 U of heparin administer 1 mg IV) available.
7. Apply pressure to all venipuncture and injection sites to prevent bleeding and hematoma formation.
8. With SC administration, do not aspirate or massage; administer in lower abdomen and rotate sites.

Client/Family Teaching

1. Take at the same time every day as prescribed; record to ensure that drug has been taken.
2. Report if dizziness, headaches, bleeding gums or wounds, or vomiting of dark material are evident; esp. important with elderly.
3. Report increased bleeding, bruising, illness, heavy menstrual flow, or blood in the urine.
4. Avoid contact sports and any unsafe situations or activities that may result in injury, falls, bumps, or cuts.
5. To prevent cuts, use an electric razor instead of a razor blade.
6. To prevent bleeding gums, use a soft bristle toothbrush and brush gently; inform dentist of drug therapy.
7. If severe sight problems, teach family that furniture should not be moved from usual places. This creates confusion for someone without full vision and can cause accidents resulting in bleeding and/or bruising; wear shoes and use a night light to prevent falls and bumps in the dark.
8. Review dietary sources of vitamin K (asparagus, spinach, broccoli, brussels sprouts, cabbage, collards, turnips, mustard greens, milk, yogurt, and cheese) that should be consumed in limited quantities; alters PT.
9. Avoid OTC drugs. Check prior to taking any nonprescription drugs that have anticoagulant-type effects such as salicylates, NSAIDs, steroids, or vitamin preparations with high levels of vitamin K, mineral preparations from health food stores, or alcohol.
10. Always carry ID, noting drug therapy, illness, the name and number of the provider so they may be contacted if excessive bleeding or emergency surgery is required.
11. Identify social/economic situations that may alter compliance; identify available resources.
12. Must return for follow-up visits and lab studies to evaluate effectiveness and to ensure proper dosage.

Outcome/Evaluate

- PT: 1.5–2 times control; INR: 2.0–3.0 (standard therapy); INR: 3–4 (valves)
- PTT: 2–2.5 times the control/normal
- Prevention of thrombus formation
- Resolution of DVT
- ↓ Risk of thromboembolism with prosthetic heart valves

ANTICONVULSANTS

See also the following individual entries:

Acetazolamide
Acetazolamide sodium
Carbamazepine
Clonazepam
Clorazepate dipotassium
Diazepam
Ethosuximide
Felbamate
Gabapentin
Lamotrigine
Methsuximide
Phenobarbital
Phenobarbital sodium
Phensuximide
Phenytoin
Phenytoin sodium extended
Phenytoin sodium parenteral
Phenytoin sodium prompt
Primidone
Tiagabine hydrochloride
Topiramate
Valproic acid

General Statement: Therapeutic agents cannot cure convulsive disorders, but do control seizures without impairing the normal functions of the CNS. This is often accomplished by selective depression of hyperactive areas of the brain responsible for the convulsions. Therefore, these drugs are taken at all times (prophylactically) to prevent the occurrence of the seizures. There are several dif-

ferent types of epileptic disorders; consult the International Classification of Epileptic Seizures. No single drug can control all types of epilepsy; thus, accurate diagnosis is important. Drugs effective against one type of epilepsy may not be effective against another. Therapy begins with a small dose of the drug, which is continuously increased until either the seizures disappear or drug toxicity occurs. If a certain drug decreases the frequency of seizures but does not completely prevent them, another drug can be added to the dosage regimen and administered concomitantly with the first. Failure of therapy most often results from the administration of doses too small to have a therapeutic effect or from failure to use two or more drugs together. With appropriate diagnosis and selection of drugs, four out of five cases of epilepsy can be controlled adequately, but it may take the provider some time to find the best drug or combination of drugs with which to treat the client.

Dosage

Dosage is highly individualized. However, trauma or emotional stress may necessitate an increase in drug dosage requirements (e.g., if the client requires surgery and starts having seizures). For details, see individual agents.

1. Shake oral suspensions thoroughly before pouring to ensure uniform mixing.
2. Drug therapy must be individualized according to client needs.
3. Do not discontinue abruptly unless provider approved. To avoid severe, prolonged convulsions, withdraw over a period of days or weeks.
4. If there is reason to substitute one anticonvulsant drug for another, withdraw the first drug at the same time the dosage of the second drug is being increased.
5. Be prepared, in case of acute oral toxicity, to assist with inducing emesis (provided the client is not comatose) and with gastric lavage, along with other supportive measures such as administration of fluids and oxygen.

HEALTH CARE CONSIDERATIONS

Assessment

1. Check medical history for hypersensitivity to anticonvulsant drugs. Note derivatives that should be avoided.
2. Assess orientation to time and place, affect, reflexes, and VS.
3. Record seizure classification (partial or generalized). Determine the frequency and severity of seizures, noting location, duration, consciousness, type, frequency and any precipitating factors, presence of an aura, and any other characteristics. Note EEG, CT/MRI results.
4. Assess skin, eyes, and mucous membranes.
5. Determine if pregnant; may cause fetal abnormalities.
6. Monitor CBC, glucose, uric acid, urinalysis, liver and renal function studies.
7. Determine why receiving therapy and when it was instituted. If no seizure experienced for over 1 year with prophylactic therapy, may try gradual drug discontinuation.

Interventions

1. Monitor VS; observe for S&S of impending seizures.
2. With IV administration, monitor closely for respiratory depression and CV collapse.
3. Note any evidence of CNS side effects, such as blurred vision, dimmed vision, slurred speech, nystagmus, or confusion; supervise ambulation until resolved.
4. Observe for muscle twitching, loss of muscle tone, episodes of bizarre behavior, and/or subsequent amnesia.
5. With phenytoin, check Ca levels; contributes to bone demineralization which can result in osteomalacia in adults and rickets in children. Risk increases with inactivity.
6. Vitamin D may be used to prevent hypocalcemia (4,000 units of vitamin D weekly); folic acid may prevent megaloblastic anemia.
7. Administer vitamin K to pregnant women 1 month before delivery to prevent postpartum hemorrhage/bleeding in the newborn and mother.

Client/Family Teaching

1. Take the prescribed amount of drug ordered. Do not increase, decrease, or discontinue without approval; convulsions may result.
2. May initially cause a decrease in mental alertness, drowsiness, headache, vertigo, and ataxia. CNS symptoms are dose-related and should subside with continued therapy; avoid hazardous tasks until symptoms resolve.
3. Lessen GI distress by taking with large amounts of fluids or with food.
4. Dosage may require adjusting if undergoing physical trauma or emotional distress.
5. Avoid alcohol and any other CNS depressants.
6. Increase fluid intake and include fruit and other foods with roughage and bulk in the diet.
7. With gingival hyperplasia, intensify oral hygiene, use a soft tooth brush, massage the

gums, use dental floss daily, and obtain routine dental checks.
8. If slurred speech develops, try to consciously slow speech patterns to avoid the problem.
9. Avoid situations/exposures that result in fever and low glucose and sodium levels; may lower seizure threshold.
10. Report if rash, fever, severe headaches, stomatitis, rhinitis, urethritis, or balanitis (inflammation of the glans penis) occur; symptoms of hypersensitivity which require change in drug.
11. Report sore throat, easy bruising, bleeding, or nosebleeds; signs of hematologic toxicity.
12. Jaundice, dark urine, anorexia, and abdominal pain may indicate liver toxicity; needs LFTs to detect for hepatitis, hepatocellular degeneration, and fatal hepatocellular necrosis.
13. Practice reliable birth control; may harm fetus.
14. If nursing, observe infant for signs of toxicity.
15. Carry ID with the form of epilepsy and prescribed therapy. Family should learn CPR and how to protect client during a seizure.
16. Identify support groups (Epilepsy Foundation; National Head Injury Group) that may assist to understand and cope with disorder.

Outcome/Evaluate

- ↓ Frequency of seizures; improved seizure control
- Serum drug levels within desired range

ANTIDEPRESSANTS, TRICYCLIC

See also the following individual entries:

Amitriptyline and Perphenazine
Amitriptyline hydrochloride
Amoxapine
Clomipramine hydrochloride
Desipramine hydrochloride
Doxepin hydrochloride
Imipramine hydrochloride
Imipramine pamoate
Nortriptyline hydrochloride
Trimipramine maleate

Action/Kinetics: It is now believed that antidepressant drugs cause adaptive changes in the serotonin and norepinephrine receptor systems, resulting in changes in the sensitivities of both presynaptic and postsynaptic receptor sites. These effects may increase the sensitivity of postsynaptic α-1 adrenergic and serotonin receptors and decrease the sensitivity of presynaptic receptor sites. The overall effect is a reregulation of the abnormal receptorneurotransmitter relationship.

The tricyclic antidepressants are chemically related to the phenothiazines; thus, they exhibit many of the same pharmacologic effects (e.g., anticholinergic, antiserotonin, sedative, antihistaminic, and hypotensive). The TCAs are less effective for depressed clients in the presence of organic brain damage or schizophrenia. Also, they can induce mania; note when given to clients with manic-depressive psychoses. Well absorbed from the GI tract. All have a long serum half-life. Up to 46 days may be required to reach steady plasma levels and maximum therapeutic effects may not be noted for 24 weeks. Because of the long half-life, single daily dosage may suffice. More than 90% bound to plasma protein. Partially metabolized in the liver and excreted primarily in the urine.

General Statement: Drugs with antidepressant effects include the tricyclic antidepressants (TCAs), selective serotonin reuptake inhibitors (SSRIs) i.e., fluoxetine, fluvoxamine, paroxetine, sertraline; and monoamine oxidase inhibitors (MAOIs) i.e., phenelzine, tranylcypromine.

Uses: Endogenous and reactive depressions. Preferred over MAO inhibitors because they are less toxic. See also individual drugs.

Contraindications: Severely impaired liver function. Use during acute recovery phase from MI. Concomitant use with MAO inhibitors.

Special Concerns: Use with caution during lactation and with epilepsy, CV diseases, glaucoma, BPH, suicidal tendencies, a history of urinary retention, and the elderly. Use during pregnancy only when benefits clearly outweigh risks. Generally not recommended for children less than 12 years of age. Geriatric clients may be more sensitive to the anticholinergic and sedative side effects.

Side Effects: Most frequent side effects are sedation and atropine-like reactions. *CNS:* Confusion, anxiety, restlessness, insomnia, nightmares, hallucinations, delusions, mania or hypomania, headache, dizziness, inability to concentrate, panic reaction, worsening of psychoses, fatigue, weakness. *Anticholinergic:* Dry mouth, blurred vision, mydriasis, constipation, paralytic ileus, urinary retention or difficulty in urination. *GI:* N&V, anorexia, gastric distress, unpleasant taste, stomatitis, glossitis, cramps, increased salivation, black tongue. *CV:* Fainting, tachycardia, hypo- or hypertension, arrhythmias, ***heart block,*** possibility of palpitations, ***MI, stroke.*** *Neurologic:* Paresthesias, numbness, incoordination, neuropathies, extrapyramidal symptoms including tardive dyskinesia, dysarthria, seizures. *Dermatologic:* Skin rashes, urticaria, flushing, pruritus, petechiae, photosensitivity, edema. *Endocrine:* Testicular swelling and gynecomastia in males, increase or decrease in libido, impotence, menstrual irregularities and galactorrhea in females, hypo- or hyperglycemia, changes in secretion of ADH. *Miscellaneous:* Sweating, alopecia, nasal congestion, lacrimation, increase in body temperature, chills, urinary frequency including nocturia. Bone marrow depression including thrombocytopenia, leukopenia, ***agranulocytosis,*** eosinophilia.

High dosage increases the frequency of seizures in epileptic clients and may cause epileptiform attacks in normal subjects.

OD Management of Overdose: *Symptoms:* CNS symptoms include agitation, confusion, hallucinations, hyperactive reflexes, choreoathetosis, ***seizures, coma.*** Anticholinergic symptoms include dilated pupils, dry mouth, flushing, and ***hyperpyrexia.*** CV toxicity includes depressed myocardial contractility, decreased HR, decreased coronary blood flow, tachycardia, intraventricular block, ***complete AV block, re-entry ventricular arrhythmias, PVCs, ventricular tachycardia or fibrillation, sudden cardiac arrest, hypotension, pulmonary edema.*** *Treatment:* Admit client to hospital and monitor ECG closely for 3 to 5 days.

- Empty stomach in alert clients by inducing vomiting followed by gastric lavage and charcoal administration **after insertion of cuffed ET tube.** Maintain respiration and avoid the use of respiratory stimulants.
- Normal or half-normal saline to prevent water intoxication.
- To reverse the CV effects (e.g., hypotension and cardiac dysrhythmias), give hypertonic sodium bicarbonate. The usual dose is 0.52 mEq/kg by IV bolus followed by IV infusion to maintain the blood at pH 7.5. If hypotension is not reversed by bicarbonate, vasopressors (e.g., dopamine) and fluid expansion may be needed. If the cardiac dysrhythmias do not respond to bicarbonate, lidocaine or phenytoin may be used.
- Isoproterenol may be effective in controlling bradyarrhythmias and torsades de pointes ventricular tachycardia. Use propranolol, 0.1 mg/kg IV (up to 0.25 mg by IV bolus), to treat life-threatening ventricular arrhythmias in children.
- Treat shock and metabolic acidosis with IV fluids, oxygen, bicarbonate, and corticosteroids.
- Control hyperpyrexia by external means (ice pack, cool baths, spongings).
- To reduce possibility of convulsions, minimize external stimulation. If necessary, use diazepam or phenytoin to control convulsions. Avoid barbiturates if MAO inhibitors have been used recently.

Drug Interactions

Acetazolamide / ↑ Effect of tricyclics by ↑ renal tubular reabsorption of the drug

Alcohol, ethyl / Simultaneous use may lead to ↑ GI complications and ↓ performance on motor skill testsdeath has been reported

Ammonium chloride / ↓ Effect of tricyclics by ↓ renal tubular reabsorption of the drug

Anticholinergic drugs / Additive anticholinergic side effects

Anticoagulants, oral / ↑ Hypoprothrombinemia due to ↓ breakdown by liver

Anticonvulsants / Tricyclics may ↑ incidence of epileptic seizures

Antihistamines / Additive anticholinergic side effects

Ascorbic acid / ↓ Effect of tricyclics by ↓ renal tubular reabsorption of the drug

Barbiturates / Additive depressant effects; also, barbiturates may ↑ breakdown of antidepressants by liver

Benzodiazepines / Tricyclic antidepressants ↑ effect of benzodiazepines

Beta-adrenergic blocking agents / Tricyclic antidepressants ↓ effect of the blocking agents

Charcoal / ↓ Absorption of tricyclic antidepressants → ↓ effectiveness (or toxicity)

Chlordiazepoxide / Concomitant use may cause additive sedative effects and/or additive atropine-like side effects

Cimetidine / ↑ Effect of tricyclics (especially serious anticholinergic symptoms) due to ↓ breakdown by liver

Clonidine / Dangerous ↑ BP and hypertensive crisis

Diazepam / Simultaneous use may cause additive sedative effects and/or additive atropine-like side effects

Dicumarol / Tricyclic antidepressants may ↑ the $t^{1/2}$ of dicumarol → ↑ anticoagulation effects

Disulfiram / ↑ Levels of tricyclic antidepressant; also, possibility of acute organic brain syndrome

Ephedrine / Tricyclics ↓ effects of ephedrine by preventing uptake at its site of action

Estrogens / Depending on the dose, estrogens may ↑ or ↓ the effects of tricyclics
Ethchlorvynol / Combination may result in transient delirium
Fluoxetine / Fluoxetine ↑ pharmacologic and toxic effects of tricyclic antidepressants (effect may persist for several weeks after fluoxetine is discontinued)
Furazolidone / Toxic psychoses possible
Glutethimide / Additive anticholinergic side effects
Guanethidine / Tricyclics ↓ antihypertensive effect of guanethidine by preventing uptake at its site of action
Haloperidol / ↑ Effect of tricyclics due to ↓ breakdown by liver
Levodopa / ↓ Effect of levodopa due to ↓ absorption
MAO inhibitors / Simultaneous use may result in excitation, increase in body temperature, delirium, tremors, and convulsions although combinations have been used successfully
Meperidine / Tricyclics enhance narcotic-induced respiratory depression; also, additive anticholinergic side effects
Methyldopa / Tricyclics may block hypotensive effects of methyldopa
Methylphenidate / ↑ Effect of tricyclics due to ↓ breakdown by liver
Narcotic analgesics / Tricyclics enhance narcotic-induced respiratory depression; also, additive anticholinergic effects
Oral contraceptives / ↑ Plasma levels of tricyclic antidepressants due to ↓ breakdown by liver
Oxazepam / Simultaneous use may cause additive sedative effects and/or atropine-like side effects
Phenothiazines / Additive anticholinergic side effects; also, phenothiazines ↑ effects of tricyclics due to ↓ breakdown by liver
Procainamide / Additive cardiac effects
Quinidine / Additive cardiac effects
Reserpine / Tricyclics ↓ hypotensive effect of reserpine
Sodium bicarbonate / ↑ Effect of tricyclics by ↑ renal tubular reabsorption of the drug
Sympathomimetics / Potentiation of sympathomimetic effects→ hypertension or cardiac arrhythmias
Tobacco (smoking) / ↓ Serum levels of tricyclic antidepressants due to ↑ breakdown by liver
Thyroid preparations / Mutually potentiating effects observed
Vasodilators / Additive hypotensive effect

Dosage

See individual drugs.

Dosage levels vary greatly in effectiveness from one client to another; therefore, carefully individualize dosage regimens.

Laboratory Test Considerations: ↑ Alkaline phosphatase, bilirubin; ↑ or ↓ blood glucose. False + or ↑ urinary catecholamines.

1. In adolescents and elderly clients, use a lower initial dosage than in adults; gradually increase the dose as required.
2. Individualize dose according to age, weight, physical and mental condition, and response to the therapy.
3. For maintenance therapy, a single daily dose may suffice.
4. Dose usually administered at bedtime, so any anticholinergic and/or sedative effects will not impact ADL.
5. To reduce incidence of sedation and anticholinergic effects, start with small doses and then gradually increase to desired dosage levels.

HEALTH CARE CONSIDERATIONS

Assessment

1. Record indications for therapy, behavioral manifestations, onset of symptoms, and any causative factors.
2. Assess for suicide ideations, extent of dysphoric mood, appetite, and excessive weight changes.
3. Note sleep disturbances, lethargy, apathy, impaired thought processes, or lack of responses.
4. List drugs currently prescribed; some that may intensify depressive reactions include antihypertensives (i.e., reserpine, methyldopa, beta blockers), antiparkinsonians, hormones, steroids, anticancers, and antituberculins (cycloserine) as well as barbiturates and alcohol.
5. Monitor CBC, liver and renal function studies.
6. Record ECG, assess heart sounds, note any CAD, and evaluate neurologic functioning. Assess for tachycardia and increase in anginal attacks; may precede MI or stroke.
7. Note eye exam; report visual changes, headaches, halos, eye pain, dilated pupils, or nausea. May require a med change, esp. with glaucoma.
8. Monitor I&O; Check for abdominal distention, urinary retention, and absence of bowel sounds (as in paralytic ileus).
9. Differentiate type of depression based on diagnostic features related to reactive, major depressive, or bipolar affective disorders. Review symptoms to determine if affective, somatic, psychomotor, or psychological.

Interventions

1. Note signs of allergic response, i.e., skin rash, alopecia, and eosinophilia.
2. Sore throat, fever, easy bruising, unusual bleeding, presence of petechiae or purpura may be symptoms of blood dyscrasias. Check for evidence of agranulocytosis, esp. common among elderly women and during the second month of drug therapy.
3. With hyperthyroidism, assess for arrhythmias precipitated by TCAs.
4. Assess for adverse endocrine disturbances such as increased or decreased libido, gynecomastia, testicular swelling, and impotence.
5. Report symptoms of cholestatic jaundice and biliary tract obstruction such as high fever, yellowing of the skin, mucous membranes and sclera, pruritus, and upper abdominal pain.
6. TCAs may alter blood sugar levels and require adjustment of hypoglycemic agent.
7. If receiving electroshock therapy, report as combination may be hazardous.
8. Discontinue several days prior to surgery; may adversely affect BP.
9. Withdraw slowly to avoid any withdrawal symptoms.
10. Assess for epileptiform seizures precipitated by the drug.

Client/Family Teaching

1. GI complaints of anorexia, N&V, epigastric distress, diarrhea, blackened tongue, or a peculiar taste require a dosage adjustment. Take with or immediately following meals to reduce gastric irritation.
2. Take sedating meds at bedtime to minimize daytime sedation; take those that cause insomnia in the a.m. or upon arising.
3. Avoid other drugs and alcohol during and for 2 weeks following TCA therapy.
4. Use caution when performing tasks requiring mental alertness or physical coordination; may cause drowsiness or ataxia.
5. Rise slowly from a supine position; do not remain standing in one place for any length of time. If feeling faint, lie down to minimize orthostatic hypotension.
6. Increase oral hygiene, take frequent sips of water, suck on hard candy, or chew sugarless gum to maintain a moist mouth. A high-fiber diet, increased fluid intake, exercise, and a stool softener may prevent constipation.
7. May affect carbohydrate metabolism; an adjustment of hypoglycemic agent and diet may be indicated.
8. If photosensitive, stay out of the sun; wear protective clothing, sunglasses, and a sunscreen.
9. May alter libido or reproductive function.
10. Practice reliable birth control; report if pregnancy suspected.
11. Report any alterations in perceptions, i.e., hallucinations, blurred vision, or excessive stimulations. Watch those recovering from depression for suicidal tendencies; remove firearms from the home.
12. May take 24 weeks to realize a maximum clinical response; stay on the treatment regimen.
13. Will see provider more often the first 23 weeks; scripts will be for only small amounts to ensure compliance and to prevent an overdose; excess consumption can be lethal. Obtain number to call for help.
14. Review how to help clients alter their behavior; meds as prescribed and active participation in psychotherapy programs.

Outcome/Evaluate

- Understand illness and need for drug therapy/medical supervision
- ↓ Depression evidenced by improved appetite, renewed interest in outside activities, ↑ socialization, improved sleeping patterns, ↑ energy, and a general sense of well being
- ↓ Anxiety; improved coping skills

ANTIDIABETIC AGENTS: HYPOGLYCEMIC AGENTS

See also *Antidiabetic Agents: Insulins. See also the following individual entries:*

Acarbose
Chlorpropamide
Glimepiride
Glipizide
Glyburide
Metformin hydrochloride
Miglitol
Tolazamide
Tolbutamide
Tolbutamide sodium

Action/Kinetics: Oral hypoglycemic drugs are classified as either first or second generation. *Generation* refers to structural changes in the basic molecule. Second-generation oral hypoglycemic drugs are more lipophilic and, as such, have greater hypoglycemic potency. Also, second-generation drugs are bound to plasma protein by covalent bonds, whereas first-generation drugs are bound to plasma protein by ionic bonds. The implication is that the second-generation drugs are potentially less susceptible to displacement from plasma protein by drugs such as salicylates and oral anticoagulants.

The oral hypoglycemics are believed to act by one or more of the following mechanisms: (1) stimulating insulin release from pancreatic beta cells, possibly due to increased intracellular cyclic AMP; (2) the peripheral tissues become more sensitive to insulin due to an increase in the number of insulin receptors or an increased ability of circulating insulin to combine with receptors; or (3) extrapancreatic effects, including decreased glucagon release and hepatic glucose production. To be effective, the client must have some ability for endogenous insulin production. Differences in oral hypoglycemic drugs are mainly in their pharmacokinetic properties and duration of action.

General Statement: The American Diabetes Association has developed standards for treating clients with diabetes. If followed, these standards will enable clients to decrease their blood glucose levels closer to normal; this will reduce the risk of complications, including blindness, kidney disease, heart disease, and amputations. The goals of these standards include establishing specific targets for control of blood glucose (usually between 80 and 120 mg/dL before meals and between 100 and 140 mg/dL at bedtime) and increased emphasis on educating clients for self-management of their disease. Targets for BP and lipid levels are also provided. If the guidelines are followed, it is estimated that the risk of development or progression of retinopathy, nephropathy, and neuropathy can be reduced by 50%–75% in clients with insulin-dependent (type I) diabetes. The guidelines suggest the following treatment modalities:

- Frequent monitoring of blood glucose.
- Regular exercise.
- Close attention to meal planning; consult a registered dietitian.
- For type I diabetics, either continuous SC insulin infusion or multiple daily insulin injections; for type II diabetics, consider insulin administration in certain situations, although dietary modification, exercise, and weight reduction are the cornerstone of treatment.
- Instruction in the prevention and treatment of hypoglycemia and other complications (both acute and chronic) of diabetes.
- Development of a process for ongoing support and continuing education for the client.
- Routine assessment of treatment goals.

Uses: Non-insulin-dependent diabetes mellitus (type II) that does not respond to diet management alone. Concurrent use of insulin and an oral hypoglycemic for type II diabetics who are difficult to control with diet and sulfonylurea therapy alone. One method used is the BIDS system: bedtime insulin (usually NPH) with daytime (morning only or morning and evening) oral hypoglycemic.

Guidelines for oral hypoglycemic therapy include onset of diabetes in clients over 40 years of age, duration of diabetes less than 5 years, absence of ketoacidosis, client is obese or has normal body weight, fasting serum glucose of 200 mg/dL or less, has a daily insulin requirement of 40 units or less, and hepatic and renal function is normal.

Contraindications: Stress before and during surgery, ketosis, severe trauma, fever, infections, pregnancy, diabetes complicated by recurrent episodes of ketoacidosis or coma; juvenile, growth-onset, insulin-dependent, or brittle diabetes; impaired endocrine, renal, or liver function. Use in diabetics who can be controlled by diet alone. Relapse may occur with the sulfonylureas in undernourished clients. Long-acting products in geriatric clients.

Special Concerns: Use with caution in debilitated and malnourished clients and during lactation since hypoglycemia may occur in the infant. Safety and effectiveness in children have not been established. Geriatric clients may be more sensitive to oral hypoglycemics and hypoglycemia may be more difficult to recognize in these clients. Use of sulfonylureas has been associated with an increased risk of CV mortality compared to treatment with either diet alone or diet plus insulin. There may be loss of blood glucose control if the client experiences stress such as infection, fever, surgery, or trauma.

Side Effects: Hypoglycemia is the most common side effect. *GI:* Nausea, heartburn, full feeling. *CNS:* Fatigue, dizziness, fever, headache, weakness, malaise, vertigo. *Hepatic:* Cholestatic jaundice, aggravation of hepatic porphyria. *Dermatologic:* Skin rashes, urticaria, erythema, pruritus, eczema, photophobia, morbilliform or maculopapular eruptions, lichenoid reactions, porphyria cutanea tardia. *Hematologic:* Thrombocytopenia, leukopenia, ***agranulocytosis, aplastic anemia,*** pancytopenia, ***hemolytic anemia.*** *Endocrine:* Inappropriate secretion of ADH resulting in excessive water retention, hyponatremia, low serum osmolality, and high urine osmolality. *Miscellaneous:* Paresthesia, tinnitus, resistance to drug action develops in a small percentage of clients.

OD **Management of Overdose:** *Symptoms:* Hypoglycemia. The following symptoms of hypoglycemia are listed in their general order of appearance: tingling of lips and tongue, hunger, nausea, decreased cerebral function (lethargy, yawning, confusion, agitation, nervousness), increased sympathetic activity (tachycardia, sweating, tremor), seizures, stupor, coma. *Treatment:* Mild hypoglycemia is treated with PO glucose and adjusting the dose of the drug or meal patterns. Severe hypoglycemia requires hospitalization. Concentrated (50%) dextrose is given by rapid IV and is followed by continuous infusion of 10% dextrose at a rate that will maintain blood glucose above 100 mg/dL. Client should be monitored for at least 24–48 hr as hypoglycemia may recur (clients with chlorpropamide toxicity should be monitored for 3–5 days due to the long duration of action of this drug).

Drug Interactions

Alcohol / Possible Antabuse-like syndrome, especially flushing of face and SOB. Also, ↓ effect of oral hypoglycemic due to ↑ breakdown by liver
Androgens/anabolic steroids / ↑ Hypoglycemic effect
Anticoagulants, oral / ↑ Effect of oral hypoglycemics by ↓ breakdown by liver and ↓ plasma protein binding
Beta-adrenergic blocking agents / ↓ Hypoglycemic effect; also, symptoms of hypoglycemia may be masked
Charcoal / ↓ Hypoglycemic effect due to ↓ absorption from GI tract
Chloramphenicol / ↑ Effect due to ↓ breakdown by liver and ↓ renal excretion
Cholestyramine / ↓ Hypoglycemic effect
Clofibrate / ↑ Hypoglycemic effect due to ↓ plasma protein binding
Diazoxide / ↓ Effects of both drugs
Digitoxin / ↑ Digitoxin serum levels
Fenfluramine / ↑ Hypoglycemic effect
Fluconazole / ↑ Hypoglycemic effect
Gemfibrozil / ↑ Hypoglycemic effect
Histamine H_2 antagonists / ↑ Hypoglycemic effect due to ↓ breakdown by liver
Hydantoins / ↓ Effect of sulfonylureas due to ↓ insulin release
Magnesium salts / ↑ Hypoglycemic effect
MAO inhibitors / ↑ Hypoglycemic effect due to ↓ breakdown by liver
Methyldopa / ↑ Hypoglycemic effect due to ↓ breakdown by liver
NSAIDs / ↑ Hypoglycemic effect of oral antidiabetics
Phenylbutazone / ↑ Effect of oral hypoglycemics due to ↓ breakdown by liver, ↓ plasma protein binding, and ↓ renal excretion
Probenecid / ↑ Hypoglycemic effect
Rifampin / ↓ Effect of sulfonylureas due to ↑ breakdown by liver
Salicylates / ↑ Effect of oral hypoglycemics by ↓ plasma protein binding
Sulfinpyrazone / ↑ Hypoglycemic effect
Sulfonamides / ↑ Effect of oral hypoglycemics by ↓ plasma protein binding and ↓ breakdown by liver
Sympathomimetics / ↑ Requirements for sulfonylureas
Thiazides / ↓ Effect of sulfonylureas
Tricyclic antidepressants / ↑ Hypoglycemic effect
Urinary acidifiers / ↑ Hypoglycemic effect due to ↓ renal excretion
Urinary alkalinizers / ↓ Hypoglycemic effect due to ↑ renal excretion

Dosage

PO. See individual preparations. Adjust dosage according to needs of client. Exercise, weight loss, and diet are of primary importance in the control of diabetes.

Laboratory Test Considerations: ↑ BUN and serum creatinine.

HEALTH CARE CONSIDERATIONS

See also *Health Care Considerations* for *Insulins*.

Administration/Storage

1. To decrease the incidence of gastric upset, take PO drugs with food.
2. If ketonuria, acidosis, increased glycosuria, or serious side effects occur, withdraw the med.
3. Transfer from insulin:
• If receiving 20 units or less of insulin daily, initiate oral hypoglycemic therapy and discontinue insulin abruptly.
• For clients receiving 20–40 units of insulin daily, initiate oral hypoglycemic therapy and reduce insulin dose by 25%–50%. Discontinue insulin gradually, using the absence of glucose in the urine as a guide. With glyburide, insulin may be discontinued abruptly.
• For clients receiving more than 40 units of insulin daily, initiate PO therapy and reduce insulin by 20%. Discontinue insulin gradually, using glucose in the urine or finger sticks as a guide. It may be advisable to hospitalize clients on such high doses of insulin while they are being transferred to oral hypoglycemic agents.
4. Transfer from one oral hypoglycemic agent to another:
• Except for chlorpropamide, no transition period is necessary. When transferring from chlorpropamide, use caution for 1–2 weeks due to the long drug half-life.

• Mild symptoms of hyperglycemia may appear during the transfer period. Perform finger sticks and test urine for ketones regularly (1–3 times daily) during the transfer period. Positive results must be reported.
5. Be prepared to treat if client develops severe hypoglycemia.
6. Review the drugs with which oral hypoglycemic agents interact and determine if client taking any.
7. Type II diabetics who do not respond to the sulfonylureas are said to be *primary failures*. Responses to the sulfonylureas during the initial months of therapy followed by failure to respond are referred to as *secondary failures*. A glucophage trial or combination therapy with insulin and oral agents may be useful in these clients.

Assessment

1. Obtain a thorough health history.
2. Record any stress. Clients about to undergo surgical procedures, who have suffered severe trauma, who have a fever and infection, or who are pregnant should generally not be placed on oral hypoglycemic agents.
3. Assess mental functions to determine if able to understand the complexities of the transfer process.
4. Note if taking oral contraceptives; effectiveness is lessened by oral hypoglycemic agents.
5. Note any previous experience with sulfonylureas and the outcome. Determine metformin trial and the outcome; elderly do better with a slower metformin titration (i.e., increase dose weekly or increase by ½ tablet instead of a whole tablet).
6. Identify clients that may benefit from ACE and vitamin E therapy.
7. Assess for Syndrome X (syndrome of insulin resistance) i.e., obesity, HTN, ASHD, dyslipidemia, hyperinsulinumia and Type II DM.
8. Monitor VS, ECG, cholesterol panel, electrolytes, CBC, HbA1c, and urine for microalbuminuria.

Client/Family Teaching

1. Use machine to test blood sugar (or urine for ketones) and record for provider review. (Urine testing is not an accurate reflection of true serum glucose levels and should not be used to modify treatment.)
2. With hypoglycemic episodes, check finger stick at the time of the reaction. Then drink 4 oz of juice (fast-acting CHO), followed by a longer acting CHO (approximately 10 g) such as half a meat sandwich or several peanut butter crackers, and recheck finger stick in 15 min. If glucose is less than 100, repeat the process, i.e., juice and a CHO and another finger stick. Report if this occurs often.
3. Medication helps to control high BS but does not cure diabetes; therapy is usually long term.
4. Must adhere to prescribed diet if drug is to be effective; most secondary failures are due to poor dietary compliance; see dietitian as needed.
5. Regular physical exercise, diet, and weight control/loss are imperative.
6. Insulin may be necessary if complications occur. Review administration of insulin and how to rotate sites. Do not change brands of insulin or syringes. Review equipment, methods of storage and discarding used syringes.
7. Report illness or if unusual itching, skin rash, jaundice, dark urine, fever, sore throat, nausea/vomiting, or diarrhea occurs.
8. With thyroid scan advise lab as sulfonylureas interfere with the uptake of radioactive iodine.
9. Avoid alcohol; a disulfuram-like reaction may occur.
10. Do not take any OTC meds without approval.
11. Need close medical supervision for the first 6 weeks and periodic lab tests; oral agents may cause blood dyscrasias.
12. Carry ID, a list of prescribed drugs, juice, and hard candy (such as Lifesavers) or a fast-acting CHO (candy bar) at all times.

Outcome/Evaluate

• Knowledge/control of diabetes; adherence with drug and dietary therapy
• ↓ Hypo/hyperglycemic episodes
• HbA1c within desired range ← 8
• Prevention of target organ damage

ANTIDIABETIC AGENTS: INSULINS

See also *Antidiabetic Agents: Hypoglycemic Agents. See also the following individual entries:*

Insulin injection
Insulin injection concentrated
Insulin lispro injection
Insulin zinc suspension (Lente)
Insulin zinc suspension, Extended (Ultralente)

Action/Kinetics: Following combination with insulin receptors on cell plasma membranes, insulin facilitates the transport of glucose into cardiac and skeletal muscle and adipose tissue. It also increases synthesis of glycogen in the liver. Insulin stimulates protein synthesis and lipogenesis and inhibits lipolysis and release of free fatty acids from fat cells.This latter effect prevents or reverses the ketoacidosis sometimes observed in the type I diabetic. Insulin also causes intracellular shifts in magnesium and potassium.

Since insulin is a protein, it is destroyed in the GI tract. Thus, it must be administered SC so that it is readily absorbed into the bloodstream and distributed throughout the extracellular fluid. Metabolized mainly by the liver.

General Statement: Insulin preparations with different times of onset, peak activity, and duration of action have been developed. Such products are prepared by precipitating insulin in the presence of zinc chloride to form zinc insulin crystals and/or by combining insulin with a protein such as protamine. Based on these modifications, insulin products are classified as fast-acting, intermediate-acting, and long-acting. These preparations permit the provider to select the preparation best suited to the life-style of the client.

RAPID-ACTING INSULIN:Insulin injection (Regular Insulin, Crystalline Zinc Insulin, Unmodified Insulin)

INTERMEDIATE-ACTING INSULIN

1. Isophane insulin suspension (NPH)
2. Insulin zinc suspension (Lente)

LONG-ACTING INSULIN: Insulin zinc suspension extended (Ultralente)

NOTE: Insulin preparations with various times of onset and duration of action are often mixed to obtain optimum control in diabetic clients.

Uses: Human insulins are being used almost exclusively. Replacement therapy in type I diabetes. Diabetic ketoacidosis or diabetic coma (use regular insulin). Insulin is also indicated in type II diabetes when other measures have failed (e.g., diet, exercise, weight reduction) or with surgery, trauma, infection, fever, endocrine dysfunction, pregnancy, gangrene, Raynaud's disease, kidney or liver dysfunction.

Regular insulin is used in IV HA solutions, in IV dextrose to treat severe hyperkalemia, and IV as a provocative test for growth hormone secretion.

Insulin and oral hypoglycemic drugs have been used in type II diabetics who are difficult to control with diet and PO therapy alone.

Contraindications: Hypersensitivity to insulin.

Special Concerns: Pregnant diabetic clients often manifest decreased insulin requirements during the first half of pregnancy and increased requirements during the latter half. Lactation may decrease insulin requirements.

Side Effects: *Hypoglycemia:* Due to insulin overdose, delayed or decreased food intake, too much exercise in relationship to insulin dose, or when transferring from one preparation to another. Even carefully controlled clients occasionally develop signs of insulin overdosage characterized by one or more of the following: hunger, weakness, fatigue, nervousness, pallor or flushing, profuse sweating, headache, palpitations, numbness of mouth, tingling in the fingers, tremors, blurred and double vision, hypothermia, excess yawning, mental confusion, incoordination, tachycardia, loss of sensitivity, and loss of consciousness. Level of awareness is markedly diminished after an attack.

Symptoms of hypoglycemia may mimic those of psychic disturbances. Severe prolonged hypoglycemia may cause brain damage, and in the elderly, may mimic stroke.

Allergic: Urticaria, angioedema, lymphadenopathy, bullae, anaphylaxis. Occurs mostly following intermittent insulin therapy or IV administration of large doses to insulin-resistant clients. Antihistamines or corticosteroids may be used to treat these symptoms. Clients who are highly allergic to insulin and cannot be treated with oral hypoglycemics may respond to human insulin products.

At site of injection: Swelling, stinging, redness, itching, warmth. These symptoms often disappear with continued use. Lipoatrophy or hypertrophy of subcutaneous fat tissue (minimize by rotating site of injection).

Insulin resistance: Usual cause is obesity. Acute resistance may occur following infections, trauma, surgery, emotional disturbances, or other endocrine disorders.

Ophthalmologic: Blurred vision, transient presbyopia. Occurs mainly during initiation of therapy or in clients who have been uncontrolled for a long period of time.

Hyperglycemic rebound (Somogyi effect): Usually in clients who receive chronic overdosage.

DIFFERENTIATION BETWEEN DIABETIC COMA AND HYPOGLYCEMIC REACTION (INSULIN SHOCK): Coma in diabetes may be caused by uncontrolled diabetes (high sugar content in blood or urine, ketoacidosis) or by too much insulin (insulin shock, hypoglycemia).

Diabetic coma and insulin shock can be differentiated in the following manner:

Drug Interactions

Alcohol, ethyl / ↑ Hypoglycemia → low blood sugar and shock

Anabolic steroids / ↑ Hypoglycemic effect of insulin

Beta-adrenergic blocking agents / ↑ Hypoglycemic effect of insulin
Chlorthalidone / ↓ Hypoglycemic effect of antidiabetics
Clofibrate / ↑ Hypoglycemic effects of insulin
Contraceptives, oral / ↑ Dosage of antidiabetic due to impairment of glucose tolerance
Corticosteroids / ↓ Effect of insulin due to corticosteroid-induced hyperglycemia
Dextrothyroxine / ↓ Effect of insulin due to dextrothyroxine-induced hyperglycemia
Diazoxide / Diazoxide-induced hyperglycemia ↓ diabetic control
Digitalis glycosides / Use with caution, as insulin affects serum potassium levels
Diltiazen / ↓ Effect of insulin
Dobutamine / ↓ Effect of insulin
Epinephrine / ↓ Effect of insulin due to epinephrine-induced hyperglycemia
Estrogens / ↓ Effect of insulin due to impairment of glucose tolerance
Ethacrynic acid / ↓ Hypoglycemic effect of antidiabetics
Fenfluramine / Additive hypoglycemic effects
Furosemide / ↓ Hypoglycemic effect of antidiabetics
Glucagon / Glucagon-induced hyperglycemia ↓ effect of antidiabetics
Guanethidine / ↑ Hypoglycemic effect of insulin
MAO inhibitors / MAO inhibitors ↑ and prolong hypoglycemic effect of antidiabetics
Oxytetracycline / ↑ Effect of insulin
Phenothiazines / ↑ Dosage of antidiabetic due to phenothiazine-induced hyperglycemia
Phenytoin / Phenytoin-induced hyperglycemia ↓ diabetic control
Propranolol / Inhibits rebound of blood glucose after insulin-induced hypoglycemia
Salicylates / ↑ Effect of hypoglycemic effect of insulin
Sulfinpyrazone / ↑ Hypoglycemic effect of insulin
Tetracyclines / May ↑ hypoglycemic effect of insulin
Thiazide diuretics / ↓ Hypoglycemic effect of antidiabetics
Thyroid preparations / ↓ Effect of antidiabetic due to thyroid-induced hyperglycemia
Triamterene / ↓ Hypoglycemic effect of antidiabetic

Dosage

Dosage highly individualized. Usually administered SC. Insulin injection (regular insulin) is the **only** preparation that may be administered IV. Give IV only for clients with severe ketoacidosis or diabetic coma. Dosage for insulin is always expressed in USP units.

Dosage is established and monitored by blood glucose (often using glucose monitoring machines in the home), urine glucose, and acetone tests. Furthermore, since requirements may change with time, dosage must be checked at regular intervals. It may be advisable to hospitalize some clients while their daily insulin and caloric requirements are being established. The main goal is to control the blood sugar and send the client home to fine tune as generally the home environment is more reliable for determining drug requirements.

In pregnancy, insulin requirements may increase suddenly during the last trimester. After delivery, requirements may suddenly drop to prepregnancy levels. To prevent the development of hypoglycemia, insulin is often discontinued on the day of delivery and glucose is administered IV.

The various insulin preparations can be mixed to obtain the combination best suited for the individual client. However, mixing must be done according to the directions received from the physician/provider and/or pharmacist.

Hypoglycemia (Insulin Shock)
Onset / Sudden (24–48 hr)
Medication / Excess insulin
Food intake / Probably too little
Overall appearance / Very weak
Skin / Moist and pale
Infection / Absent
Fever / Absent
Mouth / Drooling
Thirst / Absent
Hunger / Occasional
Vomiting / Absent
Abdominal pain / Rare
Respiration / Normal
Breath / Normal
BP / Normal
Pulse / Full and bounding
Vision / Diplopia
Tremor / Frequent
Convulsions / In late stages
Urine sugar / Absent in second specimen
Ketone bodies / Absent in second specimen
Blood sugar / Less than 60 mg/100 mL

Source: Adapted with permission from *The Merck Manual,* 11th ed.

Diabetic coma is usually precipitated by the client's failure to take insulin. Hypoglycemia is often precipitated by the client's unpredictable response, excess exertion, stress due to illness or surgery, errors in calculating dosage, or failure to eat.

TREATMENT OF DIABETIC COMA OR SEVERE ACIDOSIS: Administer 30–60 units regular insulin. This is followed by doses of 20 units or more q 30 min. To avoid a hypoglycemic state, 1 g dextrose is administered for each unit of insulin given. Treatment is often supplemented by electrolytes and fluids. Urine samples are collected for analysis, and VS are monitored as ordered.

TREATMENT OF HYPOGLYCEMIA (INSULIN SHOCK): Mild hypoglycemia can be relieved by PO administration of CHO such as orange juice, candy, or a lump of sugar. If comatose, adults may be given 10–30 mL of 50% dextrose solution IV; children should receive 0.5–1 mL/kg of 50% dextrose solution. Epinephrine, hydrocortisone, or glucagon may be used in severe cases to cause an increase in blood glucose.

Hyperglycemia (Diabetic Coma)

Onset / Gradual (days)
Medication / Insufficient insulin
Food intake / Normal or excess
Overall appearance / Extremely ill
Skin / Dry and flushed
Infection / Frequent
Fever / Frequent
Mouth / Dry
Thirst / Intense
Hunger / Absent
Vomiting / Common
Abdominal pain / Frequent
Respiration / Increased, air hunger
Breath / Acetone odor
BP / Low
Pulse / Weak and rapid
Vision / Dim
Tremor / Absent
Convulsions / None
Urine sugar / High
Ketone bodies / High (type I only)
Blood sugar / High

Diet: The dietary control of diabetes is as important as medication with appropriate drugs. The role of health care professionals and dietitian in teaching the client how to eat properly cannot be underestimated. They must teach the client how to calculate exchange values of various foods. Food lists and food-exchange values published by the American Diabetes Association and the American Dietetic Association are valuable teaching aids.

Diabetic clients should adhere to a regular meal schedule. The frequency of meals and the overall caloric intake vary with the type of drug taken and individual client needs. Close attention to meal frequency and meal planning is imperative and a registered dietitian should be consulted. Diabetic children may be on a less restricted diet, adjusting the insulin dosage according to blood and urine glucose readings. Children with negative urine glucose tend to become hypoglycemic rapidly with exercise or decrease in appetite, and many providers allow for glucose spilling.

Laboratory Test Considerations: Alters liver function tests and thyroid function tests. False + Coombs' test, ↑ serum protein, ↓ serum amino acids, calcium, cholesterol, potassium, and urine amino acids.

1. Read product information and any important notes inserted into the insulin package.
2. Discard open vials not used for several weeks or whose expiration date has passed.
3. Refrigerate stock supply of insulin but avoid freezing. Freezing destroys the manner in which insulin is suspended in the formulation.
4. Store vial in a cool place, avoiding extremes of temperature or exposure to sunlight.
5. Use the following guidelines with respect to mixing the various insulins:
   - Regular insulin may be mixed with NPH or Lente insulins. However, to avoid transfer of the longer-acting insulin into the regular insulin vial, withdraw regular insulin into the syringe first.
   - Give a mixture of regular insulin with NPH or Lente insulin within 15 min of mixing due to binding of regular insulin by excess protamine and/or zinc in the longer-acting preparations.
   - Lente or Ultralente insulins may be mixed with each other in any proportion; however, do not mix these with NPH insulins.
   - When used in an insulin infusion pump, insulin may be mixed in any proportion with either 0.9% NaCl injection or water for injection. Due to stability changes, use such mixtures within 24 hr of their preparation. Buffered insulin is usually the form prescribed and utilized with the insulin pump.
6. Store compatible insulin mixtures for no longer than 1 month at room temperature or 3 months at 2°C–8°C (36°F–46°F). However, bacterial contamination may occur.
7. To ensure a constant amount of precipitate in each dose, invert the vial several times to mix before withdrawing the material. Avoid vigorous shaking and frothing of the material. (Regular and globin insulin are the only two insulins that do not have a precipitate.)
8. Discard any vial in which the precipitate is clumped or granular in appearance or

which has formed a solid deposit of particles on the side of the vial.

9. To prevent dosage error, do not alter the order of mixing insulins or change the model or brand of syringe or needle.

10. Administer at a 90° angle with a 28- or 29-gauge needle. Syringes come in 0.3-cc (30-U), 0.5-cc (50-U) and 1-cc (100-U) sizes. Get the smallest syringe with the smallest needles to enhance dosage validity (e.g., if client is prescribed less than 30 U insulin, advise to obtain the 0.3-cc syringe).

11. Provide an automatic injector for clients fearful of injecting themselves.

12. Assist visually impaired clients to obtain information and devices for self-administration by consulting their local diabetes association or by writing to the American Diabetes Association, 149 Madison Avenue, New York, NY 10016 (telephone: 212-725-4925), for their buyer's guide, which lists numerous available products for diabetics. Clients may also contact The Lighthouse, Inc., 800 Second Avenue, New York, NY 10017 (telephone: 212-808-0077) for additional information on visual impairments.

13. Lipoatrophy may occur. This may appear as mild dimpling of the skin or as deep pits in young girls and women and lipodystrophy, appearing as well-developed muscle on the anterior and lateral thighs of young boys and men. To prevent, rotate injection sites.

- Make a chart indicating the injection sites (see Figure 1).
- Allow 3–4 cm between injection sites.
- Do not inject in the same site for at least 1–2 weeks.
- Avoid injecting within 1 cm around the umbilicus because of the high vascularity in this area.
- Avoid injections around the waistline because of the sensitive nerve supply to this area and the potential for fabric irritation.
- Use insulin at room temperature to prevent lipodystrophy.

14. Rotation of injection sites may lead to differences in blood levels of insulin. The abdomen is considered the best site due to constant insulin peak times with better gradual absorption.

15. If insulin has been refrigerated, allow it to remain at room temperature for at least 1 hr before using.

16. Apply gentle pressure after injection but do not massage since this may alter rate of absorption.

17. If breakfast is delayed for lab tests, check for dosage adjustment.

18. Care of reusable syringes and needles.

- Do not use heavily chlorinated water or water with a high chemical content for sterilizing syringes. To sterilize, boil the syringe and needle for 5 min.
- Needle and syringe can be sterilized by soaking in isopropyl alcohol for at least 5 min. The alcohol must evaporate from the equipment before use to prevent reduction in the strength (dilution) of the insulin.
- Clean syringes covered by a precipitate with a cotton-tipped swab soaked in vinegar; then thoroughly rinse syringe in water and sterilize it. Clean needles with a wire and sharpen with a pumice stone.
- Avoid alcohol when reusing disposable syringes, as it removes silicone (facilitates insertion) from the needle.
- Disposable syringes may be reused by the same individual and are generally usable for several sticks. Client will be the judge depending on comfort and experienced "dullness."

HEALTH CARE CONSIDERATIONS

Also includes general applications for all clients with diabetes controlled by medication (whether it be insulin or an oral hypoglycemic agent).

Assessment

1. Obtain a thorough history and physical exam. Note any first-degree relatives with disease.

2. Assess for S&S of hyperglycemia: thirst, polydypsia, polyuria, drowsiness, blurred vision, loss of appetite, fruity odor to the breath, and flushed dry skin. Note state of consciousness.

3. Assess for S&S of hypoglycemia: drowsiness, chills, confusion, anxiety, cold sweats, cool pale skin, excessive hunger, nausea,

Figure 1 Each injection area is divided into squares; each square is an injection site. Start in a corner of an injection area and move down or across the injection sites in order. Jumping from site to site will make it more difficult to remember where the last shot was administered. Keep track of the rotation pattern to assist in maintaining site rotation. A grid may be developed from this figure and numbered to keep track of injections. Systematically use all the sites in one area before moving to another (for example, use all the sites in both arms before moving to the legs). This will help keep the blood sugar more even from day to day. An important consideration when choosing injection sites is that insulin is absorbed into the bloodstream faster from some areas than from others; it enters the bloodstream most quickly from the abdomen (stomach), a little more slowly from the arms, even more slowly from the legs, and most slowly from the buttocks. (Courtesy Eli Lilly & Company.)

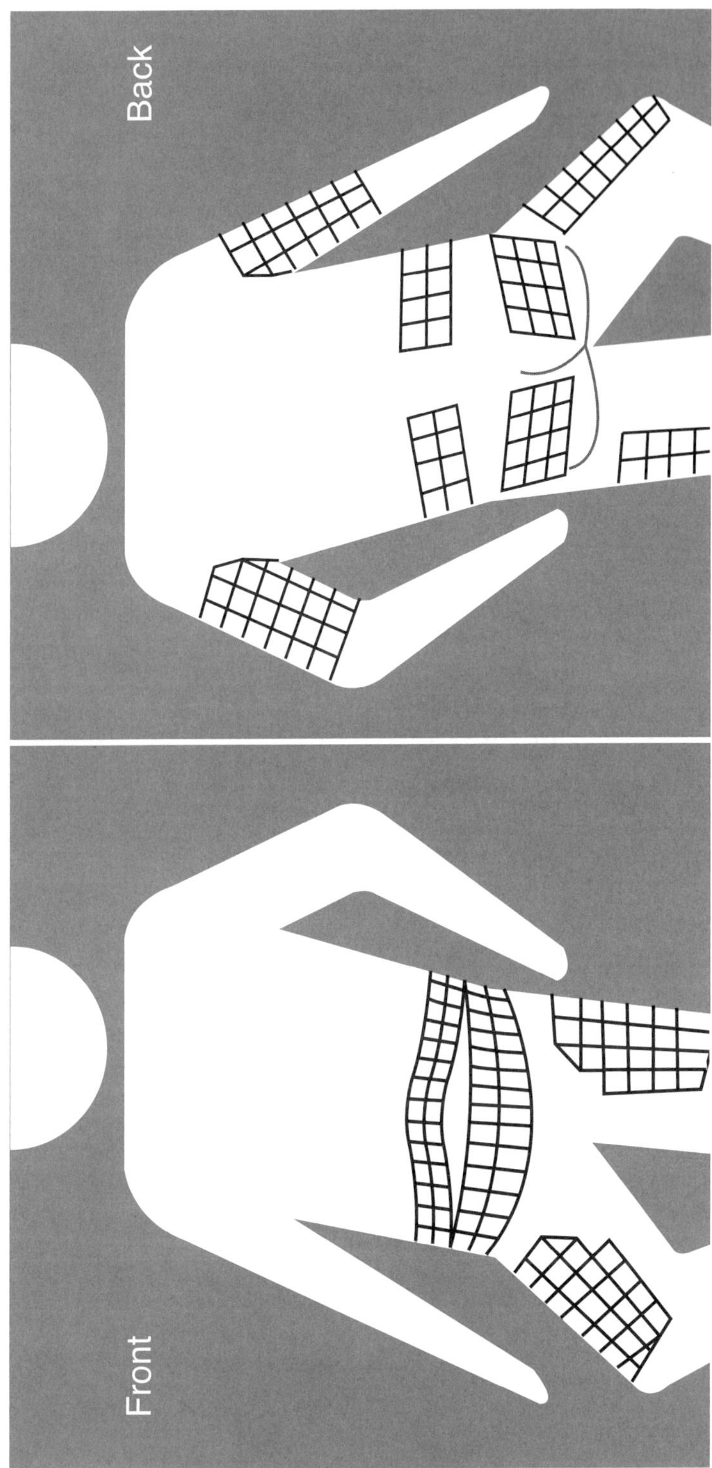
Back
Front

headache, irritability, shakiness, rapid pulse, and unusual weakness or tiredness.
4. Determine when first noticed changes in physical condition and what these changes were. Note any psychologic changes.
5. Weigh client to determine amount of hypoglycemic agent needed.
6. Monitor electrolytes, lipid profile, thyroid studies, BS, phosphate, Mg, CBC, HbA1c, and urinalysis.
7. Assess psychologic state, including disease acceptance, readiness to learn, support system, evidence of depression, or need for client/family counseling.
8. During physical exam assess DTRs; check extremities (monofilament) to assess for sensation and neuropathy.
9. Identify candidates for ACE therapy to prevent/preserve renal function and inhibit organ damage and vitamin E (400 IU) for CAD protection.
10. Assess injection sites, monitor VS, plot growth and weight every 3–4 months.
11. Schedule yearly eye exams if over 12 yrs; or younger if > 5 yrs with the disease.

Interventions

1. For a *hyperglycemic reaction:*
- Have regular insulin available.
- Obtain BS or finger stick.
- Monitor after giving insulin for further signs of hyperglycemia such as SOB, facial flushing, air hunger, and acetone breath.

2. Assess for S&S of *hypoglycemia,* such as easy fatigue, hunger, headache, cold, clammy, drowsiness, nausea, lassitude, and tremulousness. Most likely to occur before meals, during or after exercise, and at insulin peak action times (i.e., 3 a.m. with evening dosing).
- Weakness, sweating, tremors, and/or nervousness may occur later.
- Excessive restlessness and profuse sweating at night.
- Obtain BS or finger stick; promptly give 4 oz of juice and a CHO, if conscious.
- If conscious and taking long-acting insulin, also give a slowly digestible CHO, such as bread with corn syrup or honey. Give additional CHO such as crackers and milk for the next 2 hr.
- If unconscious, apply honey or Karo syrup to the buccal membrane or give glucagon.
- If hospitalized, minimally responsive or unconscious, give 10%–20% IV dextrose solution.

3. A Somogyi effect is often mistaken as client not following the prescribed therapy. This occurs when hypoglycemia triggers the release of epinephrine and glucocorticoids, which stimulates glycogenesis and results in a higher a.m. BS level. Reduction in bedtime insulin dosage is necessary to stabilize. If treated for hypoglycemia, check 3 a.m. BS; if normal and then BS rises between 3 a.m. and 7 a.m., this is related to growth hormone release—termed the Dawn Phenomenon. To control, give long-acting insulin at bedtime instead of at dinnertime.
4. Juveniles with diabetes demand closer attention and observation for infection or emotional disturbances and hypoglycemia. They are more susceptible to insulin shock and have a more limited response to glucagon. Determine if managed with intensive or conventional insulin therapy; adjust for hypoglycemia unawareness (when client passes out due to loss of catecholamine response).
5. For the newly diagnosed elderly client, start insulin doses low and gradually increase.
6. The usual dose of NPH insulin is 0.8–1.5 U/kg; give two-thirds of dose in a.m. and one-third of dose in p.m. If using regular insulin, try 1:2 in a.m. and 1:1 in p.m. with NPH.
7. Identify BS goals, i.e., young child 80–180 mg/dL premeal and 100–180 mg/dL at bedtime; adolescent 70–150 mg/dL premeal and 100–180 mg/dL at bedtime; adult 80–140 mg/dL premeal and 100–180 mg/dL at bedtime and adjust as symptoms and condition dictate.

Client/Family Teaching

1. Medications assist to control diabetes but do not cure it. Type I diabetes is usually early onset and the pancreas makes little or no insulin; individuals with type I diabetes must take insulin injections or they will die. Type II diabetes is usually later onset and the pancreas still makes insulin, but the body cannot use it (termed insulin resistance); individuals with type II diabetes can use either oral hypoglycemic agents or insulin to lower their blood sugar and to help them utilize their own insulin better.
2. Urine testing is not an accurate reflection of what the blood sugar is doing and is not generally used to adjust the treatment plan. If testing urine for sugar, review how to conduct this test. Follow instructions when testing for glycosuria with Clinitest Tablets, Tes-Tape, Diastix, or Clinistix.
- Test a fresh second-voided specimen.
- Empty bladder by voiding 1 hr before mealtime.
- As soon as able to void again, obtain and test specimen.

3. In type I diabetics, urine ketones indicate that there is not enough insulin present to get the body's sugar into the cells so it is burning body fat as an alternative and producing ketones as waste products; may lead to ketoacidosis, a life-threatening condition. Test

urine for ketones with a "dip-and-read" product when:
• Finger sticks > 240 mg/dL
• Pregnant
• Experiencing severe stress
• Vomiting or sick to stomach
• Sick with flu/cold or virus infection
• Experiencing symptoms of hyperglycemia (unusual fatigue, vision difficulty, increased thirst and/or hunger, polydipsia, unusually tired or sleepy, stomach pain, increased nausea, fruity odor to breath, rapid respirations, weight loss without altering food intake or activity patterns)

4. If performing finger sticks to monitor glucose levels, review procedure. Review instructions for technique, calibration, operation, and device maintenance. Bring in periodically to double check machine accuracy and to review data bank to ensure values coincide with client log. Some general principles may be followed.
• Rotate sites.
• Cleanse area with soap and water or alcohol prior to stabbing.
• Stab finger outside, by nail, where the capillaries are abundant and let a bead of blood form.
• Wipe off with a cotton ball.
• Let blood bead re-form and apply to the test strip.
• Follow specific guidelines for the device in use.

5. Regimens are specific to the individual, based on age, severity of diabetes, weight, any other medical problems they have, as well as the philosophy of the health care team.

6. Take insulin 30 min before a meal (exception is Humalog, which can be taken at meal time). Administer at a 90° angle with a 28- or 29-gauge needle. Syringes come in 0.3-cc (30-U), 0.5-cc (50-U) and 1-cc (100-U) sizes. Purchase the smallest syringe with the smallest needles to enhance dosage validity (e.g., if prescribed less than 30 U insulin, obtain the 0.3-cc syringe). May reuse disposable insulin syringes; based on comfort and perceived dullness.

7. Use a chart to document and rotate injection sites to avoid lipohypertrophy of injection sites (lumps from scar tissue after many injections). Avoid these areas due to unreliable absorption.
• For self-injection, brace the arm against a hard surface such as the wall or a chair.
• Cleanse the area thoroughly with alcohol, allow to dry, then, depending on the condition of the skin, either pinch between the thumb and forefingers of one hand, or spread the skin using the thumb and fingers of one hand.
• Insert into the subcutaneous tissue and aspirate to be sure needle is not in a blood vessel.
• Inject insulin and withdraw the needle.

8. Review use and care of equipment, proper disposal of needles and syringes, and provision and storage of drug.

9. *Always* check expiration dates; have an extra vial and equipment on hand for traveling, away from home, or when hospitalized.

10. Have regular insulin for emergency use.

11. Must balance food, insulin, and exercise. Exercise increases the utilization of CHO and increases CHO needs. Have snacks available; 5–8 Lifesavers, juice, or hard candy helps counteract hypoglycemia.

12. Adhere to prescribed diet, weight control, and ingestion of food relative to the peak action of insulin being used. Record weekly weights; reduce intake of animal fats and salt; select a variety of foods to meet starch and sugar, protein, and fat requirements (usual recommendation, CHO 50%; protein 20%; fat 30%). Consume the kinds of fiber that help lower BS and fat levels (breads, cereals, and crackers made from whole grains, such as whole wheat and brown rice, fresh vegetables and fruits, dried beans, and peas), as well as low cholesterol and polyunsaturated and monosaturated fats.

13. Confer with dietitian for assistance in shopping, food selection/exchanges, diet, and meal planning. Consume premeal snacks in the a.m., in the afternoon, and at bedtime.

14. If ill and omit a meal because of fever, nausea, or vomiting, replace solid foods that contain starch and sugar, such as bread and fruit, with liquids that contain sugar (fruit juice, regular sodas) and follow designated sliding scale for "sick days." Do not omit insulin or hypoglycemic agents unless instructed. Perform finger sticks q 4 hr, and with type I, also test urine for ketones; report if moderate or high.

15. Blurred vision may occur at beginning of insulin therapy; should subside in 6–8 weeks. The effect is caused by fluctuation of blood glucose levels, which produce osmotic changes in the lens of the eye and within the ocular fluids. If it does not clear up in 8 weeks, consult eye doctor.

16. May experience allergic responses: itching, redness, swelling, stinging, or warmth may occur at the injection site and usually disappears after a few weeks of therapy. Report as purified or human insulins are used for local allergy and lipohypertrophy at injection site.

17. Failure to take insulin will result in ketoacidosis. Adjust insulin based on BS and guidelines for insulin administration during sick days. Identify soft foods and liquids to consume for sick days (i.e., regular soda, apple juice, clear broth, cream soups, puddings, apple sauce, popsicle, ice cream).
18. If ill, notify provider; to prevent coma, maintain adequate hydration by drinking 1 cup or more of noncaloric fluids such as coffee, tea, water, or broth every hour. Test finger sticks and urine more; identify when to go to the emergency room.
19. If there is no insulin/equipment to administer, decrease food intake by one-third and drink plenty of fluids. Obtain supplies as soon as possible and return to prescribed diet and insulin dosage.
20. Follow good hygienic practices to prevent infection. Bathe daily with mild soap and lukewarm water. Use lotion to prevent skin dryness. Avoid injury from punctures. Avoid scratches; wear gloves when working with the hands. Always protect feet and wear shoes. Use sunscreen and protective clothing to avoid sunburn, and dress appropriately for the weather, taking care to prevent frostbite.
21. Establish a daily routine of checking and caring for the feet. Wear comfortable shoes (leather or canvas) and stockings (no garters or elastic tops) and do exercises. Clip toenails (straight across); do not undertake any self-treatment for ingrown toenails, corns, warts, or calluses. Do not use any heat treatments, hot water bottles, or heating pads, and do not smoke, as this decreases blood flow to the feet. Obtain annual foot screen.
22. Hyperglycemia compounds risk for tooth and gum problems; brush after meals, floss daily, and see dentist q 6 mo.
23. Diabetes can damage the small blood vessels to the eye; obtain yearly eye exams. Eye damage has no symptoms in the early, treatable stage. Report blurred or double vision, narrowed visual fields, increased difficulty seeing in dim light, pressure or pain in the eye, or seeing dark spots.
24. May experience decreased sensation in feet, legs, and hands; use care when handling hot or cold items, wear shoes to protect feet, and dress appropriately for the weather.
25. Carry ID and list of meds, who to notify and what to do if unable to respond.
26. Avoid alcohol; causes hypoglycemia. Excessive intake may require a reduction of insulin; also causes a disulfiram-type reaction with oral hypoglycemic agents.
27. Carry all medications, syringes, glucagon, and blood testing equipment in carry-on luggage when traveling. Always carry diabetes ID. Keep to the usual meal, exercise, and medication routines as closely as possible. Carry food and fast-acting sugar in the event meals are delayed. Request meds for vomiting/diarrhea and plan ahead for mealtimes when crossing two or more time zones. Protect insulin and test strips from extremes in heat or cold (keeping between 15°C and 30°C or 59°F and 86°F).
28. Use only the insulin prescribed; check for correct species (human, beef, pork, or mixed beef-pork), brand name (Humulin, Iletin I, Iletin II, etc.), and type (Regular, Lente, NPH, etc.).
29. Check vials before each dose is taken. Regular and Buffered Regular insulin (for pumps) should be clear and colorless, whereas other forms may be cloudy.
30. Two kinds of insulin can be mixed in the same syringe:

- Regular insulin can be mixed with any other insulin.
- Lente forms can be mixed with other Lente insulins but cannot be mixed with other insulins except regular insulin.
- A single form of insulin in a syringe can be stable for weeks or a month.
- Except for the commercially prepared mixtures, mixtures of insulin are not stable and should be administered within 5 min of preparation.
- When mixed, regular (unmodified) insulin should always be drawn up in the syringe first.

31. Impotence may be caused by damaged nerves and reduced blood flow related to diabetes; should be evaluated to find cause and best treatment.
32. Silent heart attacks may occur. Identify risk factors and alter life-style to prevent CAD (i.e., regular exercise, low-fat, low-salt, low-cholesterol diet, no tobacco or alcohol, stress reduction).
33. Identify support groups to assist in understanding and coping with this disease. The American Diabetes Association, 1660 Duke Street, Alexandria, VA 22314 (telephone: 703-549-1500 or 1-800-ADA-DISC) and local diabetes support groups offer additional information and support.

Outcome/Evaluate

- Understanding/control of DM
- Positive coping strategies
- BS, HbA1c, and renal function studies WNL
- Healthy skin at injection sites
- Prevention of target organ damage

ANTIEMETICS

See also the following individual entries:

Dimenhydrinate
Diphenhydramine hydrochloride
Dronabinol
Granisetron hydrochloride
Hydroxyzine hydrochloride
Hydroxyzine pamoate
Meclizine hydrochloride
Ondansetron hydrochloride
Phosphorated carbohydrate solution
Prochlorperazine
Prochlorperazine edisylate
Prochlorperazine maleate
Scopolamine hydrobromide
Trimethobenzamide hydrochloride

General Statement: Nausea and vomiting can be caused by a variety of conditions, such as infections, drugs, radiation, motion, organic disease, or psychologic factors. The underlying cause of the symptoms must be elicited before emesis is corrected. Many drugs used for other conditions, such as the antihistamines, phenothiazines, barbiturates, and scopolamine, have antiemetic properties and can be used. However, CNS depression make their routine use undesirable.

Drug Interactions: Because of their antiemetic and antinauseant activity, the antiemetics may mask overdosage caused by other drugs.

HEALTH CARE CONSIDERATIONS

Assessment

1. Determine if nausea is an unusual occurrence or a recurring phenomenon; establish onset, duration, and associated factors such as vertigo, chemotherapy, or illness.
2. Note past use of antiemetics; under what conditions and response.
3. Ensure no intestinal obstruction, drug overdose, or increased ICP.
4. Determine physiologic mechanism triggering N&V. Generally, if centrally mediated to the CTZ, would see nausea without vomiting, whereas if the vomiting center were triggered directly, then may see retching with vomiting.
5. Assess for other effects; antiemetics may mask signs of underlying pathology or overdosage of other drugs.
6. Monitor I&O; observe for dehydration. Offer liquids and then gradually advance to regular foods as tolerated.

Client/Family Teaching

1. Drug may cause drowsiness and dizziness. Avoid driving or other hazardous tasks til drug effects evaluated.
2. Practice measures to decrease nausea such as ice chips, sips of water, nongreasy foods, removal of noxious stimuli (odors or materials), and frequent oral hygiene. Advance diet only as tolerated.
3. Dangle legs before standing, rise slowly to prevent symptoms of orthostatic hypotension (↓ BP, ↑ dizziness).
4. Report any unresponsive N&V or abdominal pain.
5. Avoid alcohol and any other nonprescribed CNS depressants.

Outcome/Evaluate

- Control of N&V; prevention of dehydration
- Improved nutritional status evidenced by weight gain and/or ↑ caloric intake

ANTIHISTAMINES (H_1 BLOCKERS)

See also the following individual entries:

Astemizole
Brompheniramine maleate
Cetirizine hydrochloride
Chlorpheniramine maleate
Cyproheptadine hydrochloride
Dexchlorpheniramine maleate
Dimenhydrinate
Diphenhydramine hydrochloride
Emedastine difumarate
Fexofenadine hydrochloride
Levocabastine hydrochloride
Loratidine
Meclizine hydrochloride
Olopatadine hydrochloride
Promethazine hydrochloride
Tripelennamine hydrochloride

Action/Kinetics: Compete with histamine at H_1 histamine receptors (competitive inhibition), thus preventing or reversing the effects of histamine. First-generation antihistamines bind to central and peripheral H_1 receptors and can cause CNS depression or stimulation. Second-generation antihistamines are selective for peripheral H_1 receptors and cause less sedation. Antihistamines do not prevent the release of histamine, antibody production, or antigen-antibody interactions. Antihistamines prevent or reduce increased capillary permeability (i.e., decrease edema, itching) and bronchospasms. Allergic reactions unrelated to histamine release are not affected by antihistamines. Certain of the first-generation antihistamines also have anticholinergic, antiemetic, antipruritic, or antiserotonin effects. Clients unresponsive to a certain antihistamine may regain sensitivity by switching to a different antihistamine.

From a chemical point of view, the antihistamines can be divided into the following classes.

FIRST GENERATION:

1. **Ethylenediamine Derivatives.** Moderate sedative effects; almost no anticholinergic or antiemetic activity. Frequently cause GI distress. Example: Tripelennamine.
2. **Ethanolamine Derivatives.** Moderate to high sedative, anticholinergic, and antiemetic effects. Low incidence of GI side effects. Examples: Clemastine, diphenhydramine.
3. **Alkylamines.** Among the most potent antihistamines. Minimal sedation, moderate anticholinergic effects, and no antiemetic effects. Paradoxical excitation may also occur. Examples: Brompheniramine, chlorpheniramine, dexchlorpheniramine.
4. **Phenothiazines.** High antihistaminic, sedative, and anticholinergic effects; very high antiemetic effect. Example: Promethazine.
5. **Phthalazinone.** High antihistaminic effect; low to no sedative and anticholinergic effects; no antiemetic effect. Example: Azelastine.
6. **Piperazine.** High antihistaminic, sedative, and antiemetic effects; moderate anticholinergic effects. Example: Hydroxyzine.
7. **Piperidines.** Moderate antihistaminic and anticholinergic effects; low to moderate sedation; no antiemetic effects. Examples: Azatadine, cyproheptadine, phenindamine.

SECOND GENERATION:

1. **Piperazine.** Moderate to high antihistamine effect; low to no sedation or anticholinergic effects; no antiemetic activity. Example: Cetirizine.
2. **Piperidines.** Moderate to high antihistamine activity; low to no sedation and anticholinergic activity; no antiemetic action. Examples: Astemizole, fexofenadine, loratidine, terfenadine.

The kinetics of most first-generation antihistamines are similar. **Onset:** 15–30 min; **peak:** 1–2 hr; **duration:** 4–6 hr (piperidines have a longer duration). Many antihistamines are available as timed-release preparations. Most first-generation antihistamines are metabolized by the liver and excreted in the urine. The pharmacokinetics of the second-generation antihistamines vary; consult individual drugs.

See also the individual drugs.

Uses: PO: Treatment of vasomotor, perennial, or seasonal allergic rhinitis and allergic conjunctivitis. Treatment of angioedema, urticarial transfusion reactions, urticaria, pruritus. Atopic dermatitis, contact dermatitis, pruritus ani, pruritus vulvae, insect bites. Sneezing and rhinorrhea due to the common cold. Treatment of anaphylaxis, parkinsonism, drug-induced extrapyramidal reactions, vertigo. Prophylaxis and treatment of motion sickness, including N&V. Nighttime sleep aid.

Parenteral: Relief of allergic reactions due to blood or plasma. As an adjunct to epinephrine in treating anaphylaxis. Uncomplication allergic conditions when PO therapy is not possible.

Contraindications: *First-generation antihistamines.* Hypersensitivity to the drug, narrow-angle glaucoma, symptomatic prostatic hypertrophy, stenosing peptic ulcer, and pyloroduodenal or bladder neck obstruction. Use with MAO inhibitors. Pregnancy or possibility thereof (some agents), lactation, premature and newborn infants. The phenothiazine-type antihistamines are contraindicated in CNS depression from any cause, bone marrow depression, jaundice, dehydrated or acutely ill children, and in comatose clients. Use to treat lower respiratory tract symptoms such as asthma.

Second-generation antihistamines. Hypersensitivity. Astemizole and terfenadine use in significant hepatic dysfunction and concomitant use with clarithromycin, erythromycin, itraconazole, ketoconazole, quinine, and troleandomycin due to the possibility of serious CV effects (including torsades de pointes, prolongation of the QT interval, other ventricular arrhythmias, cardiac arrest, and death). Also terfenadine use with cisapride, HIV protease inhibitors, mibefradil, serotonin reuptake inhibitors, sparfloxacin, and zileuton.

Special Concerns: Administer with caution to clients with convulsive disorders and in respiratory disease. Excess dosage may cause hallucinations, convulsions, and death in infants and children. Use in geriatric clients may result in dizziness, excessive sedation, syncope, toxic confusional states, and hypotension.

Side Effects: *CNS:* Sedation ranging from mild drowsiness to deep sleep. Dizziness, incoordination, faintness, fatigue, confusion, lassitude, restlessnesss, excitation, nervousness, tremor, ***tonic-clonic seizures,*** headache, irritability, insomnia, euphoria, paresthesias, oculogyric crisis, torticollis, catatonic-like states, hallucinations, disorientation, tongue protrusion (usually with IV use or overdosage), disturbing dreams, nightmares, pseudoschizophrenia, weakness, diplopia, vertigo, hysteria, neuritis, paradoxical excitation, epileptiform seizures in clients with focal lesions. Extrapyramidal reactions include opisthotonus, dystonia, akathisia, dyskinesia, and parkinsonism. *CV:* Postural hypotension, palpitations, bradycardia, tachycardia, reflex tachycardia, extrasystoles, increased or decreased BP, ECG changes (including blunting of T waves and prolongation of the Q-T interval), ***cardiac arrest.*** *GI:* Epigastric distress, anorexia, increased appetite and weight gain, N&V, diarrhea, constipation, change in bowel habits, stomatitis. *GU:* Urinary frequency, dysuria, urinary retention, gynecomastia, inhibition of ejaculation, decreased libido, impotence, early menses, induction of lactation. *Hematologic:* Hypoplastic anemia, ***aplastic anemia, hemolytic anemia,*** thrombocytopenia, leukopenia, pancytopenia, ***agranulocytosis,*** thrombocytopenic purpura. *Respiratory:* Thickening of bronchial secretions, wheezing, nasal stuffiness, chest tightness, sore throat, ***respiratory depression;*** dry mouth, nose, and throat. *Ophthalmic:* Blurred vision, diplopia. *Miscellaneous:* Tinnitus, photosensitivity, acute labyrinthitis, obstructive jaundice, erythema, high or prolonged glucose tolerance curves, glycosuria, elevated spinal fluid proteins, increased plasma cholesterol, increased perspiration, chills; tingling, heaviness, and weakness of the hands.

Topical use: Prolonged use may result in local irritation and allergic contact dermatitis.

OD **Management of Overdose:** *Symptoms (Acute Toxicity):* Although antihistamines have a wide therapeutic range, overdosage can nevertheless be fatal. Children are particularly susceptible. Early toxic effects may be seen within 30–120 min and include drowsiness, dizziness, blurred vision, tinnitus, ataxia, and hypotension. Symptoms range from CNS depression (sedation, ***coma,*** decreased mental alertness) to ***CV collapse*** and CNS stimulation (insomnia, hallucinations, tremors, or ***seizures***). Also, ***profound hypotension, respiratory depression, coma, and death*** may occur. Anticholinergic effects include flushing, dry mouth, hypotension, fever, ***hyperthermia*** (especially in children), and fixed, dilated pupils. Body temperature may be as high as 107°F. In children, symptoms include hallucinations, toxic psychosis, delirum tremens, ataxia, incoordination, muscle twitching, excitement, athetosis, ***hyperthermia, seizures,*** and hyperreflexia followed by postictal depression and ***cardiorespiratory arrest.*** *Treatment:*

- Treat symptoms and provide supportive care.
- Vomiting is induced with syrup of ipecac (do not use for phenothiazine overdosage) followed by activated charcoal and a cathartic. If vomiting has not been induced within 3 hr of ingestion, gastric lavage can be undertaken.
- Hypotension can be treated with a vasopressor such as norepinephrine, dopamine, or phenylephrine (do not use epinephrine).
- For convulsions, use only short-acting depressants (e.g., diazepam). IV physostigmine can be used to treat centrally mediated convulsions.
- Ice packs and a cool sponge bath are effective in reducing fever in children.
- Severe cases of overdose can be treated by hemoperfusion.

Drug Interactions

Alcohol, ethyl / See *CNS depressants*

Antidepressants, tricyclic / Additive anticholinergic side effects

CNS depressants, antianxiety agents, barbiturates, narcotics, phenothiazines, procarbazine, sedative-hypnotics / Potentiation or addition of CNS depressant effects. Concomitant use may lead to drowsiness, lethargy, stupor, respiratory depression, coma, and possibly death

Heparin / Antihistamines may ↓ the anticoagulant effects

MAO inhibitors / Intensification and prolongation of anticholinergic side effects; use with phenothiazine antihistamine → hypotension and extrapyramidal reactions

NOTE: Also see *Drug Interactions* for *Phenothiazines.*

Dosage

Usually PO. Parenteral administration is seldom used because of irritating nature of drugs. Topical usage is also limited because antihistamines often cause hypersensitivity reactions. When given for motion sickness, antihistamines are usually given 30–60 min before anticipated travel. See individual drugs.

Laboratory Test Considerations: Discontinue antihistamines 4 days before skin testing to avoid false – result.

1. Inject IM preparations deep into the muscle; irritating to tissues.
2. Swallow sustained-release preparations whole. May break scored tablets before swallowing. If difficulty swallowing capsules, may open and put contents into soft food for ingestion.
3. Do not apply topical preparations to raw, blistered, or oozing areas of the skin.
4. Do not apply to the eyes, around the genitalia, or to mucous membranes.
5. PO preparations may cause gastric irritation; administer with meals, milk, or a snack.

HEALTH CARE CONSIDERATIONS

Assessment

1. Note any drug sensitivity; record known allergens and all meds prescribed.
2. Avoid with any ulcers, glaucoma, or pregnancy.
3. Record type, onset, and duration of symptoms; note triggers.
4. Stop antihistamines 2–4 days prior to skin testing to avoid false negative results.
5. Record VS, CV status, and lung sounds; note characteristics of secretions.
6. Assess extent and characteristics of any rash, if present.

Client/Family Teaching

1. Take med before or at the onset of symptoms; cannot reverse reactions but may prevent them.
2. Do not drive or operate equipment until drug effects realized or drowsiness worn off. Sedative effects may disappear after several days or may not occur at all.
3. Report sore throat, fever, unexplained bruising, bleeding, or petechiae; may cause blood dyscrasia.
4. May cause sensitivity to sun or ultraviolet light; avoid long exposures, use sunscreen, hat, sunglasses, and protective clothing when exposed.
5. For motion sickness, take 30 min before travel time.
6. Reduce symptoms of dry mouth by frequent rinsing, good oral hygiene, and sugarless gum or candies.
7. Severe CNS depression is a symptom of overdosage. Report dizziness or weakness; avoid other CNS depressants.
8. Ensure adequate hydration. If bronchial secretions are thick, increase fluids to decrease secretion viscosity; avoid milk temporarily. If voiding problems, void prior to taking the drug.
9. Exercise regularly; consume 2 L fluids/day and more fruits, fruit juices, and dietary fiber to prevent constipation. Stool softeners may be needed.
10. Recurrent reactions may be referred to an allergist. Protect self from undue exposure and create an allergen-free living area.
11. Raises BP, use with high BP only if medically supervised.
12. Avoid alcohol and OTC products.
13. Children may manifest excitation rather than sedation.
14. Clinical effectiveness may diminish with continued usage; switching to another class may restore drug effectiveness.
15. Family/significant other should learn CPR; survival is greatly increased when CPR is initiated immediately.

Outcome/Evaluate

- ↓ Frequency/intensity of allergic manifestations; ↓ itching/swelling
- Prevention of motion sickness
- Effective nighttime sedation

ANTIHYPERLIPIDEMIC AGENTS—HMG-COA REDUCTASE INHIBITORS

See also the following individual entries:

Atorvastatin calcium
Cerivastatin sodium
Fluvastatin sodium
Lovastatin
Pravastatin sodium
Simvastatin

Action/Kinetics: The HMG-CoA reductase inhibitors competitively inhibit HMG-CoA reductase; this enzyme catalyzes the early rate-limiting step in the synthesis of cholesterol. HMG-CoA reductase inhibitors increase HDL cholesterol and decrease LDL cholesterol, VLDL cholesterol, and plasma triglycerides. The mechanism to lower LDL cholesterol may be due to both a decrease in VLDL cholesterol levels and induction of the LDL receptor, leading to reduced production or increased catabolism of LDL cholesterol. The maximum therapeutic response is seen in 4–6 weeks.

General Statement: The National Cholesterol Education Program Expert Panel on Detection, Evaluation, and Treatment of High Blood Cholesterol in Adults has developed guidelines for the treatment of high cholesterol and LDL in adults. Cholesterol levels less than 200 mg/dL are desirable. Cholesterol levels between 200 and 239 mg/dL are considered borderline-high while levels greater than 240 mg/dL are considered high. With respect to LDL, levels less than 130 mg/dL are considered desirable while levels between 130 and 159 md/dL are considered borderline-high and levels greater than 160 mg/dL are considered high. Depending on the levels of cholesterol and LDL and the number of risk factors present for CAD, the provider will develop a treatment regimen.

Uses: Adjunct to diet to decrease elevated total LDL and cholesterol in clients with primary hypercholesterolemia (types IIa and IIb) when the response to diet and other nondrug approaches has not been adequate. See also individual drugs.

Contraindications: Active liver disease or unexplained persistent elevated liver function tests. Pregnancy, lactation. Use in children.

Special Concerns: Use with caution in those who ingest large quantities of alcohol or who have a history of liver disease. May cause photosensitivity. Safety and efficacy have not been established in children less than 18 years of age.

Side Effects: The following side effects are common to most HMG-CoA reductase inhibitors. Also see individual drugs. *GI:* N&V, diarrhea, constipation, abdominal cramps or pain, flatulence, dyspepsia, heartburn. *CNS:* Headache, dizziness, dysfunction of certain cranial nerves (e.g., alteration of taste, facial paresis, impairment of extraocular movement), tremor, vertigo, memory loss, paresthesia, anxiety, insomnia, depression. *Musculoskeletal:* Localized pain, myalgia, muscle cramps or pain, myopathy, rhabdomyolysis, arthralgia. *Respiratory:* URI, rhinitis, cough. *Ophthalmic:* Progression of cataracts (lens opacities), ophthalmoplegia. *Hypersensitivity:* ***Anaphylaxis, angioedema,*** vasculitis, purpura, thrombocytopenia, leukopenia, ***hemolytic anemia,*** lupus erythematosus-like syndrome, polymyalgia rheumatica, positive ANA, ESR increase, arthritis, arthralgia, eosinophilia, urticaria, photosensitivity, fever, chills, flushing, malaise, dyspnea, ***toxic dermal necrolysis, Stevens-Johnson syndrome.*** *Miscellaneous:* Rash, pruritus, cardiac chest pain, fatigue, influenza, alopecia, edema, dryness of skin and mucous membranes, changes to hair and nails, skin discoloration.

Drug Interactions: See also individual drugs.

Cyclosporine / Possibility of myopathy or severe rhabdomyolysis
Digoxin / Slight ↑ in digoxin levels
Gemfibrozil / Possibility of severe myopathy or rhabdomyolysis
Itraconazole / ↑ Levels of HMG-CoA inhibitors
Nicotinic acid / Possibility of myopathy or severe rhabdomyolysis
Propranolol / ↓ Antihyperlipidemic activity
Warfarin / ↑ Anticoagulant effect of warfarin.

Dosage

See individual drugs.

Laboratory Test Considerations: ↑ AST, ALT, CPK, alkaline phosphatase, bilirubin. Abnormal thyroid function tests.Lovastatin should be taken with meals; cerivastatin, fluvastatin, pravastatin, and simavastatin may be taken without regard to meals.

HEALTH CARE CONSIDERATIONS

Assessment

1. Review life-style, duration of illness, and attempts made to control with diet, exercise, and weight reduction.
2. Record any alcohol abuse or liver disease.
3. Perform PMH, ROS, and physical exam; record risk factors.
4. Monitor LFTs as recommended. Transaminase levels 3 times normal may precipitate severe hepatic toxicity. If CK elevated, assess renal function as rhabdomyolsis with myoglobinuria could cause renal shutdown. Stop drug therapy.
5. Note nutritional analysis by dietician; assess cholesterol profile (HDL, LDL, cholesterol, and triglycerides) after 3–6 months of exercise and diet therapy if risk factors do not require immediate drug therapy. With diabetes and coronary heart disease a more aggressive drug approach should be instituted in addition to diet therapy with goals of reducing LDL below 100.

Client/Family Teaching

1. Take only as directed.
2. May cause photosensitivity; avoid prolonged sun or UV light exposure. Use sunscreens, sunglasses, and protective clothing when exposed.
3. Report any pain in skeletal muscles or unexplained muscle pain, tenderness, or weakness promptly, especially with fever or malaise.
4. Stop drug with any major trauma, surgery, or serious illness.
5. Continue life-style modifications that include low-fat, low-cholesterol, and low-sodium diets, weight reduction with obese clients, smoking cessation, reduction of alcohol consumption, HRT with menopause, and regular aerobic exercise in the overall goal of cholesterol reduction.
6. Avoid niacin; may cause hepatic failure; may use niaspan (ER form) with careful monitoring. Use a fibrate cautiously; monitor LFTs and assess for muscle pain.
7. Avoid any unprescribed or OTC agents.
8. Report regularly for labs to prevent liver toxicity and to assess drug results.

Outcome/Evaluate

- ↓ LDL, triglycerides, and total cholesterol levels; ↓ risk of CAD and death

ANTIHYPERTENSIVE AGENTS

See also the following drug classes and individual drugs:

Agents Acting Directly on Vascular Smooth Muscle

Diazoxide IV
Hydralazine hydrochloride

Alpha-1-Adrenergic Blocking Agents

Doxazosin mesylate
Prazosin hydrochloride
Terazosin

Angiotensin-II Receptor Blockers

Candesartan cilexetil
Irbesartan
Losartan potassium
Valsartan

Angiotensin-Converting Enzyme Inhibitors

Benazepril hydrochloride
Captopril
Enalapril maleate
Fosinopril sodium
Lisinopril
Moexipril hydrochloride
Quinapril hydrochloride
Ramipril
Trandolopril

Beta-Adrenergic Blocking Agents

Calcium Channel Blocking Agents

Amlodipine
Bepridil hydrochloride
Diltiazem hydrochloride
Felodipine
Isradipine
Nicardipine hydrochloride
Nifedipine
Nimodipine
Nisoldipine
Verapamil

Centrally-Acting Agents

Clonidine hydrochloride
Guanabenz acetate
Guanfacine hydrochloride
Methyldopa
Methyldopate hydrochloride

Combination Drugs Used for Hypertension

Amiloride and Hydrochlorothiazide
Amlodipine and Benazepril hydrochloride
Bisoprolol fumarate and Hydrochlorothiazide
Enalapril maleate and Hydrochlorothiazide
Fosinopril sodium
Lisinopril and Hydrochlorothiazide
Losartan potassium and Hydrochlorothiazide
Methyldopa and Hydrochlorothiazide
Propranolol and Hydrochlorothiazide
Spironolactone and Hydrochlorothiazide
Triamterene and Hydrochlorothiazide

Miscellaneous Agents

Carvedilol
Epoprostenol sodium
Labetalol hydrochloride
Minoxidil, oral

Peripherally-Acting Agents

Guanadrel sulfate
Guanethidine monosulfate

General Statement: The Sixth Report of the Joint National Committee on Prevention, Detection, Evaluation and Treatment of High Blood Pressure classifies BP for adults aged 18 and over as follows: Optimal as <120/<80 mm Hg, Normal as <130/<85 mm Hg, High Normal as 130–139/85–89 mm Hg, Stage 1 Hypertension as 140–159/90–99 mm Hg, Stage 2 Hypertension as 160–179/100–109 mm Hg, and Stage 3 Hypertension as 180 or greater/110 or greater mm Hg. Drug therapy is recommended depending on the BP and whether certain risk factors (e.g., smoking, dyslipidemia, diabetes, age, gender, target organ damage, clinical CV disease) are present. Life-style modification is an important component of treating hypertension, including weight reduction, reduction of sodium intake, regular exercise, cessation of smoking, and moderate alcohol intake.

The goal of antihypertensive therapy is a BP of <140/90 mm Hg, except in hypertensive diabetics where the goal is <135/85 mm Hg and those with renal insufficiency where the goal is <130/85 mm Hg. Generally speaking, the primary agents for initial monotherapy to treat uncomplicated hypertension are diuretics and beta blockers. Alternative drugs include ACE inhibitors, alpha-1 blockers, alpha-beta blocker, and calcium antagonists.

HEALTH CARE CONSIDERATIONS

Assessment

1. Note any family history of hypertension, stroke, CVD, CHD, dyslipidemia, and diabetes.
2. Determine baseline BP before starting antihypertensive therapy. To ensure accuracy of baseline readings, take BP in both (bared and supported) arms (lying, standing, and sitting) 2 min apart (30 min after last cigarette or caffeine consumption) at least three times during one visit and on two subsequent visits. Record height, weight and risk factors.

3. Ascertain life-style modifications (weight reduction, ↓ alcohol intake, regular exercise, reduced sodium/fat intake, and smoking cessation) needed to achieve lowered BP. Offer a trial following these modifications and reassess in 3–6 mo before starting therapy unless BP severe.
4. Monitor ECG, chem-7, CBC, uric acid, urinalysis, cholesterol panel, and lfts.
5. Note funduscopic and neurologic exam findings.
6. Assess for thyroid enlargement and presence of target organ damage. If difficult to control, assess for renal artery stenosis or secondary causes of HTN and refer for 24-hr ambulatory BP monitoring.

Client/Family Teaching

1. Drugs control but do not cure hypertension. Take meds despite feeling fine and do not stop abruptly; may cause rebound hypertension.
2. Keep a record of BP readings; helps identify "white collar syndrome."
3. Adhere to a low-sodium, low-fat diet; see dietitian as needed for education and meal planning, preparation, and food selections.
4. Weakness, dizziness, and fainting may occur with rapid changes of position from supine to standing. Rise slowly from a lying or sitting position and dangle legs for several minutes before standing to minimize orthostatic effects. Exercising in hot weather may enhance effects.
5. If dose missed, do not double up or take two doses close together.
6. Have yearly eye exams to detect early retinal changes.
7. Avoid meds that may lower BP (e.g., alcohol, barbiturates, CNS depressants) or that could elevate BP (e.g., OTC cold remedies, oral contraceptives, steroids, NSAIDs, appetite suppressants, tricyclic antidepressants, MAO inhibitors). Sympathomimetic amines in products used to treat asthma, colds, and allergies must be used with extreme caution
8. Avoid excessive amounts of caffeine (tea, coffee, chocolate, or colas).
9. Notify provider if sexual dysfunction occurs as med can usually be changed to minimize symptoms or other options for sexual dysfunction explored.
10. Identify holistic interventions/life-style modifications necessary for BP control: dietary restrictions of fat and sodium (2–3 g/day), weight reduction, ↓ alcohol (i.e., less than 24 oz beer or less than 8 oz of wine or less than 2 oz of 100-proof whiskey per day), tobacco cessation, ↑ physical activity, regular exercise programs, proper rest, and methods to reduce and deal with stress.

Outcome/Evaluate

- Understanding of disease/compliance with prescribed therapy
- ↓ BP (SBP < 140 and DBP < 85 mm Hg)
- Control/prevent target organ damage, stroke, and death

ANTI-INFECTIVE DRUGS

See also the following individual drugs and drug classes:

Amebicides and Trichomonacides
Aminoglycosides
4-Aminoquinolines
Anthelmintics
Antimalarials
Antiviral Drugs
Bacitracin
Becaplermin
Butenafine hydrochloride
Cephalosporins
Clindamycin
Erythromycins
Fluoroquinolones
Fosfomycin tromethamine
Imipenem-Cilastatin sodium
Lincomycin hydrochloride
Loracarbef
Macrolides
Mupirocin
Penicillins
Spectinomycin hydrochloride
Sulfonamides
Tetracyclines
Vancomycin hydrochloride

Action/Kinetics: The mechanism of action of the anti-infectives varies. The following modes of action have been identified.* Note the considerable overlap among these mechanisms:

1. Inhibition of synthesis of or activation of enzymes that disrupt bacterial cell walls leading to loss of viability and possibly cell lysis (e.g., penicillins, cephalosporins, cycloserine, bacitracin, vancomycin, miconazole, ketoconazole, clotrimazole).
2. Direct effect on the microbial cell mem-

* Chambers, H.F., Sande, M.A.: Antimicrobial agents. In *Goodman and Gilman's The Pharmacological Basis of Therapeutics,* 9th ed. Edited by Hardman, J.G., Limbud, L.E., New York, McGraw-Hill, 1996, p. 1029.

brane to affect permeability and leading to leakage of intracellular components (e.g., polymyxin, colistimethate, nystatin, amphotericin).
3. Effect on the function of 30S and 50S bacterial ribosomes to cause a reversible inhibition of protein synthesis (e.g., chloramphenicol, tetracyclines, erythromycin, clindamycin).
4. Bind to the 30S ribosomal subunit that alters protein synthesis and leads to cell death (e.g., aminoglycosides).
5. Effect on nucleic acid metabolism which inhibits DNA-dependent RNA polymerase (e.g., rifampin) or inhibition of gyrase (e.g., fluoroquinolones).
6. Antimetabolites that block specific metabolic steps essential to the life of the microorganism (e.g., trimethoprim, sulfonamides).
7. Bind to viral enzymes that are essential for DNA synthesis leading to a halt of viral replication (e.g., acyclovir, ganciclovir, vidarabine, zidovudine).

General Statement

The following general guidelines apply to the use of most anti-infective drugs:
1. Anti-infective drugs can be divided into those that are *bacteriostatic,* that is, stop the multiplication and further development of the infectious agent, or *bactericidal,* that is, kill and thus eradicate all living microorganisms. Both time of administration and length of therapy may be affected by this difference.
2. Some anti-infectives halt the growth of or eradicate many different microorganisms and are termed *broad-spectrum antibiotics.* Others affect only certain specific organisms and are termed *narrow-spectrum antibiotics.*
3. Some of the anti-infectives stimulate a hypersensitivity reaction in some persons. Penicillins cause more severe and more frequent hypersensitivity reactions than any other drug.
4. Because of differences in susceptibility of infectious agents to anti-infectives, the sensitivity of the microorganism to the drug ordered should be determined before treatment is initiated. Several sensitivity tests are commonly used for this purpose.
5. Certain anti-infective agents have marked side effects, some of the more serious of which are neurotoxicity, including ototoxicity, and nephrotoxicity. Care must be taken not to administer two anti-infectives with similar side effects at the same time, or to administer these drugs to clients in whom the side effects might be damaging (e.g., a nephrotoxic drug to a client suffering from kidney disease). The choice of anti-infective also depends on its distribution in the body (i.e., whether it passes the blood-brain barrier).
6. Anti-infective drugs can also eradicate the normal intestinal flora necessary for proper digestion, synthesis of vitamin K, and control of fungi that may gain access to the GI tract (superinfection).

Uses: See individual drugs. The choice of the anti-infective depends on the nature of the illness to be treated, the sensitivity of the infecting agent, and the client's previous experience with the drug. Hypersensitivity and allergic reactions may preclude the use of the agent of choice.

Contraindications: Hypersensitivity or allergies to the drug.

Side Effects: The antibiotics and anti-infective agents have few direct toxic effects. Kidney and liver damage, deafness, and blood dyscrasias are occasionally observed.

The following undesirable manifestations, however, occur frequently:
1. Suppresion of the normal flora of the body, which in turn keeps certain pathogenic microorganisms, such as *Candida albicans, Proteus,* or *Pseudomonas,* from causing infections. If the flora is altered, *superinfections* (monilial vaginitis, enteritis, UTIs), which necessitate the discontinuation of therapy or the use of other antibiotics, can result.
2. Incomplete eradication of an infectious organism. Casual use of anti-infectives favors the emergence of *resistant* strains insensitive to a particular drug.

To minimize the chances for the development of resistant strains, anti-infectives are usually given at specified doses for a prescribed length of time after acute symptoms have subsided.

OD **Management of Overdose:** *Treatment:* Discontinue the drug and treat symptomatically. Supportive measures should be instituted as needed. Hemodialysis may be used although its effectiveness is questionable, depending on the drug and the status of the client (i.e., more effective in impaired renal function).
1. Check expiration date.
2. Store according to recommended storage method.
3. Mark date and time of reconstitution, your initials, and the solution strength. Mark expiration date; store under appropriate conditions.
4. Complete infusion (or as ordered) before the drug loses potency; check drug info.

HEALTH CARE CONSIDERATIONS

Assessment

1. Record onset and characteristics of symptoms, location and source of infection (if known).
2. Record any unusual reaction/sensitivity with any anti-infectives (usually penicillin).
3. Obtain cultures before administering empiric therapy. Use correct procedure for obtaining, storing, and transporting specimens.
4. Monitor CBC, liver and renal function studies.

Client/Family Teaching

1. Take meds at prescribed intervals; use only under medical supervision.
2. Do not share with friends or family members.Prevent recurrence by completing entire prescription, despite feeling well. This ensures that the organism is eradicated and diminishes the emergence of drug-resistant bacterial strains. Incomplete therapy may render client unresponsive to the antibiotic with the next infection.
3. Report any unusual bruising or bleeding, e.g., bleeding gums, blood in stool, urine, or other secretions; S&S of allergic reactions, including rash, fever, pruritis, and urticaria or superinfections such as pain, swelling, redness, drainage, perineal itching, diarrhea, rash, or a change in symptoms.
4. Discard any unused drug after therapy completed.
5. Take antipyretics as prescribed ATC (q 4 hr) for fever reduction when needed.

Interventions

1. In a very obvious place mark allergy in red on the medication records.
2. Assess for hives, rashes, or difficulty breathing, which may indicate a hypersensitivity or allergic response; stop drug and report.
3. Monitor VS, I&O; ensure adequate hydration.
4. If drug mainly excreted by the kidneys, reduce dose with renal dysfunction. Nephrotoxic drugs are usually contraindicated with renal dysfunction because toxic drug levels are rapidly attained with impaired renal function.
5. Verify orders when two or more anti-infectives are ordered for the same client, especially if they have similar side effects, such as nephrotoxicity and/or neurotoxicity.
6. Assess for superinfections, particularly of fungal origin, characterized by black furred tongue, nausea, and/or diarrhea. *Prevent superinfections by:*
   • Limiting exposure to persons suffering from an active infectious process
   • Rotating IV site q 72 hr; changing IV tubing q 24–48 hr
   • Providing/emphasizing good hygiene
   • Washing hands carefully before and after contact with client
7. Schedule administration throughout 24-hr period to maintain therapeutic drug levels. Administration schedule is determined by the drug half-life ($t^{1/2}$), severity of infection, evidence of organ dysfunction, and client's need for sleep. Assess drug levels (peak and trough) to ensure appropriate dosing.

Outcome/Evaluate

- Prevention/resolution of infection
- ↓ Fever, WBCs; ↑ appetite
- Negative culture reports
- Therapeutic serum drug levels

GENERAL HEALTH CARE CONSIDERATIONS FOR ALL ANTIINFECTIVES

ANTIMALARIAL DRUGS, 4-AMINOQUINOLINES

See also the following individual entries:

Chloroquine hydrochloride
Chloroquine phosphate
Hydroxychloroquine sulfate

Action/Kinetics: Several mechanisms have been proposed for the action of 4-aminoquinolines. These include (a) an active chloroquine-concentrating mechanism in the acid vesicles of the parasite causing inhibition of growth, (b) release of aggregates of ferriprotoporphyrin IX from erythrocytes in the parasite causing membrane damage and erythrocyte or parasite lysis, (c) interference with hemoglobin digestion by the parasite, and (d) interference with synthesis of nucleoprotein by the parasite. The drugs are active against the erythrocytic forms of *Plasmodium vivax* and *P. malariae* as well as most strains of *P. falciparum*. The aminoquinolines are rapidly and almost completely absorbed from the GI tract and are widely distributed throughout the body. **Peak serum levels:** 1–6 hr. Very slowly excreted; presence of drug has been demonstrated in the bloodstream weeks and even months after the drug has been discontinued. Up to 70% may be excreted unchanged. Urinary excretion is increased by acidifying the urine; excretion is slowed by alkalinization.

See also *General Health Care Considerations for All Anti-Infectives*.

Uses: Treatment or prophylaxis of acute attacks of malaria caused by *Plasmodium falciparum, P. vivax, P. ovale,* and *P. malariae.* Will cause a radical cure of vivax and malariae malaria if combined with primaquine. Effective only against the erythrocytic stages and therefore will not prevent infections. However, complete cure of infections due to sensitive strains of falciparum malaria is possible.

Extraintestinal amebiasis caused by *Entamoeba histolytica.* Discoid or lupus erythematosus, scleroderma, pemphigus, lichen planus, polymyositis, sarcoidosis, porphyria cutanea tarda.

Contraindications: Hypersensitivity. Changes in retinal or visual field. Lactation. Use in psoriasis or porphyria only if benefits clearly outweigh risks. Concomitantly with gold or phenylbutazone or in clients receiving drugs that depress blood-forming elements of bone marrow.

Special Concerns: Use with extreme caution in the presence of hepatic, severe GI, neurologic, and blood disorders. Infants and children are sensitive to the effects of 4-aminoquinolines. Certain strains of *P. falciparum* are resistant to 4-aminoquinolines.

Side Effects: *GI:* N&V, diarrhea, cramps, anorexia, epigastric distress, stomatitis, dry mouth. *CNS:* Headache, fatigue, nervousness, anxiety, irritability, agitation, apathy, confusion, personality changes, depression, psychoses, ***seizures.*** *CV:* Hypotension, ECG changes (inversion or depression of T wave, widening of QRS complex). *Dermatologic:* Pruritus, changes in pigment of skin and mucous membranes, dermatoses, bleaching of hair. *Hematologic:* Neutropenia, ***aplastic anemia,*** thrombocytopenia, ***agranulocytosis.*** *Ocular:* Retinopathy that may be permanent and may lead to blindness. Blurred vision, difficulty in focusing or in accommodation; chronic use may lead to corneal deposits or keratopathy. *Miscellaneous:* Peripheral neuritis, ototoxicity, neuromyopathy manifested by muscle weakness.

OD **Management of Overdose:** *Symptoms:* Headache, drowsiness, visual disturbances, ***CV collapse, seizures followed by sudden and early respiratory and cardiac arrest.*** Infants and children have manifested respiratory depression, ***CV collapse, shock, seizures, and death following overdoses of parenteral chloroquine.*** ECG changes include nodal rhythm, atrial standstill, prolonged intraventricular conduction, and bradycardia, which lead to ***ventricular fibrillation or arrest.*** *Treatment:* Undertake gastric lavage or emesis followed by activated charcoal. Seizures should be controlled prior to gastric lavage. Seizures due to anoxia can be treated by oxygen, mechanical ventilation, or vasopressors (in shock with hypotension). Tracheostomy or tracheal intubation may be required. Forced fluids and acidification of the urine may hasten excretion. Peritoneal dialysis and exchange transfusions may also help.

Drug Interactions

Acidifying agents, urinary (ammonium chloride, etc.) / ↑ Urinary excretion of antimalarial and thus ↓ its effectiveness

Alkalinizing agents, urinary (bicarbonate, etc.) / ↓ Excretion of antimalarial and thus ↑ amount of drug in system

Antipsoriatics / 4-Aminoquinolines inhibit antipsoriatic drugs

MAO inhibitors / ↑ Toxicity of 4-Aminoquinolines due to ↓ breakdown in liver

Dosage

See individual drug entries.

Laboratory Test Considerations: Colors urine brown.Store in amber-colored containers.

HEALTH CARE CONSIDERATIONS

Assessment

1. Note if prophylaxis or acute drug therapy; identify source and exposure dates.
2. Obtain cultures. Note any hepatic, neurologic, or blood disorders; monitor lab parameters.
3. Assess for retinopathy manifested by visual disturbances. Retinal changes are not reversible. Mandate regular eye exams during prolonged therapy.

Interventions

1. Observe for overdosage and symptoms of acute toxicity (headache, drowsiness, visual disturbances, CV collapse, convulsions, and cardiac arrest) which develop within 30 min of ingestion. Death may occur within 2 hr; see *Overdose Management.*
2. Monitor VS, I&O, and state of consciousness.
3. With some therapies, fluids will have to be forced and ammonium chloride administered for weeks to months to acidify urine and promote renal excretion of the drug.
4. Check toxic effects of other drugs being used because the combination with chloroquine may intensify toxic effects.

Client/Family Teaching

1. Take exactly as prescribed.
2. Take with the evening meal with discoid lupus erythematosus.
3. When used for suppressive therapy, take on the same day each week, immediately

before or after meals to minimize gastric irritation (e.g., hydroxychloroquine).
4. Ensure that adequate fluid intake as well as the meds to acidify urine are taken as prescribed. Some drugs may discolor urine brown.
5. Report any persistent, new, or bothersome side effects.
6. Report as scheduled for F/U and labs to prevent relapse.
7. Wear sunglasses to prevent photophobia.
8. Avoid alcohol during therapy.
9. Keep in child-proof containers and out of child's reach.

Outcome/Evaluate

- Understanding of disease/adherence with prescribed therapy
- Malaria prophylaxis
- Elimination of causative organism
- Symptomatic improvement

ANTINEOPLASTIC AGENTS

See also the following individual entries:

Altretamine
Anastrozole
Bicalutamide
Busulfan
Capecitabine
Chlorambucil
Cisplatin
Diethylstilbestrol diphosphate
Estramustine phosphate sodium
Flutamide
Goserelin acetate
Hydroxyurea
Letrozole
Leuprolide acetate
Levamisole hydrochloride
Lomustine
Mechlorethamine hydrochloride
Megestrol acetate
Mercaptopurine
Methotrexate
Methotrexate sodium
Nilutamide
Procarbazine hydrochloride
Tamoxifen
Testolactone
Thioguanine
Toremifene citrate
Trastuzumab
Valrubicin

Action/Kinetics: During division, cells go through a number of stages during which they may be susceptible to various chemotherapeutic agents (see *Action/Kinetics* of various agents). The various cell stages are described in Figure 2.

General Statement: The choice of the chemotherapeutic agent(s) depends both on the cell type of the tumor and on its site of growth. All antineoplastic agents are cytotoxic (i.e., cell poisons) and therefore interfere with normal as well as neoplastic cells. However, neoplastic cells are more active and multiply more rapidly than normal cells and are thus more affected by the antineoplastic agents. Normal, rapidly growing tissue cells, such as those of the bone marrow, the GI mucosal epithelium, and hair follicles, are particularly susceptible to antineoplastic agents. The margin between the dose of antineoplastic drug needed to destroy the neoplastic cells and that needed to cause bone marrow damage, for example, is narrow. Since WBCs or platelets show the effect of an overdose more rapidly than do erythrocytes, the platelet and WBC counts are often used as a guide to dosage. If a blood or marrow test indicates a precipitous fall in the WBC or platelet count, the antineoplastic agent may have to be discontinued or the dosage modified significantly. Drugs are frequently withheld when the WBC count falls below 2,000/mm^3 and the platelet count falls below 100,000/mm^3. With the advent of granulocyte colony-stimulating factors, providers may now utilize this to support large dosing on an aggressive cancer, thus preventing postponement of therapy until recovery of the client's hematologic parameters. Sometimes the effect of the antineoplastic drugs on the bone marrow is cumulative, with the depression of WBCs and platelets occurring weeks or months after initiation of therapy.

GI tract toxicity is manifested by development of oral ulcers, intestinal bleeding, nausea, vomiting, loss of appetite, and diarrhea. Finally, alopecia often results from antineoplastic drug therapy.

Uses: Most of the drugs discussed in this section are used exclusively for neoplastic disease. A few are used on an experimental basis for some of the rheumatic diseases.

Contraindications: Hypersensitivity to drug. Some antineoplastic agents may be contraindicated for a period of 4 weeks after radiation therapy or chemotherapy with similar drugs. During first trimester of pregnancy.

Special Concerns: Use with caution, and at reduced dosages, in clients with preexisting bone marrow depression, malignant infiltra-

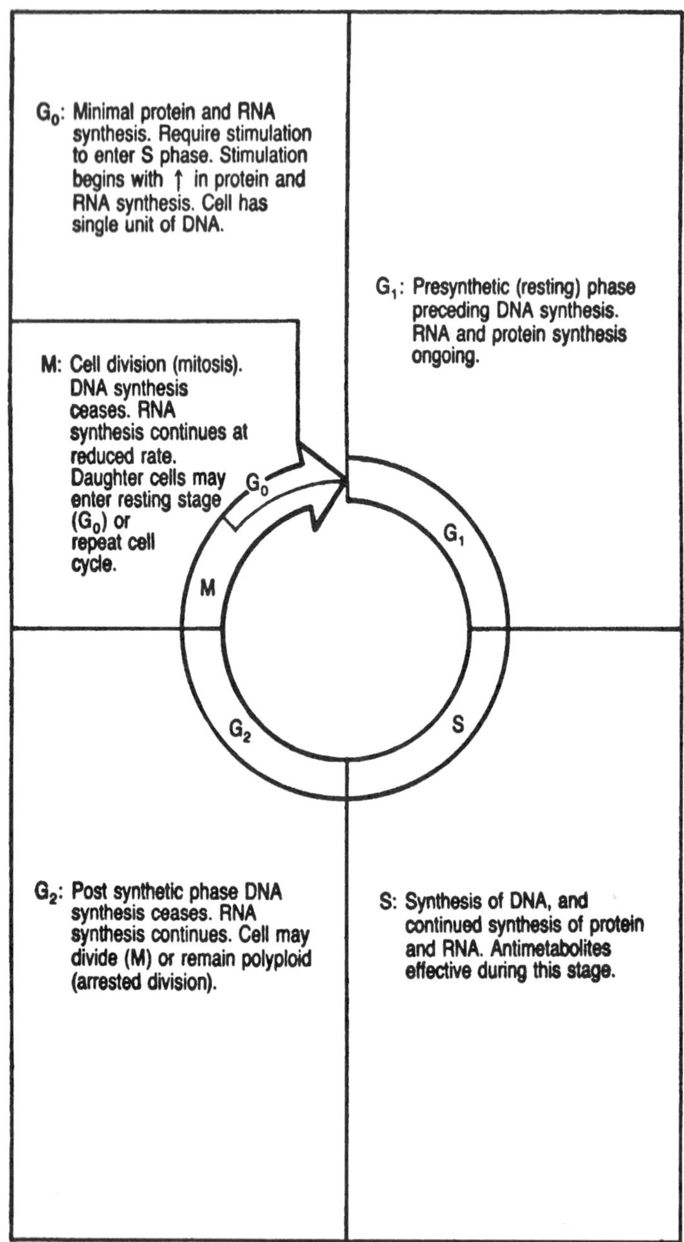

Figure 2 Cell stages

tion of bone marrow or kidney, liver dysfunction, or previous recent chemotherapy usage. The safe use of these drugs during pregnancy has not been established.

Side Effects: *Bone marrow depression* (leukopenia, thrombocytopenia, ***agranulocytosis,*** anemia) is the major danger of antineoplastic therapy. ***Bone marrow depression can sometimes be irreversible.*** *It is mandatory that the client have frequent total blood counts and periodic bone marrow examinations. Precipitous falls must be reported to a physician.* Other side effects include: *GI:* N&V (may be severe), anorexia, diarrhea (may be hemorrhagic), stomatitis, mucositis, enteritis, abdominal cramps, intestinal ulcers. *Hepatic:* Hepatic toxicity including jaundice and changes in liver enzymes. *Dermatologic:* Dermatitis, erythema, various dermatoses including maculopapular rash, alopecia (reversible), pruritus, staining of vein path with some drugs, urticaria, cheilosis. *Immunologic:* Immunosuppression with increased susceptibility to viral, bacterial, or fungal infections. *CNS:* Depression, lethargy, confusion, dizziness, headache, fatigue, malaise, fever, weakness. *GU:* ***Acute renal failure,*** reproductive abnormalities including amenorrhea and azoospermia. *NOTE:* Alkylating agents, in particular, may be both carcinogenic and mutagenic.

GENERAL HEALTH CARE CONSIDERATIONS FOR ANTINEOPLASTIC AGENTS

1. Antineoplastic drugs should be prepared only by trained personnel and avoided if pregnant.
2. Cytotoxic exposure may be through inhalation, ingestion, and absorption during preparation; prepare under a laminar flow (biologic) hood.
• If not available, prepare in a separate room in a work area away from cooling or heating vents and away from other people. Cover work table area with a disposable plastic liner.
• Use latex gloves to protect the skin when reconstituting; do not use gloves made of PVC since these are permeable to some cytotoxic drugs. Good handwashing before and after preparation is essential. Prevent drug contact with skin or mucous membranes; document occurrence and wash area immediately with copious amounts of water.
• Wear disposable, nonpermeable gown with closed front and knit cuffs that completely cover the wrists.
• Wear goggles. Should material enter eyes, wash well with isotonic saline eyewash (or water if isotonic saline is unavailable) and consult ophthalmologist.
3. Start infusion with a solution not containing the chemotherapy drug. Avoid dorsum of the hand, wrist, or antecubital fossa as infusion site.
4. Use disposable Luer-Lok fittings, protective needles, syringes, and connectors.
• If drug to be reconstituted from a vial, vent the vial at the beginning of the procedure. Venting lowers the internal pressure and reduces the risk of spilling or spraying (aerosolization) solution when the needle is withdrawn.
• Use sterile alcohol wipe around the needle and vial top when withdrawing the drug and when expelling air.
5. Wipe external surfaces of syringes and bottles with an alcohol sponge once prepared. Place all disposable equipment in a separate plastic bag specifically marked for chemotherapy and sent for incineration.
6. Report pain, redness, or edema near the injection site during or after treatment.
7. Ensure reliable contraception.
8. Wear latex gloves when disposing of vomitus, urine, or feces.
9. Record all exposure times during preparation, administration, cleanup, and spills. Follow appropriate institutional guidelines governing exposures allowed, extravasation, and periodic lab evaluations.

HEALTH CARE CONSIDERATIONS DURING INITIATION OF CHEMOTHERAPY

Assessment

1. Identify condition requiring therapy and any previous radiation, surgery, or chemotherapy treatments.
2. Assess emotional status; note any hypersensitivity to drugs or foods.
3. Assess nutritional status; note height, weight, and VS; doses are based on BSA (m^2).
4. Examine oral mucosa for any abnormalities or problems.
5. Monitor bone marrow function (CBC with differential), platelets, liver and renal function.
6. Note prescribed route of administration: oral, IV, IM, or directly at the tumor site (intracavity, intrapleural, intrathecal, intravesical, intraperitoneal, intra-arterial, or topical).
7. Depending on the route, length of therapy, frequency of access, venous integrity, and client preference, determine if venous access device would be more comfortable.
8. Assess pain control regimen to ensure

that meds are available in quantities sufficient to relieve pain.

9. Premedicate (antiemetic, antihistamine, and/or anti-inflammatory) 30–60 min before therapy and as needed.

Client/Family Teaching

1. Comply with all aspects of the therapeutic regimen.
2. Review information/literature R/T condition requiring treatment. The American Cancer Society provides many free booklets on cancers, chemotherapy, and how to deal with the side effects of treatments. Go to the library, internet, local cancer society, and provider with unanswered questions. May also call 1-800-4-CANCER, the Cancer Information Service at the National Cancer Institute, or access through the Internet for further information.
3. Review drug side effects that may occur and a means for coping with these problems.
4. Identify community support groups that may assist in coping with illness.
5. Provide a number to reach provider to report adverse side effects or to request clarification of instructions.
6. When antineoplastic agents are prepared and administered in the home, advise families how to dispose of urine, feces, vomitus, and equipment and how to handle drug spills.

Interventions

1. Monitor VS, I&O.
2. Report any pain, redness, or edema near injection site during or after treatment. If extravasation occurs, stop infusion and follow institutional protocol for minimizing effects. General guidelines for managing an extravasation include:
   - Record and report.
   - Aspirate drug through the cannula with a small syringe (tuberculin size).
   - Administer antidote when indicated.
   - Remove needle and apply ice (heat if vinca alkaloids).
   - Assess and follow-up until site is healed.
3. Chart antineoplastic drugs on the medication administration record (MAR) and according to the established protocol.
   - Record client's drug therapy on the MAR:
   - Day 1: first day of the first dose.
   - Number each day after that in sequence, even though may not receive drug daily.
   - Indicate when nadir (the time of most severe physiologic depression) is likely to occur so that possible complications, such as infection and bleeding, can be anticipated, assessed for, and treated early; note recovery time.
   - When repeating drug regimen, the first day of therapy is charted as day 1.
4. Establish interventions to promote client adherence. Keep informed and interpret complicated terminology/therapy; support client/family and help them to understand unconventional emotions and anger.
5. Identify support groups to assist in coping with illness, complex therapy, and emotional turmoil within family unit.

Outcome/Evaluate

- Understanding of illness, therapy options, drug side effects, and goals of therapy
- N&V, pain, anorexia, or diarrhea may indicate inadequate levels of prescribed agents
- Evidence of acute renal failure, hepatic toxicity, or changes in liver enzymes
- Presence and extent of psychologic depression, lethargy, or other mental status changes
- Control of pain
- Control/regression of malignant cell proliferation
- Desired cure

HEALTH CARE CONSIDERATIONS FOR BONE MARROW DEPRESSION (MYELOSUPPRESSION)

LEUKOPENIA

Assessment

1. Assess for granulocytopenia or decreased WBCs (normal values: 5,000–10,000/mm^3).
2. Review differential (normal values: neutrophils 60%–70%, lymphocytes 25%–30%, monocytes 2%–6%, eosinophils 1%–3%, basophils 0.25%–0.5%).
3. Note any sudden sharp drop in WBC count or a reduction below 2,000/mm^3; may require a dosage reduction or withdrawal of drug.
4. Determine nadir (time the blood count reaches its lowest point after chemotherapy) for prescribed agent (generally 7–14 days). This assists to predict, monitor, and respond to effects of the bone marrow depression.
5. Report fever above 38°C (100°F); limited resistance to infection due to leukopenia and immunosuppression. Assess for early signs of infection: check oral cavity for sores/ulcerated areas and urine for odor or particulate matter. With reduced or absent granulocytes, local abscesses do not form with pus; infection becomes systemic.
6. Increased weakness or fatigue may indicate anemia or electrolyte imbalance. Fatigue is a significant side effect of therapy. With cytobines, e.g., interferon, fatigue may be overwhelming.

Interventions

1. *Prevent infection by* using strict medical asepsis and frequent handwashing.

2. Provide frequent, meticulous, physical hygiene; maintain clean environment.
3. Cleanse and dry rectal area after each bowel movement. Apply ointment if irritated; use Tucks and/or Nupercainal for discomfort.
4. Use a gentle antiseptic to wash with tendency for skin eruptions.
5. Provide mouth care q 4–6 hr; otherwise mucosal deterioration occurs. Avoid lemon or glycerin; these tend to reduce saliva production and change pH of the mouth.
6. If WBC falls below 1,500–2,000/mm^3, may protect with:
• Private room; explain reasons
• Universal precautions; use gloves, masks, and gowns
• Avoid indwelling urinary catheters
• Limit articles brought into room
• Provide private bathroom or bedside commode
• Minimize traffic in and out of room
• Screen visitors for infection before they enter room; limit visitations
• Avoid exposure to dust, sprays, contaminated medical equipment
• Avoid deodorants; blocks sebaceous gland secretion
• Keep fresh fruits, vegetables, cut flowers, and any source of stagnant water (water pitcher, humidifiers, flower vases) away from client
• Review/stress kitchen hygiene and food safety at home
• Dogs, cats, birds, and other animals may carry infection; avoid contact
• Assess orders for granulocyte colony-stimulating factors and ensure availability
7. Prevent nosocomial infections from invasive procedures by:
• Washing hands before and after any contact
• Cleansing skin with antiseptic before procedure
• Changing IV tubing q 24 hr
• Changing IV site q 48 hr, if no implanted device or other designated catheter for long-term use
• Practice strict asepsis with all treatments and dressing changes

THROMBOCYTOPENIA

Assessment

1. Obtain platelet count (normal values: 150,000–400,000/mm^3). If platelet count below 50,000/mm^3 monitor closely.
2. Inspect skin for petechiae/bruising; assess all orifices for bleeding.
3. May hemorrhage spontaneously if platelets are below 20,000; transfuse platelets.

Interventions

1. Minimize SC or IM injections; apply pressure for 3–5 min to prevent leakage or hematoma.
2. Do not apply BP cuff or other tourniquet for excessive periods of time.
3. Avoid rectal temps and constipation; test all urine, GI secretions, and stool for occult blood.
4. Use safety precautions to avoid falls.
5. *Control bleeding*
• With epistaxis: pinch nose for 10 min and apply pressure to upper lip to stop; in severe cases, small sponges saturated with neosynephrine 1/4% gently inserted into affected nare, or nasal packing, may be necessary.
• With transfusions, monitor VS before and 15 min after transfusion started and after completed. Assess for histoincompatibility, indicated by chills, fever, and urticaria. Stop transfusion, provide supportive care, and follow appropriate institutional protocol for transfusion reaction.
6. Advise client to *prevent bleeding* by:
• Not picking or forcefully blowing their nose
• Avoiding contact sports and any activities that may lead to injury
• Reporting any severe frontal headaches
• Using an electric razor for shaving rather than a blade
• Using a soft-bristled toothbrush or massaging gums with fingers or a cotton ball and avoiding dental floss to limit irritation
• Avoiding rectal irritation by contact with enemas, suppositories, or thermometers
• Using a water-based lubricant before intercourse
• Consuming plenty of fluids, increasing activity, and taking stool softeners to prevent constipation
• Rearranging furniture so that area for ambulation is unimpeded and also to prevent bumping into furniture at night when getting out of bed to go to the bathroom
• Having a night light to permit visualization during the night
• Wearing shoes or slippers when ambulating

ANEMIA

Assessment

1. Monitor CBC, reticulocyte count, MCV and hemoglobin (normal values: men, 13.5–18.0 g/dL blood; women, 11.5–15.5 g/dL blood), and hematocrit (normal values: men, 40%–52%; women, 35%–46%), and iron panel.
2. Assess for pallor, lethargy, dizziness, increased SOB, or unusual fatigue.

Interventions

1. *Minimize anemia by:*
• Providing a nutritious tolerable diet
• Taking vitamins/iron supplements as ordered
2. *Assist with treatment of anemia by:*
• Administering diet high in iron
• Giving vitamins with minerals
• Administering blood transfusions
• Spacing/scheduling activities to permit frequent rest periods
• Positioning to facilitate ventilation; teaching breathing and relaxation techniques and administering oxygen
• Controlling room temperature for comfort and providing emotional support

HEALTH CARE CONSIDERATIONS FOR GI TOXICITY

NAUSEA AND VOMITING; ANOREXIA

Assessment

1. N&V may be due to either a CNS effect on the chemoreceptor trigger zone or direct irritation to the GI tract. With radiation therapy, N&V may be attributed to the accumulation of toxic waste products of cell destruction and localized damage to the lining of the throat, stomach, and intestine.
2. Anticipatory N&V is a conditioned response of unknown origin prior to chemotherapy which does respond to premedication.
3. Determine if refusing food or fluids or experiencing anorexia.
4. Monitor nutritional status and weights.
5. Examine the frequency, character, and amount of vomitus. List antiemetics prescribed and results.

Interventions

1. *Prevent N&V by:*
• Premedicating with antiemetics. Usually given 30–60 min before or just after drug therapy.
• Administering therapy on an empty stomach, with meals, or at bedtime
• Using an antiemetic suppository
• Providing ice chips at onset of nausea
• Avoiding carbonated beverages
• Ingesting dry carbohydrates such as toast and dry crackers before any activity
• Waiting for N&V to pass before serving food
• Providing small, nutritious snacks and planning meal schedules to coincide with client's best tolerance time
• Encouraging cold foods and salads with little cooking aroma to minimize N&V
• Providing nourishing foods client likes
• Encouraging intake of a high-protein diet
• Freezing and serving dietary supplements like ice cream to make them more palatable
• Avoiding foods with overpowering aroma
• Chewing foods well
• Providing good oral hygiene both before and after meals (try 1 tsp baking soda in a glass of warm water)
• Eating favorite foods
• Eating meals with others, preferably at a table. Sharing encourages some clients to eat.
2. Antiemetics that have different actions/pharmacokinetics may be administered concurrently in an effort to control severe N&V.
3. *Treat N&V by:*
• Administering antiemetic(s). Report all vomiting; a change in therapy or electrolyte correction may be needed.
• Giving other medications after meals
• Offering simple foods: rice, toast, noodles, bananas, scrambled eggs, mashed potatoes, custards, ice cream
• Offering salty foods (pretzels, crackers)
• Avoiding solid and liquid foods at the same meal
• Eliminating any room odors; avoiding malodorous foods (e.g., cabbage, sauerkraut, etc.)
• Keeping as comfortable, clean, and free from odor as possible
• Trying another or concurrent antiemetic agents
• Correcting electrolytes; providing hyperalimentation
• Screening visitors and calls until client ready
4. *Approach anorexia by:*
• Providing small, frequent meals q 2 or 3 hr on schedule
• Maximizing caloric intake by offering nutrient-dense snacks and drinks (yogurt, cheese and crackers, peanut butter and jelly sandwiches, cereal, dried fruit, fruit nectars, and instant breakfast drink mixes)
• Making nutrient-dense supplements with whole milk
• Suggesting a walk or activity before eating to boost appetite
• Concentrating on and obtaining favorite foods
5. *Increase caloric intake and protein consumption by:*
• Adding high-calorie foods such as mayonnaise, butter, and gravy to foods
• Using whole milk in puddings, cream soups, custards
• Making double-strength milk by adding powdered milk to whole milk for gravies, hot cereals, mashed potatoes, eggs, casseroles, baked things, etc.
• Adding whipped cream to frosting and desserts

• Offering milkshakes, nectar, and eggnog when thirsty
• Offering peanut butter on crackers, bagels with cream cheese, trail mix, and nuts and seeds for snacks
• Cutting up meats and cheeses and adding to salads, soups, scrambled eggs, etc.

BOWEL DYSFUNCTION (DIARRHEA/ABDOMINAL CRAMPING)

Assessment

1. Note frequency and severity of cramping caused by hypermotility.
2. Document frequency, color, consistency, and amount of diarrhea; indicates tissue destruction. Culture stool.
3. Assess for dehydration and acidosis indicating electrolyte imbalance; monitor I&O.

Interventions

1. *Prevent diarrhea/abdominal cramping by:*
• Providing small, frequent meals on a schedule
• Identifying factors that aggravate/increase incidence
• Using constipating foods, i.e., hard cheeses
2. *Treat diarrhea by:*
• Administering antidiarrheal and narcotic agent (i.e., codeine, tincture of opium, imodium, or lomotil). Report diarrhea or abdominal cramping as a change in therapy or electrolyte correction may be needed.
• Increasing fluids to avoid dehydration
• Providing foods to correct sodium and potassium losses, e.g., bananas, potatoes, fish and meat, apricot nectar, tomato juice, and sports drinks with "electrolytes"
• Avoiding high-fiber foods that contain "insoluble fiber," such as wheat bran, brown rice, and popcorn
• Administering bulk-forming agents (i.e., metamucil)
• Offering "soluble-fiber" foods, i.e., white rice, oatmeal, applesauce, mashed potatoes, and pears
• Avoiding fried foods and greasy foods
• Avoiding excessive sweets; may aggravate diarrhea due to sorbitol, found in many gums and candies
• Using alumimum-containing antacids
• Avoiding gas-forming foods, such as broccoli, corn, onion, garlic, lentils, and kidney beans
• Considering lactose-free products or Lact-Aid, which facilitates digestion of lactose
• Restricting oral intake to rest the bowel if necessary
• Providing good skin care, especially to perianal area to prevent skin breakdown. Apply A&D ointment for perianal tenderness. Change gown and bed linens frequently; use special mattresses and room deodorizers as needed.
3. *Prevent constipation by:*
• Providing a high-fiber diet
• Administering stool softeners and bulk-forming agents
• Promoting increased fluid intake
• Increasing activity levels
• Monitoring frequency, consistency, and amount of stool
4. *Prevent obstruction by:*
• Aggressive management of constipation
• Assessing for early S&S such as abdominal pain, N&V, and diminished or absent bowel sounds
• Keeping NPO, using NG suction to relieve before referring for surgical intervention

STOMATITIS (MUCOSAL ULCERATION)

Assessment

1. Assess for mouth dryness, erythema, soreness, painful swallowing, and white patchy areas of oral mucosa.
2. Symptom onset usually 5 days to 2 weeks after starting therapy; assess regularly.

Interventions

1. *Prevent stomatitis by:*
• Assessing oral cavity t.i.d. and reporting bleeding gums or burning sensation when acid liquids such as fruit juice are ingested
• Setting up a regular schedule for oral preventive care
• Providing good mouth care
• Applying lubricant (Vaseline) to lips t.i.d.
2. *Treat stomatitis by:*
• Providing good oral care
• Applying topical viscous anesthetic, such as benzocaine 20%, or a swish and gargle anesthetic dyclonine hydrochloride 0.5%, or a swish, swallow/discard agent such as lidocaine 2% (Xylocaine), before meals or as needed to anesthetize oral mucosa. May swallow lidocaine after swishing it around oral cavity but encourage to expectorate it.
• Puncture a vitamin E capsule and apply to painful lesions to promote healing
• Offering "Magic Mouthwash," which consists of 4 g (approx. ⅛ teaspoon) baking soda, 30mL viscous xylocaine, 30mL benedryl elixir, and 30mL Maalox (optional) in 1 L NSS; swish and spit out q 1–2 hr as needed
• Providing allopurinol mouthwash for fluorouracil-related stomatitis; or try sucking ice chips ½ hr before and during treatment

• Offering small, frequent meals of bland foods at medium temperatures
• Administering nystatin solution or clotrimazole troches orally for fungal infections
3. Administer medications (antifungals, antivirals) to prevent general infections.

HEALTH CARE CONSIDERATIONS FOR NEUROTOXICITY

Assessment

1. Be aware of agents causing or having the potential to cause neurotoxic effects; further administration once symptoms have become prominent may be life threatening.
2. Report symptoms of minor neuropathies, i.e., tingling in hands and feet; loss of deep tendon reflexes. Use a monofilament to measure progressive loss of sensation.
3. Report serious neuropathies, i.e., weakness of hands, ataxia, loss of coordination, foot drop, wrist drop, or paralytic ileus.

Interventions

1. *Prevent functional loss due to neurotoxicity by:*
• Identifying neuropathies early so drug regimen can be adjusted
• Practicing/teaching seizure precautions
2. *Treat neuropathies by:*
• Using safety measures with functional losses
• Maintaining good body alignment by frequent and anatomically correct repositioning; ROM exercises.
• Providing stool softeners/laxatives as needed

HEALTH CARE CONSIDERATIONS FOR OTOTOXICITY

Assessment: Assess for hearing difficulties before initiating therapy.

Interventions

1. Report tinnitus or hearing impairment.
2. Perform audiometry testing p.r.n. during therapy.

HEALTH CARE CONSIDERATIONS FOR HEPATOTOXICITY

Assessment

1. Obtain/assess the following LFTs:
• Total serum bilirubin (normal values: 0.1–1.0 mg/dL); elevations may indicate liver disease or increased rate of RBC hemolysis.
• AST (normal: 8–33 units/L). Elevations indicative of changes in liver, skeletal muscles, lungs, pancreas, and heart. Hepatitis produces striking elevations in the AST.
• ALT (normal: 8–20 units/L). Elevations may precede hepatic necrosis.
• LDH (normal: 70–250 units/L). Elevations may indicate hepatitis, pulmonary infarction, and CHF.
2. Assess for liver involvement, i.e., abdominal pain, high fever, diarrhea, and yellowing of skin/sclera.

Interventions

1. Prevent further hepatotoxicity by reporting LFT elevations and signs of liver involvement so drug regimen can be changed.
2. Assist with the treatment for hepatotoxicity by providing supportive nursing care for pain, fever, diarrhea, and symptoms associated with jaundice.

HEALTH CARE CONSIDERATIONS FOR RENAL TOXICITY

Assessment

1. Assess the following renal function tests:
• BUN (normal: 5–20 mg/dL)
• Serum uric acid (normal: men, 3.5–7.0 mg/dL; women, 2.4–6.0 mg/dL)
• C_{CR} (normal: women, 0.8–1.7 g/24 hr; men, 1.0–1.9 g/24 hr)
• Quantitative uric acid (normal: 250–750 mg/day)
2. Report stomach pain, swelling of feet or lower legs, shakiness, unusual body movement, or stomatitis.

Interventions

1. Monitor I&O.
2. Limit hyperuricemia with extra fluids to speed excretion of uric acid and to decrease hazard of crystal and urate stone formation. Administer uricosuric agents (i.e., probenecid) or antigout agents (i.e., allopurinol, colchicine) to lower uric acid levels.
3. Test pH and alkalinize urine.

HEALTH CARE CONSIDERATIONS FOR IMMUNOSUPPRESSION

Assessment

1. Assess for the presence of fever, chills, or sore throat.
2. Note any changes in CBC.

Interventions

1. Treat immunosuppression by:
• Preventing infection as noted under bone marrow depression
• Delaying active immunization for several months after therapy is completed; may experience a hypo- or hyperactive response
• Avoiding contact with children who have recently taken the oral polio vaccine
• Administering granulocyte colony-stimulating factor
2. Review food safety (e.g., storage, handling, washing, cooking meats thoroughly, avoiding raw eggs) and stress the importance of kitchen hygiene when preparing meals at home.

HEALTH CARE CONSIDERATIONS FOR GU ALTERATIONS

Assessment

1. Assess for altered GU function. Most

symptoms, such as amenorrhea, cease after med is discontinued.
2. Review risks; sterility may be a permanent result of therapy.

Client/Family Teaching

1. Certain drugs may render individuals sterile. Advise that egg/sperm harvesting may be performed prior to therapy to accommodate future pregnancies.
2. To prevent teratogenesis, teach client and partner to use reliable contraceptive measures to avoid pregnancy, both during and for several months after therapy.

HEALTH CARE CONSIDERATIONS FOR ALOPECIA

Client/Family Teaching

1. Hair loss is a normal occurrence during chemotherapy. Treatment disrupts the mitotic activity of the hair follicle which weakens the hair shaft which causes it to break off. This includes all hair, i.e., eyebrows, body, and pubic hair.
2. Alopecia may occur within 2–3 weeks after the initial treatment. Assist to understand, be prepared for, and expect this as normal with chemotherapy. People respond differently; some may lose hair with a certain agent, others may not.
3. Reinforce that hair will grow back but may be of a different texture or color. It should start to grow in again about 8 weeks after therapy is completed.
4. If receiving more than 4,500 rad to the cranium, hair loss may be permanent.
5. Alternatives for managing alopecia include:
   - Shopping for a wig before hair loss begins
   - Wearing a bandana or hat to cover head, and taking special care to protect the bare head from sun exposure
   - Shaving head, if hair starts to fall out in large clumps, and using a wig or scarf until scalp hair regrows
   - Wearing a night cap at bedtime so hair that falls out during the night will be collected in one place and not all over the bed in the morning.
   - Encouraging expression of feelings related to changes in self-image

HEALTH CARE CONSIDERATIONS FOR ALTERATIONS IN SKIN

Assessment

1. Document skin turgor and integrity.
2. Slight changes in skin color may occur during therapy.

Interventions

1. Maintain cleanliness of skin through bathing and frequent linen changes.
2. Prevent dryness and replenish skin moisture with emollient lotions.
3. Prevent excessive exposure to sun or artificial ultraviolet light; use sunscreen and protective clothing when exposed.
4. Use a special mattress or bed to redistribute weight on bony prominences and to minimize pressure and friction on pressure points.
5. Establish and document a schedule for repositioning, massaging, and assessing skin condition.
6. Ensure adequate nutritional intake.
7. Refer for assistance with makeup application.
8. With pruritus, attempt to stop scratching as this may impair skin integrity. Administer antihistamines, corticosteroids, nonirritating moisturizers, and cool/ice compresses as needed.

ANTIPARKINSON AGENTS

See also the following individual entries:

Amantadine hydrochloride
Benztropine mesylate
Biperiden hydrochloride
Bromocriptine mesylate
Carbidopa
Carbidopa/Levodopa
Diphenhydramine hydrochloride
Levodopa
Pergolide mesylate
Pramipexole
Ropinirole hydrochloride
Tolcapone
Trihexyphenidyl hydrochloride

General Statement: Parkinson's disease is a progressive disorder of the nervous system, affecting mostly people over the age of 50. Parkinsonism is a frequent side effect of certain antipsychotic drugs, including prochlorperazine, chlorpromazine, and reserpine. Drug-induced symptoms usually disappear when the responsible agent is discontinued. The cause of Parkinson's disease is unknown; however, it is associated with a depletion of the neurotransmitter dopamine in the nervous system. Administration of levodopa—the precursor of dopamine—relieves symptoms in 75%–80% of the clients. Most of the newer antiparkinson drugs must be given with levodopa. Anticholinergic agents also have a beneficial effect by reducing tremors and rigidity and improving mobility, muscular coordination, and motor performance. They are often administered together with levodopa. Certain antihistamines, notably diphenhydramine (Benadryl), are also useful in the treatment of parkinsonism. Clients suffering from Parkinson's disease need emotional support and encouragement because the debilitating nature of the disorder often causes depression. Comprehensive treatment also includes physical therapy.

See *Health Care Considerations* for individual drugs.

HEALTH CARE CONSIDERATIONS

Assessment

1. Record PMH, onset and characteristics of symptoms, and progression.
2. Determine if S&S drug induced with agents such as haldol or phenothiazines.
3. Assess for depression, behavioral changes, and suicide ideations.

Client/Family Teaching

1. Parkinson's disease is a movement disorder of unknown origin; is usually progressive and leads to disability if untreated.
2. Drug therapy is aimed at restoring normal balances of cholinergic and dopaminergic influences in the brain (basal ganglia).
3. Take only as prescribed; some have many adverse side effects.
4. Close follow-up is imperative; some drugs may lose their effectiveness.

Outcome/Evaluate

- Improved motor function/mood
- ↓ Drooling, ↓ rigidity, ↓ tremors
- Improved gait, posture, and ↓ muscle spasms

ANTIPSYCHOTIC AGENTS, PHENOTHIAZINES

See also the following individual entries:

Chlorpromazine hydrochloride
Fluphenazine decanoate
Fluphenazine enanthate
Fluphenazine hydrochloride
Mesoridazine besylate
Perphenazine
Prochlorperazine
Prochlorperazine edisylate
Prochlorperazine maleate
Promazine hydrochloride
Thioridazine hydrochloride
Trifluoperazine

Action/Kinetics: It has been postulated that excess amounts of dopamine in certain areas of the CNS cause psychoses. Phenothiazines are thought to act by blocking postsynaptic mesolimbic dopamine receptors, leading to a reduction in psychotic symptoms. Phenothiazines block both D_1 and D_2 dopamine receptors. The antiemetic effects are thought to be due to inhibition or blockade of dopamine (D_2) receptors in the chemoreceptor trigger zone in the medulla as well as by peripheral blockade of the vagus nerve in the GI tract. Relief of anxiety is manifested as a result of an indirect decrease in arousal and increased filtering of internal stimuli to the brain stem reticular system. Alpha-adrenergic blockade produces sedation. Phenothiazines also raise pain threshold and produce amnesia due to suppression of sensory impulses. In addition, these drugs produce anticholinergic and antihistaminic effects and depress the release of hypothalamic and hypophyseal hormones. Peripheral effects include anticholinergic and alpha-adrenergic blocking properties.

Peak plasma levels: 2–4 hr after PO administration. Widely distributed throughout the body. **t½ (average):** 10–20 hr. Most metabolized in the liver and excreted by the kidney.

General Statement: Antipsychotic drugs do not cure mental illness, but they calm the intractable client, relieve the despondency of the severely depressed, activate the immobile and withdrawn, and make some more accessible to psychotherapy.

Most phenothiazines induce some sedation, especially during the initial phase of the treatment. Medicated clients can, however, be easily roused. In this manner, the phenothiazines differ markedly from the narcotic analgesics and sedative hypnotics. However, phenothiazines potentiate the analgesic properties of opiates and prolong the action of CNS depressant drugs. These drugs also cause sedation, decrease spontaneous motor activity, and many lower BP.

According to their detailed chemical structure, the phenothiazines belong to three subgroups:

1. **Aliphatic compounds.** Moderate to high sedative, anticholinergic, and orthostatic hypotensive effects. Moderate extrapyramidal symptoms. Often the first choice for clients in acute excitatory states. Examples: Chlorpromazine, promazine, triflupromazine.
2. **Piperazine compounds.** Act most selectively on the subcortical sites. Low to moderate sedative effects; low anticholinergic and orthostatic hypotensive effects; high incidence of extrapyramidal symptoms. Greatest antiemetic effects because they specifically depress the CTZ of the vomiting center. Examples: Fluphenazine, perphenazine, prochlorperazine, trifluoperazine.
3. **Piperidine compounds.** Low incidence of extrapyramidal effects; high sedative and anticholinergic effects; low to moderate or-

thostatic hypotensive effect. Examples: Mesoridazine, thioridazine.

Uses: Psychoses, especially if excessive psychomotor activity manifested. Involutional, toxic, or senile psychoses. Used in combination with MAO inhibitors in depressed clients manifesting anxiety, agitation, or panic (use with caution). With lithium in acute manic phase of manic-depressive illness. As an adjunct in alcohol withdrawal to reduce anxiety, tension, depression, nausea, and/or vomiting. For severe behavioral problems in children, manifested by hyperexcitable and/ or combative behavior; also, for short-term use in hyperactive children who exhibit excess motor activity and conduct disorders.

Prophylaxis and control of severe N&V due to cancer chemotherapy, radiation therapy, postoperatively. Intractable hiccoughs, intermittent porphyria, tetanus (as adjunct). As preoperative and/or postoperative medications. Some phenothiazines are antipruritics. See also individual drugs.

Contraindications: Severe CNS depression, coma, clients with subcortical brain damage, bone marrow depression, lactation. In clients with a history of seizures and in those on anticonvulsant drugs. Geriatric or debilitated clients, hepatic or renal disease, CV disorders, glaucoma, prostatic hypertrophy. Contraindicated in children with chickenpox, CNS infections, measles, gastroenteritis, dehydration due to increased risk of extrapyramidal symptoms.

Special Concerns: Use with caution in clients exposed to extreme heat or cold and in those with asthma, emphysema, or acute respiratory tract infections. Use during pregnancy only when benefits outweigh risks. Children may be more sensitive to the neuromuscular or extrapyramidal effects (especially dystonias); those especially at risk include children with chickenpox, CNS infections, measles, dehydration, or gastroenteritis. Thus, generally, phenothiazines are not recommended for use in children less than 12 years of age. Geriatric clients often manifest higher plasma levels due to decreases in lean body mass, total body water, and albumin and an increase in total body fat. Also, geriatric clients may be more likely to manifest orthostatic hypotension, anticholinergic effects, sedative effects, and extrapyramidal side effects.

Side Effects: *CNS:* Depression, drowsiness, dizziness, lethargy, fatigue. Extrapyramidal effects, Parkinson-like symptoms including shuffling gait or tic-like movements of head and face, tardive dyskinesia (see what follows), akathisia, dystonia. ***Seizures,*** especially in clients with a history thereof. ***Neuroleptic malignant syndrome (rare).*** *CV:* Orthostatic hypotension, increase or decrease in BP, tachycardia, fainting. *GI:* Dry mouth, anorexia, constipation, paralytic ileus, diarrhea. *Endocrine:* Breast engorgement, galactorrhea, gynecomastia, increased appetite, weight gain, hyper- or hypoglycemia, glycosuria. Delayed ejaculation, increased or decreased libido. *GU:* Menstrual irregularities, loss of bladder control, urinary difficulty. *Dermatologic:* Photosensitivity, pruritus, erythema, eczema, exfoliative dermatitis, pigment changes in skin (long-term use of high doses). *Hematologic:* ***Aplastic anemia,*** leukopenia, ***agranulocytosis,*** eosinophilia, thrombocytopenia. *Ophthalmologic:* Deposition of fine particulate matter in lens and cornea leading to blurred vision, changes in vision. *Respiratory:* ***Laryngospasm, bronchospasm, laryngeal edema,*** breathing difficulties. *Miscellaneous:* Fever, muscle stiffness, decreased sweating, muscle spasm of face, neck, or back, obstructive jaundice, nasal congestion, pale skin, mydriasis, systemic lupus-like syndrome.

Tardive dyskinesia has been observed with all classes of antipsychotic drugs, although the precise cause is not known. The syndrome is most commonly seen in older clients, especially women, and in individuals with organic brain syndrome. It is often aggravated or precipitated by the sudden discontinuance of antipsychotic drugs and may persist indefinitely after the drug is discontinued. Early signs of tardive dyskinesia include fine vermicular movements of the tongue and grimacing or tic-like movements of the head and neck. Although there is no known cure for the syndrome, it may not progress if the dosage of the drug is slowly reduced. Also, a few drug-free days may unmask the symptoms of tardive dyskinesia and help in early diagnosis.

OD **Management of Overdose:** *Symptoms:* CNS depression including deep sleep and ***coma,*** hypotension, extrapyramidal symptoms, agitation, restlessness, seizures, hypothermia, ***hyperthermia,*** autonomic symptoms, ***cardiac arrhythmias,*** ECG changes. *Treatment:* Emetics are not to be used as they are of little value and may cause a dystonic reaction of the head or neck that may result in aspiration of vomitus.

- Hypotension: Volume replacement; norepinephrine or phenylephrine may be used (do not use epinephrine).

• Ventricular arrhythmias: phenytoin, 1 mg/kg IV, not to exceed 50 mg/min; may be repeated q 5 min up to 10 mg/kg.
• Seizures or hyperactivity: Diazepam or pentobarbital.
• Extrapyramidal symptoms: Antiparkinson drugs, diphenhydramine, barbiturates.

Drug Interactions
Alcohol, ethyl / Potentiation or addition of CNS depressant effects. Concomitant use may lead to drowsiness, lethargy, stupor, respiratory collapse, coma, or death
Aluminum salts (antacids) / ↓ Absorption from GI tract
Amphetamine / ↓ Effect of amphetamine by ↓ uptake of drug to the site of action
Anesthetics, general / See *Alcohol*
Antacids, oral / ↓ Effect of phenothiazines due to ↓ absorption from GI tract
Antianxiety drugs / See *Alcohol*
Anticholinergic drugs / Additive anticholinergic side effects and/or ↓ antipsychotic effect
Antidepressants, tricyclic / Additive anticholinergic side effects; also, ↑ TCA serum levels
Barbiturate anesthetics / ↑ Chance of tremor, involuntary muscle activity, and hypotension
Barbiturates / See *Alcohol;* also, barbiturates may ↓ effect due to ↑ breakdown by liver
Bromocriptine / Phenothiazines ↓ effect
Charcoal / ↓ Effect of phenothiazines due to ↓ absorption from GI tract
CNS depressants / See *Alcohol;* also, ↓ effect of phenothiazines due to ↑ breakdown by liver
Colistimethate / Additive respiratory depression
Diazoxide / Additive hyperglycemic effect
Guanethidine / ↓ Effect of guanethidine by ↓ uptake of drug at the site of action
Hydantoins / ↑ Risk of hydantoin toxicity
Lithium carbonate / ↑ Risk of extrapyramidal symptoms, disorientation, or unconsciousness
MAO inhibitors / ↑ Effect of phenothiazines due to ↓ breakdown by liver
Meperidine / ↑ Risk of hypotension and sedation
Metrizamide / ↑ Risk of seizures during subarachnoid administration of metrizamide
Narcotics / See *Alcohol*
Phenytoin / ↑ or ↓ Serum levels of phenytoin
Pimozide / Additive effect on QT interval; do not use together
Propranolol / ↑ Plasma levels of both drugs
Sedative-hypnotics, nonbarbiturate / See *Alcohol*

Dosage
See individual drugs. Effective over a wide dosage range. Dosage is usually increased gradually to minimize side effects over 7 days until the minimal effective dose is attained. Dosage is increased more gradually in elderly or debilitated clients because they are more susceptible to the effects and side effects of drugs. After symptoms are controlled, dosage is gradually reduced to maintenance levels. It is usually desirable to keep chronically ill clients on maintenance levels indefinitely. Medication, especially in clients on high dosages, should not be discontinued abruptly.

Laboratory Test Considerations: False +: Bile (urine dipstick), ferric chloride, pregnancy tests, urinary porphobilinogen, urinary steroids, urobilinogen (urine dipstick). False –: Inorganic phosphorus, urinary steroids. *Caused by pharmacologic effects:* ↑ Alkaline phosphatase, bilirubin, serum transaminases, serum cholesterol, urinary catecholamines. ↓ Glucose tolerance, serum uric acid, 5-HIAA, FSH, growth hormone, LH, vanillylmandelic acid.

Special Considerations
1. When working with the elderly, be particularly observant for symptoms of tardive dyskinesia. May exhibit puffing of the cheeks or tongue; may develop chewing movements and involuntary movements of the extremities and trunk.
2. If administering to a child, note neuromuscular reactions, especially if dehydrated or has an acute infection making more susceptible to side effects.
1. Do not interchange brands of PO form of drug or suppositories; may differ in bioavailability.
2. Do not use pink or markedly discolored solutions.
3. When preparing or administering parenteral solutions health care professional and client should avoid contact of drug with skin, eyes, and clothing to prevent contact dermatitis.
4. Do not mix antipsychotic drugs with other drugs in the same syringe.
5. Order a specific flow rate when administering parenteral solutions.
6. To lessen injection pain, dilute commercially available injectable solutions in saline or local anesthetic.
7. When administering IM, inject drug deeply into the muscle.
8. Massage area of injection site after IM administration to reduce pain.
9. Prevent extravasation of the IV solution.
10. Store solutions in a cool dry place in amber-colored containers.

HEALTH CARE CONSIDERATIONS

Assessment

1. Take a complete medical and drug history; note any drug hypersensitivity or genetic predisposition. (These agents are referred to as neuroleptics in Europe.)
2. Determine any history of seizures; this class of drugs may lower seizure threshold.
3. Record indications for therapy. Assess baseline mental status, noting mood, behavior, and any depression.
4. If administering to children, note extent of hyperexcitability.
5. Assess child for chickenpox or measles.
6. Record any history of asthma or emphysema.
7. Monitor VS; assess BP in both arms in a reclining position, standing position, and sitting position, 2 min apart.
8. Monitor hematologic profile, liver and renal function studies, urinalysis, ECG, and ocular findings.

Interventions

1. If administered IV, monitor flow rate and BP. Keep recumbent for at least 1 hr after IV completed, then slowly elevate HOB and observe for tachycardia, faintness, or dizziness; supervise ambulation.
2. If hospitalized, ensure that med has been swallowed. May give a liquid preparation to permit better control over drug taking and to improve compliance.
3. Measure I&O; report abdominal distention and urinary retention. May need to reduce dosage, add antispasmodics, or change therapy.
4. Note any changes in carbohydrate metabolism (e.g., glycosuria, weight loss, polyphagia, increased appetite, or excessive weight gain); may require a change in diet/drug therapy and can be significant with diabetes.
5. Some may develop a hypersensitivity reaction with fever, asthma, laryngeal edema, angioneurotic edema, and anaphylactic reaction. *Stop* medication, notify provider, and treat symptomatically.
6. The antiemetic effects of phenothiazines may mask other pathology such as toxicity to other drugs, intestinal obstruction, or brain lesions.
7. If receiving barbiturates to relieve anxiety, reduce barbiturate dose. If administered as an anticonvulsant, do not reduce dosage.
8. Discontinue drug gradually to minimize severe GI disturbances or tardive dyskinesia.

Client/Family Teaching

1. May take with food or milk to minimize GI upset. Take as directed, may be weeks or months before the full effects will be noticed
2. Do not stop taking abruptly. Abrupt cessation of high doses of phenothiazines can cause N&V, tremors, sensations of warmth and cold, sweating, tachycardia, headache, and insomnia.
3. Report distress when in a hot or cold room; may affect heat-regulating mechanism.
   - Provide extra blankets if feeling cold.
   - Bathe in tepid water if feeling too warm.
   - Do *NOT* use heating pads or hot water bottles if feeling cold.
   - Avoid hot tubs, hot baths/showers; low BP may occur.
4. Report if excessively active or depressed. Spasms of face, neck, back, or tongue may be treated with antihistamines, or provider may discontinue drug.
5. Report any elevation of body temperature, feeling of weakness, easy bruising, or sore throat (symptoms of blood dyscrasias).
6. Take slow, deep breaths if respiratory symptoms occur; may depress cough reflex.
7. May cause menstrual irregularity and false positive pregnancy tests; may develop engorged breasts and begin lactating. Keep accurate record of periods and report if pregnancy is suspected.
8. Males may experience decreased libido and develop breast enlargement. Report so med can be adjusted.
9. May develop photosensitivity reactions; wear protective clothing, sunglasses, sunscreen and avoid sunbathing.
10. Drug may discolor the urine pink or reddish brown. With long-term therapy may develop a yellow-brown skin reaction that may turn grayish purple.
11. Avoid driving a car or operating heavy machinery or engaging in any activities that require mental alertness until effects realized; consult provider prior to resuming.
12. Long-term therapy may affect vision; schedule regular ophthalmic exams. Report blurred vision and avoid driving.
13. Report evidence of early cholestatic jaundice, such as high fever, upper abdominal pain, nausea, diarrhea, itching, and rash.
14. Withhold drug and report if yellowing of the sclera, skin, or mucous membranes occurs; may indicate biliary obstruction.
15. To prevent dry mouth, rinse mouth frequently, increase fluid intake, chew sugarless gum, and suck on sour hard candies.
16. Increase fluids and bulk in diet to minimize constipation; may need laxatives. Report

any urinary retention or persistent constipation.
17. Rise slowly from a lying or sitting position; dangle legs before standing to avoid orthostatic symptoms.
18. Avoid alcohol, OTC drugs, and any other CNS depressants without approval.
19. Report for periodic labs and follow-up care to evaluate and adjust drug dosage.

Outcome/Evaluate

- ↓ Excitable, withdrawn, agitated, or paranoid behaviors
- Orientation to time and place, and an understanding of illness
- Adherence to prescribed drug regimen
- Relief of N&V

ANTITHYROID DRUGS

See also the following individual entries:

Methimazole
Propylthiouracil

Action/Kinetics: These drugs inhibit (partially or completely) the production of thyroid hormones by the thyroid gland by preventing the incorporation of iodide into tyrosine and coupling of iodotyrosines. They do not affect release or activity of preformed hormone; thus, it may take several weeks for the therapeutic effect to become established.
Uses: Hyperthyroidism; prior to surgery or radiotherapy. Adjunct in treatment of thyrotoxicosis or thyroid storm. Propylthiouracil is also used to reduce mortality due to alcoholic liver disease.
Contraindications: Lactation (may cause hypothyroidism in the infant).
Special Concerns: Use with caution in the presence of CV disease. PT should be monitored during therapy as propylthiouracil may cause hypoprothrombinemia and bleeding.
Side Effects: *Hematologic:* ***Agranulocytosis,*** thrombocytopenia, granulocytopenia, hypoprothrombinemia, ***aplastic anemia,*** leukopenia. *GI:* N&V, taste loss, epigastric pain, sialadenopathy. *CNS:* Headache, paresthesia, drowsiness, vertigo, depression, CNS stimulation. *Dermatologic:* Skin rash, urticaria, alopecia, skin pigmentation, pruritus, exfoliative dermatitis, erythema nodosum. *Miscellaneous:* Jaundice, arthralgia, myalgia, neuritis, edema, lymphadenopathy, vasculitis, lupus-like syndrome, drug fever, periarteritis, hepatitis, nephritis, interstitial pneumonitis, insulin autoimmune syndrome resulting in hypoglycemic coma.
OD **Management of Overdose:** *Symptoms:* N&V, headache, fever, pruritus, epigastric distress, arthralgia, pancytopenia, ***agranulocytosis*** (most serious). Rarely, exfoliative dermatitis, hepatitis, neuropathies, CNS stimulation or depression. *Treatment:* Maintain a patent airway and support ventilation and perfusion. Very carefully monitor and maintain VS, blood gases, and serum electrolytes. Monitor bone marrow function.

Dosage

See individual drugs.
Special Considerations: Children must be checked every 6 months for appropriate growth and development; plot on a graph.

HEALTH CARE CONSIDERATIONS

Assessment

1. Record onset of illness, symptoms experienced, physical presentation, and any underlying cause.
2. Determine if pregnant.
3. Monitor VS, I&O, and weights; PT, CBC, ECG, and thyroid function studies.
4. Assess thyroid gland noting any enlargement, pain, asymmetry, nodules, or bruits.

Client/Family Teaching

1. It takes 6–12 weeks for the drug to produce full effect. Take regularly and exactly as directed q 8 hr around the clock. Hyperthyroidism may recur if not taken properly.
2. Report symptoms of hyperthyroidism or thyrotoxicosis (palpitations, increased HR, nervousness, sleeplessness, sweating, diarrhea, weight loss, fever).
3. Report symptoms of hypothyroidism (weak, listless, tired, headache, dry skin, cold intolerance, constipation) as dosage may require adjustment.
4. Report any sore throat, enlargement of the cervical lymph nodes, GI disturbances, fever, skin rashes, itching, or jaundice; may require either a dosage reduction or withdrawal of the drug.
5. May alter taste perception; increase use of herbs and nonsodium seasonings.
6. Report symptoms of iodism (cold symptoms, skin lesions, stomatitis, GI upset, metallic taste)
7. Identify dietary sources of iodine (iodized salt, shellfish, turnips, cabbage, kale) that may need to be omitted from the diet.
8. Report unusual bleeding, alopecia, nausea, loss of taste, or epigastric pain.
9. When drug is taken for 1 year, more than half the clients achieve a permanent remission. Those who relapse are usually treated with radioiodine.
10. Carry ID listing medical problems and currently prescribed meds.

Outcome/Evaluate

• Thyroid function studies within desired range (euthyroid)
• Control of symptoms associated with hyperthyroidism
• ↓ Vascularity and friability of the thyroid gland in preparation for surgery
• ↓ Mortality in clients with alcoholic liver disease

ANTIVIRAL DRUGS

See also the following individual entries:

Abacavir sulfate
Acyclovir (Acycloguanosine)
Amantadine hydrochloride
Delavirdine mesylate
Didanosine (ddI, Dideoxyinosine)
Efavirenz
Famciclovir
Fomivirsen sodium
Ganciclovir sodium
Idoxuridine (IDU)
Indinavir sulfate
Lamivudine
Lamivudine and Zidovudine
Nelfinavir mesylate
Nevirapine
Penciclovir
Rimantidine hydrochloride
Ritonavir
Saquinavir mesylate
Stavudine
Valacyclovir hydrochloride
Vidarabine
Zalcitabine
Zidovudine (Azidothymidine, AZT)

Action/Kinetics: To maintain their growth and reproduce, viruses must enter living cells. Thus, it is difficult to find a drug that is specific for the virus and that does not interfere with the function of the host cell. However, there are enzymes and replicative mechanisms that are unique to viruses and an increasing number of drugs with specific antiviral activity have been developed. The antiviral drugs currently marketed act by one of the following mechanisms:
1. Inhibition of enzymes required for DNA synthesis. Example: Idoxuridine.
2. Inhibition of viral nucleic acid synthesis by interacting directly with herpes virus DNA polymerase or HIV reverse transcriptase. Example: Foscarnet.
3. Inhibition of viral DNA or protein synthesis. Examples: Acyclovir, cidofovir, famciclovir, fomivirsen, ganciclovir, penciclovir, trifluridine, valacyclovir, vidarabine.
4. Prevent penetration of the virus into cells by inhibiting uncoating of the RNA virus. Examples: Amantadine, rimantadine.
5. Protease inhibitors resulting in release of immature, noninfectious viral particles. Examples: Indinavir, nelfinavir, ritonavir, saquinavir.
6. Reverse transcriptase inhibitors (nucleoside and non-nucleoside) resulting in inhibition of replication of the virus. Examples of nucleoside inhibitors: Abacavir, didanosine, lamivudine, stavudine, zalcitabine, zidovudine. Examples of non-nucleoside inhibitors: Efavirenz, delavirdine, nevirapine. It is often necessary to combine two antiviral drugs that have the same or different mechanisms of action in order to treat HIV infections and to minimize development of resistant viruses. For example, regimens of choice include two nucleosides and one protease inhibitor or two nucleosides and one non-nucleoside.

See *General Health Care Considerations For All Anti-Infectives.*

HEALTH CARE CONSIDERATIONS

Assessment

1. Record indications for therapy, type and onset of symptoms, and exposure characteristics.
2. Monitor CBC, liver and renal function studies; also viral loads and T cells when indicated.
3. List other agents prescribed to ensure none interact unfavorably.
4. Note underlying medical conditions that may preclude drug therapy.

Client/Family Teaching

1. Review method and frequency for drug administration. Take exactly as directed; do not share meds.
2. Identify specific measures to decrease/halt disease spread.
3. Maintain adequate nutrition; consume 2–3 L/day of fluids to prevent crystalluria.
4. Report any rashes or unusual side effects of drug therapy.
5. Report if symptoms do not improve or worsen after specified time.
6. Close medical supervision/follow-up required during therapy.

Outcome/Evaluate

• Prophylaxis of viral infections
• Reduction in length and severity of symptoms of viral infections

BARBITURATES

See also the following individual entries:

Pentobarbital
Pentobarbital sodium
Phenobarbital
Phenobarbital sodium
Secobarbital sodium

Action/Kinetics: Barbiturates produce all levels of CNS depression, ranging from mild depression (sedation) following low doses to hypnotic (sleep-inducing) effects, and even coma and death, as dosage is increased. Certain barbiturates are also effective anticonvulsants. The depressant and anticonvulsant effects may be related to their ability to increase and/or mimic the inhibitory activity of the neurotransmitter GABA on nerve synapses. Importantly, barbiturates are not analgesics and therefore should not be given to clients for the purpose of ameliorating pain. Sodium salts are readily absorbed after PO, rectal, or parenteral administration. They are distributed throughout all tissues, cross the placental barrier, and appear in breast milk. The main difference between the various barbiturates is in the onset of action, which ranges from 10 to 15 min for pentobarbital and secobarbital and 60 or more minutes for phenobarbital. Metabolized almost completely in the liver (except for phenobarbital) and are excreted in the urine.

Uses: Preanesthetic medication. Sedation, hypnotic, anticonvulsant (phenobarbital) and for the control of acute convulsive conditions (only phenobarbital, mephobarbital), as in epilepsy, tetanus, meningitis, eclampsia, and toxic reactions to local anesthetics or strychnine. The benzodiazepines have replaced barbiturates for the treatment of many conditions, especially daytime sedation. See also information on individual drugs.

Contraindications: Hypersensitivity to barbiturates, severe trauma, pulmonary disease when dyspnea or obstruction is present, edema, uncontrolled diabetes, history of porphyria, and impaired liver function and for clients in whom they produce an excitatory response. Also, clients who have been addicted previously to sedative-hypnotics.

Special Concerns: Use with caution during lactation and in clients with CNS depression, hypotension, marked asthenia (characteristic of Addison's disease, hypoadrenalism, and severe myxedema), porphyria, fever, anemia, hemorrhagic shock, cardiac, hepatic or renal damage, and a history of alcoholism in suicidal clients. Geriatric clients usually manifest increased sensitivity to barbiturates, as evidenced by confusion, excitement, mental depression, and hypothermia. When given in the presence of pain, restlessness, excitement, and delirium may result. Intra-arterial use may cause symptoms from transient pain to gangrene; SC use produces tissue irritation, including tenderness and redness to necrosis.

Side Effects: *CNS:* Sleepiness, drowsiness, agitation, confusion, hyperkinesia, ataxia, CNS depression, nightmares, nervousness, psychiatric disturbances, hallucinations, insomnia, anxiety, dizziness, headache, abnormal thinking, vertigo, lethargy, hangover, excitement, appearance of being inebriated. Irritability and hyperactivity in children. *Musculoskeletal:* Localized or diffuse myalgic, neuralgic, or arthritic pain, especially in psychoneurotic clients. Pain is often most intense in the morning and is frequently located in the neck, shoulder girdle, and arms. *Respiratory:* Hypoventilation, ***apnea, respiratory depression.*** *CV:* Bradycardia, hypotension, syncope, ***circulatory collapse.*** *GI:* N&V, constipation, liver damage (especially with chronic use of phenobarbital). *Allergic:* Skin rashes, ***angioedema,*** exfoliative dermatitis (including ***Stevens-Johnson syndrome and toxic epidermal necrolysis***). Allergic reactions are most common in clients who have asthma, urticaria, angioedema, and similar conditions. Symptoms include localized swelling (especially of the lips, cheeks, or eyelids) and erythematous dermatitis).

After SC use: Tissue necrosis, pain, tenderness, redness, permanent neurologic damage if injected near peripheral nerves.

After IV use. CV: Circulatory depression, thrombophlebitis, ***peripheral vascular collapse, seizures with cardiorespiratory arrest, myocardial depression, cardiac arrhythymias.*** *Respiratory:* ***Apnea, laryngospasm, bronchospasm,*** dyspnea, rhinitis, sneezing, coughing. *CNS:* Emergence delirium, headache, anxiety, prolonged somnolence and recovery, restlessness, ***seizures.*** *GI:* N&V, abdominal pain, diarrhea, cramping. *Hypersensitivity:* ***Acute allergic reactions, including erythema, pruritus, anaphylaxis.*** *Miscellaneous:* Pain or nerve injury at injection site, salivation, hiccups, skin rashes, shivering, skeletal muscle hyperactivity, ***immune hemolytic anemia with renal failure,*** and radial nerve palsy.

After IM use: Pain at injection site.

Barbiturates can induce physical and psychologic dependence if high doses are used regularly for long periods of time. Withdrawal symptoms usually begin after 12–16 hr of abstinence. Manifestations of withdrawal include anxiety, weakness, N&V, muscle cramps, delirium, and even ***tonic-clonic seizures.***

OD Management of Overdose: *Symptoms (Acute Toxicity):* Characterized by cortical and ***respiratory depression; anoxia; peripheral vascular collapse;*** feeble, rapid pulse; pulmonary edema; decreased body temperature; clammy, cyanotic skin; depressed reflexes; stupor; and ***coma.*** After initial constriction the pupils become dilated. ***Death results from respiratory failure or arrest followed by cardiac arrest.*** *Symptoms (Chronic Toxicity):* Prolonged use of barbiturates at high doses may lead to physical and psychologic dependence, as well as tolerance. Doses of 600–800 mg daily for 8 weeks may lead to physical dependence. The addict usually ingests 1.5 g/day. Addicts prefer short-acting barbiturates. Symptoms of dependence are similar to those associated with chronic alcoholism, and withdrawal symptoms are equally severe. Withdrawal symptoms usually last for 5–10 days and are terminated by a long sleep. *Treatment (Acute Toxicity):*

- Maintenance of an adequate airway, oxygen intake, and carbon dioxide removal are essential.
- After PO ingestion, gastric lavage or gastric aspiration may delay absorption. Emesis should not be induced once the symptoms of overdosage are manifested, as the client may aspirate the vomitus into the lungs. Also, if the dose of barbiturate is high enough, the vomiting center in the brain may be depressed.
- Absorption following SC or IM administration of the drug may be delayed by the use of ice packs or tourniquets.
- Maintain renal function.
- Removal of the drug by peritoneal dialysis or an artificial kidney should be carried out.
- Supportive physiologic methods have proven superior to use of analeptics.

Treatment (Chronic Toxicity): Cautious withdrawal of the hospitalized addict over a 2–4-week period. A stabilizing dose of 200–300 mg of a short-acting barbiturate is administered q 6 hr. The dose is then reduced by 100 mg/day until the stabilizing dose is reduced by one-half. The client is then maintained on this dose for 2–3 days before further reduction. The same procedure is repeated when the initial stabilizing dose has been reduced by three-quarters. If a mixed spike and slow activity appear on the EEG, or if insomnia, anxiety, tremor, or weakness is observed, the dosage is maintained at a constant level or increased slightly until symptoms disappear.

Drug Interactions

GENERAL CONSIDERATIONS

1. Barbiturates stimulate the activity of enzymes responsible for the metabolism of a large number of other drugs by a process known as *enzyme induction.* As a result, when barbiturates are given to clients receiving such drugs, their therapeutic effectiveness is markedly reduced or even abolished.
2. The CNS depressant effect of the barbiturates is potentiated by many drugs. Simultaneous administration may result in coma or fatal CNS depression. Barbiturate dosage should either be reduced or eliminated when other CNS drugs are given.
3. Barbiturates also potentiate (increase) the toxic effects of many other agents.

Acetaminophen / ↑ Risk of hepatotoxicity when used with large or chronic doses of barbiturates
Alcohol / Potentiation or addition of CNS depressant effects. Simultaneous use may lead to drowsiness, lethargy, stupor, respiratory collapse, coma, or death
Anesthetics, general / See *Alcohol*
Anorexiants / ↓ Effect of anorexiants due to opposite activities
Antianxiety drugs / See *Alcohol*
Anticoagulants, oral / ↓ Effect of anticoagulants due to ↓ absorption from GI tract and ↑ breakdown by liver
Antidepressants, tricyclic / ↓ Effect of antidepressants due to ↑ breakdown by liver
Antidiabetic agents / Prolong the effects of barbiturates
Antihistamines / See *Alcohol*
Beta-adrenergic agents / ↓ Beta blockade due to ↑ breakdown by the liver
Carbamazepine / ↓ Serum carbazepine levels may occur
Charcoal / ↓ Absorption of barbiturates from the GI tract
Chloramphenicol / ↑ Effect of barbiturates by ↓ breakdown by the liver and ↓ effect of chloramphenicol by ↑ breakdown by liver
Clonazepam / Barbiturates may ↑ excretion of clonazepam → loss of efficacy
CNS depressants / See *Alcohol*
Corticosteroids / ↓ Effect of corticosteroids due to ↑ breakdown by liver
Digitoxin / ↓ Effect of digitoxin due to ↑ breakdown by liver
Doxorubicin / ↓ Effect of doxorubicin due to ↑ excretion
Doxycycline / ↓ Effect of doxycycline due to ↑ breakdown by liver (effect may last up to 2 weeks after barbiturates are discontinued)

Estrogens / ↓ Effect of estrogen due to ↑ breakdown by liver
Felodipine / ↓ Plasma levels of felodipine → ↓ effect
Fenoprofen / ↓ Bioavailability of fenoprofen
Furosemide / ↑ Risk or intensity of orthostatic hypotension
Griseofulvin / ↓ Effect of griseofulvin due to ↓ absorption from GI tract
Haloperidol / ↓ Effect of haloperidol due to ↑ breakdown by liver
MAO inhibitors / ↑ Effect of barbiturates due to ↓ breakdown by liver
Meperidine / CNS depressant effects may be prolonged
Methadone / ↓ Effect of methadone
Methoxyflurane / ↑ Kidney toxicity due to ↑ breakdown of methoxyflurane by liver to toxic metabolites
Metronidazole / ↓ Effect of metronidazole
Narcotic analgesics / See *Alcohol*
Oral contraceptives / ↓ Effect of contraceptives due to ↑ breakdown by liver
Phenothiazines / ↓ Effect of phenothiazines due to ↑ breakdown by liver; also see *Alcohol*
Phenylbutazone / ↓ Elimination t½ of phenylbutazone
Phenytoin / Effect variable and unpredictable; monitor carefully
Probenecid / Anesthesia with thiobarbiturates may be ↑ or achieved at lower doses
Procarbazine / ↑ Effect of barbiturates
Quinidine / ↓ Effect of quinidine due to ↑ breakdown by liver
Rifampin / ↓ Effect of barbiturates due to ↑ breakdown by liver
Sedative-hypnotics, nonbarbiturate / See *Alcohol*
Sulfisoxazole / Sulfisoxazole may ↑ the anesthetic effects of thiobarbiturates
Theophyllines / ↓ Effect of theophyllines due to ↑ breakdown by liver
Valproic acid / ↑ Effect of barbiturates due to ↓ breakdown by liver
Verapamil / ↑ Excretion of verapamil → ↓ effect
Vitamin D / Barbiturates may ↑ requirements for vitamin D due to ↑ breakdown by the liver

Dosage

See individual drugs. Aim for minimum effective dosage. As hypnotics, barbiturates should be administered intermittently because tolerance develops. Elderly clients should receive one-half of the adult dose, and children should receive one-quarter to one-half the adult dose.

Laboratory Test Considerations

1. **Interference with test method:** ↑ 17-Hydroxycorticosteroids.
2. **Caused by pharmacologic effects:** ↑ Creatinine phosphokinase, alkaline phosphatase, serum transaminase, serum testosterone (in certain women), urinary estriol, porphobilinogen, coproporphyrin, uroporphyrin. ↓ PT in clients on coumarin. ↑ or ↓ Bilirubin. False + lupus erythematosus test.

1. Aqueous solutions of sodium salts are unstable and must be used within 30 min after preparation.
2. Discard parenteral solutions that contain precipitate.
3. During IV administration:
• Closely monitor for correct flow rate. Rapid injection may produce respiratory depression, dyspnea, and shock.
• Monitor IV site closely for extravasation (fluid not infusing within the vein), which may cause pain, nerve damage, and necrosis.
• Note any redness or swelling along the site of the vein; evidence of thrombophlebitis.
4. Maintain record of the barbiturates on hand and the amounts dispensed following appropriate institutional and DEA guidelines.

HEALTH CARE CONSIDERATIONS

Assessment

1. Note any adverse reactions to any of the barbiturate family of drugs.
2. Determine any trials with non-narcotic sedatives and the outcome.
3. Identify indications for therapy, associated symptoms, and anticipated time frame for administration.
4. When used for sleep disorders, review sleeping patterns. This is important when considering the type of barbiturate to prescribe.
• Determine usual bedtime and usual wakening hours.
• Identify causes of insomnia. A person in pain who gains relief of the pain may not need sleeping medication. Note evidence of fear and anxiety that may interfere with sleep or appetite.
• Assess environmental preferences for sleep, such as room temperature, lights, and sounds.
• Note sensory alterations that could cause sleeplessness or disruptions in sleep time.
5. Determine if pregnant; identify other measures to encourage sleep if pregnancy is a probability.
6. Record any evidence or history of previous dependence on any sedative-hypnotics.

7. Assess for physical conditions that may preclude drug therapy.
8. Monitor CBC, liver and renal function studies. Many barbiturates are metabolized by the liver. Assess for hematologic disorders such as agranulocytosis, megaloblastic anemia, or thrombocytopenia.

Interventions

1. Assist during ambulation and use side rails once in bed. May become confused and unsteady; particular problem among elderly—"at risk for fall" should be prominently posted.
2. Use supportive measures such as a back rub, warm drinks, quiet atmosphere and a calm attitude to encourage relaxation.
3. When administered PO, remain with the client to determine that the drug has been swallowed. If disoriented or wearing dentures, check the buccal cavity, under the tongue, and under denture plates. Check bedside area to ensure client not hoarding medication.
4. May experience a period of transitory elation, confusion, or euphoria before sedation; provide measures to calm and to prevent injury.
5. If confused after taking the barbiturate, do not apply cuffs or other restraints. Remain and try to soothe and orient by turning on a light and talking quietly and calmly until they are relaxed.
6. If a second sleeping medication requested during the night, try to determine the cause of the sleeplessness. Institute comfort measures; relieve pain. Wait approximately 20–30 min and then give the second dose of sleeping medication if client has not yet fallen asleep.
7. Record length of therapy. Sedative doses of medication over an 8-week period will cause physical dependence. Assess for evidence of physical and/or psychologic dependence and tolerance. Document any changes in the VS and skin condition.
8. Be alert to S&S of porphyria, a metabolic disorder characterized by N&V, abdominal pain, and muscle spasms; stop drug and report.
9. With a child, supervise play activity, especially if riding a bicycle or engaging in other potentially dangerous forms of play.
10. When receiving barbiturates on an outpatient basis, be alert to the number of prescription refills. Increased frequency of refills may indicate dependency or they may be selling the drug for profit.

Client/Family Teaching

1. Review goals of therapy and estimated time frame to accomplish.
2. Do not drive a car or operate other hazardous machinery after taking drug.
3. Take only as prescribed.
4. Avoid OTC drugs or any other agents unless prescribed.
5. Avoid the alcohol; potentiates effects of barbiturates.
6. If for insomnia, take 30 min before bedtime.
7. To avoid accidental overdose, keep in a medicine closet or drawer *away from* the bedside.
8. Keep out of the reach of children. Large doses may be fatal and the potential for abuse exists.
9. If taking for 8 or more weeks, do not stop suddenly without supervision; may result in withdrawal symptoms: weakness, anxiety, delirium, and tonic-clonic seizures.
10. Report any signs of hematologic toxicity such as infections (sore throat or fever) or increased bleeding tendencies (nosebleeds or easy bruising).
11. Identify factors contributing to insomnia. Try alternative methods to promote relaxation and sleep (such as progressive muscle relaxation, guided imagery, white noise simulator, or soft music). Consider sleep disorder center.
12. Daily exercise helps promote rest; identify a program and establish a daily routine such as with daily walks in the development or mall.
13. Limit caffeine intake and avoid after midday.
14. Establish a regular bedtime routine; discourage dozing during the afternoon or early evening hours.
15. Take prescribed analgesics for adequate pain relief. Allow sufficient time to unwind from a busy or overstimulating day, before retiring.
16. With continuous use of these drugs a decrease in responsiveness (drug tolerance) may develop. Abuse and physical dependence limit the usefulness of these drugs in long-term therapy.

Outcome/Evaluate

- ↓ Muscle spasms, ↓ tremulousness, and ↓ pre-op anxiety
- Effective sedation
- Improved sleeping patterns with less frequent awakenings
- Control of seizures

BETA-ADRENERGIC BLOCKING AGENTS

See also Alpha-1-Adrenergic Blocking Agents and the following individual agents:

Acebutolol hydrochloride
Atenolol
Betaxolol hydrochloride
Bisoprolol fumarate
Carteolol hydrochloride
Levobunolol hydrochloride
Metipranolol hydrochloride
Metoprolol succinate
Metoprolol tartrate
Nadolol
Penbutolol sulfate
Pindolol
Propranolol hydrochloride
Sotalol hydrochloride
Timolol maleate

Action/Kinetics: Combine reversibly with beta-adrenergic receptors to block the response to sympathetic nerve impulses, circulating catecholamines, or adrenergic drugs. Beta-adrenergic receptors are classified as beta-1 (predominantly in the cardiac muscle) and beta-2 (mainly in the bronchi and vascular musculature). Blockade of beta-1 receptors decreases HR, myocardial contractility, and CO; in addition, AV conduction is slowed. These effects lead to a decrease in BP, as well as a reversal of cardiac arrhythmias. Blockade of beta-2 receptors increases airway resistance in the bronchioles and inhibits the vasodilating effects of catecholamines on peripheral blood vessels. The various beta-blocking agents differ in their ability to block beta-1 and beta-2 receptors (see individual drugs); also, certain of these agents have intrinsic sympathomimetic action.

Certain of these drugs (betaxolol, carteolol, levobunolol, metipranolol, and timolol) are used for glaucoma. Act by reducing production of aqueous humor; metipranolol and timolol may also increase outflow of aqueous humor. Drugs have little or no effect on the pupil size or on accommodation.

Uses: See individual drugs.

Contraindications: Sinus bradycardia, second- and third-degree AV block, cardiogenic shock, CHF unless secondary to tachyarrhythmia treatable with beta blockers, overt cardiac failure. Most are contraindicated in chronic bronchitis, bronchial asthma or history thereof, bronchospasm, emphysema, severe COPD.

Special Concerns: Use with caution in diabetes, thyrotoxicosis, cerebrovascular insufficiency, and impaired hepatic and renal function. Withdrawing beta blockers before major surgery is controversial. Safe use during pregnancy and lactation and in children has not been established. May be absorbed systemically when used for glaucoma; thus, there is the potential for an additive effect with beta blockers used systemically. Certain of the products for use in glaucoma contain sulfites, which may result in an allergic reaction. Also, see individual agents.

Side Effects: *CV:* Bradycardia, hypotension (especially following IV use), CHF, cold extremities, claudication, worsening of angina, strokes, edema, syncope, arrhythmias, chest pain, peripheral ischemia, flushing, SOB, sinoatrial block, pulmonary edema, vasodilation, increased HR, palpitations, conduction disturbances, ***first-, second-, and third-degree heart block,*** worsening of AV block, thrombosis of renal or mesenteric arteries, precipitation or worsening of Raynaud's phenomenon. Sudden withdrawal of large doses may cause angina, ventricular tachycardia, ***fatal MI, sudden death,*** or ***circulatory collapse.*** *GI:* N&V, diarrhea, flatulence, dry mouth, constipation, anorexia, cramps, bloating, gastric pain, dyspepsia, distortion of taste, weight gain or loss, retroperitoneal fibrosis, ischemic colitis. *Hepatic:* Hepatomegaly, acute pancreatitis, elevated liver enzymes, liver damage (especially with chronic use of phenobarbital). *Respiratory:* Asthma-like symptoms, ***bronchospasms, bronchial obstruction, laryngospasm with respiratory distress,*** wheeziness, worsening of chronic obstructive lung disease, dyspnea, cough, nasal stuffiness, rhinitis, pharyngitis, rales. *CNS:* Dizziness, fatigue, lethargy, vivid dreams, depression, hallucinations, delirium, psychoses, paresthesias, insomnia, nervousness, nightmares, headache, vertigo, disorientation of time and place, hypoesthesia or hyperesthesia, decreased concentration, short-term memory loss, change in behavior, emotional lability, slurred speech, lightheadedness. In the elderly, paranoia, disorientation, and combativeness have occurred. *Hematologic:* ***Agranulocytosis,*** thrombocytopenia. *Allergic:* Fever, sore throat, respiratory distress, rash, pharyngitis, ***laryngospasm, anaphylaxis.*** *Skin:* Pruritus, rashes, increased skin pigmentation, sweating, dry skin, alopecia, skin irritation, psoriasis (reversible). *Musculoskeletal:* Joint and muscle pain, arthritis, arthralgia, back pain, muscle cramps, muscle weakness when used in clients with myasthenic symptoms. *GU:* Impotence, decreased libido, dysuria, UTI, nocturia, urinary retention or frequency, pollakiuria. *Ophthalmic:* Visual disturbances, eye irritation, dry or burning eyes, blurred vision, conjunctivitis. When used ophthalmically: keratitis, blepharoptosis, diplopia, ptosis, and visual disturbances including refractive changes. *Other:* Hyperglycemia or hypoglycemia, lupus-like syndrome, Peyronie's disease, tinnitus, increase in symptoms of myasthenia gravis, facial swelling, decreased exercise tolerance, rigors, speech disorders. *Systemic effects due to ophthalmic beta-1 and beta-2 blockers:* Headache, depression, arrhythmia, heart block, CVA, syncope, CHF, palpitation, cerebral ischemia, nausea, localized and generalized rash, bronchospasm (especially in those with preexisting bronchospastic disease), respiratory failure, masked symptoms of hypoglycemia in insulin-dependent diabetics, keratitis, visual disturbances (including refractive changes), blepharoptosis, ptosis, diplopia.

OD **Management of Overdose:** *Symptoms:* CV symptoms include bradycardia, hypotension, CHF, ***cardiogenic shock,*** intraventricular conduction disturbances, ***AV block, pulmonary edema, asystole,*** and tachycardia. Also, overdosage of pindolol may cause hypertension and overdosage of propranolol may result in systemic vascular resistance. CNS symptoms include respiratory depression, decreased consciousness, ***coma, and seizures.*** Miscellaneous symptoms include ***bronchospasm*** (especially in clients with obstructive pulmonary disease), hyperkalemia, and hypoglycemia. *Treatment:*

- To improve blood supply to the brain, place client in a supine position and raise the legs.
- Measure blood glucose and serum potassium. Monitor BP and ECG continuously.
- Provide general supportive treatment such as inducing emesis or gastric lavage and artificial respiration.
- *Seizures:* Give IV diazepam or phenytoin.
- *Excessive bradycardia:* If hypotensive, give atropine, 0.6 mg; if no response, give q 3 min for a total of 2–3 mg. Cautious administration of isoproterenol may be tried. Also, glucagon, 5–10 mg rapidly over 30 sec, followed by continuous IV infusion of 5 mg/hr may reverse bradycardia. Transvenous cardiac pacing may be needed for refractory cases.
- *Cardiac failure:* Digitalis, diuretic, and oxygen; if failure is refractory, IV aminophylline or glucagon may be helpful.
- *Hypotension:* Place client in Trendelenburg position. IV fluids unless pulmonary edema is present; also vasopressors such as norepinephrine (may be drug of choice), dobutamine, dopamine with monitoring of BP. If refractory, glucagon may be helpful. In intractable cardiogenic shock, intra-aortic balloon insertion may be required.
- *Premature ventricular contractions:* Lidocaine or phenytoin. Disopyramide, quinidine, and procainamide should be avoided as they depress myocardial function further.
- *Bronchospasms:* Give a beta-2-adrenergic agonist, epinephrine, or theophylline.
- *Heart block, second or third degree:* Isoproterenol or transvenous cardiac pacing.

Drug Interactions

Anesthetics, general / Additive depression of myocardium

Anticholinergic agents / Counteract bradycardia produced by beta-adrenergic blockers

Antihypertensives / Additive hypotensive effect

Ophthalmic beta blockers / Additive systemic beta-blocking effects if used with oral beta blockers

Chlorpromazine / Additive beta-adrenergic blocking action

Cimetidine / ↑ Effect of beta blockers due to ↓ breakdown by liver

Clonidine / Paradoxical hypertension; also, ↑ severity of rebound hypertension

Disopyramide / ↑ Effect of both drugs

Epinephrine / Beta blockers prevent beta-adrenergic action of epinephrine but not alpha-adrenergic action → ↑ systolic and diastolic BP and ↓ HR

Furosemide / ↑ Beta-adrenergic blockade

Hydralazine / ↑ Beta-adrenergic blockade

Indomethacin / ↓ Effect of beta blockers possibly due to inhibition of prostaglandin synthesis

Insulin / Beta blockers ↑ hypoglycemic effect of insulin

Lidocaine / ↑ Effect of lidocaine due to ↓ breakdown by liver

Methyldopa / Possible ↑ BP to alpha-adrenergic effect

NSAIDs / ↓ Effect of beta blockers, possibly due to inhibition of prostaglandin synthesis

Oral contraceptives / ↑ Effect of beta blockers due to ↓ breakdown by liver

Phenformin / ↑ Hypoglycemia

Phenobarbital / ↓ Effect of beta blockers due to ↑ breakdown by liver

Phenothiazines / ↑ Effect of both drugs

Phenytoin / Additive depression of myocardium; also phenytoin ↓ effect of beta blockers due to ↑ breakdown by liver

Prazosin / ↑ First-dose effect of prazosin (acute postural hypotension)

Reserpine / Additive hypotensive effect

Rifampin / ↓ Effect of beta blockers due to ↑ breakdown by liver

Ritodrine / Beta blockers ↓ effect of ritodrine

Salicylates / ↓ Effect of beta blockers, possibly due to inhibition of prostaglandin synthesis
Succinylcholine / Beta blockers ↑ effects of succinylcholine
Sympathomimetics / Reverse effects of beta blockers
Theophylline / Beta blockers reverse the effect of theophylline; also, beta blockers ↓ renal clearance of theophylline
Tubocurarine / Beta blockers ↑ effects of tubocurarine
Verapamil / Possible side effects since both drugs ↓ myocardial contractility or AV conduction; bradycardia and asystole when beta blockers are used ophthalmically

Dosage

See individual drugs.

Laboratory Test Considerations: ↓ Serum glucose.

1. Sudden stopping of beta blockers may precipitate or worsen angina.
2. The lowering of intraocular pressure (IOP) may take a few weeks to stabilize when using betaxolol or timolol.
3. Due to diurnal variations in IOP, the response to b.i.d. therapy is best assessed by measuring IOP at different times during the day.
4. If IOP is not controlled using beta blockers, add additional drugs to the regimen, including pilocarpine, dipivefrin, or systemic carbonic anhydrase inhibitors.

HEALTH CARE CONSIDERATIONS

Assessment

1. Record indications for therapy and any symptoms or history of depression; assess mental status.
2. Determine pulse and BP in both arms while lying, sitting, and standing.
3. Monitor EKG, glucose, CBC, electrolytes, liver and renal function studies.
4. Record any history of asthma, diabetes, or impaired renal function.
5. With asthma, avoid nonselective beta antagonists due to beta-2 receptor blockade which may lead to increased airway resistance.
6. Review drugs currently prescribed to ensure none interact unfavorably.

Interventions

1. Monitor HR and BP; obtain written parameters for medication administration (e.g., hold for SBP < 90 or HR < 50).
2. When assessing respirations note rate and quality; may cause dyspnea and bronchospasm.
3. Monitor I&O and daily weights. Observe for increasing dyspnea, coughing, difficulty breathing, fatigue, or edema—symptoms of CHF, may require digitalization, diuretics, and/or discontinuation of drug therapy.
4. Complaints of cold S&S, easy fatigue, or feeling lightheaded may require a drug change.
5. With diabetics watch for symptoms of hypoglycemia, such as hypotension or tachycardia; most mask these signs.
6. During IV administration, monitor EKG (may slow AV conduction and increase PR interval) and activities closely until drug effects evident.

Client/Family Teaching

1. When prescribed for BP control, drug helps control hypertension but does not cure it. Must continue to take despite feeling better.
2. Record BP and take pulse immediately prior to first dose each day so medication can be adjusted.
3. Review instructions when to call provider, i.e., if HR < 50 beats/min or SBP < 80 mm Hg.
4. Review life-style changes necessary for BP control: regular exercise, low-fat and reduced-calorie diet, decreased salt and alcohol intake, smoking cessation, and relaxation techniques.
5. Always consult provider before interrupting therapy; abrupt withdrawal may precipitate angina, MI, or rebound hypertension. A 2-week taper is useful.
6. May cause blurred vision, dizziness, or drowsiness; avoid activities that require mental alertness until drug effects realized.
7. Rise from a sitting or lying position slowly and dangle legs before standing to avoid symptoms of orthostatic hypotension. Elastic support hose may help decrease symptoms.
8. Dress warmly during cold weather. Diminished blood supply to extremities may cause cold sensitivity; check extremities for warmth.
9. Avoid excessive intake of alcohol, coffee, tea, or cola. Avoid OTC agents without approval.
10. If diabetic, perform finger sticks often and report S&S of hypoglycemia.
11. Report any asthma-like symptoms, cough, or nasal stuffiness; may be symptoms of CHF.
12. Report any bothersome side effects or changes, especially new-onset depression.

Outcome/Evaluate

- ↓ BP; ↓ IOP
- ↓ Frequency/severity of anginal attacks; improved exercise tolerance
- ↓ Anxiety levels; ↓ tremors
- Migraine prophylaxis
- Control of cardiac arrhythmias

CALCIUM CHANNEL BLOCKING AGENTS

See also the following individual entries:

Amlodipine
Bepridil hydrochloride
Diltiazem hydrochloride
Felodipine
Isradipine
Nicardipine hydrochloride
Nifedipine
Nimodipine
Nisoldipine
Verapamil

Action/Kinetics: For contraction of cardiac and smooth muscle to occur, extracellular calcium must move into the cell through openings called *calcium channels*. The calcium channel blocking agents (also called *slow channel blockers* or *calcium antagonists*) inhibit the influx of calcium through the cell membrane, resulting in a depression of automaticity and conduction velocity in both smooth and cardiac muscle. This leads to a depression of contraction in these tissues. Drugs in this class have different degrees of selectivity on vascular smooth muscle, myocardium, and conduction and pacemaker tissues. In the myocardium, these drugs dilate coronary vessels in both normal and ischemic tissues and inhibit spasms of coronary arteries. They also decrease total peripheral resistance, thus reducing energy and oxygen requirements of the heart. Also effective against certain cardiac arrhythmias by slowing AV conduction and prolonging repolarization. In addition, they depress the amplitude, rate of depolarization, and conduction in atria.

Uses: See individual drugs.

Contraindications: Sick sinus syndrome, second- or third-degree AV block (except with a functioning pacemaker). Use of bepridil, diltiazem, or verapamil for hypotension (<90 mm Hg systolic pressure). Lactation.

Special Concerns: Abrupt withdrawal may result in increased frequency and duration of chest pain. Hypertensive clients treated with calcium channel blockers have a higher risk of heart attack than clients treated with diuretics or beta-adrenergic blockers. May also be an increased risk of heart attacks in diabetics (only nisoldipine studied). Safety and effectiveness of bepridil, diltiazem, felodipine, and isradipine have not been established in children.

Side Effects: Side effects vary from one calcium channel blocker to another; refer to individual drugs.

OD **Management of Overdose:** *Symptoms:* Nausea, weakness, drowsiness, dizziness, slurred speech, confusion, marked and prolonged hypotension, bradycardia, junctional rhythms, ***second- or third-degree block.*** *Treatment:*

- Treatment is supportive. Monitor cardiac and respiratory function.
- If client is seen soon after ingestion, emetics or gastric lavage should be considered followed by cathartics.
- *Hypotension:* IV calcium, dopamine, isoproterenol, metaraminol, norepinephrine. Also, provide IV fluids. Place client in Trendelenburg position.
- *Ventricular tachycardia:* IV procainamide or lidocaine; also, cardioversion may be necessary. Also, provide slow-drip IV fluids.
- *Bradycardia, asystole, AV block:* IV atropine sulfate (0.6–1 mg), calcium gluconate (10% solution), isoproterenol, norepinephrine; also, cardiac pacing may be indicated. Provide slow-drip IV fluids.

Drug Interactions

Beta-adrenergic blocking agents / Beta blockers may cause depression of myocardial contractility and AV conduction
Cimetidine / ↑ Effect of calcium channel blockers due to ↓ first-pass metabolism
Fentanyl / Severe hypotension or increased fluid volume requirements
Ranitidine / ↑ Effect of calcium channel blockers due to ↓ first-pass metabolism

Dosage

See individual drugs.

HEALTH CARE CONSIDERATIONS

Assessment

1. Record indications for therapy, type and onset of symptoms. List other agents used and the outcome.
2. Record any experience with these agents and the response.
3. Assess and document CV and mental status. These drugs cause peripheral vasodilation. Any excessive hypotensive response and increased HR may precipitate angina.
4. Record VS, weight, ECG and BP in both arms while lying, sitting, and standing. Assess for CHF (weight gain, peripheral edema, dyspnea, rales, jugular vein distention).
5. Monitor BS, electrolytes, I&O, liver and renal function studies.

Client/Family Teaching

1. These agents work by decreasing myocardial contractile force, which in turn decreases the myocardial oxygen requirements.
2. Take with meals to reduce GI irritation.
3. Review goals of therapy (e.g., ↓ DBP by 10 mm Hg, ↓ HR by 20 beats/min).
4. Take pulse and BP at the same time of day and at least twice a week as well as weights; review instructions regarding when to hold meds and contact provider.
5. Do not perform activities that require mental alertness until drug effects realized.
6. Report side effects such as dizziness, vertigo, unusual flushing, facial warmth, edema, nausea, or persistent constipation; toxic drug effects
7. If postural hypotension occurs, change positions slowly, especially when standing from a reclining position. Sit down immediately if lightheadedness occurs. Move slowly from a lying to a sitting or standing position.
8. Long periods of standing, excessive heat, hot showers or baths, and ingestion of alcohol may exacerbate postural hypotension; avoid these situations.
9. Any swelling of the hands or feet, pronounced dizziness, or chest pain accompanied by diaphoresis, SOB, or severe headaches should be reported immediately.
10. Review life-style changes for BP control, i.e., regular exercise, low-fat, low-cholesterol, reduced-calorie diet, decreased salt and alcohol consumption, smoking cessation, and stress reduction.

Outcome/Evaluate

- Control of hypertension; ↓ HR
- ↓ frequency/intensity of anginal attacks
- Stable cardiac rhythm

CALCIUM SALTS

See also the following individual entries:

Calcium carbonate
Calcium citrate
Calcium glubionate
Calcium gluconate
Calcium lactate

Action/Kinetics: Calcium is essential for maintaining normal function of nerves, muscles, the skeletal system, and permeability of cell membranes and capillaries. The normal serum calcium concentration is 9–10.4 mg/dL (4.5–5.2 mEq/L). Hypocalcemia is characterized by muscular fibrillation, twitching, skeletal muscle spasms, leg cramps, tetanic spasms, cardiac arrhythmias, smooth muscle hyperexcitability, mental depression, and anxiety states. Excessive, chronic hypocalcemia is characterized by brittle, defective nails, poor dentition, and brittle hair. Calcium is well absorbed from the upper GI tract. However, severe low-calcium tetany is best treated by IV administration of calcium gluconate. The presence of vitamin D is necessary for maximum calcium utilization. The hormone of the parathyroid gland is necessary for the regulation of the calcium level.

Uses: IV: Acute hypocalcemic tetany secondary to renal failure, hypoparathyroidism, premature delivery, maternal diabetes mellitus in infants, and poisoning due to magnesium, oxalic acid, radiophosphorus, carbon tetrachloride, fluoride, phosphate, strontium, and radium. To treat depletion of electrolytes. Also during cardiac resuscitation when epinephrine or isoproterenol has not improved myocardial contraction (may also be given into the ventricular cavity for this purpose). To reverse cardiotoxicity or hyperkalemia. **IM or IV:** Reduce spasms in renal, biliary, intestinal, or lead colic. To relieve muscle cramps due to insect bites and to decrease capillary permeability in various sensitivity reactions. **PO:** Osteoporosis, osteomalacia, chronic hypoparathyroidism, rickets, latent tetany, hypocalcemia secondary to use of anticonvulsant drugs. Myasthenia gravis, Eaton-Lambert syndrome, supplement for pregnant, postmenopausal, or nursing women. Also, prophylactically for primary osteoporosis. *Investigational:* As an infusion to diagnose Zollinger-Ellison syndrome and medullary thyroid carcinoma. To antagonize neuromuscular blockade due to aminoglycosides.

Contraindications: Digitalized clients, sarcoidosis, renal or cardiac disease, ventricular fibrillation. Cancer clients with bone metastases. Renal calculi, hypophosphatemia, hypercalcemia.

Special Concerns: Calcium requirements decrease in geriatric clients; thus, dose may have to be adjusted. Also, low levels of active vitamin D metabolites may impair calcium absorption in older clients. Use with caution in cor pulmonale, respiratory acidosis, renal disease or failure, ventricular fibrillation, hypercalcemia.

Side Effects: Following PO use: GI irritation, constipation. **Following IV use:** Venous irritation, tingling sensation, feeling of oppression or heat, chalky taste. Rapid IV administration may result in vasodilation, decreased BP and HR, ***cardiac arrhythmias,*** syncope, or ***cardiac arrest.*** **Following IM use:** Burning feeling, necrosis, tissue sloughing, cellulitis, soft tissue calcification. *NOTE:* If calcium is injected into the myocardium rather than into the ventricle, ***laceration of coronary arteries, cardiac tamponade, pneumothorax, and ventricular fibrillation*** may occur. *Symptoms due to ex-*

cess calcium (hypercalcemia): Lassitude, fatigue, GI symptoms (anorexia, N&V, abdominal pain, dry mouth, thirst), polyuria, depression of nervous and neuromuscular function (emotional disturbances, confusion, skeletal muscle weakness, and constipation), confusion, delirium, stupor, ***coma,*** impairment of renal function (polyuria, polydipsia, and azotemia), renal calculi, arrhythmias, and bradycardia.

OD **Management of Overdose:** *Symptoms:* Systemic overloading from parenteral administration can result in an acute hypercalcemic syndrome with symptoms including markedly increased plasma calcium levels, lethargy, intractable N&V, weakness, ***coma, and sudden death.*** *Treatment:* Discontinue therapy and lower serum calcium levels by giving an IV infusion of sodium chloride plus a potent diuretic such as furosemide. Consider hemodialysis.

Drug Interactions

Atenolol / ↓ Effect of atenolol due to ↓ bioavailability and plasma levels
Cephalocin / Incompatible with calcium salts
Corticosteroids / Interfere with absorption of calcium from GI tract
Digitalis / ↑ Digitalis arrhythmias and toxicity. Death has resulted from combination of digitalis and IV calcium salts
Iron salts / ↓ Absorption of iron from the GI tract
Milk / Excess of either may cause hypercalcemia, renal insufficiency with azotemia, alkalosis, and ocular lesions
Norfloxacin / ↓ Bioavailability of norfloxacin
Sodium polystyrene sulfonate / Metabolic alkalosis and ↓ binding of resin to potassium in clients with renal impairment
Tetracyclines / ↓ Effect of tetracyclines due to ↓ absorption from GI tract
Thiazide diuretics / Hypercalcemia due to thiazide-induced renal tubular reabsorption of calcium and bone release of calcium
Verapamil / Calcium antagonizes the effect of verapamil
Vitamin D / Enhances intestinal absorption of dietary calcium

Dosage

See individual agents.

HEALTH CARE CONSIDERATIONS

Administration

ORAL

1. Administer 1–1.5 hr after meals. Alkalis and large amounts of fat decrease the absorption of calcium.
2. If difficulty swallowing large tablets, obtain a calcium in water suspension. Because calcium goes into suspension six times more readily in hot water than in cold water, the solution can be prepared by diluting the medication with *hot* water. Solution may then be cooled before administering.

IV

1. Warm solutions to body temperature and give slowly (0.5–2 mL/min), stop if discomfort experienced.
2. Administer slowly, observing for bradycardia, hypotension, and cardiac arrhythmias.
3. Prevent leakage of salts into the tissues; extremely irritating.
4. Keep client recumbent for a short time following the injection.
5. Do not mix calcium salts with carbonates, phosphates, sulfates, or tartrates in parenteral admixtures.

IM

1. Rotate injection sites; calcium may cause tissue sloughing.
2. Do not administer IM calcium gluconate to children.

Assessment

1. Perform a thorough medical history, noting indications for therapy and any underlying causes.
2. Note if receiving digitalis products; drug may be contraindicated.
3. Monitor calcium levels and renal function; assess for renal disease. Administer vitamin D to facilitate absorption.
4. With hypocalcemic tetany, use safety precautions to protect from injury.
5. Assess for S&S of hypercalcemia, i.e., fatigue and CNS depression.

Client/Family Teaching

1. Calcium requirements are best met by dietary sources (including milk in the diet). Supplements need vitamin D to facilitate absorption.
2. Multivitamin and mineral preparations are expensive and do not contain sufficient calcium to meet daily requirements.
3. Consult a dietitian to assist with proper food selection and meal planning/preparation.
4. Review prescribed replacement regimen. Need follow-ups for dosage adjustments to prevent hypercalcemia and hypercalciuria.

Outcome/Evaluate

- Resolution of hypocalcemia
- Relief of muscle cramps
- Osteoporosis prophylaxis
- Serum calcium levels within desired range (8.8–10.4 mg/dL)

CARDIAC GLYCOSIDES

See also the following individual entries:

Digitoxin
Digoxin

Action/Kinetics: Cardiac glycosides increase the force and velocity of myocardial contraction (positive inotropic effect) by increasing the refractory period of the AV node and increasing total peripheral resistance. This effect is due to inhibition of sodium/potassium–ATPase in the sarcolemmal membrane, which alters excitation–contraction coupling. Inhibiting sodium, potassium–ATPase, results in an increase of calcium influx and an increased release of free calcium ions within the myocardial cells, which then potentiate the contractility of cardiac muscle fibers. The digitalis glycosides also decrease the rate of conduction and increase the refractory period of the AV node due to an increase in parasympathetic tone and a decrease in sympathetic tone. Clinical effects are not seen until steady-state plasma levels are reached. The initial dose of digitalis glycosides is larger (loading dose) and is traditionally referred to as the *digitalizing dose;* subsequent doses are referred to as *maintenance doses.*

Uses: All types of CHF, including that due to venous congestion, edema, dyspnea, orthopnea, and cardiac arrhythmia. Control of rapid ventricular contraction rate in clients with atrial fibrillation or flutter. Slow HR in sinus tachycardia due to CHF. Supraventricular tachycardia. Prophylaxis and treatment of recurrent paroxysmal atrial tachycardia with paroxysmal AV junctional rhythm. Cardiogenic shock (value not established).

Contraindications: Ventricular fibrillation or tachycardia (unless congestive failure supervenes after protracted episode not due to digitalis), in presence of digitalis toxicity, hypersensitivity to cardiac glycosides, beriberi heart disease, certain cases of hypersensitive carotid sinus syndrome.

Special Concerns: Use with caution in clients with ischemic heart disease, acute myocarditis, hypertrophic subaortic stenosis, hypoxic or myxedemic states, Adams-Stokes or carotid sinus syndromes, cardiac amyloidosis, or cyanotic heart and lung disease, including emphysema and partial heart block. Those with carditis associated with rheumatic fever or viral myocarditis are especially sensitive to digoxin-induced disturbances in rhythm. Electric pacemakers may sensitize the myocardium to cardiac glycosides. Also use with caution and at reduced dosage in elderly, debilitated clients, pregnant women and nursing mothers, and newborn, term, or premature infants who have immature renal and hepatic function and in reduced renal and/or hepatic function.

Side Effects: Cardiac glycosides are extremely toxic and have caused death even in clients who have received the drugs for long periods of time. There is a narrow margin of safety between an effective therapeutic dose and a toxic dose. Overdosage caused by the cumulative effects of the drug is a constant danger in therapy with cardiac glycosides. Digitalis toxicity is characterized by a wide variety of symptoms, which are hard to differentiate from those of the cardiac disease itself.

CV: Changes in the rate, rhythm, and irritability of the heart and the mechanism of the heartbeat. Extrasystoles, bigeminal pulse, coupled rhythm, ectopic beat, and other forms of arrhythmias have been noted. ***Death most often results from ventricular fibrillation.*** Cardiac glycosides should be discontinued in adults when pulse rate falls below 60 beats/min. All cardiac changes are best detected by the ECG, which is also most useful in clients suffering from intoxication. ***Acute hemorrhage.*** *GI:* Anorexia, N&V, excessive salivation, epigastric distress, abdominal pain, diarrhea, bowel necrosis. Clients on digitalis therapy may experience two vomiting stages. The first is an early sign of toxicity and is a direct effect of digitalis on the GI tract. Late vomiting indicates stimulation of the vomiting center of the brain, which occurs after the heart muscle has been saturated with digitalis. *CNS:* Headaches, fatigue, lassitude, irritability, malaise, muscle weakness, insomnia, stupor. Psychotomimetic effects (especially in elderly or arteriosclerotic clients or neonates) including disorientation, confusion, depression, aphasia, delirium, hallucinations, and, rarely, ***convulsions.*** *Neuromuscular:* Neurologic pain involving the lower third of the face and lumbar areas, paresthesia. *Visual disturbances:* Blurred vision, flickering dots, white halos, borders around dark objects, diplopia, amblyopia, color perception changes. *Hypersensitivity (5–7 days after starting therapy):* Skin reactions (urticaria, fever, pruritus, facial and ***angioneurotic edema***). *Other:* Chest pain, coldness of extremities.

OD **Management of Overdose:** The relationship of cardiac glycoside levels to symptoms of toxicity varies significantly from client to client; thus, it is not possible to identify glycoside levels that would define toxicity accurately. *Symptoms (Toxicity): GI:* Anorexia, N&V, diarrhea, abdominal discomfort, or pain. *CNS:* Blurred, yellow, or green vision and halo effect; headache, weakness, drowsiness, mental depression, apathy, restlessness, disorientation, confusion, ***seizures,*** EEG abnormalities, delirium, hallucinations, neuralgia, psychosis. *CV:* Ventricular tachycardia, unifocal or multiform PVCs (especially in bigeminal or trigeminal patterns), paroxysmal and nonparoxysmal nodal rhythms, AV dissociation, accelerated junctional rhythm, excessive slowing of the pulse, ***AV block (may proceed to complete block),*** atrial fibrillation, ***ventricular fibrillation (most common cause of death).*** *Children:* Visual disturbances, headache, weakness, apathy, and psychosis occur but may be difficult to recognize. *CV:* Conduction disturbances, supraventricular tachyarrhythmias (e.g., ***AV block***), atrial tachycardia with or without block, nodal tachycardia, unifocal or multiform ventricular premature contractions, ventricular tachycardia, sinus bradycardia (especially in infants). *Treatment in Adults:*

- Discontinue drug and admit to the intensive care area for continuous monitoring of ECG.
- If serum potassium is below normal, potassium chloride should be administered in divided PO doses totaling 3–6 g (40–80 mEq). Potassium should not be used when severe or complete heart block is due to digitalis and not related to tachycardia.
- *Atropine:* A dose of 0.01 mg/kg IV to treat severe sinus bradycardia or slow ventricular rate due to secondary AV block.
- *Cholestyramine, colestipol, activated charcoal:* To bind digitalis in the intestine, thus preventing enterohepatic recirculation.
- *Digoxin immune FAB:* See drug entry. Given in approximate equimolar quantities as digoxin, it reverses S&S of toxicity, often with improvement seen within 30 min.
- *Lidocaine:* A dose of 1 mg/kg given over 5 min followed by an infusion of 15–50 mcg/kg/min to maintain normal cardiac rhythm.
- *Phenytoin:* For atrial or ventricular arrhythmias unresponsive to potassium, can give a dose of 0.5 mg/kg at a rate not exceeding 50 mg/min (given at 1–2 hr intervals). The maximum dose should not exceed 10 mg/kg/day.
- *Countershock:* A direct-current countershock can be used *only as a last resort.* If required, therapy should be initiated at low voltage levels.

Treatment in Children: Give potassium in divided doses totaling 1–1.5 mEq/kg (if correction of arrhythmia is urgent, a dose of 0.5 mEq/kg/hr can be used) with careful monitoring of the ECG. The potassium IV solution should be dilute to avoid local irritation although IV fluid overload must be avoided. Digoxin immune FAB may also be used.

Digoxin is not removed effectively by dialysis, by exchange transfusion, or during cardiopulmonary bypass as most of the drug is found in tissues rather than the circulating blood. Digitoxin is not effectively removed by either peritoneal or hemodialysis due to its high degree of plasma protein binding.

Drug Interactions: One of the most serious side effects of digitalis-type drugs is hypokalemia (lowering of serum potassium levels). This may lead to cardiac arrhythmias, muscle weakness, hypotension, and respiratory distress. Other agents causing hypokalemia reinforce this effect and increase the chance of digitalis toxicity. Such reactions may occur in clients who have been on digitalis maintenance for a long time.

Albuterol / ↑ Skeletal muscle binding of digoxin
Amiloride / ↓ Inotropic effects of digoxin
Aminoglycosides / ↓ Effect of digitalis glycosides due to ↓ absorption from GI tract
Aminosalicylic acid / ↓ Effect of digitalis glycosides due to ↓ absorption from GI tract
Amphotericin B / ↑ K depletion caused by digitalis; ↑ risk of digitalis toxicity
Antacids / ↓ Effect of digitalis glycosides due to ↓ absorption from GI tract
Beta blockers / Complete heart block possible
Calcium preparations / Cardiac arrhythmias if parenteral calcium given with digitalis
Chlorthalidone / ↑ K and Mg loss with ↑ chance of digitalis toxicity
Cholestyramine / Binds digitoxin in the intestine and ↓ its absorption
Colestipol / Binds digitoxin in the intestine and ↓ its absorption
Ephedrine / ↑ Chance of cardiac arrhythmias
Epinephrine / ↑ Chance of cardiac arrhythmias
Ethacrynic acid / ↑ K and Mg loss with ↑ chance of digitalis toxicity
Furosemide / ↑ K and Mg loss with ↑ chance of digitalis toxicity
Glucose infusions / Large infusions of glucose may cause ↓ in serum potassium and ↑ chance of digitalis toxicity
Hypoglycemic drugs / ↓ Effect of digitalis glycosides due to ↑ breakdown by liver
Methimazole / ↑ Chance of toxic effects of digitalis
Metoclopramide / ↓ Effect of digitalis glycosides by ↓ absorption from GI tract

Muscle relaxants, nondepolarizing / ↑ Risk of cardiac arrhythmias
Propranolol / Potentiates digitalis-induced bradycardia
Reserpine / ↑ Chance of cardiac arrhythmias
Spironolactone / Either ↑ or ↓ toxic effects of digitalis glycosides
Succinylcholine / ↑ Chance of cardiac arrhythmias
Sulfasalazine / ↓ Effect of digitalis glycosides by ↓ absorption from GI tract
Sympathomimetics / ↑ Chance of cardiac arrhythmias
Thiazides / ↑ K and Mg loss with ↑ chance of digitalis toxicity
Thioamines / ↑ Effect and toxicity of cardiac glycosides
Thyroid / ↓ Effectiveness of digitalis glycosides
Triamterene / ↑ Pharmacologic effects of digoxin

Dosage

PO, IM, or IV. *Highly individualized.* See individual drugs: digitoxin, digoxin. The rates at which clients become digitalized vary considerably. Clients with mild signs of congestion can often be digitalized gradually over a period of several days. Clients suffering from more serious congestion, for example, those showing signs of acute LV failure, dyspnea, or lung edema, can be digitalized more rapidly by parenteral administration of a fast-acting cardiac glycoside. Once digitalization has been attained (pulse 68–80 beats/min) and symptoms of CHF have subsided, the client is put on maintenance dosage. Depending on the drug and the age of the client, the daily maintenance dose is often approximately 10% of the digitalizing dose.

Laboratory Test Considerations: May ↓ PT. Alters tests for 17-ketosteroids and 17-hydroxycorticosteroids.

Special Considerations

1. Elderly clients must be observed for early S&S of toxicity (N&V, anorexia, confusion, and visual disturbances) because their rate of drug elimination is slower.
2. The half-life of cardiac glycosides is prolonged in the elderly; anticipate smaller drug doses.
3. Be especially alert to cardiac arrhythmias in children. This sign of toxicity occurs more frequently in children than in adults.

1. The names digoxin and digitoxin are similar. However, their dosage and duration of their effect differ markedly. Check client's name, the order, the MAR, and the label of drug to be administered.
2. Measure liquids precisely, using a calibrated dropper or syringe.
3. Obtain written parameters indicating the pulse rates, both high and low, at which cardiac glycosides are to be held; changes in rate or rhythm may indicate toxicity.

FOR CLIENTS STARTING ON A DIGITALIZING DOSE

HEALTH CARE CONSIDERATIONS

Assessment

1. Record type, onset, and characteristics of symptoms. If administered for heart failure, note causes; ensure that failure not solely related to diastolic dysfunction as drug's positive inotropic effect may increase cardiac outflow obstruction with hypertrophic cardiomyopathy.
2. Record any drugs prescribed that would adversely interact with digitalis glycosides and monitor; diuretics may increase toxicity.
3. Monitor CBC, serum electrolytes, calcium, magnesium, liver and renal function tests.
4. Obtain ECG; note rhythm/rate.
5. Record cardiopulmonary findings; note presence of S3, JVD, HJR, displaced PMI, HR above 100 bpm, rales, peripheral edema, DOE, PND, and echo, MUGA, and/or cardiac cath findings. Note New York Heart Association Classification based on client symptoms.

FOR CLIENTS BEING DIGITALIZED AND FOR CLIENTS ON A MAINTENANCE DOSE OF A CARDIAC GLYCOSIDE

Interventions

1. During digitalization, monitor closely.
2. Observe monitor for bradycardia and/or arrhythmias, or count apical rate for at least 1 min before administering the drug. Obtain written parameters (e.g., HR > 50 or 60) for drug administration.
   - Document adult HR below 50 bpm or if an arrhythmia (irregular pulse) occurs.
   - If child's HR is 90–110 bpm or if an arrhythmia is present, withhold drug and report.
3. Anticipate more than once daily dosing in most children (up to age 10) due to higher metabolic activity.
4. With co-worker simultaneously take the apical and radial pulse for 1 min, and report pulse deficit (e.g., the wrist rate is less than the apical rate); may indicate an adverse drug reaction.
5. Monitor weights and I&O. Weight gain may indicate edema. Adequate intake will help prevent cumulative toxic drug effects.
6. If taking non-potassium-sparing diuretics as well as a cardiac glycoside, will need potas-

sium supplements. Provide the most palatable preparation available. (Liquid potassium preparations are usually bitter.)
7. If gastric distress experienced, use an antacid. Antacids containing aluminum or magnesium and kaolin/pectin mixtures should be given 6 hr before or 6 hr after dose of cardiac glycoside to prevent decreased therapeutic effects.
8. When given to newborns, use a cardiac monitor to identify early evidence of toxicity: excessive slowing of sinus rate, sinoatrial arrest, or prolonged PR interval.
9. Monitor digoxin levels periodically and assess for symptoms of toxicity; draw specimen more than 6 hr after last dose. Have digoxin antidote available (digoxin immune FAB) for severe toxicity.
10. Use caution; digoxin withdrawal may worsen heart failure.

Client/Family Teaching

1. Take after meals to lessen gastric irritation.
2. Maintain a written record of pulse rates and weights; review guidelines for withholding medication and reporting abnormal pulse rates.
3. Do not change brands; different preparations have variations in bioavailability and could cause toxicity or loss of effect.
4. Follow directions carefully for taking the medication. If one dose of drug is accidentally missed, do not double up on the next dose.
5. Report toxic drug symptoms: anorexia, N&V, and diarrhea are often early symptoms and are due to the toxic effects on the GI tract and CTZ stimulation. Disorientation, agitation, visual disturbances, changes in color perception, and hallucinations may also occur.
6. Maintain a sodium-restricted diet. Read labels and review foods low in sodium; consult dietitian for assistance in food selection, meal planning, and preparation.
7. Consult provider before taking any other medications, whether prescribed or OTC, because drug interactions occur frequently with cardiac glycosides.
8. Report any persistent cough, difficulty breathing, or edema (S&S of CHF).
9. Identify community health agencies available to assist in maintaining health.
10. Return for scheduled follow-up visits and lab tests.

Outcome/Evaluate

- Stable cardiac rate and rhythm, improved breathing patterns, ↓ severity of S&S of CHF, improved CO, improved activity tolerance, ↓ weight, and improved diuresis
- Serum drug levels within therapeutic range (e.g., digoxin 0.5–2.0 ng/mL)

CEPHALOSPORINS

See also the following individual entries:

Cefaclor
Cefadroxil monohydrate
Cefdinir
Cefixime oral
Cefotaxime sodium
Cefpodoxime proxetil
Cefprozil
Ceftibuten
Ceftriaxone sodium
Cefuroxime axetil
Cefuroxime sodium
Cephalexin hydrochloride monohydrate
Cephalexin monohydrate
Cephradine
Loracarbef

Action/Kinetics: The cephalosporins interfere with a final step in the formation of the bacterial cell wall (inhibition of mucopeptide biosynthesis), resulting in unstable cell membranes that undergo lysis (same mechanism of actions as penicillins). Also, cell division and growth are inhibited. The cephalosporins are most effective against young, rapidly dividing organisms and are considered bactericidal. Cephalosporins are widely distributed to most tissues and fluids. First- and second-generation drugs do not enter the CSF well but third-generation drugs enter inflamed meninges readily. Rapidly excreted by the kidneys.

General Statement: Cephalosporins are broad-spectrum antibiotics classified as first-, second-, and third-generation drugs. The difference among generations is based on pharmacokinetics and antibacterial spectra. Generally, third-generation cephalosporins have more activity against gram-negative organisms and resistant organisms and less activity against gram-positive organisms than first-generation drugs. Third-generation cephalosporins are also stable against beta-lactamases. Cephalosporins can be destroyed by cephalosporinase.

See also *General Health Care Considerations for All Anti-Infectives.*

Uses: See individual drugs. A listing of the drugs in each generation follows:

First-Generation Cephalosporins: Cefadroxil, cefazolin, cephalexin, cephapirin, cephradine.

Second-Generation Cephalosporins:

Cefaclor, cefmetazole, cefonicid, cefotetan, cefoxitin, cefprozil, cefuroxime, and loracarbef.

Third-Generation Cephalosporins: Cefdinir, cefepime, cefixime, cefoperazone, cefotaxime, cefpodoxime, ceftazidime, ceftibuten, ceftizoxime, ceftriaxone.

Contraindications: Hypersensitivity to cephalosporins or related antibiotics.

Special Concerns: Safe use in pregnancy and lactation has not been established (pregnancy category: B). Use with caution in the presence of impaired renal or hepatic function, together with other nephrotoxic drugs, and in clients over 50 years of age. Perform C_{cr} on all clients with impaired renal function who receive cephalosporins. If hypersensitive to penicillin, may occasionally cross-react to cephalosporins.

Side Effects: *GI:* N&V, diarrhea, abdominal cramps or pain, dyspepsia, glossitis, heartburn, sore mouth or tongue, dysgeusia, anorexia, flatulence, cholestasis. Pseudomembranous colitis. *Allergic:* Urticaria, rashes (maculopapular, morbilliform, or erythematous), pruritus (including anal and genital areas), fever, chills, erythema, ***angioedema,*** serum sickness, joint pain, exfoliative dermatitis, chest tightness, myalgia, erythema multiforme, edema, itching, numbness, chills, ***Stevens-Johnson syndrome, anaphylaxis.*** *NOTE:* Cross-allergy may be manifested between cephalosporins and penicillins. *Hematologic:* Leukopenia, leukocytosis, lymphocytosis, neutropenia (transient), eosinophilia, thrombocytopenia, thrombocythemia, ***agranulocytosis,*** granulocytopenia, bone marrow depression, ***hemolytic anemia,*** pancytopenia, decreased platelet function, ***aplastic anemia,*** hypoprothrombinemia (may lead to bleeding), thrombocytosis (transient). *CNS:* Headache, malaise, fatigue, vertigo, dizziness, lethargy, confusion, paresthesia, precipitation of ***seizures*** (especially in clients with impaired renal function). *Hepatic:* Hepatomegaly, hepatitis. Intrathecal use may result in hallucinations, nystagmus, or ***seizures.*** *Miscellaneous:* Superinfection including oral candidiasis and enterococcal infections, hypotension, sweating, flushing, dyspnea, interstitial pneumonitis.

IV or IM use may result in local swelling, inflammation, cellulitis, paresthesia, burning, phlebitis, thrombophlebitis. IM use may also cause pain and induration, tenderness, increased temperature. Sterile abscesses have been observed following SC use. Nephrotoxicity (↑ BUN with and without ↑ serum creatinine) may occur in clients over 50 and in young children.

OD **Management of Overdose:** *Symptoms:* Parenteral use of large doses of cephalosporins may cause seizures, especially in clients with impaired renal function. *Treatment:* If seizures occur, discontinue the drug immediately and give anticonvulsant drugs. Hemodialysis may also be effective.

Drug Interactions

Alcohol / Antabuse-like reaction if used with cefazolin, cefmetazole, cefoperazone, or cefotetan
Aminoglycosides / ↑ Risk of renal toxicity with certain cephalosporins
Antacids / ↓ Plasma levels of cefaclor, cefdinir, or cefpodoxime
Anticoagulants / ↑ Hypoprothrombinemic effects if used with cefazolin, cefmetazole, cefoperazone, or cefotetan
Colistimethate / ↑ Risk of renal toxicity
Colistin / ↑ Risk of renal toxicity
Ethacrynic acid / ↑ Risk of renal toxicity
Furosemide / ↑ Risk of renal toxicity
H_2 antagonists / ↓ Plasma levels of cefpodoxime or cefuroxime
Polymyxin B / ↑ Risk of renal toxicity
Probenecid / ↑ Effect of cephalosporins by ↓ excretion by kidneys
Vancomycin / ↑ Risk of renal toxicity

Dosage

See individual drugs.

Laboratory Test Considerations: False + for urinary glucose with Benedict's solution, Fehling's solution, or Clinitest tablets. Enzyme tests (Clinistix, Tes-Tape) are unaffected. False + Coombs' test and urinary 17-ketosteroids.

↑ AST, ALT, total bilirubin, GGTP, LDH, alkaline phosphatase.

1. Parenteral solutions infused too rapidly may cause pain and irritation; infuse over 30 min unless otherwise indicated and assess site.
2. Continue therapy for at least 2–3 days after symptoms of infection have disappeared.
3. For group A beta-hemolytic streptococcal infections, continue therapy for at least 10 days to prevent the development of glomerulonephritis or rheumatic fever.

HEALTH CARE CONSIDERATIONS

Assessment

1. With hypersensitivity reactions to penicillin, assess for cross-sensitivity to cephalosporins.
2. Many agents in this group of antibiotics are quite expensive. Clients on fixed incomes with limited health benefits may be unable to afford them.

3. Record indications for therapy and symptoms of infection; obtain baseline cultures.
4. Monitor CBC, BS, electrolytes, liver and renal function studies. With renal impairment reduce dose; for dialysis clients, administer after treatment.
5. May cause false + Coombs' test.

Interventions

1. The cephalosporins all have similar sounding and similarly spelled names. Use care when transcribing orders for administration and request clarification as needed.
2. Pseudomembranous colitis may occur. If diarrhea develops, note any fever and report immediately. Continue to monitor VS, I&O, stool C&S, and for electrolyte imbalance.
3. Persistent temperature elevations may be drug-induced fever.

Client/Family Teaching

1. Oral meds should be taken on an empty stomach but, if GI upset occurs, may be administered with meals.
2. Report any S&S that may necessitate drug withdrawal such as vaginal itching/drainage, fever, or diarrhea.
3. Yogurt or buttermilk (4 oz) may be prescribed daily for diarrhea related to intestinal superinfections (to restore intestinal flora); consult provider.
4. Report signs of superinfection (black furry tongue, vaginal itching or discharge, and loose, foul-smelling stools). Nystatin may be ordered for secondary infections.
5. Immediately report any abnormal bleeding or bruising.
6. May cause false positive Coombs' test. This would be of concern if being cross-matched for blood transfusions or in newborns whose mothers have taken cephalosporins during pregnancy.
7. Avoid alcohol and alcohol-containing products, as a disulfiram-type reaction may occur.

Outcome/Evaluate

- Negative C&S reports
- Resolution of infection
- Symptomatic improvement, i.e., ↓ WBCs, ↓ fever, improved appetite

CHOLINERGIC BLOCKING AGENTS

Atropine sulfate
Benztropine mesylate
Biperiden hydrochloride
Dicyclomine hydrochloride
Ipratropium bromide
Propantheline bromide
Scopolamine hydrobromide
Scopolamine transdermal therapeutic system
Trihexyphenidyl hydrochloride

Action/Kinetics: Cholinergic blocking agents prevent the neurotransmitter acetylcholine from combining with receptors on the postganglionic parasympathetic nerve terminal (muscarinic site). Effects include reduction of smooth muscle spasms, blockade of vagal impulses to the heart, decreased secretions (e.g., gastric, salivation, bronchial mucus, sweat glands), production of mydriasis and cycloplegia, and various CNS effects. In therapeutic doses, these drugs have little effect on transmission of nerve impulses across ganglia (nicotinic sites) or at the neuromuscular junction. Several anticholinergic drugs abolish or reduce the S&S of Parkinson's disease, such as tremors and rigidity, and result in some improvement in mobility, muscular coordination, and motor performance. These effects may be due to blockade of the effects of acetylcholine in the CNS.

Uses: See individual drugs.

Contraindications: Glaucoma, adhesions between iris and lens of the eye, tachycardia, myocardial ischemia, unstable CV state in acute hemorrhage, partial obstruction of the GI and biliary tracts, prostatic hypertrophy, renal disease, myasthenia gravis, hepatic disease, paralytic ileus, pyloroduodenal stenosis, pyloric obstruction, intestinal atony, ulcerative colitis, obstructive uropathy. Cardiac clients, especially when there is danger of tachycardia; older persons suffering from atherosclerosis or mental impairment. Lactation.

Special Concerns: Use with caution in pregnancy. Infants and young children are more susceptible to the toxic side effects of anticholinergic drugs. Use in children when the ambient temperature is high may cause a rapid increase in body temperature due to suppression of sweat glands. Geriatric clients are particularly likely to manifest anticholinergic side effects and CNS effects, including agitation, confusion, drowsiness, excitement, glaucoma, and impaired memory. Use with caution in hyperthyroidism, CHF, cardiac arrhythmias, hypertension, Down syndrome, asthma, spastic paralysis, blonde individuals, allergies, and chronic lung disease.

Side Effects: These are desirable in some conditions and undesirable in others. Thus, the anticholinergics have an antisalivary effect that is useful in parkinsonism. This same effect is unpleasant when the drug is used for spastic conditions of the GI tract. Most side effects are dose-related and decrease when dosage decreases. *GI:* N&V, dry mouth, dysphagia, constipation, heartburn, change in taste perception, bloated feeling, paralytic ileus. *CNS:* Dizziness, drowsiness, nervousness, disorientation, headache, weakness, insomnia, fever (especially in children). Large doses may produce CNS stimulation including tremor and restlessness. Anticholinergic psychoses: ataxia, euphoria, confusion, disorientation, loss of short-term memory, decreased anxiety, fatigue, insomnia, hallucinations, dysarthria, agitation. *CV:* Palpitations. *GU:* Urinary retention or hesitancy, impotence. *Ophthalmologic:* Blurred vision, dilated pupils, photophobia, cycloplegia, precipitation of acute glaucoma. *Allergic:* Urticaria, skin rashes, ***anaphylaxis.*** *Other:* Flushing, decreased sweating, nasal congestion, suppression of glandular secretions including lactation. Heat prostration (fever and heat stroke) in presence of high environmental temperatures due to decreased sweating.

OD **Management of Overdose:** *Symptoms ("Belladonna Poisoning"):* Infants and children are especially susceptible to the toxic effects of atropine and scopolamine. Poisoning (dose-dependent) is characterized by the following symptoms: dry mouth, burning sensation of the mouth, difficulty in swallowing and speaking, blurred vision, photophobia, rash, tachycardia, increased respiration, ***increased body temperature*** (up to 109°F, 42.7°C), restlessness, irritability, confusion, muscle incoordination, dilated pupils, hot dry skin, ***respiratory depression and paralysis,*** tremors, ***seizures,*** hallucinations, and ***death.*** *Treatment ("Belladonna Poisoning"):*

- Gastric lavage or induction of vomiting followed by activated charcoal. General supportive measures.
- Anticholinergic effects can be reversed by physostigmine (Eserine), 1–3 mg IV (effectiveness uncertain; thus use other agents if possible). Neostigmine methylsulfate, 0.5–2 mg IV, repeated as necessary.
- If there is excitation, diazepam, a short-acting barbiturate, IV sodium thiopental (2% solution), or chloral hydrate (100–200 mL of a 2% solution by rectal infusion) may be given.
- For fever, cool baths may be used. Keep client in a darkened room if photophobia is manifested.
- Artificial respiration should be instituted if there is paralysis of respiratory muscles.

Drug Interactions

Amantadine / Additive anticholinergic side effects
Antacids / ↓ Absorption of anticholinergics from GI tract
Antidepressants, tricyclic / Additive anticholinergic side effects
Antihistamines / Additive anticholinergic side effects
Atenolol / Anticholinergics ↑ effects of atenolol
Benzodiazepines / Additive anticholinergic side effects
Corticosteroids / Additive ↑ intraocular pressure
Cyclopropane / ↑ Chance of ventricular arrhythmias
Digoxin / ↑ Effect of digoxin due to ↑ absorption from GI tract
Disopyramide / Potentiation of anticholinergic side effects
Guanethidine / Reversal of inhibition of gastric acid secretion caused by anticholinergics
Haloperidol / Additive ↑ intraocular pressure
Histamine / Reversal of inhibition of gastric acid secretion caused by anticholinergics
Levodopa / Possible ↓ effect of levodopa due to ↑ breakdown of levodopa in stomach (due to delayed gastric emptying time)
MAO inhibitors / ↑ Effect of anticholinergics due to ↓ breakdown by liver
Meperidine / Additive anticholinergic side effects
Methylphenidate / Potentiation of anticholinergic side effects
Metoclopramide / Anticholinergics block action of metoclopramide
Nitrates, nitrites / Potentiation of anticholinergic side effects
Nitrofurantoin / ↑ Bioavailability of nitrofurantoin
Orphenadrine / Additive anticholinergic side effects
Phenothiazines / Additive anticholinergic side effects; also, effects of phenothiazines may ↓
Primidone / Potentiation of anticholinergic side effects
Procainamide / Additive anticholinergic side effects
Quinidine / Additive anticholinergic side effects
Reserpine / Reversal of inhibition of gastric acid secretion caused by anticholinergics
Sympathomimetics / ↑ Bronchial relaxation
Thiazide diuretics / ↑ Bioavailability of thiazide diuretics
Thioxanthines / Potentiation of anticholinergic side effects

Dosage

See individual drugs.Dosage is often small. To prevent overdosage, check dosage and measure the drug exactly.

HEALTH CARE CONSIDERATIONS

Assessment

1. Record indications for therapy; assess for asthma, glaucoma, or duodenal ulcer (contraindications for therapy).
2. Note any renal disease, cardiac problems, or hepatic disease.
3. Determine age; elderly clients, especially those with mental impairment or atherosclerosis, should not receive these drugs.
4. Assess for constipation and urinary retention and tolerance.

Interventions

1. If the client complains of a dry mouth, provide frequent mouth care and cold drinks, especially postoperatively. Sugarless hard candies and chewing gum may also be of some benefit.
2. Drugs such as atropine may suppress thermoregulatory sweating; counsel client concerning activity (especially in hot weather) and appropriate clothing. Also, children and infants may exhibit "atropine fever."

Client/Family Teaching

1. Certain side effects are to be expected, such as dry mouth or blurred vision, and may have to be tolerated because of the overall beneficial effects of drug therapy. These should be reported so symptoms may be alleviated by reducing the dose or temporarily stopping drug.
2. With parkinsonism, do not withdraw abruptly. If the medication is changed, one drug should be withdrawn slowly and the other started in small doses.

Assessment

1. Monitor VS and ECG. Assess for any hemodynamic changes and intraventricular conduction blocks.
2. Note any complaints of palpitations.

OCULAR

Assessment

1. Determine any experience with these drugs and results.
2. Document IOP; assess accommodation and pupillary response.

Client/Family Teaching

1. Review methods for instillation of drops or ointment.
2. Vision will be affected by the meds; temporary stinging and blurred vision will occur. Assess response and plan activities for safety.
3. Night vision may be impaired. Photophobia, which may occur, can be relieved by wearing dark glasses.
4. Report any marked changes in vision, eye irritation, or persistent headaches immediately.
5. With large doses, tears may diminish; may experience dry or "sandy" eyes.

Interventions

1. Note complaints of dizziness or blurred vision; assist with ambulation and institute safety measures.
2. Hold meds and report any complaints of eye pain after instillation.

Outcome/Evaluate

- Dilation of pupils
- ↓ Bowel motility with improved elimination patterns
- ↑ HR
- ↓ Secretion production
- ↓ Muscle tremors, rigidity, and spasticity

ADDITIONAL HEALTH CARE CONSIDERATIONS RELATED TO PATHOLOGIC CONDITIONS FOR WHICH THE DRUG IS ADMINISTERED

CARDIOVASCULAR

GASTROINTESTINAL

Client/Family Teaching

1. Take early enough before a meal (at least 20 min) so that it will be effective when needed.
2. Review printed information related to the prescribed diet; see dietitian for assistance in meal planning as needed.
3. Gastric emptying times may be prolonged and intestinal transit time lengthened. Drug-induced intestinal paralysis is temporary and should resolve after 1–3 days of therapy.

GENITOURINARY

Client/Family Teaching

1. Report any evidence of urinary retention; may be more pronounced in elderly men with BPH.
2. Monitor I&O. Report evidence of bladder distention and need for catheterization if no u.o. >8 hr.
3. Consult with the provider for medication adjustment if impotence occurs; may be drug-related.

CORTICOSTEROIDS

See also the following individual entries:

Beclomethasone dipropionate
Betamethasone
Betamethasone dipropionate
Betamethasone valerate
Budesonide

Cortisone acetate
Dexamethasone
Dexamethasone acetate
Dexamethasone sodium phosphate
Fludrocortisone acetate
Flunisolide
Fluticasone propionate
Hydrocortisone
Hydrocortisone acetate
Hydrocortisone butyrate
Hydrocortisone cypionate
Hydrocortisone sodium phosphate
Hydrocortisone sodium succinate
Hydrocortisone valerate
Loteprednol etabonate
Methylprednisolone
Methylprednisolone acetate
Methylprednisolone sodium succinate
Mometasone furoate monohydrate
Prednisolone
Prednisolone acetate
Prednisolone acetate and Prednisolone sodium phosphate
Prednisolone sodium phosphate
Prednisolone tebutate
Prednisone
Rimexolone
Triamcinolone
Triamcinolone acetonide
Triamcinolone diacetate
Triamcinolone hexacetonide

Action/Kinetics: The hormones of the adrenal gland influence many metabolic pathways and all organ systems and are essential for survival. These processes include carbohydrate metabolism (e.g., glycogen deposition in the liver and conversion of glycogen to glucose), protein metabolism (e.g., gluconeogenesis, protein catabolism), fat metabolism (e.g., deposition of fatty tissue), and water and electrolyte balance (e.g., fluid retention, excretion of potassium, calcium, and phosphorus).

According to their chemical structure and chief physiologic effect, the corticosteroids fall into two subgroups, which have considerable functional overlap. First are those, like cortisone and hydrocortisone, that mainly regulate the metabolic pathways involving protein, carbohydrate, and fat. This group is often referred to as *glucocorticoids*. In the second group are those, like aldosterone and desoxycorticosterone, that are more specifically involved in electrolyte and water balance. These are often referred to as *mineralocorticoids*. Hormones, such as cortisone and hydrocortisone, although classified as glucocorticoids, possess significant mineralocorticoid activity. Therapeutically, a distinction must be made between physiologic doses used for replacement therapy and pharmacologic doses used to treat inflammatory and other disease states.

The hormones have a marked anti-inflammatory effect because of their ability to inhibit prostaglandin synthesis. These agents also inhibit accumulation of macrophages and leukocytes at sites of inflammation as well as inhibit phagocytosis and lysosomal enzyme release. They aid the organism in coping with various stressful situations (trauma, severe illness). The immunosuppressant effect is thought to be due to a reduction of the number of T lymphocytes, monocytes, and eosinophils. Corticosteroids also decrease binding of immunoglobulin to receptors on the cell surface and inhibit the synthesis and/or release of interleukins which, in turn, decrease T-lymphocyte blastogenesis and reduce the primary immune response.

Uses: When used for anti-inflammatory or immunosuppressant therapy, the corticosteroid should possess minimal mineralocorticoid activity. Therapy with glucocorticoids is not curative and in many situations should be considered as adjunctive rather than primary therapy. The following list is not inclusive but provides examples of the physiologic and pharmacologic uses of corticosteroids.

1. **Replacement therapy.** Acute and chronic adrenal insufficiency, including Addison's disease. For replacement therapy, drugs must possess both glucocorticoid and mineralocorticoid effects.
2. **Rheumatic disorders,** including rheumatoid arthritis (including juveniles), other types of arthritis, ankylosing spondylitis, acute and subacute bursitis.
3. **Collagen diseases,** including SLE.
4. **Allergic diseases,** including control of severe allergic conditions as serum sickness, drug hypersensitivity reactions, anaphylaxis.
5. **Respiratory diseases,** including prophylaxis and treatment of bronchial asthma (and status asthmaticus), seasonal or perennial rhinitis.
6. **Ocular diseases,** including severe acute and chronic allergic and inflammatory conditions. Corneal injury.
7. **Dermatologic diseases,** including angioedema or urticaria, contact dermatitis, atopic dermatitis, severe erythema multiforme (Stevens-Johnson syndrome).
8. **Diseases of the intestinal tract,** including chronic ulcerative colitis, regional enteritis.
9. **Nervous system,** including acute exacerbations of multiple sclerosis, optic neuritis.
10. **Malignancies,** including leukemias and lymphomas in adults and acute leukemia in children.
11. **Nephrotic syndrome,** including that

due to lupus erythematosus or of the idiopathic type.

12. **Hematologic diseases,** including acquired hemolytic anemia, RBC anemia, idiopathic and secondary thrombocytopenic purpura in adults, congenital hypoplastic anemia.

13. **Intra-articular or soft tissue administration,** including acute episodes of synovitis osteoarthritis, rheumatoid arthritis, acute gouty arthritis, bursitis.

14. **Intralesional administration,** including keloids, psoriatic plaques, discoid lupus erythematosus.

Lotions are considered best for weeping eruptions, especially in areas subject to chafing (axilla, feet, and groin). Creams are suitable for most inflammations; ointments are preferred for dry, scaly lesions.

Contraindications: Suspected infection as these drugs may mask infections. Also peptic ulcer, psychoses, acute glomerulonephritis, herpes simplex infections of the eye, vaccinia or varicella, the exanthematous diseases, Cushing's syndrome, active tuberculosis, myasthenia gravis. Recent intestinal anastomoses, CHF or other cardiac disease, hypertension, systemic fungal infections, open-angle glaucoma. Also, hyperlipidemia, hyperthyroidism or hypothyroidism, osteoporosis, myasthenia gravis, tuberculosis. Lactation (if high doses are used). Inhalation products to relieve acute bronchospasms.

Topically in the eye for dendritic keratitis, vaccinia, chickenpox, other viral disease that may involve the conjunctiva or cornea, and tuberculosis and fungal or acute purulent infections of the eye. Topically in the ear in aural fungal infections and perforated eardrum. Topically in tuberculosis of the skin, herpes simplex, vaccinia, varicella, and infectious conditions in the absence of anti-infective agents.

Inhalation products for relief of acute bronchospasms, primary treatment of status asthmaticus, or other acute episodes of asthma.

Special Concerns: Use with caution in diabetes mellitus, hypertension, chronic nephritis, thrombophlebitis, convulsive disorders, infectious diseases, renal or hepatic insufficiency, pregnancy. Chronic use may inhibit the growth and development of children or adolescents. Pediatric clients are also at greater risk for developing cataracts, osteoporosis, avascular necrosis of the femoral heads, and glaucoma. Geriatric clients are more likely to develop hypertension and osteoporosis (especially postmenopausal women). Use inhalation products with caution in children less than 6 years of age.

Side Effects: Small physiologic doses given as replacement therapy or short-term high-dosage therapy during emergencies rarely cause side effects. Prolonged therapy may cause a Cushing-like syndrome with atrophy of the adrenal cortex and subsequent adrenocortical insufficiency. A steroid withdrawal syndrome may occur following prolonged use; symptoms include anorexia, N&V, lethargy, headache, fever, joint pain, desquamation, myalgia, weight loss, hypotension.

SYSTEMIC: *Fluid and electrolyte:* Edema, hypokalemic alkalosis, hypokalemia, hypocalcemia, hypotension or shock-like reaction, hypertension, CHF. *Musculoskeletal:* Muscle wasting, muscle pain or weakness, osteoporosis, spontaneous fractures including vertebral compression fractures and fractures of long bones, tendon rupture, aseptic necrosis of femoral and humeral heads. *GI:* N&V, anorexia or increased appetite, diarrhea or constipation, abdominal distention, pancreatitis, gastric irritation, ulcerative esophagitis. ***Development or exacerbation of peptic ulcers with the possibility of perforation and hemorrhage; perforation of the small and large bowel,*** especially in inflammatory bowel disease. *Endocrine:* Cushing's syndrome (e.g., central obesity, moonface, buffalo hump, enlargement of supraclavicular fat pads), amenorrhea, postmenopausal bleeding, menstrual irregularities, decreased glucose tolerance, hyperglycemia, glycosuria, increased insulin or sulfonylurea requirement in diabetics, development of diabetes mellitus, negative nitrogen balance due to protein catabolism, suppression of growth in children, secondary adrenocortical and pituitary unresponsiveness (especially during periods of stress). *CNS/Neurologic:* Headache, vertigo, insomnia, restlessness, increased motor activity, ischemic neuropathy, EEG abnormalities, ***seizures,*** pseudotumor cerebri. Also, euphoria, mood swings, depression, anxiety, personality changes, psychoses. *CV:* Thromboembolism, thrombophlebitis, ECG changes (due to potassium deficiency), fat embolism, necrotizing angiitis, cardiac arrhythmias, ***myocardial rupture following recent MI,*** syncopal episodes. *Dermatologic:* Impaired wound healing, skin atrophy and thinning, petechiae, ecchymoses, erythema, purpura, striae, hirsutism, urticaria, ***angioneurotic edema,*** acneiform eruptions, allergic dermatitis, lupus erythematosus-like lesions, suppression of skin test reactions, perineal irritation. *Ophthal-*

mic: Glaucoma, posterior subcapsular cataracts, increased intraocular pressure, exophthalmos. *Miscellaneous:* Hypercholesterolemia, atherosclerosis, aggravation or masking of infections, leukocytosis, increased or decreased motility and number of spermatozoa. **In children:** Suppression of linear growth; reversible pseudobrain tumor syndrome characterized by papilledema, oculomotor or abducens nerve paralysis, visual loss, or headache.

PARENTERAL USE: Sterile abscesses, Charcot-like arthropathy, subcutaneous and cutaneous atrophy, burning or tingling (especially in the perineal area following IV use), scarring, inflammation, paresthesia, induration, hyperpigmentation or hypopigmentation, blindness when used intralesionally around the face and head (rare), transient or delayed pain or soreness, nystagmus, ataxia, muscle twitching, hiccoughs, ***anaphylaxis with or without circulatory collapse, cardiac arrest, bronchospasm,*** arachnoiditis after intrathecal use, foreign body granulomatous reactions.

INTRA-ARTICULAR: Postinjection flare, Charcot-like arthropathy, tendon rupture, skin atrophy, facial flushing, osteonecrosis. Due to reduction in inflammation and pain, clients may overuse the joint.

INTRASPINAL: Aseptic, bacterial, chemical, cryptococcal, or tubercular meningitis; adhesive arachnoiditis, conus medullaris syndrome.

INTRAOCULAR: Increased ocular pressure, thereby inducing or aggravating simple glaucoma. Stinging, burning, dendritic keratitis (herpes simplex), corneal perforation (especially when the drugs are used for diseases that cause corneal thinning). Posterior subcapsular cataracts, especially in children. Exophthalmos, secondary fungal or viral eye infections.

TOPICAL USE: When used over large areas, when the skin is broken, or with occlusive dressings, may cause atrophy of the epidermis, drying of the skin, or atrophy of the dermal collagen. When used on the face, diffuse thinning and homogenization of the collagen, epidermal thinning, and striae formation. Occasionally, sensitization reaction may occur, which necessitates discontinuation of the drug.

OD **Management of Overdose:** *Symptoms (Continued Use of Large Doses)—Cushing's Syndrome:* Acne, hypertension, moonface, striae, hirsutism, central obesity, ecchymoses, myopathy, sexual dysfunction, osteoporosis, diabetes, hyperlipidemia, increased susceptibility to infection, peptic ulcer, electrolyte and fluid imbalance. Acute toxicity or death is rare. *Treatment of Chronic Overdose:* Gradually taper the dose of the steroid and frequently monitor lab tests. During periods of stress, steroid supplementation is necessary. Dose should be reduced to the lowest one that will control the symptoms (or discontinue the steroid completely). Recovery of normal adrenal and pituitary function may take up to 9 months. Large, acute overdoses may be treated with gastric lavage, emesis, and general supportive measures.

Drug Interactions

Acetaminophen / ↑ Risk of hepatotoxicity due to ↑ rate of formation of hepatotoxic acetaminophen metabolite
Alcohol / ↑ Risk of GI ulceration or hemorrhage
Amphotericin B / Corticosteroids ↑ K depletion caused by amphotericin B
Aminoglutethimide / ↓ Adrenal response to corticotropin
Anabolic steroids / ↑ Risk of edema
Antacids / ↓ Effect of corticosteroids due to ↓ absorption from GI tract
Antibiotics, broad-spectrum / Concomitant use may result in emergence of resistant strains, leading to severe infection
Anticholinergics / Combination ↑ intraocular pressure; will aggravate glaucoma
Anticoagulants, oral / ↓ Effect of anticoagulants by ↓ hypoprothrombinemia; also ↑ risk of hemorrhage due to vascular effects of corticosteroids
Anticholinesterases / Corticosteroids may ↓ effect of anticholinesterases when used in myasthenia gravis
Antidiabetic agents / Hyperglycemic effect of corticosteroids may necessitate an ↑ dose of antidiabetic agent
Asparaginase / ↑ Hyperglycemic effect of asparaginase and the risk of neuropathy and disturbances in erythropoiesis
Barbiturates / ↓ Effect of corticosteroids due to ↑ breakdown by liver
Bumetanide / Enhanced potassium loss due to potassium-losing properties of both drugs
Carbonic anhydrase inhibitors / Corticosteroids ↑ K depletion caused by carbonic anhydrase inhibitors
Cholestyramine / ↓ Effect of corticosteroids due to ↓ absorption from GI tract
Colestipol / ↓ Effect of corticosteroids due to ↓ absorption from GI tract
Contraceptives, oral / Estrogen ↑ anti-inflammatory effect of hydrocortisone by ↓ breakdown by liver
Cyclophosphoramide / ↑ Effect of cyclophosphoramide due to ↓ breakdown by liver

Cyclosporine / ↑ Effect of both drugs due to ↓ breakdown by liver
Digitalis glycosides / ↑ Chance of digitalis toxicity (arrhythmias) due to hypokalemia
Ephedrine / ↓ Effect of corticosteroids due to ↑ breakdown by liver
Estrogens / ↑ Anti-inflammatory effect of hydrocortisone by ↓ breakdown by liver
Ethacrynic acid / Enhanced potassium loss due to potassium-losing properties of both drugs
Folic acid / Requirements may ↑
Furosemide / Enhanced potassium loss due to potassium-losing properties of both drugs
Heparin / Ulcerogenic effects of corticosteroids may ↑ risk of hemorrhage
Immunosuppressant drugs / ↑ Risk of infection
Indomethacin / ↑ Chance of GI ulceration
Insulin / Hyperglycemic effect of corticosteroids may necessitate ↑ dose of antidiabetic agent
Isoniazid / ↓ Effect of isoniazid due to ↑ breakdown by liver and ↑ excretion
Ketoconazole / ↓ Effect of corticosteroids due to ↑ rate of clearance
Mexiletine / ↓ Effect of mexiletine due to ↑ breakdown by liver
Mitotane / ↓ Response of adrenal gland to corticotropin
Muscle relaxants, nondepolarizing / ↓ Effect of muscle relaxants
Neuromuscular blocking agents / ↑ Risk of prolonged respiratory depression or paralysis
NSAIDs / ↑ Risk of GI hemorrhage or ulceration
Phenobarbital / ↓ Effect of corticosteroids due to ↑ breakdown by liver
Phenytoin / ↓ Effect of corticosteroids due to ↑ breakdown by liver
Potassium supplements / ↓ Plasma levels of potassium
Rifampin / ↓ Effect of corticosteroids due to ↑ breakdown by liver
Ritodrine / ↑ Risk of maternal edema
Salicylates / Both are ulcerogenic; also, corticosteroids may ↓ blood salicylate levels
Somatrem, Somatropin / Glucocorticoids may inhibit effect of somatrem
Streptozocin / ↑ Risk of hyperglycemia
Theophyllines / Corticosteroids ↑ effect of theophyllines
Thiazide diuretics / Enhanced potassium loss due to potassium-losing properties of both drugs
Tricyclic antidepressants / ↑ Risk of mental disturbances
Vitamin A / Topical vitamin A can reverse impaired wound healing in clients receiving corticosteroids

Dosage

Highly individualized, according to both the condition being treated and the client's response. Therapy must not be discontinued abruptly. Except for replacement therapy, treatment should always involve the minimum effective dose and the shortest period of time. If corticosteroids are used for replacement therapy or high doses are used for prolonged periods of time, the dose must be *increased* if surgery is required.

Laboratory Test Considerations: ↑ Urine glucose, serum cholesterol, serum amylase. ↓ Serum potassium, triiodothyronine, serum uric acid. Alteration of electrolyte balance.

Special Considerations

1. Check child's height and weight regularly and graph; growth suppression may occur with corticosteroid therapy; not prevented by growth hormone administration.
2. Large doses of glucocorticoids in children may increase intracranial pressure (pseudotumor cerebri); report symptoms: vertigo, headache, and convulsions. These should disappear once therapy discontinued.

1. Administer PO forms of drug with food to minimize ulcerogenic effect.
2. At frequent intervals, reduce the dose gradually to determine if symptoms of the disease can be effectively controlled by smaller drug dose.
3. When treating clients with conditions such as asthma, ulcerative colitis, and rheumatoid arthritis, corticosteroids, given every other day, provide the beneficial effect of the steroid while minimizing pituitary-adrenal suppression. With this therapy, twice the usual daily dose of an intermediate-acting steroid is given every other morning.
4. Local administration of corticosteroids is preferred over systemic therapy to minimize systemic side effects.
5. Discontinue gradually if used chronically.

HEALTH CARE CONSIDERATIONS

Administration of Topical Corticosteroids

1. Cleanse area before applying the medication.
2. Wear gloves, apply sparingly, and rub gently into the area.
3. When prescribed, apply an occlusive dressing (not to be used if an infection is present) to promote hydration of the stra-

tum corneum and increase the absorption of the medication.The following are two methods of applying an occlusive type dressing:

- Apply a large amount of medication to the cleansed area. Cover with a thin, pliable, nonflammable plastic film, which is then sealed to the surrounding tissue with skin tape or held in place with gauze. Change the dressing q 3–4 days.
- Apply a small amount of medication to the area and cover with a damp cloth. Then cover with a thin, pliable, nonflammable plastic film and seal to the surrounding tissue with tape, or hold in place with gauze. Change dressing b.i.d.

Assessment: (General)

1. Record indications for therapy, type, onset, and characteristics of symptoms; note underlying cause: adrenal or nonadrenal disorder.
2. Note mental status (i.e., mood, affect, aggression, behavioral changes, depression) and neurologic function.
3. Check for evidence of allergic reactions to corticosteroids or tartrazine.
4. Monitor ECG, electrolytes, BS, urinalysis, renal and LFTs.
5. Record VS and weight. Obtain CXR and PPD if therapy prolonged.
6. Note childhood illnesses and immunization status.
7. List medications taking and identify those that may interact with corticosteroids. These include antidiabetic agents, cardiac glycosides, oral contraceptives, anticoagulants, and drugs influenced by liver enzymes.
8. If female, determine if pregnant.

Interventions

TOPICAL CORTICOSTEROIDS

1. Assess for local sensitivity reaction at the site of application.
2. Absorption varies regionally with the highest absorption in scrotal skin and the lowest on the foot. Inflamed skin enhances absorption several-fold.
3. Better action has been noted with the ointment bases than with the lotion or cream vehicles.
4. Observe for signs of infections since corticosteroids tend to mask. Avoid occlusive dressing when an infection is present. Document the site of the infection, the nature of the infection, and characteristics (e.g., redness, swelling, odor, or drainage).
5. With large occlusive dressing, take temperatures q 4 hr. Report if elevated and remove the dressing.
6. Assess for evidence of systemic absorption. Longterm use of large quantities of potent topical corticosteroids to large BSAs may precipitate iatrogenic Cushing's syndrome. Symptoms may include edema and transient inhibition of pituitary-adrenal cortical function as manifested by muscular pain, lassitude, depression, hypotension, and weight loss.
7. Advise family members applying the topical ointment to wash their hands and to wear gloves or to apply with a sterile applicator (e.g., tongue blade).
8. Report erythema, telangiectases, purpura, bruising, pustules, and depressed shiny, wrinkled skin. Prolonged use of potent topical corticosteroids may increase incidence of systemic side effects.

Interventions

ORAL CORTICOSTEROIDS

1. When first placed on corticosteroids, check BP b.i.d. until maintenance dose established; report increases.
2. Short-term oral therapy (e.g., 60 mg PO for 5 days) does not require divided doses or titration. With long-term therapy, continuously monitor for symptoms of adrenal insufficiency, which include hypotension, confusion, restlessness, lethargy, weakness, N&V, anorexia, and weight loss; titrate dose to withdraw.
3. Evaluate for increased sodium and fluid retention. Monitor weight and observe for edema. If noted, adjust the diet to one low in sodium and high in potassium. Anticipate a small weight gain due to increased appetite, but sudden increases are probably due to edema. Edema occurs most frequently with cortisone or desoxycorticosterone acetate and less frequently with the synthetic agents.
4. Assess for SOB, distended neck veins, edema, and easy fatigue; S&S of CHF. Obtain a CXR and ECG.
5. Monitor serum glucose, electrolytes, and platelet counts with long-term therapy. Report any unusual bleeding, bruising, the presence of petechiae, symptoms of diabetes, and any other skin changes.
6. Assess muscles for weakness and wasting; signs of a negative nitrogen balance.
7. Report changes in appearance, especially those resembling Cushing's syndrome (such as rounding of the face, hirsutism, presence of acne, and thinning of the hair and nails) so dosage can be adjusted.
8. With diabetes, may develop hyperglycemia necessitating a change in diet and insulin dosage.
9. Assess for signs of depression, lack of interest in personal appearance, insomnia or anorexia.
10. Discuss potential for menstrual difficulties and amenorrhea related to long-term therapy.

11. Observe for S&S of other illnesses as these drugs tend to mask the severity of most illnesses.
12. GI bleeding may occur; periodically test stools for occult blood and monitor hematologic profile.

Client/Family Teaching

1. These agents generally work by inhibiting or decreasing the inflammatory response.
2. Take the oral medication with food and report any symptoms of gastric distress. To prevent gastric irritation, may use antacids and eat frequent small meals. If the symptoms persist, diagnostic X rays may be indicated.
3. High doses of glucocorticoids stimulate the stomach to produce excess acid and pepsin and may cause peptic ulcers. Antacids 3–4 times/day may relieve epigastric distress.
4. Report changes in mood or affect.
5. Obtain weight daily at the same time, wearing clothing of approximately the same weight, and using the same scales. Consistent weight gain may reflect fluid retention; initiate caloric management to prevent obesity.
6. Identify foods high in potassium and low in sodium to prevent electrolyte disturbances. Supplement diet with potassium-rich foods such as citrus juices, collard greens, or bananas. Read labels of canned or processed foods and consult dietician for assistance in shopping and meal preparation.
7. Eat a diet high in protein to compensate for the loss due to protein breakdown from gluconeogenesis.
8. Exercise daily and consume foods high in calcium to decrease possibility of osteoporosis (due to catabolic bone effects). Consume adequate protein, calcium, and vitamin D to minimize bone loss. On-going bone resorption with depressed bone formation is the cause of osteoporosis.
9. Avoid falls and accidents. Steroids may cause osteoporosis, which makes the bones more susceptible to fractures. Use a night light and a hand rail or other device for support if need to get up at night.
10. Corticosteroids can cause a loss of contraceptive action with oral contraceptives. Keep accurate menstrual records and consider alternative methods of birth control. May also have an adverse effect on sperm production and count.
11. Weight gain, acne, and excess hair growth may occur.
12. Need to gradually withdraw the medication when therapy has exceeded 7 consecutive days. This should proceed slowly so that the adrenal cortex will gradually be reactivated and take over the production of hormones. Sudden withdrawal may be life-threatening. Any sudden change will provoke symptoms of adrenal insufficiency.
13. With dosage reduction, flare-ups may occur; these are caused by the reduction.
14. With arthritis, do not overuse the joint once injected and painless. Permanent joint damage may result from overuse, because underlying pathology is still present.
15. With diabetes, monitor glucose levels frequently and report changes as insulin dose and diet may require adjustment.
16. Wounds may heal slowly because steroid therapy causes a delay in development of granulation tissue, increasing potential for infection. Observe any healing process for signs of infection and report any injury or postoperative separation of wound or suture line.
17. These drugs mask symptoms of infection and cause immunosuppression. Because antibody production is decreased by corticosteroids, clients are at risk for infection. Must maintain general hygiene and scrupulous cleanliness to avoid infection. Report if sore throat, cough, fever, malaise, or an injury that does not heal occurs. Avoid contact with persons with contagious diseases.
18. Delay any vaccinations, immunizations, or skin testing while receiving corticosteroid therapy because there is limited immune response.
19. Clients on long-term eye therapy are prone to developing cataracts, exophthalmus, and increased IOP. Schedule routine eye exams.
20. Avoid OTC meds, including aspirin and ibuprofen compounds, as well as alcohol, since these may aggravate gastric irritation and bleeding.
21. Carry ID, listing drugs and dosage, condition being treated, and who to contact in the event of an emergency.

Outcome/Evaluate

- Effective wound healing
- Suppression of inflammatory/immune responses or disease manifestation in allergic reactions, autoimmune diseases, and organ transplants
- Serum cortisol levels within desired range in adrenal deficiency states (8 a.m. level 110–520 nmol/L)

DIURETICS, LOOP

See also the following individual entries:

Bumetanide
Ethacrynate sodium

Ethacrynic acid
Furosemide
Torsemide

Action/Kinetics: Loop diuretics inhibit reabsorption of sodium and chloride in the proximal and distal tubules and the loop of Henle. Metabolized in the liver and excreted primarily through the urine. Significantly bound to plasma protein.

See also *Diuretics, Thiazides.*

Uses: See individual drugs.

Contraindications: Hypersensitivity to loop diruetics or to sulfonylureas. In hepatic coma or severe electrolyte depletion (until condition improves or is corrected). Lactation.

Special Concerns: Sudden alterations of electrolytes in hepatic cirrhosis and ascites may precipitate hepatic encephalopathy and coma. SLE may be activated or worsened. Ototoxicity is most common with rapid injection, in severe renal impairment, with doses several times the usual dose, and with concurrent use of other ototoxic drugs. The risk of hospitalization is doubled in geriatric clients who take diuretics and NSAIDs. Safety and efficacy of most loop diuretics have not been determined in children or infants.

Side Effects: See individual drugs. Excessive diuresis may cause dehydration with the possibility of ***circulatory collapse and vascular thrombosis or embolism.*** Ototoxicity including tinnitus, hearing impairment, deafness (usually reversible), and vertigo with a sense of fullness are possible. Electrolyte imbalance, especially in clients with restricted salt intake. Photosensitivity. Changes include hypokalemia, hypomagnesemia, and hypocalcemia.

OD **Management of Overdose:** *Symptoms:* Acute profound water loss, volume and electrolyte depletion, dehydration, decreased blood volume, and ***circulatory collapse with possibility of fascicular thrombosis and embolism.*** *Treatment:* Replace fluid and electrolyte loss. Carefully monitor urine and plasma electrolyte levels. Emesis and gastric lavage may be useful. Supportive measures may include oxygen or artificial respiration.

Drug Interactions

Aminoglycosides / ↑ Ototoxicity with hearing loss
Anticoagulants / ↑ Anticoagulant activity
Chloral hydrate / Transient diaphoresis, hot flashes, hypertension, tachycardia, weakness and nausea
Cisplatin / Additive ototoxicity
Digitalis glycosides / ↑ Risk of arrhythmias due to diuretic-induced electrolyte disturbances
Lithium / ↑ Plasma levels of lithium → toxicity
Muscle relaxants, nondepolarizing / Effect of muscle relaxants may be either ↑ or ↓, depending on the dose of diuretic
Nonsteroidal anti-inflammatory drugs / ↓ Effect of loop diuretics
Probenecid / ↓ Effect of loop diuretics
Salicylates / Diuretic effect may be ↓ in clients with cirrhosis and ascites
Sulfonylureas/ Loop diuretics may ↓ glucose tolerance
Theophyllines / Action of theophyllines may be ↑ or ↓
Thiazide diuretics / Additive effects with loop diuretics → profound diuresis and serious electrolyte abnormalities

Dosage

See individual drugs.

HEALTH CARE CONSIDERATIONS

See also *Diuretics, Thiazides.*

Assessment

1. Record indications for therapy. Note other agents prescribed and the outcome.
2. Monitor CBC, electrolytes, Mg, Ca, glucose, uric acid, renal and LFTs.
3. Note any sensitivity to sulfonamides. May exhibit cross-reactivity with furosemide.
4. Determine presence of SLE; drug may worsen condition.
5. Assess auditory function carefully when large doses are anticipated or when used concurrently with other ototoxic agents. Ototoxicity is dose related and generally reversible.

Interventions

1. Record weights I&O; keep bedpan or urinal within reach. Report absence/decrease in diuresis and note changes in lung sounds.
2. When ambulatory, check for edema in the extremities; if on bed rest, check for edema in the sacral area.
3. Monitor for serum electrolyte levels, pH, and the following *signs of electrolyte imbalance:*

- *Hyponatremia* (low-salt syndrome)—characterized by muscle weakness, leg cramps, dryness of mouth, dizziness, and GI upset.
- *Hypernatremia* (excessive sodium retention)—characterized by CNS disturbances, i.e., confusion, loss of sensorium, stupor, and coma. Poor skin turgor and postural hypotension not as prominent as with combined sodium and water deficits.
- *Water intoxication* (caused by defective water diuresis)—characterized by lethargy,

confusion, stupor, and coma. Neuromuscular hyperexcitability with increased reflexes, muscular twitching, and convulsions if acute.

- *Metabolic acidosis*—characterized by weakness, headache, malaise, abdominal pain, and N&V. Hyperpnea occurs in severe metabolic acidosis. S&S of volume depletion: poor skin turgor, soft eyeballs, and dry tongue may be observed.
- *Metabolic alkalosis*—characterized by irritability, neuromuscular hyperexcitability, tetany if severe.
- *Hypokalemia (potassium deficiency)*—characterized by muscular weakness, peristalsis failure, postural hypotension, respiratory embarrassment, and cardiac arrhythmias.
- *Hyperkalemia (excess potassium)*—characterized by early signs of irritability, nausea, intestinal colic, and diarrhea; and by later signs of weakness, flaccid paralysis, dyspnea, dysphagia, and arrhythmias.

4. With high doses monitor for hyperlipidemia and hyperuricemia; precipitating a gout attack.
5. With liver dysfunction, assess for electrolyte imbalances, which could cause stupor, coma, and death.
6. If receiving EC potassium tablets, assess for abdominal pain, distention, or GI bleeding; can cause small bowel ulceration. Check stool for intact tablets.
7. Diuretics potentiate the effects of antihypertensive agents; monitor BP.
8. May precipitate symptoms of diabetes with latent or mild diabetes. Test urine or perform finger sticks and monitor chemisty studies.
9. Hyper- or hypokalemia associated with diuretic therapy may potentiate the toxic effects of digitalis and precipitate arrhythmias.
10. Assess for sore throat, skin rash, and yellowing of the skin or sclera; may be blood dyscrasias.

Client/Family Teaching

1. May cause frequent, copious voiding. Plan activities and take in the morning to prevent sleep disruption.
2. Take with food or milk to decrease GI upset.
3. Weakness and/or dizziness may occur. Rise slowly from bed and sit down or lie down if evident. Use caution in driving a car or operating other hazardous machinery until drug effects apparent.
4. The use of alcohol, standing for prolonged periods, and exercise in hot weather may enhance/lower BP.
5. Ensure adequate fluids; monitor BP and weight. Report excessive weight loss, loss of skin turgor or if dizziness, nausea, muscle weakness, cramps, or tingling of the extremities occurs.
6. Wear protective clothing, sunscreens, and sunglasses to prevent photosensitivity reactions.
7. Include foods high in potassium, such as citrus, grape, cranberry, apple, pear, and apricot juices; bananas; meat, fish, or fowl; cereals; and tea and cola beverages. This is preferable to taking potassium chloride supplements but potassium supplements are usually prescribed with non-potassium-sparing diuretics. Unless conditions such as gastric ulcer or diabetes exists, drink a large glass of orange juice daily. Consult dietitian as needed, for assistance in shopping, planning, selecting, and preparing foods.
8. Avoid all OTC preparations without approval.

Outcome/Evaluate

- Symptomatic relief (↓ weight, ↓ swelling/edema, ↑ diuresis)
- Clinical improvement in S&S associated with CHF and renal failure

DIURETICS, THIAZIDES

See also the following individual entries:

Chlorothiazide
Chlorthalidone
Hydrochlorothiazide
Indapamide

Action/Kinetics: Thiazides promote diuresis by decreasing the rate at which sodium and chloride are reabsorbed by the distal renal tubules of the kidney. By increasing the excretion of sodium and chloride, they force excretion of additional water. They also increase the excretion of potassium and, to a lesser extent, bicarbonate, as well as decrease the excretion of calcium and uric acid. Sodium and chloride are excreted in approximately equal amounts. Thiazides do not affect the glomerular filtration rate. Thiazides also have an antihypertensive effect which is attributed to direct dilation of the arterioles, as well as to a reduction in the total fluid volume of the body and altered sodium balance. The thiazide diuretics are related chemically to the sulfonamides. Although devoid of anti-infective activity, the thiazides can cause the same hypersensitivity reactions as the sulfonamides. A large fraction is excreted unchanged in urine.

Uses: Edema, CHF, hypertension, pregnancy, and premenstrual tension. Thiazides are used for edema due to CHF, nephrosis, nephritis, renal failure, PMS, hepatic cirrhosis, corticosteroid or estrogen therapy. Hypertension. *Investigational:* Thiazides are used alone or in combination with allopurinol (or amiloride) for prophylaxis of calcium nephrolithiasis. Nephrogenic diabetes insipidus.

Contraindications: Hypersensitivity to drug, anuria, renal decompensation. Impaired renal function and advanced hepatic cirrhosis. Do not use indiscriminately in clients with edema and toxemia of pregnancy, even though they may be therapeutically useful, because the thiazides may have adverse effects on the newborn (thrombocytopenia and jaundice).

Special Concerns: Geriatric clients may manifest an increased risk of hypotension and changes in electrolyte levels. The risk of hospitalization is doubled in geriatric clients who take diuretics and NSAIDs. Administer with caution to debilitated clients or to those with a history of hepatic coma or precoma, gout, diabetes mellitus, or during pregnancy and lactation. Particular care must be exercised when thiazides are administered concomitantly with drugs that also cause potassium loss, such as digitalis, corticosteroids, and some estrogens. Clients with advanced heart failure, renal disease, or hepatic cirrhosis are most likely to develop hypokalemia. May activate or worsen SLE.

Side Effects: The following side effects may be observed with most thiazides. See also individual drugs. *Electrolyte imbalance:* Hypokalemia (most frequent) characterized by cardiac arrhythmias. Hyponatremia characterized by weakness, lethargy, epigastric distress, N&V. Hypokalemic alkalosis. *GI:* Anorexia, epigastric distress or irritation, N&V, cramping, bloating, abdominal pain, diarrhea, constipation, jaundice, pancreatitis. *CNS:* Dizziness, lightheadedness, headache, vertigo, xanthopsia, paresthesias, weakness, insomnia, restlessness. *CV:* Orthostatic hypotension, MIs in elderly clients with advanced arteriosclerosis, especially if the client is also receiving therapy with other antihypertensive agents. *Hematologic:* ***Agranulocytosis, aplastic or hypoplastic anemia, hemolytic anemia,*** leukopenia, thrombocytopenia. *Dermatologic:* Purpura, photosensitivity, photosensitivity dermatitis, rash, urticaria, necrotizing angiitis, vasculitis, cutaneous vasculitis. *Metabolic:* neutropenia, hemolytic anemia. *Endocrine:* Hyperglycemia, glycosuria, hyperuricemia. *Miscellaneous:* Blurred vision, impotence, reduced libido, fever, muscle cramps, muscle spasm, respiratory distress.

OD **Management of Overdose:** *Symptoms:* Symptoms of plasma volume depletion, including orthostatic hypotension, dizziness, drowsiness, syncope, electrolyte abnormalities, hemoconcentration, hemodynamic changes. Signs of potassium depletion, including confusion, dizziness, muscle weakness, and GI disturbances. Also, N&V, GI irritation, GI hypermotility, CNS effects, cardiac abnormalities, ***seizures, hypotension, decreased respiration, and coma.*** *Treatment:*

- Induce emesis or perform gastric lavage followed by activated charcoal. Undertake measures to prevent aspiration.
- Electrolyte balance, hydration, respiration, CV, and renal function must be maintained. Cathartics should be avoided, as use may enhance fluid loss.
- Although GI effects are usually of short duration, treatment may be required.

Drug Interactions

Allopurinol / ↑ Risk of hypersensitivity reactions to allopurinol
Amphotericin B / Enhanced loss of electrolytes, especially potassium
Anesthetics / Thiazides may ↑ effects of anesthetics
Anticholinergic agents / ↑ Effect of thiazides due to ↑ amount absorbed from GI tract
Anticoagulants, oral / Anticoagulant effects may be decreased
Antidiabetic agents / Thiazides antagonize hypoglycemic effect of antidiabetic agents
Antigout agents / Thiazides may ↑ uric acid levels; thus, ↑ dose of antigout drug may be necessary
Antihypertensive agents / Thiazides potentiate the effect of antihypertensive agents
Antineoplastic agents / Thiazides may prolong leukopenia induced by antineoplastic agents
Calcium salts / Hypercalcemia due to renal tubular reabsorption or bone release may be ↑ by exogenous calcium
Cholestyramine / ↓ Effect of thiazides due to ↓ absorption from GI tract
Colestipol / ↓ Effect of thiazides due to ↓ absorption from GI tract
Corticosteroids / Enhanced potassium loss due to potassium-losing properties of both drugs
Diazoxide / Enhanced hypotensive effect. Also, ↑ hyperglycemic response
Digitalis glycosides / Thiazides produce ↑ potassium and magnesium loss with ↑ chance of digitalis-induced arrhythmias
Ethanol / Additive orthostatic hypotension
Fenfluramine / ↑ Antihypertensive effect of thiazides

Furosemide / Profound diuresis and electrolyte loss
Guanethidine / Additive hypotensive effect
Indomethacin / ↓ Effect of thiazides, possibly by inhibition of prostaglandins
Insulin / ↓ Effect due to thiazide-induced hyperglycemia
Lithium / ↑ Risk of lithium toxicity due to ↓ renal excretion; may be used together but use should be carefully monitored
Loop diuretics / Additive effect to cause profound diuresis and serious electrolyte losses
Methenamine / ↓ Effect of thiazides due to alkalinization of urine by methenamine
Methyldopa / ↑ Risk of hemolytic anemia (rare)
Muscle relaxants, nondepolarizing / ↑ Effect of muscle relaxants due to hypokalemia
Norepinephrine / Thiazides ↓ arterial response to norepinephrine
Quinidine / ↑ Effect of quinidine due to ↑ renal tubular reabsorption
Reserpine / Additive hypotensive effect
Sulfonamides / ↑ Effect of thiazides due to ↓ plasma protein binding
Sulfonylureas / ↓ Effect due to thiazide-induced hyperglycemia
Tetracyclines / ↑ Risk of azotemia
Tubocurarine / ↑ Muscle relaxation and ↑ hypokalemia
Vasopressors (sympathomimetics) / Thiazides ↓ responsiveness of arterioles to vasopressors
Vitamin D / ↑ Effect of vitamin D due to thiazide-induced hypercalcemia

Dosage

See individual drugs.

Laboratory Test Considerations: Hypokalemia, hypercalcemia, hyponatremia, hypomagnesemia, hypochloremia, hypophosphatemia, hyperuricemia. ↑ BUN, creatinine, glucose in blood and urine. ↓ Serum PBI levels (no signs of thyroid disturbance). Initial ↑ total cholesterol, LDL cholesterol, and triglycerides.

1. Clients resistant to one type of thiazide may respond to another.
2. Liquid potassium preparations are bitter. Administer with fruit juice or milk to enhance palatability.
3. To minimize electrolyte imbalance, thiazides may be taken every other day or on a 3–5-day basis for treatment of edema.
4. To prevent excess hypotension, reduce dose of other antihypertensive agents when beginning therapy.

HEALTH CARE CONSIDERATIONS

Assessment

1. Record any drug hypersensitivity. Record indications for therapy and any experience with these drugs.
2. Monitor CBC, glucose, electrolytes, Ca, Mg, renal and LFTs.
3. Note any history of heart disease or gout; check uric acid levels.
4. Determine extent of edema; assess skin turgor, mucous membranes, extremities, and lung fields.
5. With cirrhosis, avoid K^+ depletion and hepatic encephalopathy.

Interventions

1. Stop drug at least 48 hr before surgery. Thiazide inhibits pressor effects of epinephrine.
2. Potassium supplements should be given only when dietary measures are inadequate. If required, use liquid preparations to avoid ulcerations that may be produced by potassium salts in the solid dosage form. Exceptions include slow-K forms (potassium salt imbedded in a wax matrix) and micro-K forms (microencapsulated potassium salt).

Client/Family Teaching

1. Administer in the morning so that the major diuretic effect will occur before bedtime.
2. Take with food or milk if GI upset occurs.
3. Eat a diet high in potassium. Include orange juice, bananas, citrus fruits, broccoli, spinach, tomato juice, cucumbers, beets, dried fruits, or apricots. Avoid black licorice; may precipitate severe hypokalemia.
4. Rise slowly and dangle legs before standing to minimize orthostatic effects. Sit or lie down if feeling faint or dizzy.
5. With gout, avoid foods high in purines and continue antigout agents as prescribed.
6. With diabetes, monitor finger sticks more frequently; may need adjustment of insulin or oral hypoglycemic agent.
7. Avoid alcohol; causes severe hypotension.
8. Do not take any other medication (including OTC drugs for asthma, cough and colds, hay fever, weight control) unless approved.
9. Report any severe weight loss, muscle weakness, cramps, dizziness, or fatigue.
10. Skin rashes may occur but severe symptoms R/T allergic reactions include acute pulmonary edema, acute pancreatitis, thrombocytopenia, cholestatic jaundice, and hemolytic anemia; report immediately.

Outcome/Evaluate

- Control of hypertension; ↓ BP
- ↑ Urine output; ↓ edema; ↓ weight

• Adequate tissue perfusion with warm dry skin and good pulses
• Normal electrolyte levels and fluid balance

ESTROGENS

See also the following individual entries:

Diethylstilbestrol diphosphate
Esterified estrogens
Estradiol transdermal system
Estrogens conjugated, oral
Estrogens conjugated, parenteral
Estrogens conjugated, vaginal
Estropipate
Oral Contraceptives

Action/Kinetics: The three primary estrogens in the human female are estradiol 17–β, estrone, and estriol, which are steroids. Nonsteroidal estrogens include diethylstilbestrol. Estrogens combine with receptors in the cytoplasm of the cell, resulting in an increase in protein synthesis. For example, estrogens are required for development of secondary sex characteristics, development and maintenance of the female genital system and breasts. They also produce effects in the pituitary and hypothalamus. In adult women, estrogens participate in bone maintenance by aiding the deposition of calcium in the protein matrix of bones. They increase elastic elements in the skin, tend to cause sodium and fluid retention, and produce an anabolic effect by enhancing the turnover of dietary nitrogen and other elements into protein. Furthermore, they tend to keep plasma cholesterol at relatively low levels. Natural estrogens have a significant first-pass effect; thus, they are given parenterally. Synthetic derivatives can be given PO and are rapidly absorbed, distributed, and excreted. Estrogens are metabolized in the liver and excreted in urine (major portion) and feces. When given transdermally, the skin metabolizes estradiol only to a small extent.

Uses: Uses include hormone replacement therapy in postmenopausal women and as a component of combination oral contraceptives. See individual drugs. Estrogens are used both systemically and vaginally.

Contraindications: Breast cancer, except in those clients being treated for metastatic disease. Cancer of the genital tract and other estrogen-dependent neoplasms. Undiagnosed abnormal genital bleeding. History of thrombophlebitis, thrombosis, or thromboembolic disorders associated with previous estrogen use (except when used to treat breast or prostatic cancer). Known or suspected pregnancy. Prolonged therapy in women who plan to become pregnant. Use during lactation. May be contraindicated in clients with blood dyscrasias, hepatic disease, or thyroid dysfunction.

Special Concerns: Use with caution, if at all, in those with asthma, epilepsy, migraine, cardiac failure, renal insufficiency, diseases involving calcium or phosphorous metabolism, or a family history of mammary or genital tract cancer. Increased risk of endometrial carcinoma in postmenopausal women. Safety and effectiveness have not been determined in children and should be used with caution in adolescents in whom bone growth is incomplete.

Side Effects: Systemic use. Side effects to estrogens are dose dependent. *CV:* Potentially, the most serious side effects involve the CV system. ***Thromboembolism,*** thrombophlebitis, ***MI, pulmonary embolism,*** retinal thrombosis, ***mesenteric thrombosis, subarachnoid hemorrhage, postsurgical thromboembolism.*** Hypertension, edema, ***stroke.*** *GI:* N&V, abdominal cramps, bloating, cholestatic jaundice, colitis, acute pancreatitis, changes in appetite. *Dermatologic:* Most common are chloasma or melasma. Also, erythema multiforme, erythema nodosum, hemorrhagic eruptions, urticaria, dermatitis, photosensitivity. *Hepatic:* Cholestatic jaundice, aggravation of porphyria, benign (most common) or malignant liver tumors. *GU:* Breakthrough bleeding, spotting, changes in amount and/or duration of menstrual flow, amenorrhea during and after use, dysmenorrhea, premenstrual-like syndrome, change in cervical eversion and degree of cervical secretion, cystitis-like syndrome, hemolytic uremic syndrome, endometrial cystic hyperplasia, increased incidence of *Candida* vaginitis. *CNS:* Mental depression, dizziness, changes in libido, chorea, headache, aggravation of migraine headaches, fatigue, nervousness, ***convulsions.*** *Ocular:* Steepening of corneal curvature resulting in intolerance of contact lenses. Optic neuritis or retinal thrombosis, resulting in sudden or gradual, partial or complete loss of vision, double vision, papilledema. *Hematologic:* Increase in prothrombin and blood coagulation factors VII, VIII, IX, and X. Decrease in antithrombin III. *Local:* Pain at injection site, sterile abscesses, postinjection flare, redness and irritation at site of application of transdermal system. *Miscellaneous:* Breast tenderness, enlargement, or secretions. Increased risk of gallbladder disease (with high doses). Premature closure of epiphyses in children. Increased frequency of benign or malignant tumors of the cervix, uterus, vagina, and other organs. Weight gain. Increased risk of congenital abnormalities. Hypercalcemia in clients with metastatic breast carcinoma. In males, estrogens may cause gynecomastia, loss of libido, decreased spermatogenesis, testicular atrophy, and feminization. Prolonged use of high doses may inhibit the function of the anterior pituitary. Estrogen therapy affects many laboratory tests. **Vaginal use.** *GU:* Vaginal bleeding, vaginal discharge, endometrial withdrawal bleeding, serious bleeding in ovariectomized women with endometriosis. *Miscellaneous:* Breast tenderness.

Drug Interactions

Anticoagulants, oral / ↓ Anticoagulant response by ↑ activity of certain clotting factors

Anticonvulsants / Estrogen-induced fluid retention may precipitate seizures. Also, contraceptive steroids ↑ effect of anticonvulsants by ↓ breakdown in liver and ↓ plasma protein binding

Antidiabetic agents / Estrogens may impair glucose tolerance and thus change requirements for antidiabetic agent

Barbiturates / ↓ Effect of estrogen by ↑ breakdown by liver

Corticosteroids / ↑ Pharmacologic and toxicologic effects of corticosteroids

Phenytoin / See *Anticonvulsants*

Rifampin / ↓ Effect of estrogen due to ↑ breakdown by liver

Succinylcholine / Estrogens may ↑ effects of succinylcholine

Tricyclic antidepressants / Possible ↑ effects of tricyclic antidepressants

Dosage

PO, IM, SC, vaginal, topical, or by implantation. The dosage of estrogens is highly individualized and is aimed at the minimal effective amount.

Laboratory Test Considerations: Alter LFTs and thyroid function tests. False + urine glucose test. ↓ Serum cholesterol, total serum lipids, pregnanediol excretion, serum folate, antithrombin III, antifactor Xa. ↑ Serum triglyceride levels, thyroxine-binding globulin, sulfobromophthalein retention. ↑ PT, partial thromboplastin time, platelet aggregation time, platelet count, fibrinogen, plasminogen, norepinephrine-induced platelet aggregability, and factors II, VII, IX, X, XI, VII-X complex, II-VII-X complex, and β–thromboglobulin. Impaired glucose tolerance, reduced response to metyrapone.

1. Most PO administered estrogens are metabolized rapidly and must be administered daily.
2. Parenterally administered estrogens are released more slowly from aqueous suspensions or oily solutions; give slowly and deeply.
3. To avoid continuous stimulation of reproductive tissue, cyclic therapy consisting of 3 weeks on and 1 week off is usually recommended for most uses.
4. To reduce postpartum breast engorgement, give during the first few days after delivery.

HEALTH CARE CONSIDERATIONS

Assessment

1. Record indications for therapy, type and onset of symptoms. List other agents prescribed and the outcome.
2. Note any history of thromboembolic problems as estrogens enhance blood coagulability; monitor coagulation factors/ PT and for thromboembolic disorders.
3. Assess mental status; note any history of depression, migraine headaches, or suicide attempts.
4. Determine any undiagnosed genital bleeding, liver disease, asthma, migraines, epilepsy, or cancer of the endometrium or breast (estrogen-dependent neoplasms), as these preclude drug therapy.
5. Monitor ECG, VS, glucose, triglycerides, electrolytes, renal and LFTs.

Client/Family Teaching

1. Review the dose, form, and frequency of prescribed agent.
2. Taking oral medications with meals or a light snack will prevent gastric irritation and may eliminate nausea. With once-a-day therapy, taking at bedtime may eliminate problems. Nausea, bloating, abdominal cramping, changes in appetite, and vomiting may occur and usually disappear with continued therapy.
3. Report any alterations in mental attitude: depression or withdrawal, insomnia or anorexia, or a lack of attention to personal appearance.
4. With cyclical therapy, take meds for 3 weeks and then omit for 1 week. Menstruation may then occur, but pregnancy will not because ovulation is suppressed. Keep a record of periods and problems, such as missed menses, unusual vaginal bleeding, spotting, or irregularity. Report if pregnancy suspected.
5. Breast tenderness, enlargement, or secretion may occur. Perform BSE monthly (usually 2 weeks after menses) and report changes.

6. Report immediately: leg pains, sudden onset of chest pain, dizziness, SOB, weakness of the arms or legs, or any numbness (S&S of thromboembolic problems).
7. Changes in the curvature of the cornea may make it difficult to wear contact lenses; consult ophthalmologist.
8. Report any skin changes, such as alopecia or discoloration.
9. May alter glucose tolerance. Monitor sugars and report increases as dose of antidiabetic drug may need to be changed.
10. Males may develop feminine characteristics or suffer from impotence; usually disappear once therapy completed.
11. Insert suppositories high into the vault. Apply vaginal preparations at bedtime. Wear a sanitary napkin and avoid the use of tampons. Store suppositories in the refrigerator.
12. Report if estrogen ointments cause systemic reactions.
13. If pregnant and planning to breast-feed, do not take estrogens. Consult provider for alternative forms of contraception; breastfeeding does not provide contraception.
14. *Do not smoke*. Attend formal smoking cessation programs.
15. Some potential risks, related to endometrial cancer, have been associated with estrogen therapy. Therapy requires close medical follow-up.

Outcome/Evaluate

- Control of estrogen imbalance
- Effective contraceptive agent
- Slowing of postmenopausal osteoporosis; ↓ risk of ASHD
- Relief of menopausal S&S
- Control of tumor size/spread in metastatic breast and prostate cancer

FLUOROQUINOLONES

See also the following individual entries:

Ciprofloxacin hydrochloride
Enoxacin
Levofloxacin
Lomefloxacin hydrochloride
Norfloxacin
Ofloxacin
Sparfloxacin

Action/Kinetics: Synthetic, broad-spectrum antibacterial agents. The fluorine molecule confers increased activity against gram-negative organisms as well as broadens the spectrum against gram-positive organisms. Are bactericidal agents by interfering with DNA gyrase, an enzyme needed for the synthesis of bacterial DNA. Food may delay the absorption of ciprofloxacin, lomefloxacin, and norfloxacin. Ciprofloxacin, levofloxacin, ofloxacin, and trovafloxacin may be given IV; all fluoroquinolones may be given PO.

See also *General Nursing Considerations for All Anti-Infectives.*

Uses: See individual drugs. Used for a large number of gram-positive and gram-negative infections.

Contraindications: Hypersensitivity to the quinolone group of antibiotics, including cinoxacin and nalidixic acid. Lactation. Use in children less than 18 years of age.

Special Concerns: Use lower doses in impaired renal function. There may be differences in CNS toxicity between the various fluoroquinolones. Use may increase the risk of Achilles and other tendon inflammation and rupture.

Side Effects: See individual drugs. The following side effects are common to each of the fluoroquinolone antibiotics. *GI:* N&V, diarrhea, abdominal pain or discomfort, dry or painful mouth, heartburn, dyspepsia, flatulence, constipation, pseudomembranous colitis. *CNS:* Headache, dizziness, malaise, lethargy, fatigue, drowsiness, somnolence, depression, insomnia, ***seizures,*** paresthesia. *Dermatologic:* Rash, photosensitivity, pruritus (except for ciprofloxacin). *Hypersensitivity reactions:* Facial or ***pharyngeal edema,*** dyspnea, urticaria, itching, tingling, loss of consciousness, ***CV collapse.*** *Other:* Visual disturbances and ophthalmologic abnormalities, hearing loss, superinfection, phototoxicity, eosinophilia, crystalluria, Achilles and other tendon inflammation and rupture. Fluoroquinolones, except norfloxacin, may also cause vaginitis, syncope, chills, and edema.

OD **Management of Overdose:** *Symptoms:* Extension of side effects. *Treatment:* For acute overdose, vomiting should be induced or gastric lavage performed. The client should be carefully observed and, if necessary, symptomatic and supportive treatment given. Hydration should be maintained.

Drug Interactions

Antacids / ↓ Serum levels of fluoroquinolones due to ↓ absorption from the GI tract
Anticoagulants / ↑ Effect of anticoagulant
Antineoplastic agents / ↓ Serum levels of fluoroquinolones
Cimetidine / ↓ Elimination of fluoroquinolones
Cyclosporine / ↑ Risk of nephrotoxicity
Didanosine / ↓ Serum levels of fluoroquinolones due to ↓ absorption from the GI tract
Iron salts / ↓ Serum levels of fluoroquinolones due to ↓ absorption from the GI tract

Probenecid / ↑ Serum levels of fluoroquinolones due to ↓ renal clearance
Sucralfate / ↓ Serum levels of fluoroquinolones due to ↓ absorption from the GI tract
Theophylline / ↑ Plasma levels and ↑ toxicity of theophylline due to ↓ clearance
Zinc salts / ↓ Serum levels of fluoroquinolones due to ↓ absorption from the GI tract

Dosage

See individual drugs.

Laboratory Test Considerations: ↑ ALT, AST. See also individual drugs.

HEALTH CARE CONSIDERATIONS

Assessment

1. Record type, onset, and characteristics of symptoms.
2. Note any previous experiences with these antibiotics. Discontinue at first sign of rash or other allergic manifestations. Hypersensitivity reactions may occur latently.
3. Assess for soft tissue/extremity injury; note instability, pain, or swelling.
4. Monitor VS, I&O, CBC, cultures, liver and renal function studies.
5. If receiving anticoagulants and theophyllines, monitor closely; quinolones can cause increased drug levels with toxic drug effects i.e., bleeding or seizures.

Client/Family Teaching

1. Take only as directed.
2. Consume >2.5 L/day of fluids.
3. Do not take any mineral supplements (i.e., iron or zinc) or antacids containing magnesium or aluminum simultaneously or 4 hr before or 2 hr after dosing with fluoroquinolones.
4. Do not perform hazardous tasks until drug effects realized; may experience dizziness.
5. Report any bothersome symptoms; N&V and diarrhea are most frequently reported side effects.
6. Report symptoms of superinfection (furry tongue, vaginal or rectal itching, diarrhea).
7. Stop drug and report any new onset tendon pain or inflammation as tendon rupture may occur.
8. Wear protective clothing and sunscreens; avoid excessive sunlight or artificial ultraviolet light. Photosensitivity reactions may occur up to several weeks after stopping therapy.

Outcome/Evaluate

- Symptomatic improvement
- Resolution of infection (↓ WBCs, ↓ temperature, ↑ appetite)
- Negative culture reports

HISTAMINE H_2 ANTAGONISTS

See also the following individual entries:

Cimetidine
Famotidine
Nizatidine
Ranitidine bismuth citrate
Ranitidine hydrochloride

Action/Kinetics: Histamine H_2 antagonists are competitive blockers of histamine. As such they inhibit all phases of gastric acid secretion including that caused by histamine, gastrin, and muscarinic agents. Both fasting and nocturnal acid secretion are inhibited. In addition, the volume and hydrogen ion concentration of gastric juice are decreased. Cimetidine, famotidine, and ranitidine have no effect on gastric emptying; cimetidine and famitidine have no effect on lower esophageal pressure. Fasting or postprandial serum gastrin is not affected by famotidine, nizatidine, or ranitidine. Cimetidine is known to affect the cytochrome P-450 drug metabolizing system for other drugs. Ranitidine also affects the P-450 enzyme system, but its effect on elimination of other drugs is not significant. Neither famotidine nor nizatidine affects the P-450 enzyme system.

Uses: See individual drugs. Also, these drugs are used as part of combination therapy to treat *Helicobacter pylori*–associated duodenal ulcer and maintenance therapy after healing of the active ulcer.

Contraindications: Hypersensitivity. Use of cimetidine, famotidine, and nizatidine during lactation.

Special Concerns: Use with caution in impaired hepatic and renal function. Symptomatic response to these drugs does not preclude gastric malignancy. Use ranitidine with caution during lactation. Safety and effectiveness have not been established for use in children. Use of cimetidine in children less than 16 years of age unless benefits outweigh risks.

Side Effects: The following side effects are common to all or most of the H_2-histamine antagonists. See individual drugs for complete listing. *GI:* N&V, abdominal discomfort, diarrhea, constipation, hepatocellular effects. *CNS:* Headache, fatigue, somnolence, dizziness, confusion, hallucinations, insomnia. *Dermatologic:* Rash, urticaria, pruritus, alopecia (rare), erythema multiforme (rare). *Hematologic:* Rarely, thrombocytopenia, agranulocytosis, granulocytopenia. *Other:* Gynecomastia, impotence, loss of libido, arthralgia, bronchospasm, transient pain at injection site, cardiac arrhythmias following rapid IV use (rare), arthralgia (rare), ***anaphylaxis*** (rare).

OD **Management of Overdose:** *Symptoms:* No experience is available for deliberate overdose. *Treatment:* Induce vomiting or perform gastric lavage to remove any unabsorbed drug. Monitor the client and undertake supportive therapy.

Dosage

See individual drugs.

HEALTH CARE CONSIDERATIONS

Assessment

1. Record symptoms noting onset, duration, intensity, and any previous treatment.
2. Assess for number of reflux occurrences. Chronic treatment usually initiated after two to three recurrences.
3. Monitor CBC, liver and renal function studies.
4. Perform CNS assessment noting level of orientation.
5. Note results of radiographic/endoscopic procedures; document *H. pylori* results.
6. Determine gastric pH; maintain greater than 5.

Client/Family Teaching

1. May be taken without regard for meals.
2. Stagger doses of antacids if used with cimetidine or ranitidine.
3. Do not take the maximum dose of OTC products for more than 2 weeks continuously without medical supervision.
4. Take as prescribed; do not stop if pain subsides or if "feeling better" as drug is necessary to inhibit gastric acid secretion.
5. These agents reduce the secretion of gastric acid and are usually prescribed for 4–8 weeks initially to control symptoms and promote ulcer healing.
6. Report any confusion or disorientation immediately.
7. Avoid alcohol, caffeine, aspirin-containing products (cough and cold products), and foods that may cause GI irritation, i.e., harsh spices.
8. Stop 24–72 hr before skin testing begins; may cause false negative response in tests with allergen extracts.
9. Smoking may interfere with drug's action. Stop smoking and do not smoke following the last dose of the day.
10. Any blood-tinged emesis or dark tarry stools as well as dizziness or rash, require immediate reporting.
11. Review GERD instructions i.e., ↑ HOB, avoid lying down after eating and dietary restrictions.
12. Report for all scheduled follow-up studies; a response to these agents does not preclude gastric malignancy.

Outcome/Evaluate

- Duodenal ulcer healing
- ↓ Gastric irritation/bleeding; ↓ abdominal pain/discomfort
- Gastric pH > 5
- Stabilization of H&H

See *Antidiabetic Agents: Insulins.*

LAXATIVES

See also the following individual entries:

Docusate calcium
Docusate potassium
Docusate sodium
Lactulose
Psyllium hydrophilic muciloid

Action/Kinetics: Laxatives act locally, either by stimulating the smooth muscles of the bowel or by changing the bulk or consistency of the stools. Laxatives can be divided into five categories.

1. *Stimulant laxatives:* Substances that chemically stimulate the smooth muscles of the bowel to increase contractions. Examples: Bisacodyl, cascara, danthron, and senna.
2. *Saline laxatives:* Substances that increase the bulk of the stools by retaining water. Examples: Magnesium salts and sodium phosphate.
3. *Bulk-forming laxatives:* Nondigestible substances that pass through the stomach and then increase the bulk of the stools. Examples: Methylcellulose and psyllium.
4. *Emollient and lubricant laxatives:* Agents that soften hardened feces and facilitate their passage through the lower intestine. Examples: Docusate and mineral oil.
5. *Miscellaneous:* Includes glycerin suppositories and lactulose.

Uses: See individual agents. Short-term treatment of constipation. Prophylaxis in clients who should not strain during defecation, i.e., following anorectal surgery or after MI (fecal softeners or lubricant laxatives). To evacuate the colon for rectal and bowel examinations (certain lubricant, saline, and stimulant laxatives). In conjunction with surgery or anthelmintic therapy. The underlying cause of constipation should be determined since a marked change in bowel habits may be a symptom of a pathologic condition.

Contraindications: Severe abdominal pain that *might* be caused by appendicitis, enteritis, ulcerative colitis, diverticulitis, intestinal obstruction. Laxative use in these conditions may cause rupture of the abdomen or intes-

tinal hemorrhage. Undiagnosed abdominal pain. Children under the age of 2. Castor oil is contraindicated during pregnancy as the irritant effects may result in premature labor.
Side Effects: *GI:* Excess activity of the colon resulting in nausea, diarrhea, griping, or vomiting. Perianal irritation, bloating, flatulence. *Electrolyte Balance:* Dehydration, disturbance of the electrolyte balance. *Miscellaneous:* Dizziness, fainting, weakness, sweating, palpitations.

Bulk laxatives: Obstruction in the esophagus, stomach, small intestine, or rectum. *Stimulant laxatives:* Chronic abuse may lead to malfunctioning colon. *Mineral Oil:* Large doses may cause anal seepage resulting in itching, irritation, hemorrhoids, and perianal discomfort.

Chronic use of laxatives may cause laxative dependency and result in chronic constipation and other intestinal disorders because the client may start to depend on the psychologic effect and physical stimulus of the drug rather than on the body's own natural reflexes.

Drug Interactions

Anticoagulants, oral / ↓ Absorption of vitamin K from GI tract induced by laxatives may ↑ effects of anticoagulants and result in bleeding

Digitalis / Cathartics may ↓ absorption of digitalis

Tetracyclines / Laxatives containing Al, Ca, or Mg may ↓ effect of tetracyclines due to ↓ absorption from GI tract

Dosage

See individual drugs.

1. When administering a laxative, note the length of time it takes for the laxative to take effect and give it so that the result of the laxative will not interfere with the client's rest or digestion and absorption of nutrients.
2. Administer liquid laxatives at a temperature that makes them more agreeable.
3. If laxative is to be administered in a liquid, select one that the client finds palatable.
4. If ordered to prepare for a diagnostic exam, check directions carefully to ensure accurate administration.

HEALTH CARE CONSIDERATIONS

Assessment

1. Determine length of use and the underlying causes; note type of laxative taking and effectiveness.
2. With abdominal pain and discomfort, note exact location and type of discomfort experiencing. R/O other intestinal disorders where laxatives should not be used.
3. Determine stool character and frequency of bowel movements. The client's definition of constipation may determine if, in fact, constipation exists.
4. Note age, state of health, activity level, and general nutritional status.
5. Identify any special restriction or limitation due to illness; may include fluid/sodium restrictions.
6. List other drugs that may contribute to constipation (i.e., diuretics, anticholinergics, antihistamines, antidepressants, iron products, and some antihypertensive agents, especially verapamil).
7. Identify recent life-style changes that may contribute to problem.

Client/Family Teaching

1. Have a regular schedule for defecation; keep record of bowel function and response to all laxatives taken.
2. Laxatives reduce the amount of time other drugs remain in the intestine and may diminish effectiveness.
3. If taken in prep for a diagnostic study, review instructions. If unable to read, find someone to review directions to ensure an accurate test.
4. Review techniques that facilitate elimination; sitting with legs slightly elevated and leaning forward to increase abdominal pressure often encourages elimination. If ill at home, consider a commode at the bedside. This will promote better bowel function by encouraging client to move about and ensure privacy.
5. Bowel tone will be lost with long-term use of laxatives; bowel movements do not have to occur daily. Use diet to achieve same purpose; two or three prunes a day are preferable to laxatives.
6. Frequent use of any type of enemas may cause damage to the rectum and small bowel as well as inhibit bowel tone and may cause electrolyte abnormalities.
7. Review importance of diet high in fiber foods (and juices such as prune) and daily exercise and benefits in maintaining proper bowel function. Include bulk foods and sufficient fluids in diet to enhance elimination. Consult dietitian for assistance in meal planning/preparation and food selections.
8. Report if constipation persists because there could be a physiologic problem that requires attention.
9. If pregnant, consult with provider before taking any laxatives to treat constipation.
10. Nursing mothers should avoid laxatives unless prescribed as many are excreted in breast milk and can cause infant diarrhea.

Outcome/Evaluate

- Relief of constipation; evacuation of a soft, formed stool
- Effective colon prep for diagnostic procedures (no stool in bowel)

NARCOTIC ANALGESICS

See also the following individual entries:

Codeine phosphate
Codeine sulfate
Fentanyl transdermal system
Fiorinal
Fiorinal with Codeine
Hydrocodone bitartrate and Acetaminophen
Hydromorphone hydrochloride
Meperidine hydrochloride
Methadone hydrochloride
Morphine hydrochloride
Morphine sulfate
Oxycodone hydrochloride
Oxymorphone hydrochloride
Paregoric
Pentazocine hydrochloride with Naloxone hydrochloride
Pentazocine lactate
Percocet
Propoxyphene hydrochloride
Propoxyphene napsylate
Tramadol hydrochloride
Tylenol with Codeine

Action/Kinetics

Narcotic analgesics are classified as agonists, mixed agonist-antagonists, or partial agonists depending on their activity at opiate receptors.The narcotic analgesics attach to specific receptors located in the CNS (cortex, brain stem, and spinal cord) resulting in various CNS effects. The mechanism is believed to involve decreased permeability of the cell membrane to sodium, which results in diminished transmission of pain impulses. Five categories of opioid receptors have been identified: mu, kappa, sigma, delta, and epsilon. Narcotic analgesics are believed to exert their activity at mu, kappa, and sigma receptors. Mu receptors are thought to mediate supraspinal analgesia, euphoria, and respiratory and physical depression. Pentazocine-like spinal analgesia, miosis, and sedation are mediated by kappa receptors while sigma receptors mediate dysphoria, hallucinations, as well as respiratory and vasomotor stimulation (caused by drugs with antagonist activity). In addition to an alteration of pain perception (analgesia), the drugs, especially at higher doses, induce euphoria, drowsiness, changes in mood, mental clouding, and deep sleep.

The narcotic analgesics also depress respiration. Death by overdosage is almost always the result of respiratory arrest. These drugs cause nausea and emesis due to direct stimulation of the CTZ. They depress the cough reflex, and small doses of narcotic analgesics (e.g., codeine) are found in certain antitussive products. Little effect on BP when the client is in a supine position. Most narcotics decrease the capacity of the client to respond to stress. Morphine and other narcotic analgesics induce peripheral vasodilation, which may result in hypotension. Many narcotic analgesics constrict the pupil, a sign of dependence with such drugs. They also decrease peristaltic motility causing constipation. The constipating effects (e.g., Paregoric) are sometimes used therapeutically in diarrhea. The narcotic analgesics also increase the pressure within the biliary tract. See also individual agents.

Uses: See individual drugs. Generally are used to treat pain due to various causes (e.g., MI, carcinoma, surgery, burns, postpartum), as preanesthetic medication, as adjuncts to anesthesia, acute vascular occlusion, diarrhea, and coughs. Methadone is used for heroin withdrawal and maintenance.

Contraindications: Asthma, emphysema, kyphoscoliosis, severe obesity, convulsive states as in epilepsy, delirium tremens, tetanus and strychnine poisoning, diabetic acidosis, myxedema, Addison's disease, hepatic cirrhosis, and children under 6 months.

Special Concerns: Use with caution in clients with head injury or after head surgery because of morphine's capacity to elevate ICP and mask the pupillary response. Use with caution in the elderly, in the debilitated, in young children, in individuals with increased ICP, in obstetrics, and with clients in shock or during acute alcoholic intoxication.

Use morphine with extreme caution in pulmonary heart disease (cor pulmonale). Deaths following ordinary therapeutic doses have been reported. Use cautiously in prostatic hypertrophy, because it may precipitate acute urinary retention. Use cautiously in clients with reduced blood volume, such as in hemorrhaging clients who are more susceptible to the hypotensive effects of morphine.

Since the drugs depress the respiratory center, give early in labor, at least 2 hr before delivery, to reduce the danger of respiratory depression in the newborn. When given before surgery, give at least 1–2 hr preoperatively so that the danger of maximum depression of respiratory function will have passed before anesthesia is initiated. These drugs may need to be withheld prior to diagnostic procedures so that the physician can use pain to locate dysfunction.

Side Effects: *Respiratory:* ***Respiratory depression, apnea.*** *CNS:* Dizziness, lightheadedness, sedation, lethargy, headache, euphoria, mental clouding, fainting. Idiosyncratic effects including excitement, restlessness, tremors, delirium, insomnia. *GI:* N&V, vomiting, constipation, increased pressure in biliary tract, dry mouth, anorexia. *CV:* Flushing, changes in HR and BP, circulatory collapse. *Allergic:* Skin rashes including pruritus and urticaria. Sweating, ***laryngospasm,*** edema. *Miscellaneous:* Urinary retention, oliguria, reduced libido, changes in body temperature. Narcotics cross the placental barrier and depress respiration of the fetus or newborn.

DEPENDENCE AND TOLERANCE: All drugs of this group are addictive. Psychologic and physical dependence and tolerance develop even when clients use clinical doses. Tolerance is characterized by the fact that the client requires shorter periods of time between doses or larger doses for relief of pain. Tolerance usually develops faster when the narcotic analgesic is administered regularly and when the dose is large.

OD **Management of Overdose:** *Symptoms (Acute Toxicity):* Severe toxicity is characterized by ***profound respiratory depression, apnea, deep sleep, stupor or coma, circulatory collapse, seizures, cardiopulmonary arrest, and death.*** Less severe toxicity results in symptoms including CNS depression, miosis, respiratory depression, deep sleep, flaccidity of skeletal muscles, hypotension, bradycardia, hypothermia, pulmonary edema, pneumonia, shock. The respiratory rate may be as low as 2–4 breaths/min. The client may be cyanotic. Urine output is decreased, the skin feels clammy, and body temperature decreases. If death occurs, it almost always results from ***respiratory depression.*** *Symptoms (Chronic Toxicity):* The problem of chronic dependence on narcotics occurs not only as a result of "street" use but is also found often among those who have easy access to narcotics (physicians, nurses, pharmacists). All the principal narcotic analgesics (morphine, opium, heroin, codeine, meperidine, and others) have, at times, been used for nontherapeutic purposes.

The nurse must be aware of the problem and be able to recognize signs of chronic dependence. These are constricted pupils, GI effects (constipation), skin infections, needle scars, abscesses, and itching, especially on the anterior surfaces of the body, where the client may inject the drug.

Withdrawal signs appear after drug is withheld for 4–12 hr. They are characterized by intense craving for the drug, insomnia, yawning, sneezing, vomiting, diarrhea, tremors, sweating, mental depression, muscular aches and pains, chills, and anxiety. Although the symptoms of narcotic withdrawal are uncomfortable, they are rarely life-threatening. This is in contrast to the withdrawal syndrome from depressants, where the life of the individual may be endangered because of the possibility of tonic-clonic seizures.

Treatment (Acute Overdose): Initial treatment is aimed at combating progressive respiratory depression by maintaining a patent airway and by artificial respiration. Gastric lavage and induced emesis are indicated in case of oral poisoning. The narcotic antagonist naloxone (Narcan), 0.4 mg IV, is effective in the treatment of acute overdosage. Respiratory stimulants (e.g., caffeine) should not be used to treat depression from the narcotic overdosage.

Drug Interactions

Alcohol, ethyl / Potentiation or addition of CNS depressant effects; concomitant use may lead to drowsiness, lethargy, stupor, respiratory collapse, coma, or death
Anesthetics, general / See *Alcohol*
Antianxiety drugs / See *Alcohol*
Antidepressants, tricyclic / ↑ Narcotic-induced respiratory depression
Antihistamines / See *Alcohol*
Barbiturates / See *Alcohol*
Cimetidine / ↑ CNS toxicity (e.g., disorientation, confusion, respiratory depression, apnea, seizures) with narcotics
CNS depressants / See *Alcohol*
MAO inhibitors / Possible potentiation of either MAO inhibitor (excitation, hypertension) or narcotic (hypotension, coma) effects; death has resulted
Methotrimeprazine / Potentiation of CNS depression
Phenothiazines / See *Alcohol*
Sedative-hypnotics, nonbarbiturate / See *Alcohol*
Skeletal muscle relaxants (surgical) / ↑ Respiratory depression and ↑ muscle relaxation

Dosage

See individual drugs.

Laboratory Test Considerations: Altered liver function tests. False + or ↑ urinary glucose test (Benedict's). ↑ Plasma amylase or lipase.

Special Considerations: For the elderly, blood levels of narcotic may be higher, resulting in longer periods of pain relief. Assess physical parameters and client complaints carefully before readministering narcotic for short-term pain control on the prescribed as-needed frequency.

1. Review list of drugs with which narcotics interact and effects.
2. Request that orders be rewritten at timed intervals as required for continued administration.
3. Record amount of narcotic used on the narcotic inventory sheet, noting drug, date, time, dose, and to whom, or if the drug was wasted; include appropriate witness as necessary, addressing all requirements for documentation.

HEALTH CARE CONSIDERATIONS

Assessment

1. Record indications for therapy, type and onset of symptoms; differentiate acute vs. chronic syndromes and rate pain levels.
2. Note any prior experience with narcotic analgesics or adverse reactions.
3. Identify clinical conditions that would precipitate pain syndromes, i.e., cancer, neuropathic, postherpetic neuralgia, or musculoskeletal injury.
4. Determine cause and record amount of pain or discomfort, its location, intensity, and duration, frequency of occurrence, and what drug has been effective in the past.
5. Use a pain rating scale (e.g., 0–10) to assess pain quantitatively so clients can accurately describe their level of pain and measure effectiveness of therapy.
6. Obtain baseline VS; generally, if the respiratory rate < 12/min or the SBP < 90 mm Hg, a narcotic should not be administered unless there is ventilatory support or specific written guidelines, with parameters for administration.
7. Note weight, age, and general body size. Too large a dosage for the client's weight and age can result in serious side effects.
8. Record amount of time elapsed between doses for relief from recurring pain.
9. Note precipitating factors as well as the impact of the pain on the client's ability to function.
10. Record asthma or other conditions that compromise respirations.
11. Determine if pregnant. Narcotics cross the placental barrier and depress fetal respirations.
12. Monitor CBC, electrolytes, liver and renal function studies.

Interventions

1. Determine when to use supportive measures, such as relaxation techniques, repositioning, and reassurance to assist in relieving pain.
2. Explore source of pain; use nonnarcotic analgesics when possible. Coadministration (such as with NSAIDs) may increase analgesic effects and permit lower doses of the narcotic.
3. Administer when needed; *prolonging until the maximum amount of pain experienced reduces drugs' effectiveness.*
4. Monitor VS and mental status. During parenteral therapy:
   - Monitor for respiratory depression.
   - Narcotics depress the cough reflex. Turn q 2 hr; cough and deep breathe to prevent atelectasis. Splinting incisions and painful areas may assist in compliance. Administer narcotic at least 30–60 min prior to activities or painful procedures.
   - Monitor for hypotension.
   - If HR below 60 beats/min in the adult or 110 beats/min in an infant, withhold and report.
   - Observe for decrease in BP, deep sleep, or constricted pupils.
   - Assess during meals to prevent choking and aspiration.
   - Monitor closely when administered as sedation for a procedure.
   - Note effects on mental status. One who has experienced pain, fear, or anxiety may become euphoric and excited. Note dizziness, drowsiness, pupil reactions, or hallucinations.
5. Report if N&V occurs; may need an antiemetic or change in therapy.
6. A snack or milk may decrease gastric irritation and lessen nausea when taken orally.
7. Monitor bowel function; narcotics, especially morphine, can have a depressant effect on the GI tract and may promote constipation. Increase fluid intake to 2.5–3 L/day; consume fruit juices, fruits, and fiber. Increase level and frequency of exercise.
8. Narcotics may cause urinary retention. Monitor I&O; palpate abdomen for distention; empty bladder q 3–4 hr. Question about difficulty voiding, pain in the bladder area, sensation of not emptying the bladder, dysuria, or any unusual odors.
9. Note difficulty with vision. Check pupillary response to light; report if pupils remain constricted.
10. Monitor mental status. If bedridden, use side rails and safety measures; assist with ambulation, BR, and transfers.
11. Reassure that flushing and a feeling of warmth may occur with therapeutic doses.
12. May perspire profusely; be prepared to bathe; change clothes and linens frequently.
13. Assess for evidence of tolerance and addiction with ATC therapy.
14. With terminal diseases and chronic debilitating pain, dependence on drug therapy is

not a consideration, whereas *adequate pain control is of the utmost concern.*

Client/Family Teaching

1. Drug may become habit forming; explore alternative methods for pain control.
2. Take as prescribed before the pain becomes too severe.
3. Avoid alcohol in any form.
4. Do not take OTC drugs without approval. Many contain small amounts of alcohol and some may interact unfavorably with the prescribed drug.
5. For fecal impaction, use preventive actions, such as increased fluid intake, increased use of fruit and fruit juices, and a stool softener.
6. Drug can cause drowsiness and dizziness; use caution when operating a motor vehicle or performing other tasks that require mental alertness.
7. Rise slowly from a lying to sitting position and dangle legs before standing, to minimize orthostatic effects.
8. When used as sedation for outpatient procedures, someone must accompany client. Expect a recovery period (to assess for any adverse side effects) of up to several hours before release.
9. Store all drugs in a safe place, out of the reach of children and away from the bedside to prevent accidental overdosage.
10. During prolonged usage, do not stop abruptly; withdrawal symptoms may occur.
11. Determine extent of relief achieved with each dosage (e.g., pain level decreased from a level 5 to a level 2, 20 min after administration of medication). Keep a record of narcotic use for breakthrough pain so that maintenance dose can be adjusted.
12. Review techniques to enhance pain relief such as relaxation techniques, splinting incision, supporting painful areas, and taking medication before strenuous activities and before pain becomes severe.
13. Identify appropriate support groups for assistance with understanding, accepting, and managing chronic pain. Seek locale of regional pain management center.
14. For those with terminal diseases, identify local support groups to provide contact with those experiencing similar symptoms and treatments.

Outcome/Evaluate

- Control of severe pain without altered hemodynamics or impaired level of consciousness
- Absence of acute toxicity, tolerance, or addiction, during short-term therapy

NARCOTIC ANTAGONISTS

See also the following individual entries:

Nalmefene hydrochloride
Naloxone hydrochloride
Naltrexone

Action/Kinetics: Narcotic antagonists competitively block the action of narcotic analgesics by displacing previously given narcotics from their receptor sites or by preventing narcotics from attaching to the opiate receptors, thereby preventing access by the analgesic. Not effective in reversing the respiratory depression induced by barbiturates, anesthetics, or other nonnarcotic agents. These drugs almost immediately induce withdrawal symptoms in narcotic addicts and are sometimes used to unmask dependence.

HEALTH CARE CONSIDERATIONS

Assessment

1. Determine etiology of respiratory depression. Narcotic antagonists do not relieve the toxicity of nonnarcotic CNS depressants.
2. Note mental status and VS.

Interventions

1. Note agent being reversed. If narcotic is long acting or sustained release, repeated doses will be required in order to continue to counteract drug effects. Monitor VS and respirations closely after duration of action of antagonist; additional doses may be necessary.
2. Observe for appearance of withdrawal symptoms characterized by restlessness, crying out due to sudden loss of pain control, lacrimation, rhinorrhea, yawning, perspiration, vomiting, diarrhea, sweating, writhing, anxiety, pain, chills, and an intense craving for the drug.
3. Observe for symptoms of airway obstruction; if comatose, turn frequently and position on side to prevent aspiration.
4. Maintain a safe, protective environment. Use side rails, supervise ambulation, and use soft supports as needed.
5. If used to diagnose narcotic use or dependence, observe for initial dilation of the pupils, followed by constriction.
6. Anticipate readministration of smaller doses of narcotic (once depressant symptoms reversed) with terminal pain and conditions that warrant narcotic pain management.

Outcome/Evaluate

- Reversal of toxic effects of narcotic analgesic evidenced by ↑ level of consciousness and improved breathing patterns
- Confirmation of narcotic dependence evidenced by withdrawal symptoms

NASAL DECONGESTANTS

See also the following individual entries:

Ephedrine sulfate
Epinephrine hydrochloride
Phenylephrine hydrochloride
Pseudoephedrine hydrochloride

Action/Kinetics: The most commonly used agents for relief of nasal congestion are the adrenergic drugs. They act by stimulating alpha-adrenergic receptors, thereby constricting the arterioles in the nasal mucosa; this reduces blood flow to the area, decreasing congestion. However, drugs such as ephedrine and pseudoephedrine also have beta-adrenergic effects. Both topical (sprays, drops) and oral agents may be used, although oral agents are not as effective.

Uses: PO. Nasal congestion due to hay fever, common cold, allergies, or sinusitis. To help sinus or nasal drainage. To relieve congestion of eustachian tubes. **Topical.** Nasal and nasopharyngeal mucosal congestion due to hay fever, common cold, allergies, or sinusitis. With other therapy to decrease congestion around the eustachian tubes. Relieve ear block and pressure pain during air travel.

Contraindications: Oral use in severe hypertension or CAD. Use with MAO inhibitors. Oral use of pseudoephedrine and phenylpropanolamine during lactation.

Special Concerns: Use with caution in hyperthyroidism, arteriosclerosis, increased intraocular pressure, prostatic hypertrophy, angina, diabetes, ischemic heart disease, hypertension. Also, clients receiving MAO inhibitors may manifest hypertensive crisis following the use of oral nasal decongestants. Use with caution in geriatric clients and during pregnancy and lactation. Rebound congestion may occur after topical use. OTC products containing ephedrine have been abused.

Side Effects: *Topical use:* Stinging and burning, mucosal dryness, sneezing, local irritation, rebound congestion (rhinitis medicamentosa). Systemic use may produce the following symptoms. *CV:* ***CV collapse with hypotension,*** arrhythmias, palpitations, precordial pain, tachycardia, transient hypertension, bradycardia. *CNS:* Anxiety, dizziness, headache, fear, restlessness, tremors, insomnia, tenseness, lightheadedness, drowsiness, psychologic disturbances, weakness, psychoses, hallucinations, ***seizures,*** depression. *GI:* N&V, anorexia. *Ophthalmologic:* Irritation, photophobia, tearing, blurred vision, blepharospasm. *Other:* Dysuria, sweating, pallor, breathing difficulties, orofacial dystonia.

NOTE: Ephedrine may also produce anorexia and urinary retention in men with prostatic hypertrophy.

OD Management of Overdose: *Symptoms:* Somnolence, sedation, ***coma,*** profuse sweating, ***hypotension, shock. Severe hypertension,*** bradycardia, and rebound hypotension may occur with naphazoline and tetrahydrozoline. *Treatment:* Supportive therapy. IV phentolamine may be used in severe cases.

Drug Interactions

Furazolidone / ↑ Pressor sensitivity to drugs with both alpha- and beta-adrenergic effects (e.g., ephedrine)
Guanethidine / ↑ Effect of direct-acting agents (e.g., epinephrine) and ↓ effect of mixed-acting drugs; also, ↓ hypotensive effect of guanethidine
MAO inhibitors / Use with mixed-acting drugs (e.g., ephedrine) → severe headache, hypertension, hyperpyrexia, and possibly hypertensive crisis
Methyldopa / ↑ Risk of a pressor response
Phenothiazines / May ↓ or reverse action of nasal decongestants
Reserpine / ↑ Pressor effect of direct-acting drugs and ↓ effect of mixed-acting drugs
Theophyllines / Enhanced toxicity
Tricyclic antidepressants / ↑ Pressor effect of direct-acting agents → possibility of dysrhythmias; ↓ pressor effect of mixed-acting drugs
Urinary acidifiers / ↑ Excretion of nasal decongestants → ↓ effect
Urinary alkalinizers / ↓ Excretion of nasal decongestants → ↑ effect

Dosage

See individual drugs.

1. Most nasal decongestants are used topically in the form of sprays, drops, or solutions.
2. Solutions may become contaminated with use, resulting in the growth of bacteria and fungi. Thus, the dropper or spray tip should be rinsed in hot water after each use and covered.
3. Use separate equipment with topical administration to prevent the spread of infection. If only one container of medication is available, use an individual dropper for each client and rinse thoroughly with hot water after each use.
4. During administration, have facial tissues and a receptacle available for used tissues.
5. Topical decongestants should not be used longer than 3–5 days and should be used sparingly, especially in infants, children, and clients with CV disease.

HEALTH CARE CONSIDERATIONS

Client/Family Teaching

1. Blow the nose gently before administering therapy. If unable to blow the nose, clear

the nasal passages with a bulb-type aspirator as needed.
2. Review the prescribed method of administration, whether drops, spray, or jelly and the goals of therapy.
3. After completing therapy, rinse the dropper or tip of spray container with hot water. Dry with a tissue and cover, using care not to introduce water into the spray container. Wipe the tip of the nasal jelly tube with a damp tissue and replace the cap.
4. Seek medical assistance if symptoms worsen or do not improve after 3–5 days of therapy.
5. Overuse or misuse of these agents may cause significant medical problems; i.e., a nasal spray used regularly for more than 3 or 4 days may precipitate rebound congestion.
6. Many OTC agents contain sympathomimetics; these should be avoided with hypertension, hyperthyroidism, angina, and insulin-dependent diabetes.

Outcome/Evaluate

- ↓ Nasal congestion
- Resolution of eustachian tube congestion/pain
- ↓ Duration/intensity of allergic manifestations

NONSTEROIDAL ANTI-INFLAMMATORY DRUGS

See also the following individual entries:

Auranofin
Aurothioglucose
Celecoxib
Diclofenac potassium
Diclofenac sodium
Diclofenac sodium/Misoprostol
Diflunisal
Etodolac
Fenoprofen calcium
Flurbiprofen
Flurbiprofen sodium
Gold sodium thiomalate
Ibuprofen
Indomethacin
Indomethacin sodium trihydrate
Ketoprofen
Ketorolac tromethamine
Meclofenamate sodium
Mefenamic acid
Nabumetone
Naproxen
Naproxen sodium
Oxaprozin
Piroxicam
Sulindac
Suprofen
Tolmetin sodium

Action/Kinetics: The anti-inflammatory effect is likely due to inhibition of the enzyme cyclooxygenase, resulting in decreased prostaglandin synthesis. Effective in reducing joint swelling, pain, and morning stiffness, as well as in increasing mobility in individuals with inflammatory disease. They do not alter the course of the disease, however. Their anti-inflammatory activity is comparable to that of aspirin. The analgesic activity is due, in part, to relief of inflammation. Also, the drugs may inhibit lipoxygenase, inhibit synthesis of leukotrienes, inhibit release of lysosomal enzymes, and inhibit neutrophil aggregation. Rheumatoid factor production may also be inhibited. The antipyretic action occurs by decreasing prostaglandin synthesis in the hypothalamus, resulting in an increase in peripheral blood flow and heat loss as well as promoting sweating. NSAIDs also inhibit miosis induced by prostaglandins during the course of cataract surgery; thus, these drugs are useful for a number of ophthalmic inflammatory conditions.

The NSAIDs differ from one another with respect to their rate of absorption, length of action, anti-inflammatory activity, and effect on the GI mucosa. Most are rapidly and completely absorbed from the GI tract; food delays the rate, but not the total amount, of drug absorbed. These drugs are metabolized in the kidney and are excreted through the urine, mainly as metabolites.

Uses: See individual drugs. Generally are used to treat inflammatory disease, including rheumatoid arthritis, osteoarthritis, ankylosing spondylitis, gout, and other musculoskeletal diseases. Treatment of nonrheumatic inflammatory conditions including bursitis, acute painful shoulder, synovitis, tendinitis, or tenosynovitis. Mild to moderate pain including primary dysmenorrhea, episiotomy pain, strains and sprains, postextraction dental pain. Primary dysmenorrhea. Ophthalmically to inhibit intraoperative miosis, for postoperative inflammation after cataract surgery, and for relief of ocular itching due to seasonal allergic conjunctivitis.

Contraindications: Most for children under 14 years of age. Lactation. Individuals in whom aspirin, NSAIDs, or iodides have caused hypersensitivity, including acute asthma, rhinitis, urticaria, nasal polyps, bronchospasm, angioedema or other symptoms of allergy or anaphylaxis.

Special Concerns: Clients intolerant to one of the NSAIDs may be intolerant to others in this group. Use with caution in clients with a history of GI disease, reduced renal function, in geriatric clients, in clients with intrinsic coagulation defects or those on anticoagulant therapy, in compromised cardiac function, in hypertension, in conditions predisposing to fluid retention, and in the presence of existing controlled infection. The risk of hospitalization is doubled in geriatric clients taking NSAIDs and diuretics. The safety and efficacy of most NSAIDs have not been determined in children or in functional class IV rheumatoid arthritis (i.e., clients incapacitated, bedridden, or confined to a wheelchair).

Side Effects: *GI (most common):* Peptic or duodenal ulceration and GI bleeding, intestinal ulceration with obstruction and stenosis, reactivation of preexisting ulcers. Heartburn, dyspepsia, N&V, anorexia, diarrhea, constipation, increased or decreased appetite, indigestion, stomatitis, epigastric pain, abdominal cramps or pain, gastroenteritis, paralytic ileus, salivation, dry mouth, glossitis, pyrosis, icterus, rectal irritation, gingival ulcer, occult blood in stool, hematemesis, gastritis, proctitis, eructation, sore or dry mucous membranes, ulcerative colitis, rectal bleeding, melena, ***perforation and hemorrhage of esophagus, stomach, duodenum, small or large intestine.*** *CNS:* Dizziness, drowsiness, vertigo, headaches, nervousness, migraine, anxiety, mental confusion, aggravation of parkinsonism and epilepsy, lightheadedness, paresthesia, peripheral neuropathy, akathisia, excitation, tremor, ***seizures,*** myalgia, asthenia, malaise, insomnia, fatigue, drowsiness, confusion, emotional lability, depression, inability to concentrate, psychoses, hallucinations, depersonalization, amnesia, ***coma,*** syncope. *CV:* CHF, hypotension, hypertension, arrhythmias, peripheral edema and fluid retention, vasodilation, exacerbation of angiitis, palpitations, tachycardia, chest pain, sinus bradycardia, peripheral vascular disease, peripheral edema. *Respiratory:* ***Bronchospasm, laryngeal edema,*** rhinitis, dyspnea, pharyngitis, hemoptysis, SOB, eosinophilic pneumonitis. *Hematologic:* Bone marrow depression, neutropenia, leukopenia, pancytopenia, eosinophila, thrombocytopenia, granulocytopenia, ***agranulocytosis, aplastic anemia, hemolytic anemia,*** decreased H&H, hypocoagulability, epistaxis. *Ophthalmologic:* Amblyopia, visual disturbances, corneal deposits, retinal hemorrhage, scotomata, retinal pigmentation changes or degeneration, blurred vision, photophobia, diplopia, iritis, loss of color vision (reversible), optic neuritis, cataracts, swollen, dry, or irritated eyes. *Dermatologic:* Pruritus, skin eruptions, sweating, erythema, eczema, hyperpigmentation, ecchymoses, petechiae, rashes, urticaria, purpura, onycholysis, vesiculobullous eruptions, cutaneous vasculitis, ***toxic epidermal necrolysis, angioneurotic edema,*** erythema nodosum, ***Stevens-Johnson syndrome,*** exfoliative dermatitis, photosensitivity, alopecia, skin irritation, peeling, erythema multiforme, desquamation, skin discoloration. *GU:* Menometrorrhagia, menorrhagia, impotence, menstrual disorders, hematuria, cystitis, azotemia, nocturia, proteinuria, UTIs, polyuria, dysuria, urinary frequency, oliguria, pyuria, anuria, renal insufficiency, nephrosis, nephrotic syndrome, glomerular and interstitial nephritis, urinary casts, acute renal failure in clients with impaired renal function, renal papillary necrosis *Metabolic:* Hyperglycemia, hypoglycemia, glycosuria, hyperkalemia, hyponatremia, diabetes mellitus. *Other:* Tinnitus, hearing loss or disturbances, ear pain, deafness, metallic or bitter taste in mouth, thirst, chills, fever, flushing, jaundice, sweating, breast changes, gynecomastia, muscle cramps, dyspnea, involuntary muscle movements, muscle weakness, facial edema, pain, serum sickness, aseptic meningitis, hypersensitivity reactions including asthma, acute respiratory distress, ***shock-like syndrome, angioedema,*** angiitis, dyspnea, ***anaphylaxis.***

Following ophthalmic use: Transient burning and stinging upon installation, ocular irritation.

OD **Management of Overdose:** *Symptoms:* CNS symptoms include dizziness, drowsiness, mental confusion, lethargy, disorientation, intense headache, paresthesia, and ***seizures.*** GI symptoms include N&V, gastric irritation, and abdominal pain. Miscellaneous symptoms include tinnitus, sweating, blurred vision, increased serum creatinine and BUN, and acute renal failure. *Treatment:* There are no antidotes; treatment includes general supportive measures. Since the drugs are acidic, it may be beneficial to alkalinize the urine and induce diuresis to hasten excretion.

Drug Interactions

Anticoagulants / Concomitant use results in ↑ PT

Aspirin / ↓ Effect of NSAIDs due to ↓ blood levels; also, ↑ risk of adverse GI effects

Beta-adrenergic blocking agents / ↓ Antihypertensive effect of blocking agents

Cimetidine / ↑ or ↓ Plasma levels of NSAIDs

Cyclosporine / ↑ Risk of nephrotoxicity

Lithium / ↑ Serum lithium levels
Loop diuretics / ↓ Effect of loop diuretics
Methotrexate / ↑ Risk of methotrexate toxicity (i.e., bone marrow suppression, nephrotoxicity, stomatitis)
Phenobarbital / ↓ Effect of NSAIDs due to ↑ breakdown by liver
Phenytoin / ↑ Effect of phenytoin due to ↓ plasma protein binding
Probenecid / ↑ Effect of NSAIDs due to ↑ plasma levels
Salicylates / Plasma levels of NSAIDs may be ↓ ; also, ↑ risk of GI side effects
Sulfonamides / ↑ Effect of sulfonamides due to ↓ plasma protein binding
Sulfonylureas / ↑ Effect of sulfonylureas due to ↓ plasma protein binding

Dosage

See individual drugs.
1. Do not take alcohol or aspirin together with NSAIDs.
2. Should GI upset occur, take with food, milk, or antacids.
3. NSAIDs may have an additive analgesic effect when administered with narcotic analgesics, thus permitting lower narcotic dosages.
4. Clients who do not respond clinically to one NSAID may respond to another.

HEALTH CARE CONSIDERATIONS

Assessment

1. Note allergic responses to aspirin or other anti-inflammatory agents.
2. Note location, intensity, and type of pain experienced. Assess joint mobility and ROM.
3. Review indications and dosage prescribed. For anti-inflammatory effects, high doses are required whereas analgesia and pain relief may be achieved with much lower dosages.
4. Asthma or nasal polyps may be exacerbated by NSAIDs.
5. Children under 14 years of age generally should not receive drugs in this category.
6. Monitor CBC, liver and renal function studies; causes platelet inhibition which is reversible in 24–48 hr, whereas aspirin requires 4–5 days to reverse antiplatelet effects.

Client/Family Teaching

1. Take NSAIDs with a full glass of water or milk, with meals, or with a prescribed antacid and remain upright 30 min following administration to reduce gastric irritation or ulcer formation.
2. Consume 2–3 L/day of water.
3. Report any changes in stool consistency or symptoms of GI irritation. Sustained GI effects may require misoprostol.
4. Regular intake of drug needed to sustain anti-inflammatory effects. If not obtained, another NSAID may provide desired response.
5. Report any episodes of bleeding, eye symptoms, tinnitus, skin rashes, purpura, weight gain, edema, decreased urine output, fever, or increased joint pain.
6. Use caution in operating machinery or in driving a car; may cause dizziness or drowsiness.
7. Avoid alcohol, aspirin, acetaminophen, and any other OTC preparations; may cause GI bleeding.
8. If diabetic, be aware of hypoglycemic effect of NSAIDs on hypoglycemic agents; dosage of agent and NSAID may need to be adjusted.
9. Record weights periodically and report any significant changes. NSAIDs cause Na and water retention; avoid with CHF.
10. Notify all providers of meds being taken to avoid drugs that would interact unfavorably with NSAIDs.

Outcome/Evaluate

- ↑ Joint mobility and ROM
- ↓ Discomfort and pain
- Improvement in symptoms

OPHTHALMIC CHOLINERGIC (MIOTIC) AGENTS

See also the following individual entries:

Physostigmine salicylate
Physostigmine sulfate
Pilocarpine hydrochloride
Pilocarpine ocular therapeutic system

Action/Kinetics: The ophthalmic cholinergic drugs fall into two classes: direct-acting (carbachol, pilocarpine) and indirect-acting (demecarium, echothiophate, isoflurophate, neostigmine, physostigmine), which inhibit the enzyme acetylcholinesterase. In the treatment of glaucoma, the drugs lead to an accumulation of acetylcholine, which stimulates the ciliary muscles and increases contraction of the iris sphincter muscle. This opens the angle of the eye and results in increased outflow of aqueous humor and consequently in a decrease of intraocular pressure. This effect is of particular importance in narrow-angle glaucoma. The drugs also cause spasms of accommodation.

Uses: See individual drugs.

Contraindications: *Direct-acting drugs:* Inflammatory eye disease (iritis), asthma, hypertension. *Indirect-acting drugs:* Same as for *direct-acting drugs,* as well as acute-angle glaucoma, history of retinal detachment, ocular hypotension accompanied by intraocular inflammatory processes, intestinal or urinary obstruction, peptic ulcer, epilepsy, parkinsonism, spastic GI conditions, vasomotor instability, severe bradycardia or hypotension, and recent MIs. Lactation.

Side Effects: *Local:* Painful contraction of ciliary muscle, pain in eye, blurred vision, spasms of accommodation, darkened vision, failure to accommodate to darkness, twitching, headaches, painful brow. Most of these symptoms lessen with prolonged usage. Iris cysts and retinal detachment (indirect-acting drugs only).

Systemic: Systemic absorption of drug may cause nausea, GI discomfort, diarrhea, hypotension, bronchial constriction, and increased salivation.

Dosage

See individual drugs.Have epinephrine and atropine available for emergency treatment of increased intraocular pressure.

HEALTH CARE CONSIDERATIONS

Assessment

1. Record indications for therapy, onset and characteristics of symptoms. List other agents prescribed and the outcome.
2. Record fundoscopic exam.
3. Review drugs and existing medical conditions that may preclude drug therapy.
4. Carefully monitor geriatric clients.
5. Hourly tonometric measurements are recommended during initiation of therapy.
6. Assess for redness around the cornea. Epinephrine or phenylephrine hydrochloride (10%) may be ordered with demecarium bromide, echothiophate iodide, or isoflurophate to minimize this reaction.

Client/Family Teaching

1. Drug must be used as ordered to maintain vision by reducing intraocular pressures.
2. Wash hands before and after therapy. Review appropriate method for instilling eye drops or ointment and frequency/duration of therapy.
3. Take eye drops exactly as prescribed. Minimize side effects by taking one dose at bedtime.
4. To prevent overflow into the nasopharynx after instillation of drops, exert pressure on the nasolacrimal duct for 1–2 min before closing eyelids.
5. Do not drive for 1–2 hr after instilling cholinergic agents. Night vision may also be impaired.
6. Pain and blurred vision may occur; should diminish with continued use of the drug.
7. Report any changes in vision, eye irritation, or evidence of severe headaches.
8. Painful eye spasms may be relieved by applying cold compresses.
9. Report for exams as scheduled and refill prescriptions as needed.

Outcome/Evaluate

- Improved visual fields and tonometric measurements
- ↓ Intraocular pressures

ORAL CONTRACEPTIVES: ESTROGEN-PROGESTERONE COMBINATIONS

See Table 1.

Action/Kinetics: The combination oral contraceptives act by inhibiting ovulation due to an inhibition (through negative-feedback mechanism) of LH and FSH, which are required for development of ova. These products also alter the cervical mucus so that it is not conducive to sperm penetration, render the endometrium less suitable for implantation of the blastocyst should fertilization occur, and inhibit enzymes required by sperm to enter the ovum.

The estrogen used in combination oral contraceptives is either ethinyl estradiol or mestranol. Mestranol is demethylated to ethinyl estradiol in the liver. **t½:** 6–20 hr. The progestin used in combination oral contraceptives is either desogestrel, ethynodiol diacetate, levonorgestrel, norethindrone, norethindrone acetate, norgestimate, or norgestrel.

The progestin-only products do not consistently inhibit ovulation. However, these products also alter the cervical mucus and render the endometrium unsuitable for implantation. These products contain either norethindrone or norgestrel. This method of contraception is less reliable than combination therapy.

Although oral contraceptives may be associated with serious side effects, a number of noncontraceptive health benefits have been confirmed. These include increased regularity of the menstrual cycle, decreased incidence of dysmenorrhea, decreased blood loss, decreased incidence of functional ovarian cysts and ectopic pregnancies, and decreased incidence of diseases such as fibroadenomas, fibrocystic disease, acute pelvic inflammatory disease, endometrial cancer, and ovarian cancer.

General Statement: There are three types of combination (i.e., both an estrogen and progestin in each tablet) oral contraceptives: (1) monophasic—contain the same amount of estrogen and progestin in each tablet; (2) biphasic—contain the same amount of estrogen in each tablet but the progestin content is lower for the first part of the cycle and higher for the last part of the cycle; (3) triphasic—the estrogen content may be the same or may vary throughout the medication cycle; the progestin content may be the same or varies, depending on the part of the cycle. The purpose of the biphasic and triphasic products is to provide hormones in a manner similar to that occurring physiologically. This is said to decrease breakthrough bleeding during the medication cycle. The other type of oral contraceptive is the progestin-only ("minipill") product, which contains a small amount of a progestin in each tablet.

Also available is an emergency contraceptive kit (Preven) containing just four tablets of ethinyl estradiol and levonorgestrel. It is intended to be used after unprotected intercourse.

See also *Health Care Considerations* for *Estrogens*, and *Progesterone and Progestins*.

Uses: Contraception, prevent pregnancy after unprotected intercourse, menstrual irregularities, menopausal symptoms. High doses are used for endometriosis and hypermenorrhea. *Investigational:* High doses of Ovral (ethinyl estradiol and norgestrel) have been used as a postcoital contraceptive.

Contraindications: Thrombophlebitis, history of deep-vein thrombophlebitis, thromboembolic disorders, cerebral vascular disease, CAD, MI, current or past angina, known or suspected breast cancer or estrogen-dependent neoplasm, endometrial carcinoma, hepatic adenoma or carcinoma, undiagnosed abnormal genital bleeding, known or suspected pregnancy, cholestatic jaundice of pregnancy. Smoking.

Special Concerns: Cigarette smoking increases the risk of cardiovascular side effects from use of oral contraceptives. Low estrogen-containing oral contraceptives do not increase the risk of stroke in women. Use with caution in clients with a history of hypertension, preexisting renal disease, hypertension-related diseases during pregnancy, familial tendency to hypertension or its consequences, a history of excessive weight gain or fluid retention during the menstrual cycle; these individuals are more likely to develop elevated BP. Use with caution in clients with asthma, epilepsy, migraine, diabetes, metabolic bone disease, renal or cardiac disease, and a history of mental depression. Use with drugs (e.g., barbiturates, hydantoins, rifampin) that increase the hepatic metabolism of oral contraceptives may result in breakthrough bleeding and an increased risk of pregnancy. Use combination products during lactation only if absolutely necessary; progestin-only products do not appear to have any adverse effects on breastfeeding performance or on the health, growth, or development of the infant.

Side Effects: The oral contraceptives have wide-ranging effects. These are particularly important, since the drugs may be given for several years to healthy women. Many authorities have voiced concern about the long-term safety of these agents. Some advise discontinuing therapy after 18–24 months of continuous use. The majority of side effects of oral contraceptives are due to the estrogen component. *CV:* ***MI, thrombophlebitis, venous thrombosis with or without embolism, pulmonary embolism, coronary thrombosis, cerebral thrombosis, arterial thromboembolism, mesenteric thrombosis, thrombotic and hemorrhagic strokes, postsurgical thromboembolism, subarachnoid hemorrhage,*** elevated BP, hypertension. *CNS:* Onset or exacerbation of migraine headaches, depression. *GI:* N&V, bloating, abdominal cramps. *Ophthalmic:* Optic neuritis, retinal thrombosis, steepening of the corneal curvature, contact lens intolerance. *Hepatic:* ***Benign and malignant hepatic adenomas,*** focal nodular hyperplasia, ***hepatocellular carcinoma,*** gallbladder disease, cholestatic jaundice. *GU:* Breakthrough bleeding, spotting, amenorrhea, change in menstrual flow, change in cervical erosion and cervical secretions, ***invasive cervical cancer,*** bleeding irregularities (more common with progestin-only products), vaginal candidiasis, ***ectopic pregnancies in contraceptive failures,*** breast tenderness, breast enlargement. *Miscellaneous:* Acute intermittent porphyria, photosensitivity, congenital anomalies, melasma, skin rash, edema, increase or decrease in weight, decreased carbohydrate tolerance, increased incidence of cervical *Chlamydia trachomatis,* decrease in the quantity and quality of breast milk.

Drug Interactions

Acetaminophen / ↓ Effect of acetaminophen due to ↑ breakdown by liver

Anticoagulants, oral / ↓ Effect of anticoagulants by ↑ levels of certain clotting factors (however, an ↑ effect of anticoagulants has also been noted in some clients)

Table 1 Injectable and Oral Contraceptive Preparations and Hormone Replacement Combinations Available in the United States

Trade Name	Estrogen	Progestin
	ORAL MONOPHASIC PRODUCTS	
Alesse 21-Day and 28-Day	Ethinyl estradiol (20 mcg)	Levonorgestrel (0.1 mg)
Apri	Ethinyl estradiol (30 mcg)	Desogestrel (0.15 mg)
Brevicon 21-Day and 28-Day	Ethinyl estradiol (35 mcg)	Norethindrone (0.5 mg)
Demulen 1/35–21 and 1/35–28	Ethinyl estradiol (35 mcg)	Ethynodiol diacetate (1 mg)
Demulen 1/50–21 and 1/50–28	Ethinyl estradiol (50 mcg)	Ethynodiol diacetate (1 mg)
Desogen (28 day)	Ethinyl estradiol (30 mcg)	Desogestrel (0.15 mg)
Levlen 21 and 28	Ethinyl estradiol (30 mcg)	Levonorgestrel (0.15 mg)
Levlite 21 and 28	Ethinyl estradiol (20 mcg)	Levonorgestrel (0.1 mg)
Levora 0.15/30-21 and -28	Ethinyl estradiol (30 mcg)	Levonorgestrel (0.15 mg)
Loestrin 21 1/20	Ethinyl estradiol (20 mcg)	Norethindrone acetate (1 mg)
Loestrin 21 1.5/30	Ethinyl estradiol (30 mcg)	Norethindrone acetate (1.5 mg)
Loestrin Fe 1/20 (28 day)	Ethinyl estradiol (20 mcg)	Norethindrone acetate (1 mg)
Loestrin Fe 1.5/30 (28 day)	Ethinyl estradiol (30 mcg)	Norethindrone acetate (1.5 mg)
Lo/Ovral-21 and -28	Ethinyl estradiol (30 mcg)	Norgestrel (0.3 mg)
Modicon 21 and 28	Ethinyl estradiol (35 mcg)	Norethindrone (0.5 mg)
Necon 0.5/35-21 Day and 28 Day	Ethinyl estradiol (35 mcg)	Norethindrone (0.5 mg)
Necon 1/35-21 Day and 28 Day	Ethinyl estradiol (35 mcg)	Norethindrone (1 mg)
Necon 1/50-21 Day and 28 Day	Mestranol (50 mcg)	Norethindrone (1 mg)
Nelova 0.5/35E 21 Day and 28 Day	Ethinyl estradiol (35 mcg)	Norethindrone (0.5 mg)
Nelova 1/35E 21 Day and 28 Day	Ethinyl estradiol (35 mcg)	Norethindrone (1 mg)
Nelova 1/50M 21 Day and 28 Day	Mestranol (50 mcg)	Norethindrone (1 mg)
Nordette-21 and -28	Ethinyl estradiol (30 mcg)	Levonorgestrel (0.15 mg)
Norinyl 1 + 35 21-Day and 28-Day	Ethinyl estradiol (35 mcg)	Norethindrone (1 mg)
Norinyl 1 + 50 21-Day and 28-Day	Mestranol (50 mcg)	Norethindrone (1 mg)

Trade Name	Estrogen	Progestin
	ORAL MONOPHASIC PRODUCTS	
Ortho-Cept 21 Day and 28 Day	Ethinyl estradiol (30 mcg)	Desogestrel (0.15 mg)
Ortho-Cyclen-21 and -28	Ethinyl estradiol (35 mcg)	Norgestimate (0.25 mg)
Ortho Novum 1/35–21 and –28	Ethinyl estradiol (35 mcg)	Norethindrone (1 mg)
Ortho Novum 1/50–21 and –28	Mestranol (50 mcg)	Norethindrone (1 mg)
Ovcon-35 21 Day and 28 Day	Ethinyl estradiol (35 mcg)	Norethindrone (0.4 mg)
Ovcon-50 21 Day and 28 Day	Ethinyl estradiol (50 mcg)	Norethindrone (1 mg)
Ovral 28 Day	Ethinyl estradiol (50 mcg)	Norgestrel (0.5 mg)
Zovia 1/35E-21 and -28	Ethinyl estradiol (35 mcg)	Ethynodiol diacetate (1 mg)
Zovia 1/50E-21 and -28	Ethinyl estradiol (50 mcg)	Ethynodiol diacetate (1 mg)
	ORAL BIPHASIC PRODUCTS	
Jenest-28	Ethinyl estradiol (35 mcg in each tablet)	Norethindrone (10 tablets of 0.5 mg followed by 11 tablets of 1 mg)
Mircette	Ethinyl estradiol (20 mcg for Days 1 - 21; 10 mcg for Days 24 - 28)	Desogestrel (150 mg for Days 1 - 21)
Necon 10/11 21 Day and 28 Day	Ethinyl estradiol (35 mcg in each tablet)	Norethindrone (10 tablets of 0.5 mg followed by 11 tablets of 1 mg)
Nelova 10/11–21 and –28	Ethinyl estradiol (35 mcg in each tablet)	Norethindrone (10 tablets of 0.5 mg followed by 11 tablets of 1 mg)
Ortho-Novum 10/11–21 and –28	Ethinyl estradiol (35 mcg in each tablet)	Norethindrone (10 tablets of 0.5 mg followed by 11 tablets of 1 mg)
	ORAL TRIPHASIC PRODUCTS	
Estrostep 21 and Estrostep Fe	Ethinyl estradiol (20 mcg for 5 days, 30 mcg for 7 days, and 35 mcg for 9 days)	Norethindrone (1 mg in each table)

Table 1 *(continued)*

Trade Name	Estrogen	Progestin
	ORAL TRIPHASIC PRODUCTS	
Ortho-Novum 7/7/7 (21 or 28 days)	Ethinyl estradiol (35 mcg in each tablet)	Norethindrone (0.5 mg the first 7 days, 0.75 the next 7 days, and 1 mg the last 7 days)
Ortho-Tri-Cyclen (21 or 28 days)	Ethinyl estradiol (35 mcg in each tablet)	Norgestimate (0.18 mg the first 7 days, 0.215 mg the next 7 days, and 0.25 mg the last seven days)
Tri-Levlen 21 or 28 Days Tri-Levlen 28 Day	First 6 days: Ethinyl estradiol (30 mcg) Next 5 days: Ethinyl estradiol (40 mcg) Last 10 days: Ethinyl estradiol (30 mcg)	Levonogestrel (0.05 mg) Levonorgestrel (0.075 mg) Levonorgestrel (0.125 mg)
Tri-Norinyl (21 or 28 day)	Ethinyl estradiol (35 mcg in each tablet)	Norethindrone (0.5 mg the first 7 days, 1 mg the next 9 days, and 0.5 mg the last 5 days)
Triphasil 21 or 28 day	First 6 days: Ethinyl estradiol (30 mcg) Next 5 days: Ethinyl estradiol (40 mcg) Last 10 days: Ethinyl estradiol (30 mcg)	Levonorgestrel (0.05 mg) Levonorgestrel (0.075 mg) Levonorgestrel (0.125 mg)
Trivora-28 day	First 6 days: Ethinyl estradiol (30 mcg) Next 5 days: Ethinyl estradiol (40 mcg) Last 10 days: Ethinyl estradiol (30 mcg)	Levonorgestrel (0.05 mg) Levonorgestrel (0.075 mg) Levonorgestrel (0.125 mg)
EMERGENCY CONTRACEPTIVE KIT		
Plan B A total of 2 tablets containing levonorgestrel.	No estrogen	Levonorgestrel (0.75 mg)
Preven A total of four tablets containing the above hormones	Ethinyl estradiol (50 mcg)	Levonorgestrel (0.25 mg)

Trade Name	Contents	Administration
	HORMONE REPLACEMENT COMBINATION	
Activella	Estradiol 17-B, 1 mg Norethindrone, 0.5 mg	One tablet daily. To treat vasomotor symptoms in menopause, vulvar and vaginal atrophy, prevention of osteoporosis
Ortho-Prefest	Estradiol 17-B, 1 mg Norgestimate, 0.09 mg	Single tablet of estradiol, 1 mg, for 3 days followed by a single tablet of estradiol, 1 mg, and norgestimate, 0.09 mg, for 3 days. Repeat regimen continuously without interruption. To treat vasomotor symptoms in menopause, vulvar and vaginal atrophy, prevention of osteoporosis.
	INJECTABLE CONTRACEPTIVE	
Lunelle	Medroxyprogesterone, 25 mg Estradiol cypionate, 5 mg	Inject 0.5 mL IM once a month, in cycles not to exceed 33 days.

All combination oral contraceptives and hormone replacement combinations are Rx and Pregnancy category: X.

Antidepressants, tricyclic / ↑ Effect of antidepressants due to ↓ breakdown by liver
Benzodiazepines / ↑ or ↓ Effect of benzodiazepines due to changes in breakdown by liver
Beta-adrenergic blockers / ↑ Effect of beta blockers due to ↓ breakdown by liver
Carbamazepine / ↓ Effect of oral contraceptives due to ↑ breakdown by liver
Corticosteroids / ↑ Effect of corticosteroids due to ↓ breakdown by liver
Erythromycins / ↓ Effect of oral contraceptives due to altered enterohepatic absorption
Griseofulvin / May ↓ effect of oral contraceptives due to ↑ breakdown
Hypoglycemics / Oral contraceptives ↓ effect of hypoglycemics due to their effect on carbohydrate metabolism
Insulin / Oral contraceptives may ↑ insulin requirements
Penicillins, oral / ↓ Effect of oral contraceptives due to altered enterohepatic absorption
Phenobarbital / ↓ Effect of oral contraceptives due to ↑ breakdown by liver
Phenytoin / ↓ Effect of oral contraceptives due to ↑ breakdown by liver
Rifampin / ↓ Effect of contraceptives due to ↑ breakdown by liver
Tetracyclines / ↓ Effect of contraceptives due to altered enterohepatic absorption
Theophyllines / ↑ Effect of theophyllines due to ↓ breakdown by liver
Troleandomycin / ↑ Chance of jaundice

Dosage

See *Administration/Storage*.

Laboratory Test Considerations: Altered liver and thyroid function tests. ↓ PT, 17-hydroxycorticosteroids, 17-ketosteroids, and 17-ketogenic steroids. ↑ Factors I (prothrombin), VII, VIII, IX, and X. (Therapy with ovarian hormones should be discontinued 60 days before performance of laboratory tests.) ↑ Gamma globulins.

1. Take tablets at approximately the same time each day.
2. Spotting or breakthrough bleeding may occur for the first 1–2 cycles; report if it continues past this time.
3. For the initial cycle, use an **additional** form of contraception the first week.
4. The type of oral contraceptive preparation will determine the precise manner in which the drug is taken:

• For the 21-day regimen, 1 tablet is taken daily beginning on day 5 of menses (day 1 is the first day of menstrual flow). No tablets are taken for 7 days.

• For a 28-day regimen, hormone-containing tablets are taken for the first 21 days, followed by 7 days of inert or iron-containing tablets.

• Certain products, including the biphasic and selected triphasic oral contraceptives, are termed *Sunday start*. The first tablet should be taken the Sunday following the beginning of menses (if menses begins on Sunday, the first tablet should be taken that day). *NOTE:* The biphasic and triphasic products have varying amounts of estrogen and/or progestin, depending on the stage of the cycle; the client should understand fully how these preparations are to be taken and which tablets are to be taken at various times during the medication cycle. Often tablets are different shapes and/or colors to help with compliance.

• For progestin-only products, the first tablet is taken on the first day of menses; thereafter, 1 tablet is taken every day of the year.

• For the contraceptive emergency kit, two tablets are taken within the first 72 hr after unprotected intercourse and the other two tablets 12 hr later. The kit also contains a pregnancy test which must be used prior to taking the tablets.

5. It is recommended that when beginning combination oral contraceptive therapy, chose a product that contains the least amount of estrogen.
6. If it is necessary to switch brands of oral contraceptives, wait 7 days to start the new pack if on a 21-day regimen or the day after the last tablet if on a 28-day regimen.
7. Non-nursing mothers may begin oral contraceptive therapy at the first postpartum exam (i.e., 4–6 weeks), regardless of whether spontaneous menstruation has occurred. Nursing mothers should not take oral contraceptives until the infant's weaned.

HEALTH CARE CONSIDERATIONS

Assessment

1. Record annual physical, internal exams, and Pap smears.
2. Determine any previous experience with these agents and results.
3. Note any family history of breast or uterine cancer or any existing medical condition that may preclude this drug therapy; note smoking history.

Client/Family Teaching

1. Take tablets exactly as prescribed to prevent pregnancy.
2. If 1 tablet is missed, take as soon as remembered.
3. If 2 tablets have been missed, the dosage

must be doubled for the next 2 consecutive days. The regular schedule may then be resumed; use additional contraceptive measures for the remainder of the cycle.
4. If 3 tablets are missed, discontinue the therapy and start a new course as indicated by the type of medication. Alternative contraceptive measures should be used when the tablets are not taken and should be continued for 7 days after starting a new course.
5. Report any missed menstrual periods. If two consecutive periods missed, discontinue therapy until pregnancy ruled out.
6. Report if pain in the legs or chest, respiratory distress, unexplained cough, severe headaches, dizziness, or blurred vision occurs, stop therapy and notify provider immediately.
7. Headaches, dizziness, blurred vision, or partial loss of sight, should be reported immediately.
8. Oral contraceptives decrease the viscosity of cervical mucus, increasing the susceptibility to vaginal infections which are difficult to treat; good hygienic practice is essential.
9. If persistent nausea, edema, and skin eruptions develop and last beyond the four cycles, a dose adjustment or different combination may be needed.
10. Alterations in thought processes, depression, or fatigue should be reported; preparations with less progesterone may be needed.
11. Androgenic effects, such as weight gain, increased oiliness of the skin, acne, or hirsutism, may require a change in medication or dosage.
12. Do not take longer than 18 months without medical consultation. Report for yearly Pap smear and physical examination; perform regular BSE (1 week after or 2 weeks before menstrual cycle).
13. Practice another form of contraception if receiving ampicillin, anticonvulsants, phenylbutazone, rifampin, or tetracycline. These may cause intermittent bleeding and interactions could result in pregnancy.
14. Contraceptives interfere with the elimination of caffeine. Limit caffeine consumption to prevent insomnia, irritability, tremors, and cardiac irregularities.
15. If breast-feeding infant, another form of contraception should be used until lactation is well established.
16. **Do not smoke.** Attend formal smoking cessation program.
17. Oral contraceptives do not provide any protection against STDs; use appropriate barrier protection with intercourse.
18. With the contraceptive emergency kit, two tablets are taken within the first 72 hr after unprotected intercourse and the other two tablets 12 hr later. The kit also contains a pregnancy test which must be used prior to taking the tablets.

Outcome/Evaluate

- Contraception
- Menstrual regularity
- ↓ Blood loss resulting from hormone imbalances

PENICILLINS

See also the following individual entries:

Amoxicillin
Amoxicillin and Potassium clavulanate
Ampicillin oral
Bacampicillin hydrochloride
Carbenicillin indanyl sodium
Cloxacillin sodium
Dicloxacillin sodium
Oxacillin sodium
Penicillin G sodium for injection
Penicillin G benzathine and procaine combined, intramuscular
Penicillin G benzathine, intramuscular
Penicillin G potassium for injection
Penicillin G procaine, intramuscular
Penicillin V potassium

Action/Kinetics: The bactericidal action of penicillins depends on their ability to bind penicillin-binding proteins (PBP-1 and PBP-3) in the cytoplasmic membranes of bacteria, thus inhibiting cell wall synthesis. Some penicillins act by acylation of membrane-bound transpeptidase enzymes, thereby preventing cross-linkage of peptidoglycan chains, which are necessary for bacterial cell wall strength and rigidity. Cell division and growth are inhibited and often lysis and elongation of susceptible bacteria occur. Penicillin is most effective against young, rapidly dividing organisms and has little effect on mature resting cells. Depending on the concentration of the drug at the site of infection and the susceptibility of the infectious microorganism, penicillin is either bacteriostatic or bactericidal. Penicillins are distributed throughout most of the body and pass the placental barrier. They also pass into synovial, pleural, pericardial, peritoneal, ascitic, and spinal fluids. Although normal meninges and the eyes are relatively impermeable to penicillins, they are better absorbed by inflamed meninges and eyes. **Peak serum levels, after PO:** 1 hr. **t½:** 30–110 min; protein binding: 20%–98% (see individual agents). Excreted largely unchanged by the urine as a result of glomerular filtration and active tubular secretion.

General Statement: Penicillins may be classifed as: (1) Natural: Penicillin G, Penicillin V. (2) Aminopenicillins: Amoxicillin, Amoxicillin/potassium clavulanate, Ampicillin, Ampicillin/sulbactam, Bacampicillin. (3) Penicillinase-resistant: Cloxacillin, Dicloxacillin, Nafcillin, Oxacillin. (4) Extended spectrum: Carbenicillin, Mezlocillin, Piperacillin, Piperacillin/tazobactam sodium, Ticarcillin, Ticarcillin/potassium clavulanate.

See also *General Nursing Considerations for All Anti-Infectives*.

Uses: See individual drugs. Effective against a variety of gram-positive, gram-negative, and anaerobic organisms.

Contraindications: Hypersensitivity to penicillins, imipenem, β–lactamase inhibitors, and cephalosporins. PO use of penicillins during the acute stages of empyema, bacteremia, pneumonia, meningitis, pericarditis, and purulent or septic arthritis. Use with a history of amoxicillin/clavulanate–associated cholestatic jaundice or hepatic dysfunction. Lactation.

Special Concerns: Use of penicillins during lactation may lead to sensitization, diarrhea, candidiasis, and skin rash in the infant. Use with caution in clients with a history of asthma, hay fever, or urticaria. Clients with cystic fibrosis have a higher incidence of side effects with broad spectrum penicillins. Safety and effectiveness of carbenicillin, piperacillin, and the beta-lactamase inhibitor/penicillin combinations (e.g., amoxicillin/potassium clavulanate, ticarcillin/ potassium clavulanate) have not been determined in children less than 12 years of age. The incidence of resistant strains of staphylococci to penicillinase-resistant penicillins is increasing. Use of prolonged therapy may lead to superinfection (i.e., bacterial or fungal overgrowth of nonsusceptible organisms). Cystic fibrosis clients have a higher incidence of side effects if given extended spectrum penicillins.

Side Effects: Penicillins are potent sensitizing agents; it is estimated that up to 10% of the US population is allergic to the antibiotic. Hypersensitivity reactions are reported to be on the increase in pediatric populations. Sensitivity reactions may be immediate (within 20 min) or delayed (as long as several days or weeks after initiation of therapy). *Allergic:* Skin rashes (including maculopapular and exanthematous), exfoliative dermatitis, erythema multiforme (rarely, ***Stevens-Johnson syndrome***), hives, pruritus, wheezing, ***anaphylaxis,*** fever, eosinophilia, hypersensitivity myocarditis, ***angioedema,*** serum sickness, ***laryngeal edema, laryngospasm, prostration, angioneurotic edema, bronchospasm, hypotension, vascular collapse, death.*** *GI:* Diarrhea (may be severe), abdominal cramps or pain, N&V, bloating, flatulence, increased thirst, bitter/unpleasant taste, glossitis, gastritis, stomatitis, dry mouth, sore mouth or tongue, furry tongue, black "hairy" tongue, bloody diarrhea, rectal bleeding, enterocolitis, pseudomembranous colitis. *CNS:* Dizziness, insomnia, hyperactivity, fatigue, prolonged muscle relaxation. Neurotoxicity including lethargy, neuromuscular irritability, ***seizures,*** hallucinations following large IV doses (especially in clients with renal failure). *Hematologic:* Thrombocytopenia, leukopenia, ***agranulocytosis,*** anemia, thrombocytopenic purpura, ***hemolytic anemia,*** granulocytopenia, neutropenia, bone marrow depression. *Renal:* Oliguria, hematuria, hyaline casts, proteinuria, pyuria (all symptoms of interstitial nephritis), nephropathy. Electrolyte imbalance following IV use. *Miscellaneous:* Hepatotoxicity (cholestatic jaundice), superinfection, swelling of face and ankles, anorexia, hyperthermia, transient hepatitis, vaginitis, itchy eyes. IM injection may cause pain and induration at the injection site, ecchymosis, and hematomas. IV use may cause vein irritation, deep vein thrombosis, and thrombophlebitis.

OD Management of Overdose: *Symptoms:* Neuromuscular hyperexcitability, convulsive seizures. Massive IV doses may cause agitation, asterixis, hallucinations, confusion, stupor, multifocal myoclonus, seizures, coma, hyperkalemia, and encephalopathy. *Treatment (Severe Allergic or Anaphylactic Reactions):* Administer epinephrine (0.3–0.5 mL of a 1:1,000 solution SC or IM, or 0.2–0.3 mL diluted in 10 mL saline, given slowly by IV). Corticosteroids should be on hand. In those instances where penicillin is the drug of choice, the physician may decide to use it even though the client is allergic, adding a medication to the regimen to control the allergic response.

Drug Interactions

Aminoglycosides / Penicillins ↓ effect of aminoglycosides, although they are used together

Antacids / ↓ Effect of penicillins due to ↓ absorption from GI tract

Antibiotics, Chloramphenicol, Erythromycins, Tetracyclines / ↓ Effect of penicillins, although synergism has also been seen

Anticoagulants / ↑ Bleeding risk by prolonging bleeding time if used with parenteral penicillins

Aspirin / ↑ Effect of penicillins by ↓ plasma protein binding
Chloramphenicol / Either ↑ or ↓ effects
Erythromycins / Either ↑ or ↓ effects
Heparin / ↑ Risk of bleeding following parenteral penicillins
Oral contraceptives / ↓ Effect of oral contraceptives
Probenecid / ↑ Effect of penicillins by ↓ excretion
Tetracyclines / ↓ Effect of penicillins

Dosage

See individual drugs. Penicillins are available in a variety of dosage forms for PO, parenteral, inhalation, and intrathecal administration. PO doses must be higher than IM or SC doses because a large fraction of penicillin given PO may be destroyed in the stomach.

Laboratory Test Considerations: ↓ Hematocrit, hemoglobin, WBC lymphocytes, serum potassium, albumin, total proteins, uric acid. ↑ Basophils, lymphocytes, monocytes, platelets, serum alkaline phosphatase, serum sodium. ↑ AST, ALT, bilirubin, LDH following semisynthetic penicillins.

1. IM and IV administration of penicillin causes a great deal of local irritation; thus, inject slowly.
2. IM injections are made deeply into the gluteal muscle. IV injections are usually diluted with an IV infusion.

HEALTH CARE CONSIDERATIONS

Assessment: Assess for allergic reactions; if reaction occurs, stop drug immediately. Allergic reactions are more likely to occur with a history of asthma, hay fever, urticaria, or allergy to cephalosporins.

Interventions

1. Detain in an ambulatory care site for at least 20 min after administering to assess for anaphylaxis.
2. Long-acting types of penicillin are for IM use only; may cause emboli, CNS pathology, or cardiac pathology if administered IV.
3. Do not massage repository (long-acting) penicillin products after injection; rate of absorption should not be increased.
4. Rapid administration of IV penicillin may cause local irritation and may precipitate convulsions. With some agents, high-dose therapy may precipitate aplastic anemia.
5. The elderly may be more sensitive to the effects of penicillin than younger people. Calculate dose based on weight and height.
6. Most penicillins are excreted in breast milk and should be prescribed cautiously to nursing mothers.

Client/Family Teaching

1. Review drugs prescribed, method and frequency of administration, side effects, and expected outcome/goals of therapy.
2. Stop medication and report any S&S of allergic reactions, i.e., rashes, fever, joint swelling, angioneurotic edema, intense itching, and respiratory distress (during therapy and in some cases 7–12 days after therapy).
3. Oral penicillins may cause GI upset. Take with a glass of water 1 hr before or 2 hr after meals to minimize binding to foods.
4. Return for repository penicillin injections as scheduled.
5. Complete the entire prescribed course of therapy, even if feeling well. Incomplete therapy will predispose client to development of resistant bacterial strains. With α-hemolytic *Streptococcus* infection, must take for a minimum of 10 days, and preferably 14 days, to prevent development of rheumatic fever or glomerulonephritis.
6. Report S&S of superinfections (furry tongue, vaginal or rectal itching, diarrhea).
7. Report if S&S do not improve or get worse after 48–72 hr of therapy.

Outcome/Evaluate

- Symptomatic improvement
- Resolution of infection (↓ fever, ↓ WBCs, ↑ appetite, negative cultures)

PROGESTERONE AND PROGESTINS

See also the following individual entries:

Levonorgestrel implants
Medroxyprogesterone acetate
Megestrol acetate
Oral Contraceptives
Progesterone gel

Action/Kinetics: Progesterone is the primary endogenous progestin. Progesterone inhibits, through positive feedback, the secretion of pituitary gonadotropins; in turn, this prevents follicular maturation and ovulation or alternatively promotes it for the "primed" follicle. It is required to prepare the endometrium for implantation of the embryo. Once implanted, progesterone is required to maintain pregnancy. Progestins inhibit spontaneous uterine contractions; certain progestins may cause androgenic or anabolic effects. Progestins given PO are rapidly absorbed and quickly metabolized in the liver. **Peak levels, after PO:** 1–2 hr. **t½, after PO:** 2–3 hr during the first 6 hr after ingestion; thereafter, 8–9 hr. **After IM,** effective levels can be maintained for 3–6 months with a **t½** of about 10 weeks. **t½, elimination, gel:** 5–20 min. A major portion is excreted in the urine with a small amount in the bile and feces.

Uses: Abnormal uterine bleeding, primary or secondary amenorrhea (used with an estrogen), endometriosis. Alone or with an estrogen for contraception. May also be used in combination with an estrogen for endometriosis and hypermenorrhea. Certain types of cancer. AIDS wasting syndrome (megestrol acetate). Infertility (progesterone gel). *NOTE:* Not to be used to prevent habitual abortion or to treat threatened abortion. *Investigational:* Medroxyprogesterone has been used to treat menopausal symptoms.

Contraindications: Carcinoma of the breast or genital organs, thromboembolic disease, thrombophlebitis, vaginal bleeding of unknown origin, impaired liver function, cerebral hemorrhage or those with a history of such, missed abortion, as a diagnostic test for pregnancy. Pregnancy, especially during the first 4 months.

Special Concerns: Use with caution in case of asthma, epilepsy, depression, migraine, and cardiac or renal dysfunction.

Side Effects: See also individual drugs. Occasionally noted with short-term dosage, frequently observed with prolonged high dosage. *CNS:* Depression, insomnia, somnolence. *GU:* Breakthrough bleeding, spotting, amenorrhea, changes in amount and/or duration of menstrual flow, changes in cervical secretions and cervical erosion, breast tenderness or secretions. *Dermatologic:* Allergic rashes with and without pruritus, acne, melasma, chloasma, photosensitivity, local reactions at the site of injection. *Note:* Progesterone is especially irritating at the site of injection, especially aqueous products. *Miscellaneous:* Weight gain or loss, cholestatic jaundice, masculinization of the female fetus, nausea, edema, precipitation of acute intermittent porphyria, pyrexia, hirsutism.

Dosage

See individual drugs. The usual schedule of administration for *functional uterine bleeding, amenorrhea, infertility, dysmenorrhea, premenstrual tension, and contraception* is days 5 through 25 of the menstrual cycle, with day 1 being the first day of menstrual flow.

Laboratory Test Considerations: Progestins may affect laboratory test results of hepatic function, thyroid, pregnanediol determination, and endocrine function. ↑ Prothrombin and Factors VII, VIII, IX, and X. ↓ Glucose tolerance (especially in diabetic clients).

HEALTH CARE CONSIDERATIONS

Assessment

1. Identify indications for therapy. Assess for any thrombophlebitis, pulmonary embolism, cardiac, liver, or renal dysfunction, cerebral hemorrhage, breast or genital cancers.
2. Monitor VS, ECG, weight, and labs.
3. Note any history of psychic depression or diabetes mellitus.
4. Record last menstrual period and absence of pregnancy.

Client/Family Teaching

1. To avoid gastric irritation and nausea, take with a light snack, in the evening. Take at the same time each day.
2. Gastric distress usually subsides after the first few cycles of the drug; report if these symptoms persist.
3. Report any symptoms of thrombic disorders such as pains in the legs, sudden onset of chest pain, SOB, and coughing.
4. Weigh twice a week and report any unusual weight gain/edema.
5. Report any yellowing of the skin or sclera (jaundice) which may necessitate discontinuation of the medication, evaluation of LFTs, and possibly a dosage change.
6. Report any unusual bleeding.
7. Progestins may reactivate or worsen psychic depression. Report any mental status changes and the circumstance of the depression.
8. With diabetes, progesterone may alter glucose tolerance and the dosage of antidiabetic medication may need to be adjusted.
9. Report early symptoms of ophthalmic pathology, such as headaches, dizziness, blurred vision, or partial loss of vision, and get a thorough eye exam.
10. Stop smoking; enroll in a formal smoking cessation program.
11. With birth control, injections must be administered every 3 mo to ensure adequate protection.
12. Progestin-only oral contraceptives may be used as early as 3 weeks after delivery in women who partially breast feed and within 6 weeks after delivery in women who fully breast feed.

Outcome/Evaluate

- Control of abnormal menstrual bleeding; menstrual regularity
- Weight gain with AIDS clients
- Effective contraceptive agent
- Symptomatic improvement in menstrual pain and flow
- ↓ Size/resolution ovarian cyst(s)

SKELETAL MUSCLE RELAXANTS, CENTRALLY ACTING

See also the following individual entries:

Baclofen
Carisoprodol
Chlorzoxazone
Cyclobenzaprine hydrochloride
Diazepam
Methocarbamol
Tizanidine

Action/Kinetics: These drugs decrease muscle tone and involuntary movement. Many relieve anxiety and tension as well. Although the precise mechanism of action is unknown, most of these agents depress spinal polysynaptic reflexes. Their beneficial effects may also be attributable to their antianxiety activity. Several of the drugs in this group also manifest analgesic properties.

Uses: Musculoskeletal and neurologic disorders associated with muscle spasms, hyperreflexia, and hypertonia, including parkinsonism, tetanus, tension headaches, acute muscle spasms caused by trauma, and inflammation (e.g., low back syndrome, sprains, arthritis, bursitis). They also may be useful in the management of cerebral palsy and multiple sclerosis.

Side Effects: See individual drugs.

OD **Management of Overdose:** *Symptoms:* Often extensions of the side effects. Stupor, ***coma, shock-like syndrome, respiratory depression,*** loss of muscle tone, and impaired deep tendon reflexes may also occur. *Treatment:* Symptomatic. Emesis or gastric lavage (followed by activated charcoal). If necessary, artificial respiration, oxygen administration, pressor agents, and IV fluids may be used. It may be possible to increase the rate of excretion of selected drugs by diuretics (including mannitol), peritoneal dialysis, or hemodialysis.

Drug Interactions: Centrally acting muscle relaxants may increase the sedative and respiratory depressant effects of CNS depressants (e.g., alcohol, barbiturates, sedatives and hypnotics, and antianxiety agents).

Dosage

See individual agents.

1. If unable to swallow, crush tablets or empty capsules into a small amount of fruit juice.
2. If skeletal muscle relaxant is to be discontinued after long-term use, taper the dose to prevent rebound spasticity, hallucinations, or other withdrawal symptoms.
3. Determine the lowest dosage to treat symptoms.

HEALTH CARE CONSIDERATIONS

Assessment

1. Record indications for therapy. List other agents prescribed and the outcome.
2. Note any prior seizures; may cause loss of seizure control.
3. Assess extent of musculoskeletal and neurologic disorders associated with muscle spasm. Note muscle stiffness, pain, and extent of ROM.
4. Record baseline mental status.

Interventions

1. Monitor BP q 4 hr. Supervise ambulation/transfers and ensure safe environment. Sedentary or immobilized clients are more prone to hypotension upon ambulation.
2. Monitor urinary output; evaluate need for drugs to increase excretion rate.
3. Record level of mobility (ROM) and comfort (pain) prior to and following drug administration.
4. Check muscle responses and DTRs for evidence of drug overdosage.

Client/Family Teaching

1. Take with meals to reduce GI upset.
2. These drugs may impair mental alertness; do not operate dangerous machinery or drive a car.
3. Do not stop abruptly; may precipitate withdrawal symptoms, rebound spasticity, and hallucinations.
4. Review additional therapies that may be prescribed for muscle spasm (heat, rest, exercise, physical therapy) and adhering to prescribed regimen.
5. Increase fluids and bulk in diet to prevent constipation.
6. Report if the urine becomes dark, the skin or sclera appears yellow, or itching develops.
7. Avoid alcohol and any other CNS depressants. Antihistamines may cause an additive depressant effect.
8. Report persistent nausea, anorexia, or changes in taste perception, as nutritional state may become impaired.
9. Report as scheduled for all lab and medical visits so therapy can be evaluated and drug dosage adjusted.

Outcome/Evaluate

- Improvement in extent/intensity of muscle spasm and pain

- ↑ ROM with measurable improvement in muscle tone, mobility, and involuntary movements
- Relief of tension headaches

SUCCINIMIDE ANTICONVULSANTS

See also the following individual entries:

Ethosuximide
Methsuximide
Phensuximide

Action/Kinetics: Suppress the paroxysmal 3-cycle/sec spike and wave activity that is associated with lapses of consciousness seen in absence seizures. Act by depressing the motor cortex and by raising the threshold of the CNS to convulsive stimuli. Rapidly absorbed from the GI tract.

See also *Health Care Considerations* for *Anticonvulsants.*

Uses: Primarily absence seizures (petit mal). May be given concomitantly with other anticonvulsants if other types of epilepsy are manifested with absence seizures.

Contraindications: Hypersensitivity to succinimides.

Special Concerns: Safe use during pregnancy has not been established. Use with caution in clients with abnormal liver and kidney function.

Side Effects: *CNS:* Drowsiness, ataxia, dizziness, headaches, euphoria, lethargy, fatigue, insomnia, irritability, nervousness, dreamlike state, hyperactivity. Psychiatric or psychologic aberrations such as mental slowing, hypochondriasis, sleep disturbances, inability to concentrate, depression, night terrors, instability, confusion, aggressiveness. Rarely, auditory hallucinations, paranoid psychosis, increased libido, suicidal behavior. *GI:* N&V, hiccoughs, anorexia, diarrhea, gastric distress, weight loss, abdominal and epigastric pain, cramps, constipation. *Hematologic:* Leukopenia, granulocytopenia, eosinophilia, ***agranulocytosis,*** pancytopenia with or without bone marrow suppression, monocytosis. *Dermatologic:* Pruritus, urticaria, erythema multiforme, lupus erythematosus, ***Stevens-Johnson syndrome,*** pruritic erythematous rashes, skin eruptions, alopecia, hirsutism, photophobia. *GU:* Urinary frequency, vaginal bleeding, renal damage, microscopic hematuria. *Miscellaneous:* Blurred vision, muscle weakness, hyperemia, hypertrophy of gums, swollen tongue, myopia, periorbital edema.

OD Management of Overdose: *Symptoms (Acute Overdose):* Confusion, sleepiness, slow shallow respiration, N&V, ***CNS depression with coma and respiratory depression,*** hypotension, cyanosis, hyper- or hypothermia, absence of reflexes, unsteadiness, flaccid muscles. *Symptoms (Chronic Overdose):* Ataxia, dizziness, drowsiness, confusion, depression, proteinuria, skin rashes, hangover, irritability, poor judgment, N&V, muscle weakness, periorbital edema, hepatic dysfunction, ***fatal bone marrow aplasia, delayed onset of coma,*** nephrosis, hematuria, casts. *Treatment:* General supportive measures. Charcoal hemoperfusion may be helpful.

Drug Interactions: Succinimides may ↑ effects of hydantoins by ↓ breakdown by the liver.

Dosage

Individualized. See individual agents.

HEALTH CARE CONSIDERATIONS

Client/Family Teaching

1. Take as directed and do not stop abruptly; may cause an increase in the severity and frequency of seizures.
2. Caution should be exercised while driving or performing other tasks requiring alertness and coordination; initially may cause, dizziness, blurred vision, headaches, N&V, and drowsiness.
3. Alert family to the possibility of transient personality changes, hypochondriacal behavior, and aggressiveness, which should be reported.
4. Report any increase in frequency of tonic-clonic (grand mal) seizures.
5. Any persistent fever, swollen glands, and bleeding gums may signal a blood dyscrasia.
6. May discolor urine pinkish brown.
7. Report for CBC, liver and renal function studies as scheduled.

Outcome/Evaluate: Control/ ↓ frequency of seizure activity

SULFONAMIDES

See also the following individual entries:

Mafenide acetate
Pediazole
Sulfacetamide sodium
Sulfadiazine
Sulfamethoxazole
Sulfasalazine
Sulfisoxazole
Sulfisoxazole diolamine
Trimethoprim and Sulfamethoxazole

Action/Kinetics: Structurally related to PABA and, as such, competitively inhibit the enzyme dihydropteroate synthetase, which is responsible for incorporating PABA into dihydrofolic acid. Thus, the synthesis of dihydrofolic acid is inhibited, resulting in a decrease in tetrahydrofolic acid, which is required for synthesis of DNA, purines, and thymidine. Are bacteriostatic. Readily absorbed from the GI tract. Distributed throughout all tissues, including the CSF, where concentrations attain 50%–80% of those found in the blood. Metabolized in the liver and primarily excreted by the kidneys. Small amounts are found in the feces, bile, breast milk, and other secretions.

See also *General Nursing Considerations for All Anti-Infectives.*

Uses: PO, Parenteral. See individual drugs. Uses include urinary tract infections, chancroid, meningitis caused by *Hemophilus influenzae,* meningogoccal meningitis, rheumatic fever, nocardiosis, trachoma, with pyrimethamine for toxoplasmosis, with quinine sulfate and pyrimethamine for chloroquine-resistant *Plasmodium falciparum,* and with penicillin for otitis media.

Ophthalmic. Conjunctivitis, corneal ulcer, and other superficial ocular infections due to susceptible organisms. Adjunct to systemic sulfonamides to treat trachoma.

Vaginal. Sulfanilamide is used to treat *Candida albicans* vulvovaginitis only.

Contraindications: Hypersensitivity reactions to sulfonamides and chemically related drugs (e.g., thiazides, sulfonylureas, loop diuretics, carbonic anhydrase inhibitors, local anesthetics, PABA-containing sunscreens). Use in infants less than 2 years of age, except with pyrimethamine to treat congenital toxoplasmosis. Use at term during pregnancy. Use in premature infants who are nursing or those with hyperbilirubinemia or G6PD deficiency. Group A beta-hemolytic streptococcal infections.

Special Concerns: Use with caution, and in reduced dosage, in clients with impaired liver or renal function, intestinal or urinary tract obstructions, blood dyscrasias, allergies, asthma, and hereditary G6PD deficiency. Use with caution if exposed to sunlight or ultraviolet light as photosensitivity may occur. Superinfection is a possibility. Use ophthalmic products with caution in clients with dry eye. Safety and efficacy of ophthalmic use in children have not been determined.

Side Effects: Systemic. *GI:* N&V, diarrhea, abdominal pain, glossitis, stomatitis, anorexia, pseudomembranous enterocolitis, pancreatitis, hepatitis, ***hepatocellular necrosis.*** *Allergic:* Rash, pruritus, photosensitivity, erythema nodosum or multiforme, generalized skin eruptions, ***Stevens-Johnson syndrome,*** conjunctivitis, rhinitis, balanitis. Serum sickness, urticaria, pruritus, exfoliative dermatitis, ***anaphylaxis, toxic epidermal necrolysis*** with or without corneal damage, periorbital edema, conjunctival and scleral injection, allergic myocarditis, decreased pulmonary function with eosinophila, disseminated lupus erythematosus, periarteritis nodosa, arteritis. *CNS:* Headaches, mental depression, ***seizures,*** hallucinations, vertigo, insomnia, apathy, ataxia, drowsiness, restlessness. *Renal:* Crystalluria, toxic nephrosis with oliguria and anuria, elevated creatinine. *Hematologic:* ***Aplastic anemia,*** leukopenia, neutropenia, ***agranulocytosis,*** thrombocytopenia, hemolytic anemia, methemoglobinemia, purpura, hypoprothrombinemia. *Neurologic:* Peripheral neuropathy, polyneuritis, neuritis, optic neuritis. *Miscellaneous:* Jaundice, tinnitus, arthralgia, superinfection, hearing loss, drug fever, pyrexia, chills, lupus erythematosus phenomenon, transient myopia.

By killing the intestinal flora, the sulfonamides also reduce the bacterial synthesis of vitamin K. This may result in ***hemorrhage.*** Administration of vitamin K to clients on long-term sulfonamide therapy is recommended.

Ophthalmic Use. Headache, browache. Blurred vision, eye irritation, itching, transient epithelial keratitis, reactive hyperemia, conjunctival edema, burning and transient stinging. Rarely, ***Stevens-Johnson syndrome,*** exfoliative dermatitis, ***toxic epidermal necrolysis,*** photosensitivity, fever, skin rash, GI disturbances, and bone marrow depression.

OD **Management of Overdose:** *Symptoms:* N&V, anorexia, colic, dizziness, drowsiness, headache, unconsciousness, vertigo, toxic fever. More serious manifestations include ***acute hemolytic anemia, agranulocytosis,*** acidosis, maculopapular dermatitis, hepatic jaundice, sensitivity reactions, toxic neuritis, ***death*** (several days after the first dose). *Treatment:* Immediately discontinue the drug.

- Induce emesis or perform gastric lavage, especially if large doses were taken.
- To hasten excretion, alkalinize the urine and force fluids (if kidney function is normal). If there is renal blockage due to sulfonamide crystals, catheterization of the ureters may be needed.
- In the event of agranulocytosis, antibiotic therapy is needed to combat infection.
- To treat severe anemia or thrombocytopenia, blood or platelet transfusions are required.

Drug Interactions

Anticoagulants, oral / ↑ Effect of anticoagulants due to ↓ plasma protein binding

Antidiabetics, oral / ↑ Hypoglycemic effect due to ↓ plasma protein binding
Cyclosporine / ↓ Effect of cyclosporine and ↑ nephrotoxicity
Diuretics, thiazide / ↑ Risk of thrombocytopenia with purpura
Indomethacin / ↑ Effect of sulfonamides due to ↓ plasma protein binding
Methenamine / ↑ Chance of sulfonamide crystalluria due to acid urine
Methotrexate / ↑ Risk of methotrexate-induced bone marrow suppression
Phenytoin / ↑ Effect of phenytoin due to ↓ breakdown in liver
Probenecid / ↑ Effect of sulfonamides due to ↓ plasma protein binding
Salicylates / ↑ Effect of sulfonamides due to ↓ plasma protein binding
Silver products / Incompatible with ophthalmic products
Uricosuric agents / Potentiation of uricosuric action

Dosage

See individual drugs.

Laboratory Test Considerations: False + or ↑ LFTs (amino acids, bilirubin, BSP), renal function (BUN, NPN, C_{CR}), blood counts, PT, Coombs' test. False + or ↑ urine glucose (copper reduction methods, such as Benedict's solution or Clinitest), protein, urobilinogen.

1. Do not use ophthalmic solutions if they have darkened or contain a precipitate.
2. Take care to avoid contamination of ophthalmic products.

HEALTH CARE CONSIDERATIONS

Assessment

1. Obtain a thorough medical and drug history. Note previous sulfonamide therapy and response.
2. Record indications for therapy, type, onset, and characteristics of symptoms. List other agents prescribed and the outcome.
3. Question concerning any conditions that may preclude drug therapy, i.e., intestinal problems, urinary tract obstructions, G6PD deficiency (may precipitate hemolysis), or allergies.
4. Determine if pregnant; drug may be harmful to developing fetus.
5. Monitor CBC, blood sugars, bleeding times, cultures, liver and renal function studies.

Interventions

1. During drug therapy, assess for any of the following reactions that may require drug withdrawal:
• Skin rashes, abdominal pain, anorexia, irritation of the mouth or tingling of the extremities
• Blood dyscrasias (characterized by sore throat, fever, pallor, purpura, jaundice, or weakness)
• Serum sickness (characterized by eruptions of purpuric spots and pain in limbs and joints); onset 7–10 days after initiation of therapy.
• Early S&S of Stevens-Johnson syndrome (characterized by high fever, severe headaches, stomatitis, conjunctivitis, rhinitis, urethritis, and balanitis [inflammation of the tip of the penis])
• Jaundice, indicating hepatic involvement; onset 3–5 days after initiation of therapy
• Renal involvement (characterized by renal colic, oliguria, anuria, hematuria, and proteinuria)
• Ecchymosis and hemorrhage (caused by decreased synthesis of vitamin K by intestinal bacteria)
• Hemolytic anemia especially in the elderly
• Behavioral changes or acute mental disturbances
2. Monitor I&O and record. Encourage adequate fluid intake to prevent crystalluria. Observe urinalysis for evidence of crystals. Minimum urine output should be 1.5 L/day. Test urine pH to determine excess acidity. Administration of a particularly insoluble sulfonamide may require urine alkalinization (i.e., $NaHCO_3$).
3. If administering long-acting sulfonamides, adequate fluid intake must be maintained for 24–48 hr after the drug has been discontinued.

Client/Family Teaching

1. Take on time and as prescribed despite feeling better.
2. May color urine orange-red or brown; not cause for alarm but report.
3. Take with 6–8 oz (180–240 mL) of water and maintain adequate fluid intake for 24–48 hr after therapy.
4. May cause N&V and loss of appetite. Monitor I&O and consume > 2.5 L/day of fluids.
5. Test urine pH and report changes in acidity as additional drug therapy may be necessary.
6. Avoid Vitamin C; may make the urine more acidic and contribute to crystal formation.
7. If also taking anticoagulants, report increased bleeding tendencies.
8. Avoid prolonged exposure to sunlight; may cause a photosensitivity reaction. Wear protective clothing, sunglasses, and sunscreen.
9. Report any changes in vision or hearing. With ophthalmic use, report if no improve-

ment in 5–7 days, if condition worsens, or if pain, redness, itching, or eye swelling occurs.
10. Do not perform activities that require mental alertness until drug effects realized.
11. Vaginal intercourse should be avoided when using vaginal products.
12. Report for labs as scheduled; notify provider if symptoms do not improve or worsen after 48–72 hr.

Outcome/Evaluate

- Negative C&S results (note any organism resistance to sulfonamide)
- Resolution of infection; symptomatic improvement

SYMPATHOMIMETIC DRUGS

See also the following individual entries:

Albuterol
Bitolterol mesylate
Brimonidine tartrate
Ephedrine sulfate
Epinephrine
Epinephrine bitartrate
Epinephrine borate
Epinephrine hydrochloride
Isoetharine hydrochloride
Isoproterenol sulfate
Metaproterenol sulfate
Phenylephrine hydrochloride
Pirbuterol acetate
Pseudoephedrine hydrochloride
Pseudoephedrine sulfate
Salmeterol xinafoate
Terbutaline sulfate

Action/Kinetics: Adrenergic drugs act: (1) by mimicking the action of norepinephrine or epinephrine by combining with alpha and/or beta receptors (directly acting sympathomimetics) or (2) by causing or regulating the release of the natural neurohormones from their storage sites at the nerve terminals (indirectly acting sympathomimetics). Some drugs exhibit a combination of both effects.

Adrenergic stimulation of receptors will manifest the following general effects:
Alpha-1-adrenergic: / Vasoconstriction, decongestion, constriction of the pupil of the eye, contraction of splenic capsule, contraction of the trigone-sphincter muscle of the urinary bladder.
Alpha-2-adrenergic: / Presynaptic to regulate amount of transmitter released; decrease tone, motility, and secretory activity of the GI tract (possibly involved in hypersecretory response also); decrease insulin secretion.
Beta-1-adrenergic: / Myocardial contraction (inotropic), regulation of heartbeat (chronotropic), improved impulse conduction, ↑ lipolysis.
Beta-2-adrenergic: / Peripheral vasodilation, bronchial dilation; ↓ tone, motility, and secretory activity of the GI tract; ↑ renin secretion.

Uses: See individual drugs.

Contraindications: Tachycardia due to arrhythmias; tachycardia or heart block caused by digitalis toxicity.

Special Concerns: Use with caution in hyperthyroidism, diabetes, prostatic hypertrophy, seizures, degenerative heart disease, especially in geriatric clients or those with asthma, emphysema, or psychoneuroses. Also, use with caution in clients with coronary insufficiency, CAD, ischemic heart disease, CHF, cardiac arrhythmias, hypertension, or history of stroke. Asthma clients who rely heavily on inhaled beta-2-agonist bronchodilators may increase their chances of death. Thus, use to "rescue" clients but do not prescribe for regular long-term use. Beta-2 agonists may inhibit uterine contractions.

Side Effects: See individual drugs; side effects common to most sympathomimetics are listed. *CV:* Tachycardia, arrhythmias, palpitations, BP changes, anginal pain, precordial pain, pallor, skipped beats, chest tightness, hypertension. *GI:* N&V, heartburn, anorexia, altered taste or bad taste, GI distress, dry mouth, diarrhea. *CNS:* Restlessness, anxiety, tension, insomnia, hyperkinesis, drowsiness, weakness, vertigo, irritability, dizziness, headache, tremors, general CNS stimulation, nervousness, shakiness, hyperactivity. *Respiratory:* Cough, dyspnea, dry throat, pharyngitis, ***paradoxical bronchospasm,*** irritation. *Other:* Flushing, sweating, ***allergic reactions***.

OD **Management of Overdose:** *Symptoms:* Following inhalation: Exaggeration of side effects resulting in anginal pain, hypertension, hypokalemia, ***seizures.*** Following systemic use: CV symptoms include bradycardia, tachycardia, palpitations, extrasystoles, ***heart block,*** elevated BP, chest pain, hypokalemia. CNS symptoms include anxiety, insomnia, tremor, delirium, ***convulsions, collapse, and coma.*** Also, fever, chills, cold perspiration, N&V, mydriasis, and blanching of the skin. *Treatment:*

- For overdosage due to inhalation: General supportive measures with sedatives given for restlessness. Use metoprolol or atenolol cautiously as they may induce an asthmatic attack in clients with asthma.

• For systemic overdosage: Discontinue or decrease dose. General supportive measures. For overdose due to PO agents, emesis, gastric lavage, or charcoal may be helpful. In severe cases, propranolol may be used but this may cause airway obstruction. Phentolamine may be given to block strong alpha-adrenergic effects.

Drug Interactions

Beta-adrenergic blocking agents / Inhibit adrenergic stimulation of the heart and bronchial tree; cause bronchial constriction; hypertension, asthma, not relieved by adrenergic agents
Ammonium chloride / ↓ Effect of sympathomimetics due to ↑ excretion by kidney
Anesthetics / Halogenated anesthetics sensitize heart to adrenergics—causes cardiac arrhythmias
Anticholinergics / Concomitant use aggravates glaucoma
Antidiabetics / Hyperglycemic effect of epinephrine may necessitate ↑ dosage of insulin or oral hypoglycemic agents
Corticosteroids / Chronic use with sympathomimetics may result in or aggravate glaucoma; aerosols containing sympathomimetics and corticosteroids may be lethal in asthmatic children
Digitalis glycosides / Combination may cause cardiac arrhythmias
Furazolidone / Furazolidone ↑ effects of mixed-acting sympathomimetics
Guanethidine / Direct-acting sympathomimetics ↑ effects of guanethidine, while indirect-acting sympathomimetics ↓ effects of guanethidine; also reversal of hypotensive effects of guanethidine
Lithium / ↓ Pressor effect of direct-acting sympathomimetics
MAO inhibitors / All effects of sympathomimetics are potentiated; symptoms include hypertensive crisis with possible intracranial hemorrhage, hyperthermia, convulsions, coma; death may occur
Methyldopa / ↑ Pressor response
Methylphenidate / Potentiates pressor effect of sympathomimetics; combination hazardous in glaucoma
Oxytocics / ↑ Chance of severe hypertension
Phenothiazines / ↑ Risk of cardiac arrhythmias
Reserpine / ↑ Risk of hypertension following use of direct-acting sympathomimetics and ↓ effect of indirect-acting sympathomimetics
Sodium bicarbonate / ↑ Effect of sympathomimetics due to ↓ excretion by kidney
Theophylline / Enhanced toxicity (especially cardiotoxicity); also ↓ theophylline levels
Thyroxine / Potentiation of pressor response of sympathomimetics
Tricyclic antidepressants / ↑ Effect of direct-acting sympathomimetics and ↓ effect of indirect-acting sympathomimetics

Dosage

See individual drugs.Discard colored solutions.

HEALTH CARE CONSIDERATIONS

Assessment

1. Determine any sensitivity to adrenergic drugs.
2. Note previous experience with drugs in this class and the outcome.
3. Record any history of CAD, tachycardia, endocrine disturbances, or respiratory tract problems.
4. Obtain baseline data regarding general physical condition and hemodynamic status including ECG, VS, and lab data and monitor.
5. Record indications for therapy, contributing factors, and anticipated response.

Client/Family Teaching

1. Review prescribed drug therapy and potential drug side effects.
2. Take exactly as directed. Do not increase the dosage and do not take more frequently than prescribed. Consult provider if symptoms become more severe.
3. Take early in the day to prevent insomnia.
4. Feelings/symptoms of fear or anxiety may be evident; these drugs mimic body's stress response.
5. Avoid all OTC preparations.
6. Stop smoking to preserve current lung function. Attend formal smoking cessation classes.

SPECIAL HEALTH CARE CONSIDERATIONS FOR ADRENERGIC BRONCHODILATORS

Assessment

1. Obtain history and PE prior to starting drug therapy.
2. Note any experience with this class of drugs.
3. Monitor VS to assess CV response.
4. Record lung assessment, ABGs (or O_2 saturation), and pulmonary function tests. Note characteristics of cough and sputum production.

Client/Family Teaching

1. Review technique for use and care of prescribed inhalers and respiratory equipment. Rinsing of equipment and of mouth after use is imperative in preventing oral fungal infections. Maintain record of peak flow

readings and seek medical attention at identified levels.
2. If postural drainage prescribed, review how to cough productively and show family how to clap and vibrate the chest to promote good respiratory hygiene.
3. Regular, consistent use of the drug is essential for maximum benefit, but overuse can be life-threatening.
4. To improve lung ventilation and reduce fatigue during eating, start inhalation therapy upon arising in the morning and before meals.
5. A single aerosol treatment is usually enough to control an asthma attack. Overuse of adrenergic bronchodilators may result in reduced effectiveness, paradoxical reaction, and death from cardiac arrest.
6. Increased fluid intake will aid in liquefying secretions and removal.
7. Consult provider if dizziness or chest pain occurs, or if there is no relief when the usual dose is used.
8. Avoid OTC preparations and any other unprescribed adrenergic meds.
9. Consult provider if more than three aerosol treatments in a 24-hr period are required for relief.
10. If using inhalable meds and bronchodilators, use the bronchodilator first and wait 5 min before using the other medication.
11. **Stop smoking,** avoid crowds during "flu seasons," dress warmly in cold weather, receive the pneumonia vaccine and seasonal flu shot, and stay in air conditioning during hot, humid days to prevent exacerbations of illness.
12. Have family/significant other learn CPR.

Interventions

1. Observe effects on CNS; if pronounced, adjust dosage and frequency of administration.
2. With status asthmaticus and abnormal ABGs, continue to provide oxygen and ventilating assistance even though the symptoms appear to be relieved by the bronchodilator.
3. To prevent depression of respiratory effort, administer oxygen based on client's clinical symptoms and ABGs or O_2 saturations.
4. If three to five aerosol treatments of the same agent have been administered within the last 6–12 hr, with no relief, further evaluation is warranted.
5. If dyspnea worsens after repeated excessive use of the inhaler, paradoxical airway resistance may occur. Be prepared to assist with alternative therapy and respiratory support.

Outcome/Evaluate

- Knowledge/understanding of disease; adherence with prescribed medication regimen
- A positive clinical response evidenced by ↓ symptoms for which the therapy was prescribed

TETRACYCLINES

See also the following individual entries:

Doxycycline calcium
Doxycycline hyclate
Doxycycline monohydrate
Tetracycline

Action/Kinetics: Tetracyclines inhibit protein synthesis by microorganisms by binding to the ribosomal 50S subunit, thereby interfering with protein synthesis. They block the binding of aminoacyl transfer RNA to the messenger RNA complex. Cell wall synthesis is not inhibited. Are mostly bacteriostatic and are effective only against multiplying bacteria. Well absorbed from the stomach and upper small intestine. Well distributed throughout all tissues and fluids and diffuse through noninflamed meninges and the placental barrier. Are deposited in the fetal skeleton and calcifying teeth. **t½:** 7–18.6 hr (see individual agents); increased in the presence of renal impairment. They bind to serum protein (range: 20%–93%; see individual agents). Concentrated in the liver in the bile; excreted mostly unchanged in the urine and feces.

See also *General Nursing Considerations for All Anti-Infectives.*

Uses: See individual drugs. Used mainly for infections caused by *Rickettsia, Chlamydia,* and *Mycoplasma.* Due to development of resistance, tetracyclines are usually not used for infections by common gram-negative or gram-positive organisms. Atypical pneumonia caused by *Mycoplasma pneumoniae.* Adjunct in the treatment of trachoma.

As an alternative to penicillin for uncomplicated gonorrhea or disseminated gonococcal infections, especially with penicillin allergy. Acute pelvic inflammatory disease. Useful as an alternative to penicillin for early syphilis.

Although not generally used for gram-positive infections, may be beneficial in anthrax, *Listeria* infections, and actinomycosis. Have also been used in conjunction with quinine sulfate for chloroquine-resistant *Plasmodium falciparum* malaria and as an intracavitary injection to control pleural or pericardial effusions caused by metastatic carcinoma. As an adjunct to amebicides in acute intestinal amebiasis. Used PO to treat uncomplicated endocervical, rectal, or urethral *Chlamydia* infections.

Topical uses include skin granulomas caused by *Mycobacterium marinum;* ophthalmic bacterial infections causing blepharitis, conjunctivitis, or keratitis; and as an adjunct in the treatment of ophthalmic chlamydial infections such as trachoma or inclusion conjunctivitis. As an alternative to silver nitrate for prophylaxis of neonatal gonococcal ophthalmia. Vaginitis. Severe acne.

Contraindications: Hypersensitivity. Use during tooth development stage (last trimester of pregnancy, neonatal period, during breast-feeding, and during childhood up to 8 years) because tetracyclines interfere with enamel formation and dental pigmentation. Never administer intrathecally.

Special Concerns: Use with caution and at reduced dosage in clients with impaired kidney function.

Side Effects: *GI* (most common): N&V, thirst, diarrhea, anorexia, sore throat, flatulence, epigastric distress, bulky loose stools. Less commonly, stomatitis, dysphagia, black hairy tongue, glossitis, or inflammatory lesions of the anogenital area. Rarely, pseudomembranous colitis. PO dosage forms may cause esophageal ulcers, especially in clients with esophageal obstructive element or hiatal hernia. *Allergic* (rare): Urticaria, pericarditis, polyarthralgia, fever, rash, pulmonary infiltrates with eosinophilia, ***angioneurotic edema,*** worsening of SLE, ***anaphylaxis,*** purpura. *Skin:* Photosensitivity, maculopapular and erythematous rashes, exfoliative dermatitis (rare), onycholysis, discoloration of nails. *CNS:* Dizziness, lightheadedness, unsteadiness, paresthesias. *Hematologic:* Eosinophilia, ***hemolytic anemia,*** neutropenia, thrombocytopenia, thrombocytopenic purpura. *Hepatic:* Fatty liver, increases in liver enzymes; rarely, hepatotoxicity, hepatitis, hepatic cholestasis. *Miscellaneous:* Candidal superinfections including oral and vaginal candidiasis, discoloration of infants' and children's teeth, bone lesions, delayed bone growth, abnormal pigmentation of the conjunctiva, pseudotumor cerebri in adults and bulging fontanels in infants.

IV administration may cause thrombophlebitis; IM injections are painful and may cause induration at the injection site.

Use of deteriorated tetracyclines may result in Fanconi-like syndrome characterized by N&V, acidosis, proteinuria, glycosuria, aminoaciduria, polydipsia, polyuria, hypokalemia.

Drug Interactions

Aluminum salts / ↓ Effect of tetracyclines due to ↓ absorption from GI tract
Antacids, oral / ↓ Effect of tetracyclines due to ↓ absorption from GI tract
Anticoagulants, oral / IV tetracyclines ↑ hypoprothrombinemia
Bismuth salts / ↓ Effect of tetracyclines due to ↓ absorption from GI tract
Bumetanide / ↑ Risk of kidney toxicity
Calcium salts / ↓ Effect of tetracyclines due to ↓ absorption from GI tract
Cimetidine / ↓ Effect of tetracyclines due to ↓ absorption from GI tract
Contraceptives, oral / ↓ Effect of oral contraceptives
Digoxin / Tetracyclines ↑ bioavailability of digoxin
Diuretics, thiazide / ↑ Risk of kidney toxicity
Ethacrynic acid / ↑ Risk of kidney toxicity
Furosemide / ↑ Risk of kidney toxicity
Insulin / Tetracyclines may ↓ insulin requirement
Iron preparations / ↓ Effect of tetracyclines due to ↓ absorption from GI tract
Lithium / Either ↑ or ↓ levels of lithium
Magnesium salts / ↓ Effect of tetracyclines due to ↓ absorption from GI tract
Methoxyflurane / ↑ Risk of kidney toxicity
Penicillins / Tetracyclines may mask bactericidal effect of penicillins
Sodium bicarbonate / ↓ Effect of tetracyclines due to ↓ absorption from GI tract
Zinc salts / ↓ Effect of tetracyclines due to ↓ absorption from GI tract

Dosage

See individual drugs.

Laboratory Test Considerations: False + or ↑ urinary catecholamines and urinary protein (degraded); ↑ coagulation time. False – or ↓ urinary urobilinogen, glucose tests (see *Health Care Considerations*). Prolonged use or high doses may change liver function tests and WBC counts.

1. Do not use outdated or deteriorated drugs as a Fanconi-like syndrome may occur (see *Side Effects*).
2. Administer IM into large muscle mass to avoid extravasation into subcutaneous or fatty tissue.

HEALTH CARE CONSIDERATIONS

Assessment

1. Determine any drug allergens or sensitivity. IM form contains procaine HCl.
2. Document indications for therapy, type, onset, and characteristics of symptoms. List other agents trialed and the outcome.
3. Note any colitis or other bowel problems.
4. If pregnant, document trimester.
5. Monitor VS, weight, CBC, BUN, creati-

nine, electrolytes, and cultures. Assess for impaired kidney function.

Interventions

1. Monitor VS and I&O. Maintain adequate I&O because renal dysfunction may result in drug accumulation, leading to toxicity. With impaired renal function assess for increased BUN, acidosis, anorexia, N&V, weight loss, and dehydration; latent symptoms may appear.
2. To prevent or treat pruritus ani, cleanse anal area with water several times a day and/or after each bowel movement. Observe for symptoms of enterocolitis, such as diarrhea, pyrexia, abdominal distention, and scanty urine; may need to discontinue drug and try another antibiotic.
3. If GI disturbances occur, avoid antacids that contain calcium, magnesium, or aluminum. May take with a light meal to reduce distress. An alternative would be to reduce the dose but increase the frequency of administration.
4. Assess with IV therapy for N&V, chills, fever, and hypertension resulting from too rapid administration or an excessively high dose; slow rate and report. Observe infant for bulging fontanelle, which may also be caused by a too rapid infusion rate.
5. Side effects such as sore throat, dysphagia, fever, dizziness, hoarseness, and inflammation of mucous membranes or candidal superinfections may occur.
6. Assess for altered level of consciousness or other CNS disturbances with impaired hepatic or renal function; may cause toxicity.
7. May cause onycholysis (loosening or detachment of the nail from the nail bed) or discoloration.

Client/Family Teaching

1. Take on an empty stomach at least 1 hr before or 2 hr after meals. Withhold antacids, iron salts, dairy foods, and other foods high in calcium for at least 2 hr after PO administration. Do not take with milk, cheese, ice cream or yogurt.
2. Zinc tablets or vitamin preparations containing zinc may interfere with drug absorption. Food sources high in zinc that should be avoided include oysters, fresh and raw; cooked lobster; dry oat flakes; steamed crabs; veal; and liver.
3. Avoid direct or artificial sunlight, which can cause a severe sunburn-like reaction; report if erythema occurs. Wear protective clothing, sunglasses, and a sunscreen for up to 3 weeks following therapy.
4. Tetracyclines interfere with formation of tooth enamel and dental pigmentation from the third trimester of pregnancy through age 8.
5. Prevent or treat pruritus ani by cleansing the anal area with water several times a day and/or after each bowel movement.
6. Use alternative method of birth control, as drug may interfere with oral contraceptives; may also cause a vaginal infection.
7. Take only as directed and complete full prescription. Discard any unused capsules to prevent reaction from deteriorated drugs.

Outcome/Evaluate

- Resolution of infection (↓ temperature, ↓ WBCs, ↑ appetite)
- Symptomatic improvement
- Negative culture reports

THEOPHYLLINE DERIVATIVES

See also the following individual entries:

Aminophylline
Theophylline

Action/Kinetics: Theophyllines stimulate the CNS, directly relax the smooth muscles of the bronchi and pulmonary blood vessels (relieve bronchospasms), produce diuresis, inhibit uterine contractions, stimulate gastric acid secretion, and increase the rate and force of contraction of the heart. The bronchodilator activity is due to direct relaxation of the bronchiolar smooth muscle and pulmonary blood vessels, which relieves bronchospasm. Although the exact mechanism is not known, theophyllines may act by altering the calcium levels of smooth muscle, blocking adenosine receptors, inhibiting the effect of prostaglandins on smooth muscle, and inhibiting the release of slow-reacting substance of anaphylaxis and histamine. Aminophylline releases free theophylline in vivo. Response to the drugs is highly individualized. Theophylline is well absorbed from uncoated plain tablets and PO liquids. *Theophylline salts:* **Onset:** 1–5 hr, depending on route and formulation. **Therapeutic plasma levels:** 10–20 mcg/mL. **t½:** 3–15 hr in nonsmoking adults, 4–5 hr in adult heavy smokers, 1–9 hr in children, and 20–30 hr for premature neonates. An increased t½ may be seen in individuals with CHF, alcoholism, liver dysfunction, or respiratory infections. Because of great variations in the rate of absorption (due to dosage form, food, dose level) as well as its extremely narrow therapeutic range, theophylline therapy is best monitored by determination of the serum levels. If these determinations cannot be obtained, saliva (contains 60% of corresponding theophylline serum levels) determinations can be used. Eighty-five percent to 90% metabolized in the liver and various metabolites, including the active 3-methylxanthine. Theophylline is metabolized partially to caffeine in the neonate. The premature neonate excretes 50% unchanged theophylline and may accumulate the caffeine metabolite. Excretion is through the kidneys (about 10% unchanged in adults).

Uses: Prophylaxis and treatment of bronchial asthma. Reversible bronchospasms associated with chronic bronchitis, emphysema, and COPD. *Investigational:* Treatment of neonatal apnea and Cheyne-Stokes respiration.

Contraindications: Hypersensitivity to any xanthine, peptic ulcer, seizure disorders (unless on medication), hypotension, CAD, angina pectoris.

Special Concerns: Use during lactation may result in irritability, insomnia, and fretfulness in the infant. Use with caution in premature infants due to the possible accumulation of caffeine. Xanthines are not usually tolerated by small children because of excessive CNS stimulation. Geriatric clients may manifest an increased risk of toxicity. Use with caution in the presence of gastritis, alcoholism, acute cardiac diseases, hypoxemia, severe renal and hepatic disease, severe hypertension, severe myocardial damage, hyperthyroidism, glaucoma.

Side Effects: Side effects are uncommon at serum theophylline levels less than 20 mcg/mL. At levels greater than 20 mcg/mL, 75% of individuals experience side effects including N&V, diarrhea, irritability, insomnia, and headache. At levels of 35 mcg/mL or greater, individuals may manifest ***cardiac arrhythmias,*** hypotension, tachycardia, hyperglycemia, ***seizures, brain damage, or death.*** *GI:* N&V, diarrhea, anorexia, epigastric pain, hematemesis, dyspepsia, rectal irritation (following use of suppositories), rectal bleeding, gastroesophageal reflux during sleep or while recumbent (theophylline). *CNS:* Headache, insomnia, irritability, fever, dizziness, lightheadedness, vertigo, reflex hyperexcitability, ***seizures,*** depression, speech abnormalities, alternating periods of mutism and hyperactivity, ***brain damage, death.*** *CV:* Hypotension, ***life-threatening ventricular arrhythmias,*** palpitations, tachycardia, ***peripheral vascular collapse,*** extrasystoles. *Renal:* Proteinuria, excretion of erythrocytes and renal tubular cells, dehydration due to diuresis, urinary retention (men with prostatic hypertrophy). *Other:* Tachypnea, ***respiratory arrest,*** fever, flushing, hyperglycemia, antidiuretic hormone syndrome, leukocytosis, rash, alopecia.

NOTE: Aminophylline given by rapid IV may produce hypotension, flushing, palpitations, precordial pain, headache, dizziness, or hyperventilation. Also, the ethylenediamine in aminophylline may cause allergic reactions, including urticaria and skin rashes.

OD **Management of Overdose:** *Symptoms:* Agitation, headache, nervousness, insomnia, tachycardia, extrasystoles, anorexia, N&V, fasciculations, tachypnea, ***tonic-clonic seizures.*** The first signs of toxicity may be seizures or ventricular arrhythmias. Toxicity is usually associated with parenteral administration but can be observed after PO administration, especially in children. *Treatment:*

- Have ipecac syrup, gastric lavage equipment, and cathartics available to treat overdose if the client is conscious and not having seizures. Otherwise a mechanical ventilator, oxygen, diazepam, and IV fluids may be necessary for the treatment of overdosage.
- For postseizure coma, maintain an airway and oxygenate the client. To remove the drug, perform only gastric lavage and give the cathartic and activated charcoal by a large-bore gastric lavage tube. Charcoal hemoperfusion may be necessary.
- Treat atrial arrhythmias with verapamil and treat ventricular arrhythmias with lidocaine or procainamide.
- Use IV fluids to treat acid-base imbalance, hypotension, and dehydration. Hypotension may also be treated with vasopressors.
- To treat hyperpyrexia, use a tepid water sponge bath or a hypothermic blanket.
- Treat apnea with artificial respiration.
- Monitor serum levels of theophylline until they fall below 20 mcg/mL as secondary rises of theophylline may occur, especially with sustained-release products.

Drug Interactions

Allopurinol / ↑ Theophylline levels
Aminoglutbethimide / ↓ Theophylline levels
Barbiturates / ↓ Theophylline levels
Benzodiazepines / Sedative effect may be antagonized by theophylline
Beta-adrenergic agonists / Additive effects
Beta-adrenergic blocking agents / ↑ Theophylline levels
Calcium channel blocking drugs / ↑ Theophylline levels
Carbamazepine / Either ↑ or ↓ theophylline levels
Charcoal / ↓ Theophylline levels
Cimetidine / ↑ Theophylline levels
Ciprofloxacin / ↑ Plasma levels of theophylline with ↑ possibility of side effects
Corticosteroids / ↑ Theophylline levels
Digitalis / Theophylline ↑ toxicity of digitalis
Disulfiram / ↑ Theophylline levels

Ephedrine and other sympathomimetics / ↑ Theophylline levels
Erythromycin / ↑ Effect of theophylline due to ↓ breakdown by liver
Ethacrynic acid / Either ↑ or ↓ theophylline levels
Furosemide / Either ↑ or ↓ theophylline levels
Halothane / ↑ Risk of cardiac arrhythmias
Interferon / ↑ Theophylline levels
Isoniazid / Either ↑ or ↓ theophylline levels
Ketamine / Seizures of the extensor-type
Ketoconazole / ↓ Theophylline levels
Lithium / ↓ Effect of lithium due to ↑ rate of excretion
Loop diuretics / ↓ Theophylline levels
Mexiletine / ↑ Theophylline levels
Muscle relaxants, nondepolarizing / Theophylline ↓ effect of these drugs
Oral contraceptives / ↑ Effect of theophyllines due to ↓ breakdown by liver
Phenytoin / ↓ Theophylline levels
Propofol / Theophyllines ↓ sedative effect of propofol
Quinolones / ↑ Theophylline levels
Reserpine / ↑ Risk of tachycardia
Rifampin / ↓ Theophylline levels
Sulfinpyrazone / ↓ Theophylline levels
Sympathomimetics / ↓ Theophylline levels
Tetracyclines / ↑ Risk of theophylline toxicity
Thiabendazole / ↑ Theophylline levels
Thyroid hormones / ↓ Theophylline levels in hypothyroid clients
Tobacco smoking / ↓ Effect of theophylline due to ↑ breakdown by liver
Troleandomycin / ↑ Effect of theophylline due to ↓ breakdown by liver
Verapamil / ↑ Effect of theophylline

Dosage

Individualized. Initially, adjust dosage according to plasma level of drug. Usual: 10–20 mcg theophylline/mL plasma. The dose of the various salts should be equivalent based on the content of anhydrous theophylline. See individual agents.

Laboratory Test Considerations: ↑ Plasma free fatty acids, bilirubin, urinary catecholamines, ESR. Interference with uric acid tests and tests for furosemide, probenecid, theobromine, and phenylbutazone.

1. Review list of agents with which theophylline derivatives interact.
2. Dilute drugs and maintain proper infusion rates to minimize problems of overdosage.
3. Wait to initiate PO therapy for at least 4–6 hr after switching from IV therapy.

HEALTH CARE CONSIDERATIONS

Assessment

1. Assess for any hypersensitivity to xanthine compounds. Note any experience with this class of drugs.
2. Record indications for therapy, type, onset, and characteristics of symptoms.
3. Note any history of hypotension, CAD, angina, PUD, or seizure disorders; avoid drug or use very cautiously in these conditions.
4. Assess for cigarette/marijuana use; induces hepatic metabolism of drug and require increase in dosage from 50% to 100%.
5. Assess diet habits which can influence the excretion of theophylline. A high-protein and/or low-carbohydrate diet will cause an increased drug excretion. A low-protein and/or high-carbohydrate diet will decrease excretion of drug.
6. Assess lung fields closely. Note characteristics of sputum and cough; assess CXR, ABGs, and PFTs.

Interventions

1. Observe for S&S of toxicity such as nausea, anorexia, insomnia, irritability, hyperexcitability, or cardiac arrhythmias; monitor serum levels.
2. Observe small children for excessive CNS stimulation; children often are unable to report side effects.

Client/Family Teaching

1. To avoid epigastric pain, take with a snack or with meals. Avoid or minimize consumption of charbroiled foods (e.g., burgers).
2. Take ATC and only as prescribed; more is *not* better. Report nausea, vomiting, GI pain, or restlessness.
3. Do not smoke; may aggravate underlying medical conditions as well as interfere with drug absorption. Attend smoking cessation program.
4. Protect from acute exacerbations of illness by avoiding crowds, dressing warmly in cold weather, obtaining the pneumonia vaccine and seasonal flu shot, covering mouth and nose so cold air is not directly inhaled, staying in air conditioning during excessively hot and humid weather, maintaining proper diet and nutrition, exercising daily, and consuming adequate fluids.
5. Report S&S of infections, adverse drug effects, difficulty breathing, and significant peak flows.
6. When secretions become thick and tacky, increase intake of fluids, avoiding milk/milk

products. This thins secretions and assists in their removal.
7. Learn to pace activity and avoid overexertion at all times.
8. Hold medication and report any side effects or CNS depression in children and infants.
9. Review dietary restrictions and limit intake of xanthine-containing products such as coffee, colas, and chocolate.
10. Identify local support groups that may assist in understanding and coping with chronic respiratory dysfunction.

Outcome/Evaluate

- Knowledge/understanding of disease management; compliance with prescribed regimen
- Improved airway exchange and breathing patterns; ↓ wheezing
- Therapeutic drug levels (10–20 mcg/mL)

TRANQUILIZERS/ANTIMANIC DRUGS/HYPNOTICS

See also the following individual entries:

Alprazolam
Barbiturates
Buspirone hydrochloride
Chlordiazepoxide
Clorazepate dipotassium
Diazepam
Estazolam
Flurazepam hydrochloride
Hydroxyzine hydrochloride
Hydroxyzine pamoate
Lithium carbonate
Lithium citrate
Lorazepam
Meprobamate
Midazolam hydrochloride
Oxazepam
Temazepam
Triazolam
Zolpidem tartrate

Action/Kinetics: Benzodiazepines are the major antianxiety agents. They are thought to affect the limbic system and reticular formation to reduce anxiety by increasing or facilitating the inhibitory neurotransmitter activity of GABA. Two benzodiazepine receptor subtypes have been identified in the brain–BZ_1 and BZ_2. Receptor subtype BZ_1 is believed to be associated with sleep mechanisms, whereas receptor subtype BZ_2 is associated with memory, motor, sensory, and cognitive function. When used for 3–4 weeks for sleep, certain benzodiazepines may cause REM rebound when discontinued. Meprobamate and the benzodiazepines also possess varying degrees of anticonvulsant activity, skeletal muscle relaxation, and the ability to alleviate tension. The benzodiazepines generally have long half-lives (1–8 days); thus cumulative effects can occur. Several of the benzodiazepines are metabolized to active metabolites in the liver, which prolongs their duration of action. Benzodiazepines are widely distributed throughout the body. Approximately 70%–99% of an administered dose is bound to plasma protein. Metabolites of benzodiazepines are excreted through the kidneys. All tranquilizers have the ability to cause psychologic and physical dependence.

Contraindications: Hypersensitivity, acute narrow-angle glaucoma, psychoses, primary depressive disorder, psychiatric disorders in which anxiety is not a signficiant symptom.

Special Concerns: Use with caution in impaired hepatic or renal function and in the geriatric or debilitated client. Use during lactation may cause sedation, weight loss, and possibly feeding difficulties in the infant. Geriatric clients may be more sensitive to the effects of benzodiazepines; symptoms may include oversedation, dizziness, confusion, or ataxia. When used for insomnia, rebound sleep disorders may occur following abrupt withdrawal of certain benzodiazepines.

Side Effects: *CNS:* Drowsiness, fatigue, confusion, ataxia, sedation, dizziness, vertigo, depression, apathy, lightheadedness, delirium, headache, lethargy, disorientation, hypoactivity, crying, anterograde amnesia, slurred speech, stupor, ***coma,*** fainting, difficulty in concentration, euphoria, nervousness, irritability, akathisia, hypotonia, vivid dreams, "glassy-eyed," hysteria, ***suicide attempt,*** psychosis. Paradoxical excitement manifested by anxiety, acute hyperexcitability, increased muscle spasticity, insomnia, hallucinations, sleep disturbances, rage, and stimulation. *GI:* Increased appetite, constipation, diarrhea, anorexia, N&V, weight gain or loss, dry mouth, bitter or metallic taste, increased salivation, coated tongue, sore gums, difficulty in swallowing, gastritis, fecal incontinence. *Respiratory:* ***Respiratory depression and sleep apnea,*** especially in clients with compromised respiratory function. *Dermatologic:* Urticaria, rash, pruritus, alopecia, hirsutism, dermatitis, edema of ankles and face. *Endocrine:* Increased or decreased libido, gynecomastia, menstrual irregularities. *GU:* Difficulty in urination, urinary retention, incontinence, dysuria, enuresis. *CV:* Hypertension, hypotension, bradycardia, tachycardia, palpitations, edema, ***CV collapse.*** *Hematologic:* Anemia, ***agranulocytosis,*** leukopenia, eosinophilia, thrombocytopenia. *Ophthalmologic:*

Diplopia, conjunctivitis, nystagmus, blurred vision. *Miscellaneous:* Joint pain, lymphadenopathy, muscle cramps, paresthesia, dehydration, lupus-like symptoms, sweating, SOB, flushing, hiccoughs, fever, hepatic dysfunction. *Following IM use:* Redness, pain, burning. *Following IV use:* Thrombosis and phlebitis at site.

OD **Management of Overdose:** *Symptoms:* Severe drowsiness, confusion with reduced or absent reflexes, tremors, slurred speech, staggering, hypotension, SOB, labored breathing, ***respiratory depression,*** impaired coordination, ***seizures,*** weakness, slow HR, ***coma.*** *NOTE:* Geriatric clients, debilitated clients, young children, and clients with liver disease are more sensitive to the CNS effects of benzodiazepines. *Treatment:* Supportive therapy. In the event of an overdose of a benzodizepine, have a benzodiazepine antagonist (flumazenil) readily available. Gastric lavage, provided that an ET tube with an inflated cuff is used to prevent aspiration of vomitus. Emesis only if drug ingestion was recent and client is fully conscious. Activated charcoal and saline cathartic may be given after emesis or lavage. Maintain adequate respiratory function. Reverse hypotension by IV fluids, norepinephrine, or metaraminol. **Do not** treat excitation with barbiturates.

Drug Interactions

Alcohol / Potentiation or addition of CNS depressant effects. Concomitant use may lead to drowsiness, lethargy, stupor, respiratory collapse, coma, or death
Anesthetics, general / See *Alcohol*
Antacids / ↓ Rate of absorption of benzodiazepines
Antidepressants, tricyclic / Concomitant use with benzodiazepines may cause additive sedative effect and/or atropine-like side effects
Antihistamines / See *Alcohol*
Barbiturates / See *Alcohol*
Cimetidine / ↑ Effect of benzodiazepines by ↓ breakdown in liver
CNS depressants / See *Alcohol*
Digoxin / Benzodiazepines ↑ effect of digoxin by ↑ serum levels
Disulfiram / ↑ Effect of benzodiazepines by ↓ breakdown in liver
Erythromycin / ↑ Effect of benzodiazepines by ↓ breakdown in liver
Fluoxetine / ↑ Effect of benzodiazepines due to ↓ breakdown in liver
Isoniazid / ↑ Effect of benzodiazepines due to ↓ breakdown in liver
Ketoconazole / ↑ Effect of benzodiazepines due to ↓ breakdown in liver
Levodopa / Effect may be ↓ by benzodiazepines
Metoprolol / ↑ Effect of benzodiazepines due to ↓ breakdown in liver
Narcotics / See *Alcohol*
Neuromuscular blocking agents / Benzodiazepines may ↑ , ↓ , or have no effect on the action of neuromuscular blocking agents
Oral contraceptives / ↑ Effect of benzodiazepines due to ↓ breakdown in liver; or, ↑ rate of clearance of benzodiazepines that undergo glucuronidation (e.g., lorazepam, oxazepam)
Phenothiazines / See *Alcohol*
Phenytoin / Concomitant use with benzodiazepines may cause ↑ effect of phenytoin due to ↓ breakdown by liver
Probenecid / ↑ Effect of selected benzodiazepines due to ↓ breakdown by liver
Propoxyphene / ↑ Effect of benzodiazepines due to ↓ breakdown by liver
Propranolol / ↑ Effect of benzodiazepines due to ↓ breakdown by liver
Ranitidine / May ↓ absorption of benzodiazepines from the GI tract
Rifampin / ↓ Effect of benzodiazepines due to ↑ breakdown by liver
Sedative-hypnotics, nonbarbiturate / See *Alcohol*
Theophyllines / ↓ Sedative effect of benzodiazepines
Valproic acid / ↑ Effect of benzodiazepines due to ↓ breakdown by liver

Dosage

See individual drugs.

Laboratory Test Considerations: ↑ AST, ALT, LDH, alkaline phosphatase.

1. Persistent drowsiness, ataxia, or visual disturbances may require dosage adjustment.
2. Lower dosage is usually indicated for older clients.
3. GI effects are decreased when drugs are given with meals or shortly afterward.
4. Withdraw drugs gradually.

HEALTH CARE CONSIDERATIONS

Assessment

1. Record indications for therapy, onset of symptoms, and behavioral manifestations. Note any prior treatments, what was used, for how long, and the outcome.
2. List drugs currently prescribed to ensure none interact unfavorably. Note any adverse reactions to this class of drugs.

3. Assess life-style and general level of health; note any situations that may contribute to these symptoms.
4. Assess the manner in which client responds to questions and discusses problems.
5. Monitor CBC, liver and renal function studies; assess for blood dyscrasias or impaired function.
6. Review physical and history for any contraindications to therapy.

Interventions

1. Record any symptoms consistent with overdosage.
2. Report any complaints of sore throat (other than those caused by NG or ET tubes), fever, or weakness and assess for blood dyscrasias; check CBC.
3. Monitor BP before and after IV dose of antianxiety medication. Keep recumbent for 2–3 hr after IV administration.
4. Administer the lowest possible effective dose, especially if elderly or debilitated.
5. When hospitalized and administered PO, remain until swallowed.
6. If client exhibits ataxia, or weakness or lack of coordination when ambulating, provide supervision/assistance. Use side rails once in bed and identify at risk for falls.
7. Note any S&S of cholestatic jaundice: nausea, diarrhea, upper abdominal pain, or the presence of high fever or rash; check LFTs.
8. Report if yellowing of sclera, skin, or mucous membranes evident (late sign of cholestatic jaundice and biliary tract obstruction); hold if overly sleepy/confused or becomes comatose.
9. With suicidal tendencies, anticipate drug will be prescribed in small doses. Report signs of increased depression immediately.
10. If history of alcoholism or if taking excessive quantities of drug, carefully supervise amount of drug prescribed and dispensed. Assess for manifestations of ataxia, slurred speech, and vertigo (symptoms of chronic intoxication and that client may be exceeding dose).
11. Note any evidence of physical or psychologic dependence. Assess frequency and quantity of refills.

Client/Family Teaching

1. These drugs may reduce ability to handle potentially dangerous equipment, such as cars and machinery.
2. Take most of daily dose at bedtime, with smaller doses during the waking hours to minimize mental and motor impairment.
3. Avoid alcohol while taking antianxiety agents. Alcohol potentiates the depressant effects of both the alcohol and the medication.
4. Do not take any unprescribed or OTC medications without approval.
5. Arise slowly from a supine position and dangle legs over side of the bed before standing. If feeling faint sit or lie down immediately and lower the head.
6. Allow extra time to prepare for daily activities; take precautions before arising, to reduce one source of anxiety and stress.
7. Do not stop taking drug suddenly. Any sudden withdrawal after prolonged therapy or after excessive use may cause a recurrence of the preexisting symptoms of anxiety. It may also cause a withdrawal syndrome, manifested by increased anxiety, anorexia, insomnia, vomiting, ataxia, muscle twitching, confusion, and hallucinations. May also develop seizures and convulsions.
8. Identify/practice relaxation techniques that may assist in lowering anxiety levels.
9. These drugs are generally for short-term therapy; follow-up is imperative to evaluate response and the need for continued therapy.
10. Attend appropriate counselling sessions as condition and length of therapy dictate.

Outcome/Evaluate

- Symptomatic improvement with ↓ anxiety/tension episodes
- Effective coping
- ↓ Frequency and intensity of muscle spasms and tremor
- Improved sleeping patterns; less frequent early morning awakenings
- Control of seizures
- Control of alcohol withdrawal symptoms

VACCINES

See Tables 2, 3, and 4.

General Statement: Vaccines have played an important role in the health and life span of our population. They have been in use over 200 years, but since World War II, once the importance of disease prevention became evident, research into the area of vaccine development exploded.

Use of a vaccine (or actually contracting the disease) usually renders one temporary or permanent resistance to an infectious disease. Vaccines and toxoids promote the type of antibody production one would see if they had experienced the natural infection. This active immunization involves the direct administration of antigens to the host to cause them to produce the desired antibodies and cell-mediated immunity. These

Table 2 Common Diseases, General Recommended Immunization Schedule, and Length of Immunity

DISEASE	IMMUNIZATION SCHEDULE	LENGTH OF IMMUNITY
Cholera	Two doses 1 week to 1 month apart	6 months
Diphtheria	Given as DPT; four doses at ages 2, 4, 6, and 15–18 months	10 years
Haemophilus influenzae (Hib)	Four doses at ages 2, 4, 6, and 15 months	Unknown
Hepatitis B	Three doses: at birth (or initial dose), 1 month later, and 6 months after second dose	Unknown
Influenza	One dose (or two doses of split virus if under 13 years)	1–3 years
Lyme Disease	Three doses at ages 15–70 years old; at 0, 1, and 12 months; plan 3rd dose just before tick season	1 yr; yearly booster
Measles	Given as MMR at ages 12–15 months and 4–6 years	Lifetime
Meningococcal meningitis	One dose (antibody response requires 5 days); antibiotic prophylaxis (Rifampin 600 mg or 10 mg/kg q 12 hr for four doses should be given to all contacts per exposure)	?Lifetime; not consistently effective in those <2 years of age
Mumps	Given as MMR at ages 12–15 months and 4–6 years	Lifetime
Pertussis	Given as DPT; four doses at ages 2, 4, 6, and 15–18 months	10 years
Pneumococcus	One dose (0.5 mL)	Approx. 5-10 years
Poliomyelitis	Four doses at ages 2, 4, and 6 months, then at age 4–6 years	Lifetime
Rabies	Postexposure: five doses on days 0, 3, 7, 14, and 28 with the rabies immune globulin; pre-exposure: two doses 1 week apart, third dose 2–3 weeks later	Approx. 2 years
Rubella	Given as MMR at ages 12–15 months and 4–6 years	Lifetime

Table 2 *(continued)*

DISEASE	IMMUNIZATION SCHEDULE	LENGTH OF IMMUNITY
Smallpox	One dose; this disease has been eradicated and vaccine is used only with military personnel and lab workers using pox viruses	3 years
Tetanus	Given initially as DPT; four doses at ages 2, 4, 6, and 15–18 months	10 years; a tetanus booster is required q 10 years
VZV (varicellazoster virus; chicken pox)	One dose (0.5 mL) age 12 months to 12 years; two injections of 0.5 mL 4–8 weeks apart in age 13 and older	?Lifetime
Yellow fever	One dose	10 years

Table 3 Active Childhood Immunization Schedule

	#1	#2	#3	#4
DPT	2 months	4 months	6 months	15–18 months
OPV	2 months	4 months	6 months	4–6 years
Hib	2 months	4 months	6 months	15–18 months
MMR	12 months	4 years		
Hep B	birth or initial dose	1 month after first dose	6 months or more after second dose	

Table 4 Active Adult Immunization Schedule

Tetanus	Tetanus booster every 10 years; with injury obtain one in 5 yrs
Pneumococcus	Every 5 years
Influenza	Every year
Lyme	Yearly booster in endemic areas after series completed
Travel outside USA call CDC: 1-877-394-8747	International Traveller's Immunization Hotline

agents may consist of live attenuated agents or killed (inactivated) agents. Immunizations confer resistance without actually producing disease.

Passive immunization occurs when immunologic agents are administered. Immunoglobulins and antivenins only offer passive short-term immunity and are usually administered for a specific exposure.

Aggressive pediatric immunization programs have helped reduce preventable infections and death in children worldwide. This focus should continue and be expanded to the adult population, many of whom have missed the natural infection and their past immunizations. A careful immunization history should be documented for every client, regardless of age. When in doubt or if unknown if had infection or immunization, appropriate titers may be drawn. Table 2 lists some of the more common diseases, the general recommended schedule to confer immunization, and the length of immunity conferred; Table 3 outlines the active childhood immunization schedule.

VITAMINS

See Tables 5, 6, and 7.

General Statement: Vitamins are essential, carbon-containing, noncaloric substances that are required for normal metabolism. They are produced by living materials such as plants and animals and they are generally obtained from the diet. Vitamin D is synthesized in the diet to a limited extent and Vitamin B–12 is synthesized in the intestinal tract by bacterial flora.

Vitamins are essential for promoting growth, health, and life. They are necessary for the metabolic processes responsible for transforming foods into tissue or energy. Vitamins are also involved in the formation and maintenance of blood cells, chemicals supporting the nervous system, hormones, and genetic materials. Vitamins do not provide energy because they contain no calories. Yet, some do help convert the calories in fats, carbohydrates, and proteins into usable body energy.

Disease states caused by severe nutritional deficiencies prompted the discovery of vitamins because scientists were able to reverse the signs and symptoms of these disease states with vitamins. Severe deficiencies include scurvy, rickets, pellagra, pernicious anemia, xerophthalmia, beriberi, osteomalacia, infantile hemolytic anemia, and hemorrhagic diseases of the newborn. Moderate vitamin deficiencies may also produce symptoms of impaired health.

Environmental factors and genetic predisposition may influence individual requirements for specific vitamins. Disease processes, growth, hormone balance, and drugs may also alter the dietary requirements and function of vitamins.

Many deficiency states can be traced to special circumstances such as pernicious anemia after gastrectomy; pellagra in corn–eating populations, and scurvy in the elderly subsisting on soft foods (e.g., eggs, bread, milk) while neglecting citrus fruits. Generally, although not common in the United States, vitamin deficiency usually involves multiple rather than single deficiencies and usually can be attributed to poor lifestyle choices and poor dietary habits with an inadequate intake of many nutrients, including all vitamins.

There are two categories of vitamins: fat soluble and water soluble. Fat soluble viatmins A, D, E, and K are found in the fat or oil of foods and require digestible fat and bile salts for absorption in the small intestine. The water-soluble vitamins, C and B complex (B-1, B-2, niacin, B-6, folic acid, B-12, pantothenic acid, and biotin) are found in the watery portion of foods and are well absorbed by the GI tract. They are easily lost through overcooking and do not require fat for absorption. Water soluble vitamins mix easily in the blood, are excreted by the kidneys, and only small amounts are stored in the tissues, so regular daily intake is essential. Fat soluble vitamins are stored in the body after binding to specific plasma globulins in fat parts of the body.

Recommended Dietary Allowances (RDAs) are the recommended human vitamin and mineral intake requirements. These were developed by the Food and Nutrition Board, National Research Council of the National Academy of Sciences and have evolved over the past 50 years and are updated every 5 years. They are based on age, height, weight, and gender. These are only estimates of nutrient needs; each client and the surrounding factors warrant individualized evaluation when replacement is being considered.

Table 5 Common Vitamin Requirements

Vitamin	RDA	Physiologic Effects Essential for:
A (retinol, retinaldehyde, retonic acid)	1400-6000 IU	Growth & development epithelial tissue maintenance; reproduction prevents night blindness
B complex:		
B-1 (thiamine)	0.3–1.5 mg	Energy metabolism: normal nerve function
B-2 (riboflavin)	0.4–1.8 mg	Reactions in energy cycle that produce ATP; oxidation of amino acids and hydroxy acids; oxidation of purines
B-3 Niacin (nicotinic acid, nicotinamide)	5–19 mg	Synthesis of fatty acids and cholesterol; blocks FFA; conversion of phenylalanine to tyrosine
B-6 (pyridoxine, pyridoxal, pyridoxamine)	0.3–2.5 mg	Amino acid metabolism; glycogenolysis, RBC/Hb synthesis; formation of neurotransmitters; formation of antibodies
Folacin (folic acid, pteroylglutamic acid)	50–800 mcg	DNA synthesis, formation of RBCs in bone marrow with cyanocobalamine
Pantothenic acid (calcium pantothenate, dexpanthenol)	10 mg	Synthesis of sterols, steroid hormones, porphyrins; synthesis and degradation of fatty acids; oxidative metabolism of carbohydrates, gluconeogenesis
B-12 (cyanocobalamin, hydroxocobalamin, extrinsic factor)	0.3–4.0 mcg	DNA synthesis in bone marrow; RBC production with folacin; nerve tissue maintenance
B-7 (Biotin)	No recommendation	Synthesis of fatty acids, generation of tricarboxylic acid cycle; formation of purines Coenzyme in CHO metabolism
C (ascorbic acid, ascorbate)	60 mg	Formation of collagen; conversion of cholesterol to bile acids; protects A and E and polyunsaturated fats from excessive oxidation; absorption and utilization of iron; converts folacin to folinic acid; some role in clotting, adrenocortical hormones, and resistance to cancer and infections

Table 5 *(continued)*

Vitamin	RDA	Physiologic Effects Essential for:
D (calcitriol, cholecalciferol, dihydrotachysterol, ergocalciferol, viosterol)	400 IU	Intestinal absorption and metabolism of calcium and phosphorus as well as renal reabsorption; release of calcium from bone and resorption
E (tocopherol)	4–15 IU	May oppose destruction of Vit. A and fats by oxygen fragments called free radicals; antioxidant; may affect production of prostaglandins which regulate a variety of body processes
K (menadione, phytonadione)	No recommendation	Formation of prothrombin and other clotting proteins by the liver; blood coagulation

Table 6 Vitamins and Uses

Vitamin	Effect	Uses
A (retinoic acid)	Reduces formation of comedones; keratin production suppression	Acne, psoriasis, ichthyosis, Darier's disease xerophthalmia, intestinal infections, prevents night blindness
Niacin	Reduction of blood cholesterol and triglycerides blocks FFA release	Hypercholesterolemia, hyperbetalipoproteinemia
D (dihydrotachysterol)	Maintains calcium and phosphorus levels in bone and blood	Hypoparathyroidism: increase intestinal absorption of calcium
C	Reduces urine pH; converts methemoglobin to hemoglobin	Idiopathic methemoglobin; recurrent UTIs in high risk clients aids in iron absorption
E	Reduces endogenous peroxidases	Hemolytic anemia in premature infants protects cell membranes from oxidation
K	Increases liver production of thrombin	Warfarin toxicity essential for blood coagulation

Table 7 Vitamin Deficiency States

Vitamin	Deficiency	Signs & Symptoms
A	Xerophthalmia	Progressive eye changes: night blindness to xerosis of conjunctiva and cornea with scarring
	Keratomalacia	Degeneration of epithelial cells with hardening and shrinking
B-6	Beriberi	Fatigue, weight loss, weakness, irritability; headaches, insomnia, peripheral neuropathy, CHF, cardiomyopathy
Niacin	Pellagra	Depression, anorexia, beefy red glossitis, cheilosis, dermatitis
B-12	Pernicious anemia	Macrocytic, megaloblastic anemia; progressive neuropathy R/T demyelination
C	Scurvy	Joint pain, growth retardation, anemia, poor wound healing with increased susceptibility to infection; petechial hemorrhages
D	Rickets (child) Osteomalacia (adult)	Demineralization of bones and teeth with bone pain and skeletal muscle deformities
E	Hemolytic anemia in low birth weight infants	Macrocytic anemia; increased hemolysis of RBC's and increased capillarity fragility
K	Hemorrhagic disease in newborns	Increase tendency to hemorrhage **[Rx]**

CHAPTER THREE
A-Z Listing of Drugs

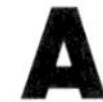

A

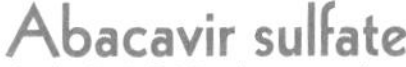

Abacavir sulfate

(uh-**BACK**-ah-veer)
Pregnancy Category: C
Ziagen **(Rx)**
Classification: Antiviral, antiretroviral drug

See also *Antiviral Drugs*.

Action/Kinetics: Synthetic nucleoside analog. Converted intracellularly to the active carbovir triphosphate. Carbovir triphosphate inhibits the activity of HIV-1 reverse transcriptase by competing with the natural substrate deoxyguanosine-5'-triphosphate and by incorporation into viral DNA. The lack of a 3'-OH group in the incorporated nucleoside analog prevents the formation of the 5' to 3' phosphodiester linkage essential for DNA chain elongation. Thus, viral DNA growth is terminated. Cross resistance in vitro has been seen to lamivudine, didanosine, and zalcitabine. Rapidly absorbed after PO use. Metabolized in the liver and excreted in both the urine and feces.

Uses: In combination with other antiretroviral drugs to treat HIV-1 infection. Do not add as a single agent when antiretroviral regimens are changed due to loss of virologic response.

Special Concerns: Fatal hypersensitivity reactions are possible (See *Side Effects*). Efficacy for long-term suppression of HIV RNA or disease progression has not been determined. Abacavir is not a cure for HIV infection; clients may continue to show illnesses associated with HIV infection, including opportunistic infections. The drug has not been shown to reduce the risk of transmission of HIV to others through sexual contact or blood.

Side Effects: *Hypersensitivity:* Fever, skin rash, fatigue, N&V, diarrhea, abdominal pain, malaise, lethargy, myalgia, arthralgia, edema, SOB, paresthesia, lymphadenopathy, conjunctivitis, mouth ulcerations, maculopapular or urticarial rash, ***life-threatening hypotension, liver failure, renal failure, death***. *GI:* N&V, diarrhea, loss of appetite, pancreatitis. *Miscellaneous:* Severe hepatomegaly with steatosis (may be fatal), insomnia, other sleep disorders, headache, fever, skin rashes.

Laboratory Test Considerations: ↑ LFTs, CPK, GGT, creatinine. Lymphopenia, anemia, neutropenia.

Drug Interactions: Ethanol ↓ excretion of abacavir → ↑ exposure.

How Supplied: *Oral Solution:* 20 mg/mL; *Tablets:* 300 mg

Dosage

- **Oral Solution, Tablets**

  Treat HIV-1 infection.

Adults: 300 mg b.i.d. with other antiretroviral drugs. **Pediatric, 3 months to 16 years:** 8 mg/kg b.i.d., not to exceed 30 mg b.i.d., in combination with other antiretroviral drugs.

HEALTH CARE CONSIDERATIONS

See also *Health Care Considerations* for *Antiviral Drugs*.

Administration/Storage

1. May be given with or without food.
2. Do not restart abacavir therapy following a hypersensitivity reaction. More severe symptoms will occur within hours and may include life-threatening hypotension or death.
3. Store at 20°C-25°C (68°F-77°F). Do not freeze, although may be refrigerated.

Assessment

1. Note indications for therapy and other agents trialed.
2. Obtain electrolytes and LFTs; assess for liver enlargement and lactic acidosis.
3. Assess for any hypersensitivity reactions; once experienced may not ever resume therapy with this drug.
4. Providers must report hypersensitivity reactions to the registry: 1-800-270-0425.

Client/Family Teaching

1. Take drug orally as directed and with other antiretroviral agents. May take with or without food.

A

2. Review medication guide that accompanies this product.
3. Drug does not cure disease but works to lower viral count.
4. Immediately report any S&S of allergic reactions (fever, severe fatigue, skin rash, N &V, diarrhea or abdominal pain) and stop drug.
5. If allergic reaction is experienced with this drug do not ever restart therapy as it may be fatal.
6. Practice safe sex, drug does not prevent disease transmission.
7. Use reliable birth control; do not breast feed.

Outcome/Evaluate: Suppression of HIV RNA

Acarbose

(ah-**KAR**-bohs)

Pregnancy Category: B

Prandase ✦, Precose **(Rx)**

Classification: Antidiabetic agent

Action/Kinetics: An oligosaccharide obtained from a fermentation process using the microorganism *Actinoplans utahensis*. Causes a competitive, reversible inhibition of pancreatic alpha-amylase and membrane-bound intestinal alpha-glucosidase hydrolase enzymes. This causes delayed glucose absorption resulting in a smaller increase in blood glucose following meals. Glycosylated hemoglobin levels are decreased in those with non-insulin-dependent diabetes mellitus. Because the mechanism of action is different from sulfonylureas (i.e., enhance insulin secretion), acarbose is additive to the effect of sulfonylureas. Approximately 65% of an oral dose of acarbose remains in the GI tract, which is the site of action. Metabolized in the GI tract by both intestinal bacteria and intestinal enzymes. The acarbose and metabolites that are absorbed are excreted in the urine.

Uses: Used alone, with diet control, to decrease blood glucose in type 2 diabetes mellitus. Also, used with a sulfonylurea when diet plus either acarbose or a sulfonylurea alone do not control blood glucose adequately.

Contraindications: Diabetic ketoacidosis, cirrhosis, inflammatory bowel disease, colonic ulceration, partial intestinal obstruction or predisposition to intestinal obstruction, chronic intestinal diseases associated with marked disorders of digestion or absorption, conditions that may deteriorate as a result of increased gas formation in the intestine. In significant renal dysfunction. Severe, persistent bradycardia. Lactation.

Special Concerns: Safety and efficacy have not been determined in children. Acarbose does not cause hypoglycemia; however, sulfonylureas and insulin can lower blood glucose sufficiently to cause symptoms or even life-threatening hypoglycemia.

Side Effects: *GI:* Abdominal pain, diarrhea, flatulence. GI side effects may be severe and be confused with paralytic ileus.

Laboratory Test Considerations: ↑ Serum transaminases (especially with doses greater than 50 mg t.i.d.). Small ↓ in hematocrit. Low plasma B_6 levels.

OD Management of Overdose: *Symptoms:* Flatulence, diarrhea, abdominal discomfort. *Treatment:* Reduce dose; symptoms will subside.

Drug Interactions

Charcoal / ↓ Effect of acarbose
Digestive enzymes / ↓ Effect of acarbose
Digoxin / ↓ Serum digoxin levels
Insulin / ↑ Hypoglycemia which may cause severe hypoglycemia
Sulfonylureas / ↑ Hypoglycemia which may cause severe hypoglycemia

How Supplied: *Tablet:* 25 mg, 50 mg, 100 mg

Dosage

- **Tablets**

Type 2 diabetes mellitus.

Individualized, depending on effectiveness and tolerance. **Initial:** 25 mg (one-half of a 50-mg tablet) t.i.d. with the first bite of each main meal. **Maintenance:** After the initial dose of 25 mg t.i.d., the dose can be increased to 50 mg t.i.d. Some may benefit from 100 mg t.i.d. The dosage can be adjusted at 4- to 8-week intervals. **Recommended maximum daily dose:** 50 mg t.i.d. for clients weighing less than 60 kg and 100 mg t.i.d. for those weighing more than 60 kg.

HEALTH CARE CONSIDERATIONS

Administration/Storage

1. Start with a low dose to reduce GI side effects and to help determine the minimum effective dose.
2. If a dose is missed, take the usual dose at the start of the next main meal.

Assessment

1. Record indications for therapy, age at symptom onset, other agents trialed and the outcome.
2. Note any cirrhosis or chronic intestinal diseases with disorders of digestion or absorption.
3. Obtain baseline CBC, HbA1c, blood sugar, electrolytes, urinalysis, liver and renal function tests; assess for B_6 deficiency. Monitor HbA1c and LFTs q 3 mo.

4. Start and titrate acarbose based on blood glucose results. Ideally, a 1-hr postprandial plasma glucose level should be measured to determine the effective dose.
5. Acarbose may enhance glycemic control with a sulfonylurea, but it may also be used alone.

Client/Family Teaching
1. Take as prescribed, three times a day with the first bite of main meals.
2. Acarbose delays digestion of ingested carbohydrates (glucose) and is a treatment in addition to diet and not instead of.
3. Caloric restrictions and weight loss, especially in the obese client, must be continued to control blood sugar and to prevent complications of diabetes; continue regular physical exercise.
4. The most common side effects are of GI origin (abdominal discomfort, diarrhea, gas); should subside in frequency and intensity.
5. Do frequent monitoring of glucose (finger sticks) and record to assess the therapeutic response.
6. Loss of glucose control may result when exposed to stress, such as fever, trauma, infection, or surgery. In these instances, temporary insulin therapy may be needed.
7. Candy bars should not be used to counteract hypoglycemia; use glucose tablets or gel or lactose.

Outcome/Evaluate: Control of blood sugar with NIDDM

Acebutolol hydrochloride

(ays-**BYOU**-toe-lohl)

Pregnancy Category: B

Apo-Acebutolol ✦, Monitan ✦, Novo-Acebutolol ✦, Nu-Acebutolol ✦, Rhotral ✦, Sectral **(Rx)**

Classification: Beta-adrenergic blocking agent

See also *Beta-Adrenergic Blocking Agents.*

Action/Kinetics: Predominantly beta-1 blocking activity but will inhibit beta-2 receptors at higher doses. Some intrinsic sympathomimetic activity. **t½:** 3-4 hr. Low lipid solubility. **Duration:** 24-30 hr. Metabolized in liver and excreted in urine and bile. Fifteen to 20% excreted unchanged.

Uses: Hypertension (either alone or with other antihypertensive agents such as thiazide diuretics). Premature ventricular contractions.

Additional Contraindications: Severe, persistent bradycardia.

Special Concerns: Dosage not established in children.

How Supplied: *Capsule:* 200 mg, 400 mg

Dosage

- **Capsules**

Hypertension.

Initial: 400 mg/day (although 200 mg b.i.d. may be needed for optimum control; **then,** 400-800 mg/day (range: 200-1,200 mg/day).

Premature ventricular contractions.

Initial: 200 mg b.i.d.; **then,** increase dose gradually to reach 600-1,200 mg/day.

Dosage should not exceed 800 mg/day in geriatric clients. In those with impaired kidney or liver function, decrease dose by 50% when C_{CR} is 50 mL/min/1.73 m² and by 75% when it is less than 25 mL/min/1.73 m².

HEALTH CARE CONSIDERATIONS

See also *Health Care Considerations* for *Beta-Adrenergic Blocking Agents* and *Antihypertensive Agents.*

Administration/Storage
1. When discontinued, gradually withdraw drug over a 2-week period.
2. Bioavailability increases in elderly clients; may require lower maintenance doses (no more than 800 mg/day).
3. May be combined with another antihypertensive agent.
4. Reduce dosage with impaired liver and renal function.

Client/Family Teaching
1. Drug may cause drowsiness; do not perform tasks that require mental alertness until drug effects realized.
2. May cause an increased sensitivity to cold; dress appropriately.
3. Report any evidence of sudden weight gain, edema, or SOB.
4. Do not stop abruptly without provider approval.

Outcome/Evaluate: ↓ BP; control of PVCs

Acetaminophen (Apap, Paracetamol)

(ah-**SEAT**-ah-**MIN**-oh-fen)

Caplets: Arthritis Foundation Pain Reliever Aspirin Free, Aspirin Free Anacid Maximum Strength, Aspirin Free Pain Relief, Atasol ✦, Atasol Forte ✦, Genapap Extra Strength, Genebs Extra Strength Caplets, Panadol, Panadol Junior Strength, Tapanol Extra Strength, Tylenol Arthritis Extended Relief, Tylenol Caplets, **Capsules:** Dapacin, Meda Cap, **Elixir:** Aceta, Genapap Children's, Mapap Children's, Oraphen-PD, Ridenol, Silapap Children's, Tylenol Children's, **Gelcaps:** Aspirin Free Anacid Maximum Strength, Tapanol Extra Strength, Tylenol Extra Strength, **Oral Liquid/Syrup:** Atasol ✦, Children's Acetaminophen Elixir Drops ✦, Halenol Children's, Panadol Children's, Pediatrix ✦, Tempra ✦, Tempra 2 Syrup, Tempra Children's Syrup ✦, Tylenol Extra Strength, **Oral Solution:** Acetaminophen Drops, Apacet, Atasol ✦, Children's Acetaminophen Oral Solution ✦, Genapap Infants' Drops, Mapap Infant Drops, Panadol Infants' Drops, Pediatrix ✦, PMS-Acetaminophen ✦, Silapap Infants, Tempra 1, Tylenol Infants' Drops, Uni-Ace, **Oral Suspension:** Tylenol Children's Suspension ✦, Tylenol Infants' Suspension ✦, **Sprinkle Capsules:** Feverall Children's, Feverall Junior Strength, **Suppositories:** Abenol 120, 325, 650 mg ✦, Acephen, Acetaminophen Uniserts, Children's Feverall, Infant's Feverall, Junior Strength Feverall, Neopap, **Tablets:** Aceta, A.F. Anacin ✦, A.F. Anacin Extra Strength ✦, Apo-Acetaminophen ✦, Aspirin Free Anacin Maximum Strength, Aspirin Free Pain Relief, Atasol ✦, Atasol Forte ✦, Extra Strength Acetaminophen ✦, Fem-Etts, Genapap, Genapap Extra Strength, Genebs, Genebs Extra Strength, Mapap Regular Strength, Mapap Extra Strength, Maranox, Meda Tab, Panadol, Redutemp, Regular Strength Acetaminophen ✦, Tapanol Extra Strength, Tapanol Regular Strength, Tempra, Tylenol Regular Strength, Tylenol Extra Strength, Tylenol Junior Strength, Tylenol Tablets 325 mg, 500 mg ✦, **Tablets, Chewable:** Apacet, Children's Chewable Acetaminophen ✦, Children's Genapap, Children's Panadol, Children's Tylenol, Tempra ✦, Tempra 3, Tylenol Chewable Tablets Fruit, Tylenol Junior Strength Chewable Tablets Fruit ✦ **(OTC)**

Acetaminophen, buffered

(ah-**SEAT**-ah-**MIN**-oh-fen)

Alka-Seltzer, Bromo Seltzer **(OTC)**

Classification: Nonnarcotic analgesic, para-aminophenol type

Action/Kinetics: Decreases fever by an effect on the hypothalamus leading to sweating and vasodilation. It also inhibits the effect of pyrogens on the hypothalamic heat-regulating centers. May cause analgesia by inhibiting CNS prostaglandin synthesis; however, due to minimal effects on peripheral prostaglandin synthesis, acetaminophen has no anti-inflammatory or uricosuric effects. Does not cause any anticoagulant effect or ulceration of the GI tract. Antipyretic and analgesic effects are comparable to those of aspirin.

Peak plasma levels: 30-120 min. **t½:** 45 min-3 hr. **Therapeutic serum levels** (analgesia): 5-20 mcg/mL. **Plasma protein binding:** Approximately 25%. Metabolized in the liver and excreted in the urine as glucuronide and sulfate conjugates. However, an intermediate hydroxylated metabolite is hepatotoxic following large doses of acetaminophen.

The extended-relief product uses a bilayer system that allows the outer layer to release acetaminophen rapidly while the inner layer is designed to release the remainder of the dose more slowly. This allows prolonged relief of symptoms.

The buffered product is a mixture of acetaminophen, sodium bicarbonate, and citric acid that effervesces when placed in water. This product has a high sodium content (0.76 g/¾ capful).

Uses: Control of pain due to headache, earache, dysmenorrhea, arthralgia, myalgia, musculoskeletal pain, arthritis, immunizations, teething, tonsillectomy. To reduce fever in bacterial or viral infections. As a substitute for aspirin in upper GI disease, aspirin allergy, bleeding disorders, clients on anticoagulant therapy, and gouty arthritis. *Investigational:* In children receiving diptheria-pertussis-tetanus vaccination to decrease incidence of fever and pain at injection site.

Contraindications: Renal insufficiency, anemia. Clients with cardiac or pulmonary disease are more susceptible to toxic effects of acetaminophen.

Special Concerns: May have to be used with caution in pregnancy. Heavy drinking and fasting may be risk factors for acetaminophen toxicity, especially if larger than recommended doses of acetaminophen are used. As little as twice the recommended dosage, over time, can lead to serious liver damage.

Side Effects: Few when taken in usual therapeutic doses. Chronic and even acute toxicity can develop after long symptom-free usage. *Hematologic:* Methemoglobinemia, **hemolytic anemia,** neutropenia, thrombocytopenia, pancytopenia, leukopenia. *Allergic:* Urticarial and erythematous skin reactions, skin eruptions, fever. *Miscellaneous:* CNS stimulation, hypoglycemic coma, jaundice, drowsiness, glossitis.

OD **Management of Overdose:** *Symptoms:* May be no early specific symptoms. Within first 24 hr: N&V, diaphoresis, anorexia, drowsiness, confusion, liver tenderness, cardiac arrhythmias, low BP, jaundice, acute hepatic and renal failure. Within 24-48 hr, increased AST, ALT, bilibrubin, prothrombin levels. After 72-96 hr, peak hepatotoxicity with death possible due to liver necrosis. *Treatment:* Initially, induction of emesis, gastric lavage, activated charcoal. Oral *N*-acetylcysteine is said to reduce or prevent hepatic damage by inactivating acetaminophen metabolites, which cause liver toxicity.

Drug Interactions

Alcohol, ethyl / Chronic use of alcohol ↑ toxicity of larger therapeutic doses of acetaminophen

Barbiturates / ↑ Potential of hepatotoxicity due to ↑ breakdown of acetaminophen by liver
Carbamazepine / ↑ Potential of hepatotoxicity due to ↑ breakdown of acetaminophen by liver
Charcoal, activated / ↓ Absorption of acetaminophen when given as soon as possible after overdose
Diuretics, loop / ↓ Effect of diuretic due to ↓ renal prostaglandin excretion and ↓ plasma renin activity
Hydantoins (including Phenytoin) / ↑ Potential of hepatotoxicity due to ↑ breakdown of acetaminophen by liver
Isoniazid / ↑ Potential of hepatotoxicity due to ↑ breakdown of acetaminophen by liver
Lamotrigine / ↓ Serum lamotrigine levels → ↓ effect
Oral contraceptives / ↑ Breakdown of acetaminophen by liver → ↓ t½
Propranolol / ↑ Effect due to ↓ breakdown by liver
Rifampin / ↑ Potential of hepatotoxicity due to ↑ breakdown of acetaminophen by liver
Sulfinpyrazone / ↑ Potential of hepatotoxicity due to ↑ breakdown of acetaminophen by liver
Zidovudine (AZT) / ↓ Effect of AZT due to ↑ nonhepatic or renal clearance

How Supplied: Acetominophen: *Capsule:* 80 mg, 160 mg, 325 mg, 500 mg, 650 mg; *Chew tablet:* 80 mg, 160 mg; *Elixir:* 120 mg/5 mL, 160 mg/5 mL; *Liquid:* 160 mg/5 mL, 325 mg/5 mL, 500 mg/15 mL, 500 mg/5 mL; *Powder for reconstitution:* 950 mg; *Solution:* 80 mg/0.8 mL, 120 mg/2.5 mL, 160 mg/mL; *Suppository:* 80 mg, 120 mg, 325 mg, 650 mg; *Suspension:* 160 mg/5 mL, 80 mg/0.8 mL; *Tablet:* 160 mg, 325 mg, 500 mg, 648 mg, 650 mg; *Tablet, Extended Release:* 650 mg. Acetaminophen, buffered: *Granule, effervescent*

Dosage

• **Caplets, Capsules, Chewable Tablets, Gelcaps, Elixir, Oral Liquid, Oral Solution, Oral Suspension, Sprinkle Capsules, Syrup, Tablets**

Analgesic, antipyretic.

Adults: 325-650 mg q 4 hr; doses up to 1 g q.i.d. may be used. Daily dosage should not exceed 4 g. **Pediatric:** Doses given 4-5 times/day. **Up to 3 months:** 40 mg/dose; **4-11 months:** 80 mg/dose; **1-2 years:** 120 mg/dose; **2-3 years:** 160 mg/dose; **4-5 years:** 240 mg/dose; **6-8 years:** 320 mg/dose; **9-10 years:** 400 mg/dose; **11 years:** 480 mg/dose. **12-14 years:** 640 mg/dose. **Over 14 years:** 650 mg/dose. *Alternative pediatric dose:* 10-15 mg/kg q 4 hr.

• **Extended Relief Caplets**

Analgesic, antipyretic.

Adults: 2 caplets (1,300 mg) q 8 hr.

• **Suppositories**

Analgesic, antipyretic.

Adults: 650 mg q 4 hr, not to exceed 4 g/day for up to 10 days. Clients on long-term therapy should not exceed 2.6 g/day. **Pediatric, 3-11 months:** 80 mg q 6 hr. **1-3 years:** 80 mg q 4 hr; **3-6 years:** 120-125 mg q 4-6 hr, with no more than 720 mg in 24 hr. **6-12 years:** 325 mg q 4-6 hr with no more than 2.6 g in 24 hr. Dosage should be given as needed while symptoms persist.

BUFFERED

Analgesic, antipyretic.

Adult, usual: 1 or 2 three-quarter capfuls are placed into an empty glass; add half a glass of cool water. May be taken while fizzing or after settling. Can be repeated q 4 hr as required or directed by provider.

HEALTH CARE CONSIDERATIONS

Administration/Storage

1. Store suppositories below 80°F (27°C).
2. Take the extended-relief product with water; do not crush, chew, or dissolve before swallowing.
3. Do not take acetaminophen for more than 5 days for pain in children, 10 days for pain in adults, or more than 3 days for fever in adults or children without consulting provider.
4. Bubble gum flavored OTC pediatric products (suspension liquid and chewable tablet) are available for children to treat fever and/or pain.

Assessment

1. Identify indications for therapy and expected outcomes.
2. If for long-term therapy, monitor CBC, liver and renal function studies.
3. Record presence of fever. Rate pain, noting type, onset, location, duration, and intensity.
4. Check urine for occult blood and albumin to assess for nephritis.

Client/Family Teaching

1. Take only as directed and with food or milk to minimize GI upset.
2. S&S of acute toxicity that require immediate reporting include N&V or abdominal pain. Any bluish coloration of the mucosa and nailbeds or complaints of dyspnea, weak-

ness, headache, or vertigo are S&S of methemoglobinemia caused by anoxia and require immediate attention.
3. Report pallor, weakness, and heart palpitations; S&S of hemolytic anemia.
4. Dyspnea, rapid, weak pulse; cold extremities; unexplained bleeding, bruising, sore throat, malaise, feeling clammy or sweaty; or subnormal temperatures may also be symptoms of chronic poisoning and should be reported.
5. Abdominal pain, yellow discoloration of skin and sclera, dark urine, itching, or clay-colored stools may indicate hepatotoxity.
6. Phenacetin, the major active metabolite, may cause urine to become dark brown or wine-colored.
7. Read labels on all OTC products consumed. Many contain acetaminophen and can produce toxic reactions if taken with the prescribed drug.
8. Headache and minor pain relievers containing combinations of salicylates, acetaminophen, and caffeine may be no more beneficial than aspirin alone; such combinations may be more dangerous.
9. Any unexplained pain or fever that persists for longer than 3-5 days requires medical evaluation.

Outcome/Evaluate

- ↓ Fever
- Relief of pain

Acetazolamide

(ah-set-ah-**ZOE**-la-myd)

Pregnancy Category: C

Acetazolam ✱, Apo-Acetazolamide ✱, Dazamide, Diamox, Diamox Sequels, Novo-Zolamide ✱ **(Rx)**

Acetazolamide sodium

(ah-**see**-tah-**ZOE**-la-myd)

Diamox **(Rx)**

Classification: Anticonvulsant, carbonic anhydrase inhibitor

See also *Anticonvulsants*.

Action/Kinetics: Sulfonamide derivative possessing carbonic anhydrase inhibitor activity. As an anticonvulsant, beneficial effects may be due to inhibition of carbonic anhydrase in the CNS, which increases carbon dioxide tension resulting in a decrease in neuronal conduction. Systemic acidosis may also be involved. As a diuretic, the drug inhibits carbonic anhydrase in the kidney, which decreases formation of bicarbonate and hydrogen ions from carbon dioxide, thus reducing the availability of these ions for active transport. Use as a diuretic is limited because the drug promotes metabolic acidosis, which inhibits diuretic activity. This may be partially circumvented by giving acetazolamide on alternate days. Acetazolamide also reduces IOP.

Absorbed from the GI tract and widely distributed throughout the body, including the CNS. Excreted unchanged in the urine. **Tablets: Onset,** 60-90 min; **peak:** 1-4 hr; **duration:** 8-12 hr. **Sustained-release capsules: Onset,** 2 hr; **peak:** 3-6 hr; **duration:** 18-24 hr. **Injection (IV): Onset,** 2 min; **peak:** 15 min; **duration:** 4-5 hr. Eliminated mainly unchanged through the kidneys.

Uses: Adjunct in the treatment of edema due to congestive heart failure or drug-induced edema. Absence (petit mal) and unlocalized seizures. Open-angle, secondary, or acute-angle closure glaucoma when delay of surgery is desired to lower intraocular pressure. Prophylaxis or treatment of acute mountain sickness in climbers attempting a rapid ascent or in those who are susceptible to mountain sickness even with gradual ascent.

Contraindications: Low serum sodium and potassium levels. Renal and hepatic dysfunction. Hyperchloremic acidosis, adrenal insufficiency, suprarenal gland failure, hypersensitivity to thiazide diuretics, cirrhosis. Chronic use in presence of noncongestive angle-closure glaucoma.

Special Concerns: Use with caution in the presence of mild acidosis and advanced pulmonary disease and during lactation. Increasing the dose does not increase effectiveness and may increase the risk of drowsiness or paresthesia. Safety and efficacy have not been established in children.

Side Effects: *GI:* Anorexia, N&V, melena, constipation, alteration in taste, diarrhea. *GU:* Hematuria, glycosuria, urinary frequency, renal colic, renal calculi, crystalluria, polyuria, phosphaturia, decreased or absent libido, impotence. *CNS:* ***Seizures,*** weakness, malaise, fatigue, nervousness, drowsiness, depression, dizziness, disorientation, confusion, ataxia, tremor, headache, tinnitus, flaccid paralysis, lassitude, paresthesia of the extremities. *Hematologic:* ***Bone marrow depression,*** thrombocytopenic purpura, thrombocytopenia, ***hemolytic anemia,*** leukopenia, pancytopenia, agranulocytosis. *Dermatologic:* Pruritus, urticaria, skin rashes, erythema multiforme, ***Stevens-Johnson syndrome, toxic epidermal necrolysis,*** photosensitivity. *Other:* Weight loss, fever, acidosis, electrolyte imbalance, transient myopia, hepatic insufficiency. *NOTE:* Side effects similar to those produced by sulfonamides may also occur.

OD **Management of Overdose:** *Symptoms:* Drowsiness, anorexia, N&V, dizziness, ataxia, tremor, paresthesias, tinnitus. *Treatment:* Emesis or gastric lavage. Hyperchloremic acidosis may respond to bicarbonate. Administration of potassium may also be necessary. Observe carefully and give supportive treatment.

Drug Interactions

Also see *Diuretics.*
Amphetamine / ↑ Effect of amphetamine by ↑ renal tubular reabsorption
Cyclosporine / ↑ Levels of cyclosporine → possible nephrotoxicity and neurotoxicity
Diflunisal / Significant ↓ in intraocular pressure with ↑ side effects
Ephedrine / ↑ Effect of ephedrine by ↑ renal tubular reabsorption
Lithium carbonate / ↓ Effect of lithium by ↑ renal excretion
Methotrexate / ↓ Effect of methotrexate due to ↑ renal excretion
Primidone / ↓ Effect of primidone due to ↓ GI absorption
Pseudoephedrine / ↑ Effect of pseudoephedrine by ↑ renal tubular reabsorption
Quinidine / ↑ Effect of quinidine by ↑ renal tubular reabsorption
Salicylates / Accumulation and toxicity of acetazolamide (including CNS depression and metabolic acidosis). Also, acidosis due to acetazolamide may ↑ CNS penetration of salicylates

How Supplied: Acetazolamide: *Capsule, Extended Release:* 500 mg; *Tablet:* 125 mg, 250 mg. Acetazolamide sodium: *Powder for injection:* 500 mg

Dosage

• **Extended-Release Capsules, Tablets, IV**

Epilepsy.

Adults/children: 8-30 mg/kg/day in divided doses. Optimum daily dosage: 375-1,000 mg (doses higher than 1,000 mg do not increase therapeutic effect).

Adjunct to other anticonvulsants.

Initial: 250 mg/day; dose can be increased up to 1,000 mg/day in divided doses if necessary.

Glaucoma, simple open-angle.

Adults: 250-1,000 mg/day in divided doses. Doses greater than 1 g/day do not increase the effect.

Glaucoma, closed-angle prior to surgery or secondary.

Adults, short-term therapy: 250 mg q 4 hr or 250 mg b.i.d. **Adults, acute therapy:** 500 mg followed by 125-250 mg q 4 hr using tablets. For extended-release capsules, give 500 mg b.i.d. in the morning and evening. IV therapy may be used for rapid decrease in intraocular pressure. **Pediatric:** 5-10 mg/kg/dose IM or IV q 6 hr or 10-15 mg/kg/day in divided doses q 6-8 hr using tablets.

Acute mountain sickness.

Adults: 250 mg b.i.d.-q.i.d. (500 mg 1-2 times/day of extended-release capsules). During rapid ascent, 1 g/day is recommended.

Diuresis in CHF.

Adults, initial: 250-375 mg (5 mg/kg) once daily in the morning. If the client stops losing edema fluid after an initial response, the dose should not be increased; rather, medication should be skipped for a day to allow the kidney to recover. The best diuretic effect occurs when the drug is given on alternate days or for 2 days alternative with a day of rest.

Drug-induced edema.

Adults: 250-375 mg once daily for 1 or 2 days. The drug is most effective if given every other day or for 2 days followed by a day of rest. **Children:** 5 mg/kg/dose PO or IV once daily in the morning.

HEALTH CARE CONSIDERATIONS

See also *Health Care Considerations* for *Anticonvulsants.*

Administration/Storage

1. Change over from other anticonvulsant therapy to acetazolamide should be gradual.
2. Acetazolamide tablets may be crushed and suspended in a cherry, chocolate, raspberry, or other sweet syrup. Do not use vehicles containing glycerin or alcohol. As an alternative, 1 tablet may be submerged in 10 mL of hot water and added to 10 mL of honey or syrup.
3. Tolerance after prolonged use may necessitate dosage increase.
4. Do not administer the sustained-release dosage form as an anticonvulsant; it should be used only for glaucoma and acute mountain sickness.
5. When used for prophylaxis of mountain sickness, initiate dosage 1-2 days before ascent and continue for at least 2 days while at high altitudes.
6. Due to possible differences in bioavailability, do not interchange brands.
IV 7. IV administration is preferred; IM administration is painful due to alkalinity of solution.
8. For parenteral use, reconstitute each 500-

A

mg vial with at least 5 mL of sterile water for injection. Use parenteral solutions within 24 hr after reconstitution, although reconstituted solutions retain potency for 1 week if refrigerated.
9. Reconstitute each 500-mg vial with at least 5 mL of sterile water for injection. For direct IV use, administer over at least 1 min. For intermittent IV use, further dilute in dextrose or saline solution and infuse over 4-8 hr.

Assessment

1. Record indications for therapy, type and onset of symptoms.
2. Review electrolytes, uric acid, and glucose. Note any liver and renal dysfunction prior to administering.
3. List drugs currently prescribed to ensure none interacts unfavorably.
4. With glaucoma, note baseline ophthalmic exam and intraocular pressures; assess for visual effects.
5. Perform a thorough CV and pulmonary assessment in clients with CHF.

Client/Family Teaching

1. Taking drug with food may decrease gastric irritation and GI upset.
2. Determine drug effects before undertaking tasks that require mental alertness.
3. Drug increases the frequency of voiding; take early in the day to avoid interrupting sleep.
4. Take only as directed. If prescribed every other day, document administration to enhance adherence.
5. Increase fluids (2-3 L/day) to prevent crystalluria and stone formation.
6. Drug may increase blood glucose levels. Monitor and report increases; dose of hypoglycemic agent may require adjustment.
7. Report if nausea, dizziness, rapid weight gain, muscle weakness, or cramps occur or any changes in the color/consistency of stools.
8. Report for labs to determine need for potassium replacement.

Outcome/Evaluate

- ↓ Seizure activity
- ↓ Intraocular pressure
- ↓ CHF-associated edema
- Prevention of mountain sickness

Acetylcysteine

(ah-see-till-**SIS**-tay-een)

Pregnancy Category: B

Mucomyst, Mucosil, Parvolex **(Rx)**

Classification: Mucolytic

Action/Kinetics: Reduces the viscosity of purulent and nonpurulent pulmonary secretions and facilitates their removal by splitting disulfide bonds. Action increases with increasing pH (peak: pH 7-9). **Onset, inhalation:** Within 1 min; **by direct instillation:** immediate. **Time to peak effect:** 5-10 min.

Uses: Adjunct in the treatment of acute and chronic bronchitis, emphysema, tuberculosis, pneumonia, bronchiectasis, atelectasis. Routine care of clients with tracheostomy, pulmonary complications after thoracic or CV surgery, or in posttraumatic chest conditions. Pulmonary complications of cystic fibrosis. Diagnostic bronchial asthma. Antidote in acetaminophen poisoning to reduce hepatotoxicity. *Investigational:* As an ophthalmic solution for dry eye.

Contraindications: Sensitivity to drug.

Special Concerns: Use with caution during lactation, in the elderly, and in clients with asthma.

Side Effects: *Respiratory:* Increased incidence of bronchospasm in clients with asthma. Increased amount of liquefied bronchial secretions, which must be removed by suction if cough is inadequate. Bronchial and tracheal irritation, tightness in chest, bronchoconstriction. *GI:* N&V, stomatitis. *Other:* Rashes, fever, drowsiness, rhinorrhea.

Drug Interactions: Acetylcysteine is incompatible with antibiotics and should be administered separately.

How Supplied: *Solution:* 10%, 20%

Dosage

- **10% or 20% Solution: Nebulization, Direct Application, or Direct Intratracheal Instillation**

Nebulization into face mask, tracheostomy, mouth piece.

1-10 mL of 20% solution or 2-10 mL of 10% solution 3-4 times/day.

Closed tent or croupette.

Up to 300 mL of 10% or 20% solution/treatment.

Direct instillation into tracheostomy.

1-2 mL of 10%-20% solution q 1-4 hr.

Percutaneous intratracheal catheter.

1-2 mL of 20% solution or 2-4 mL of 10% solution q 1-4 hr by syringe attached to catheter.

Instillation to particular portion of bronchopulmonary tree using small plastic catheter into the trachea.

2-5 mL of 20% solution instilled into the trachea by means of a syringe connected to a catheter.

Diagnostic procedures.

2-3 doses of 1-2 mL of 20% or 2-4 mL of 10% solution by nebulization or intratracheal instillation before the procedure.

Acetaminophen overdose.

Given PO, initial: 140 mg/kg; **then,** 70 mg/kg q 4 hr for a total of 17 doses.

HEALTH CARE CONSIDERATIONS

Administration/Storage

1. Use nonreactive plastic, glass, or stainless steel equipment for administration.
2. May use the 10% solution undiluted.
3. Use either water for injection or saline to dilute the 20% solution.
4. May administer via face mask, face tent, oxygen tent, head tent, or by positive-pressure apparatus.
5. Administer with compressed air for nebulization. Hand nebulizers are contraindicated.
6. After prolonged nebulization, dilute the last fourth of the medication with sterile water for injection to prevent drug concentration.
7. Solution may develop a light purple color; does not affect action.
8. Closed bottles of solution remain stable for 2 years when stored at 20°C (68°F). Store open bottles at 2°C-8°C (35°F-46°F) and use within 96 hr. Once opened, record time/ date to prevent use beyond 96-hr.
9. Incompatible with antibiotics; administer separately.
10. Have ET tube and suction available at the bedside for removal of increased secretions.

Assessment

1. Determine when spasms occur.
2. Record conditions likely to cause congestion and wheezing.
3. Identify previous approaches (successful and unsuccessful) used to treat symptoms.
4. Determine smoking status and if currently taking antibiotics.
5. With acetaminophen overdosage document time of ingestion. Administer drug within 8-10 hr following overdose to protect from hepatoxicity and death. Monitor LFTs and acetaminophen levels.

Interventions

1. If bronchospasm occurs, have a bronchodilator, such as isoproterenol for aerosol inhalation, readily available.
2. Position to facilitate removal of secretions. If unable to cough up secretions, provide suction.
3. Monitor VS and I&O.
4. Wash face following nebulization treatments; medication may cause the face to become sticky.
5. Administration route for acetaminophen toxicity is oral and will consist of 17 doses.

Client/Family Teaching:

1. Use only as directed; do not exceed prescribed dosage.
2. Report any unusual changes in color, consistency, or characteristics of sputum.
3. The nauseous odor present when the treatment begins will likely become less noticeable as therapy continues.
4. Avoid any triggers that may stimulate bronchospasm (i.e., cigarette smoke, dust, chemicals, cold air).
5. Promote smoking cessation classes and support groups to help stop smoking.

Outcome/Evaluate

- Improved airway exchange with ↓ viscosity and mobilization and expectoration of secretions
- ↓ Acetaminophen levels and associated liver toxicity

Acetylsalicylic acid (ASA, Aspirin)

(ah-**SEE**-till-sal-ih-**SILL**-ick **AH**-sid)

Pregnancy Category: C

Apo-Asa ✱, Asaphen ✱, Aspergum, Aspirin, Aspirin Regimen Bayer 81 mg with Calcium, Bayer Children's Aspirin, Easprin, Ecotrin Caplets and Tablets, Ecotrin Maximum Strength Caplets and Tablets, Empirin, Entrophen ✱, Excedrin Geltabs, Genprin, Genuine Bayer Aspirin Caplets and Tablets, Halfprin, 8-Hour Bayer Timed-Release Caplets, Maximum Bayer Aspirin Caplets and Tablets, MSD Enteric Coated ASA ✱, Norwich Extra Strength, Novasen ✱, St. Joseph Adult Chewable Aspirin, Therapy Bayer Caplets, ZOR-prin **(OTC)** (Easprin and ZOR-prin are **Rx**)

Acetylsalicylic acid, buffered

(ah-**SEE**-till-sal-ih-**SILL**-ick **AH**-sid)

Pregnancy Category: C

Alka-Seltzer Extra Strength with Aspirin, Alka-Seltzer with Aspirin, Alka-Seltzer with Aspirin (flavored), Arthritis Pain Formula, Ascriptin A/D, Ascriptin Regular Strength, Bayer Buffered, Buffered Aspirin, Bufferin, Buffex, Cama Arthritis Pain Reliever, Magnaprin, Magnaprin Arthritis Strength Captabs, Tri-Buffered Bufferin Caplets and Tablets **(OTC)**

Classification: Nonnarcotic analgesic, antipyretic, anti-inflammatory agent

Action/Kinetics: Exhibits antipyretic, anti-inflammatory, and analgesic effects. The antipyretic effect is due to an action on the hypothalamus, resulting in heat loss by vasodilation of peripheral blood vessels and promoting sweating. Prostaglandins have been implicated in the inflammatory process, as well as in mediation of pain. Thus, if levels are decreased, the inflammatory reaction may subside.The anti-inflammatory effects are probably mediated through inhibition of cyclo-oxygenase, which results in a decrease in prostaglan-

A

din synthesis and other mediators of the pain response. The mechanism of action for the analgesic effects of aspirin is not known fully but is partly attributable to improvement of the inflammatory condition. Aspirin also produces inhibition of platelet aggregation by decreasing the synthesis of endoperoxides and thromboxanes—substances that mediate platelet aggregation.

Large doses of aspirin (5 g/day or more) increase uric acid secretion, while low doses (2 g/day or less) decrease uric acid secretion. However, aspirin antagonizes drugs used to treat gout.

Rapidly absorbed after PO administration. Is hydrolyzed to the active salicylic acid, which is 70%-90% protein bound. For arthritis and rheumatic disease, blood levels of 150-300 mcg/mL should be maintained. For analgesic and antipyretic, achieve blood levels of 25-50 mcg/mL. For acute rheumatic fever, achieve blood levels of 150-300 mcg/mL. **Therapeutic salicylic acid serum levels:** 150-300 mcg/mL, although tinnitus occurs at serum levels above 200 mcg/mL and serious toxicity above 400 mcg/mL. **t½:** aspirin, 15-20 min; salicylic acid, 2-20 hr, depending on the dose. Salicylic acid and metabolites are excreted by the kidney. The bioavailability of enteric-coated salicylate products may be poor. The addition of antacids (buffered aspirin) may decrease GI irritation and increase the dissolution and absorption of such products.

Uses: Analgesic: Pain arising from integumental structures, myalgias, neuralgias, arthralgias, headache, dysmenorrhea, and similar types of pain. Antipyretic. **Anti-Inflammatory:** Arthritis, osteoarthritis, SLE, acute rheumatic fever, gout, and many other conditions. Mucocutaneous lymph node syndrome (Kawasaki disease). Reduce the risk of recurrent transient ischemic attacks and strokes in men. Decrease risk of death from nonfatal MI in clients who have a history of infarction or who manifest unstable angina; aortocoronary bypass surgery. Gout. May be effective in less severe postoperative and postpartum pain; pain secondary to trauma and cancer. *Investigational:* Chronic use to prevent cataract formation; low doses to prevent toxemia of pregnancy; in pregnant women with inadequate uteroplacental blood flow. Reduce colon cancer mortality (low doses). Low doses of aspirin and warfarin to reduce the risk of a second heart attack.

Contraindications: Hypersensitivity to salicylates. Clients with asthma, hay fever, or nasal polyps have a higher incidence of hypersensitivity reactions. Severe anemia, history of blood coagulation defects, in conjunction with anticoagulant therapy. Salicylates can cause congestive failure when taken in the large doses used for rheumatic diseases. Vitamin K deficiency; 1 week before and after surgery. In pregnancy, especially the last trimester as the drug may cause problems in the newborn child or complications during delivery. In children or teenagers with chicken-pox or flu due to possibility of development of Reye's syndrome.

Controlled-release aspirin is not recommended for use as an antipyretic or short-term analgesic because adequate blood levels may not be reached. Also, controlled-release products are not recommended for children less than 12 years of age and in children with fever accompanied by dehydration.

Special Concerns: Use with caution during lactation and in the presence of gastric or peptic ulcers, in mild diabetes, erosive gastritis, bleeding tendencies, in cardiac disease, and in liver or kidney disease. Aspirin products now carry the following labeling: "It is especially important not to use aspirin during the last three months of pregnancy unless specifically directed to do so by a doctor because it may cause problems in the newborn child or complications during delivery."

Side Effects: The toxic effects of the salicylates are dose-related. *GI:* Dyspepsia, heartburn, anorexia, nausea, occult blood loss, epigastric discomfort, ***massive GI bleeding, potentiation of peptic ulcer***. *Allergic:* ***Bronchospasm, asthma-like symptoms, anaphylaxis,*** skin rashes, angioedema, urticaria, rhinitis, nasal polyps. *Hematologic:* Prolongation of bleeding time, thrombocytopenia, leukopenia, purpura, shortened erythrocyte survival time, decreased plasma iron levels. *Miscellaneous:* Thirst, fever, dimness of vision.

NOTE: Use of aspirin in children and teenagers with flu or chickenpox may result in the development of ***Reye's syndrome***. Also, dehydrated, febrile children are more prone to salicylate intoxication.

Laboratory Test Considerations: False + or ↑ : Amylase, AST, ALT, uric acid, PBI, urinary VMA (most tests), catecholamines, urinary glucose (Benedict's, Clinitest), and urinary uric acid (at high doses) values. False - or ↓ : CO_2 content, glucose (fasting), potassium, urinary VMA (Pisano method), and thrombocyte values.

OD **Management of Overdose:** *Symptoms of Mild Salicylate Toxicity (Salicylism):* At serum levels between 150 and 200 mcg/mL. *GI:* N&V, diarrhea, thirst. *CNS:* Tinnitus (most common), dizziness, difficulty in hearing, mental confusion, lassitude. *Miscellaneous:* Flushing, sweating, tachycardia.

Symptoms of salicylism may be observed with doses used for inflammatory disease or rheumatic fever. *Symptoms of Severe Salicylate Poisoning:* At serum levels over 400 mcg/mL. *CNS:* Excitement, confusion, disorientation, irritability, hallucinations, lethargy, stupor, ***coma, respiratory failure, seizures.*** *Metabolic:* Respiratory alkalosis (initially), respiratory acidosis and metabolic acidosis, dehydration. *GI:* N&V. *Hematologic:* Platelet dysfunction, hypoprothrombinemia, increased capillary fragility. *Miscellaneous:* ***Hyperthermia, hemorrhage, CV collapse, renal failure,*** hyperventilation, pulmonary edema, tetany, hypoglycemia (late). *Treatment (Toxicity):*

1. If the client has had repeated administration of large doses of salicylates, document and report evidence of hyperventilation or complaints of auditory or visual disturbances (symptoms of salicylism).
2. Severe salicylate poisoning, whether due to overdose or accumulation, will have an exaggerated effect on the CNS and the metabolic system:
   - Clients may develop a salicylate jag characterized by garrulous behavior. They may act as if they were inebriated.
   - Convulsions and coma may follow.
3. When working with febrile children or the elderly who have been treated with aspirin, maintain adequate fluid intake. These clients are more susceptible to salicylate intoxication if they are dehydrated.
4. The following treatment approaches may be considered for treatment of *acute salicylate toxicity:*
   - Initially induce vomiting or perform gastric lavage followed by activated charcoal (most effective if given within 2 hr of ingestion).
   - Monitor salicylate levels and acid-base and fluid and electrolyte balance. If required, administer IV solutions of dextrose, saline, potassium, and sodium bicarbonate as well as vitamin K.
   - Seizures may be treated with diazepam.
   - Treat hyperthermia if present.
   - Alkaline diuresis will enhance renal excretion. Hemodialysis is effective but should be reserved for severe poisonings.
   - If necessary, administer oxygen and artificial ventilation

Drug Interactions

ACE inhibitors / ↓ Effect of ACE inhibitors possibly due to prostaglandin inhibition
Acetazolamide / ↑ CNS toxicity of salicylates; also, ↑ excretion of salicylic acid if urine kept alkaline
Alcohol, ethyl / ↑ Chance of GI bleeding caused by salicylates
Alteplase, recombinant / ↑ Risk of bleeding
Ammonium chloride / ↑ Effect of salicylates by ↑ renal tubular reabsorption
Antacids / ↓ Salicylate levels in plasma due to ↑ rate of renal excretion
Anticoagulants, oral / ↑ Effect of anticoagulant by ↓ plasma protein binding and plasma prothrombin
Antirheumatics / Both are ulcerogenic and may cause ↑ GI bleeding
Ascorbic acid / ↑ Effect of salicylates by ↑ renal tubular reabsorption
Beta-adrenergic blocking agents / Salicylates ↓ action of beta-blockers, possibly due to prostaglandin inhibition
Charcoal, activated / ↓ Absorption of salicylates from GI tract
Corticosteroids / Both are ulcerogenic; also, corticosteroids may ↓ blood salicylate levels by ↑ breakdown by liver and ↑ excretion
Dipyridamole / Additive anticoagulant effects
Furosemide / ↑ Chance of salicylate toxicity due to ↓ renal excretion; also, salicylates may ↓ effect of furosemide in clients with impaired renal function or cirrhosis with ascites
Heparin / Inhibition of platelet adhesiveness by aspirin may result in bleeding tendencies
Hypoglycemics, oral / ↑ Hypoglycemia due to ↓ plasma protein binding and ↓ excretion
Indomethacin / Both are ulcerogenic and may cause ↑ GI bleeding
Insulin / Salicylates ↑ hypoglycemic effect of insulin
Methionine / ↑ Effect of salicylates by ↑ renal tubular reabsorption
Methotrexate / ↑ Effect of methotrexate by ↓ plasma protein binding; also, salicylates block renal excretion of methotrexate
Nitroglycerin / Combination may result in unexpected hypotension
Nizatidine / ↑ Serum levels of salicylates
NSAIDs / Additive ulcerogenic effects; also, aspirin may ↓ serum levels of NSAIDs
Para-aminosalicylic acid (PAS) / Possible ↑ effect of PAS due to ↓ excretion by kidney or ↓ plasma protein binding
Phenylbutazone / Combination may produce hyperuricemia
Phenytoin / ↑ Effect of phenytoin by ↓ plasma protein binding
Probenecid / Salicylates inhibit uricosuric activity of probenecid

Sodium bicarbonate / ↓ Effect of salicylates by ↑ rate of excretion
Spironolactone / Aspirin ↓ diuretic effect of spironolactone
Sulfinpyrazone / Salicylates inhibit uricosuric activity of sulfinpyrazone
Sulfonamides / ↑ Effect of sulfonamides by ↑ blood levels of salicylates
Valproic acid / ↑ Effect of valproic acid due to ↓ plasma protein binding

How Supplied: *Chew tablet:* 80 mg, 81 mg; *Enteric coated tablet:* 81 mg, 162 mg, 324 mg, 325 mg, 500 mg, 650 mg, 975 mg; *Gum:* 227 mg; *Suppository:* 60 mg, 120 mg, 125 mg, 200 mg, 300 mg, 325 mg, 600 mg, 650 mg; *Tablet:* 81 mg, 324 mg, 325 mg, 486 mg, 500 mg, 650 mg; *Tablet, Extended Release:* 650 mg, 800 mg

Dosage

• **Gum, Chewable Tablets, Coated Tablets, Effervescent Tablets, Enteric-Coated Tablets, Suppositories, Tablets, Extended Release Tablets**

Analgesic, antipyretic.

Adults: 325-500 mg q 3 hr, 325-600 mg q 4 hr, or 650-1,000 mg q 6 hr. As an alternative, the adult chewable tablet (81 mg each) may be used in doses of 4-8 tablets q 4 hr as needed. **Pediatric:** 65 mg/kg/day (alternate dose: 1.5 g/m^2/day) in divided doses q 4-6 hr, not to exceed 3.6 g/day. Alternatively, the following dosage regimen can be used: **Pediatric, 2-3 years:** 162 mg q 4 hr as needed; **4-5 years:** 243 mg q 4 hr as needed; **6-8 years:** 320-325 mg q 4 hr as needed; **9-10 years:** 405 mg q 4 hr as needed; **11 years:** 486 mg q 4 hr as needed; **12-14 years:** 648 mg q 4 hr.

Arthritis, rheumatic diseases.

Adults: 3.2-6 g/day in divided doses.

Juvenile rheumatoid arthritis.

60-110 mg/kg/day (alternate dose: 3 g/m^2) in divided doses q 6-8 hr. When initiating therapy at 60 mg/kg/day, dose may be increased by 20 mg/kg/day after 5-7 days and by 10 mg/kg/day after another 5-7 days.

Acute rheumatic fever.

Adults, initial: 5-8 g/day. **Pediatric, initial,** 100 mg/kg/day (3 g/m^2/day) for 2 weeks; **then,** decrease to 75 mg/kg/day for 4-6 weeks.

TIAs in men.

Adults: 650 mg b.i.d. or 325 mg q.i.d. A dose of 300 mg/day may be as effective and with fewer side effects.

Prophylaxis of MI.

Adults: 300 or 325 mg/day (both solid PO dosage forms-regular and buffered as well as buffered aspirin in solution). The adult chewable tablets can also be used.

Kawasaki disease.

Adults: 80-180 mg/kg/day during the febrile period. After the fever resolves, the dose may be adjusted to 10 mg/kg/day.

NOTE: Doses as low as 80-100 mg/day are being studied for use in unstable angina, MI, and aortocoronary bypass surgery. Aspirin Regimen Bayer 81 mg with Calcium contains 250 mg calcium carbonate (10% of RDA) and 81 mg of acetylsalicylic acid for individuals who require aspirin to prevent recurrent heart attacks and strokes.

HEALTH CARE CONSIDERATIONS

Administration/Storage

1. Enteric-coated tablets or buffered tablets are better tolerated by some.
2. Take with a full glass of water to prevent lodging of the drug in the esophagus.
3. Have epinephrine available to counteract hypersensitivity reactions should they occur. Asthma caused by hypersensitive reaction to salicylates may be refractory to epinephrine, so antihistamines should also be available for parenteral and PO use.

Assessment

1. Take a complete drug history and note any evidence of hypersensitivity. Individuals allergic to tartrazine should not take aspirin. Clients who have tolerated salicylates well in the past may suddenly have an allergic or anaphylactoid reaction.
2. If administered for pain, rate and determine the type and pattern of pain, if the pain is unusual, or if it is recurring. Note the effectiveness of aspirin if previously used for pain.
3. Note if client has asthma, hay fever, ulcer disease or nasal polyps.
4. Record age; drug is discouraged in those under 12. Assess for chickenpox or the flu.
5. Test stool and urine for blood; monitor CBC routinely during high-dose and chronic therapy.
6. Determine if diagnostic tests scheduled. Drug causes irreversible platelet effects. Anticipate 4-7 days for the body to replace these once drug discontinued; hence no salicylates one week prior to procedure.
7. Determine any history of peptic ulcers or bleeding tendencies. Obtain bleeding parameters with prolonged use.
8. Review drugs currently prescribed for drug interactions.
9. The therapeutic serum level of salicylate is 150-300 mcg/mL for adult and juvenile rheumatoid arthritis and acute rheumatic fever. Reassure that the higher dosage is necessary for anti-inflammatory effects.

Client/Family Teaching
1. Take only as directed. To reduce gastric irritation, administer with meals, milk, a full glass of water, or crackers.
2. Do not take salicylates if product is off-color or has a strange odor. Note expiration date.
3. Report any toxic effects: ringing in the ears, difficulty hearing, dizziness or fainting spells, unusual increase in sweating, severe abdominal pain, or mental confusion.
4. Salicylates potentiate the effects of antidiabetic drugs. Monitor glucose levels and report hypoglycemia.
5. When administering for antipyretic effect, follow temperature administration parameters.
• Obtain temperature 1 hr after administering to assess outcome.
• With marked diaphoresis, dry client, change linens, provide fluids, and prevent chilling.
6. Cardiac clients on large doses should report symptoms of CHF.
7. Tell dentist and other HCPs you are taking salicylates.
8. Before purchasing other OTC preparations, notify provider and note the quantity used per day.
9. Salicylates should be administered to children only upon specific medical recommendation due to increased risk of Reye's syndrome.
10. If child refuses medication or vomits it, consider aspirin suppositories or acetaminophen.
11. Children who are dehydrated and who have a fever are especially susceptible to aspirin intoxication from even small doses. Report any gastric irritation/pain; may be S&S of hypersensitivity or toxicity.
12. Sodium bicarbonate may decrease the serum level of aspirin, reducing its effectiveness.
13. Report any unusual bruising or bleeding. Large doses may increase PT and should be avoided. Aspirin and NSAIDs may interfere with blood-clotting mechanisms (antiplatelet effects) and are usually discontinued 1 week before surgery to prevent increased risk of bleeding.
14. Avoid indiscriminate use.

Outcome/Evaluate
• Relief of pain/discomfort; Improved joint mobility/function
• ↓ Fever
• Prophylaxis of MI/TIA

Acitretin
(ah-sih-**TREH**-tin)
Pregnancy Category: X
Soriatane **(Rx)**
Classification: Antipsoriasis product.

Action/Kinetics: Retinoic acid derivative that is the main metabolite of etretinate. Mechanism is not known. Absorption optimal when given with food. **t½, terminal:** 49 hr. Extensively metabolized; excreted through feces and urine.

Uses: Severe psoriasis, including erythrodermic and generalized pustular types. *Investigational:* Darier's disease, palmoplantar pustulosis, lichen planus, children with lamellar ichthyosis, non-bullous and bullous ichthyosiform erythroderma, Sjögren-Larsson syndrome, lichen sclerosus et atrophicus of the vulva and palmoplantar lichen nitidus.

Contraindications: Use during pregnancy or in those who intend to become pregnant during therapy or at any time for at least 3 years following discontinuation of therapy. Use by females who may not use reliable contraception during treatment or for at least 3 years following treatment. Use of ethanol in women either during treatment or for 2 months after cessation of treatment. Lactation.

Special Concerns: Use with caution in those with severely impaired liver or kidney function. Safety and efficacy have not been determined in children.

Side Effects: *Dermatologic:* Alopecia, skin peeling, dry skin, nail disorder, pruritus, erythematous rash, hyperesthesia, paresthesia, paronychia, skin atrophy, sticky skin, abnormal skin odor, abnormal hair texture, bullous eruption, cold/clammy skin, dermatitis, increased sweating, infection, psoriasis-like rash, purpura, pyogenic granuloma, rash, seborrhea, skin fissures, skin ulceration, sunburn. *CNS:* Rigors, headache, pain, depression, insomnia, somnolence. *GI:* Abdominal pain, nausea, diarrhea, tongue disorder, altered taste, hepatotoxicity. *Ophthalmic:* Xerophthalmia, blurred vision, abnormal vision, blepharitis, irritation, conjunctivitis, corneal epithelial abnormality, decreased night vision, blindness, eye abnormality, eye pain, photophobia. *Musculoskeletal:* Arthralgia, spinal hyperostosis, arthritis, arthrosis, back pain, hypertonia, myalgia, osteodynia, peripheral joint hyperostosis. *Mucous membranes:* Cheilitis, rhinitis, epistaxis, dry mouth, gingival bleeding, gingivitis, increased salivation, stomatitis, thirst, ulcera-

tive stomatitis. *Body as a whole:* Anorexia, edema, fatigue, hot flashes, increased appetite, flushing, sinusitis. *Otic:* Earache, tinnitus.
Laboratory Test Considerations: ↑ AST, ALT, GGT, LDH, triglyceride, cholesterol. ↓ HDL.

Drug Interactions

Ethanol / Possible formation of etretinate which has a longer half-life than acitretin
Glyburide / Enhanced clearance of blood glucose
Methotrexate / ↑ Risk of hepatotoxicity
Oral contraceptives, "minipill" / Acitretin interferes with the contraceptive effect
How Supplied: *Capsules:* 10 mg, 25 mg

Dosage

- **Capsules**

Psoriasis.

Must individualize dosage. **Initial:** 25 or 50 mg/day given as a single dose with main meal. **Maintenance:** 25 to 50 mg/day.

HEALTH CARE CONSIDERATIONS

Administration/Storage: Terminate therapy when lesions have sufficiently resolved. Treat relapses as described for initial therapy.

Assessment

1. Describe, record and photograph condition requiring therapy; note other treatments trialed and outcome.
2. Determine if pregnant. Females must undergo pregnancy testing and receive contraceptive counselling due to risk of fetal abnormalities.
3. Monitor lipids and LFTs at 1-2 week intervals until drug response obtained (4-8 weeks).

Client/Family Teaching

1. Take with food to enhance absorption.
2. Do not consume vit A supplements; avoid sun lamps and excess sun exposure.
3. Females should avoid all alcohol products during and for 2 mo following therapy.
4. Practice reliable contraception 1 mo prior to and during therapy; avoid pregnancy for at least 3 yrs following therapy due to risk of severe fetal malformations.
5. Tubal ligation and microdose progestin "minipill" products may fail; use alternative forms of birth control.
6. May experience worsening of psoriasis during initial treatment period; may take 2-3 mo to see improvement.
7. Do not donate blood during and for up to 3 yr following therapy.

Outcome/Evaluate: Healing/clearing of lesions

Acyclovir (Acycloguanosine)

(ay-**SYE**-kloh-veer, ay-**SYE**-kloh-**GWON**-oh-seen)

Pregnancy Category: C
Alti-Acyclovir ✱, Apo-Acyclovir ✱, Avirax ✱, Nu-Acyclovir ✱, Zovirax **(Rx)**
Classification: Antiviral anti-infective

See also *Antiviral Drugs.*
Action/Kinetics: A synthetic acyclic purine nucleoside analog converted by HSV-infected cells to acyclovir triphosphate, which interferes with HSV DNA polymerase, thereby inhibiting DNA replication. Systemic absorption is slow from the GI tract (although therapeutic levels are reached) and following topical administration. It is preferentially taken up and converted to the active triphosphate form by herpes virus-infected cells. Food does not affect absorption. **Peak levels after PO:** 1.5-2 hr. Widely distributed in tissues and body fluids. The half-life and total body clearance depend on renal function. **t½, PO, C_{CR}, greater than 80 mL/min/1.73 m²:** 2.5 hr. Metabolites and unchanged drug (up to 85%) are excreted through the kidney. Reduce dosage in clients with impaired renal function. Clients who take acyclovir (600-800 mg/day) with AZT had a significantly prolonged survival rate compared with clients taking only acyclovir.
Uses: PO. Initial and recurrent genital herpes in immunocompromised and nonimmunocompromised clients. Prophylaxis of frequently recurrent genital herpes infections in nonimmunocompromised clients. Treatment of chickenpox in children ranging from 2 to 18 years of age. Acute treatment of herpes zoster (shingles).

Parenteral. Initial therapy for severe genital herpes in clients who are not immunocompromised; initial and recurrent mucosal and cutaneous HSV-1 and HSV-2 infections in immunocompromised individuals. Varicella zoster infections (shingles) in immunocompromised clients. HSE in clients over 6 months of age. Neonatal herpes simplex infections.

Topical. To decrease healing time and duration of viral shedding in initial herpes genitalis. Limited non-life-threatening mucocutaneous HSV infections in immunocompromised clients. No beneficial effect in recurrent herpes genitalis or in herpes labialis in nonimmunocompromised clients.

Investigational: Cytomegalovirus and HSV infection following bone marrow or renal transplantation; herpes simplex ocular infections; herpes simplex proctitis; herpes simplex labialis; herpes simplex whitlow; herpes zoster encephalitis; disseminated primary eczema herpeticum; herpes simplex-associated erythema multiforme; infectious mononucleosis; and varicella pneumonia.

Contraindications: Hypersensitivity to formulation. Use in the eye. Use to prevent recurrent HSV infections.

Special Concerns: Use with caution during lactation or with concomitant intrathecal methotrexate or interferon. Safety and efficacy of PO form not established in children less than 2 years of age. Prolonged or repeated doses in immunocompromised clients may result in emergence of resistant viruses. Use of oral acyclovir does not eliminate latent HSV and is not a cure.

Side Effects: PO. *Short-term treatment of herpes simplex. GI:* N&V, diarrhea, anorexia, sore throat, taste of drug. *CNS:* Headache, dizziness, fatigue. *Miscellaneous:* Edema, skin rashes, leg pain, inguinal adenopathy.

Long-term treatment of herpes simplex. GI: Nausea, diarrhea. *CNS:* Headache. *Other:* Skin rash, asthenia, paresthesia.

Treatment of herpes zoster. GI: N&V, diarrhea, constipation. *CNS:* Headache, malaise.

Treatment of chickenpox. GI: Vomiting, diarrhea, abdominal pain, flatulence. *Dermatologic:* Rash.

Parenteral (frequency greater than 1%). A*t injection site:* Phlebitis, inflammation. *GI:* N&V. *CNS:* Encephalopathic changes, including lethargy, obtundation, tremors, agitation, confusion, hallucination, ***seizures, coma***, jitters, headache. *Miscellaneous:* Skin rashes, urticaria, itching, transient elevation of serum creatinine or BUN (most often following rapid IV infusion), elevation of transaminases, ***fatal renal failure, fatal thrombotic thrombocytopenic purpura or hemolytic uremic syndrome in immunocompromised clients***.

Topical. Transient burning, stinging, pain. Pruritus, rash, vulvitis, local edema. *NOTE:* All of these effects have also been reported with the use of a placebo preparation.

OD Management of Overdose: *Symptoms:* Increased BUN and serum creatinine, ***renal failure following parenteral overdose.*** *Treatment:* Hemodialysis (peritoneal dialysis is less effective).

Drug Interactions

Probenecid / ↑ Bioavailability and half-life of acyclovir → ↑ effect

Zidovudine / Severe lethargy and drowsiness

How Supplied: *Capsule:* 200 mg; *Injection:* 5 mg/mL, 25 mg/mL, 50 mg/ml; *Ointment:* 5%; *Powder for injection:* 500 mg, 1000 mg; *Suspension:* 200 mg/5 mL; *Tablet:* 400 mg, 800 mg

Dosage

- **Capsules, Suspension, Tablets**

Initial genital herpes.

200 mg q 4 hr, 5 times/day for 10 days.

Chronic genital herpes.

400 mg b.i.d., 200 mg t.i.d., or 200 mg 5 times/day for up to 12 months.

Intermittent therapy for genital herpes.

200 mg q 4 hr, 5 times/day for 5 days. Start therapy at the first symptom/sign of recurrence.

Herpes zoster, acute treatment.

800 mg q 4 hr, 5 times/day for 7-10 days.

Chickenpox.

20 mg/kg (of the suspension) q.i.d. for 5 days. A single dose should not exceed 800 mg. Begin therapy at the earliest sign/symptom.

- **IV Infusion**

Mucosal and cutaneous herpes simplex in immunocompromised clients.

Adults: 5 mg/kg infused at a constant rate over 1 hr, q 8 hr (15 mg/kg/day) for 7 days. **Children less than 12 years of age:** 250 mg/m^2 infused at a constant rate over 1 hr, q 8 hr for 7 days.

Varicella-zoster infections (shingles) in immunocompromised clients.

Adults: 10 mg/kg infused at a constant rate over 1 hr, q 8 hr for 7 days (not to exceed 500 mg/m^2 q 8 hr). **Children less than 12 years of age:** 500 mg/m^2 infused at a constant rate over at least 1 hr, q 8 hr for 7 days.

Herpes simplex encephalitis.

Adults: 10 mg/kg infused at a constant rate over at least 1 hr, q 8 hr for 10 days. **Children less than 12 years of age and greater than 6 months of age:** 500 mg/m^2 infused at a constant rate over at least 1 hr, q 8 hr for 10 days.

- **Topical (5% Ointment)**

Adults and children: Lesion should be covered with sufficient amount of ointment (0.5-in. ribbon/4 in.^{2} of surface area) q 3 hr, 6 times/day for 7 days. Initiate treatment as soon as possible after onset of symptoms.

HEALTH CARE CONSIDERATIONS

See also *General Health Care Considerations for All Anti-Infectives* and *Antiviral Drugs*.

Administration/Storage

1. Store ointment in a dry place at room temperature.
2. Adjust both the PO and parenteral dose

and/or dosing interval in acute or chronic renal impairment.
3. The suspension may be used to treat varicella zoster infections.
IV 4. Prepare IV solution by dissolving the contents of the 500- or 1000-mg vial in 10 or 20 mL sterile water for injection, respectively (final concentration of 50 mg/mL). Infusion concentrations of 7 mg/mL or lower are recommended; thus, the calculated dose must be added to an appropriate IV solution at the correct volume. Reconstituted solution should be used within 12 hr. Bacteriostatic water containing benzyl alcohol or parabens should not be used as it will cause a precipitate.
5. Accompany IV infusion by hydration (3 L/day) to prevent precipitation in renal tubules (crystalluria).
6. Administer infusion over 1 hr to prevent renal tubular damage; do not administer by rapid or bolus IV, IM, or SC injections.
7. If refrigerated, reconstituted solution may show a precipitate which dissolves at room temperature.

Assessment

1. Record indications for therapy and assess all skin lesions.
2. Monitor CBC, electrolytes, renal and LFTs; closely with IV therapy and if immunocompromised.
3. With chickenpox or herpes zoster, institute appropriate precautions for all susceptible individuals [i.e., pregnant women, immunocompromised clients, and those who have not had chickenpox (may check titer if unknown)].

Client/Family Teaching

1. Drug is not a cure; only used to help manage symptoms. It will not prevent disease transmission to others or prevent reinfection.
2. Adequately cover all lesions with topical acyclovir as ordered; do not exceed dosage, frequency of application or treatment time.
3. Report any burning, stinging, itching, and rash when applying.
4. Complete all exams/tests to rule out presence of other STDs.
5. Acyclovir is ineffective for treatment of reinfection; return to provider if HSV recurs.
6. Apply ointment as directed with a finger cot or rubber glove to prevent transmission of infection to other body sites.
7. Use condoms for sexual intercourse to prevent reinfections while undergoing treatment. Abstain during acute outbreaks (lesions present) and use condoms at all other times.
8. The total dose and dosage schedule differ depending on whether the infection is initial or chronic and whether intermittent therapy regimen is being used. Therefore, follow prescribed dosage, dosage combinations (i.e., with AZT) and duration of treatment.
9. Consume 2-3 L/day of fluids, especially during parenteral therapy, to prevent renal toxicity/crystalluria.
10. Females should have an annual Pap test; an increased risk of cervical cancer may be associated with genital herpes.
11. Do not exceed dosage and do not share meds.

Outcome/Evaluate

- Less severe and less frequent herpes outbreaks
- Crusting and healing of herpetic lesions

Adapalene

(ah-**DAP**-ah-leen)
Pregnancy Category: C
Differin **(Rx)**
Classification: Topical acne product

Action/Kinetics: Binds to specific retinoic acid receptors which may normalize the differentiation of follicular epithelial cells resulting in decreased microcomedone formation. Trace amounts absorbed through the skin.
Uses: Topical treatment of acne vulgaris.
Contraindications: Hypersensitivity to adapalene or any components of the vehicle gel. Use in sunburn until fully recovered.
Special Concerns: Use with caution in those who normally have high levels of sun exposure or in those sensitive to the sun. Use with caution with medicated or abrasive soaps and cleaners, with soaps and cosmetics that have a strong drying effect, and with products that have high concentrations of alcohol, stringents, spices, or lime. Also use particular caution with products containing sulfur, resorcinol, or salicylic acid. Use with caution during lactation. Safety and efficacy have not been determined in children less than 12 years of age.
Side Effects: *Dermatologic:* Erythema, scaling, dryness, pruritus, burning, pruritus or burning immediately after application, skin irritation, stinging sunburn, acne flares.
How Supplied: *Gel:* 0.1%; *Topical Solution:* 0.1%.

Dosage

- **Topical Gel**

Treatment of acne vulgaris.

Adults and children over 12 years of age: Apply a thin film once a day to affected areas after washing in the evening prior to going to bed.

HEALTH CARE CONSIDERATIONS

Administration/Storage

1. Avoid contact with eyes, lips, and mucous membranes.
2. During early weeks of therapy, acne may worsen due to action of the drug on previously unseen lesions—not a reason to discontinue therapy.
3. Beneficial effects should be seen after 8 to 12 weeks of treatment.
4. Store at controlled room temperatures of 20°C to 25°C (68°F to 77°F).

Assessment

1. Record indications for therapy, noting onset, duration, and location of acne lesions.
2. List other agents trialed and the outcome; note any family history with condition.
3. Determine skin type and any sensitivity reactions to soaps, sun, or other agents or conditions.
4. Describe clinical presentation; use photographs to document condition and extent of lesions.

Client/Family Teaching

1. Apply only as directed and avoid contact with cut, irritated, or sunburned skin. Avoid contact with eyes, lips, and mucous membranes.
2. Excessive application will cause increased peeling, discomfort, and redness.
3. Avoid prolonged sun exposure and weather extremes (i.e., wind, cold). Use sunscreen and protective clothing when exposed.
4. Condition may worsen before improving; don't be discouraged.
5. Expect itching, burning, scaling, and erythema during the first 2 to 4 weeks of therapy; these should lessen with continued use. If severe discomfort is experienced, reduce frequency of application or stop therapy and report.

Outcome/Evaluate: Clearing and healing of acne lesions in 8 to 12 weeks

Albendazole

(al-**BEN**-dah-zohl)

Pregnancy Category: C

Albenza **(Rx)**

Classification: Anthelmintic

Action/Kinetics: Acts by inhibiting tubular polymerization, resulting in the loss of cytoplasmic microtubules and inability of the cell to function. Poorly absorbed from the GI tract; enhance absorption by ingesting a meal containing at least 40 g of fat. Rapidly converted to albendazole sulfoxide, the active metabolite. **Peak plasma levels, sulfoxide:** 2-5 hr. **t½, terminal, of sulfoxide:** 8-12 hr. Further metabolized to other metabolites with excretion through the bile, accounting for a portion of elimination.

Uses: Treatment of parenchymal neurocysticercosis due to *Taenia solium*. Treatment of cystic hydatid disease of the liver, lung, and peritoneum caused by the larval form of the dog tapeworm, *Echinococcus granulosus*.

Contraindications: Hypersensitivity to benzimidazole compounds.

Special Concerns: Use with caution during lactation. Clients should not become pregnant for at least 1 month following termination of albendazole therapy.

Side Effects: *GI:* N&V, abdominal pain. *CNS:* Headache, dizziness, vertigo, increased ICP, meningeal signs. *Hematologic:* Leukopenia, granulocytopenia, pancytopenia, agranulocytosis, thrombocytopenia (rare). *Dermatologic:* Reversible alopecia, rash, urticaria. *Miscellaneous:* Fever, allergic reactions, acute renal failure.

Drug Interactions

Cimetidine / ↑ Levels of albendazole sulfoxide in bile and cystic fluid in hydatid cyst clients

Dexamethasone / Possible ↑ plasma levels of albendazole sulfoxide

Praziquantel / ↑ Plasma levels of albendazole sulfoxide

How Supplied: *Tablet:* 200 mg

Dosage

- **Tablets**

Hydatid disease.

Those weighing 60 kg or more: 400 mg b.i.d. with meals for a 28-day cycle followed by a 14-day albendazole-free interval, for a total of three cycles. **Those weighing less than 60 kg:** 15 mg/kg/day given in divided doses b.i.d. with meals, up to a maximum of 800 mg/day, using the same duration as for those weighing 60 kg or more.

Neurocysticercosis.

Those weighing 60 kg or more: 400 mg b.i.d. with meals for 8 to 30 days. **Those weighing less than 60 kg:** 15 mg/kg/day given in divided doses b.i.d. with meals, up to a maximum dose of 800 mg/day, for 8 to 30 days.

HEALTH CARE CONSIDERATIONS

Administration/Storage: Clients being treated for neurocysticercosis should receive corticosteroid and anticonvulsant therapy as needed. Consider PO or IV steroids for the first week of treatment to prevent cerebral hypertensive episodes.

Assessment

1. Record indications for therapy as length of therapy is based on condition requiring treatment.
2. Obtain negative pregnancy test, baseline cultures, and neurologic assessment.
3. Determine baseline CBC and check every 2 weeks during each 28-day cycle.
4. Obtain LFTs and monitor for significant enzyme elevations which may necessitate interruption of drug therapy until return to baseline.
5. Assess for retinal lesions with cysticercosis. The need for anticysticeral therapy should be weighed against the possibility of retinal damage due to albendazole-induced changes to the retinal lesion.

Interventions

1. Anticipate coadministration of PO or IV corticosteroids during the first week of therapy to prevent cerebral hypertensive episodes.
2. Monitor neurologic status carefully. Administer steroids and anticonvulsants with neurocysticerosis.

Client/Family Teaching

1. Review the prescribed dosage, frequency, and cycle or length of therapy required.
2. Take as directed with food.
3. Use reliable birth control during and for 4-6 weeks following completion of drug therapy; drug may cause fetal harm.
4. Avoid crowds and persons with contagious diseases; report any S&S of infection.

Outcome/Evaluate: Symptomatic improvement with resolution of infective organisms

---

Albuterol (Salbutamol)

(al-**BYOU**-ter-ohl)

Pregnancy Category: C

Alti-Salbutamol Sulfate ✦, Asmavent ✦, Dom-Salbutamol ✦, Gen-Salbutamol Sterinebs P.F. ✦, Med-Salbutamol ✦, Novo-Salmol Inhaler ✦, PMS-Salbutamol Respirator Solution ✦, Proventil, Proventil HFA—3M, Proventil Repetabs, Rho-Salbutamol ✦, Salbu-2 and -4 ✦, Salbutamol Nebuamp ✦, Salmol ✦, Ventodisk Disk/Diskhaler ✦, Ventolin, Ventolin Rotacaps, Volmax **(Rx)**

Classification: Direct-acting adrenergic (sympathomimetic) agent

---

See also *Sympathomimetic Drugs*.

Action/Kinetics: Stimulates beta-2 receptors of the bronchi, leading to bronchodilation. Causes less tachycardia and is longer-acting than isoproterenol. Has minimal beta-1 activity. Available as an inhaler that contains no chlorofluorocarbons (Proventil HFA-3M). **Onset, PO:** 15-30 min; **inhalation,** 5-15 min. **Peak effect, PO:** 2-3 hr; **inhalation,** 60-90 min (after 2 inhalations). **Duration, PO:** 8 hr (up to 12 hr for extended-release); **inhalation,** 3-6 hr. Metabolites and unchanged drug excreted in urine and feces. Do not use tablets in children less than 12 years of age.

Uses: Bronchial asthma; bronchospasm due to bronchitis or emphysema; bronchitis; reversible obstructive pulmonary disease in those 4 years of age and older; exercise-induced bronchospasm. Prophylaxis of bronchial asthma or bronchospasms. Parenteral for treatment of status asthmaticus. *Investigational:* Nebulized albuterol may be useful as an adjunct to treat serious acute hyperkalemia in hemodialysis clients.

Contraindications: Aerosol for prevention of exercise-induced bronchospasm is not recommended for children less than 12 years of age. Use during lactation.

Special Concerns: Dosage has not been established for the syrup in children less than 2 years of age, for tablets in children less than 6 years of age, and for extended-release tablets in children less than 12 years of age. Albuterol may delay preterm labor.

Additional Side Effects: *GI:* Diarrhea, dry mouth, increased appetite, epigastric pain. *CNS:* CNS stimulation, malaise, emotional lability, fatigue, lightheadedness, nightmares, disturbed sleep, aggressive behavior, irritability. *Respiratory:* Bronchitis, epistaxis, hoarseness (especially in children), nasal congestion, increase in sputum. *Hypersensitivity (may be immediate):* Urticaria, ***angioedema,*** rash, ***bronchospasm.*** *Miscellaneous:* Muscle cramps, pallor, teeth discoloration, conjunctivitis, dilated pupils, difficulty in urination, muscle spasm, voice changes, oropharyngeal edema.

OD Management of Overdose: *Symptoms:* Seizures, anginal pain, hypertension, hypokalemia, tachycardia (rate may increase to 200 beats/min).

See *Sympathomimetic Drugs*.

How Supplied: *Metered dose inhaler:* 0.09 mg/inh; *Capsule:* 200 mcg; *Solution:* 0.083%, 0.5%; *Syrup:* 2 mg/5 mL; *Tablet:* 2 mg, 4 mg; *Tablet, Extended Release:* 4 mg, 8 mg

Dosage

- **Metered Dose Inhaler**

  Bronchodilation.

Adults and children over 12 years of age: 180 mcg (2 inhalations) q 4-6 hr (Ventolin aerosol may be used in children over 4 years of age). In some clients 1 inhalation (90 mcg) q 4 hr may be sufficient.

Prophylaxis of exercise-induced bronchospasm.

Adults and children over 12 years of age: 180 mcg (2 inhalations) 15 min before exercise.

• **Solution for Inhalation**

Bronchodilation.

Adults and children over 12 years of age: 2.5 mg t.i.d.-q.i.d. by nebulization (dilute 0.5 mL of the 0.5% solution with 2.5 mL sterile NSS and deliver over 5-15 min).

• **Capsule for Inhalation**

Bronchodilation.

Adults and children over 4 years of age: 200 mcg q 4-6 hr using a Rotahaler inhalation device. In some clients, 400 mcg q 4-6 hr may be required.

Prophylaxis of exercise-induced bronchospasm.

Adults and children over 12 years: 200 mcg 15 min before exercise using a Rotahaler inhalation device.

• **Syrup**

Bronchodilation.

Adults and children over 14 years of age: 2-4 mg t.i.d.-q.i.d., up to a maximum of 8 mg q.i.d. **Children, 6-14 years, initial:** 2 mg (base) t.i.d.-q.i.d.; **then,** increase as necessary to a maximum of 24 mg/day in divided doses. **Children, 2-6 years, initial:** 0.1 mg/kg t.i.d.; **then,** increase as necessary up to 0.2 mg/kg, not to exceed 4 mg t.i.d.

• **Tablets**

Bronchodilation.

Adults and children over 12 years of age, initial: 2-4 mg (of the base) t.i.d.-q.i.d.; **then,** increase dose as needed up to a maximum of 8 mg t.i.d.-q.i.d. In geriatric clients or those sensitive to beta agonists, start with 2 mg t.i.d.-q.i.d. and then increase dose gradually, if needed, to a maximum of 8 mg t.i.d.-q.i.d. **Children, 6-12 years of age, usual, initial:** 2 mg t.i.d.-q.i.d.; **then,** if necessary, increase the dose in a stepwise fashion to a maximum of 24 mg/day in divided doses.

• **Extended-Release Tablets**

Bronchodilation.

Adults and children over 12 years of age: 4 or 8 mg (of the base) q 12 hr up to a maximum of 32 mg/day. Clients on regular-release albuterol can be switched to the Repetabs in that a 4-mg extended-release tablet q 12 hr is equivalent to a regular 2-mg tablet q 6 hr.

HEALTH CARE CONSIDERATIONS

See also *Health Care Considerations* for *Sympathomimetic Drugs.*

Administration/Storage

1. When given by nebulization, either a face mask or mouthpiece may be used. Use compressed air or oxygen with a gas flow of 6-10 L/min; a single treatment lasts from 5 to 15 min.
2. When given by IPPB, the inspiratory pressure should be from 10 to 20 cm water, with the duration of treatment ranging from 5 to 20 min depending on the client and instrument control.
3. The MDI may also be administered on a mechanical ventilator through an adapter.
4. Take extended-release tablets whole with the aid of liquids; do not chew or crush. The outer coating of Volmax Extended-Release Tablets is not absorbed and is excreted in the feces; empty outer coating may be seen in the stool.
5. The contents of the MDI container are under pressure. Do not store near heat or open flames and do not puncture the container.

Assessment

1. Obtain medical history and assess CNS status.
2. Record PFTs, CXR, and lung sounds. Note anxiety; may contribute to air hunger.
3. Record symptom characteristics, onset, duration, frequency, and any precipitating factors.
4. Determine if able to self-administer medication.

Interventions

1. Maintain a calm, reassuring approach. Do not leave unattended if acutely short of breath.
2. Instruct how to inhale through nose and exhale with pursed lips or diaphragmatic breathing in order to prolong expiration and keep the airways open longer, thus reducing the work of breathing.
3. Monitor pulmonary status (i.e., breath sounds, VS, peak flow, or ABGs) for effects of the therapy.
4. Observe for evidence of allergic responses.

Client/Family Teaching

1. Take only as directed; do not exceed prescribed dose.
2. Do not put lips around inhaler; go two fingerbreadths away before attempting to activate and inhale. Attend instruction on the correct method for administration.

A

3. When using albuterol inhalers, do not use other inhalation medication unless specifically prescribed.
4. A spacer used with the MDI may enhance drug dispersion. Always thoroughly rinse mouth and equipment with water following each use to prevent oral fungal infections.
5. Establish dosing regimens that fit lifestyle, i.e., 1-2 puffs q 6 hr or 4 puffs 4 times/day; the usual dosing is q 4-6 hr with an as-needed order. Check peak flows, call if requiring more puffs more frequently than prescribed or if dose of drug used previously does not provide relief.

Outcome/Evaluate: Improved breathing patterns/airway exchange. Improved peak expiratory flow (PEF) readings.

Alendronate sodium

(ay-**LEN**-droh-nayt)
Pregnancy Category: C
Fosamax **(Rx)**
Classification: Bone growth regulator (biphosphonate)

Action/Kinetics: Binds to bone hydroxyapatite and inhibits osteoclast activity, thereby preventing bone resorption. Appears to reduce fracture risk and reverse the progression of osteoporosis. Does not inhibit bone mineralization. Well absorbed orally and initially distributed to soft tissues, but then quickly redistributed to bone. Not metabolized; excreted through the urine. **t½, terminal** believed to be more than 10 years, due to slow release from the skeleton.

Uses: Prevention and treatment of osteoporosis in postmenopausal women. Paget's disease of bone in those with alkaline phosphatase at least two times the upper limit of normal or for those who are symptomatic or at risk for future complications from the disease.

Contraindications: In hypocalcemia. Severe renal insufficiency (C_{CR} less than 35 mL/min). Use of hormone replacement therapy with alendronate for osteoporosis in postmenopausal women. Lactation.

Special Concerns: Use with caution in those with upper GI problems, such as dysphagia, symptomatic esophageal diseases, gastritis, duodenitis, or ulcers. Safety and effectiveness have not been determined in children or for use in male osteoporosis.

Side Effects: *GI:* Flatulence, acid regurgitation, esophageal ulcer, dysphagia, abdominal distention, gastritis, abdominal pain, constipation, diarrhea, dyspepsia, N&V. *Miscellaneous:* Musculoskeletal pain, pain, headache, taste perversion, rash and erythema (rare), back pain, glaucoma, accidental injury, edema, flu-like symptoms.

Laboratory Test Considerations: ↓ Serum calcium and phosphate.

OD Management of Overdose: *Symptoms:* Hypocalcemia, hypophosphatemia, upset stomach, heartburn, esophagitis, gastritis, ulcer. *Treatment:* Administration of milk or antacids to bind the drug should be considered.

Drug Interactions
Antacids / ↓ Absorption of alendronate
Aspirin / ↑ Risk of upper GI side effects
Calcium supplements / ↓ Absorption of alendronate
Ranitidine / ↑ Bioavailability of alendronate (significance not known)

How Supplied: *Tablet:* 5 mg, 10 mg, 40 mg

Dosage

• **Tablets**

Prevention of osteoporosis in postmenopausal women.

5 mg once a day in the morning ½ hr before the first food, beverage, or medication of the day with 6-8 oz of plain water.

Treatment of osteoporosis or prevention of fractures in postmenopausal women with osteoporosis.

10 mg once a day in the morning ½ hr before the first food, beverage, or medication of the day with 6-8 oz of plain water. Safety of treatment for more than 4 years has not been determined.

Paget's disease of bone.

40 mg once a day for 6 months taken as for osteoporosis.

HEALTH CARE CONSIDERATIONS

Administration/Storage

1. To improve delivery to the stomach and reduce the potential for irritation of the esophagus, do not lie down for at least 30 min following administration.
2. Due to possible interference with absorption, at least 30 min should elapse before taking antacids or calcium supplements.
3. Retreatment for Paget's disease may be considered following a 6-month posttreatment evaluation in clients who have relapsed, based on increases in serum alkaline phosphatase. Retreatment may also be appropriate for those who failed to normalize their serum alkaline phosphatase.

Assessment

1. Record indications for therapy: osteoporosis prevention or treatment in postmenopausal women or Paget's disease. Note symptoms, age at onset, and physical changes.

2. Obtain baseline calcium, liver and renal function studies and correct any calcium or vitamin D deficiencies.
3. Note any history of upper GI problems such as gastritis, dysphagia, duodenitis, or ulcers.
4. All bone mineral density studies and/or skeletal X rays reports should be placed in the patient's chart and results noted in progress notes.
5. Assess for fractures and manage appropriately to prevent further injury and loss of function.
6. With Paget's disease, document baseline alkaline phosphatase and monitor periodically during therapy.

Client/Family Teaching

1. Osteoporosis occurs usually after age 40 and is a systemic skeletal disease characterized by low bone mass due to a higher amount of bone resorbed than formed.
2. Take only as prescribed. Benefit will be seen only when each tablet is taken with plain water the first thing in the morning at least 30 min before the first food, beverage, or medication of the day. Waiting > 30 min will improve absorption. Taking with juice or coffee will markedly reduce absorption.
3. Do not lie down after taking drug; wait at least 30 min.
4. Take calcium (500 mg) and vitamin D daily, especially if dietary intake or sun exposure is inadequate.

Outcome/Evaluate

- Prevention of osteoporosis and bone resorption (↓ bone turnover)
- Inhibition of kyphosis and pain due to bone fracture or deformity
- ↓ Pain; ↓ Serum alkaline phosphatase levels with Paget's disease

Allopurinol

(al-oh-**PYOUR**-ih-nohl)

Pregnancy Category: C

Alloprin ✱, Apo-Allopurinol ✱, Novo-Purol ✱, Purinol ✱, Zyloprim **(Rx)**

Classification: Antigout agent

Action/Kinetics: Allopurinol and its major metabolite, oxipurinol, are potent inhibitors of xanthine oxidase, an enzyme involved in the synthesis of uric acid, without disrupting the biosynthesis of essential purine. This results in decreased levels of uric acid. The drug also increases reutilization of xanthine and hypoxanthine for synthesis of nucleotide and nucleic acid synthesis by acting on the enzyme hypoxanthine-guanine phosphoribosyltransferase. The resultant increases in nucleotides cause a negative feedback to inhibit synthesis of purines and a decrease in uric acid levels. **Peak plasma levels:** 1.5 hr for allopurinol and 4.5 hr for oxipurinol. **Onset:** 2-3 days. **t½** (allopurinol); 1-3 hr; **t½** (oxipurinol): 12-30 hr. **Peak serum levels, allopurinol:** 2-3 mcg/mL; **oxipurinol:** 5-6.5 mcg/mL (up to 50 mcg/mL in clients with impaired renal function). **Maximum therapeutic effect:** 1-3 weeks. Well absorbed from GI tract, metabolized in liver, excreted in urine and feces (20%).

Uses: Primary or secondary gout (acute attacks, tophi, joint destruction, nephropathy, uric acid lithiasis). Clients with leukemia, lymphoma, or other malignancies in whom drug therapy causes elevations of serum and urinary uric acid. Recurrent calcium oxalate calculi where daily uric acid excretion exceed 800 mg/day in males and 750 mg/day in females. *Investigational:* Mixed with methylcellulose as a mouthwash to prevent stomatitis following fluorouracil administration. Reduce the granulocyte suppressant effect of fluorouracil. Prevent ischemic reperfusion tissue damage. Reduce the incidence of perioperative mortality and postoperative arrhythmias in coronary artery bypass surgery. Reduce the rates of *Helicobacter pylori*-induced duodenal ulcers and treatment of hematemesis from NSAID-induced erosive esophagitis. Alleviate pain due to acute pancreatitis. Treatment of American cutaneous leishmaniasis and against *Trypanosoma cruzi*. Treat Chagas' disease. As an alternative in epileptic seizures refractory to standard therapy.

Contraindications: Hypersensitivity to drug. Clients with idiopathic hemochromatosis or relatives of clients suffering from this condition. Children except as an adjunct in treatment of neoplastic disease. Severe skin reactions on previous exposure. To treat asymptomatic hyperuricemia.

Special Concerns: Use with caution during lactation and in clients with liver or renal disease. In children use has been limited to rare inborn errors of purine metabolism or hyperuricemia as a result of malignancy or cancer therapy.

Side Effects: *Dermatologic* (most frequent): Pruritic maculopapular skin rash (may be accompanied by fever and malaise). Vesicular bullous dermatitis, eczematoid dermatitis, pruritus, urticaria, onycholysis, purpura, lichen planus, ***Stevens-Johnson syndrome, toxic epidermal necrolysis.*** Skin rash has been accompanied by hypertension and cataract development. *Allergy:* Fever, chills, leukopenia, eosinophilia, arthralgia, skin rash, pruritus, N&V, nephritis. *GI:* N&V, diarrhea, gastritis, dyspepsia, abdominal pain (intermittent). *Hematologic:* Leukopenia, eosinophilia, thrombocytopenia, leukocytosis. *Hepatic:* Hepatomegaly, cholestatic jaundice, ***hepatic necrosis,*** granulomatous hepatitis. *Neurologic:* Headache, peripheral neuropathy, paresthesia, somnolence, neuritis. *CV:* Necrotizing angiitis, hypersensitivity vasculitis. *Miscellaneous:* Ecchymosis, epistaxis, taste loss, arthralgia, acute attacks of gout, fever, myopathy, renal failure, uremia, alopecia.

Laboratory Test Considerations: ↑ ALT, AST, alkaline phosphatase. ↑ Serum cholesterol. ↓ Serum glucose levels.

Drug Interactions

ACE inhibitors / ↑ Risk of hypersensitivity reactions
Aluminum salts / ↓ Effect of allopurinol
Ampicillin / ↑ Risk of ampicillin-induced skin rashes
Anticoagulants, oral / ↑ Effect of anticoagulant due to ↓ breakdown by liver
Azathioprine / ↑ Effect of azathioprine due to ↓ breakdown by liver
Cyclophosphamide / ↑ Risk of bleeding or infection due to ↑ myelosuppressive effects of cyclophosphamide
Iron preparations / Allopurinol ↑ hepatic iron concentrations
Mercaptopurine / ↑ Effect of mercaptopurine due to ↓ breakdown by liver
Theophylline / Allopurinol ↑ plasma theophylline levels → possible toxicity
Thiazide diuretics / ↑ Risk of hypersensitivity reactions to allopurinol
Uricosuric agents / ↓ Effect of oxipurinol due to ↑ rate of excretion

How Supplied: *Tablet:* 100 mg, 300 mg

Dosage

• **Tablets**

Gout/hyperuricemia.

Adults: 200-600 mg/day, depending on severity (minimum effective dose: 100-200 mg/day). Maximum daily dose should not exceed 800 mg.

Prevention of uric acid nephropathy during treatment of neoplasms.

Adults: 600-800 mg/day for 2-3 days (with high fluid intake).

Prophylaxis of acute gout.

Initial: 100 mg/day; increase by 100 mg at weekly intervals until serum uric acid level of 6 mg/100 mL or less is reached.

Hyperuricemia associated with malignancy.

Pediatric, 6-10 years of age: 300 mg/day either as a single dose or 100 mg t.i.d.; **under 6 years of age:** 150 mg/day in three divided doses.

Recurrent calcium oxalate calculi.

200-300 mg/day in one or more doses (dose may be adjusted according to urinary levels of uric acid).

To ameliorate granulocyte suppressant effect of fluorouracil.

600 mg/day.

Reduce perioperative mortality and postoperative arrhythmias in coronary artery bypass surgery.

300 mg 12 hr and 1 hr before surgery.

Reduce relapse rates of H. pylori*-induced duodenal ulcers; treat hematemesis from NSAID-induced erosive gastritis.*

50 mg q.i.d.

Alleviate pain due to acute pancreatitis.

50 mg q.i.d.

Treat American cutaneous leishmaniasis and T. cruzi.

20 mg/kg for 15 days.

Treat Chagas' disease.

600-900 mg/day for 60 days.

Alternative to treat epileptic seizures refractory to standard therapy.

300 mg/day, except use 150 mg/day in those less than 20 kg.

• **Mouthwash**

Prevent fluorouracil-induced stomatitis.

20 mg in 3% methylcellulose (1 mg/mL).

HEALTH CARE CONSIDERATIONS

Administration/Storage

1. Keep urine slightly alkaline to prevent formation of uric acid stones.
2. Transfer from colchicine, uricosuric agents, and/or anti-inflammatory agents to allopurinol should be made gradually by decreasing the dosage of one and increasing the dosage of allopurinol until a normal serum uric acid level is achieved.
3. Reduce the dose as follows in impaired renal function: creatinine clearance (C_{CR}) less than 10 mL/min: 100 mg 3 times a week; C_{CR}, 10 mL/min: 100 mg every other day; C_{CR} 20 mL/min: 100 mg/day; C_{CR}, 40 mL/min: 150 mg/day; C_{CR}, 60 mL/min: 200 mg/day.

Assessment

1. Take a complete drug history, noting any that may interact unfavorably.
2. Record indications for therapy, type and onset of symptoms and any previous allopurinol use. Note location, severity, and frequency of attacks and joint deformity.
3. If female and of childbearing age, or if nursing, allopurinol is contraindicated.
4. Determine any history of idiopathic hemochromatosis.
5. Monitor CBC, uric acid, liver and renal function studies. Reduce dose with renal dysfunction.

Client/Family Teaching
1. Take with food or immediately after meals to lessen gastric irritation. Consume at least 10-12 8-oz glasses of fluid/day to prevent stone formation.
2. Monitor weight if experiencing N&V or other signs of gastric irritation. Report persistent weight loss.
3. Skin rashes may start after months of therapy. If drug related, must discontinue drug.
4. Do not take iron salts as high iron concentrations may occur in the liver.
5. Avoid excessive intake of vitamin C; may lead to formation of kidney stones.
6. Avoid caffeine and alcoholic beverages; decreases allopurinol effect.
7. Avoid foods high in purine; these may include sardines, roe, salmon, scallops, anchovies, organ meats, and mincemeat.
8. Minimize exposure to UV light due to increased risk of cataracts. Report vision changes.

Outcome/Evaluate
- ↓ Uric acid levels (6 mg/dL)
- ↓ Joint pain and inflammation
- ↓ Frequency of gout attacks
- Inhibition of stomatitis following fluorouracil therapy

Alprazolam
(al-PRAYZ-oh-lam)
Pregnancy Category: D
Alti-Alprazolam ✱, Apo-Alpraz ✱, Gen-Alprazolam ✱, Novo-Alprazol ✱, Nu-Alpraz ✱, Xanax, Xanax TS ✱ **(C-IV) (Rx)**
Classification: Antianxiety agent

See also *Tranquilizers/Antimanic Drugs/Hypnotics.*
Action/Kinetics: Peak plasma levels: PO, 8-37 ng/mL after 1-2 hr. **t½:** 12-15 hr. 80% plasma protein bound. Metabolized to alpha-hydroxyalprazolam, an active metabolite. **t½:** 12-15 hr. Excreted in urine.
Uses: Anxiety. Anxiety associated with depression with or without agoraphobia. *Investigational:* Agoraphobia with social phobia, depression, PMS.
Contraindications: Use with itraconazole or ketoconazole.
How Supplied: *Tablet:* 0.25 mg, 0.5 mg, 1 mg, 2 mg

Dosage
- **Tablets**

Anxiety disorder.
Adults, initial: 0.25-0.5 mg t.i.d.; **then,** titrate to needs of client, with total daily dosage not to exceed 4 mg. **In elderly or debilitated: initial;** 0.25 mg b.i.d.-t.i.d.; **then,** adjust dosage to needs of client.

Antipanic agent.
Adults: 0.5 mg t.i.d.; increase dose as needed up to a maximum of 10 mg/day.

Agoraphobia with social phobia.
Adults: 2-8 mg/day.

PMS.
0.25 mg t.i.d.

HEALTH CARE CONSIDERATIONS

See also *Health Care Considerations* for *Tranquilizers/Antimanic Drugs/Hypnotics.*

Administration/Storage
1. Do not decrease the daily dose more than 0.5 mg over 3 days if therapy is terminated or the dose decreased.
2. Reduce dosage in elderly and debilitated clients.

Assessment
1. Take a thorough history of the presenting complaints to determine if the patient is a candidate for this particular drug. IBS is a diagnosis of exclusion and may present with either constipation or diarrhea as the major symptom. Persons who have diarrhea as their predominating symptom may be treated with alosetron but those experiencing constipation as their primary symptom are **not** candiates for starting this medication.
2. Just as important is to obtain a thorough past medication history to determine that the patient does not have a history of constipation and/or other intestinal disease for which alosetron is contraindicated.

Client/Family Teaching
1. May take with milk or food to decrease GI upset.
2. Include extra fluids and bulk in the diet to minimize constipation.
3. Use support devices as needed, especially at night; elderly tend to become confused. Store drug away from bedside.

Outcome/Evaluate
- Positive behaviors with phobias
- ↓ Anxiety/restlessness; Control of panic disorder
- Improvement in PMS symptoms

Altretamine (Hexylmethylmelamine)
(all-TRET-ah-meen)
Pregnancy Category: D
Hexalen **(Rx)**
Classification: Antineoplastic, miscellaneous

A

See also *Antineoplastic Agents.*
Action/Kinetics: The mechanism of action is unknown, although metabolism of the drug is required for cytotoxicity. Well absorbed following PO ingestion; undergoes rapid demethylation in the liver, yielding the principal metabolites-pentamethylmelamine and tetramethylmelamine. **Peak plasma levels:** 0.5-3 hr. **t½:** 4.7-10.2 hr. Metabolites are excreted mainly through the kidney.
Uses: Used alone in the palliative treatment of persistent or recur-rent ovarian cancer after first-line cisplatin- or alkylating agent-based combination therapy.
Contraindications: Preexisting bone marrow depression or severe neurologic toxicity, although the drug has been used safely in clients with preexisting cisplatin neuropathies. Lactation.
Special Concerns: Safety and effectiveness have not been determined in children. High daily doses may result in gradual onset of N&V.
Side Effects: *GI:* N&V (most common). *Neurologic:* Peripheral sensory neuropathy, fatigue, anorexia, seizures. *CNS:* Mood disorders, disorders of consciousness, ataxia, dizziness, vertigo. *Hematologic:* Leukopenia, thrombocytopenia, anemia. *Miscellaneous:* ***Hepatic toxicity,*** skin rash, pruritus, alopecia.
Laboratory Test Considerations: ↑ Serum creatinine, BUN, alkaline phosphatase.
Drug Interactions: Use with MAO inhibitors may cause severe orthostatic hypotension, especially in clients over the age of 60 years.
How Supplied: *Capsule:* 50 mg

Dosage

- **Capsules**

Ovarian cancer.

260 mg/m²/day given either for 14 or 21 consecutive days in a 28-day cycle. The total daily dose is given as four divided doses PO after meals and at bedtime.

HEALTH CARE CONSIDERATIONS

See also *Health Care Considerations* for *Antineoplastic Agents.*

Assessment

1. Record onset of symptoms and note all previous therapies.
2. Note baseline neurologic findings.
3. Obtain baseline hematologic and liver function studies.

Interventions

1. Anticipate neurotoxicity as a side effect of drug therapy. Assess neuro status prior to starting therapy and before each subsequent course.
2. Give pyridoxine with altretamine to reduce the severity of the neurotoxic effects.
3. Monitor peripheral blood counts monthly, prior to the initiation of each course of therapy and as clinically indicated.

Client/Family Teaching

1. Report any adverse symptoms, such as tingling, decreased sensation, dizziness, and N&V. Dose may need to be decreased or therapy discontinued.
2. Practice barrier contraception; may cause fetal damage.
3. Report for monthly hematologic studies.

Outcome/Evaluate: Control of tumor growth and spread

Amantadine hydrochloride

(ah-**MAN**-tah-deen)
Pregnancy Category: C
Endantadine ✤, Gen-Amantadine ✤, PMS-Amantadine ✤, Symadine, Symmetrel **(Rx)**
Classification: Antiviral and antiparkinson agent

See also *Antiviral Drugs.*
Action/Kinetics: Amantadine is believed to prevent penetration of the virus into cells, possibly by inhibiting uncoating of the RNA virus. The reaction appears to be virus specific for influenza A but not host specific. It may also prevent the release of infectious viral nucleic acid into the host cell. The drug reduces symptoms of viral infections if given within 24-48 hr after onset of illness. For the treatment of parkinsonism, amantadine may increase the release of dopamine from dopaminergic nerve terminals in the substantia nigra of parkinson clients, resulting in an increase in dopamine levels in dopaminergic synapses. The drug decreases extrapyramidal symptoms, including akinesia, rigidity, tremors, excessive salivation, gait disturbances, and total functional disability. Well absorbed from GI tract. **Onset:** 48 hr. **Peak serum concentration:** 0.2 mcg/mL after 1-4 hr. **t½:** Approximately 15 hr; elimination half-life increases two- to threefold when C_{CR} is less than 40 mL/min/1.73 m². Ninety percent excreted unchanged in urine.
Uses: Influenza A viral infections of the respiratory tract (prophylaxis and treatment of high-risk clients with immunodeficiency, CV, metabolic, neuromuscular, or pulmonary disease). Symptomatic treatment of idiopathic parkinsonism and parkinsonism syndrome resulting from encephalitis, carbon monoxide intoxication, drugs, or cerebral arteriosclerosis. Favorable results have been obtained in about 50% of the clients. Improvements can last for up to 30 months, al-

though some clients report that the effect of the drug wears off in 1-3 months. A rest period or an increased dosage may reestablish effectiveness. For parkinsonism, amantadine hydrochloride is usually used concomitantly with other agents, such as levodopa and anticholinergic agents.

Amantadine is recommended for prophylaxis in the following situations:

- Short-term prophylaxis during the course of a presumed outbreak of influenza A
- Adjunct to late immunization in high-risk clients
- To reduce disruption of medical care and to decrease spread of virus in high-risk clients when influenza A virus outbreaks occur
- To supplement vaccination protection in clients with impaired immune responses
- As chemoprophylaxis during flu season for those high-risk clients for whom influenza vaccine is contraindicated due to anaphylactic response to egg protein or prior severe reactions associated with flu vaccination

Contraindications: Hypersensitivity to drug.

Special Concerns: Use with caution in clients with liver and renal disease, history of epilepsy, CHF, peripheral edema, orthostatic hypotension, recurrent eczematoid dermatitis, or severe psychosis, in clients taking CNS stimulant drugs, to those exposed to rubella, and to nursing mothers. Safe use in lactating mothers and in children less than 1 year has not been established.

Side Effects: *GI:* N&V, constipation, anorexia, xerostomia. *CNS:* Depression, psychosis, ***convulsions,*** hallucinations, lightheadedness, confusion, ataxia, irritability, anxiety, headache, dizziness, fatigue, insomnia. *CV:* ***CHF,*** orthostatic hypotension, peripheral edema. *Miscellaneous:* Urinary retention, leukopenia, neutropenia, mottling of skin of the extremities due to poor peripheral circulation (livedo reticularis), skin rashes, visual problems, slurred speech, oculogyric episodes, dyspnea, weakness, eczematoid dermatitis.

OD **Management of Overdose:** *Symptoms:* Anorexia, N&V, CNS effects. *Treatment:* Gastric lavage or induction of emesis followed by supportive measures. Ensure that client is well hydrated; give IV fluids if necessary. To treat CNS toxicity: IV physostigmine, 1-2 mg given q 1-2 hr in adults or 0.5 mg at 5-10-min intervals (maximum of 2 mg/hr) in children. Sedatives and anticonvulsants may be given if needed; antiarrhythmics and vasopressors may also be required.

Drug Interactions

Anticholinergics / Additive anticholinergic effects (including hallucinations, confusion), especially with trihexyphenidyl and benztropine

CNS stimulants / May ↑ CNS and psychic effects of amantadine; use cautiously together

Hydrochlorothiazide/triamterene combination / ↓ Urinary excretion of amantadine → ↑ plasma levels

Levodopa / Potentiated by amantadine

How Supplied: *Capsule:* 100 mg; *Syrup:* 50 mg/5 mL; *Tablet:* 100 mg

Dosage

- **Capsules, Syrup, Tablets**

Antiviral.

Adults: 200 mg/day as a single or divided dose. **Children, 1-9 years:** 4.4-8.8 mg/kg/day up to a maximum of 150 mg/day in one or two divided doses (use syrup); **9-12 years:** 100 mg b.i.d.

Prophylactic treatment.

Institute before or immediately after exposure and continue for 10-21 days if used concurrently with vaccine or for 90 days without vaccine.

Symptomatic management.

Initiate as soon as possible and continue for 24-48 hr after disappearance of symptoms. Decrease dose in renal impairment (see package insert). Reduce dose to 100 mg/day for persons with active seizure disorders due to the increased risk of seizure frequency using daily doses of 200 mg.

Parkinsonism.

Use as sole agent, usual: 100 mg b.i.d., up to 400 mg/day in divided doses, if necesssary. **Use with other antiparkinson drugs:** 100 mg 1-2 times/day.

Drug-induced extrapyramidal symptoms.

100 mg b.i.d. (up to 300 mg/day may be required in some). Reduce dose in impaired renal function.

HEALTH CARE CONSIDERATIONS

See also *General Health Care Considerations for All Anti-Infectives* and *Antiviral Drugs.*

Administration/Storage

1. Protect capsules from moisture.
2. Initiate therapy for viral illness as soon as possible after symptoms begin and for 24-48 hr after symptoms disappear.

Assessment

1. Obtain medical history and note any evidence of seizures, CHF, and renal insufficiency.

2. With active seizure disorder reduce drug dosage to prevent breakthrough seizures. With an increase in seizure activity, take appropriate precautions and ensure that dosage is reduced to 100 mg/day to prevent loss of seizure control.
3. Monitor I&O; observe clients with renal impairment for crystalluria, oliguria, and increased BUN or creatinine levels.
4. With Parkinson's disease, following loss of drug effectiveness, benefits may be regained by increasing the dosage or discontinuing the drug for several weeks and then reinstituting it.

Client/Family Teaching

1. Administer last daily dose several hours before retiring to prevent insomnia.
2. Do not drive a car or work in a situation where alertness is important until drug effects are realized; can affect vision, concentration, and coordination.
3. Rise slowly from a prone position because orthostatic hypotension may occur. Lie down if dizzy or weak to relieve these symptoms.
4. Report diffuse patchy discoloration or mottling of the skin. Discoloration lessens when legs are elevated and usually fades completely within weeks after discontinuing drug.
5. Report any exposure to rubella; drug may increase susceptibility to disease.
6. Susceptible individuals (elderly, immunocompromised) should avoid crowds during "flu" season and receive annual flu shot and pneumonia vaccine.
7. Psychologic changes such as confusion, mental status changes, nervousness, or depression should be reported as well as any persistent, or new symptoms.
8. Avoid alcohol or any other unprescribed OTC products.
9. Clients with parkinsonism should not stop drug abruptly.
10. Clients with seizure disorders should be advised to report any early signs or symptoms of seizure activity as dosage may require adjustment.

Outcome/Evaluate

- ↓ Drug-induced extrapyramidal S&S
- Improved motor control; ↓ tremor
- Influenza A prophylaxis; ↓ spread of infection to high-risk individuals during outbreaks

COMBINATION DRUG

Amiloride and Hydrochlorothiazide

(ah-**MILL**-oh-ryd, hy-droh-klor-oh-**THIGH**-ah-zyd)

Pregnancy Category: C

Alti-Amiloride HCTZ ✱, Ami-Hydro ✱, Apo-Amilzide, Moduret ✱, Moduretic, Novamilor ✱, Nu-Amilzide ✱ **(Rx)**

Classification: Antihypertensive

See also *Amiloride* and *Hydrochlorothiazide*.

Content: *Diuretic, potassium-sparing:* Amiloride HCl, 5 mg. *Antihypertensive/diuretic:* Hydrochlorothiazide, 50 mg.

Uses: Hypertension or CHF, especially when hypokalemia occurs. Used alone or with other antihypertensive drugs, such as beta-adrenergic blocking drugs and methyldopa.

Special Concerns: Use with caution during lactation. Geriatric clients may be more sensitive to the hypotensive and electrolyte effects of this combination; also, age-related decreases in renal function may require a decrease in dosage.

How Supplied: See Content

Dosage

- **Tablets**

  All uses.

Initial: 1 tablet/day; **then,** dosage may be increased to 2 tablets/day.

HEALTH CARE CONSIDERATIONS

See *Health Care Considerations for Antihypertensive Agents* and individual agents.

Assessment

1. Record indications for therapy and assess appropriate parameters.
2. Record age; obtain baseline electrolytes and renal function studies.

Client/Family Teaching

1. Take with food.
2. May take the daily dose as a single dose or in divided doses.
3. More than 2 tablets/day are not usually necessary.
4. Maintenance therapy may be intermittent.

Outcome/Evaluate

- Control of hypertension
- Desired diuresis

Amiloride hydrochloride

(ah-**MILL**-oh-ryd)

Pregnancy Category: B

Midamor **(Rx)**

Classification: Diuretic, potassium-sparing

Action/Kinetics: Acts on the distal tubule to inhibit Na^+, K^+-ATPase, thereby inhibiting sodium exchange for potassium; this results in increased secretion of sodium and water and conservation of potassium. In the proximal tubule, amiloride inhibits the Na^+/H^+

exchange mechanism. Has weak diuretic and antihypertensive activity. **Onset:** 2 hr. **Peak effect:** 6-10 hr. **Peak plasma levels:** 3-4 hr. **Duration:** 24 hr. **t½:** 6-9 hr. Twenty-three percent is bound to plasma protein. Approximately 50% is excreted unchanged by kidney and 40% unchanged by the feces.
Uses: Adjunct with thiazides or loop diuretics in the treatment of hypertension or edema due to CHF, hepatic cirrhosis, and nephrotic syndrome to help restore normal serum potassium or prevent hypokalemia. Prophylaxis of hypokalemia in clients who would be at risk if hypokalemia developed (e.g., digitalized clients or clients with significant cardiac arrhythmias). *Investigational:* To reduce lithium-induced polyuria. Aerosolized amiloride may slow the progression of pulmonary function reduction in adults with cystic fibrosis.
Contraindications: Hyperkalemia (>5.5 mEq potassium/L). In clients receiving other potassium-sparing diuretics or potassium supplements. Impaired renal function. Diabetes mellitus. Use during lactation.
Special Concerns: Use with caution in metabolic or respiratory acidosis; during lactation. Geriatric clients may have a greater risk of developing hyperkalemia. Safety and efficacy have not been determined in children.
Side Effects: *Electrolyte:* Hyperkalemia, hyponatremia, and hypochloremia if used with other diuretics. *CNS:* Headache, dizziness, encephalopathy, tremors, paresthesias, mental confusion, insomnia, decreased libido, depression, sleepiness, vertigo, nervousness. *GI:* Nausea, anorexia, vomiting, diarrhea, changes in appetite, gas and abdominal pain, dry mouth, flatulence, abdominal fullness, GI bleeding, GI disturbance, thirst, dyspepsia, heartburn, jaundice, constipation, activation of preexisting peptic ulcer. *Respiratory:* Dyspnea, cough, SOB. *Musculoskeletal:* Weakness; muscle cramps; fatigue; joint, chest and back pain; neck or shoulder ache; pain in extremities. *GU:* Impotence, polyuria, dysuria, bladder spasms, urinary frequency. *CV:* Angina, palpitations, ***arrhythmias,*** orthostatic hypotension. *Hematologic:* ***Aplastic anemia,*** neutropenia. *Dermatologic:* Skin rash, itching, pruritus, alopecia. *Miscellaneous:* Visual disturbances, nasal congestion, tinnitus, increased intraocular pressure, abnormal liver function.
OD **Management of Overdose:** *Symptoms:* Electrolyte imbalance, ***dehydration.*** *Treatment:* Induce emesis or gastric lavage. Treat hyperkalemia by IV sodium bicarbonate or oral or parenteral glucose with a rapid-acting insulin. Sodium polystyrene sulfonate, oral or by enema, may also be used.
Drug Interactions
ACE inhibitors / ↑ Risk of significant hyperkalemia
Digoxin / Possible ↑ renal clearance and ↓ nonrenal clearance of digoxin. Possible ↑ inotropic effect of digoxin
Lithium / ↓ Renal excretion of lithium → ↑ chance of toxicity
NSAIDs / ↓ Therapeutic effect of amiloride
Potassium products / Hyperkalemia with possibility of cardiac arrhythmias or cardiac arrest
Spironolactone, Triamterene / Hyperkalemia, hyponatremia, hypochloremia
How Supplied: *Tablet:* 5 mg

Dosage

- **Tablets**

As single agent or with other diuretics.
Adults, initial: 5 mg/day; 10 mg/day may be necessary in some clients. Doses as high as 20 mg/day may be used, if needed, with careful monitoring of electrolytes.

Reduce lithium-induced polyuria.
10-20 mg/day.

Slow progression of pulmonary function reduction in cystic fibrosis.
Adults: Drug is dissolved in 0.3% saline and delivered by nebulizer.

HEALTH CARE CONSIDERATIONS

See also *Health Care Considerations* for *Diuretics.*

Assessment

1. Monitor renal function studies, I&O, and weights.
2. Obtain serum electrolytes. Assess for hyperkalemia and for indications to withdraw drug; cardiac irregularities may be precipitated.

Client/Family Teaching

1. Administer with food to reduce chance of GI upset.
2. Avoid potassium supplementation or foods rich in potassium because drug does not promote potassium excretion. Do not take with other potassium-sparing diuretics.

Outcome/Evaluate

- ↓ BP and enhanced diuresis
- Conservation of potassium
- ↓ Lithium-induced polyuria
- Maintenance of pulmonary function with cystic fibrosis

A

Aminolevulinic acid

(ah-**MEEN**-oh-lev-you-**lin**ick **AH**-sid)

Pregnancy Category: C

Levulan Kerastick **(Rx)**

Classification: Topical photosensitizing agent, topical prophyrin agent

Action/Kinetics: Useful in the detection and/or treatment of a variety of superficial skin conditions such as early cancers, pre-cancers and skin conditions. When delivered to target tissues, aminolevulinic acid is taken up and converted by fast growing cells into protoporphyrin IX (PpIX), a potent photosensitizer, which can then be activated by an appropriate light source.

Uses: Treatment of non-hyperkeratotic actinic keratoses of the face or scalp: use in combination with blue light illumination.

Side Effects: Transient stinging, burning, itching, erythema and edema due to the photosensitizingproperties of this agent. Symptoms stop between 1 minute and 24 hours after turningoff the blue light illuminator. Scaling, hyperpigmentation/hypopigmentation have been reported.

Drug Interactions: Theoretically, photosensitizing agents including griseofulvin, thiazide diuretics, sulfonamides, sulfonylureas, phenothiazines, and tetracyclines may increase the photosensitizing activity of aminolevulinic acid.

How Supplied: *Solution:* 20%

Dosage

- **Topical 20% solution with applicator**

Non-hyperkeratotic actinic keratoses.

Adults: Apply solution with the applicator provided to actinic keratoses (not surrounding skin) followed 14-18 hours later by blue light illumination. Application may be repeated after 8 weeks.

HEALTH CARE CONSIDERATIONS

Administration/Storage

1. Store at 25°C (77°F).
2. Topical solution should be used immediately; completed within 2 hours of solution preparation.
3. Lesions to be treated should be clean and dry.
4. Solution is applied directly to the lesion, but not the surrounding skin using the applicator provided.
5. Solution should not be applied to the area around the eyes or come in contact with ocular or mucous membranes.
6. After application, blue light exposure should follow between 14 and 18 hours.

Assessment: Record client complaints, location, size, color, asymmetry of the lesion.

Client/Family Teaching

1. Avoid exposure to sunlight, bright indoor light, or tanning beds during the period between application and prior to blue light treatment.
2. Wear a wide-brimmed hat to protect from exposure.
3. Sunscreens do not protect against photosensitization by this agent.

Outcome/Evaluate: Healed skin in lesion area with no remaining signs or symptoms of lesion.

Aminophylline

(am-in-**OFF**-ih-lin)

Pregnancy Category: C

Aminophyllin, Jaa Aminophylline ✦, Phyllocontin, Phyllocontin-350 ✦, Truphyllin **(Rx)**

Classification: Bronchodilator

Action/Kinetics: Contains 79% theophylline.

Additional Uses: Neonatal apnea, respiratory stimulant in Cheyne-Stokes respiration. Parenteral form has been used for biliary colic and as a cardiac stimulant, a diuretic, and an adjunct in treating CHF, although such uses have been replaced by more effective drugs.

Special Concerns: Use with caution when aminophylline and sodium chloride are used with corticosteroids or in clients with edema.

Additional Side Effects: The ethylenediamine in the product may cause exfoliative dermatitis or urticaria.

How Supplied: *Injection:* 25 mg/mL; *Oral Solution:* 105 mg/5 mL; *Suppository:* 250 mg, 500 mg; *Tablet:* 100 mg, 200 mg

Dosage

- **Oral Solution, Tablets**

Bronchodilator, acute attacks, in clients not currently on theophylline therapy.

Adults and children up to 16 years of age, loading dose: Equivalent of 5-6 mg of anhydrous theophylline/kg.

Bronchodilator, acute attacks, in clients currently receiving theophylline.

Adults and children up to 16 years of age: If possible, a serum theophylline level should be obtained first. Then, base loading dose on the premise that each 0.5 mg theophylline/kg lean body weight will result in a 0.5-1.6-mcg/mL increase in serum theophylline levels. If immediate therapy is needed and a serum level cannot be obtained, a single dose of the equivalent of 2.5 mg/kg of anhydrous theophylline can be given.

Maintenance in acute attack, based on equivalent of anhydrous theophylline.

Young adult smokers: 4 mg/kg q 6 hr; **healthy, nonsmoking adults:** 3 mg/kg q 8 hr; **geriatric clients or clients with cor pulmonale:** 2 mg/kg q 8 hr; **clients with CHF or liver failure:** 2 mg/kg q 8-12 hr. **Pediatric, 12-16 years:** 3 mg/kg q 6 hr; **9-12 years:** 4 mg/kg q 6 hr; **1-9 years:** 5 mg/kg q 6 hr; **6-12 months:** Use the formula: dose (mg/kg q 8 hr) = (0.05) (age in weeks) + 1.25; **up to 6 months:** Use the formula: dose (mg/kg q 8 hr) = (0.07) (age in weeks) + 1.7.

Chronic therapy, based on equivalent of anhydrous theophylline.

Adults, initial: 6-8 mg/kg up to a maximum of 400 mg/day in three to four divided doses at 6-8-hr intervals; **then,** dose can be increased in 25% increments at 2-3 day intervals up to a maximum of 13 mg/kg or 900 mg/day, whichever is less. **Pediatric, initial:** 16 mg/kg up to a maximum of 400 mg/day in three to four divided doses at 6-8 hr intervals; **then,** dose may be increased in 25% increments at 2-3 day intervals up to the following maximum doses (without measuring serum theophylline): **16 years and older:** 13 mg/kg or 900 mg/day, whichever is less; **12-16 years:** 18 mg/kg/day; **9-12 years:** 20 mg/kg/day; **1-9 years:** 24 mg/kg/day; **up to 12 months,** Use the following formula: dose (mg/kg/day) = (0.3) (age in weeks) + 8.0.

• **Enteric-Coated Tablets**

Bronchodilator, chronic therapy, based on equivalent of anhydrous theophylline.

Adults, initial: 6-8 mg/kg up to a maximum of 400 mg/day in three to four divided doses at 6-8-hr intervals; **then,** dose may be increased, if needed and tolerated, by increments of 25% at 2-3 day intervals up to a maximum of 13 mg/kg/day or 900 mg/day, whichever is less, without measuring serum theophylline. **Pediatric, over 12 years of age, initial:** 4 mg/kg q 8-12 hr; **then,** dose may be increased by 2-3 mg/kg/day at 3-day intervals up to the following maximum doses (without measuring serum levels): **16 years and older:** 13 mg/kg/day or 900 mg/day, whichever is less; **12-16 years:** 18 mg/kg/day.

• **Enema**

For use as a bronchodilator for loading doses and for maintenance in acute attacks, see doses for oral solution and tablets.

• **IV Infusion**

Bronchodilator, acute attacks, for clients not currently on theophylline.

Adults and children up to 16 years, loading dose based on anhydrous theophylline: 5 mg/kg given over a period of 20 min.

Bronchodilator, acute attack, for clients currently on theophylline.

Adults and children up to 16 years, loading dose based on anhydrous theophylline: If possible, a serum theophylline level should be obtained first. Then, base loading dose on the premise that each 0.5 mg theophylline/kg lean body weight will result in a 0.5-1.6 mcg/mL increase in serum theophylline levels. If immediate therapy is needed and a serum level cannot be obtained, a single dose of the equivalent of 2.5 mg/kg of anhydrous theophylline can be given.

Maintenance for acute attacks, based on equivalent of anhydrous theophylline.

Young adult smokers: 0.7 mg/kg/hr; **nonsmoking, healthy adults:** 0.43 mg/kg/hr; **geriatric clients or clients with cor pulmonale:** 0.26 mg/kg/hr; **clients with CHF or liver failure:** 0.2 mg/kg/hr. **Pediatric, 12-16 years, nonsmokers:** 0.5 mg/kg/hr; **9-12 years,** 0.7 mg/kg/hr; **1-9 years,** 0.8 mg/kg/hr; **up to 1 year,** Based on the following formula: dose (mg/kg/hr) = (0.008) (age in weeks) + 0.21.

HEALTH CARE CONSIDERATIONS

Administration/Storage

1. IM injection is not recommended due to severe, persistent pain at the site of injection.
2. Enteric-coated tablets may be incompletely and slowly absorbed.
3. Enteric-coated tablets are not recommended for children less than 12 years of age.
4. Use of aminophylline suppositories is not recommended due to the possibility of slow and unreliable absorption.

IV 5. To avoid hypotension, administer IV doses at a rate not to exceed 25 mg/min.

6. Use only the 25 mg/mL injection (which should be further diluted) for IV administration. Use an infusion pump or device to regulate infusion rates.
7. A minimum of 4-6 hr should elapse when switching from IV to the first dose of PO therapy.

Assessment

1. Record indications for therapy, onset, duration, and symptom characteristics; note other therapies tried.
2. List medications currently prescribed to ensure that none interact unfavorably.
3. Perform baseline lung assessments and PFTs; note ABGs and ECG.
4. Monitor VS closely during IV administration; may cause a transitory lowering of BP.

If evident, adjust the drug dosage and rate of flow.
5. Monitor clients with a history of CAD for chest pain and ECG changes.
6. Report serum levels greater than 20 mcg/mL or symptoms of toxicity.

Client/Family Teaching

1. Drug acts by relaxation of muscles of bronchi and pulmonary blood vessels to relieve bronchospasm.
2. Take with a snack or meal to prevent GI upset; avoid coffee, cola, and chocolate.
3. Practice pursed-lip and diaphragmatic breathing to help reduce the work of breathing by prolonging expiration and keeping the airways open longer.
4. Report symptoms of toxicity, i.e., N&V, restlessness, convulsions, and arrhythmias.
5. Stop smoking; attend a formal smoking cessation program if unable to quit.

Outcome/Evaluate

- Improved airway exchange
- ↓ SOB; relief of PND
- Termination of asthma attack
- Therapeutic serum drug levels (10-20 mcg/mL)

COMBINATION DRUG

Amitriptyline and Perphenazine

(ah-me-**TRIP**-tih-leen, per-**FEN**-ah-zeen)

Apo-Peram ✱, Elavil Plus ✱, Etrafon 2-10 ✱, Etrafon-A ✱, Etrafon-D ✱, Etrafon-F ✱, PMS-Levazine 2/25 ✱, PMS-Levazine 4/25 ✱, Proavil ✱, Triavil 2-10, 2-25, 4-10, 4-25, and 4-50 **(Rx)**

Classification: Antidepressant

Content: See also information on individual components.

Antidepressant: Amitriptyline HCl, 10, 25, or 50 mg. *Antipsychotic:* Perphenazine, 2 or 4 mg.

There are five different strengths of Triavil: Triavil 2-10, Triavil 2-25, Triavil 4-10, Triavil 4-25, and Triavil 4-50. *NOTE:* The first number refers to the number of milligrams of perphenazine and the second number refers to the number of milligrams of amitriptyline.

Uses: Depression with moderate to severe anxiety and/or agitation. Depression and anxiety in clients with chronic physical disease. Also schizophrenic clients with symptoms of depression.

Contraindications: Use during pregnancy. CNS depression due to drugs. In presence of bone marrow depression. Concomitant use with MAO inhibitors. During acute recovery phase from MI. Use in children.

How Supplied: See Content

Dosage

- **Tablets**

Antidepressant.

Adults, initial: One tablet of Triavil 2-25 or 4-25 t.i.d.-q.i.d. or 1 tablet of Triavil 4-50 b.i.d. Schizophrenic clients should receive an initial dose of 2 tablets of Triavil 4-50 t.i.d., with a fourth dose at bedtime, if necessary. Initial dosage for geriatric or adolescent clients in whom anxiety dominates is Triavil 4-10 t.i.d.-q.i.d., with dosage adjusted as required. **Maintenance:** One tablet Triavil 2-25 or 4-25 b.i.d.-q.i.d. or 1 tablet Triavil 4-50 b.i.d.

HEALTH CARE CONSIDERATIONS

See also *Health Care Considerations* for *Antidepressants, Tricyclic.*

Administration/Storage

1. Do not exceed a total daily dosage with Triavil of 4 of the 4-50 tablets or 8 tablets of all other dosage strengths.
2. The therapeutic effect may take up to several weeks to be manifested.
3. Once a satisfactory response has been observed, reduce the dose to the smallest amount required for relief of symptoms.

Outcome/Evaluate: Relief of S&S of depression and associated anxiety.

Amitriptyline hydrochloride

(ah-me-**TRIP**-tih-leen)

Pregnancy Category: C

Apo-Amitriptyline ✱, Elavil, Levate ✱ **(Rx)**, Novo-Tryptin ✱

Classification: Antidepressant, tricyclic

See also *Antidepressants, Tricyclic.*

Action/Kinetics: Amitriptyline is metabolized to an active metabolite, nortriptyline. Has significant anticholinergic and sedative effects with moderate orthostatic hypotension. Very high ability to block serotonin uptake and moderate activity with respect to norepinephrine uptake. **Effective plasma levels of amitriptyline and nortriptyline:** Approximately 110-250 ng/mL. **Time to reach steady state:** 4-10 days. **t½:** 31-46 hr. Up to 1 month may be required for beneficial effects to be manifested.

Uses: Relief of symptoms of depression, including depression accompanied by anxiety and insomnia. Chronic pain due to cancer or other pain syndromes. Prophylaxis of cluster and migraine headaches. *Investigational:* Pathologic laughing and crying secondary to forebrain disease, bulimia nervosa, antiulcer agent, enuresis.

Contraindications: Use in children less than 12 years of age.

How Supplied: *Injection:* 10 mg/mL; *Tablet:* 10 mg, 25 mg, 50 mg, 75 mg, 100 mg, 150 mg

Dosage

- **Tablets**

Antidepressant.

Adults (outpatients): 75 mg/day in divided doses; may be increased to 150 mg/day. *Alternate dosage:* **Initial,** 50-100 mg at bedtime; **then,** increase by 25-50 mg, if necessary, up to 150 mg/day. **Hospitalized clients: initial,** 100 mg/day; may be increased to 200-300 mg/day. **Maintenance: usual,** 40-100 mg/day (may be given as a single dose at bedtime). **Adolescent and geriatric:** 10 mg t.i.d. and 20 mg at bedtime up to a maximum of 100 mg/day. **Pediatric, 6-12 years:** 10-30 mg (1-5 mg/kg) daily in two divided doses.

Chronic pain.

50-100 mg/day.

Enuresis.

Pediatric, over 6 years: 10 mg/day as a single dose at bedtime; dose may be increased up to a maximum of 25 mg. **Less than 6 years:** 10 mg/day as a single dose at bedtime.

- **IM Only**

Antidepressant.

Adults: 20-30 mg q.i.d.; switch to **PO** therapy as soon as possible.

HEALTH CARE CONSIDERATIONS

See also *Health Care Considerations* for *Antidepressants, Tricyclic.*

Administration/Storage

1. Initiate dosage increases late in the afternoon or at bedtime.
2. Sedative effects may be manifested prior to antidepressant effects.

Client/Family Teaching

1. Take with food to minimize gastric upset.
2. Do not drive a car or operate hazardous machinery until drug effects realized; drug causes a high degree of sedation.
3. May take entire dose at bedtime if sedation is manifested during waking hours.
4. Rise slowly from a lying to a sitting position to reduce orthostatic drug effects.
5. Urine may appear blue-green in color; this is harmless.
6. Beneficial antidepressant effects may not be noted for 30 days.

Outcome/Evaluate

- ↓ Symptoms of depression
- Control of incontinence
- Enhanced pain control with chronic pain management
- Relief of insomnia

Amlexanox

(am-**LEX**-an-ox)

Pregnancy Category: B

Aphthasol **(Rx)**

Classification: Aphthous ulcer product.

Action/Kinetics: Mechanism not known. May be absorbed through GI tract.

Uses: Treat aphthous ulcers in those with normal immune systems.

Special Concerns: Use with caution during lactation. Safety and efficacy in children have not been determined.

Side Effects: Transient pain, burning, or stinging at application site. Contact mucositis, nausea, diarrhea.

How Supplied: *Paste:* 5%

Dosage

- **Paste**

Aphthous ulcers.

Squeeze about 0.25 inch of paste onto fingertip and, with gentle pressure, dab onto each mouth ulcer. Apply following oral hygiene after breakfast, lunch, dinner, and at bedtime. Start as soon as possible after symptoms of aphthous ulcer noted and continue until ulcer heals.

HEALTH CARE CONSIDERATIONS

Administration/Storage

1. If significant healing has not occurred within 10 days, consult physician or dentist.
2. Wash hands immediately after applying paste.

Client/Family Teaching

1. Apply paste as soon as ulcers appear; rinse mouth thoroughly and use after each meal and at bedtime.
2. Place a small amount of paste on fingertip and gently dab onto each oral ulcer.
3. Wash hands after applying; avoid contact with eyes and wash promptly if eye contact occurs.
4. Continue to apply paste until healing takes place. Report if pain or ulcers persist after 10 days.

Outcome/Evaluate: Pain relief; ulcer healing

Amlodipine

(am-**LOH**-dih-peen)

Pregnancy Category: C

Norvasc **(Rx)**

Classification: Antihypertensive, antianginal (calcium channel blocking agent)

See also *Calcium Channel Blocking Agents.*

A

Action/Kinetics: Increases myocardial contractility although this effect may be counteracted by reflex activity. CO is increased and there is a pronounced decrease in peripheral vascular resistance. **Peak plasma levels:** 6-12 hr. **t½, elimination:** 30-50 hr. 90% metabolized in the liver to inactive metabolites; 10% excreted unchanged in the urine.
Uses: Hypertension alone or in combination with other antihypertensives. Chronic stable angina alone or in combination with other antianginal drugs. Confirmed or suspected Prinzmetal's or variant angina alone or in combination with other antianginal drugs.
Special Concerns: Use with caution in clients with CHF and in those with impaired hepatic function or reduced hepatic blood flow. Safety and efficacy have not been determined in children.
Side Effects: *CNS:* Headache, fatigue, lethargy, somnolence, dizziness, lightheadedness, sleep disturbances, depression, amnesia, psychosis, hallucinations, paresthesia, asthenia, insomnia, abnormal dreams, malaise, anxiety, tremor, hand tremor, hypoesthesia, vertigo, depersonalization, migraine, apathy, agitation, amnesia. *GI:* Nausea, abdominal discomfort, cramps, dyspepsia, diarrhea, constipation, vomiting, dry mouth, thirst, flatulence, dysphagia, loose stools. *CV:* Peripheral edema, palpitations, hypotension, syncope, bradycardia, unspecified arrhythmias, tachycardia, ventricular extrasystoles, peripheral ischemia, ***cardiac failure,*** pulse irregularity, increased risk of MI. *Dermatologic:* Dermatitis, rash, pruritus, urticaria, photosensitivity, petechiae, ecchymosis, purpura, bruising, hematoma, cold/clammy skin, skin discoloration, dry skin. *Musculoskeletal:* Muscle cramps, pain, or inflammation; joint stiffness or pain, arthritis, twitching, ataxia, hypertonia. *GU:* Polyuria, dysuria, urinary frequency, nocturia, sexual difficulties. *Respiratory:* Nasal or chest congestion, sinusitis, rhinitis, SOB, dyspnea, wheezing, cough, chest pain. *Ophthalmologic:* Diplopia, abnormal vision, conjunctivitis, eye pain, abnormal visual accommodation, xerophthalmia. *Miscellaneous:* Tinnitus, flushing, sweating, weight gain, epistaxis, anorexia, increased appetite, taste perversion, parosmia.
How Supplied: *Tablet:* 2.5 mg, 5 mg, 10 mg

Dosage

- **Tablets**

Hypertension.

Adults, usual, individualized: 5 mg/day, up to a maximum of 10 mg/day. Titrate the dose over 7-14 days.

Chronic stable or vasospastic angina.

Adults: 5-10 mg, using the lower dose for elderly clients and those with hepatic insufficiency. Most clients require 10 mg.

HEALTH CARE CONSIDERATIONS

See also *Health Care Considerations* for *Calcium Channel Blocking Agents.*

Administration/Storage

1. Food does not affect the bioavailability of amlodipine. Thus, may be taken without regard to meals.
2. Elderly clients, small/fragile clients, or those with hepatic insufficiency may be started on 2.5 mg/day. This dose may also be used when adding amlodipine to other antihypertensive therapy.

Assessment

1. Record any history of CAD or CHF.
2. Review list of drugs currently prescribed to prevent any unfavorable interactions.
3. Record baseline VS, ECG, CBC, and liver and renal function studies and monitor. Reduce dose with cirrhosis.

Client/Family Teaching

1. Take only as directed, once daily. May take with or without food.
2. Report any symptoms of chest pain, SOB, dizziness, swelling of extremities, irregular pulse, or altered vision immediately.

Outcome/Evaluate

- Desired BP control
- ↓ Frequency/intensity of angina

COMBINATION DRUG

Amlodipine and Benazepril hydrochloride

(am-**LOH**-dih-peen, beh-**NAYZ**-eh- prill)
Pregnancy Category: C (first trimester), D (second and third trimesters)
Lotrel **(Rx)**
Classification: Antihypertensive

See also *Amlodipine* and *Benazepril hydrochloride.*
Content: Lotrel 2.5/10: *Calcium channel blocking agent:* Amlodipine, 2.5 mg. *ACE inhibitor:* Benazepril hydrochloride, 10 mg. Lotrel 5/10 and Lotrel 5/20 contain 5 mg of amlodipine and either 10 or 20 mg of benazepril hydrochloride.
Action/Kinetics: The incidence of edema is significantly reduced with this combination product. **Peak plasma levels, benazepril:** 0.5-2 hr (1.5-4 hr for benazeprilat, the active metabolite). **Peak plasma levels, amlodipine:** 6-12 hr. **Elimination t½, benazeprilat:** 10-11 hr; **elimination t½, amlodipine:** 2 days.

Uses: Treatment of hypertension. Therapy with this combination is suggested when the client either has failed to achieve the desired antihypertensive effect with either drug alone or has demonstrated inability to achieve an adequate antihypertensive effect with amlodipine without developing edema.
Contraindications: Initial treatment of hypertension. Hypersensitivity to amlodipine or benazepril. Lactation.
Special Concerns: Discontinue ACE inhibitors as soon as pregnancy is determined. The addition of benazepril to amlodipine should not be expected to provide additional antihypertensive effects in African-Americans, although there will be less edema. Use with caution in those with severe renal disease, in CHF, and in severe hepatic impairment. Safety and efficacy have not been determined in children.
Side Effects: See individual drugs. Side effects include angioedema, cough, headache, and edema.
How Supplied: See Content

Dosage

- **Capsules**

  Hypertension.

One 2.5/10 mg, 5/10 mg, or 5/20 mg capsule once daily. In those with severe renal impairment, the recommended initial dose of benazepril is 5 mg (Lotrel is not recommended in these clients). In small, elderly, frail, or hepatically impaired clients, the recommended initial dose of amlodipine (either as monotherapy or in combination) is 2.5 mg.

HEALTH CARE CONSIDERATIONS

See also *Health Care Considerations* for *Antihypertensive Agents*, *Amlodipine*, and *Benazepril hydrochloride.*

Assessment

1. Record indications for therapy, onset, duration of symptoms, and other agents trialed.
2. Obtain baseline ECG, electrolytes, and liver and renal function studies and monitor. Anticipate reduced dosage with organ impairment and with the frail, elderly client.

Client/Family Teaching

1. Take exactly as directed, at the same time each day.
2. Continue regular exercise, diet, rest, and stress reduction in the overall goal of BP control.
3. Avoid alcohol and tobacco use; attend counseling.
4. Practice reliable contraception; stop drug and notify provider if pregnancy is suspected.
5. Report any persistent headaches, cough, or extremity swelling.
6. Maintain a BP record and bring to each provider visit.

Outcome/Evaluate: Desired BP control

Amoxapine

(ah-**MOX**-ah-peen)
Pregnancy Category: C
Asendin **(Rx)**
Classification: Antidepressant, tricyclic

See also *Antidepressants, Tricyclic.*
Action/Kinetics: In addition to its effect on monoamines, this drug also blocks dopamine receptors. Significant anticholinergic effects, moderate sedation, and slight orthostatic hypotensive effect. Metabolized to the active metabolites 7-hydroxy- and 8-hydroxyamoxapine. **Peak blood levels:** 90 min. **Effective plasma levels:** 200-500 ng/mL. **Time to reach steady state:** 2-7 days. **t½:** 8 hr; **t½ of major metabolite:** 30 hr. Excreted in urine.
Uses: Endogenous and reactive depression. Antianxiety agent.
Contraindications: Avoid high dose levels in clients with a history of convulsive seizures. During acute recovery period after MI.
Special Concerns: Safe use in children under 16 years of age and during lactation not established.
Additional Side Effects: Tardive dyskinesia. ***Overdosage may cause seizures (common), neuroleptic malignant syndrome,*** testicular swelling, impairment of sexual function, and breast enlargement in males and females. Also, renal failure may be seen 2-5 days after overdosage.
How Supplied: *Tablet:* 25 mg, 50 mg, 100 mg, 150 mg

Dosage

- **Tablets**

  Antidepressant.

Adults, individualized, initial: 50 mg t.i.d. Can be increased to 100 mg t.i.d. during first week. Do not use doses greater than 300 mg/day unless this dose has been ineffective for at least 14 days. **Maintenance:** 300 mg as a single dose at bedtime. **Hospitalized clients:** Up to 150 mg q.i.d. **Geriatric, initial:** 25 mg b.i.d.-t.i.d. If necessary, increase to 50 mg b.i.d.-t.i.d. after first week. **Maintenance:** Up to 300 mg/day at bedtime.

A

HEALTH CARE CONSIDERATIONS

See also *Health Care Considerations* for *Antidepressants, Tricyclic.*

Client/Family Teaching

1. Take with food to minimize gastric upset.
2. Administer entire dose at bedtime if daytime sedation experienced.
3. Report early CNS manifestations of tardive dyskinesia, i.e., slow repetitive movements.
4. Report any side effects R/T overdosage, especially seizures, that require immediate medical care.

Outcome/Evaluate

- Improved coping mechanisms
- Control of depression; ↓ anxiety

Amoxicillin (amoxycillin)

(ah-mox-ih-**SILL**-in)

Amox ✱, Amoxil, Amoxil Pediatric Drops, Apo-Amoxi ✱, Novamoxin ✱, Nu-Amoxi ✱, Pro-Amox ✱, Trimox, Trimox Pediatric Drops, Wymox **(Rx)**

NOTE: All products are amoxicillin trihydrate.

Classification: Antibiotic, penicillin

See also *Anti-Infectives* and *Penicillins.*

Action/Kinetics: Semisynthetic broad-spectrum penicillin closely related to ampicillin. Destroyed by penicillinase, acid stable, and better absorbed than ampicillin. From 50% to 80% of a PO dose is absorbed from the GI tract. **Peak serum levels: PO:** 4-11 mcg/mL after 1-2 hr. **t½:** 60 min. Mostly excreted unchanged in urine.

Uses: Gram-positive streptococcal infections including *Streptococcus faecalis, S. pneumoniae,* and non-penicillinase-producing staphylococci. Gram-negative infections due to *Hemophilus influenzae, Proteus mirabilis, Escherichia coli,* and *Neisseria gonorrhoeae.* In combination with omeprazole and clarithromycin to treat duodenal ulcers by eradicating *Helicobacter pylori.*

Special Concerns: Safe use during pregnancy has not been established.

How Supplied: *Capsule:* 250 mg, 500 mg; *Chew tablet:* 125 mg, 250 mg; *Powder for oral suspension:* 50 mg/mL, 125 mg/5 mL, 250 mg/5 mL; *Tablet:* 500 mg, 875 mg

Dosage

- **Capsules, Oral Suspension, Chewable Tablets, Tablets**

Susceptible infections of ear, nose, throat, GU tract, skin and soft tissues.

Adults and children over 20 kg: 250-500 mg q 8 hr; alternatively, 500 mg or 875 mg q 12 hr. **Children under 20 kg:** 20-40 (or more) mg/kg/day in three equal doses. The pediatric dose should not exceed the maximum adult dose.

Infections of the lower respiratory tract.

Adults and children over 20 kg: 500 mg q 8 hr. **Children under 20 kg:** 40 mg/kg/day in divided doses q 8 hr.

Prophylaxis of bacterial endocarditis: dental, oral, or upper respiratory tract procedures in those at risk.

Adults: 2 g (50 mg/kg for children) PO 1 hr prior to procedure.

Prophylaxis of bacterial endocarditis: GU or GI procedures.

Adults, standard regimen: 2 g ampicillin plus 1.5 mg/kg gentamicin not to exceed 80 mg, either IM or IV, 30 min prior to procedure, followed by 1.5 g amoxicillin. **Children, standard regimen:** 50 mg/kg ampicillin plus 2 mg/kg gentamicin 30 min prior to procedure, followed by 25 mg/kg amoxcillin.. **Adults, moderate risk:** 2 g PO 1 hr prior to procedure. **Children, moderate risk:** 50 mg/kg PO 1 hr pior to procedure. **Adults, alternate low-risk regimen:** 3 g 1 hr before procedure, followed by 1.5 g 6 hr after the initial dose.

Treat duodenal ulcers due to H. pylori.

A ten day course of therapy consisting of amoxicillin, 1,000 mg b.i.d.; omeprazole, 20 mg b.i.d.; and, clarithromycin, 500 mg b.i.d.

Gonococcal infections,uncomplicated urethral, endocervical, or rectal infections.

Adults: 3 g as a single PO dose. **Children, over 2 years (prepubertal):** 50 mg/kg amoxicillin combined with 25 mg/kg probenecid as a single dose.

Chlamydia trachomatis during pregnancy (as an alternative to erythromycin).

0.5 g t.i.d. for 7 days.

HEALTH CARE CONSIDERATIONS

See also *Health Care Considerations* for *Penicillins.*

Administration/Storage

1. The children's dose should not exceed the maximum adult dose.
2. Dry powder is stable at room temperature for 18-30 months. Reconstituted suspension is stable for 1 week at room temperature and for 2 weeks at 2°C-8°C (36°F-46°F).

Client/Family Teaching

1. Take entire prescription; do not stop when feeling "better" as this creates antibiotic resistance.

2. With school-age child space medication evenly over the 24-hr period. Give suspension or tablet before school, upon arrival home, and at bedtime.
3. Chewable tablets are available for pediatric use and may be administered with food.
4. Pediatric drops are placed directly on the child's tongue for swallowing. Alternatively, the drops may be added to formula, milk, fruit juice, water, gingerale or cold drinks. The beverage must be taken immediately and consumed completely.
5. Report any unusual rash or lack of response.

Outcome/Evaluate

- Resolution of infection; symptomatic improvement
- Therapeutic peak serum drug levels (4-11 mcg/mL)

COMBINATION DRUG

Amoxicillin and Potassium clavulanate

(ah-mox-ih-**SILL**-in, poh-**TASS**-ee-um klav-you-**LAN**-ayt)

Pregnancy Category: B

Augmentin, Clavulin ✤ **(Rx)**

Classification: Antibiotic, penicillin

See also *Anti-Infectives* and *Penicillins.*

Content: Each '250' Tablet contains: 250 mg amoxicillin and 125 mg potassium clavulanate. Each '500' Tablet contains 500 mg amoxicillin and 125 mg potassium clavulanate. Each '875' tablet contains: 875 mg amoxicillin and 125 mg potassium clavulanate

Each '125' Chewable Tablet contains 125 mg amoxicillin and 31.25 mg potassium clavulanate. Each '200' Chewable Tablet contains 200 mg amoxicillin and 28.5 mg potassium clavulanate. Each '250' Chewable Tablet contains 250 mg amoxicillin and 62.5 mg potassium clavulanate. Each '400' Chewable Tablet contains 400 mg amoxicillin and 57 mg potassium clavulanate.

Each 5 mL of the '125' Powder for Oral Suspension contains 125 mg amoxicillin and 31.25 mg potassium clavulanate. Each 5 mL of the '200' Powder for Oral Suspension contains 200 mg amoxicillin and 28.5 mg potassium clavulanate. Each 5 mL of the '250' Powder for Oral Suspension contains 250 mg amoxicillin and 62.5 mg potassium clavulanate. Each 5 mL of the '400' Powder for Oral Suspension contains 400 mg amoxicillin and 57 mg potassium clavulanate.

Action/Kinetics: *For details, see amoxicillin.* Potassium clavulanate inactivates lactamase enzymes, which are responsible for resistance to penicillins. Effective against microorganisms that have manifested resistance to amoxicillin. For potassium clavulanate: **Peak serum levels:** 1-2 hr. **t¹/₂:** 1 hr.

Uses: For beta-lactamase-producing strains of the following organisms: Lower respiratory tract infections, otitis media, and sinusitis caused by *Hemophilus influenzae* and *Moraxella catarrhalis*; skin and skin structure infections caused by *Staphylococcus aureus, Escherichia coli,* and *Klebsiella*; UTI caused by *E. coli, Klebsiella,* and *Enterobacter. NOTE:* Mixed infections caused by organisms susceptible to ampicillin and organisms susceptible to amoxicillin/potassium clavulanate should not require an additional antibiotic.

How Supplied: See Content.

Dosage

- **Oral Suspension, Chewable Tablets, Tablets**

Susceptible infections.

Adults, usual: One 500-mg tablet q 12 hr or one 250-mg tablet q 8 hr. Adults unable to take tablets can be given the 125-mg/5 mL or the 250-mg/5 mL suspension in place of the 500-mg tablet or the 200-mg/5 mL or 400-mg/5 mL suspension can be given in place of the 875-mg tablet. **Children less than 3 months old:** 30 mg/kg/day amoxicillin in divided doses q 12 hr. Use of the 125-mg/5 mL suspension is recommended. **Children over 3 months old:** 25 mg/kg/day amoxicillin in divided doses q 12 hr or 20 mg/kg/day in divided doses q 8 hr.

Respiratory tract and severe infections.

Adults: One 875-mg tablet q 12 hr or one 500-mg tablet q 8 hr. **Children over 3 months old:** 45 mg/kg/day of amoxicillin in divided doses q 12 hr or 40 mg/kg/day amoxicillin in divided doses q 8 hr (these doses are used in children for otitis media, lower respiratory tract infections, or sinusitis). Treatment duration for otitis media is 10 days.

HEALTH CARE CONSIDERATIONS

See also *Health Care Considerations* for *Penicillins.*

Administration/Storage

1. Both the '250' and '500' tablets contain 125 mg potassium clavulanate; therefore, two '250' tablets are not the same as one '500' tablet. Also, the 250-mg tablet and the 250-mg chewable tablet do not contain the same amount of potassium clavulanate and are not interchangeable. The 250-mg tablet should not be used until children are over 40 kg.

A

2. Pediatric formulations are now available in fruit flavors for the oral suspension and chewable tablets. These formulations allow twice-daily dosing, which is more convenient than three-times daily dosing and, importantly, the incidence of diarrhea is significantly reduced.
3. The 200- and 400-mg suspensions and chewable tablets contain aspartame and should not be used by clients with phenylketonuria.

Client/Family Teaching

1. Take exactly as directed and complete entire prescription.
2. May be taken without regard for meals; however, absorption is enhanced if taken at the beginning of a meal.
3. Report any rash, persistent diarrhea, lack of response or worsening of symptoms after 48-72 hr of therapy.
4. Refrigerate the reconstituted suspension and discard after 10 days.
5. Return as scheduled for follow-up evaluation.

Outcome/Evaluate: Resolution of infection; symptomatic improvement

Amphetamine sulfate

(am-**FET**-ah-meen)
Pregnancy Category: C
Adderall, Dexedrine ✱ **(C-II) (Rx)**
Classification: CNS stimulant

See also *Amphetamines and Derivatives.*
Action/Kinetics: Completely absorbed in 3 hr. **Peak effects:** 2-3 hr. **Duration:** 4-24 hr; **t½:** 10-30 hr, depending on urinary pH. Excreted in urine. Acidification increases excretion, whereas alkalinization decreases it. For every one unit increase in pH, the plasma half-life will increase by 7 hr.
Uses: Attention deficit hyperactivity disorder in children, narcolepsy. Adderall contains dextroamphetamine sulfate, dextroamphetamine saccharate, amphetamine sulfate, and amphetamine aspartate and is used in children aged three years and older who have attention deficit hyperactivity disorder or narcolepsy.
Special Concerns: Use in children less than 3 years of age for attention deficit disorders and in children less than 6 years of age for narcolepsy. Not recommended as an appetite suppressant.
How Supplied: *Tablet:* 5 mg, 10 mg. *Adderall:* 5 mg, 10 mg, 20 mg, 30 mg.

Dosage

- **Tablets**

Narcolepsy.

Adults: 5-20 mg 1-3 times/day. **Children over 12 years, initial:** 5 mg b.i.d.; increase in increments of 10 mg/day at weekly intervals until optimum dose is reached. **Children, 6-12 years, initial:** 2.5 mg b.i.d.; increase in increments of 5 mg at weekly intervals until optimum dose is reached (maximum is 60 mg/day).

Attention deficit disorders in children. **3-6 years, initial:** 2.5 mg/day; increase by 2.5 mg/day at weekly intervals until optimum dose is achieved (usual range 0.1-0.5 mg/kg/dose each morning). **6 years and older, initial:** 5 mg 1-2 times/day; increase in increments of 5 mg/week until optimum dose is achieved (rarely over 40 mg/day). The dose of Adderall is 5-30 mg per day.

HEALTH CARE CONSIDERATIONS

See also *Health Care Considerations* for *Amphetamines and Derivatives.*

Assessment

1. Review CNS/neurologic status prior to initiating therapy.
2. Record type and onset of symptoms and pretreatment findings.
3. Determine if pregnant.
4. Monitor weight, CBC, chemistry profile, urinalysis, and ECG.

Client/Family Teaching

1. When used for attention deficit disorders or narcolepsy, give the first dose on awakening with an additional one or two doses given at intervals of 4-6 hr. Give the last dose 6 hr before bedtime.
2. Report any changes in mood or affect, including symptoms of impaired mental processes.
3. Do not use caffeine or caffeine-containing products. Avoid any OTC preparations that contain caffeine, or other agents that affect CV system.
4. Avoid using heavy machinery or driving until drug effects realized.
5. Monitor weight and record.
6. Drink at least 2.5 L/day of fluids; increase intake of high-fiber foods/fruits to prevent constipation.
7. Chew sugarless gum/candies and rinse mouth frequently with nonalcoholic mouth rinses for dry mouth.
8. Children receiving amphetamines may have their growth retarded. Drug should periodically be discontinued by provider to allow growth to proceed normally and to evaluate the need for continued drug therapy.

Outcome/Evaluate

- Improved attention span
- ↓ Episodes of narcolepsy

A

Amphotericin B (Deoxycholate)

(am-foe-TER-ih-sin)

Pregnancy Category: B

Fungizone ✱

Amphotericin B Lipid Complex (Amphotericin B Cholesteryl Sulfate Complex)

(am-foe-TER-ih-sin)

Pregnancy Category: B

Abelcet, AmBisome, Amphotec **(Rx)**

Classification: Antibiotic, antifungal

See also *Anti-Infectives.*

Action/Kinetics: This antibiotic is produced by *Streptomyces nodosus;* it is fungistatic or fungicidal depending on the concentration of the drug in body fluids and the susceptibility of the fungus. Amphotericin B binds to specific chemical structures—sterols—of the fungal cellular membrane, increasing cellular permeability and promoting loss of potassium and other substances. Liposomal encapsulation or incorporation in a lipid complex can significantly affect the functional properties of the drug compared with those of the unencapsulated or nonlipid-associated drug. The liposomal amphotericin B product causes less nephrotoxicity. Amphotericin B is used either IV or topically. It is highly bound to serum protein (90%) **Peak plasma levels:** 0.5-2 mcg/mL. **t½, initial:** 24 hr; **second phase:** 15 days. Slowly excreted by kidneys.The kinetics of the drug differ in adults and children and are also dependent on the product used.

Uses: The drug is toxic and should be used only for clients under close medical supervision with progressive or potentially fatal fungal infections. **Systemic Amphotericin B (deoxycholate):** Disseminated North American blastomycosis, cryptococcosis, and other systemic fungal infections, including coccidioidomycosis, histoplasmosis, aspergillosis, sporotrichosis, disseminated candidiasis, and monilial overgrowth resulting from oral antibiotic therapy. Zygomycosis, including mucormycosis due to *Mucor, Rhizopus,* and *Absidia* species. Infections due to susceptible species of *Conidiobolus* and *Basidiobolus.* Secondary therapy to treat American mucocutaneous leishmaniasis.

Topical: Cutaneous and mucocutaneous infections of *Candida (Monilia)* infections, especially in children, adults, and AIDS clients with thrush.

Contraindications: Hypersensitivity to drug unless the condition is life-threatening and amenable only to amphotericin B therapy. Use to treat common forms of fungal diseases showing only positive skin or serologic tests. Use to treat noninvasive forms of fungal disease such as oral thrush, vaginal candidiasis, and esophageal candidiasis in clients with normal neutrophil counts. Lactation.

Special Concerns: The bone marrow depressant effects may result in increased incidence of microbial infection, delayed healing, and gingival bleeding. Although used in children, safety and efficacy have not been determined. Use with caution in clients receiving leukocyte transfusions.

Side Effects: After topical use. Irritation, pruritus, dry skin. Redness, itching, or burning especially in skin folds.

Laboratory Test Considerations: ↑ AST, ALT, GGT, LDH, alkaline phosphatase, serum creatinine, BUN, bilirubin, BSP retention values, PT. Hypomagnesemia, hyperkalemia, hypocalcemia, hypercalcemia, acidosis, hypoglycemia, hyperglycemia, hypermyalesmia, hyperuricemia, hypophosphatemia.

OD **Management of Overdose:** *Symptoms:* Cardiopulmonary arrest. *Treatment:* Discontinue therapy, monitor clinical status, and provide supportive therapy.

Drug Interactions

Aminoglycosides / Additive nephrotoxicity and/or ototoxicity

Antineoplastic drugs / ↑ Risk for renal toxicity, bronchospasm, and hypotension

Corticosteroids, Corticotropin / ↑ Potassium depletion caused by amphotericin B → cardiac dysfunction

Cyclosporine / ↑ Renal toxicity

Digitalis glycosides / ↑ Potassium depletion caused by amphotericin B → ↑ incidence of digitalis toxicity

Flucytosine / ↑ Risk of flucytosine toxicity due to ↑ cellular uptake or ↓ renal excretion

Nephrotoxic drugs / ↑ Risk of nephrotoxicity

Skeletal muscle relaxants, surgical (e.g., succinylcholine, *d*-tubocurarine) / ↑ Muscle relaxation due to amphotericin B-induced hypokalemia

Tacrolimus / ↑ Serum creatinine levels

Thiazides / ↑ Electrolyte depletion, especially potassium

Zidovudine (AZT) / ↑ Risk of myelotoxicity and nephrotoxicity

How Supplied: *Cream:* 3%; *Lotion:* 3%. Oral Suspension.

Dosage

- **Amphotericin B deoxycholate,**
- **Amphotericin B Deoxycholate Suspension**

Oral candidiasis.

Swish the suspension in the mouth and then swallow.

- **Topical (Lotion, Cream, Ointment—Each 3%)**

Apply liberally to affected areas b.i.d.-q.i.d. Depending on the type of lesion, up to 4 weeks of therapy may be necessary.

HEALTH CARE CONSIDERATIONS

See also *General Health Care Considerations for All Anti-Infectives.*

Administration/Storage

1. Rub creams and lotions into lesion.
2. The cream may cause drying and slight skin discoloration; the lotion and ointment may cause staining of nail lesions, but not skin.

Assessment

1. Assess for any adverse effects and hypersensitivity reactions.
2. Note mental status and age.
3. Describe characteristics of any lesions requiring therapy.
4. Review list of drugs prescribed to ensure none interact unfavorably.
5. Obtain CBC, liver and renal function, and cultures.

Interventions

1. Ensure prescribed form is prepared correctly for administration.
2. Premedicate with antipyretics, antihistamines, corticosteroids, and/or antiemetic drugs to reduce side effects. Rashes, fevers, and chills may occur with this therapy.

Client/Family Teaching

1. Report any anorexia, N&V, headache, rashes, fever, or chills.
2. Amphotericin therapy usually requires long-term treatments (6-11 weeks) to ensure an adequate response and to prevent any relapse.
3. Neurologic symptoms such as tinnitus, blurred vision, or vertigo should be reported immediately.
4. Guidelines for therapy with creams and lotions:
- Does not stain skin when rubbed into lesion.
- Any discoloration of fabric caused by cream or lotion may be removed by washing with soap and water.
- Discoloration of clothing caused by ointment may be removed with a standard cleaning fluid.
- Report any worsening of condition, lack of response, itching, burning, or rash.
- Do not apply an occlusive dressing as this may promote yeast growth.

Outcome/Evaluate

- Resolution of fungal infection
- Reduction in number of lesions
- Symptomatic improvement

Ampicillin oral

(am-pih-**SILL**-in)

Pregnancy Category: B

Jaa Amp ✱, Marcillin, Novo-Ampicillin ✱, Omnipen, Penbritin ✱, Principen, Totacillin **(Rx)**

NOTE: The following Canadian drugs are ampicillin trihydrate: Apo-Ampi, Jaa Amp, Nu-Ampi, Pro-Ampi, Taro-Ampicillin.

—COMBINATION DRUG—

Ampicillin with Probenecid

(am-pih-**SILL**-in, proh-**BEN**-ih-sid)

Pro-Biosan ✱ **(Rx)**

Ampicillin sodium, parenteral

(am-pih-**SILL**-in)

Pregnancy Category: B

Ampicin ✱, Omnipen-N **(Rx)**

Classification: Antibiotic, penicillin

See also *Anti-Infectives* and *Penicillins.*

Content: The Powder for Oral Suspension of Ampicillin with Probenecid contains 3.5 g ampicillin and 1 g probenecid per bottle.

Action/Kinetics: Synthetic, broad-spectrum antibiotic suitable for gram-negative bacteria. Acid resistant, destroyed by penicillinase. Absorbed more slowly than other penicillins. From 30% to 60% of PO dose absorbed from GI tract. **Peak serum levels: PO:** 1.8-2.9 mcg/mL after 2 hr; **IM,** 4.5-7 mcg/mL. **t½:** 80 min—range 50-110 min. Partially inactivated in liver; 25%-85% excreted unchanged in urine.

Uses: Infections of respiratory, GI, and GU tracts caused by *Shigella, Salmonella, Escherichia coli, Hemophilus influenzae, Proteus* strains, *Neisseria gonorrhoeae, N. meningitidis,* and *Enterococcus.* Also, otitis media in children, bronchitis, rat-bite fever, and whooping cough. Penicillin G-sensitive staphylococci, streptococci, pneumococci.

Additional Drug Interactions

Allopurinol / ↑ Incidence of skin rashes

Ampicillin / ↓ Effect of oral contraceptives

How Supplied: Ampicillin oral: *Capsule:* 250 mg, 500 mg; *Powder for reconstitution:* 125 mg/5 mL, 250 mg/5 mL. Ampicillin with Probenecid: See Content. Ampicillin sodium, parenteral: *Powder for injection:* 125 mg, 250 mg, 500 mg, 1 g, 2 g, 10 g

Dosage

• **Ampicillin: Capsules, Oral Suspension; Ampicillin Sodium: IV, IM**

Respiratory tract and soft tissue infections. **PO: 20 kg or more:** 250 mg q 6 hr; **less than 20 kg:** 50 mg/kg/day in equally divided doses q 6-8 hr. **IV, IM: 40 kg or more:** 250-500 mg q 6 hr; **less than 40 kg:** 25-50 mg/kg/day in equally divided doses q 6-8 hr.

Bacterial meningitis.
Adults and children: 150-200 mg/kg/day in divided doses q 3 to 4 hr. Initially give IV drip, followed by IM q 3 to 4 hr.

Bacterial endocarditis prophylaxis (dental, oral, or upper respiratory tract procedures).
Clients at moderate risk or those unable to take PO medications: **Adults, IM, IV:** 2 g 30 min prior to procedure; **children:** 50 mg/kg, 30 min prior to procedure. Clients at high risk: **Adults, IM, IV:** 2 g ampicillin plus gentamicin, 1.5 mg/kg, given 30 min before procedure followed in 6 hr by ampicillin, 1 g IM or IV, or amoxicillin, 1 g PO. **Children, IM, IV:** Ampicillin, 50 mg/kg, plus gentamicin, 1.5 mg/kg, 30 min prior to procedure followed in 6 hr by ampicillin, 25 mg/kg IM or IV, or amoxicillin, 25 mg/kg PO.

Septicemia.
Adults/children: 150-200 mg/kg/day, IV for first 3 days, then IM q 3-4 hr.

GI and GU infections, other than N. gonorrhea.
Adults/children, more than 20 kg: 500 mg PO q 6 hr. Use larger doses, if needed, for severe or chronic infections. **Children, less than 20 kg:** 100 mg/kg/day q 6 hr.

N. gonorrhea infections.
PO: Single dose of 3.5 g given together with probenecid, 1 g. **Parenteral, Adults/children over 40 kg:** 500 mg IV or IM q 6 hr. **Children, less than 40 kg:** 50 mg/kg/day IV or IM in equally divided doses q 6 to 8 hr.

Urethritis in males caused by N. gonorrhea.
Parenteral, males over 40 kg: Two 500 mg doses IV or IM at an interval of 8 to 12 hr. Repeat treatment if necessary. In complicated gonorrheal urethritis, prolonged and intensive therapy is recommended.

• **Ampicillin with Probenecid: Oral Suspension**

Urethral, endocervical, or rectal infections due to N. gonorrhoeae.
Adults: 3.5 g ampicillin and 1 g probenecid as a single dose.

Prophylaxis of infection in rape victims.
3.5 g with 1 g probenecid.

HEALTH CARE CONSIDERATIONS

See also *Health Care Considerations* for *Penicillins.*

Administration/Storage

1. Reconstituted PO solution is stable for 7 days at room temperature, not exceeding 25°C (77°F) or 14 days refrigerated.
2. For IM use, dilute only with sterile water for injection or bacteriostatic water for injection.
3. If the C_{CR} is less than 10 mL/min, the dosing interval should be increased to 12 hr.
IV 4. After reconstitution for IM or direct IV administration, the solution **must be used within the hour**.
5. For IVPB, ampicillin may be reconstituted with NaCl injection.
6. Give IV injections of reconstituted sodium ampicillin slowly over at least 10-15 min.
7. For administration by IV drip, check compatibility and length of time that drug retains potency in a particular solution.

Assessment

1. Record indications for therapy, type, onset, and duration of symptoms.
2. Note history of sensitivity/reactions to this drug or related drugs.
3. Monitor CBC, cultures, liver and renal function studies.
4. Advise that IM route may be painful; rotate and document injection sites.
5. Monitor urinary output and serum K^+ levels, especially in the elderly.

Client/Family Teaching

1. Take medication 1 hr before or 2 hr after meals.
2. Review the appropriate method for administration and storage.
3. Take for the prescribed number of days even if the symptoms subside.
4. Ampicillin chewable tablets should not be swallowed whole.
5. Do not save for future use or share with family members/friends who have similar symptoms.
6. May decrease effectiveness of oral contraceptives; use additional contraception during therapy.
7. Report any "ampicillin rashes"; a dull, red, itchy, flat or raised rash occurs more often with this drug than with other penicillins and is usually benign. If a late skin rash develops with symptoms of fever, fatigue, sore throat, generalized lymphadenopathy, and

A

enlarged spleen, a heterophil antibody test may be considered to rule out mononucleosis.

Outcome/Evaluate

- Resolution of S&S of infection; symptomatic improvement
- Negative culture reports

Amyl nitrite

(AM-ill)

Pregnancy Category: X

Amyl Nitrite Aspirols, Amyl Nitrite Vaporole **(Rx)**

Classification: Coronary vasodilator, antidote for cyanide poisoning

See also *Antianginal Drugs—Nitrates/Nitrites.*

Action/Kinetics: Believed to act by reducing systemic and PA pressure (afterload) and by decreasing CO due to peripheral vasodilation. Vascular relaxation occurs due to stimulation of intracellular cyclic guanosine monophosphate. As an antidote to cyanide poisoning, amyl nitrite promotes formation of methemoglobin which combines with cyanide to form the nontoxic cyanmethemoglobin. **Onset (inhalation):** 30 sec. **Duration:** 3-5 min. About 33% is excreted through the kidneys.

Uses: Prophylaxis or relief of acute attacks of angina pectoris; acute cyanide poisoning. *Investigational:* Diagnostic aid to assess reserve cardiac function.

Contraindications: Lactation.

Special Concerns: Use in children has not been studied. Hypotensive effects are more likely to occur in geriatric clients.

How Supplied: *Solution*

Dosage

- **Inhalation**

Angina pectoris.

Usual: 0.3 mL (1 container crushed). Usually, 1-6 inhalations from one container produces relief. Dosage may be repeated after 3-5 min.

Antidote for cyanide poisoning.

Administer for 30-60 sec q 5 min until client is conscious; is then repeated at longer intervals for up to 24 hr.

HEALTH CARE CONSIDERATIONS

See also *Health Care Considerations* for *Antianginal Drugs—Nitrates/Nitrites.*

Administration/Storage

1. Administer only by inhalation.
2. Protect containers from light, store at 15°C-30°C (59°F-86°F).
3. *Amyl nitrite vapors are highly flammable. Do not use near flame or intense heat.*

Assessment

1. List precipitating incidents that precede onset of chest pain.
2. Record degree, location, radiation, type, and duration of pain.
3. Identify cardiac risk factors.
4. With cyanide poisoning, note source and presenting symptoms.

Client/Family Teaching

1. Mutually set goals of therapy.
2. Identify changes in lifestyle that may reduce need for drug.
3. Enclose fabric-covered ampule in a handkerchief or piece of cloth and crush by hand.
4. Sit or lie down during inhalation to avoid hypotension.
5. Drug has a pungent odor, but several deep breaths must nevertheless be taken to attain drug effects.
6. Drug is inactivated when exposed to heat.
7. Always store medication out of reach of children.
8. The medication has the potential for abuse (sexual stimulant) and must be stored appropriately.

Outcome/Evaluate

- Improved tissue perfusion with termination of angina attack
- Antidote for cyanide poisoning

Anagrelide hydrochloride

(an-AG-greh-lyd)

Pregnancy Category: C

Agrylin **(Rx)**

Classification: Antiplatelet drug

Action/Kinetics: May act to reduce platelets by decreasing megakaryocyte hypermaturation. Does not cause significant changes in white cell counts or coagulation parameters. Inhibits platelet aggregation at higher doses than needed to reduce platelet count. **Peak plasma levels:** 5 ng/mL at 1 hr. **t½:** 1.3 hr; **terminal t½:** About 3 days. Metabolized in liver and excreted in urine and feces.

Uses: Reduce platelet count in essential thrombocythemia.

Contraindications: Lactation.

Special Concerns: Use with caution in known or suspected heart disease and in impaired renal or hepatic function. Safety and efficacy have not been determined in those less than 16 years of age.

Side Effects: *CV:* CHF, palpitations, chest pain, tachycardia, arrhythmias, angina, postural hypotension, hypertension, cardiovascular disease, vasodilation, migraine, syncope, ***MI,***

cardiomyopathy, complete heart block, fibrillation, CVA, pericarditis, hemorrhage, heart failure, cardiomegaly, atrial fibrillation. *GI:* Diarrhea, abdominal pain, pancreatitis, gastric/duodenal ulcers, N&V, flatulence, anorexia, constipation, GI distress, ***GI hemorrhage,*** gastritis, melena, aphthous stomatitis, eructations. *Respiratory:* Rhinitis, epistaxis, respiratory disease, sinusitis, pneumonia, bronchitis, asthma, pulmonary infiltrate, ***pulmonary fibrosis, pulmonary hypertension,*** dyspnea. *CNS:* Headache, ***seizures,*** dizziness, paresthesia, depression, somnolence, confusion, insomnia, nervousness, amnesia. *Musculoskeletal:* Arthralgia, myalgia, leg cramps. *Dermatologic:* Pruritus, skin disease, alopecia, rash, urticaria. *Hematologic:* Anemia, thrombocytopenia, ecchymosis, lymphadenoma. *Body as a whole:* Fever, flu symptoms, chills, photosensitivity, dehydration, malaise, asthenia, edema, pain. *Ophthalmic:* Amblyopia, abnormal vision, visual field abnormality, diplopia. *Miscellaneous:* Back pain, tinnitus.

Laboratory Test Considerations: ↑ Liver enzymes.

OD **Management of Overdose:** *Symptoms:* Thrombocytopenia. *Treatment:* Close clinical monitoring. Decrease or stop dose until platelet count returns to within the normal range.

How Supplied: *Capsules:* 0.5 mg

Dosage

- **Capsules**

  Essential thrombocythemia.

Initial: 0.5 mg q.i.d. or 1 mg b.i.d. Maintain for one week or more. **Then,** adjust to lowest effective dose to maintain platelet count less than 600,000/mcL. Can increase the dose by 0.5 mg or less/day in any 1 week. **Maximum dose:** 10 mg/day or 2.5 mg in single dose. Most respond at a dose of 1.5 to 3 mg/day.

HEALTH CARE CONSIDERATIONS

Assessment

1. Record cause; record onset and duration of thrombocythemia.
2. Note any CAD, liver or renal dysfunction; document cardiovascular assessment and monitor closely.
3. Monitor VS, CBC, liver and renal function; check platelets every 2 days during first week and then weekly thereafter until stabilized.
4. Determine if pregnant.

Client/Family Teaching

1. Take exactly as directed.
2. Drug is used to lower platelet counts. Increases usually occur within 4 days after interruption of therapy.
3. Practice reliable contraception; may cause fetal harm.
4. Report any palpitations, SOB, dizziness, chest or abdominal pain or unusual bleeding.

Outcome/Evaluate: Reduction in platelet counts; ↓ risk of thrombosis

Anastrozole

((an-**AS**-troh-zohl))

Pregnancy Category: D

Arimidex **(Rx)**

Classification: Antineoplastic, hormone

See also *Antineoplastic Agents*.

Action/Kinetics: Growth of many breast cancers is due to stimulation of estrogen receptors by estrogens. In postmenopausal women the main source of circulating estrogen is conversion of androstenedione to estrone by aromatase in peripheral tissues with further conversion to estradiol. Anastrozole is a nonsteroidal aromatase inhibitor that significantly decreases serum estradiol levels. Has no effect on formation of adrenal corticosteroids or aldosterone. Well absorbed from the GI tract; food does not affect the extent of absorption. **t½, terminal:** 50 hr. Metabolized by the liver and both unchanged drug (about 10%) and metabolites are excreted through the urine.

Uses: Advanced breast cancer in postmenopausal women with progression of the disease following tamoxifen therapy. *NOTE:* Clients with negative tumor estrogen receptors and those who do not respond to tamoxifen are rarely helped by anastrozole.

Special Concerns: Use with caution during lactation. Safety and efficacy have not been determined in children.

Side Effects: *GI:* N&V, diarrhea, constipation, abdominal pain, anorexia, dry mouth, increased appetite. *CNS:* Headache, paresthesia, dizziness, depression, somnolence, confusion, insomnia, anxiety, nervousness. *CV:* Hypertension, thromboembolic disease, thrombophlebitis. *Musculoskeletal:* Asthenia, back pain, bone pain, myalgia, arthralgia, pathological fracture. *Respiratory:* Dyspnea, increased cough, pharyngitis, sinusitis, bronchitis, rhinitis. *Dermatologic:* Hot flushes, rash, sweating, hair thinning, pruritus. *GU:* Vaginal hemorrhage, UTI, breast pain, vaginal dryness, vaginal bleeding during first few weeks after changing from hormone therapy. *Hematologic:* Anemia, leukopenia.

A

Miscellaneous: Pain, peripheral edema, pelvic pain, chest pain, weight gain or loss, flu syndrome, fever, neck pain, malaise, accidental injury, infection.
Laboratory Test Considerations: ↑ GGT, AST, ALT, alkaline phosphatase, total cholesterol, LDL cholesterol.
How Supplied: *Tablet:* 1 mg

Dosage

- **Tablets**

Advanced breast cancer.
1 mg daily.

HEALTH CARE CONSIDERATIONS

See also *Health Care Considerations* for *Antineoplastic Agents.*
Administration/Storage: Glucocorticoid or mineralocorticoid therapy is not required.
Assessment
1. Record and record disease progression and last tamoxifen therapy.
2. Obtain baseline CBC, liver and renal function studies and negative pregnancy test.
Client/Family Teaching
1. Take as directed at the same time each day.
2. Use reliable birth control; drug may cause fetal harm and impair fertility.
Outcome/Evaluate: Control of malignant cell proliferation

Atenolol

(ah-TEN-oh-lohl)
Pregnancy Category: C
Apo-Atenol ✱, Dom-Atenolol ✱, Gen-Atenolol ✱, Med-Atenolol ✱, Novo-Atenol ✱, Nu-Atenol ✱, Scheinpharm Atenolol ✱, Taro-Atenolol ✱, Tenolin ✱, Tenormin **(Rx)**
Classification: Beta-adrenergic blocking agent

See also *Beta-Adrenergic Blocking Agents.*
Action/Kinetics: Predominantly beta-1 blocking activity. Has no membrane stabilizing activity or intrinsic sympathomimetic activity. Low lipid solubility. **Peak blood levels:** 2-4 hr. **t½:** 6-9 hr. 50% eliminated unchanged in the feces.
Uses: Hypertension (either alone or with other antihypertensives such as thiazide diuretics). Angina pectoris due to hypertension, coronary atherosclerosis, and AMI. *Investigational:* Prophylaxis of migraine, alcohol withdrawal syndrome, situational anxiety, ventricular arrhythmias, prophylactically to reduce incidence of supraventricular arrhythmias in coronary artery bypass surgery.
Special Concerns: Dosage not established in children.
How Supplied: *Injection:* 0.5 mg/mL; *Tablet:* 25 mg, 50 mg, 100 mg

Dosage

- **Tablets**

Hypertension.
Initial: 50 mg/day, either alone or with diuretics; if response is inadequate, 100 mg/day. Doses higher than 100 mg/day will not produce further beneficial effects. Maximum effects usually seen within 1-2 weeks.
Angina.
Initial: 50 mg/day; if maximum response is not seen in 1 week, increase dose to 100 mg/day (some clients require 200 mg/day).
Alcohol withdrawal syndrome.
50-100 mg/day.
Prophylaxis of migraine.
50-100 mg/day.
Ventricular arrhythmias.
50-100 mg/day.
Prior to coronary artery bypass surgery.
50 mg/day started 72 hr prior to surgery.
Adjust dosage in cases of renal failure to 50 mg/day if C_{CR} is 15-35 mL/min/1.73 m² and to 50 mg every other day if C_{CR} is less than 15 mL/min/1.73 m².

- **IV**

Acute myocardial infarction.
Initial: 5 mg over 5 min followed by a second 5-mg dose 10 min later. Begin treatment as soon as possible after client arrives at the hospital. In clients who tolerate the full 10-mg dose, give a 50-mg tablet 10 min after the last IV dose followed by another 50-mg dose 12 hr later. **Then,** 100 mg/day or 50 mg b.i.d. for 6-9 days (or until discharge from the hospital).

HEALTH CARE CONSIDERATIONS

See also *Health Care Considerations* for *Antihypertensive Agents* and *Beta-Adrenergic Blocking Agents.*
Administration/Storage
1. For hemodialysis clients, give 50 mg in the hospital after each dialysis.
IV 2. For IV use, the drug may be diluted in NaCl injection, dextrose injection, or both.
Assessment
1. Record indications for therapy, type, and onset of symptoms.
2. Note any history of diabetes, pulmonary disease, or cardiac failure.
Client/Family Teaching
1. With angina, do not stop abruptly; may cause an anginal attack.
2. Report any changes in mood or affect, especially severe depression.
3. May enhance sensitivity to cold.
4. With initiation of therapy or change in

dosage stress importance of returning as scheduled for evaluation of drug response.

Outcome/Evaluate

- ↓ BP; ↓ HR
- ↓ Frequency of anginal attacks
- Prevention of reinfarction

Atorvastatin calcium

((ah-**TORE**-vah-**stah**-tin))

Pregnancy Category: X

Lipitor **(Rx)**

Classification: Antihyperlipidemic, HMG-CoA reductase inhibitor

See also *Antihyperlipidemic Agents—HMG-CoA Reductase Inhibitors.*

Action/Kinetics: Undergoes first-pass metabolism. **t½:** 14 hr. Over 98% bound to plasma proteins. Plasma levels are not affected by renal disease but they are markedly increased with chronic alcoholic liver disease.

Uses: Adjunct to diet to reduce elevated total and LDL cholesterol levels in primary hypercholesterolemia (Types IIa and IIb) when the response to diet and other nondrug measures alone have been inadequate. With changes in diet in clients with high triglyceride or fat levels. Treat dysbetalipoproteinemia in those with inadequate response to diet changes.

Contraindications: Active liver disease or unexplained persistently high liver function tests. Pregnancy, lactation.

Special Concerns: Safety and efficacy have not been determined in children less than 18 years of age.

Side Effects: See also *Antihyperlipidemic Agents—HMG-CoA Reductase Inhibitors. GI:* Altered liver function tests (usually within the first 3 months of therapy), flatulence, dyspepsia. *CNS:* Headache. *Musculoskeletal:* Myalgia. *Miscellaneous:* Infection, rash, pruritus, allergy.

Laboratory Test Considerations: ↑ CPK (due to myalgia).

Drug Interactions

Antacids / ↓ Atorvastatin plasma levels
Colestipol / ↓ Plasma levels of atorvastatin
Erythromycin / ↑ Plasma levels of atorvastatin; possibility of severe myopathy or rhabdomyolysis
Oral contraceptives / ↑ Plasma levels of norethindrone and ethinyl estradiol

How Supplied: *Tablets:* 10 mg, 20 mg, 40 mg

Dosage

- **Tablets**

  Hyperlipidemia.

  Initial: 10 mg/day; **then,** a dose range of 10-80 mg/day may be used.

HEALTH CARE CONSIDERATIONS

See also *Health Care Considerations* for *Antihyperlipidemic Agents—HMG-CoA Reductase Inhibitors.*

Administration/Storage

1. Give as a single dose at any time of the day, with or without food.
2. Determine lipid levels within 2-4 weeks; adjust dosage accordingly.
3. For an additive effect, may be used in combination with a bile acid binding resin. Do not use atorvastatin with fibrates.

Assessment

1. Record indications for therapy, onset and duration of disease, and other agents and measures trialed.
2. Obtain baseline cholesterol profile and LFTs. Monitor LFTs at 6 and 12 weeks after starting therapy and with any dosage change then semiannually thereafter. If ALT or AST exceed 3 times the normal level, reduce dose or withdraw drug. Assess need for liver biopsy if elevations remain after stopping drug therapy.
3. Review dietary habits, weight, and exercise patterns; identify life-style changes needed.

Client/Family Teaching

1. These drugs help to lower blood cholesterol and fat levels, which have been proven to promote CAD.
2. Drug may be taken with or without food.
3. Continue dietary restrictions of saturated fat and cholesterol, regular exercise and weight loss in the overall goal of lowering cholesterol levels. See dietician for additional dietary recommendations.
4. Report immediately any unexplained muscle pain, weakness, or tenderness, especially if accompanied by fever or malaise.
5. Use UV protection (i.e., sunglasses, sunscreens, clothing/hat) to prevent photosensitivity.
6. Report for lab studies to evaluate effectiveness and need for dosage adjustments.

Outcome/Evaluate: Reduction in total and LDL cholesterol levels

Atovaquone

(ah-**TOV**-ah-kwohn)

Pregnancy Category: C

Mepron **(Rx)**

Classification: Antiprotozoal agent

A

Action/Kinetics: The mechanism of action of atovaquone against *Pneumocystis carinii* is not known. However, in *Plasmodium,* appears to act by inhibiting electron transport resulting in inhibition of nucleic acid and ATP synthesis. The bioavailability of the drug is increased twofold when taken with food. Plasma levels in AIDS clients are about one-third to one-half the levels achieved in asymptomatic HIV-infected volunteers. **t½:** 2.2 days in AIDS clients due to enterohepatic cycling and eventually fecal elimination. Not metabolized in the liver; over 94% is excreted unchanged in the feces.
Uses: Acute oral treatment of mild to moderate *P. carinii* in clients who are intolerant to trimethoprim-sulfamethoxazole. Has not been evaluated as an agent for prophylaxis of *P. carinii.* Not effective for concurrent pulmonary diseases such as bacterial, viral, or fungal pneumonia or in mycobacterial diseases.
Contraindications: Hypersensitivity to atovaquone or any components of the formulation; potentially life-threatening allergic reactions are possible.
Special Concerns: Use with caution during lactation and in elderly clients. There are no efficacy studies in children. GI disorders may limit absorption of atovaquone.
Side Effects: Since many clients taking atovaquone have complications of HIV disease, it is often difficult to distinguish side effects caused by atovaquone from symptoms caused by the underlying medical condition. *Dermatologic:* Rash (including maculopapular), pruritus. *GI:* Nausea, diarrhea, vomiting, abdominal pain, constipation, dyspepsia, taste perversion. *CNS:* Headache, fever, insomnia, dizziness, anxiety, anorexia. *Respiratory:* Cough, sinusitis, rhinitis. *Hematologic:* Anemia, neutropenia. *Miscellaneous:* Asthenia, oral monilia, pain, sweating, hypoglycemia, hypotension, hyperglycemia, hyponatremia.
Laboratory Test Considerations: ↑ ALT, AST, alkaline phosphatase, amylase.
Drug Interactions: Since atovaquone is highly bound to plasma proteins (>99.9%), caution should be exercised when giving the drug with other highly plasma protein-bound drugs with narrow therapeutic indices as competition for binding may occur.
How Supplied: *Suspension:* 750 mg/5 mL

Dosage

- **Suspension**

Adults: 750 mg (5 mL) given with food b.i.d. for 21 days (total daily dose: 1,500 mg).

HEALTH CARE CONSIDERATIONS

Administration/Storage

1. Failure to give the drug with food may result in lower plasma levels and may limit the response to therapy.
2. Dispense drug in a well-closed container and store at 15°C -25°C (59°F -77°F).

Assessment

1. Record previous therapy for *P. carinii,* drugs used, and results.
2. Assess baseline pulmonary status, CBC, and pulmonary culture results.
3. Clients with acute *P. carinii* must be carefully evaluated/screened for other related pulmonary diseases of viral, bacterial, or fungal origin and treated with additional drugs as appropriate.

Client/Family Teaching

1. This is not a cure but alleviates symptoms of *P. carinii.*
2. Take only as directed and with meals as food enhances absorption.
3. Review side effects noting those that require immediate reporting.
4. Do not exceed prescribed dose and do not share medication.
5. Continue precautions for safe sex, as the risk of HIV transmission is not reduced.
6. Identify appropriate support groups and individuals to assist the client/family to understand and cope with disease.

Outcome/Evaluate: Relief of symptoms R/T *Pneumocystis carinii*; three consecutive negative sputum cultures

COMBINATION DRUG

Atovaquone and proguanil

(ah-**TOH**-vah-kwohn and proh-**GWAHN**-ill)

Pregnancy Category: C
Malarone **(Rx)**
Classification: Antimalarial agent

Content: Adult Tablet contains atovaquone 250 mg and proguanil hydrochloride 100 mg. Pediatric tablet contains atovaquone 62.5 mg and proguanil hydrochloride 25 mg
Action/Kinetics: Atovaquone: Selectively inhibits parasite mitochondrial electron transport. Proguanil: The metabolite cycloguanil inhibits dihydrofolate reductase, disrupting deoxythymidylate synthesis. Atovaquone/cycloquanil, together, affect the erythrocytic and exoerythrocytic stages of development. Proguanil is metabolized in the liver to an active metabolite, cycloguanil (via CYP2C19) and 4-chlorophenylbiguanide. **t½:** Atovaquone: 2-3 days in adults, 1-2 days in children; proguanil: 12-21 hours. Elimination: atova-

quone 94% in feces: proguanil 40 to 60% in kidneys.

Uses: Prevention or treatment of acute, uncomplicated *P. falciparum* malaria.

Contraindications: Known hypersensitivity to atovaquone, proguanil, or any component.

Special Concerns: Not indicated for severe or complicated malaria. Patients experiencing diarrhea or vomiting may have decreased absorption of atovaquone: monitor closely and consider use of an antiemetic. If severe GI upset, consider use of another antimalarial medication. Do not use with other medications containing proguanil. Give with caution to patients having pre-existing renal disease. Not for use in patients weighing <11 kg. Delayed cases of *P. falciparum* malaria may occur after stopping preventive treatment; travelers returning from malaria endemic areas who develop febrile illnesses should be evaluated for malaria. Recurrent infections or infections following preventive treatment with this medication should be treated with alternative medication(s).

Side Effects: The following adverse reactions were reported in >5% of adults taking atovaquone/proguanil in treatment doses: *GI:* Abdominal pain (17%), nausea (12%), vomiting (12% in adults, 10% to 13% in children), diarrhea (8%), anorexia (5%). *CNS:* Headache (10%), dizziness (5%). *Dermatologic:* Pruritus (6% children). *Musculoskeletal:* Weakness (8%).

Drug Interactions

Proguanil: CYP2C19 substrate, Metoclopramide / ↓ bioavailability of atovaquone

Rifampin / ↓ atovaquone levels by 50%

Tetracycline / ↓ atovaquone by 40%.

How Supplied: See Content.

Dosage

- **Tablet**

Prevention of malaria.

Children (dosage based on body weight): Start 1-2 days prior to entering a malaria-endemic area. Continue throughout the stay and for 7 days after returning. Take as a single dose, once daily. *11-20 kg:* Atovaquone/proguanil 62.5 mg/25 mg; *21-30 kg:* Atovaquone/proguanil 125 mg/50 mg; *31-40 kg:* Atovaquone/proguanil 187.5 mg/75 mg; *>40 kg:* Atovaquone/proguanil 250 mg/100 mg. **Adults:** Atovaquone/proguanil 250 mg/100 mg once daily. Start 1-2 days prior to entering a malaria-endemic area. Continue throughout the stay and for 7 days after returning.

Treatment of acute malaria.

Children: Take as a single dose, once daily for 3 consecutive days. *11-20 kg:* Atovaquone/proguanil 250 mg/100 mg; *21-30 kg:* Atovaquone/proguanil 500 mg/200 mg; *31-40 kg:* Atovaquone/proguanil 750 mg/300 mg; *>40 kg:* Atovaquone/proguanil 1 g/400 mg. **Adults:** Atovaquone/proguanil 1 g/400 mg as a single dose, once daily for 3 consecutive days. *NOTE:* See administration category.

HEALTH CARE CONSIDERATIONS

Administration/Storage

1. Store at 25°C (77°F).
2. This medication should be taken with food or milk at the same time each day.
3. If the patient vomits within 1 hour of taking the medicine, repeat the dose.

Assessment

1. Record reasons for treatment.
2. If due to actual onset of malaria, record onset of signs and symtoms, duration of illness, and any previous drugs taken.
3. This drug should not be used if previously used for prevention of malaria.

Client/Family Teaching

1. This medication is used to treat or prevent malaria.
2. This medication should be taken with food or milk at the same time each day. If vomiting occurs within one hour of taking the medicine, the dose should be repeated.
3. When traveling to malaria-endemic areas, wear protective clothing and use insect repellents and bednets to help prevent exposure to mosquitos.
4. Patients should notify their healthcare provider if a fever develops during or after travel to a malaria-endemic area.

Outcome/Evaluate: In preventive treatment, patient does not develop signs or symptoms of malaria. In use for treatment of active malaria, improvement of signs and symptoms within 4 to 5 days after starting therapy.

Atropine sulfate

(AH-troh-peen)

Pregnancy Category: C

Atropair, Atropine-1 Ophthalmic, Atropine Sulfate Ophthalmic, Atropine-Care Ophthalmic, Atropisol Ophthalmic, Isopto Atropine Ophthalmic, Minims Atropine ✦ **(Rx)**

Classification: Cholinergic blocking agent

See also *Cholinergic Blocking Agents.*

Action/Kinetics: Atropine blocks the action of acetylcholine on postganglionic cholinergic receptors in smooth muscle, cardiac muscle, exocrine glands, urinary bladder, and the AV and SA nodes in the heart. Ophthalmologically, atropine blocks the effect of acetylcholine on the sphincter muscle of the iris and the accommodative muscle of the ciliary body. This results in dilation of the pupil (mydriasis) and paralysis of the muscles required to accommodate for close vision (cycloplegia). **Peak effect:** *Mydriasis,* 30-40 min; *cycloplegia,* 1-3 hr. **Recovery:** Up to 12 days. **Duration, PO:** 4-6 hr. **t½:** 2.5 hr. Metabolized by the liver although 30%-50% is excreted through the kidneys unchanged.

Uses: PO: Adjunct in peptic ulcer treatment. Irritable bowel syndrome. Adjunct in treatment of spastic disorders of the biliary tract. Urologic disorders, urinary incontinence. During anesthesia to control salivation and bronchial secretions. Has been used for parkinsonism but more effective drugs are available.

Parenteral: Antiarrhythmic, adjunct in GI radiography. Prophylaxis of arrhythmias induced by succinylcholine or surgical procedures. Reduce sinus bradycardia (severe) and syncope in hyperactive carotid sinus reflex. Prophylaxis and treatment of toxicity due to cholinesterase inhibitors, including organophosphate pesticides. Treatment of curariform block. As a preanesthetic or in dentistry to decrease secretions.

Ophthalmologic: Cycloplegic refraction or pupillary dilation in acute inflammatory conditions of the iris and uveal tract. *Investigational:* Treatment and prophylaxis of posterior synechiae; pre- and postoperative mydriasis; treatment of malignant glaucoma.

Additional Contraindications: Ophthalmic use: Infants less than 3 months of age, primary glaucoma or a tendency toward glaucoma, adhesions between the iris and the lens, geriatric clients and others where undiagnosed glaucoma or excessive pressure in the eye may be present, in children who have had a previous severe systemic reaction to atropine.

Special Concerns: Use with caution in infants, small children, geriatric clients, diabetes, hypo- or hyperthyroidism, narrow anterior chamber angle, individuals with Down syndrome.

Additional Side Effects: *Ophthalmologic:* Blurred vision, stinging, increased intraocular pressure, contact dermatitis. Long-term use may cause irritation, photophobia, eczematoid dermatitis, conjunctivitis, hyperemia, or edema.

OD **Management of Overdose:** *Treatment of Ocular Overdose:* Eyes should be flushed with water or normal saline. A topical miotic may be necessary.

How Supplied: *Injection:* 0.05 mg/mL, 0.1 mg/mL, 0.4 mg/mL, 0.5 mg/mL, 0.8 mg/mL, 1 mg/mL; *Ophthalmic Ointment:* 1%; *Ophthalmic Solution:* 0.5%, 1%; *Tablet:* 0.4 mg

Dosage

- **Tablets**

Anticholinergic or antispasmodic.

Adults: 0.3-1.2 mg q 4-6 hr. **Pediatric, over 41 kg:** same as adult; **29.5-41 kg:** 0.4 mg q 4-6 hr; **18.2-29.5 kg:** 0.3 mg q 4-6 hr; **10.9-18.2 kg:** 0.2 mg q 4-6 hr; **7.3-10.9 kg:** 0.15 mg q 4-6 hr; **3.2-7.3 kg:** 0.1 mg q 4-6 hr.

Prophylaxis of respiratory tract secretions and excess salivation during anesthesia.

Adults: 2 mg.

Parkinsonism.

Adults: 0.1-0.25 mg q.i.d.

- **IM, IV, SC**

Anticholinergic.

Adults, IM, IV, SC: 0.4-0.6 mg q 4-6 hr. **Pediatric, SC:** 0.01 mg/kg, not to exceed 0.4 mg (or 0.3 mg/m^2).

To reverse curariform blockade.

Adults, IV: 0.6-1.2 mg given at the same time or a few minutes before 0.5-2 mg neostigmine methylsulfate (use separate syringes).

Treatment of toxicity from cholinesterase inhibitors.

Adults, IV, initial: 2-4 mg; **then,** 2 mg repeated q 5-10 min until muscarinic symptoms disappear and signs of atropine toxicity begin to appear. **Pediatric, IM, IV, initial:** 1 mg; **then,** 0.5-1 mg q 5-10 min until muscarinic symptoms disappear and signs of atropine toxicity appear.

Treatment of mushroom poisoning due to muscarine.

Adults, IM, IV: 1-2 mg q hr until respiratory effects decrease.

Treatment of organophosphate poisoning.

Adults, IM, IV, initial: 1-2 mg; **then,** repeat in 20-30 min (as soon as cyanosis has disappeared). Dosage may be continued for up to 2 days until symptoms improve.

Arrhythmias.

Pediatric, IV: 0.01-0.03 mg/kg.

Prophylaxis of respiratory tract secretions, excessive salivation, succinylcholine- or surgical procedure-induced arrhythmias.

Pediatric, up to 3 kg, SC: 0.1 mg; **7-9 kg:** 0.2 mg; **12-16 kg:** 0.3 mg; **20-27 kg:** 0.4 mg; **32 kg:** 0.5 mg; **41 kg:** 0.6 mg.

- **Ophthalmic Solution**

Uveitis.

Adults: 1-2 gtt instilled into the eye(s) up to q.i.d. **Children:** 1-2 gtt of the 0.5% solution into the eye(s) up to t.i.d.

Refraction.

Adults: 1-2 gtt of the 1% solution into the eye(s) 1 hr before refracting. **Children:** 1-2 gtt of the 0.5% solution into the eye(s) b.i.d. for 1-3 days before refraction.

• **Ophthalmic Ointment**

Instill a small amount into the conjunctival sac up to t.i.d.

HEALTH CARE CONSIDERATIONS

See also *Health Care Considerations* for *Cholinergic Blocking Agents.*

Administration/Storage

1. After instillation of the ophthalmic ointment, compress the lacrimal sac by digital pressure for 1-3 min. to decrease systemic effects.
2. Have physostigmine available in the event of overdose.

Assessment

1. Record indications for therapy and any presenting symptoms.
2. Check for any history of glaucoma before ophthalmic administration; may precipitate an acute crisis.
3. Obtain VS and ECG; monitor CP status during IV therapy.

Client/Family Teaching

1. When used in the eye, vision will be temporarily impaired. Close work, operating machinery, or driving a car should be avoided until drug effects have worn off.
2. Do not blink excessively; wait 5 min before instilling other drops.
3. Drug impairs heat regulation; avoid strenuous activity in hot environments; wear sunglasses.
4. Males with BPH may experience urinary retention and hesitancy.
5. Increase fluids and add bulk to diet to diminish constipating effects.
6. Use sugarless candies and gums to decrease dry mouth symptoms.

Outcome/Evaluate

- ↑ HR
- Desired pupillary dilatation
- ↓ GI activity; ↓ Salivation
- Reversal of muscarinic effects of anticholinesterase agents

Auranofin

(or-**AN**-oh-fin)

Pregnancy Category: C

Ridaura **(Rx)**

Classification: Antiarthritic, oral gold compound

Action/Kinetics: Auranofin is a gold-containing (29%) compound for PO administration. It has fewer side effects than injectable gold products. Although the mechanism is not known, auranofin will improve symptoms of rheumatoid arthritis; it is most effective in the early stages of active synovitis and may act by inhibiting sulfhydryl systems. Other possible mechanisms include inhibition of phagocytic activity of macrophages and polymorphonuclear leukocytes, alteration of biosynthesis of collagen, and alteration of the immune response. Gold will not reverse damage to joints caused by disease. Approximately 25% of an oral dose is absorbed. **Plasma t½ of auranofin gold:** 26 days. **Onset:** 3-4 months (up to 6 months in certain clients). Approximately 3 months are required for steady-state blood levels to be achieved. The drug is metabolized and excreted in both the urine and feces.

Uses: Adults and children with rheumatoid arthritis that have not responded to other drugs. Up to 6 months may be required for beneficial effects to occur. Auranofin should be part of a total treatment regimen for rheumatoid arthritis, including nondrug treatments.

Contraindications: History of gold-induced disorders including necrotizing enterocolitis, pulmonary fibrosis, exfoliative dermatitis, bone marrow aplasia, or other hematologic severe disorders. Use during lactation.

Special Concerns: Use with extreme caution in renal or hepatic disease, skin rashes, marked hypertension, compromised cerebral or CV circulation, or history of bone marrow depression (e.g., agranulocytopenia, anemia). Gold dermatitis may be aggravated by exposure to sunlight. Although used in children, a recommended dosage has not been established. Tolerance to gold is often decreased in geriatric clients.

Side Effects: *GI:* N&V, diarrhea (common), abdominal pain, metallic taste, stomatitis, glossitis, gingivitis, anorexia, constipation, flatulence, dyspepsia, dysgeusia, melena. Rarely, dysphagia, ***GI bleeding, ulcerative enterocolitis.*** *Dermatologic:* Skin rashes, pruritus, alopecia, urticaria, angioedema, actinic rash. *Hematologic:* Leukopenia, anemia, thrombocytopenia (with or without purpura), neutropenia, agranulocytosis, eosinophilia, pancytopenia, hypoplastic anemia, ***aplastic anemia,*** pure red cell aplasia. *Renal:* Proteinuria, hematuria. *Hepatic:* Jaundice (with or without cholestasis, hepatitis with jaundice, ***toxic hepatitis,*** intrahepatic cholestasis. *Other:* Conjunctivitis, cholestatic jaundice, fever, interstitial pneumonia and fibrosis, peripheral neuropathy.

Laboratory Test Considerations: ↑ Liver enzymes.

A

OD **Management of Overdose:** *Symptoms:* Rapid appearance of hematuria, proteinuria, thrombocytopenia, granulocytopenia. Also, N&V, diarrhea, fever, urticaria, papulovesicular lesions, urticaria, exfoliative dermatitis, pruritus. *Treatment:* Discontinue promptly and give dimercaprol. Supportive therapy should be provided for renal and hematologic symptoms. Treat moderately severe skin and mucous membrane symptoms with topical corticosteroids, oral antihistamines, and anesthetic lotions. Treat severe stomatitis or dermatitis with prednisone, 10-40 mg daily. Treat serious renal, hematologic, pulmonary, and enterocolitic complications with prednisone, 40-100 mg daily in divided doses. The duration of treatment varies, depending on the severity of symptoms and the response to steroids. In acute overdosage, induce emesis or perform gastric lavage immediately.

How Supplied: *Capsule:* 3 mg

Dosage

- **Capsules**

Rheumatoid arthritis.

Adults, initial: Either 6 mg/day or 3 mg b.i.d. If response is unsatisfactory after 6 months, increase to 3 mg t.i.d. If response is still inadequate after 3 additional months, discontinue the drug. Dosages greater than 9 mg/day are not recommended.

Children, initial: 0.1 mg/kg/day; **maintenance:** 0.15 mg/kg/day, not to exceed 0.2 mg/kg/day.

Transfer from injectable gold.

Discontinue injectable gold and begin auranofin at a dose of 6 mg/day.

HEALTH CARE CONSIDERATIONS

Administration/Storage: A positive response should be noted after 6 months of therapy.

Assessment

1. Review history, note any other severe systemic diseases such as renal, hepatic, or cardiac dysfunction.
2. Record extent of debilitation (functional class), pain level, ROM, and active synovitis.
3. Note onset, course of disease, other agents used, including disease-modifying agents, and results.
4. Assess for any skin eruptions.
5. Check gums and oral mucosa; note lesions or treatment needs.
6. Obtain baseline CBC, ESR, X rays, and liver and renal function studies.
7. Clients with diabetes mellitus or CHF should be well controlled before beginning gold therapy.

Interventions:

1. Determine if a dermal test dose has ever been performed with a gold salt.
2. Record I&O and weight.
3. If diarrhea develops, check electrolytes, report abnormalities.
4. Monitor renal and LFTs; check urine for protein and blood.
5. Observe for peripheral neuropathy.
6. Encourage to return for follow-up evaluation; provide a 2-week supply.

Client/Family Teaching

1. Avoid sunlight. If exposed, wear long sleeves, pants, hat, glasses, and apply sunscreen.
2. Practice regular oral hygiene, including regular tooth brushing, daily flossing, checkups and mouth washes, avoiding those with alcohol or other drying ingredients.
3. Report S&S of toxicity (skin rash, pruritus, metallic taste, stomatitis, diarrhea, leukopenia, and thrombocytopenia).
4. Women should use a reliable form of contraception.
5. Skin irritation (puritic dermatitis) and mouth ulcers may persist for months after stopping medication.
6. Expect to continue anti-inflammatory doses of NSAIDs for several weeks to months until auranofin takes effect. It may take up to 6 months of therapy before improvement will be noticed.

Outcome/Evaluate

- Improved mobility and ROM
- ↓ Pain, swelling, and stiffness in joints
- Slowing of the progression and degenerative effects of RA

Aurothioglucose

(or-oh-thigh-oh-**GLOO**-kohz)

Pregnancy Category: C

Solganol **(Rx)**

Classification: Antiarthritic

For additional information regarding aurothioglucose, see *Gold Sodium Thiomalate.*

Action/Kinetics: The gold content of aurothioglucose is 50%. **Time to peak effect:** 4-6 hr. **Mean steady-state plasma levels:** 1-6 mcg/mL. Is 95%-99% protein bound. **t½, after 11th dose:** Up to 168 days. Seventy percent is excreted in the urine and 30% is excreted through the feces.

Side Effects: *GI:* N&V, anorexia, abdominal cramps, metallic taste, gastritis, ***ulcerative enterocolitis,*** colitis. *Dermatologic:* Dermatitis (papular, vesicular, exfoliative), rash, urticaria, angioedema, chrysiasis. *Renal:* Nephrotic syndrome, glomerulonephritis with proteinuria and hematuria, acute renal failure secondary to acute tubular necrosis, acute nephritis, degeneration of proximal tubular epithelium. *Hematologic:* ***Granulocytopenia, panmyelopathy, hemorrhagic diathesis***. *Respiratory:* Inflammation of upper respiratory tract, pharyngitis, tracheitis, bold bronchitis, interstitial pneumonitis, fibrosis. *CNS:* Confusion, hallucinations, ***seizures***. *Mucous membranes:* Stomatitis, diffuse glossitis, gingivitis. *Reactions of the nitroid type:* Anaphylactoid symptoms, flushing, fainting, dizziness, sweating, N&V, malaise, headache, weakness. *Ophthalmologic:* Iritis, corneal ulcers, gold deposits in ocular tissues. *Miscellaneous:* Vaginitis.

OD **Management of Overdose:** *Treatment:* Discontinue and give dimercaprol. Provide supportive therapy for renal and hematologic symptoms. In acute overdose, induce emesis or gastric lavage immediately.

How Supplied: *Injection:* 50 mg/mL

Dosage

- **IM Only**

  Rheumatoid arthritis.

Adults: *Week 1:* 10 mg; *weeks 2 and 3:* 25 mg; **then,** 25-50 (maximum) mg/week until a total of 0.8-1 g has been administered. If client tolerates the dose and has improved, 50 mg may be given q 3-4 weeks for several months. **Pediatric, 6-12 years:** *Week 1:* 2.5 mg; *weeks 2 and 3:* 6.25 mg; **then,** 12.5 mg/week until a total dose of 200-250 mg has been administered. **Maintenance:** 6.25-12.5 mg q 3-4 weeks.

HEALTH CARE CONSIDERATIONS

See also *Health Care Considerations* for *Gold Sodium Thiomalate.*

Administration/Storage

1. Give IM injections only in the upper outer quadrant of the gluteal region using an 18-gauge, 1½-in. needle (or 2 in. for obese clients).
2. To obtain a uniform suspension, shake the vial carefully before the dose is withdrawn.
3. Both the syringe and needle used to withdraw the dose should be dry.
4. To assist with withdrawing the appropriate dose of the suspension, immerse the vial in warm water.

Assessment

1. Record any sensitivity to sesame oil and determine if a dermal test dose has been performed.
2. Monitor CBC, liver and renal function studies. Assess for blood dyscrasias, photosensitivity reactions, hepatic dysfunction, nephrotoxicity, and fibrosis of the lungs (pneumonitis).
3. Keep supine for 10 min after injection and observe for 15 min following administration for evidence of flushing, dizziness, sweating, and hypotension (nitroid reaction).
4. Carefully determine dosage and track until maximum level is administered.
5. Assess mobility and stress the need to continue anti-inflammatory doses of NSAIDs for several more months.

Outcome/Evaluate

- ↓ Joint pain, swelling, and stiffness with improved ROM
- Slowing of the progression and degenerative effects of arthritis

Azathioprine

(ay-zah-**THIGH**-oh-preen)

Pregnancy Category: D

Gen-Azathioprine ✱, Imuran **(Rx)**

Classification: Immunosuppressant

Action/Kinetics: Antimetabolite that is quickly split to form mercaptopurine. To be effective, the drug must be given during the induction period of the antibody response. The precise mechanism in depressing the immune response is unknown, but it suppresses cell-mediated hypersensitivities and alters antibody production. Inhibits synthesis of DNA, RNA, and proteins and may interfere with meiosis and cellular metabolism. The mechanism for its effect on autoimmune diseases is not known. Is readily absorbed from the GI tract. The anuric client manifests increased effectiveness and toxicity (up to twofold). **Onset:** 6-8 weeks for rheumatoid arthritis. **t½:** 3 hr.

Uses: As an adjunct to prevent rejection in renal homotransplantation. In adult clients meeting criteria for classic or definite rheumatoid arthritis as defined by the American Rheumatism Association. Restrict use to clients with severe, active, and erosive disease that is not responsive to conventional therapy. *Investigational:* Chronic ulcerative colitis, generalized myasthenia gravis, to control the progression of Behçet's syndrome (especially eye disease), Crohn's disease (low doses).

Contraindications: Treatment of rheumatoid arthritis in pregnancy or in clients previously treated with alkylating agents. Pregnancy and lactation.

Special Concerns: Hematologic toxicity is dose-related and may occur late in the course of therapy; may be more severe in renal transplant clients undergoing rejection. Although used in children, safety and efficacy have not been established.

Side Effects: *Hematologic:* Leukopenia, thrombocytopenia, macrocytic anemia, ***severe bone marrow depression,*** selective erythrocyte aplasia. *GI:* N&V, diarrhea, abdominal pain, steatorrhea. *CNS:* Fever, malaise. *Other:* ***Increased risk of carcinoma,*** severe infections (fungal, viral, bacterial, and protozoal), and ***hepatotoxicity*** are major side effects. Also, skin rashes, alopecia, myalgias, increase in liver enzymes, hypotension, negative nitrogen balance.

OD **Management of Overdose:** *Symptoms:* Large doses may result in ***bone marrow hypoplasia,*** bleeding, infection, and death. *Treatment:* Approximately 45% can be removed from the body following 8 hr of hemodialysis.

Drug Interactions

ACE inhibitors / ↑ Risk of severe leukopenia

Allopurinol / ↑ Pharmacologic effect of azathioprine due to ↓ breakdown in liver

Anticoagulants / ↓ Effect of anticoagulants

Corticosteroids / With azathioprine, it may cause muscle wasting after prolonged therapy

Cyclosporine / ↑ Plasma levels of cyclosporine

Methotrexate / ↑ Plasma levels of the active metabolite, 6-mercaptopurine

Tubocurarine / Azathioprine ↓ effect of tubocurarine and other nondepolarizing neuromuscular blocking agents

How Supplied: *Powder For Injection:* 100 mg; *Tablet:* 50 mg

Dosage

- **Tablets, IV**

Use in renal homotransplantation.

Adults and children, initial: 3-5 mg/kg (120 mg/m^2), 1-3 days before or on the day of transplantation; **maintenance:** 1-3 mg/kg (45 mg/m^2) daily.

Rheumatoid arthritis, SLE.

Adults and children, tablets, initial: 1 mg/kg (50-100 mg); **then,** increase dose by 0.5 mg/kg/day after 6-8 weeks and thereafter q 4 weeks, up to maximum of 2.5 mg/kg/day; **maintenance:** lowest effective dose. Dosage should be reduced in clients with renal dysfunction.

Myasthenia gravis.

2-3 mg/kg/day. However, side effects occur in more than 35% of clients.

To control progression of Behçet's syndrome.

2.5 mg/kg/day.

To treat Crohn's disease.

75-100 mg/day.

HEALTH CARE CONSIDERATIONS

Administration/Storage

1. When used for rheumatoid arthritis, a therapeutic response may not be observed for 6-8 weeks.
2. May be discontinued abruptly, but delayed effects are possible.
3. When used with allopurinol, reduce dose of azathioprine by 25%-33% of the usual dose.
4. IV Reconstitute drug (100 mg) with 10 mL of sterile water for injection and use within 24 hr. Further dilution with NSS or dextrose is usually made and infusion time ranges from 5 min to 8 hr.

Assessment

1. Record indications for therapy and include preassessment data.
2. Assess for drug interactions.
3. Monitor CBC and liver and renal function studies. Observe for symptoms of hepatic dysfunction. Stop drug and report if jaundiced or develops abnormal LFTs.
4. Assess I&O and weigh daily. Report any decreases in urine volume and C_{cr} or oliguria; symptoms of kidney transplant rejection.

Client/Family Teaching

1. If GI upset occurs, give in divided doses or take with food.
2. Take only as directed and do not skip or stop medication without approval; increase fluid intake.
3. Practice reliable contraception during and for 4 months following therapy.
4. Report any bruising, bleeding, S&S of infection, fever, rash, abdominal pain, yellow eyes or skin, itching, and/or clay-colored stools.
5. Must take this medication for life to prevent transplant rejection .
6. Avoid crowds or contact with any person who has taken oral poliovirus vaccine recently or persons with active infections.
7. When used for RA, improvement in joint pain, swelling, and stiffness may take 6-12 weeks. Client should be considered refractory if no beneficial effect is noted after 12 weeks of therapy.

Outcome/Evaluate

- Prevention of transplant rejection
- Suppression of cell-mediated immunity
- With RA ↓ joint pain and inflammation with improved mobility

Azelaic acid

(ah-zih-**LAY**-ic ah-**SID**)

Pregnancy Category: B
Azelex **(Rx)**
Classification: Antiacne drug

Action/Kinetics: The precise mechanism of action in treating acne is not known, but the drug possesses antimicrobial activity against *Propionibacterium acnes* and *Staphylococcus epidermidis.* Causes a decrease in the thickness of the stratum corneum, a reduction in the number and size of keratohyalin granules, and a reduction in the amount and distribution of filaggrin in epidermal layers. After application, the drug penetrates to the stratum corneum, epidermis, and dermis. A small amount of the drug (4%) is absorbed into the systemic circulation.
Uses: Treatment of mild to moderate inflammatory acne vulgaris.
Contraindications: Ophthalmic use.
Special Concerns: Use with caution during lactation. Safety and efficacy have not been determined in children less than 12 years of age.
Side Effects: *Dermatologic:* Pruritus, burning, stinging, tingling, erythema, dryness, rash, peeling, irritation, dermatitis, contact dermatitis, vitiligo depigmentation, small depigmented spots, hypertrichosis, reddening (sign of keratosis pilaris), exacerbation of recurrent herpes labialis (rare). *Miscellaneous:* ***Worsening of asthma, allergic reactions.***
How Supplied: *Cream:* 20%

Dosage

- **Cream**

Acne vulgaris.

Gently but thoroughly massage a thin film into the affected areas b.i.d., in the morning and evening, after the skin is thoroughly washed and patted dry.

HEALTH CARE CONSIDERATIONS

Administration/Storage

1. The duration of treatment depends on the severity of the acne. Most improve within 4 weeks.
2. Protect the cream from freezing and store between 15°C and 30°C (59°F and 86°F).

Assessment

1. Record indications for therapy, onset and duration of symptoms, and other agents/therapies trialed.
2. Assess severity of acne and the number of inflammatory lesions. Obtain pretreatment photos.

Client/Family Teaching

1. Use only as directed; after thorough cleansing and drying of skin, massage a small amount of cream into affected areas every morning and every evening. Improvement should be evident within 4 weeks.
2. Wash hands thoroughly before and after use. Keep cream away from mouth, eyes, and other mucous membranes.
3. Do not cover area with any wrappings or occlusive dressings.
4. Cream may cause temporary skin irritation (due to low pH) when applied to broken or inflamed skin; this should subside with continued therapy. If rash is persistent, apply the drug only once a day or stop treatment until symptoms improve. Discontinue treatment if sensitivity or severe irritation develops.
5. Report any alterations in skin color with dark complexions.

Outcome/Evaluate: Clearing and healing of acne and inflammatory lesions

Azithromycin

(az-**zith**-roh-**MY**-sin)
Pregnancy Category: B
Zithromax **(Rx)**
Classification: Antibiotic, macrolide

Action/Kinetics: A macrolide antibiotic derived from erythromycin. The drug acts by binding to the P site of the 50S ribosomal subunit and may inhibit RNA-dependent protein synthesis by stimulating the dissociation of peptidyl t-RNA from ribosomes. Rapidly absorbed and distributed widely throughout the body. Food increases the absorption of azithromycin. **Time to reach maximum concentration:** 2.2 hr. **t½, terminal:** 68 hr. A loading dose will achieve steady-state levels more quickly. Mainly excreted unchanged through the bile with a small amount being excreted through the kidneys.
Uses: Adults: Acute bacterial exacerbations of COPD due to *Hemophilus influenzae, Moraxella catarrhalis,* or *Streptococcus pneumoniae.* Required initial IV therapy in community-acquired pneumonia due to *S. pneumoniae, Chlamydia pneumoniae, Mycoplasma pneumoniae, H. influenzae, M. catarrhalis, Legionella pneumophila,* and *Staphylococcus aureus.* Those who can take PO therapy in community-acquired pneumonia due to *C. pneumoniae, M. pneumoniae, S. pneumoniae, or H. influenzae.* PO for genital ulcer disease in men due to *Haemophilus ducreyi.* Initial IV therapy in pelvic inflammatory disease due to *Chlamydia trachomatis, Neisseria gonorrhoeae,* or *Mycoplasma hominis.* As an alternative to first-line therapy to treat streptococcal pharyn-

A

gitis or tonsillitis due to *Streptococcus pyogenes*. PO for uncomplicated skin and skin structure infections due to *S. aureus, Staphyloccus pyogenes,* or *Streptococcus agalactiae*. Abscesses usually require surgical drainage. PO for urethritis and cervicitis due to *C. trachomatis* or *N. gonorrhoeae*.

Children: PO for acute otitis media due to *H. influenzae, M. catarrhalis,* or *S. pneumoniae* in children over 6 months of age. PO for community-acquired pneumonia due to *C. pneumoniae, H. influenzae, M. pneumoniae,* or *S. pneumoniae* in children over 6 months of age. Pharyngitis/tonsillitis due to *S. pyogenes* in children over 2 years of age who cannot use first-line therapy.

Investigational: Uncomplicated gonococcal pharyngitis of the cervix, urethra, and rectum caused by *N. gonorrhoeae*. Gonococcal pharyngitis due to *N. gonorrhoeae*. Chlamydial infections due to *C. trachomatis*.

Contraindications: Hypersensitivity to azithromycin, any macrolide antibiotic, or erythromycin. In clients who are not eligible for outpatient PO therapy (e.g., known or suspected bacteremia, immunodeficiency, functional asplenia, nosocomially acquired infections, geriatric or debilitated clients). Use with astemizole, cisapride, or pimozide.

Special Concerns: Use with caution in clients with impaired hepatic or renal function and during lactation. Safety and efficacy for acute otitis media have not been determined in children less than 6 months of age or for pharyngitis/tonsillitis in children less than 2 years of age.

Side Effects: *GI:* N&V, diarrhea, loose stools, abdominal pain, dyspepsia, anorexia, gastritis, flatulence, melena, mucositis, oral moniliasis, taste perversion, cholestatic jaundice, pseudomembranous colitis. In children, gastritis, constipation, and anorexia have also been noted. *CNS:* Dizziness, headache, somnolence, fatigue, vertigo. In children, hyperkinesia, agitation, nervousness, insomnia, fever, and malaise have also been noted. *CV:* Chest pain, palpitations, ***ventricular arrhythmias (including ventricular tachycardia and torsades de pointes in clients with prolonged QT intervals observed with other macrolides).*** *GU:* Monilia, nephritis, vaginitis. *Allergic:* Angioedema, photosensitivity, rash, ***anaphylaxis.*** *Hematologic:* Leukopenia, neutropenia, decreased platelet count. *Miscellaneous:* Superinfection, bronchospasm, local IV site reactions. In children, pruritus, urticaria, conjunctivitis, and chest pain have been noted.

Laboratory Test Considerations: ↑ Serum CPK, potassium, ALT, GGT, AST, serum alkaline phosphatase, bilirubin, BUN, creatinine, blood glucose, LDH, and phosphate.

Drug Interactions:

Aluminum- and magnesium-containing antacids / ↓ Peak serum levels of azithromycin but not the total amount absorbed
Cyclosporine / ↑ Serum levels of cyclosporine due to ↓ metabolism → ↑ risk of nephrotoxicity and neurotoxicity
HMG-CoA reductase inhibitors / ↑ Risk of severe myopathy or rhabdomyolysis
Phenytoin / ↑ Serum levels of phenytoin due to ↓ metabolism
Pimozide / Possibility of sudden death

How Supplied: *Powder for Injection:* 500 mg; *Powder for Oral Suspension:* 100 mg/5mL, 200 mg/5mL, 1 gm/packet; *Tablet:* 250 mg, 600 mg

Dosage

- **Suspension, Tablets**

Adults: Mild to moderate acute bacterial exacerbations of COPD, mild community-acquired pneumonia, second-line therapy for pharyngitis/tonsillitis; uncomplicated skin and skin structure infections.

Adults and children over 16 years of age: 500 mg as a single dose on day 1 followed by 250 mg once daily on days 2-5 for a total dose of 1.5 g.

Nongonococcal urethritis and cervicitis due to C. trachomatis *or genital ulcer disease due to* H. ducreyi.

1 g given as a single dose.

Gonococcal urethritis/cervicitis due to N. gonorrhoeae.

2 g given as a single dose.

Uncomplicated gonococcal infections due to N. gonorrhoeae.

1 g given as a single dose plus a single dose of 400 mg PO cefixime, 125 mg IM ceftriaxone, 500 mg PO ciprofloxacin, or 400 mg PO ofloxacin.

Gonococcal pharyngitis.

1 g given as a single dose plus a single dose of 125 mg IM ceftriaxone, 500 mg ciprofloxacin, or 400 mg ofloxacin.

Chlamydial infections caused by C. trachomatis.

1 g given as a single dose.

- **Oral Suspension**

Pediatric: Otitis media or community-acquired pneumonia.

10 mg/kg (not to exceed 500 mg) on day 1, followed by 5 mg/kg (not to exceed 250 mg/day) on days 2 through 5.

Pediatric: Pharyngitis/tonsillitis.

12 mg/kg once daily for 5 days, not to exceed 500 mg/day.

Chlamydial infections in children caused by C. trachomatis.

Children 45 kg or more and less than 8 years of age or over 8 years of age: 1 g given as a single dose.

HEALTH CARE CONSIDERATIONS

Administration/Storage

1. Give suspension at least 1 hr prior to or at least 2 hr after a meal.
2. Tablets may be taken with or without food, although increased tolerability if taken with food. May be taken with milk.

Assessment

1. Determine any history of sensitivity to erythromycins and note any previous therapy.
2. Determine other drugs prescribed; may cause an increase in serum concentrations of certain drugs (digoxin, carbamazepine, cyclosporine, dilantin).
3. Obtain documentation (labs, discharge summaries, etc.) that clients with sexually transmitted cervicitis or urethritis are tested for gonorrhea and syphilis at the time of diagnosis. Ensure that appropriate drug therapy is instituted if necessary.
4. Obtain liver and renal function studies and cultures when warranted.

Client/Family Teaching

1. Do not administer capsules with meals; food decreases absorption.
2. Avoid ingesting aluminum- or magnesium-containing antacids simultaneously with azithromycin.
3. Notify provider if N&V or diarrhea is excessive.
4. Avoid sun exposure and use protection when needed.
5. With STDs, encourage sexual partner to seek medical evaluation and treatment to prevent reinfections. Use condoms during intercourse throughout therapy.

Outcome/Evaluate: Resolution of S&S of infection; Negative cultures

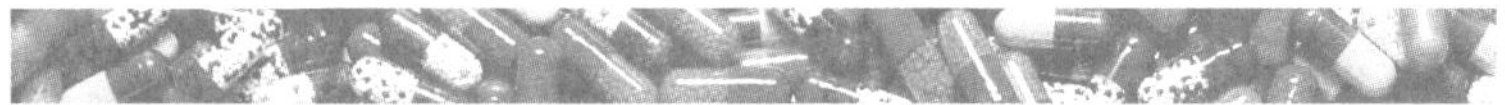

Bacampicillin hydrochloride

(bah-kam-pih-**SILL**-in)

Pregnancy Category: B

Penglobe ✱, Spectrobid **(Rx)**

Classification: Antibiotic, penicillin

See also *Anti-Infectives* and *Penicillins*.

Action/Kinetics: Semisynthetic, acid-resistant penicillin that is hydrolyzed to the active ampicillin in the GI tract. Food does not affect absorption. 98% absorbed from the GI tract and approximately 20% plasma protein bound. **Peak serum levels:** About 3 times equivalent doses of ampicillin after 0.9 hr. Seventy-five percent is excreted in the urine as active ampicillin within 8 hr.

Uses: Upper and lower respiratory tract infections (including acute exacerbations of chronic bronchitis) caused by beta-hemolytic streptococcus, *Staphylococcus pyogenes*, pneumococci, non-penicillinase-producing staphylococci, and *Haemophilus influenzae*. UTIs caused by *Escherichia coli, Proteus mirabilis,* and enterococci. Skin and skin structure infections caused by streptococci and susceptible staphylococci. Acute uncomplicated urogenital infections caused by *Neisseria gonorrhoeae*.

Contraindications: History of penicillin allergy. Concomitant use with disulfiram (Antabuse).

Laboratory Test Considerations: False + reaction to Clinitest, Benedict's solution, and Fehling's solution. ↑ AST.

Drug Interactions: Bacampicillin should not be used concomitantly with disulfiram.

How Supplied: *Tablet:* 400 mg; *Injection:* 0.3 mg/mL

Dosage

- **Tablets**

Upper respiratory tract infections, otitis media, UTIs, skin and skin structure infections.

Adults: 400 mg q 12 hr; **pediatric, over 25 kg:** 25 mg/kg/day in equally divided doses q 12 hr. Dose may be doubled in cases of lower respiratory tract infections, severe infections, or in treating less susceptible organisms.

Gonorrhea.

Males and females: 1.6 g with 1 g probenecid as a single dose. No pediatric dosage has been established.

HEALTH CARE CONSIDERATIONS

See also *General Health Care Considerations for All Anti-Infectives*.

Administration/Storage: May be taken with meals.

Client/Family Teaching

1. May take on an empty stomach or with meals.
2. Do not start disulfiram while taking bacampicillin.
3. Diabetics should monitor fingersticks to assess replacement needs.
4. With allopurinol therapy, report any skin rash.

Outcome/Evaluate: Resolution of infection; negative C&S results

Bacitracin intramuscular

(bass-ih-TRAY-sin)

Bacitracin Sterile **(Rx)**

Bacitracin ointment

(bass-ih-TRAY-sin)

Baciguent, Bacitin ✱ **(OTC)**

Bacitracin ophthalmic ointment

(bass-ih-TRAY-sin)

AK-Tracin, Bacitracin Ophthalmic Ointment **(Rx)**

Classification: Antibiotic, miscellaneous

See also *Anti-Infectives*.

Action/Kinetics: Produced by *Bacillus subtilis*. Interferes with synthesis of cell wall, preventing incorporation of amino acids and nucleotides. Is bactericidal, bacteriostatic, and active against protoplasts. Not absorbed from the GI tract. When given parenterally, drug is well distributed in pleural and ascitic fluids. High nephrotoxicity. Systemic use is restricted to infants (see *Uses*). Carefully evaluate renal function prior to, and daily, during use. **Peak plasma levels: IM,** 0.2-2 mcg/mL after 2 hr. From 10% to 40% is excreted in the urine after IM administration.

Uses: Parenteral: Limited to the treatment of staphylococcal pneumonia and staphylococcus-induced empyema in infants. **Topical:** Prophylaxis or treatment of infections in minor cuts, wounds, burns, and skin abrasions. As an aid to healing and for treating superficial infections of the skin due to susceptible organisms. **Ophthalmic:** Effective against species of *Staphylococcus, S. aureus, Streptococcus, S. pneumoniae, S. pyogenes, Corynebacterium, Neisseria, N. gonorrhoeae,* and beta-hemolytic streptococci. Do not use topical antibiotics in deep-seated ocular infections or in those that are likely to become systemic.

Contraindications: Hypersensitivity or toxic reaction to bacitracin. Pregnancy. Epithelial herpes simplex keratitis, vaccinia, varicella, mycobacterial eye infections, fungal diseases of the eye.

Special Concerns: Ophthalmic ointments may retard corneal epithelial healing. Prolonged or repeated use may result in bacterial or fungal overgrowth of nonsusceptible organisms leading to a secondary infection.

Side Effects: Parenteral use: ***Nephrotoxicity due to tubular and glomerular necrosis, renal failure;*** toxic reactions; N&V. **Topical use:** Allergic contact dermatitis, superinfection. **Ophthalmic use:** Transient burning, stinging, itching, irritation, inflammation, angioneurotic edema, urticaria, vesicular and maculopapular dermatitis.

Drug Interactions

Aminoglycosides / Additive nephrotoxicity and neuromuscular blocking activity

Anesthetics / ↑ Neuromuscular blockade → possible muscle paralysis

Neuromuscular blocking agents / Additive neuromuscular blockade → possible muscle paralysis

How Supplied: Bacitracin intramuscular: *Powder for Injection:* 50,000 u/vial Bacitracin ointment: *Ophthalmic Ointment:* 500 U/g; *Topical Ointment:* 500 U/g

Dosage

- **IM Only**

Infants, 2.5 kg and below: 900 units/kg/day in two to three divided doses; **infants over 2.5 kg:** 1,000 units/kg/day in two to three divided doses.

- **Ophthalmic Ointment (500 units/g)**

Acute infections.

½ in. in lower conjunctival sac q 3-4 hr until improvement occurs. Reduce treatment before the drug is discontinued.

Mild to moderate infections.

½ in. b.i.d.-t.i.d.

- **Topical Ointment (500 units/g)**

Apply a small amount equal to the surface area of a fingertip 1-3 times/day after cleaning the affected area. Do not use for more than 1 week.

HEALTH CARE CONSIDERATIONS

See also *General Health Care Considerations for All Anti-Infectives*.

Administration/Storage: Do not mix bacitracin with glycerin or other polyalcohols that cause drug to deteriorate. When used topically, the affected area may be covered with a sterile bandage.

Assessment

1. Record indications for therapy, type, onset, and duration of symptoms.
2. List any previous experiences with this type of infection (especially ocular), agents used, and results.

3. Recurrent ophthalmic infections should be cultured and carefully assessed by an ophthalmologist.

Interventions

1. Monitor renal function studies and maintain adequate I&O with parenteral therapy.
2. Test urine pH daily; pH should be kept at 6 or greater to decrease renal irritation. Have $NaHCO_3$ or other alkali available if pH < 6.
3. Do not administer with a topical or systemic nephrotoxic drug.

Client/Family Teaching

1. Apply as directed. Cleanse area thoroughly before applying bacitracin as a wet dressing or ointment.
2. Report any lack of response, rash, or unusual symptoms.

Outcome/Evaluate

- Resolution of S&S of infection
- Restoration of skin integrity

Baclofen

(BAK-low-fen)

Pregnancy Category: C

Apo-Baclofen ✱, Dom-Baclofen ✱, Gen-Baclofen ✱, Lioresal, Lioresal Intrathecal ✱, Med-Baclofen ✱, Novo-Baclofen ✱, Nu-Baclo ✱, PMS-Baclofen ✱ **(Rx)**

Classification: Skeletal muscle relaxant, centrally acting

See also *Skeletal Muscle Relaxants, Centrally Acting.*

Action/Kinetics: Related chemically to GABA, an inhibitory neurotransmitter. May act by combining with the $GABA_B$ receptor subtype. It increases threshold for excitation of primary afferent nerves and decreases the release of excitatory amino acids from presynaptic sites. May also act at certain brain sites. Has CNS depressant effects. After PO use, baclofen is rapidly and extensively absorbed. **Peak serum levels, PO:** 2-3 hr. **Therapeutic serum levels:** 80-400 ng/mL. **t½, PO:** 3-4 hr. **Onset after intrathecal bolus:** 30-60 min; **peak effect after intrathecal bolus:** 4 hr; **duration after intrathecal bolus:** 4-8 hr. **t½ after bolus lumbar injection of 50 or 100 mcg:** 1.5 hr over the first 4 hr. **Onset after intrathecal continuous infusion:** 6-8 hr; **peak effect after intrathecal continuous infusion:** 24-48 hr. Seventy percent to 80% of the drug is eliminated unchanged by the kidney.

Uses: PO. Multiple sclerosis (flexor spasms, pain, clonus, and muscular rigidity) and diseases and injuries of the spinal cord associated with spasticity. Not effective for the treatment of cerebral palsy, stroke, parkinsonism, or rheumatic disorders. *Investigational:* Trigeminal neuralgia, tardive dyskinesia, intractable hiccoughs.

Intrathecal. Severe spasticity of spinal cord of cerebral origin in clients unresponsive to PO baclofen therapy or who have intolerable CNS side effects. *Investigational:* Reduce spasticity in children with cerebral palsy.

Contraindications: Hypersensitivity. PO used to treat rheumatic disorders, spasm resulting from Parkinson's disease, stroke, cerebral palsy. Intrathecal product for IV, IM, SC, or epidural use.

Special Concerns: Use during lactation only if potential benefit outweighs the potential risk. Safe use of the oral product for children under 12 years of age and of the intrathecal product for children under 4 years of age has not been established. Use with caution in impaired renal function, in those with autonomic dysreflexia and where spasticity is used to sustain an upright posture and balance in locomotion; in those with psychotic disorders, schizophrenia, or confusional states as worsening of these conditions has occurred following PO use. Geriatric clients may be at higher risk for developing CNS toxicity, including mental depression, confusion, hallucinations, and significant sedation. Due to serious, life-threatening side effects after intrathecal use, physicians must be trained and educated in chronic intrathecal infusion therapy. Abrupt drug withdrawal may cause hallucinations and seizures.

Side Effects: PO. *CNS:* Drowsiness, dizziness, lightheadedness, weakness, lethargy, fatigue, confusion, headaches, insomnia, euphoria, excitement, depression, paresthesia, muscle pain, coordination disorder, tremor, rigidity, dystonia, ataxia, strabismus, dysarthria. Hallucinations following abrupt withdrawal. *CV:* Hypotension. Rarely, chest pain, syncope, palpitations. *GI:* N&V, constipation, dry mouth, anorexia, taste disorder, abdominal pain, diarrhea. *GU:* Urinary frequency, enuresis, urinary retention, dysuria, impotence, inability to ejaculate, nocturia. *Ophthalmic:* Nystagmus, miosis, mydriasis, diplopia. *Miscellaneous:* Rash, pruritus, ankle edema, increased perspiration, weight gain, dyspnea, nasal congestion.

Intrathecal, spasticity of spinal origin. *CNS:* Dizziness, somnolence, paresthesia, headache, ***convulsion,*** confusion, speech disorder, coma, ***death,*** insomnia, anxiety, depression, hallucinations. *GI:* N&V, constipa-

B

tion, dry mouth, diarrhea, anorexia. *GU:* Urinary retention, impotence, urinary incontinence, urinary frequency. *CV:* Hypotension, hypertension. *Miscellaneous:* Accidental injury, asthenia, amblyopia, pain, peripheral edema, dyspnea, hypoventilation, fever, urticaria, anorexia, diplopia, dysautonomia.

Intrathecal, spasticity of cerebral origin. *CNS:* Somnolence, headache, ***convulsion,*** dizziness, paresthesia, abnormal thinking, agitation, coma, speech disorder, tremor. *GI:* N&V, increased salivation, constipation, dry mouth. *GU:* Urinary retention, urinary incontinence, impaired urination. *Miscellaneous:* Hypertonia, hypoventilation, hypotension, back pain, pain, pruritus, peripheral edema, asthenia, chills, pneumonia.

Laboratory Test Considerations: ↑ AST, alkaline phosphatase, blood glucose.

OD **Management of Overdose:** *Symptoms:* Symptoms after PO use include vomiting, drowsiness, muscular hypotonia, muscle twitching, accommodation disorders, respiratory depression, seizures, coma. Symptoms after intrathecal use include drowsiness, dizziness, lightheadedness, somnolence, respiratory depression, rostral progression of hypotonia, ***seizures, loss of consciousness leading to coma (for up to 24 hr).*** *Treatment:*

1. After PO use:
- Induce vomiting (only if the client is alert and conscious) followed by gastric lavage.
- If the client is not alert and conscious, undertake only gastric lavage making sure the airway is secured with a cuffed ET tube.
- Maintain an adequate airway.
- Atropine may be used to improve HR, BP, ventilation, and core body temperature.

2. After intrathecal use:
- The residual solution is to be removed from the pump as soon as possible.
- Intubate the client with respiratory depression until the drug is eliminated.
- IV physostigmine (total dose of 1-2 mg given over 5-10 min) may be tried, with caution.
- Consideration can also be given to withdrawing 30-60 mL of CSF to decrease baclofen levels (provided that lumbar puncture is not contraindicated).

Drug Interactions

CNS depressants / Additive CNS depression
MAO inhibitors / ↑ CNS depression and hypotension
Ticyclic antidepressants / Muscle hypotonia

How Supplied: *Kit:* 0.05 mg/mL, 0.5 mg/mL, 2 mg/mL; *Tablet:* 10 mg, 20 mg

Dosage

- **Tablets**

Muscle relaxant, spasticity.

Adults, initial: 5 mg t.i.d. for 3 days; **then,** 10 mg t.i.d. for 3 days, 15 mg t.i.d. for 3 days, and 20 mg t.i.d. Additional increases in dose may be required but should not exceed 20 mg q.i.d. Maximum daily dose for spasticity should not exceed 260 mg. **Children (treatment of spasticity), initial:** 10-15 mg/kg/day in 3 divided doses. Titrate to a maximum of 40 mg/day if less than 8 years of age and to a maximum of 80 mg/day if more than 8 years of age.

Trigeminal neuralgia.

50-60 mg/day.

Tardive dyskinesia.

40 mg/day used in combination with neuroleptics.

- **Intrathecal**

Initial screening bolus.

50 mcg/mL given into the intrathecal space by barbotage over a period of not less than 1 min. The client is observed for 4-8 hr for a positive response consisting of a decrease in muscle tone, frequency, and/or severity of muscle spasms. If the response is not adequate, a second bolus dose of 75 mcg/1.5 mL, 24 hr after the first bolus dose, can be given with the client observed for 4-8 hr. If the response is still inadequate, a final bolus screening dose of 100 mcg/2 mL can be given 24 hr later.

Postimplant dose titration.

To determine the initial daily dose of baclofen following the implant for intrathecal use, the screening dose that gave a positive response should be doubled and given over a 24-hr period. However, if the effectiveness of the bolus dose lasted for more than 12 hr, the daily dose should be the same as the screening dose but delivered over a period of 24 hr. After the first 24 hr, the dose can be increased slowly by 10%-30% increments only once each 24 hr until the desired effect is reached.

Maintenance therapy.

The maintenance dose may need to be adjusted during the first few months of intrathecal therapy. The daily dose may be increased by 10% to no more than 40% daily. If side effects occur, the daily dose may be decreased by 10%-20%. Daily doses for long-term continuous infusion have ranged from 12 to 1,500 mcg (usual maintenance is 300-800 mcg/day). The lowest dose producing optimal control should be used.

Reduce spasticity of cerebral palsy in children.

25, 50, or 100 mcg.

HEALTH CARE CONSIDERATIONS

See also *Health Care Considerations* for *Skeletal Muscle Relaxants, Centrally Acting,*.

Administration/Storage

1. If beneficial effects are not noted, withdraw the drug slowly.
2. Check the manufacturer's manual for specific instructions and precautions for programming the implantable intrathecal infusion pump and refilling the reservoir.
3. Prior to intrathecal implantation of the pump, clients must show a positive response to a bolus dose of baclofen in a screening trial.
4. If there is not a significant clinical response to increases in the daily dose given intrathecally, check the pump for proper function and the catheter for patency.
5. During long-term intrathecal treatment, approximately 10% of clients become tolerant to increasing doses. If this occurs, a drug "holiday" consisting of a gradual decrease of intrathecal baclofen over a 2-week period can be considered. Alternate methods to treat spasticity must be undertaken. After a few days, sensitivity to baclofen may return. However, to avoid possible side effects or overdose, the alternative medication should be discontinued slowly.
6. Filling of the reservoir for intrathecal use must be performed only by fully trained and qualified personnel. Refill intervals must be carefully calculated to avoid depletion of the reservoir.
7. Use extreme caution when filling an FDA-approved implantable pump equipped with an injection port (i.e., that allows direct access to the intrathecal catheter). Direct injection into the catheter through the access port may result in a life-threatening overdose of baclofen.
8. For screening purposes, intrathecal baclofen, either 10 mg/20 mL or 10 mg/5 mL, must be diluted with sterile preservative-free NaCl for injection, to a concentration of 50 mcg/mL for bolus administration. For maintenance, baclofen must be diluted with sterile preservative-free NaCl for injection USP for clients who require concentrations other than 500 mcg/mL (i.e., the 10 mg/20 mL product) or 2,000 mcg/mL (i.e., the 10 mg/5 mL product).

Assessment

1. Record indications for therapy; note pretreatment findings.
2. With epilepsy assess for clinical S&S of disease. Obtain EEG at regular intervals to assess for reduced seizure control.
3. Obtain initial renal and LFTs.
4. Note if client has diabetes.
5. Clients must be closely monitored in a fully equipped and staffed facility during both the intrathecal screening phase and dose-titration period following the intrathecal implant. Resuscitative equipment should be readily available.
6. Ensure client is free from S&S of infection. Systemic infection may alter response to screening trials and (during pump implantation) may lead to surgical complications and interfere with the pump dosing rate.
7. Assess for level of useful spasticity (e.g., to aid in transfers or to maintain posture) as rigidity is important for gait in some clients.
8. In those who require hypertonicity to stand upright, to maintain balance when walking, or to increase functionality, baclofen may be contraindicated because it interferes with this coping mechanism.

Interventions

1. Note any evidence of hypersensitivity reaction and report.
2. Monitor urine output; test for blood.
3. If improvement in condition does not occur within 6-8 weeks, the drug should be withdrawn gradually.
4. For clients with an intrathecal pump:
   - Calculate pump refill interval to prevent an empty reservoir and return of severe spasticity.
   - Access the pump reservoir percutaneously. Refill and program by one specifically trained in this procedure.
   - When filling pumps with injection ports that permit direct access to the catheter, use care as an injection directly into the catheter can cause a lethal overdose. And, in this event, immediately remove any residual drug from the pump and follow guidelines for Treatment under Management of Overdose.
   - When the dose requirements suddenly escalate, assess for catheter kinks or dislodgement.
   - When programming for increased dosage, e.g., at bedtime, the flow rate should be programmed to change 2 hr before desired effect.

Client/Family Teaching

1. Take oral medication with meals or a snack to avoid gastric irritation. Report if GI S&S are severe/persistent.
2. To prevent constipation, increase fluids and roughage in diet.
3. It may take several weeks of therapy before improvement occurs.

B

4. Monitor and record weight and I&O; note frequency and amount of each voiding; report any edema.
5. May alter insulin requirements.
6. Report impotence as a change of drug or dosage may be required. Do not stop abruptly.
7. With the intrathecal pump:
• Once screening trials completed, the "baclofen pump" will be surgically placed in the abdominal wall and attached to an implanted lumbar intrathecal catheter. Demonstrate proper postop site care and review S&S of infection that require immediate reporting.
• Maintain a log identifying when the spasms are greatest. This facilitates proper pump programming to ensure optimal control of spasticity and discomfort.
• Identify symptoms that require immediate medical intervention.
• Report as scheduled (usually monthly with maintenance) to ensure proper reservoir drug levels and to prevent loss of effect or air entering the reservoir.
• Drowsiness, dizziness, and lower extremity weakness may occur; report if persistent or progressive as dose may require adjustment.
• Those who become refractory to increasing doses may require hospitalization for a "drug holiday." This would consist of a *gradual reduction* of intrathecal baclofen over a 2-week period and alternative therapy with other agents. Sensitivity to baclofen usually returns after several days and may be resumed intrathecally at the initial continuous dose.

Outcome/Evaluate

• Improved muscle tone and involuntary movements; ↓ muscle spasticity and pain
• ↓ Painful/disabling symptoms permitting ↑ functioning level

Becaplermin

(beh-**KAP**-ler-min)
Pregnancy Category: C
Regranex **(Rx)**
Classification: Topical wound healing drug

Action/Kinetics: Topical recombinant human platelet-derived growth factor. Promotes chemotactic recruitment and proliferation of cells involved in wound repair and enhances formation of granulation tissue.
Uses: As adjunct to good ulcer care practices to treat lower extremity diabetic neuropathic ulcers that extend into SC tissue or beyond and have adequate blood supply. Use for diabetic neuropathic ulcers that do not extend through dermis into SC tissue or ischemic ulcers has not been studied.
Contraindications: Known neoplasms at application site. Use in wounds that close by primary intention.
Special Concerns: Effect on exposed joints, tendons, ligaments, and bone has not been established. Use with other topical drugs has not been studied. Use with caution during lactation. Safety and efficacy have not been determined in children less than 16 years of age.
Side Effects: *General:* Infection, cellulitis, osteomyelitis, erythematous rashes.
How Supplied: *Gel:* 0.01%

Dosage

• **Gel, 0.01%**

Lower extremity diabetic neuropathic ulcers. Dose depends on size of ulcer area. To determine length of gel to be applied, measure greatest length of ulcer by greatest width of ulcer in either inches or centimeters. To calculate length of gel in inches:
7.5 g or 15 g tube: length x width x 0.6
2 g tube: length x width x 1.3
Generally, each square inch of ulcer surface will require about ⅔ inch from 7.5 g or 15 g tube and about 1¼ inches from 2 g tube. To calculate length of gel in centimeters:
7.5 g or 15 g tube: length x width divided by 4
2 g tube: length x width divided by 2
Generally, each square centimeter of ulcer surface will require about 0.25 cm of gel from 7.5 or 15 g tube or about 0.5 cm of gel from 2 g tube. Calculate amount to be applied at weekly or biweekly intervals depending on rate of change in ulcer area.

HEALTH CARE CONSIDERATIONS

Administration/Storage

1. Squeeze calculated length of gel onto a clean measuring surface (e.g., wax paper). Gel is transferred from clean measuring surface using an application aid and then spread over entire ulcer area. This should yield thin continuous layer of about 1/16 inch thickness.
2. Cover site with saline moistened dressing and leave in place about 12 hr.
3. Remove dressing after 12 hr and rinse ulcer with saline or water to remove residual gel. Cover again with second moist dressing without gel for remainder of day.
4. Apply once daily until complete ulcer healing has occurred.
5. If ulcer does not decrease in size by about 30% after 10 weeks of therapy or complete healing has not occurred in 20 weeks, reassess treatment.

6. Refrigerate gel but do not freeze. Do not use gel after expiration date at bottom of tube.

Assessment

1. Record onset, duration, size, and characteristics of area requiring treatment. May record initial wound assessment with photographs.
2. Assess area to ensure it is free from infection, cellulitis, rash, and osteomyelitis.
3. Ensure client is enrolled in active wound management program with ongoing debridement, relief of pressure (e.g., wheel chair, wedge shoe), systemic management of infections, and moist dressings changed b.i.d.

Client/Family Teaching

1. Wash hands before application.
2. Apply gel with cotton swab or tongue depressor; do not let tube tip come in contact with wound or skin surfaces and cap tightly.
3. Squeeze calculated length of gel on firm, dry, surface. Spread gel over area requiring treatment and cover with saline moistened gauze dressing.
4. Gently rinse wound after 12 hr with saline or water to remove gel; cover wound with saline moistened dressing.
5. Report any changes in wound that resemble infection, such as purulent drainage, odor, swelling, redness, or increased pain.

Outcome/Evaluate: Healing of diabetic neuropathic foot ulcers.

Beclomethasone dipropionate

(be-kloh-**METH**-ah-zohn)

Pregnancy Category: C

Aerosol Inhaler: Alti-Beclomethasone Dipropionate ✱, Beclodisk Diskhaler ✱, Becloforte Inhaler ✱, Beclovent, Beclovent Rotacaps or Rotahaler ✱, Vanceril, Vanceril DS **(Rx)**, **Intranasal:** Beclodisk for Oral Inhalation ✱, Beconase AQ Nasal, Beconase Inhalation, Gen-Beclo Aq. ✱, Vancenase AQ 84 mcg Double Strength, Vancenase AQ Forte, Vancenase AQ Nasal, Vancenase Nasal Inhaler **(Rx)**, **Topical:** Propaderm ✱

Classification: Glucocorticoid

See also *Corticosteroids.*

Action/Kinetics: t½: 15 hr. Rapidly inactivated, thereby resulting in few systemic effects.

Uses: Relief of symptoms of seasonal or perennial rhinitis in clients not responsive to more conventional therapy, to prevent recurrence of nasal polyps following surgical removal, and to treat allergic or nonallergic (vasomotor) rhinitis (spray formulations). Inhalation therapy for chronic use in bronchial asthma. In glucocorticoid-dependent clients, beclomethasone often permits a decrease in the dosage of the systemic agent. Withdrawal of systemic corticosteroids must be done gradually.

Contraindications: Status asthmaticus, acute episodes of asthma, hypersensitivity to drug or aerosol ingredients.

Special Concerns: Safe use during lactation and in children under 6 years of age not established.

Side Effects: *Intranasal:* Headache, pharyngitis, coughing, epistaxis, nasal burning, pain, conjunctivitis, myalgia, tinnitus. Rarely, ulceration of the nasal mucosa and nasal septum perforation.

How Supplied: *Metered dose inhaler:* 0.042 mg/inh, 0.084 mg/inh; *Nasal Spray:* 0.042 mg/inh, 0.084 mg/inh

Dosage

- **Metered Dose Inhaler**

Asthma.

Beclovent. **Adults:** 2 inhalations (total of 84 mcg beclomethasone) t.i.d.-q.i.d. In some clients, 4 inhalations (168 mcg) b.i.d. have been effective. Do not exceed 20 inhalations (840 mcg) daily. **Pediatric, 6-12 years:** 1-2 inhalations (42-84 mcg) t.i.d.-q.i.d. In some, 4 inhalations (168 mcg) b.i.d. have been effective. Do not to exceed 10 inhalations (420 mcg) daily. Dosage has not been determined in children less than 6 years of age.

Vanceril. **Adults:** 2 inhalations (total of 168 mcg) b.i.d. In those with severe asthma, start with 6-8 inhalations/day and adjust dose downward as determined by client response. Do not exceed 10 inhalations (840 mcg) daily. **Children, 6-12 years:** 2 inhalations (168 mcg) b.i.d. Do not exceed 5 inhalations (420 mcg) daily. Dosage has not been determined in children less than 6 years of age.

NOTE: Vanceril DS can be used once daily for treatment of asthma.

In clients also receiving systemic glucocorticosteroids, beclomethasone should be started when client's condition is relatively stable.

- **Nasal Aerosol or Spray**

Allergic or nonallergic rhinitis, Prophylaxis of nasal polyps.

Adults and children over 12 years: 1 inhalation (42 mcg) in each nostril b.i.d.-q.i.d. (i.e., total daily dose: 168-336 mcg). If no response after 3 weeks, discontinue therapy. **Maintenance, usual:** 1 inhalation in each nostril t.i.d. (252 mcg/day). For nasal polyps, treatment may be required for several weeks or more before a therapeutic effect can be assessed fully. Two sprays of the double-strength product (Vancenase AQ 84 mcg Double Strength) are administered once daily.

Vancenase AQ Forte may be used once daily for treatment of rhinitis.

HEALTH CARE CONSIDERATIONS

See also *Health Care Considerations* for *Corticosteroids*.

Administration/Storage

1. To prevent explosion of contents under pressure, do not store or use near heat or open flame, or throw into a fire or incinerator. Keep secure from children.
2. If the cansister is cold, the therapeutic effect may be decreased.
3. If a client is on systemic steroids, transfer to beclomethasone may be difficult because recovery from impaired renal function may be slow.

Assessment

1. Note any history of sensitivity to corticosteroids or fluorocarbon propellants.
2. Record indications for therapy, pretreatment pulmonary assessments, presenting symptoms, and PFT's.

Client/Family Teaching

1. Review use, care, and storage of inhaler. Rinse out mouth and wash the mouth piece, spacer, sprayer and dry after each use.
2. A spacer may facilitate administration. With nasal administration aim toward the outer eye and not the septum to decrease nasal irritation. Review video/instruction to ensure proper use.
3. To administer with an inhaler:
• Shake metal canister thoroughly immediately prior to use.
• Exhale as completely as possible.
• Place the mouthpiece of the inhaler into the mouth and tighten lips around it.
• Inhale deeply through the mouth while pressing the metal canister down with forefinger.
• Hold breath for as long as possible (or 10 seconds).
• Remove mouthpiece.
• Exhale slowly.
• A minimum of 60 sec must elapse between inhalations.
4. Inhaler is not to be used for acute asthma attacks but should be used regularly to prevent the occurrence of these attacks.
5. Comply with prescribed drug therapy even though it may take 1-4 weeks for any improvement to be realized.
6. Report signs of adrenal insufficiency (i.e., muscular pain, lassitude, and depression) even if respiratory function has improved. Symptoms such as hypotension and weight loss are indications that the dosage of systemic steroid should be boosted temporarily, and then withdrawn more gradually.
7. More than 1 mg in adults or more than 500 mcg in children may precipitate hypothalamic-pituitary axis depression, resulting in adrenal insufficiency. Do not overuse inhaler or exceed prescribed dosage.
8. Report any symptoms of localized oral fungal infections. Gargling and rinsing after treatments and rinsing of the spacer and/or administration port may help prevent these infections. Report immediately; will require antifungal meds and possibly discontinuation of drug.
9. If also receiving bronchodilators by inhalation (i.e., Albuterol) use the bronchodilator first to open the airways and then use beclomethasone. This increases penetration of steroid and reduces potential toxicity from inhaled fluorocarbon propellants of both inhalers.
10. For those receiving systemic steroid therapy, initiate beclomethasone therapy *very* slowly, withdrawing the systemic steroids as ordered. The benefit of inhaled steroids is that it requires a much lower dose since it goes to the target organ and does not require weaning. Once systemic steroid withdrawn, keep a supply of PO glucocorticoids and take immediately if subjected to unusual stress.
11. Carry ID with diagnosis, treatment, and possible need for systemic glucocorticoids, in the event of exposure to unusual stress.
12. Identify and practice relaxation techniques during stressful situations.

Outcome/Evaluate

• Control of asthma
• Relief of rhinitis
• Prophylaxis of nasal polyp recurrence

Benazepril hydrochloride

(beh-**NAYZ**-eh-prill)
Pregnancy Category: D
Lotensin **(Rx)**
Classification: Antihypertensive, ACE inhibitor

See also *Angiotensin-Converting Enzyme Inhibitors*.

Action/Kinetics: Both supine and standing BPs are reduced with mild-to-moderate hypertension and no compensatory tachycardia. Also an antihypertensive effect in clients with low-renin hypertension. Food does not affect the extent of absorption. Almost completely converted to the active benazeprilat,

which has greater ACE inhibitor activity. **Onset:** 1 hr. **Duration:** 24 hr. **Peak plasma levels, benazepril:** 30-60 min. **Peak plasma levels, benazeprilat:** 1-2 hr if fasting and 2-4 hr if not fasting. **t½, benazeprilat:** 10-11 hr. **Peak reduction in BP:** 2-4 hr after dosing. **Peak effect with chronic therapy:** 1-2 weeks. Highly bound to plasma protein and excreted through the urine with about 20% of a dose excreted as benazeprilat.
Uses: Alone or in combination with thiazide diuretics to treat hypertension.
Contraindications: Hypersensitivity to benazepril or any other ACE inhibitor.
Special Concerns: Use with caution during lactation. Safety and effectiveness have not been determined in children.
Side Effects: *CNS:* Headache, dizziness, fatigue, anxiety, insomnia, drowsiness, nervousness. *GI:* N&V, constipation, abdominal pain, gastritis, melena, pancreatitis. *CV:* Symptomatic hypotension, postural hypotension, syncope, angina pectoris, palpitations, peripheral edema, ECG changes. *Dermatologic:* Flushing, photosensitivity, pruritus, rash, diaphoresis. *GU:* Decreased libido, impotence, UTI. *Respiratory:* Cough, asthma, bronchitis, dyspnea, sinusitis, bronchospasm. *Neuromuscular:* Paresthesias, arthralgia, arthritis, asthenia, myalgia. *Hematologic:* Occasionally, eosinophilia, leukopenia, neutropenia, decreased hemoglobin. *Miscellaneous:* Angioedema, which may be associated with involvement of the tongue, glottis, or larynx; hypertonia; proteinuria; hyponatremia; infection.
Laboratory Test Considerations: ↑ Serum creatinine, BUN, serum potassium. ↓ Hemoglobin. ECG changes.
Drug Interactions
Diuretics / Excessive ↓ in BP
Lithium / ↑ Serum lithium levels with ↑ risk of lithium toxicity
Potassium-sparing diuretics, potassium supplements / ↑ Risk of hyperkalemia
How Supplied: *Tablet:* 5 mg, 10 mg, 20 mg, 40 mg

Dosage

- **Tablets**

Clients not receiving a diuretic.
Initial: 10 mg once daily; **maintenance:** 20-40 mg/day given as a single dose or in two equally divided doses. Total daily doses greater than 80 mg have not been evaluated.
Clients receiving a diuretic.
Initial: 5 mg/day.
$C_{CR} < 30$ *mL/min/1.73 m²*. The recommended starting dose is 5 mg/day; **maintenance:** titrate dose upward until BP is controlled or to a maximum total daily dose of 40 mg.

HEALTH CARE CONSIDERATIONS

See also *Health Care Considerations* for *Angiotensin-Converting Enzyme Inhibitors* and *Antihypertensive Agents.*

Administration/Storage
1. Base dosage adjustment on measuring peak (2-6 hr after dosing) and trough responses. Consider increasing the dose or give divided doses if once-daily dosing does not provide an adequate trough response.
2. If BP not controlled by benazepril alone, add a diuretic.
3. If receiving a diuretic, discontinue the diuretic, if possible, 2-3 days before beginning benazepril therapy.

Assessment
1. Note any previous experience with this class of drugs.
2. Review diet, weight loss, exercise, and life-style changes necessary to control BP.
3. Monitor electrolytes, liver and renal function studies.

Client/Family Teaching
1. Take only as directed. May be taken with or without food.
2. Avoid concomitant administration of potassium supplements, or potassium-sparing diuretics; may lead to increased K^+ levels.
3. Side effects such as headache, fatigue, dizziness, and cough have been associated with this drug therapy; report if persistent/bothersome.

Outcome/Evaluate: Control of hypertension

Benzonatate

(ben-**ZOH**-nah-tayt)
Pregnancy Category: C
Tessalon Perles **(Rx)**
Classification: Antitussive, nonnarcotic

Action/Kinetics: Acts peripherally by anesthetizing stretch receptors in the respiratory passages, lungs, and pleura, thus depressing the cough reflex at its source. No effect on the respiratory center in the doses recommended. **Onset:** 15-20 min. **Duration:** 3-8 hr.
Uses: Symptomatic relief of cough.
Contraindications: Sensitivity to benzonatate or related drugs such as procaine and tetracaine.
Special Concerns: Use with caution during lactation. Safety and efficacy have not been determined in children less than 10 years of age.

B

Side Effects: *Hypersensitivity reactions:* ***Bronchospasm, laryngospasm, CV collapse.*** *GI:* Nausea, GI upset, constipation. *CNS:* Sedation, headache, dizziness, mental confusion, visual hallucinations. *Dermatologic:* Pruritus, skin eruptions. *Miscellaneous:* Nasal congestion, sensation of burning in the eyes, "chilly" sensation, numbness of the chest.

OD **Management of Overdose:** *Symptoms:* Oropharyngeal anesthesia if capsules are chewed or dissolved in the mouth. CNS stimulation, including restlessness, tremors, and clonic convulsions followed by profound CNS depression. *Treatment:* Evacuate gastric contents followed by copious amounts of activated charcoal slurry. Due to depressed cough and gag reflexes, efforts may be needed to protect against aspiration of gastric contents and orally administered substances. Treat convulsions with a short-acting IV barbiturate. Do not use CNS stimulants. Support of respiration and CV-renal function.

How Supplied: *Perles:* 100 mg.

Dosage

- **Capsules (Perles)**

  Antitussive.

Adults and children over 10 years of age: 100 mg t.i.d., up to a maximum of 600 mg/day.

HEALTH CARE CONSIDERATIONS

Assessment

1. Record indications for therapy, onset, duration, and characteristics of symptoms.
2. Note any sensitivity to benzonatate or tetracaine.
3. Not for use during pregnancy.

Client/Family Teaching

1. Take only as directed and with plenty of fluids. Swallow perles without chewing to avoid the local anesthetic effect on the oral mucosa and to prevent choking.
2. Do not perform tasks that require alertness until drug effects realized.
3. Do not change positions suddenly due to postural effects; take appropriate precautions if dizziness or drowsiness occur.
4. Report if symptoms intensify or do not improve after 5 days.

Outcome/Evaluate: Control of persistent coughing episodes.

Benztropine mesylate

(BENS-troh-peen)

Pregnancy Category: C

Apo-Benztropine ✤, Benzylate ✤, Cogentin, PMS-Benztropine ✤ **(Rx)**

Classification: Synthetic anticholinergic, antiparkinson agent

See also *Cholinergic Blocking Agents.*

Action/Kinetics: Synthetic anticholinergic possessing antihistamine and local anesthetic properties. **Onset, PO:** 1-2 hr; **IM, IV:** Within a few minutes. Effects are cumulative; is long-acting (24 hr). **Full effects:** 2-3 days. Low incidence of side effects.

Uses: Adjunct in the treatment of parkinsonism (all types). To reduce severity of extrapyramidal effects in phenothiazine or other antipsychotic drug therapy (not effective in tardive dyskinesia).

Contraindications: Use in children under 3 years of age.

Special Concerns: Geriatric and emaciated clients cannot tolerate large doses. Certain drug-induced extrapyramidal symptoms may not respond to benztropine.

How Supplied: *Injection:* 1 mg/mL; *Tablet:* 0.5 mg, 1 mg, 2 mg

Dosage

- **Tablets**

  Parkinsonism.

Adults: 1-2 mg/day (range: 0.5-6 mg/day).

Idiopathic parkinsonism.

Adults, initial: 0.5-1 mg/day, increased gradually to 4-6 mg/day, if necessary.

Postencephalitic parkinsonism.

Adults: 2 mg/day in one or more doses.

Drug-induced extrapyramidal effects.

Adults: 1-4 mg 1-2 times/day.

- **IM, IV (Rarely)**

  Acute dystonic reactions.

Adults, initial: 1-2 mg; **then,** 1-2 mg PO b.i.d. usually prevents recurrence. Clients can rarely tolerate full dosage.

HEALTH CARE CONSIDERATIONS

See also *Health Care Considerations* for *Cholinergic Blocking Agents.*

Administration/Storage

1. When used as replacement for or supplement to other antiparkinsonism drugs, substitute or add gradually.
2. For difficulty swallowing tablets, may crush tabs and mix with a small amount of food or liquid.
3. Some may benefit by taking the entire dose at bedtime while others are best treated by taking divided doses, b.i.d.-q.i.d.
4. Start therapy with a low dose (e.g., 0.5 mg) and then increase in increments of 0.5 mg at 5-6-day intervals. Do not exceed 6 mg/day.
5. IV If administered IV, may give undiluted at a rate of 1 mg over 1 min.

Assessment
1. Note if phenothiazines or TCAs are being used; may cause a paralytic ileus.
2. Note age; elderly clients require a lower dosage.

Interventions
1. Monitor I&O. Assess for urinary retention and bowel sounds; especially important with limited mobility.
2. Inspect skin at regular intervals for evidence of skin changes.
3. Observe for extrapyramidal symptoms, i.e., drooling, muscle spasms, shuffling gait, muscle rigidity, and pill rolling.
4. If excitation or vomiting occurs, withdraw drug temporarily and resume at a lower dose.

Client/Family Teaching
1. Review goals of therapy (control of parkinsonian symptoms, i.e., improved gait and balance and less rigidity and involuntary movements; control of extrapyramidal symptoms, i.e., less drooling, muscle spasms, shuffling gait, or pill rolling).
2. Use caution when performing tasks that require mental alertness; drug has a sedative effect and may also cause postural hypotension.
3. It usually takes 2-3 days for drug to exert a desired effect. Take as ordered unless side effects occur; these usually subside with continued drug use.
4. Avoid strenuous activity and increased heat exposure. Plan rest periods during the day as ability to tolerate heat will be reduced and heat stroke may occur.
5. Report any difficulty in voiding or inadequate emptying of the bladder.
6. Avoid alcohol and any other CNS depressants.

Outcome/Evaluate
- ↓ Involuntary movements and rigidity with improved gait and balance
- Control of extrapyramidal side effects of antipsychotic agents

Bepridil hydrochloride
(BEH-prih-dill)
Pregnancy Category: C
Vascor **(Rx)**
Classification: Antianginal, calcium channel blocking drug

See also *Calcium Channel Blocking Agents*.
Action/Kinetics: Inhibits the transmembrane influx of calcium ions into cardiac and vascular smooth muscle. Increases the effective refractory period of the atria, AV node, His-Purkinje fibers, and ventricles. Dilates peripheral arterioles and reduces total peripheral resistance; reduces HR and arterial pressure at rest and at a given level of exercise. Rapidly and completely absorbed following PO use. **Onset:** 60 min. **Time to peak plasma levels:** 2-3 hr. Greater than 99% bound to plasma protein. Food does not affect either the peak plasma levels or the extent of absorption. **Therapeutic serum levels:** 1-2 ng/mL. **t½, distribution:** 2 hr; **terminal elimination:** 24 hr. Steady-state blood levels do not occur for 8 days. Metabolized in the liver and metabolites are excreted through both the kidney (70%) and the feces (22%).
Uses: Chronic stable angina (classic effort-associated angina) in clients who have failed to respond to other antianginal medications or who are intolerant to such medications. May be used alone or with beta blockers or nitrates. An additive effect occurs if used with propranolol.
Contraindications: Clients with a history of serious ventricular arrhythmias, sick sinus syndrome, second- or third-degree heart block (except in the presence of a functioning ventricular pacemaker), hypotension (less than 90 mm Hg systolic), uncompensated cardiac insufficiency, congenital QT interval prolongation, and in those taking other drugs that prolong the QT interval (e.g., quinidine, procainamide, tricyclic antidepressants). Use in clients with MI during the previous 3 months. Lactation.
Special Concerns: Safety and effectiveness have not been determined in children. Use with caution in clients with CHF, left bundle block, sinus bradycardia (less than 50 beats/min), serious hepatic or renal disorders. New arrhythmias can be induced. Geriatric clients may require more frequent monitoring.
Side Effects: *CV: **Induction of new serious arrhythmias such as torsades de pointes type ventricular tachycardia, prolongation of QTc and QT interval, increased PVC rates, new sustained VT and VT/VF,*** sinus tachycardia, sinus bradycardia, hypertension vasodilation, palpitations. *GI:* Nausea (common), dyspepsia, GI distress, diarrhea, dry mouth, anorexia, abdominal pain, constipation, flatulence, gastritis, increased appetite. *CNS:* Nervousness, dizziness, drowsiness, insomnia, depression, vertigo, akathisia, anxiousness, tremor, hand tremor, syncope, paresthesia. *Respiratory:* Cough, pharyngitis, rhinitis, dyspnea, respiratory infection. *Body as a whole:* Asthenia, headache, flu syndrome, fever, pain, superinfection. *Dermatologic:* Rash, skin irritation, sweating. *Miscellaneous:* Tinnitus, arthritis,

blurred vision, taste change, loss of libido, impotence, agranulocytosis.

Laboratory Test Considerations: ↑ ALT, transaminase. Abnormal liver function tests.

Drug Interactions

Cardiac glycosides / Exaggeration of the depression of AV nodal conduction

Digoxin / Possible ↑ serum digoxin levels

Potassium-wasting diuretics / Hypokalemia, which causes an ↑ risk of serious ventricular arrhythmias

Procainamide / ↑ Risk of serious side effects due to exaggerated prolongation of the QT interval

Quinidine / ↑ Risk of serious side effects due to exaggerated prolongation of the QT interval

Tricyclic antidepressants / ↑ Risk of serious side effects due to exaggerated prolongation of the QT interval

How Supplied: *Tablet:* 200 mg, 300 mg

Dosage

- **Tablets**

  Chronic stable angina.

Adults, initial: 200 mg once daily; after 10 days the dosage may be adjusted upward depending on the response of the client (e.g., ability to perform ADL, QT interval, HR, frequency and severity of angina). **Maintenance:** 300 mg/day, not to exceed 400 mg/day. The minimum effective dose is 200 mg.

HEALTH CARE CONSIDERATIONS

See also *Health Care Considerations* for *Calcium Channel Blocking Agents.*

Assessment

1. Note antianginal agents used previously and their effects.
2. Monitor VS, CBC, K^+, and ECG.
3. List drugs currently prescribed; note any that may prolong the QT interval (e.g., procainamide, quinidine, tricyclic antidepressants). QT intervals should be checked prior to initiating therapy with bepridil, 1 to 3 weeks after beginning therapy, and periodically thereafter; especially after any dosage adjustment. Prolongation may lead to serious ventricular arrhythmias, especially torsades de pointes.
4. Note any evidence of AV block, new arrhythmias, or history of MI, and/or implanted ventricular pacemaker.
5. Geriatric clients require more frequent monitoring.
6. If diuretics required, use a potassium-sparing agent.

Client/Family Teaching

1. Can be taken with meals or at bedtime if nausea occurs.
2. Take at about the same time each day. If a dose is missed, the next dose should *not* be doubled.
3. Continue taking nitroglycerin if prescribed.
4. Report dizziness, chest pain, altered mental status, ↑ SOB, or fainting.

Outcome/Evaluate

- Prophylaxis/control of angina
- Therapeutic levels (1-2 ng/mL)

Betamethasone

(bay-tah-**METH**-ah-zohn)
Celestone **(Rx)**

Betamethasone dipropionate

(bay-tah-**METH**-ah-zohn)
Topical: Alphatrex, Betaprone ✱, Diprolene, Diprolene Glycol ✱, Diprosone, Maxivate, Occlucort ✱, Pro-Lene Glycol ✱, Pro-Sone ✱, Rolene ✱, Rosone ✱, Taro-Sone ✱, Topilene ✱, Topisone ✱ **(Rx)**

Betamethasone sodium phosphate

(bay-tah-**METH**-ah-zohn)
Betnesol ✱, Celestone Phosphate, Cel-U-Jec **(Rx)**

Betamethasone sodium phosphate and Betamethasone acetate

(bay-tah-**METH**-ah-zohn)
Celestone Soluspan **(Rx)**

Betamethasone valerate

(bay-tah-**METH**-ah-zohn)
Topical: Betacort ✱, Betaderm ✱, Betatrex, Betnovate ✱, Betnovate-1/2 ✱, Celestoderm-V ✱, Celestoderm-V/2 ✱, Dermabet, Ectosone Mild ✱, Ectosone Regular, Ectosone Scalp Lotion ✱, Prevex B ✱, Rivasone ✱, Valisone, Valisone Reduced Strength, Valnac **(Rx)**

Classification: Glucocorticoid

See also *Corticosteroids.*

Action/Kinetics: Causes low degree of sodium and water retention, as well as potassium depletion. The injectable form contains both rapid-acting and repository forms of betamethasone (mixture of betamethasone sodium phosphate and betamethasone acetate). Long-acting. **t½:** over 300 min.

Additional Uses: Prevention of respiratory distress syndrome in premature infants.

Contraindications: Not recommended for replacement therapy in any acute or chronic adrenal cortical insufficiency because it does not have strong sodium-retaining effects.
Special Concerns: Safe use during pregnancy and lactation has not been established.
How Supplied: Betamethasone: *Syrup:* 0.6 mg/5 mL; *Tablet:* 0.6 mg. Betamethasone dipropionate: *Cream:* 0.05%; *Lotion:* 0.05%; *Ointment:* 0.05%; *Spray:* 0.1%. Betamethasone sodium phosphate: *Injection:* 3 mg/mL, 4 mg/mL. Betamethasone sodium phosphate and betamethasone acetate: *Injection:* 3 mg/mL. Betamethasone valerate: *Cream:* 0.1%; *Lotion:* 0.1%; *Ointment:* 0.1%

Dosage

BETAMETHASONE
- **Syrup, Tablets**

0.6-7.2 mg/day.

BETAMETHASONE SODIUM PHOSPHATE
- **IV, Intra-articular, Intralesional, Soft Tissue Injection**

Initial: up to 9 mg/day; **then,** adjust dosage at minimal level to reduce symptoms.

BETAMETHASONE SODIUM PHOSPHATE AND BETAMETHASONE ACETATE(contains 3 mg/mL each of the acetate and sodium phosphate)
- **IM**

Initial: 0.5-9 mg/day (dose ranges are 1/3-1/2 the PO dose given q 12 hr.)
- **Intra-articular, Intrabursal, Intradermal, Intralesional**

Bursitis, peritendinitis, tenosynovitis.
1 mL.
Rheumatoid arthritis and osteoarthritis.
0.25-2 mL, depending on size of the joint.
Foot disorders, bursitis.
0.25-0.5 mL under heloma durum or heloma molle; 0.5 mL under calcaneal spur or over hallux rigidus or digiti quinti varus. Tenosynovitis or periostitis of cuboid: 0.5 mL.
Acute gouty arthritis.
0.5-1 mL.
- **Intradermal**

0.2 mL/cm^2 not to exceed 1 mL/week.

BETAMETHASONE DIPROPIONATE, BETAMETHASONE VALERATE
- **Topical Aerosol, Cream, Lotion, Ointment**

Apply sparingly to affected areas and rub in lightly.

HEALTH CARE CONSIDERATIONS

See also *Health Care Considerations* for *Corticosteroids.*

Administration/Storage: Avoid injection into deltoid muscle because SC tissue atrophy may occur.
Assessment: Record indications for therapy, type, onset, and duration of symptoms; list agents trialed with the outcome.
Client/Family Teaching
1. Report any S&S of infection, i.e., increased fever, any redness, odor, or purulent wound drainage.
2. Cover topically to avoid sun burn.
3. Do not overuse joint after injection; this may further injure joint.
4. Record weight; report any sudden weight gain or edema.

Outcome/Evaluate
- ↓ Pain/inflammation; ↑ mobility
- Prevention of respiratory distress syndrome in premies
- Improved skin integrity; healing of lesions

Betaxolol hydrochloride
(beh-TAX-oh-lohl)
Pregnancy Category: C
Betoptic, Betoptic S, Kerlone **(Rx)**
Classification: Beta-adrenergic blocking agent

See also *Beta-Adrenergic Blocking Agents.*
Action/Kinetics: Inhibits beta-1-adrenergic receptors although beta-2 receptors will be inhibited at high doses. Has some membrane stabilizing activity but no intrinsic sympathomimetic activity. Low lipid solubility. Reduces the production of aqueous humor, thus, reducing intraocular pressure. No effect on pupil size or accommodation. **t1/2:** 14-22 hr. Metabolized in the liver with most excreted through the urine; about 15% is excreted unchanged.
Uses: PO: Hypertension, alone or with other antihypertensive agents (especially diuretics). **Ophthalmic:** Ocular hypertension and chronic open-angle glaucoma (used alone or in combination with other antiglaucoma drugs).
Special Concerns: Use with caution during lactation. Safety and effectiveness have not been determined in children. Geriatric clients are at greater risk of developing bradycardia.
How Supplied: *Ophthalmic Solution:* 0.5%; *Ophthalmic Suspension:* 0.25%; *Tablet:* 10 mg, 20 mg

Dosage
- **Tablets**

Hypertension.

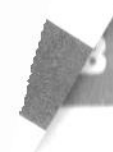

Initial: 10 mg once daily either alone or with a diuretic. If the desired effect is not reached, the dose can be increased to 20 mg although doses higher than 20 mg will not increase the therapeutic effect. In geriatric clients the initial dose should be 5 mg/day.

• **Ophthalmic Solution, Suspension**

Adults: 1-2 gtt b.i.d. If used to replace another drug, continue the drug being used and add 1 gtt of betaxolol b.i.d. The previous drug should be discontinued the following day. If transferring from several antiglaucoma drugs being used together, adjust one drug at a time at intervals of not less than 1 week. The agents being used can be continued and add 1 gtt betaxolol b.i.d. The next day, another agent should be discontinued. The remaining antiglaucoma drug dosage can be decreased or discontinued depending on the response of the client.

HEALTH CARE CONSIDERATIONS

See also *Health Care Considerations* for *Beta-Adrenergic Blocking Agents* and *Antihypertensive Agents*,

Administration/Storage

1. Full antihypertensive effect usually observed within 7 to 14 days.
2. As the PO dose is increased, the HR decreases.
3. Discontinue PO therapy gradually over a 2-week period.
4. Shake ophthalmic suspension well before use.
5. Store ophthalmic products at room temperature not to exceed 30°C (86°F).

Outcome/Evaluate

- ↓ BP (PO)
- ↓ Intraocular pressure

Bethanechol chloride

(beh-**THAN**-eh-kohl)

Pregnancy Category: C

Duvoid, Myotonachol, PMS-Bethanechol Chloride ✱, Urecholine **(Rx)**

Classification: Cholinergic (parasympathomimetic), direct-acting

Action/Kinetics: Directly stimulates cholinergic receptors, primarily muscarinic type. This results in stimulation of gastric motility, increases gastric tone, and stimulates the detrusor muscle of the urinary bladder. Produces a slight transient fall of DBP, accompanied by minor reflex tachycardia. Is resistant to hydrolysis by acetylcholinesterase, which increases its duration of action. **PO: Onset,** 30-90 min; **maximum:** 60-90 min; **duration:** 1 hr (large doses up to 6 hr). **SC: Onset,** 5-15 min; **maximum:** 15-30 min; **duration:** 2 hr.

Uses: Postpartum or postoperative urinary retention, neurogenic atony of the bladder with urinary retention. *Investigational:* Reflux esophagitis in adults and gastroesophageal reflux in infants and children.

Contraindications: Hypotension, hypertension, CAD, coronary occlusion, AV conduction defects, vasomotor instability, pronounced bradycardia, peptic ulcer, bronchial asthma (latent or active), hyperthyroidism, parkinsonism, epilepsy, obstruction of the bladder or bladder neck, if the strength or integrity of the GI or bladder wall is questionable, peritonitis, GI spastic disease, acute inflammatory lesions of the GI tract, when increased muscular activity of the GI tract or urinary bladder might be harmful (e.g., following recent urinary bladder surgery), GI resection and anastomosis, GI obstruction, marked vagotonia. Lactation. Not to be used IM or IV.

Special Concerns: Safety and effectiveness have not been determined in children.

Side Effects: Serious side effects are uncommon with PO dosage but more common following SC use. *GI:* Nausea, diarrhea, salivation, GI upset, involuntary defecation, cramps, colic, belching, rumbling/gurgling of stomach. *CV:* Hypotension with reflex tachycardia, vasomotor response. *CNS:* Headache, malaise. *Other:* Flushing, sensation of heat about the face, sweating, urinary urgency, attacks of asthma, bronchial constriction, miosis, lacrimation.

OD **Management of Overdose:** *Symptoms:* Early signs include N&V, abdominal discomfort, salivation, sweating, flushing. *Treatment:* Atropine, 0.6 mg SC for adults; a dose of 0.01 mg/kg atropine SC (up to a maximum of 0.4 mg) is recommended for infants and children up to 12 years of age. IV atropine may be used in emergency situations.

Drug Interactions

Cholinergic inhibitors / Additive cholinergic effects

Ganglionic blocking agents / Critical hypotensive response preceded by severe abdominal symptoms

Procainamide / Antagonism of cholinergic effects

Quinidine / Antagonism of cholinergic effects

How Supplied: *Injection:* 5 mg/mL; *Tablet:* 5 mg, 10 mg, 25 mg, 50 mg

Dosage

• **Tablets**

Urinary retention.

Adults, usual: 10-50 mg t.i.d.-q.i.d. The minimum effective dose can be determined by giving 5-10 mg initially and repeating this dose q 1-2 hr until a satisfactory response is observed or a maximum of 50 mg has been given.

Treat reflux esophagitis in adults.
25 mg q.i.d.

Gastroesophageal reflex in infants and children.
3 mg/m²/dose t.i.d.

• **SC**

Urinary retention.
Adults, usual: 5 mg t.i.d.-q.i.d. The minimum effective dose is determined by giving 2.5 mg initially and repeating this dose at 15-30-min intervals to a maximum of four doses or until a satisfactory response is obtained.

Diagnosis of reflux esophagitis in adults.
Two 50-mcg/kg doses 15 min apart.

HEALTH CARE CONSIDERATIONS

Administration/Storage

1. Administer only PO or SC.
2. Observe closely 30 to 60 min after drug administration for possible severe side effects. Have atropine available during SC therapy to counteract manifestations of acute toxicity.

Assessment

1. Take a complete medical history.
2. Note drugs currently prescribed to ensure none interact unfavorably.
3. Assess I&O with urinary tract problems.
4. With GI atony, assess bowel sounds, function and habits.
5. If taking antacids, assess for peptic ulcers.

Client/Family Teaching

1. Take tablets on an empty stomach (1 hr before or 2 hr after meals) to avoid N&V. Take exactly as prescribed for maximum effect.
2. With SC therapy, administer 2 hr before eating to reduce the potential for nausea.
3. Report decreased bowel activity when used for GI atony.
4. Any marked decrease in urine output, any gnawing, aching, burning, or epigastric pain in the left epigastric area should be reported.

Outcome/Evaluate

• Improved bladder tone and function without retention
• ↑ GI tract motility with ↓ abdominal distension

Bexarotene

(bex-**AIR**-oh-teen)
Pregnancy Category: X
Targretin **(Rx)**
Classification: Antineoplastic, retinoid

See also *Antineoplastic Agents.*
Action/Kinetics: Binds with and activates retinoid X receptor subtypes. Once activated, these receptors act as transcription factors that regulate the expression of genes that control cell differentiation and proliferation. Exact mechanism to treat cutaneous T-cell lymphoma is not known but the drug inhibits growth of some tumor cell lines, in vitro, of hematopoietic and squamous cell origin and induces tumor regression, in vitro, in some animal models. Maximum absorption within 2 hr. More than 99% bound to plasma proteins. Metabolized in the liver and excreted through the hepatobiliary system. **t½, terminal:** 7 hr.
Uses: Cutaneous T-cell lymphoma in clients refractory to 1 or more prior systemic treatments.
Contraindications: Pregnancy, lactation.
Special Concerns: Use with caution in clients using insulin, sulfonylureas, or insulin-sensitizers due to possible enhanced hypoglycemic effect. Safety and efficacy have not been determined in children.
Side Effects: Use induces major lipid abnormalities (e.g., ↑ fasting triglycerides, total and LDL cholesterol; ↓ HDL). *GI:* Acute pancreatitis, impaired hepatic function, abdominal pain, N&V, diarrhea, anorexia, constipation, dry mouth, flatulence, colitis, dyspepsia, cheilitis, gastroenteritis, gingivitis, ***liver failure,*** melena. *CNS:* Headache, insomnia, depression, agitation, ataxia, confusion, dizziness, hyperesthesia, hypesthesia, neuropathy. *CV:* ***CVA, hemorrhage,*** hypertension, angina pectoris, chest pain, syncope, tachycardia. *Hematologic:* Leukopenia, anemia, hypochromic anemia, eosinophilia, thrombocythemia, lymphocytosis, thrombocytopenia. *Dermatologic:* Dry skin, rash, exfoliative dermatitis, alopecia, skin ulcer, acne, skin nodule, maculopapular rash, pustular rash, serous drainage, vesicular bullous rash. *Respiratory:* Pharyngitis, rhinitis, dyspnea, pleural effusion, bronchitis, increased cough, lung edema, hemoptysis, hypoxia. *GU:* Urinary incontinence, UTI, urinary urgency, dysuria, abnormal kidney function, breast pain. *Musculoskeletal:* Arthralgia, myalgia, bone pain, myasthenia, arthrosis. *Ophthalmic:* Dry eyes, conjunctivitis, blepharitis, corneal lesion, keratitis, visual field defect. *Body as a whole:* Asthenia, bacterial infection, pneumonia, chills, fever, flu syndrome, peripheral edema, increase or decrease in weight,

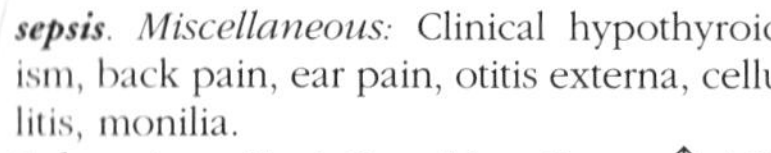

sepsis. *Miscellaneous:* Clinical hypothyroidism, back pain, ear pain, otitis externa, cellulitis, monilia.
Laboratory Test Considerations: ↑ AST, ALT, alkaline phosphatase, LDH, creatinine, amylase. Bilirubinemia, hypercholesterolemia, hyperlipemia, hyperglycemia, hypocalcemia, hyponatremia, hypoproteinemia.
Drug Interactions
Antidiabetic drugs (insulin, sulfonylureas) ↑ Risk of hypoglycemia
Erythromycin / ↑ Plasma bexarotene levels R/T ↓ liver metabolism
Gemfibrozil / Significant ↑ in plasma bexarotene levels
Grapefruit juice / ↑ Plasma bexarotene levels R/T ↓ liver metabolism
Itraconazole / ↑ Plasma bexarotene levels R/T ↓ liver metabolism
Ketoconazole / ↑ Plasma bexarotene levels R/T ↓ liver metabolism
Phenobarbital / ↓ Plasma bexarotene levels R/T ↑ liver metabolism
Phenytoin / ↓ Plasma bexarotene levels R/T ↑ liver metabolism
Rifampin / ↓ Plasma bexarotene levels R/T ↑ liver metabolism
Vitamin A / Additive toxic effects
How Supplied: *Capsules:* 75 mg

Dosage

- **Capsules**

Cutaneous T-cell lymphoma.

Initial: 300 mg/m²/day; **then,** adjust for body surface area as a single PO daily dose taken with a meal as follows: **0.88-1.12 m²:** 300 mg/day; **1.13-1.37 m²:** 375 mg/day; **1.38-1.62 m²:** 450 mg/day; **1.63-1.87 m²:** 525 mg/day; **1.88-2.12 m²:** 600 mg/day; **2.13-2.37 m²:** 675 mg/day; **2.38-2.62 m²:** 750 mg/day. *NOTE:* If there is no response after 8 weeks of therapy and if the initial dose of 300 mg/m²/day is well tolerated, the dose can be increased to 400 mg/m²/day; monitor carefully. If toxic effects occur, the 300 mg/m²/day may be decreased to 200 mg/m²/day or 100 mg/m²/day. When toxicity is controlled, the dose can be readjusted upward.

HEALTH CARE CONSIDERATIONS

See also *Health Care Considerations* for *Antineoplastic Agents*.

Assessment

1. Record onset and characteristics of disease; list other agents/therapies trialed.
2. List drugs prescribed to ensure none interact; enhances effects of hypoglycemic agents.
3. Monitor renal and LFTs. Use cautiously with impaired function as drug is metabolized in liver.

Client/Family Teaching

1. Take as directed; avoid grapefruit juice.
2. May experience flu-like symptoms. Report any unusual side effects including rashes, abnormal bruising/bleeding, UTI/URI, unsteady gait, confusion, dizziness/drowsiness, abdominal pain, yellow skin discoloration, depression or pain in extremities.
3. Practice reliable birth control.
4. Identify local support groups to assist with disease understanding/management.

Outcome/Evaluate: Inhibition of malignant cell proliferation

Bicalutamide

(buy-kah-LOO-tah-myd)
Pregnancy Category: X
Casodex **(Rx)**
Classification: Antineoplastic, antiandrogen

See also *Antineoplastic Agents,*.
Action/Kinetics: A nonsteroidal antiandrogen that competitively inhibits the action of androgens by binding to androgen receptors in the cytosol in target tissues. Well absorbed after PO administration; food does not affect the rate or amount absorbed. Metabolized in the liver, and both parent drug and metabolites are eliminated in the urine and feces. **t½:** 5.8 days. **Mean steady-state concentration in prostatic cancer:** 8.9 mcg/mL.
Uses: In combination therapy with a leutinizing hormone-releasing hormone analog for the treatment of advanced prostate cancer.
Contraindications: Pregnancy.
Special Concerns: Use with caution in clients with moderate to severe hepatic impairment and during lactation. Safety and efficacy have not been established in children.
Side Effects: *GI:* Constipation, N&V, diarrhea, anorexia, dyspepsia, rectal hemorrhage, dry mouth, melena. *CNS:* Dizziness, paresthesia, insomnia, anxiety, depression, decreased libido, hypertonia, confusion, neuropathy, somnolence, nervousness. *GU:* Gynecomastia, nocturia, hematuria, UTI, impotence, urinary incontinence, urinary frequency, impaired urination, dysuria, urinary retention, urinary urgency. *CV:* Hot flashes (most common), hypertension, angina pectoris, CHF. *Metabolic:* Peripheral edema, hyperglycemia, weight loss or gain, dehydration, gout. *Musculoskeletal:* Myasthenia, arthritis, myalgia, leg cramps, pathologic fracture. *Respiratory:* Dyspnea, increased cough, pharyngitis, bronchitis, pneumonia, rhinitis, lung disorder. *Dermatologic:* Rash, sweating, dry skin, prur-

itus, alopecia. *Hematologic:* Anemia, hypochromic and iron deficiency anemia. *Body as a whole:* General pain, back pain, asthenia, pelvic pain, abdominal pain, chest pain, flu syndrome, edema, neoplasm, fever, neck pain, chills, ***sepsis.*** *Miscellaneous:* Infection, bone pain, headache, breast pain, diabetes mellitus.
Laboratory Test Considerations: ↑ Alkaline phosphatase, creatinine, AST, ALT, bilirubin, BUN, liver enzyme tests. ↓ Hemoglobin, white cell count.
Drug Interactions: Bicalutamide may displace coumarin anticoagulants from their protein-binding sites, resulting in an increased anticoagulant effect.
How Supplied: *Tablet:* 50 mg

Dosage
- **Tablets**

Prostatic carcinoma.

50 mg (1 tablet) once daily (morning or evening) in combination with an LHRH analog with or without food.

HEALTH CARE CONSIDERATIONS

See also *Health Care Considerations* for *Antineoplastic Agents.*

Administration/Storage

1. Take at the same time each day.
2. Start treatment at the same time as LHRH analog.

Assessment

1. Note indications for therapy, onset, duration of symptoms, and any other agents/therapies trialed.
2. Monitor liver and renal function studies, CBC, and PSA. (If transaminases increase over two times the ULN, discontinue drug.)
3. If prescribed warfarin, monitor PT/INR closely; can displace from protein binding sites.

Client/Family Teaching

1. Take as directed, at the same time each day, with prescribed LHRH analog drug (i.e., goserelin implant or leuprolide depot).
2. Side effects that require immediate attention include hemorrhage, urinary retention, yellow skin, fracture, and respiratory distress.
3. Periodic lab studies for PSA, CBC, liver and renal function will be required to assess response.

Outcome/Evaluate

- Symptomatic improvement
- Reductions of serum PSA and inhibition of tumor growth

Biperiden hydrochloride

(bye-**PER**-ih-den)
Pregnancy Category: C
Akineton Hydrochloride **(Rx)**
Classification: Synthetic anticholinergic, antiparkinson agent

See also *Antiparkinson Drugs* and *Cholinergic Blocking Agents.*
Action/Kinetics: Synthetic anticholinergic. Tremor may increase as spasticity is relieved. Slight respiratory and CV effects. **Time to peak levels:** 60-90 min. **Peak levels:** 4-5 mcg/L. **t½:** About 18-24 hr. Tolerance may develop.
Uses: Parkinsonism, especially of the postencephalitic, arteriosclerotic, and idiopathic types. Drug-induced (e.g., phenothiazines) extrapyramidal manifestations.
Additional Contraindications: Children under the age of 3 years.
Special Concerns: Use with caution in older children.
Additional Side Effects: Muscle weakness, inability to move certain muscles.
How Supplied: *Injection:* 5 mg/mL (as lactate) *Tablet:* 2 mg.

Dosage
- **Tablets**

Parkinsonism.

Adults: 2 mg t.i.d.-q.i.d., to a maximum of 16 mg/day.

Drug-induced extrapyramidal effects.

Adults: 2 mg 1-3 times/day. Maximum daily dose: 16 mg.
- **IM, IV**

Drug-induced extrapyramidal effects.

Adults: 2 mg; repeat q 30 min until symptoms improve, but not more than four consecutive doses/24 hr.
- **IM**

Drug-induced extrapyramidal effects.

Pediatric: 0.04 mg/kg (1.2 mg/m²); repeat q 30 min until symptoms improve, but not more than four doses daily.

HEALTH CARE CONSIDERATIONS

See also *Health Care Considerations* for *Antiparkinson Drugs* and *Cholinergic Blocking Agents.*

Assessment

1. Note age; older clients should receive lower doses of biperiden.
2. Record drugs client taking to prevent any unfavorable interactions.

Interventions

1. If administered IM, supervise and assist in walking; may cause transient incoordination.
2. If administered IV, have client remain recumbent during and for 15 min after administration. Dangle legs at the bedside prior to standing and walking, to prevent hypotension, syncope, and falling.

Client/Family Teaching

1. Take after meals to avoid gastric irritation.
2. Do not use antacids or antidiarrheal for 1-2 hr after taking drug.
3. Record stools; increase intake of fluids, fruit juices, and fiber to avoid constipation.
4. Avoid overheating; drug decreases perspiration.
5. Record I&O; report urinary difficulty.
6. Use sugarless gum or candies and rinse mouth often to control dry mouth effects.

Outcome/Evaluate: Control of drug-induced (phenothiazine) extrapyramidal manifestations (i.e., ↓ muscle rigidity and drooling)

Bismuth subsalicylate, Metronidazole, Tetracycline hydrochloride

(**BIS**-muth, meh-troh-**NYE**-dah-zohl, teh-trah-**SYE**-kleen)

Pregnancy Category: B (Metronidazole), D (Tetracycline)

Helidac **(Rx)**

Classification: Agent to treat *Helicobacter pylori* infections

See also *Metronidazole* and *Tetracycline hydrochloride.*

Action/Kinetics: The information to follow was derived from each drug being given alone and not in the combination in this product. Bismuth subsalicylate is hydrolyzed in the GI tract to bismuth and salicylic acid. Less than 1% of bismuth from PO doses of bismuth subsalicylate is absorbed into the general circulation. However, more than 80% of salicylic acid is absorbed. Metronidazole is well absorbed from the GI tract. **Peak plasma levels, metronidazole:** 1-2 hr; **t½, elimination:** 8 hr. Metronidazole is metabolized by the liver and is excreted through both the urine (60% to 80%) and the feces (6% to 15%). Tetracyclines are readily absorbed from the GI tract. The relative contributions of systemic versus local antimicrobial activity against *H. pylori* for agents used in eradication therapy have not been determined.

Uses: In combination with an H_2 antagonist to treat active duodenal ulcer associated with *H. pylori* infection.

Contraindications: Use during pregnancy or lactation, in children, or in renal or hepatic impairment. Hypersensitivity to bismuth subsalicylate, metronidazole or other imidazole derivatives, and any tetracycline. Use in those allergic to aspirin or salicylates. Children and teenagers who have or who are recovering from chicken pox or the flu should not take bismuth subsalicylate due to the possibility of Reye's syndrome. Tetracyclines should not be used during tooth development in children (i.e., last half of pregnancy, infancy, and childhood to 8 years of age) due to the possibility of permanent tooth discoloration.

Special Concerns: Use with caution in elderly clients and in clients with evidence or history of blood dyscrasias. Safety and efficacy have not been determined in children.

Side Effects: See also *Metronidazole* and *Tetracyclines* for specific side effects for these drugs. The following side effects were noted when the three drugs were given concomitantly. *GI:* N&V, diarrhea, abdominal pain, melena, anal discomfort, anorexia, constipation. *CNS:* Dizziness, paresthesia, insomnia. *Miscellaneous:* Asthenia, pain, upper respiratory infection.

Excessive doses of bismuth subsalicylate may cause neurotoxicity, which is reversible if therapy is terminated. Large doses of metronidazole have been associated with seizures and peripheral neuropathy (characterized by numbness or paresthesia of an extremity). Metronidazole may exacerbate candidiasis. Tetracycline use may cause superinfection, benign intracranial hypertension (pseudotumor cerebri), and photosensitivity.

Drug Interactions: See also *Metronidazole,* and *Tetracyclines.* There may be a decrease in absorption of tetracycline due to the presence of bismuth or calcium carbonate (an excipient in bismuth subsalicylate tablets).

How Supplied: *Patient Pak. Capsule:* Tetracycline hydrochloride, 500 mg; *Tablets:* Bismuth subsalicylate, 262.4 mg; Metronidzole, 250 mg.

Dosage

• **Tablets (Bismuth Subsalicylate, Metronidazole) and Capsules (Tetracycline Hydrochloride)**

Treatment of H. pylori.

Each dose includes two pink, round chewable tablets (525 mg bismuth subsalicylate), one white tablet (250 mg metronidazole), and one pale orange and white capsule (500 mg tetracycline hydrochloride). Each dose is taken q.i.d. with meals and at bedtime for 14 days. *NOTE:* Concomitant therapy with an H_2 antagonist is also required.

HEALTH CARE CONSIDERATIONS

See also *Health Care Considerations* for *Metronidazole* and *Tetracycline hydrochloride*.

Administration/Storage

1. Bismuth subsalicylate may cause darkening of the tongue and black stools, do not confuse with melena.
2. The bismuth subsalicylate tablets should be chewed and swallowed. Take metronidazole and tetracycline whole with 8 oz of water.
3. Ingest adequate fluids, especially with the bedtime dose, in order to decrease the risk of esophageal irritation and ulceration.
4. If a dose is missed, it can be made up by continuing the normal dosage schedule until the medication is gone. Double doses are not to be taken. Report if more than four doses are missed.

Assessment

1. Note clinical presentation and characteristics of symptoms, including onset and duration.
2. Record any allergy to aspirin or salicylates.
3. Determine women of child-bearing age are not pregnant. Do not use in children under age 8.
4. Obtain CBC, liver and renal function studies; note dysfunction.
5. Record serum and/or endoscopic confirmation of organism.
6. Note H_2 agent prescribed; therapy requires an H_2 antagonist.

Client/Family Teaching

1. Review the tablets: 2 pink round chewable (bismuth), 1 white tablet (metronidazole), and 1 pale orange and white capsule (tetracycline). All must be taken 4 times a day with meals and at bedtime for 14 days total. Chew and swallow the pink chewables (bismuth); swallow the others with a full glass of water. Consume plenty of fluids to prevent esophageal irritation. Avoid milk/dairy products; may alter tetracycline absorption. Take H_2 antagonist as prescribed.
2. Do not double up on missed doses; take next dose and continue prescription as directed until completed. Frequent multiple missed doses should be reported.
3. Avoid alcohol during and for 24 hr following completion of therapy.
4. Use additional contraception with birth control pills; tetracycline may lower effectiveness.
5. Avoid prolonged sun exposure to prevent a photosensitivity reaction. Use sunglasses, sun screen, and protective clothing when exposed.
6. Tongue may darken and stools may appear black; this is only temporary. Report any unusual or persistent side effects.

Outcome/Evaluate

- Eradication of *H. pylori* infection
- ↓ Recurrence of duodenal ulcers

Bisoprolol fumarate

(BUY-soh-proh-lol)

Pregnancy Category: C

Zebeta **(Rx)**

Classification: Beta-adrenergic blocking agent

See also *Beta-Adrenergic Blocking Agents.*

Action/Kinetics: Inhibits beta-1-adrenergic receptors and, at higher doses, beta-2 receptors. No intrinsic sympathomimetic activity and no membrane-stabilizing activity. **t½:** 9-12 hr. Over 90% of PO dose is absorbed. Approximately 50% is excreted unchanged through the urine and the remainder as inactive metabolites; a small amount (less than 2%) is excreted through the feces.

Uses: Hypertension alone or in combination with other antihypertensive agents. *Investigational:* Angina pectoris, SVTs, PVCs.

Special Concerns: Use with caution during lactation. Safety and efficacy have not been determined in children. Since bisoprolol is selective for beta-1 receptors, it may be used with caution in clients with bronchospastic disease who do not respond to, or who cannot tolerate, other antihypertensive therapy.

Laboratory Test Considerations: ↑ AST, ALT, uric acid, creatinine, BUN, serum potassium, glucose, and phosphorus. ↓ WBCs and platelets.

How Supplied: *Tablet:* 5 mg, 10 mg

Dosage

- **Tablets**

Antihypertensive.

Dose must be individualized. **Adults, initial:** 5 mg once daily (in some clients, 2.5 mg/day may be appropriate). **Maintenance:** If the 5-mg dose is inadequate, the dose may be increased to 10 mg/day and then, if needed, to 20 mg once daily. In clients with impaired renal or hepatic function, the initial daily dose should be 2.5 mg with caution used in titrating the dose upward.

ALTH CARE ONSIDERATIONS

See also *Health Care Considerations* for *Beta-Adrenergic Blocking Agents.*

Administration/Storage

1. Food does not affect the bioavailability of bisoprolol; may be given without regard to meals.
2. The half-life of bisoprolol is increased in clients with a C_{CR} below 40 mL/min and in those with cirrhosis; adjust dose.
3. Bisoprolol is not dialyzable so dose adjustments are not required in clients undergoing hemodialysis.

Assessment

1. Record indications for therapy, previous agents used, and the outcome.
2. Monitor CBC, electrolytes, liver and renal function studies. Reduce dose with dysfunction.
3. Once baseline parameters have been determined, continue to monitor BP in both arms with client lying, sitting, and standing.
4. Record cardiac rhythm; note any arrhythmias.

Outcome/Evaluate

- ↓ BP; relief of angina
- Stable cardiac rhythm

—COMBINATION DRUG—

Bisoprolol fumarate and Hydrochlorothiazide

(**BUY**-soh-**proh**-lol, **high**-droh-**klor**-oh-**THIGH**-ah-zyd)

Pregnancy Category: C

Ziac **(Rx)**

Classification: Antihypertensive

See also *Bisoprolol fumarate* and *Hydrochlorothiazide,*.

Content: *Beta-adrenergic blocking agent:* Bisoprolol fumarate: 2.5, 5, or 10 mg. *Diuretic/antihypertensive:* Hydrochlorothiazide: 6.25 mg in all tablets.

Uses: First-line therapy in mild to moderate hypertension.

Contraindications: Use in bronchospastic pulmonary disease, cardiogenic shock, overt CHF, second- or third-degree AV block, marked sinus bradycardia, anuria, hypersensitivity to either drug or to other sulfonamide-derived drugs, during lactation.

Special Concerns: Use with caution in clients with peripheral vascular disease, impaired renal or hepatic function, and progressive liver disease and in clients also receiving myocardial depressants or inhibitors of AV conduction such as verapamil, diltiazem, and disopyramide. Elderly clients may be more sensitive to the effects of this drug product. Safety and effectiveness have not been determined in children.

Side Effects: See individual drugs. Most commonly, dizziness and fatigue. At higher doses, bisoprolol inhibits beta-2-adrenergic receptors located in bronchial and vascular muscle.

Drug Interactions

Antihypertensives / Additive effect to decrease BP

Cyclopropane / Additive depression of myocardium

Trichloroethylene / Additive depression of myocardium

How Supplied: See Content

Dosage

- **Tablets**

  Antihypertensive.

Adults, initial: One 2.5/6.25-mg tablet given once daily. If needed, the dose may be increased q 14 days to a maximum of two 10/6.25-mg tablets given once daily.

HEALTH CARE CONSIDERATIONS

See also *Health Care Considerations* for *Beta-Adrenergic Blocking Agents, Antihypertensive Agents,* and *Diuretics, Thiazides.*

Administration/Storage

1. The combination may be substituted for the titrated individual components.
2. If withdrawal is necessary, undertake gradually over a 2 week period with careful monitoring.
3. Clients whose BP is controlled adequately with 50 mg hydrochlorothiazide but who experience significant potassium loss may achieve similar control of BP without the electrolyte disturbances by using the combination of bisoprolol and hydrochlorothiazide.

Assessment

1. Record indications for therapy, other agents used, and outcome.
2. Determine any sensitivity to drug components.
3. List all drugs prescribed to ensure none interact unfavorably.
4. Obtain baseline electrolytes, liver and renal function studies.
5. Screen client carefully as drug is not for use with bronchospastic pulmonary disease, PVD, diabetes, thyrotoxicosis, compensated cardiac failure, liver or renal disease.
6. Assess ECG to ensure no dysrhythmias (second- or third-degree AV block or bradycardia) that would preclude drug therapy.

Interventions

1. Monitor VS carefully; drug will cause a reduction in SBP and DBP and HR. Request

parameters for administration (e.g., hold if SBP < 90; HR < 50) when necessary.
2. Monitor I&O and serum electrolytes; observe for S&S of fluid and electrolyte imbalance.
3. To withdraw therapy, taper dosages over 2 weeks to prevent any adverse sequelae.
4. If therapy is to be discontinued in clients receiving both clonidine and Ziac, the Ziac should be withdrawn several days before withdrawal of clonidine.

Client/Family Teaching

1. Do not stop abruptly. With CAD, a heart attack or ventricular arrhythmia may be precipitated.
2. Do not perform activities that require mental alertness until drug effects realized.
3. Report S&S of heart failure (↑ SOB, edema, fatigue) as alternative therapy may be indicated.
4. Diabetics should monitor sugars carefully as beta blockers may mask symptoms of hypoglycemia.
5. Report any persistent or bothersome side effects.
6. Monitor BP and pulse regularly.
7. Continue diet restrictions (e.g., low salt, low fat, low calorie), weight reduction, and a regular exercise routine.

Outcome/Evaluate: Control of BP

Bitolterol mesylate

(bye-**TOHL**-ter-ohl)
Pregnancy Category: C
Tornalate Aerosol **(Rx)**
Classification: Bronchodilator

See also *Sympathomimetic Drugs*.
Action/Kinetics: Bitolterol is a prodrug in that it is converted by esterases in the body to the active colterol. Colterol combines with beta-2-adrenergic receptors, producing dilation of bronchioles. Minimal beta-1-adrenergic activity. **Onset following inhalation:** 3-4 min. **Time to peak effect:** 30-60 min. **Duration:** 5-8 hr.
Uses: Prophylaxis and treatment of bronchial asthma and bronchospasms. Treatment of bronchitis, emphysema, bronchiectasis, and COPD. May be used with theophylline and/or steroids.
Special Concerns: Safety has not been established for use during lactation and in children less than 12 years of age. Use with caution in ischemic heart disease, hypertension, hyperthyroidism, diabetes mellitus, cardiac arrhythmias, seizure disorders, or in those who respond unusually to beta-adrenergic agonists. There may be decreased effectiveness in steroid-dependent asthmatic clients. Hypersensitivity reactions may occur.
Laboratory Test Considerations: ↑ AST. ↓ Platelets, WBCs. Proteinuria.
Additional Side Effects: *CNS:* Hyperactivity, hyperkinesia, lightheadedness. *CV:* Premature ventricular contractions. *Other:* Throat irritation.
Drug Interactions: Additive effects with other beta-adrenergic bronchodilators.
How Supplied: *Metered dose inhaler:* 0.37 mg/inh; *Solution:* 0.2%

Dosage

- **Metered Dose Inhaler**

Bronchodilation.
Adults and children over 12 years: 2 inhalations at an interval of 1-3 min q 8 hr (if necessary, a third inhalation may be taken). The dose should not exceed 3 inhalations q 6 hr or 2 inhalations q 4 hr.
Prophylaxis of bronchospasm.
Adults and children over 12 years: 2 inhalations q 8 hr.

HEALTH CARE CONSIDERATIONS

See also *Health Care Considerations* for *Sympathomimetic Drugs*.

Administration/Storage

1. Bitolterol is available in a MDI. The inhaler delivers 0.37 mg bitolterol per actuation.
2. Do not store the medication above 120°F (49°C).

Client/Family Teaching

1. With the inhaler in an upright position, breathe out completely in a normal fashion. Breathe in slowly and deeply, squeeze the canister and mouthpiece between the thumb and forefinger to activate the medication. Hold the breath for 10 sec and then slowly exhale. A spacer may facilitate drug dispersion. Review video/instruction for proper administration guidelines.
2. Do not exceed prescribed dosage; seek medical assistance if symptoms worsen.

Outcome/Evaluate

- Improved airway exchange with ↓ airway resistance
- Asthma/bronchospasm prophylaxis

Bivalirudin

(by-val-ih-**ROO**-din)
Pregnancy Category:
Hirulog **(Rx)**
Classification: Anticoagulant

Action/Kinetics: Direct-acting thrombin inhibitor. Can inactivate both soluble and clot-bound thrombin. Binding to thrombin is reversible and occurs in a 1:1 relationship. When bound to thrombin, all effects of thrombin are inhibited, including activation of platelets, cleavage of fibrinogen, and activation of the positive amplification reactions of thrombin. Advantages over heparin include activity against clot-bound thrombin, more predictable anticoagulation, and no inhibition by components of the platelet release reaction. **Onset after IV bolus during cardiac catheterization:** 2 min; **peak response:** 15 min; **duration:** 2 hr. **Peak plasma levels, after SC:** 2 hr. **t½, after IV:** Less than 1 hr. Metabolized in the liver with about 20% excreted unchanged in the urine.
Uses: IV: Adjunct to streptokinase in acute MI. To reduce ischemic complications in postinfarction MI clients undergoing coronary angioplasty. Unstable angina. **SC:** Prevent DVT in orthopedic surgery.
Contraindications: Use in cerebral aneurysm, intracranial hemorrhage, or general uncontrollable hemorrhage.
Special Concerns: Dose may have to be reduced in impaired renal function. Increased risk of hemorrhage with GI ulceration or hepatic disease. Hypertension may increase risk of cerebral hemorrhage. Use with caution following recent surgery or trauma and during lactation.
Side Effects: Major side effect is bleeding with possiblity (infrequent) of major hemorrhage, including intracranial hemorrhage and retroperitoneal hemorrhage. *GI:* N&V, abdominal cramps, diarrhea. *CNS:* Headache. *Dermatologic:* Hematoma at IV infusion site, pain at SC injection site.
Laboratory Test Considerations: Prolongation of APTT, activated clotting time, thrombin time, and PT.
How Supplied: *Injection, lyophilized:* 250 mg/vial

Dosage

• **IV**

MI clients undergoing coronary angioplasty.
Initial bolus: 1 mg/kg; **then,** 2.5 mg/kg/hr for 4 hr by continuous IV infusion followed by 0.2 mg/kg/hr for 14-20 hr. Initiate immediately before angioplasty. Also give aspirin 300-325 mg.

Unstable angina.
0.2 mg/kg/hr by continuous IV infusion for up to 5 days. Use in addition to aspirin, nitrates, or calcium channel blockers.

Adjunct to streptokinase in acute MI.
0.5 mg/kg/hr by IV infusion decreasing to 0.1 mg/kg/hr after 12 hr. Start infusion immediately before or with streptokinase, 1.5 million units IV over 45 -60 min. Continue infusion until 1 hr before second angiogram (average of 4.7 days). Aspirin, 325 mg, is given before bivalirudin/streptokinase.

• **SC**

Prophylaxis of DVT in orthopedic surgery.
1 mg/kg q 8 hr for up to 14 days.

HEALTH CARE CONSIDERATIONS

Assessment

1. Record indications for and method of therapy.
2. Note any history of cerebral aneurysm or intracranial hemorrhage.
3. Monitor ECG, CBC, bleeding parameters, renal and LFTs; reduce dose with renal dysfunction.
4. Assess carefully for any evidence of bleeding abnormalities.

Client/Family Teaching

1. Review procedure, dosage and frequency of administration. Rotate sites.
2. Report any adverse side effects or unusual bruising or bleeding. New onset SOB, chest pain or edema warrant evaluation.
3. Incorporate life style changes related to smoking, alcohol, diet and exercise into daily routine.
4. Encourage family member to learn CPR.

Outcome/Evaluate

• ↓ Ischemic complications during angioplasty
• DVT prophylaxis

Brimonidine tartrate

(brih-**MOH**-nih-deen)
Pregnancy Category: B
Alphagan **(Rx)**
Classification: Sympathomimetic

See also *Sympathomimetic Drugs.*
Action/Kinetics: An alpha-2 adrenergic receptor agonist that reduces aqueous humor production and increases uveoscleral outflow. **Peak plasma levels after intraocular administration:** 1-4 hr. **t½, systemic:** About 3 hr. Metabolized by the liver and excreted through the urine as unchanged drug and metabolites.
Uses: Lower IOP in open-angle glaucoma or ocular hypertension.
Contraindications: Use in clients on MAO inhibitor therapy. Lactation.
Special Concerns: Use with caution in those with renal or hepatic impairment; in severe CV disease, depression, cerebral or cor-

onary insufficiency, Raynaud's phenomenon, orthostatic hypotension, or thromboangiitis obliterans. Safety and efficacy have not been determined in children. Benzylkonium chloride, a preservative in the product, may be absorbed by soft contact lenses.
Side Effects: *Ophthalmic:* Ocular hyperemia, burning and stinging, blurring, foreign body sensation, conjunctival follicles, ocular allergic reactions, ocular pruritus, corneal staining or erosion, photophobia, eyelid erythema, ocular ache or pain, ocular dryness, tearing, eyelid edema, conjunctival edema, blepharitis, ocular irritation, conjunctival blanching, abnormal vision, lid crusting, conjunctival hemorrhage, conjunctival discharge. *CNS:* Headache, fatigue, drowsiness, dizziness, insomnia, depression, anxiety. *Miscellaneous:* Upper respiratory symptoms, GI symptoms, asthenia, muscle pain, abnormal taste, hypertension, palpitations, nasal dryness, syncope.
How Supplied: *Solution:* 0.2%

Dosage

- **Solution, 0.2%**

  Open-angle glaucoma or ocular hypertension.

Adults: 1 gtt in the affected eye(s) t.i.d., with doses about 8 hr apart.

HEALTH CARE CONSIDERATIONS

See also *Health Care Considerations* for *Sympathomimetic Drugs.*
Administration/Storage: Store at or below 25°C (77°F).
Assessment
1. Record ophthalmic findings and ensure routine screenings.
2. Note if MAO inhibitor ordered as this precludes drug therapy.

Client/Family Teaching
1. Wash hands before and after instillation. Use as directed: 1 gtt every 8 hr to affected eye(s).
2. Remove and do not reinsert soft contact lenses for at least 15 min following instillation of drops.
3. Use caution when performing activities that require mental alertness as drug may cause fatigue and drowsiness. Report any unusual or intolerable side effects.
4. Avoid alcohol and any other CNS depressants.
5. Report for follow-up ophthalmic evaluations.

Outcome/Evaluate: Reduction in intraocular pressures

Brinzolamide ophthalmic suspension

(brin-**ZOH**-lah-myd)
Pregnancy Category: C
Azopt **(Rx)**
Classification: Antiglaucoma drug

Action/Kinetics: Inhibits carbonic hydrase in the ciliary processes of the eye, thus decreasing aqueous humor production and reducing IOP. Is absorbed into the systemic circulation following ocular use. It can then distribute to RBCs. Eliminated unchanged mainly through the urine.
Uses: Treatment of elevated IOP in ocular hypertension or open-angle glaucoma.
Contraindications: Use in those with severe renal impairment (C_{CR} less than 30 mL/min). Concomitant use with oral carbonic anhydrase inhibitors. Lactation.
Special Concerns: Is a sulfonamide; thus, similar side effects can occur. Use with caution in hepatic impairment. Safety and efficacy have not been determined in children.
Side Effects: *Ophthalmic:* Blurred vision following dosing, blepharitis, dry eye, foreign body sensation, hyperemia, ocular discharge, ocular discomfort, ocular keratitis, ocular pain, ocular pruritus, rhinitis, conjunctivitis, diplopia, eye fatigue, keratoconjunctivitis, keratopathy, lid margin crusting or sticky sensation, tearing, hypertonia. *GI:* Bitter, sour, or unusual taste; nausea, diarrhea, dry mouth, dyspepsia. *CNS:* Headache, dizziness. *Miscellaneous:* Dermatitis, allergic reactions, alopecia, chest pain, dyspnea, kidney pain, pharyngitis, urticaria.
Drug Interactions: Possible additive effects with oral carbonic anhydrase inhibitors.
How Supplied: *Ophthalmic Suspension:* 1%

Dosage

- **Ophthalmic suspension**

  Increased intraocular pressure.

1 gtt in the affected eye(s) t.i.d.

HEALTH CARE CONSIDERATIONS

Administration/Storage: Shake well before use. Benzalkonium chloride, the preservative in the product, may be absorbed by soft contact lenses. Remove lenses during administration; reinsert 15 min after administration.
Assessment
1. Note any sulfonamide sensitivity.
2. Obtain renal and LFTs; do not use with severe impairment.

B

Client/Family Teaching
1. Shake well and administer as directed.
2. Avoid allowing the tip of the container to touch the eye or surrounding structures, since contamination may occur.
3. Use care operating machinery or car; may temporarily cause blurred vision after dosing.
4. If more than one topical ophthalmic drug is being used, administer at least 10 min apart.
5. Report any S&S of infection, eye trauma or surgery.
6. Benzalkonium chloride, the preservative in the product, may be absorbed by soft contact lenses. Remove lenses during administration; reinsert 15 min after administration.

Outcome/Evaluate: ↓ IOP

Bromocriptine mesylate

(broh-moh-**KRIP**-teen)
Pregnancy Category: B
Apo-Bromocriptine ✦, Parlodel **(Rx)**
Classification: Prolactin secretion inhibitor; antiparkinson agent

Action/Kinetics: Nonhormonal agent that inhibits the release of the hormone prolactin by the pituitary. Use only when prolactin production by pituitary tumors has been ruled out. Effect in parkinsonism is due to a direct stimulating effect on dopamine type 2 receptors in the corpus striatum. Use for parkinsonism may allow the dose of levodopa to be decreased, thus decreasing the incidence of severe side effects following long-term levodopa therapy. Less than 30% of the drug is absorbed from the GI tract. **Onset, lower prolactin:** 2 hr; **antiparkinson:** 30-90 min; **decrease growth hormone:** 1-2 hr. **Peak plasma concentration:** 1-3 hr. **t½, plasma:** 6-8 hr; **terminal:** 15 hr. **Duration, lower prolactin:** 24 hr (after a single dose); **decrease growth hormone:** 4-8 hr. Significant first-pass effect. Metabolized in liver, excreted mainly through bile and thus the feces.

Uses: Short-term treatment of amenorrhea with or without galactorrhea, infertilitiy, or hypogonadism. Alone or as an adjunct in the treatment of acromegaly. As adjunctive therapy with levodopa in the treatment of idiopathic or postencephalitic Parkinson's disease. May provide additional benefit in clients who are taking optimal doses of levodopa, in those who are developing tolerance to levodopa therapy, or in those who are manifesting levodopa "end of dose failure." Clients unresponsive to levodopa are not good candidates for bromocriptine therapy. No longer recommended to suppress postpartum lactation. *Investigational:* Hyperprolactinemia due to pituitary adenoma, neuroleptic malignant syndrome, cocaine dependence, cyclical mastalgia.

Contraindications: Sensitivity to ergot alkaloids. Pregnancy, lactation, children under 15 years of age. Peripheral vascular disease, ischemic heart disease.

Special Concerns: Geriatric clients may manifest more CNS effects. Use with caution in liver or kidney disease.

Side Effects: The type and incidence of side effects depend on the use of the drug. *When used for hyperprolactinemia. GI:* N&V, abdominal cramps, diarrhea, constipation. *CNS:* Headache, dizziness, fatigue, drowsiness, lightheadedness, psychoses. *Other:* Nasal congestion, hypotension, CSF rhinorrhea.

When used for acromegaly. GI: N&V, anorexia, dry mouth, dyspepsia, indigestion, GI bleeding. *CNS:* Dizziness, syncope, drowsiness, tiredness, headache, lightheadedness, lassitude, vertigo, sluggishness, paranoia, insomnia, heavy headedness, decreased sleep requirement, delusional psychosis, visual hallucinations. *CV:* Orthostatic hypotension, digital vasospasm, Raynaud's syndrome; rarely, arrhythmias, ventricular tachycardia, bradycardia, vasovagal attack. *Respiratory:* Nasal stuffiness, SOB. *Other:* Potentiation of effects of alcohol, hair loss, paresthesia, tingling of ears, muscle cramps, facial pallor, reduced tolerance to cold.

When used for parkinsonism. GI: N&V, abdominal discomfort, constipation, anorexia, dry mouth, dysphagia. *CNS:* Confusion, hallucinations, fainting, drowsiness, dizziness, insomnia, depression, vertigo, anxiety, fatigue, headache, lethargy, nightmares. *GU:* Urinary incontinence, urinary retention, urinary frequency. *Other:* Abnormal involuntary movements, asthenia, visual disturbances, ataxia, hypotension, SOB, edema of feet and ankles, blepharospasm, erythromelalgia, skin mottling, nasal stuffiness, paresthesia, skin rash.

Laboratory Test Considerations: ↑ BUN, AST, ALT, GGPT, CPT, alkaline phosphatase, uric acid.

Drug Interactions
Alcohol / ↑ Chance of GI toxicity; alcohol intolerance
Antihypertensives / Additive ↓ BP
Butyrophenones / ↓ Effect of bromocriptine because butyrophenones are dopamine antagonists
Diuretics / Should be avoided during bromocriptine therapy
Erythromycins / ↑ Levels of bromocriptine → ↑ pharmacologic and toxic effects

Phenothiazines / ↓ Effect of bromocriptine because phenothiazines are dopamine antagonists
Sympathomimetics / ↑ Side effects of bromocriptine, including ventricular tachycardia and cardiac dysfunction
How Supplied: *Capsule:* 5 mg; *Tablet:* 2.5 mg

Dosage

- **Capsules, Tablets**

For hyperprolactinemic conditions.
Adults, initial: 0.5-2.5 mg/day with meals; **then,** increase dose by 2.5 mg q 3-7 days until optimum response observed (usual: 5-7.5 mg/day; range: 2.5-15 mg/day). For amenorrhea/galactorrhea, do not use for more than 6 months. Side effects may be reduced by temporarily decreasing the dose to ½ tablet 2-3 times/day.

Parkinsonism.
Initial: 1.25 mg (½ tablet) b.i.d. with meals while maintaining dose of levodopa, if possible. Dosage may be increased q 14-28 days by 2.5 mg/day with meals. The usual dosage range is 10-40 mg/day. Any decrease in dosage should be done gradually in 2.5-mg decrements.

Acromegaly.
Initial: 1.25-2.5 mg for 3 days with food and on retiring; **then,** increased by 1.25-2.5 mg q 3-7 days until optimum response observed. Usual optimum therapeutic range: 20-30 mg/day, not to exceed 100 mg/day. Clients should be reevaluated monthly and dosage adjusted accordingly.

Hyperprolactinemia associated with pituitary adenomas.
Maintenance: 0.625-10 mg/day for 6 to 52 months.

HEALTH CARE CONSIDERATIONS

Administration/Storage
1. Before administering first dose, have client lie down because of the possibility of fainting or dizziness.
2. Use tablets for doses less than 5 mg.

Assessment
1. Note sensitivity to ergot alkaloids.
2. Record indications for therapy, onset and type of symptoms, other agents used, and the outcome.
3. Note if female, sexually active and likely to become pregnant.
4. Monitor liver and renal function studies; note any dysfunction.
5. With Parkinson's disease, assess and document physical ability and areas of disability to distinguish between desired response and drug-induced side effects, which may be severe initially before subsiding with therapy. List drugs currently prescribed.

Client/Family Teaching
1. Take with food to minimize GI upset.
2. May cause dizziness, drowsiness, or syncope; lie down if evident and avoid activities that require mental alertness.
3. Report any complaints of fatigue, headache, nausea, drowsiness, cramps, or diarrhea.
4. With oral contraceptives, use additional nonhormonal method.
5. When menstrual period is missed, should receive pregnancy tests q 4 weeks during amenorrhea and after resumption of menses.
6. If pregnancy is likely, withhold drug and report. Pregnancy tests may fail to diagnose early pregnancy; drug may harm the fetus.
7. Report unusal or persistant side effects.

Outcome/Evaluate
- Normal menstrual cycle
- ↓ Growth hormone with acromegaly
- ↓ Muscle rigidity/tremor

Brompheniramine maleate

(brohm-fen-**EAR**-ah-meen)
Pregnancy Category: B
Brombay, Chlorphed, Conjec-B, Cophene-B, Diamine T.D., Dimetane Extentabs, Dimetane-Ten, Histaject Modified, Nasahist B, ND Stat Revised, Oraminic II, Sinusol-B, Veltane (Rx; Dimetane and Dimetane Extentabs are OTC)
Classification: Antihistamine, alkylamine type

See also *Antihistamines.*
Action/Kinetics: Fewer sedative effects. **t½:** 25 hr. **Time to peak effect:** 3-9 hr. **Duration:** 4-25 hr.
Uses: Allergic rhinitis (oral). Parenterally to treat allergic reactions to blood or plasma; adjunct to treat anaphylaxis; uncomplicated allergic conditions when PO therapy is not possible or is contraindicated.
Contraindications: Use in neonates.
Special Concerns: Geriatric clients may be more sensitive to the usual adult dose.
How Supplied: *Injection:* 10 mg/mL; *Liqui-Gels:* 4 mg

Dosage

- **Liqui-Gels**

Allergic rhinitis.
Adults and children over 12 years: 4 mg q 4-6 hr, not to exceed 24 mg/day.

- **IM, IV, SC**

Adults: usual, 10 mg (range: 5-20 mg) b.i.d. (maximum daily dose: 40 mg); **pediatric,**

under 12 years: 0.5 mg/kg/day (15 mg/m^2/day) divided into three or four doses.

B

HEALTH CARE CONSIDERATIONS

See also *Health Care Considerations* for *Antihistamines*.

Administration/Storage

1. For IM or SC use undiluted or diluted 1:10 with NSS.

IV 2. Do not use solutions containing preservatives for IV injection.

3. For IV, the 10-mg/mL preparations may be used undiluted or diluted 1:10 with sterile saline for injection. Administer over 1 min.

4. Give IV slowly preferably to a recumbent client.

5. May be added to 0.9% NSS, 5% dextrose, or whole blood for IV administration.

6. The 100-mg/mL preparation is not recommended for IV use.

Client/Family Teaching

1. Drug may cause drowsiness.

2. Consume 1.5-2 L of fluids/day to decrease secretion viscosity.

3. Avoid alcohol.

4. Report any persistent or bothersome side effects and loss of drug responsiveness.

Outcome/Evaluate: Relief of allergic manifestations; ↓ congestion

Budesonide

(byou-**DES**-oh-nyd)

Pregnancy Category: C

Entocort ✱, Gen-Budesonide Aq. ✱, Pulmicort Nebuamp ✱, Pulmicort Turbuhaler, Rhinocort, Rhinocort Aqua or Turbuhaler ✱ **(Rx)**

Classification: Corticosteroid

See also *Corticosteroids*.

Action/Kinetics: Exerts a direct local anti-inflammatory effect with minimal systemic effects when used intranasally. Exceeding the recommended dose may result in suppression of hypothalamic-pituitary-adrenal function. **t½:** 2-3 hr. Metabolism of absorbed drug is rapid.

Uses: Treat symptoms of seasonal or perennial allergic rhinitis in both adults and children. Also, nonallergic perennial rhinitis in adults.The Turbuhaler is used for maintenance and prophylaxis of asthma in adults and children 6 years of age and older; also for those requiring oral corticosteroid therapy for asthma.

Contraindications: Hypersensitivity to the drug. Untreated localized nasal mucosa infections. Lactation. Use in children less than 6 years of age or for acute or life-threatening asthma attacks, including status asthmaticus.

Special Concerns: Use with caution in clients already on alternate day corticosteroids (e.g., prednisone), in clients with active or quiescent tuberculosis infections of the respiratory tract, or in untreated fungal, bacterial, or systemic viral infections or ocular herpes simplex. Use with caution in clients with recent nasal septal ulcers, recurrent epistaxis, nasal surgery, or trauma. Exposure to chicken pox or measles should be avoided.

Side Effects: *Respiratory:* Nasopharyngeal irritation, nasal irritation, pharyngitis, increased cough, hoarseness, nasal pain,burning, stinging, dryness, epistaxis, bloody mucus, rebound congestion, ***bronchial asthma,*** occasional sneezing attacks (especially in children), rhinorrhea, reduced sense of smell, throat discomfort, ulceration of the nasal mucosa, sore throat, dyspnea, localized infections of nose and pharynx with *Candida albicans*, wheezing (rare). *CNS:* Lightheadedness, headache, nervousness. *GI:* Nausea, loss of sense of taste, bad taste in mouth, dry mouth, dyspepsia. *Miscellaneous:* Watery eyes, ***immediate and delayed hypersensitivity reactions,*** moniliasis, facial edema, rash, pruritus, herpes simplex, alopecia, arthralgia, myalgia, contact dermatitis (rare).

OD **Management of Overdose:** *Symptoms:* Symptoms of hypercorticism, including menstrual irregularities, acneiform lesions, and cushingoid features (all are rarely seen, however). *Treatment:* Discontinue the drug slowly using procedures that are acceptable for discontinuing oral corticosteroids.

How Supplied: *Inhalation Powder:* 200 mcg/inh

Dosage

- **Inhalation Aerosol**

  Seasonal or perennial rhinitis.

Adults and children 6 years of age and older, initial: 256 mcg/day given as either 2 sprays in each nostril in the morning and evening or 4 sprays in each nostril in the morning. Doses greater than 256 mcg/day are not recommended. **Maintenance:** Reduce initial dose to the smallest amount necessary to control symptoms; decrease dose q 2-4 weeks as long as desired effect is maintained. If symptoms return, the dose may be increased briefly to the initial dose.

- **Pulmicort Turbuhaler**

  Prevention or treatment of asthma.

Adults: 200-400 mcg b.i.d. **Children, over 6 years of age:** 200 mcg b.i.d. 200 mcg released with each actuation actually delivers about 160 mcg to the client.

HEALTH CARE CONSIDERATIONS

See also *Health Care Considerations* for *Corticosteroids.*

Administration/Storage

1. The Turbuhaler contains no chlorofluorocarbons as propellants; the medication is delivered by the client's own inhalation.
2. The Turbuhaler does not require a spacer; the device delivers about twice the amount of drug per inhalation to the airway as metered dose inhalers.

Assessment

1. Record indications for therapy, onset and frequency of symptoms.
2. List drugs prescribed to ensure that none interact unfavorably.

Client/Family Teaching

1. Review the appropriate method and frequency for administration. A spacer may enhance drug dispersion. Review video/instruction for proper administration guidelines.
2. Rinse mouth and equipment thoroughly after each use to prevent oral fungal infections.
3. Prior to using, clear nasal passages of secretions. If nasal passages are blocked, use decongestant first.
4. Maximum benefit is usually not seen for 3-7 days, although a decrease in symptoms can be seen within 24 hr. Report if no improvement noted within 3 weeks.
5. Shake canister well before administering. Store valve down and away from areas of high humidity. Once aluminum pouch is opened, use or discard within 6 months.
6. Avoid persons with chicken pox or communicable diseases.
7. Symptoms of hoarseness may be evident but should subside upon completion of therapy.
8. Drug is a steroid; chronic use in excessive amounts may lead to adverse systemic reactions.
9. Identify triggers and avoid irritants to control symptoms.

Outcome/Evaluate: Relief of nasal congestion/allergic manifestations

---

Bumetanide

(byou-**MET**-ah-nyd)

Pregnancy Category: C

Bumex, Burinex ✱ **(Rx)**

Classification: Loop diuretic

See also *Diuretics, Loop.*

Action/Kinetics: Inhibits reabsorption of both sodium and chloride in the proximal tubule as well as the ascending loop of Henle. Possible activity in the proximal tubule to promote phosphate excretion. **Onset, PO:** 30-60 min. **Peak effect, PO:** 1-2 hr. **Duration, PO:** 4-6 hr (dose-dependent). **Onset, IV:** Several minutes. **Peak effect, IV:** 15-30 min. **Duration, IV:** 3.5-4 hr. **t½:** 1-1.5 hr. Metabolized in the liver although 45% excreted unchanged in the urine.

Uses: Edema associated with CHF, nephrotic syndrome, hepatic disease. Adjunct to treat acute pulmonary edema. Especially useful in clients refractory to other diuretics. *Investigational:* Treatment of adult nocturia. Not effective in males with prostatic hypertrophy.

Contraindications: Anuria. Hepatic coma or severe electrolyte depletion until the condition is improved or corrected. Hypersensitivity to the drug. Lactation.

Special Concerns: Safety and efficacy in children under 18 have not been established. Geriatric clients may be more sensitive to the hypotensive and electrolyte effects and are at greater risk in developing thromboembolic problems and circulatory collapse. SLE may be activated or made worse. Clients allergic to sulfonamides may show cross sensitivity to bumetanide. Sudden changes in electrolyte balance may cause hepatic encephalopathy and coma in clients with hepatic cirrhosis and ascites.

Side Effects: *Electrolyte and fluid changes:* Excess water loss, ***dehydration,*** electrolyte depletion including hypokalemia, hypochloremia, hyponatremia; hypovolemia, thromboembolism, ***circulatory collapse.*** *Otic:* Tinnitus, reversible and irreversible hearing impairment, deafness, vertigo (with a sense of fullness in the ears). *CV:* ***Reduction in blood volume may cause circulatory collapse and vascular thrombosis and embolism, especially in geriatric clients.*** Hypotension, ECG changes, chest pain. *CNS:* Asterixis, encephalopathy with preexisting liver disease, vertigo, headache, dizziness. *GI:* Upset stomach, dry mouth, N&V, diarrhea, GI pain. *GU:* Premature ejaculation, difficulty maintaining erection, renal failure. *Musculoskeletal:* Arthritic pain, weakness, muscle cramps, fatigue. *Hematologic:* Agranulocytosis, thrombocytopenia. *Allergic:* Pruritus, urticaria, rashes. *Miscellaneous:* Sweating, hyperventilation, rash, nipple tenderness, photosensitivity, pain following parenteral use.

Laboratory Test Considerations: Alterations in LDH, AST, ALT, alkaline phosphatase,

B

creatinine clearance, total serum bilirubin, serum proteins, cholesterol. Changes in hemoglobin, PT, hematocrit, WBCs, platelet and differential counts, phosphorus, carbon dioxide content, bicarbonate, and calcium. ↑ Urinary glucose and protein, serum creatinine. Also, hyperuricemia, hypochloremia, hypokalemia, azotemia, hyponatremia, hyperglycemia.

OD **Management of Overdose:** *Symptoms: **Profound loss of water, electrolyte depletion, dehydration, decreased blood volume, circulatory collapse (possibility of vascular thrombosis and embolism).*** Symptoms of electrolyte depletion include: anorexia, cramps, weakness, dizziness, vomiting, and mental confusion. *Treatment:* Replace electrolyte and fluid losses and monitor urinary electrolyte levels as well as serum electrolytes. Emesis or gastric lavage. Oxygen or artificial respiration may be necessary. General supportive measures.

How Supplied: *Injection:* 0.25 mg/mL; *Tablet:* 0.5 mg, 1 mg, 2 mg

Dosage

- **Tablets**

Adults: 0.5-2 mg once daily; if response is inadequate, a second or third dose may be given at 4-5-hr intervals up to a maximum of 10 mg/day.

- **IV, IM**

Adults: 0.5-1 mg; if response is inadequate, a second or third dose may be given at 2-3-hr intervals up to a maximum of 10 mg/day. Initiate PO dosing as soon as possible.

HEALTH CARE CONSIDERATIONS

See also *Health Care Considerations* for *Diuretics, Loop*.

Administration/Storage

1. The recommended PO medication schedule is on alternate days or for 3-4 days with a 1-2-day rest period in between.
2. Bumetanide, at a 1:40 ratio of bumetanide:furosemide, may be ordered if allergic to furosemide.
3. Reserve IV or IM administration for clients in whom PO use is not practical or absorption from the GI tract is impaired.
4. **IV** In severe chronic renal insufficiency, a continuous infusion (12 mg over 12 hr) may be more effective and cause fewer side effects than intermittent bolus therapy.
5. Prepare solutions fresh for IM or IV; use within 24 hr.
6. Ampules may be reconstituted with D5W, 0.9% NaCl, or RL solution.
7. Administer IV solutions slowly over 1-2 min.

Assessment

1. Record indications for therapy and pretreatment findings.
2. Note any sulfonamide allergy; may be cross sensitivity.
3. Monitor electrolytes, liver and renal function studies; assess for ↓ K^+.
4. Review history; note any hearing impairment, lupus, or thromboembolic events.
5. *NOTE:* 1 mg of bumetanide is equivalent to 40 mg of furosemide.
6. Monitor VS. Rapid diuresis may cause dehydration and circulatory collapse (especially in the elderly). Hypotension may occur when administered with antihypertensives.
7. Assess hearing and for ototoxicity, especially if receiving other ototoxic drugs

Client/Family Teaching

1. Take early in the day to prevent nighttime voidings.
2. Do not perform activities that require mental alertness until drug effects realized.
3. Review dietary requirements such as reduced sodium and high potassium; may see dietitian.
4. Record weights; report any sudden weight gain or evidence of swelling in the hands or feet.
5. Report any unusual side effects.

Outcome/Evaluate: ↓ Peripheral and sacral edema; Enhanced diuresis

Bupropion hydrochloride

(byou-**PROH**-pee-on)

Pregnancy Category: B

Wellbutrin, Wellbutrin SR, Zyban **(Rx)**

Classification: Antidepressant, miscellaneous

Action/Kinetics: Bupropion is an antidepressant whose mechanism of action is not known; the drug does not inhibit MAO and it only weakly blocks neuronal uptake of epinephrine, serotonin, and dopamine. Exerts moderate anticholinergic and sedative effects, but only slight orthostatic hypotension. **Peak plasma levels:** 2-3 hr. **t½:** 8-24 hr. **Time to steady state:** 1.5-5 days. Significantly metabolized by a first-pass effect through the liver to both active and inactive metabolites. During chronic use the plasma levels of two active metabolites may be higher than bupropion. Excreted through both the urine (87%) and the feces (10%). Zyban is a sustained-release formulation.

Uses: Short-term (6 weeks or less) treatment of depression. Aid to stop smoking (may be combined with a nicotine transdermal system).

Contraindications: Seizure disorders; presence or history of bulimia or anorexia nervosa due to the higher incidence of seizures in such clients. Concomitant use of an MAO inhibitor. Wellbutrin, Wellbutrin SR, and Zyban all contain bupropion; do not use together.

Special Concerns: Use with caution in clients with a history of seizures, cranial trauma, with drugs that lower the seizure threshold, and other situations that might cause seizures (e.g., abrupt cessation of a benzodiazepine). Use with caution and in lower doses in clients with liver or kidney disease and in those with a recent history of MI or unstable heart disease. Assess benefits versus risks during lactation. Safety and efficacy have not been established in clients less than 18 years of age.

Side Effects: Listed are side effects with an incidence of 0.1% or greater. *CNS:* Insomnia, abnormal dreams, dizziness, disturbed concentration, nervousness, tremor, dysphoria, somnolence, agitation, abnormal thinking, depression, irritability, CNS stimulation, confusion, decreased libido, decreased memory, depersonalization, emotional lability, hostility, hyperkinesia, hypertonia, hypesthesia, paresthesia, suicidal ideation, vertigo. *GI:* Nausea, dry mouth, constipation, diarrhea, anorexia, mouth ulcer, thirst, increased appetite, dyspepsia, flatulence, vomiting, abnormal liver function, bruxism, dysphagia, gastric reflux, gingivitis, glossitis, jaundice, stomatitis. *CV:* Palpitations, hypertension, flushing, mi-graine, postural hypotension, hot flashes, ***stroke,*** tachycardia, vasodilation. *Body as a whole:* Abdominal pain, accidental injury, neck pain, chest pain, facial edema, asthenia, fever, headache, back pain, chills, inguinal hernia, musculoskeletal chest pain, pain, photosensitivity. *Dermatologic:* Rash, pruritus, urticaria, dry skin, sweating, acne, dry skin. *Musculoskeletal:* Arthralgia, myalgia, leg cramps. *Respiratory:* Rhinitis, bronchitis, increased cough, pharyngitis, sinusitis, epistaxis, dyspnea. *GU:* Urinary frequency, impotence, polyuria, urinary urgency. *Ophthalmic:* Amblyopia, abnormal accommodation, dry eye. *Miscellaneous:* Taste perversion, tinnitus, ecchymosis, edema, increased weight, peripheral edema.

OD Management of Overdose: *Symptoms:* Seizures, hallucinations, loss of consciousness, tachycardia, multiple uncontrolled seizures, bradycardia, fever, muscle rigidity, hypotension, rhabdomyolosis, stupor, coma, respiratory failure, cardiac failure and cardiac arrest prior to death. *Treatment:* Client should be hospitalized. If conscious, syrup of ipecac is given to induce vomiting followed by activated charcoal q 6 hr during the first 12 hr after ingestion. Monitor both ECG and EEG for 48 hr; fluid intake must be adequate. If the client is in a stupor, is comatose, or is convulsing, gastric lavage may be undertaken provided intubation of the airway has been performed. Seizures may be treated with IV benzodiazepines and other supportive procedures.

Drug Interactions

Alcohol / Alcohol ↓ seizure threshold; use with bupropion may precipitate seizures
Amantadine / Psychotic reactions
Carbamazepine / ↑ Bupropion metabolism → ↓ plasma levels
Cimetidine / Cimetidine inhibits the metabolism of bupropion
Fluoxetine / Panic symptoms and psychotic reactions
Levodopa / ↑ Risk of side effects
MAO inhibitors / Acute toxicity to bupropion may ↑ , especially if used with phenelzine
Phenobarbital / ↑ Bupropion metabolism → ↓ plasma levels
Phenytoin / ↑ Bupropion metabolism → ↓ plasma levels
Retonavir / ↑ Risk of bupropion toxicity

How Supplied: *Tablet:* 75 mg, 100 mg; *Tablet Extended Release:* 100 mg, 150 mg

Dosage

- **Tablets**

Antidepressant.

Adults, initial: 100 mg in the morning and evening for the first 3 days; **then,** 100 mg t.i.d., given in the morning, midday, and in the evening (6 hr should elapse between doses). If no response is observed after 4 weeks or longer, the dose may be increased to 450 mg/day with individual doses not to exceed 150 mg. Doses higher than 450 mg should not be administered. The sustained-release dosage form may be used for twice-daily dosing. **Maintenance:** Lowest dose to control depression.

Smoking deterrent.

Begin dosing at 150 mg/day for the first 3 days followed by 150 mg b.i.d. Eight hours or more should elapse between successive doses.

HEALTH CARE CONSIDERATIONS

Administration/Storage

1. To reduce risk of seizures, the total daily dose should not exceed 450 mg to treat depression or 300 mg as a smoking deterrent; each single dose should not exceed 150 mg, and increase doses gradually.
2. Several months of treatment may be necessary to control acute depression.

B

3. Intitiate treatment while the client is still smoking since about 1 week of treatment is needed to reach steady-state blood levels. A "target quit date," usually in the second week, should be set. Continue treatment for 7 to 12 weeks. If significant progress has not been made by week 7 of treatment, it is not likely the client will stop smoking during this attempt. Thus, discontinue treatment.

Assessment

1. Record indications for therapy, presenting behaviors, and duration of symptoms.
2. Note any history of seizures, recent MI, bulimia or anorexia nervosa.
3. Determine if client of childbearing age and lactating.
4. Monitor weight, ECG, liver and renal function studies; reduce dose with renal and/or liver dysfunction.
5. Assess mental stability and potential for compliance. Fewer side effects (no CV effects, drug interactions, sedation, and weight gain) with bupropion than other antidepressants.
6. With tobacco abuse, ensure client is ready to quit; note numbers of cigarettes smoked per day, nicotine content, other failures, and date desired to quit so that treatment can be started 1 week prior.

Client/Family Teaching

1. May experience a change in taste perceptions which could result in appetite and weight loss. Record weights and report changes.
2. May cause menstrual irregularities and impotence. Any changes in urinary output should be reported.
3. Beneficial drug effects may not be evident for 5-21 days. Continue taking and do not be discouraged by the delayed response.
4. Dizziness may occur. Do not arise from a supine position suddenly. If dizziness occurs during the day, sit until subsides.
5. Report for follow-up so that drug therapy and dosage may be evaluated and adjusted as needed.
6. Report any mood swings or suicidal ideations immediately.
7. May cause drowsiness, hyperactivity, GI upset, diarrhea, constipation, and dry mouth.
8. With the sustained-released formulation, for smoking cessation, drug will be started in low dose for b.i.d. consumption. Take last dose 4 to 6 hr before bedtime to prevent insomnia. GlaxoWellcome operates a toll- free number (1-800-u can quit, 822-6784) for assistance and support during withdrawal of nicotine; they can also be reached on the Internet at www.glaxowellcome.com.

Outcome/Evaluate

- Improvement in symptoms of depression such as ↓ fatigue, improved eating and sleeping patterns, and ↑ socialization
- Successful nicotine withdrawal

Buspirone hydrochloride

(byou-**SPYE**-rohn)

Pregnancy Category: B

Apo-Buspirone ✱, BuSpar, Bustab ✱, Gen-Buspirone ✱, Linbuspirone ✱, Novo-Buspirone ✱, Nu-Buspirone ✱, PMS-Buspirone ✱ **(Rx)**

Classification: Nonbenzodiazepine antianxiety agent

Action/Kinetics: The mechanism of action is unknown. Not chemically related to the benzodiazepines; no anticonvulsant, muscle relaxant properties, or significant sedation has been observed. Binds to serotonin (5-HT_{1A}) and dopamine (D_2) receptors in the CNS; it is thus possible that dopamine-mediated neurologic disorders may occur. These include dystonia, Parkinson-like symptoms, akathisia, and tardive dyskinesia. **Peak plasma levels:** 1-6 ng/mL 40-90 min after a single PO dose of 20 mg. **t½:** 2-3 hr. Extensive first-pass metabolism; active and inactive metabolites excreted in the urine and through the feces.

Uses: Anxiety disorders, short-term use to relieve symptoms of anxiety due to motor tension, apprehension, autonomic hyperactivity, or hyperattentiveness.

Contraindications: Psychoses, severe liver or kidney impairment, lactation. Not usually indicated for treatment of anxiety and tension due to stress of everyday living.

Special Concerns: Safety and efficacy in children less than 18 years of age not established. A decrease in dose may be necessary in geriatric clients due to age-related impairment of renal function.

Side Effects: *CNS:* Dizziness, drowsiness, insomnia, fatigue, nervousness, excitement, dream disturbances, dysphoria, noise intolerance, euphoria, depersonalization, akathisia, hallucinations, suicidal ideation, seizures, decreased concentration, confusion, anger or hostility, depression. *CV:* Nonspecific chest pain, hypotension, palpitations, tachycardia, syncope, hypertension. *GI:* N&V, diarrhea, constipation, abdominal distress, dry mouth, altered taste, increased appetite, irritable colon. *Ophthalmologic:* Redness and itching of eyes, conjunctivitis, photophobia, eye pain. *Dermatologic:* Skin rash, pruritus, dry skin, edema of face, acne, easy bruising, flushing. *Neurologic:* Paresthesia, tremor, numbness, incoordination. *GU:* Urinary hesitancy or frequency, enuresis, amenorrhea, pelvic inflammatory disease. *Miscellaneous:* Tinnitus, sore throat, nasal congestion, altered smell, muscle aches or pains, skin rash, headache, sweating, hyperventilation, SOB, hair loss, galactorrhea, decreased or increased libido, delayed ejaculation.

OD **Management of Overdose:** *Symptoms:* Dizziness, drowsiness, N&V, gastric distress, miosis. *Treatment:* Immediate gastric lavage; general symptomatic and supportive measures.

Drug Interactions: Use with MAO inhibitors may cause an increase in BP.

How Supplied: *Tablet:* 5 mg, 10 mg, 15 mg

Dosage

- **Tablets**

Adults: 5 mg t.i.d. Dosage may be increased in increments of 5 mg/day q 2-3 days to achieve optimum effects; the total daily dose should not exceed 60 mg. BuSpar is available in a 15-mg tablet that is scored in 5-mg increments and notched in 7.5-mg increments so clients can take the drug b.i.d. rather than t.i.d.

HEALTH CARE CONSIDERATIONS

Administration/Storage

1. No cross-tolerance with other sedative-hypnotic drugs, including benzodiazepines.
2. Buspirone will not block the withdrawal syndrome, which may occur following cessation of sedative-hypnotics. Thus, withdraw clients on chronic sedative-hypnotic therapy gradually prior to beginning buspirone therapy.
3. To date, no potential for abuse, tolerance, or either physical or psychologic dependence.
4. Up to 2 weeks may be required before beneficial antianxiety effects are manifested.

Assessment

1. Record indications for therapy and note pretreatment findings.
2. Determine support systems and encourage active family involvement in treatment plan.
3. Assess for recent benzodiazepine therapy; drug may be less effective.
4. Record mental status and note age; good agent to use in elderly because of less CNS suppression.
5. Determine causative factor/event that precipitated disorder.

Client/Family Teaching

1. Take with food or snack to decrease nausea, a common side effect; report if persistant/severe.
2. May cause drowsiness or dizziness. Use caution when operating a motor vehicle or performing tasks that require mental alertness.
3. Avoid the use of alcohol.
4. Do not stop suddenly as withdrawal symptoms such as N&V, dry mouth, nasal congestion, or sore throat may occur.
5. Report any weakness, restlessness, nervousness, headaches, or feelings of depression.
6. Report any involuntary, repetitive movements of the face or neck muscles, Parkinson-like symptoms or suicide ideations immediately.
7. Avoid all OTC agents.

Outcome/Evaluate: Relief of agitated depressive S&S; ↓ anxiety

COMBINATION DRUG

Butalbital and Acetaminophen

(byou-**TAL**-bih-tall, ah-**SEAT**-ah-**MIN**-oh-fen)

Pregnancy Category: C

Axocet **(Rx)**

Classification: Sedative, analgesic

See also *Pentobarbital Sodium* and *Acetaminophen.*

Content: Each capsule contains: *Sedative/hypnotic:* Butalbital, 50 mg, and *analgesic:* acetaminophen, 650 mg.

Uses: Treatment of tension headaches.

Contraindications: Hypersensitivity to butalbital or acetaminophen. Clients with porphyria.

Special Concerns: Use with caution as butalbital is habit-forming and has the potential to be abused. Use with caution in geriatric or debilitated clients, those with severe renal or hepatic dysfunction, and clients with acute abdominal conditions. Safety and efficacy have not been determined in children less than 12 years of age.

Side Effects: See also *Sedative-hypnotics* and *Acetaminophen.* The most frequently reported side effects are drowsiness, lightheadedness, sedation, dizziness, SOB, N&V, abdominal pain, and an intoxicated feeling.

Drug Interactions

CNS depressants (including alcohol, general anesthetics, narcotic analgesics, sedative-hypnotics, tranquilizers) / Additive CNS depression

MAO inhibitors / MAO inhibitors ↑ the CNS effects of butalbital

How Supplied: See Content

Dosage

- **Capsules**

Treatment of tension headaches.

1 capsule q 4 hr, not to exceed 6 capsules daily.

B

HEALTH CARE CONSIDERATIONS

See also *Health Care Considerations* for *Acetaminophen* and *Pentobarbital Sodium*.

Administration/Storage: Should not be used for extended periods of time due to the potential for development of physical dependence.

Assessment

1. Record onset of symptoms, frequency of occurrence, what usually works, and what other agents used for headaches.
2. Identify triggers; tension headaches usually respond to NSAIDs or acetaminophen if taken at the first symptom.
3. Note any liver or renal dysfunction or acute abdomen; these preclude use of this drug.
4. Obtain neurologic evaluation.

Client/Family Teaching

1. Take only as directed and do not exceed 6 capsules daily.
2. Do not drive or perform activities that require mental alertness during therapy.
3. Avoid alcohol and CNS depressants.
4. Keep a journal of foods, activities, and any other factors that surround headaches to identify triggers.

Outcome/Evaluate: Relief of tension headaches

Butenafine hydrochloride

(byou-**TEN**-ah-feen)
Pregnancy Category: B
Mentax **(Rx)**
Classification: Antifungal drug

See also Anti-Infectives.

Action/Kinetics: Acts by inhibiting epoxidation of squalene, thus blocking the synthesis of ergosterol, an essential component of fungal cell membranes. Depending on the concentration and the fungal species, the drug may be fungicidal. Although applied topically, some of the drug is absorbed into the general circulation.

Uses: Treatment of interdigital tinea pedia (athlete's foot) due to *Epidermophyton floccosum, Trichophyton mentagrophytes,* or *T. rubrum*.

Special Concerns: Use with caution during lactation and in clients sensitive to allylamine antifungal drugs as the drugs may be cross-reactive. Safety and efficacy have not been determined in children less than 12 years of age.

Side Effects: *Dermatologic:* Contact dermatitis, burning or stinging, worsening of the condition, erythema, irritation, itching.

How Supplied: *Cream:* 1%

Dosage

- **Cream, 1%**
  Athlete's foot.

Apply the cream to cover the affected area and immediate surrounding skin once daily for 4 weeks. Review the diagnosis if no beneficial effects are noted after the treatment period.

HEALTH CARE CONSIDERATIONS

See also *General Health Care Considerations for All Anti-Infectives*.

Administration/Storage

1. For external use only; not for ophthalmic, PO, or intravaginal use.
2. Store the drug between 5°C and 30°C (41°F-86°F).

Assessment: Record indications for therapy, onset, duration, and characteristics of symptoms; describe clinical presentation.

Client/Family Teaching

1. Review method for site preparation and application of cream; wash hands before and after applying.
2. After bathing, dry feet thoroughly and carefully between each toe before applying. Avoid occlusive dressings.
3. Avoid contact with the eyes, nose, mouth, and other mucous membranes.
4. Do not stop therapy when condition shows improvement; continue for full prescribed time.
5. Report any increased swelling, itching, burning, blistering, drainage, irritation, or lack of improvement.

Outcome/Evaluate: Resolution of fungal infection

Butoconazole nitrate

(byou-toe-**KON**-ah-zohl)
Pregnancy Category: C
Femstat 1 **(Rx)**, Femstat 3 **(OTC)**
Classification: Antifungal agent

Action/Kinetics: By permeating chitin in the fungal cell wall, butoconazole increases membrane permeability to intracellular substances, leading to reduced osmotic resistance and viability of the fungus. Approximately 5.5% of drug is absorbed following vaginal administration; plasma. **t½:** 21-24 hr.

Uses: Vulvovaginal fungal infections caused by *Candida* species.

Contraindications: Use during first trimester of pregnancy.
Special Concerns: Pediatric dosage has not been established. Use with caution during lactation.
Side Effects: *GU:* Vaginal burning, vulvar burning or itching, discharge; soreness, swelling, and itching of the fingers.
How Supplied: *Vaginal cream:* 2%

Dosage

- **Vaginal Cream (2%)**

During pregnancy, second and third trimesters only.
One full applicator (about 5 g) of the cream intravaginally at bedtime for 6 days.
Nonpregnant.
One full applicator (about 5 g) intravaginally at bedtime for 3 days (if necessary, may be used for up to 6 days). *NOTE:* Vaginal infections may also be treated by one dose of butoconazole.

HEALTH CARE CONSIDERATIONS

Administration/Storage
1. During pregnancy, use of a vaginal applicator may be contraindicated.
2. If there is no response, repeat studies to confirm the diagnosis before reinstituting antifungal therapy.
3. Not to be stored above 40°C (104°F).

Assessment
1. Record onset and symptoms requiring treatment.
2. Determine if pregnant.
3. Obtain appropriate cultures and pretreatment lab studies.

Client/Family Teaching
1. Review technique for administration; insert cream high into the vagina.
2. Use as prescribed and continue during menstrual cycle.
3. Report any irritation or burning.
4. Use sanitary napkins to prevent soiling and staining of undergarments and clothing.
5. To prevent reinfection, partner should use a condom during intercourse and seek treatment if symptomatic.
6. If having recurrent vaginal infections and exposed to HIV, consult provider to determine the cause of symptoms. If the symptoms return within 2 months, R/O pregnancy or a serious underlying medical cause (e.g., diabetes, HIV infection).

Outcome/Evaluate: Eradication of fungal infection; symptomatic improvement

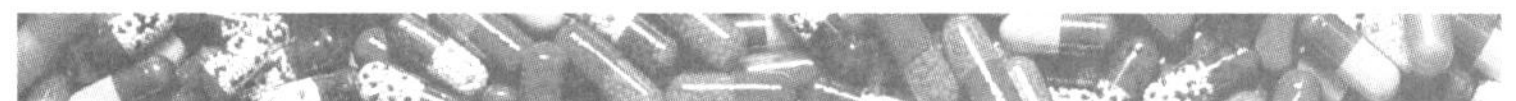

Cabergoline

(cah-**BER**-goh-leen)
Pregnancy Category: B
Dostinex **(Rx)**
Classification: Drug to treat hyperprolactinemia

Action/Kinetics: Synthetic ergot derivative that is a dopamine receptor agonist at D_2 receptors. Secretion of prolactin occurs through the release of dopamine from tuberofundibular neurons. Inhibits basal and metoclopramide-induced prolactin secretion. **Peak plasma levels:** 2–3 hr. Significant first-pass effect. Extensively metabolized in the liver and excreted in both the urine and feces. **t½, elimination**: 63–69 hr.
Uses: Treatment of hyperprolactinemia, either idiopathic or due to pituitary adenomas. *Investigational:* Shrink tumors in clients with microprolactinoma or macroprolactinoma. Parkinson's disease. Normalize androgen levels and improve menstrual cyclicity in polycystic ovary syndrome.
Contraindications: Uncontrolled hypertension or in pregnancy-induced hypertension (i.e., preeclampsia, eclampsia). Hypersensitivity to ergot alkaloids. Lactation. Not to be used to inhibit or suppress physiologic lactation.
Special Concerns: Use with caution in those with impaired hepatic function or with other drugs that lower BP. Safety and efficacy have not been determined in children.
Side Effects: *GI:* N&V, constipation, abdominal pain, dyspepsia, dry mouth, diarrhea, flatulence, throat irritation, toothache, anorexia, weight loss or gain. *CNS:* Headache, dizziness, somnolence, vertigo, paresthesia, depression, nervousness, anxiety, insomnia. *CV:* Postural hypotension, hypotension, palpitations. *GU:* Breast pain, dysmenorrhea, increased libido. *Body as a whole:* Asthenia, fatigue, syncope, flu-like symptoms, malaise, periorbital edema, peripheral edema, hot flashes. *Miscellaneous:* Nasal stuffiness, abnormal vision, acne, epistaxis, pruritus.
OD Management of Overdose: *Symptoms:* Nasal congestion, syncope, hallucinations. *Treatment:* Support BP, if necessary.

Drug Interactions
Antihypertensive drugs / Additive hypotension
Butyrophenones / ↓ Effects of cabergoline
Metoclopramide / Effects of cabergoline
Phenothiazines / Effects of cabergoline
Thioxanthenes / Effects of cabergoline
How Supplied: *Tablets:* 0.5 mg.

Dosage

- **Tablets**

Hyperprolactinemia.
Adults, initial: 0.5 mg twice a week. Dose may be increased by 0.25 mg twice weekly to less than or equal to 1 mg twice a week, depending on the serum prolactin level. Do not increase dose more often than every 4 weeks.
Parkinson's disease.
Adults: 7.5 mg/day.
Improve menstrual cyclicity in polycystic ovary syndrome.
Adults: 0.5 mg/week.

HEALTH CARE CONSIDERATIONS

Administration/Storage

1. If the client does not respond adequately and higher doses do not result in additional beneficial effects, use the lowest dose that achieved maximal response. Consideration should be given to other approaches.
2. May be discontinued if prolactin levels are normal for 6 months.
3. Efficacy of treatment for > 24 mo has not been determined.

Assessment

1. Record indications for therapy, onset, duration, and characteristics of symptoms. List other agents trialed and the outcome.
2. Any sensitivity to ergot derivatives precludes drug use, as does lactation and uncontrolled HTN.
3. Monitor VS, serum prolactin level, renal and LFTs; use cautiously with impairment and HTN.
4. Determine if pregnant; review the risks and do not administer if client plans to become pregnant.
5. With adenomas, review pituitary scans to assess tumor size.
6. With polycystic ovary conditions, review record of menstrual cycles.

Client/Family Teaching

1. Take as directed; do not exceed prescribed dose and frequency.
2. Sudden changes in position, especially standing up, may cause dizziness or lightheadedness.
3. Use reliable birth control; report immediately if pregnancy suspected.
4. Drug dosage is dependent on serum prolactin levels with hyperprolactinemic disorders; once prolactin levels are normal for 6 months, drug may be discontinued and levels monitored periodically to determine when or if drug needs to be reinstituted.

Outcome/Evaluate

- ↓ Serum prolactin levels to within desired range (< 20 mcg/L in women; < 15 mcg/L in men)
- Normalization of androgen levels and improved menstrual cycling with polycystic ovary syndrome

Calcipotriene (Calcipotriol)

(kal-**SIH**-poh-tren)
Pregnancy Category: C
Dovonex **(Rx)**
Classification: Topical antipsoriatic

Action/Kinetics: Synthetic vitamin D_3 analog. Vitamin D_3 receptors are located in skin cells known as keratinocytes. Abnormal growth and production of keratinocytes cause the scaly red patches of psoriasis. Calcipotriene regulates production and development of these skin cells. About 6% of a topically applied dose is absorbed into the systemic circulation where it is converted to inactive metabolites.
Uses: *Cream, Ointment:* Treatment of moderate plaque psoriasis. *Solution:* Control moderately severe scalp psoriasis.
Contraindications: Demonstrated hypercalcemia or evidence of vitamin D toxicity. Use on the face; oral, ophthalmic, intravaginal use.
Special Concerns: Side effects are more common in geriatric clients. Use with caution during lactation. Safety and efficacy for use of topical calcipotriene in dermatoses other than psoriasis have not been studied. Safety and efficacy have not been determined in children. Children have a higher ratio of skin surface to body mass; thus, children are at a greater risk than adults of systemic side effects following use of topical medication.
Side Effects: *Topical:* Most commonly burning, itching, skin irritation. Also, erythema, dry skin, peeling, rash, worsening of psoriasis, dermatitis, skin atrophy, hyperpigmentation, hypercalcemia, folliculitis. Irritation of lesions and surrounding uninvolved skin. *Systemic:* Transient, rapidly reversible hypercalcemia.
OD **Management of Overdose:** *Symptoms:* Hypercalcemia and other systemic effects. *Treatment:* Discontinue use of the medication until normal calcium levels are restored.

How Supplied: *Cream:* 0.005%; *Ointment:* 0.005%; *Solution:* 0.005%

Dosage

- **Ointment, Cream, Solution (each 0.005%)**

Treatment of psoriasis.

A thin layer is applied to the affected skin b.i.d. and rubbed in gently and completely.

HEALTH CARE CONSIDERATIONS

Administration/Storage

1. For external use only. Avoid contact with the face and eyes.
2. Safety and efficacy have been shown for use up to 8 weeks.

Assessment

1. Describe psoriatic lesions requiring therapy; assess extent, location/characteristics.
2. Monitor calcium levels with extended use.

Client/Family Teaching

1. Apply a thin layer directly to psoriatic lesions; wash hands before and after application.
2. Use only as directed and do not exceed prescribed dosage; avoid contact with face and eyes.
3. Do not mix or apply at the same time as other topical products.
4. Transient burning and stinging may occur. Avoid use on the face if possible; report if erythema and facial dermatitis occur.

Outcome/Evaluate: Clearing and healing of psoriatic lesions

Calcitonin-human

(kal-sih-**TOH**-nin)

Pregnancy Category: C

(Rx)

Calcitonin-salmon

(kal-sih-**TOH**-nin)

Pregnancy Category: C

Calcimar, Caltine ✱, Miacalcin, Osteocalcin, Salmonine **(Rx)**

Classification: Calcium regulator

Action/Kinetics: Calcitonins are polypeptide hormones produced in mammals by the parafollicular cells of the thyroid gland. Calcitonin isolated from salmon has the same therapeutic effect as the human hormone, except for a greater potency per milligram and a somewhat longer duration of action. Calcitonin-human is a synthetic product that has the same sequence of amino acids as the naturally occurring calcitonin found in human beings. Ineffective when administered PO. Beneficial in Paget's disease of bone by reducing the rate of turnover of bone; the drug acts to both block initial bone resorption, decreasing alkaline phosphatase levels in the serum, and urinary hydroxyproline excretion. Its effectiveness in treating osteoporosis or hypercalcemia is due to decreased serum calcium levels from direct inhibition of bone resorption. Use of the nasal spray for osteoporosis results in significant increases in bone mass density within 6 months. **Time to peak plasma levels, calcitonin-salmon:** 16–25 min for the injection and 31–39 min for the spray. **Duration, calcitonin-salmon:** 6–8 hr for hypercalcemia. **t½:** 60 min for calcitonin-human and 43 min for calcitonin-salmon. The onset of calcitonin-human in reducing serum alkaline phosphatase level and urinary hydroxyproline excretion in Paget's disease may take 6–24 months. Metabolized to inactive compounds in the kidneys, blood, and peripheral tissues.

Uses: Injection: Prevention of progressive loss of bone mass in postmenopausal osteoporosis in women who are more than 5 years past menopause and who have low bone mass compared with women before menopause. Also, for women who cannot or will not take estrogens. Moderate to severe Paget's disease characterized by polyostotic involvement with elevated serum alkaline phosphatase and urinary hydroxyproline excretion. With other therapies for early treatment of hypercalcemic emergencies. *NOTE:* Calcitonin human is now an orphan drug. **Nasal:** Postmenopausal osteoporosis.

Contraindications: Allergy to calcitonin-salmon or its gelatin diluent.

Special Concerns: Use with caution during lactation. Safe use in children not established.

Side Effects: Side effects listed are for calcitonin-salmon. *GI:* N&V, anorexia, epigastric discomfort, salty taste, flatulence, increased appetite, gastritis, diarrhea, dry mouth, abdominal pain, dyspepsia, constipation. *CNS:* Dizziness, paresthesia, insomnia, anxiety, vertigo, migraine, neuralgia, agitation, depression (rare). *CV:* Hypertension, tachycardia, palpitation, bundle branch block, ***MI, CVA, thrombophlebitis,*** angina pectoris (rare). *Respiratory:* Sinusitis, URTI, pharyngitis, bronchitis, pneumonia, coughing, dyspnea, taste perversion, parosmia, ***bronchospasm.*** *Musculoskeletal:* Arthrosis, arthritis, polymyalgia rheumatica, stiffness, myalgia. *Dermatologic:* Inflammatory reactions at the injection site, flushing of face or hands, pruritus of ear lobes, edema of feet, skin rash, skin ulceration, eczema, alopecia, increased sweating. *Endocrine:* Goiter, hyperthyroidism. *Ophthalmic:* Abnormal lacrimation, conjunctivitis, eye pain, blurred vision, vitreous floater. *Otic:* Tinnitus, hearing loss, earache. *Hematologic:* Lymphadenopathy, anemia, infection. *Metabolic:* Mild tetanic symptoms, asymptomatic mild hypercalcemia, cholelithiasis, thirst, hepatitis, weight increase. *Miscellaneous:* Flu-like symptoms, fatigue, nocturia, feverish sensation. Use of the nasal spray may cause rhinitis, nasal irritation, redness, nasal sores, back pain, arthralgia, epistaxis, and headache.

Laboratory Test Considerations: Reduction of alkaline phosphatase and 24-hr urinary excretion of hydroxyproline are indicative of successful therapy. Monitor urine for casts (indicative of kidney damage).

OD **Management of Overdose:** *Symptoms:* N&V.

How Supplied: Calcitonin-salmon: *Injection:* 200 IU/mL; *Nasal Spray:* 200 IU/inh

Dosage

CALCITONIN-HUMAN

- **SC**

Paget's disease.

Adults, initial: 0.5 mg/day; **then,** depending on severity of disease, dosage may range from 0.5 mg 2–3 times/week to 0.25 mg/day.

CALCITONIN-SALMON

- **IM, SC**

Paget's disease.

Adults, initial: 100 IU/day; **maintenance, usual:** 50 IU/day, every other day, or 3 times/week.

Hypercalcemia.

Adults, initial: 4 IU/kg q 12 hr; **then,** increase the dose, if necessary after 1 or 2 days (i.e., if unsatisfactory response), to 8 IU/kg q 12 hr up to a maximum of 8 IU/kg q 6 hr. If the volume to be injected exceeds 2 mL by the SC route, the dose should be given IM with multiple sites used.

Postmenopausal osteoporosis.

Adults: 100 IU/day given with calcium carbonate (1.5 g/day) and vitamin D (400 units/day).

- **Nasal Spray**

Adults: 200 IU/day, alternating nostrils daily given with calcium carbonate (1.5 g/day) and vitamin D (400 units/day).

HEALTH CARE CONSIDERATIONS

Administration/Storage

1. Before initiating therapy, determine serum alkaline phosphatase level and urinary hydroxyproline excretion. Repeat at the end of 3 months and q 3–6 months thereafter.
2. Activate the pump for the nasal spray before use. To do this, hold the bottle upright and depress the two white side arms toward the bottle six times, until a faint spray is emitted. The pump has been activated once the first faint spray is emitted. Place the nozzle firmly into the nostril with the head in the upright position and depress the pump toward the bottle. It is not necessary to reactivate the pump before each dose.
3. Store calcitonin-salmon injection at a temperature between 2°C and 6°C (36°F and 43°F).
4. *Store the unopened calcitonin nasal spray between 2°C and 8°C* (36°F and 46°F). Once pump is activated, may be stored at room temperature.
5. With Paget's disease, more than 1 year of therapy may be required to treat neurologic lesions.
6. Check for hypersensitivity reactions before administering either medication. Administer 1 IU intracutaneously in the inner forearm and observe for 15 min to ensure test is negative.
7. Have emergency drugs for a hypersensitivity reaction.

Assessment

1. Note any hypersensitivity to drug or its gelatin diluent.
2. Record indications for therapy, noting baseline assessments.
3. Review diet and intake of calcium and vitamin D; obtain levels.

Interventions

1. Perform test dose; note local inflammatory reactions at site; assess for systemic allergic reactions.
2. Observe for hypocalcemic tetany, i.e., muscular fibrillation, twitching, tetanic spasms, and convulsions. Check at least q 10 min for the next 30 min following injection; have IV calcium available.
3. Check for evidence of hypercalcemia and report, i.e., increased thirst, anorexia, polyuria, and N&V.
4. Assess for facial flushing, abdominal distress, anorexia, diarrhea, epigastric distress, or changes in taste perception. Record weights, I&O, and report if symptoms persist.
5. If client has initial good clinical response, then has a relapse, check for antibody formation to drug.

Client/Family Teaching

1. Identify what to observe for with Pagent's disease and how to assess the response to therapy.
2. Review aseptic methods of reconstituting solution, proper injection technique, and importance of alternating injection sites.

3. With the spray: take with vitamin D (400 IU) and calcium (1,000 mg) daily, alternate nostrils, and do not exceed prescribed dosage.
4. N&V may occur at the onset of therapy, but should subside as treatment continues; report if persists.
5. Report increased urine sediment; have periodic urine tests to assess for kidney damage.
6. Continue regular exercise/activity to minimize bone loss.
7. May take in the evening to minimize flushing.
8. See dietitian for adjustments in the diet.

Outcome/Evaluate

- ↓ Serum calcium, ↓ alkaline phosphatase, and ↓ 24-hr urinary excretion of hydroxyproline
- Promotion of bone formation with ↑ bone mass density
- ↓ Bone pain
- Halt in postmenopausal osteoporosis

Calcium carbonate

(KAL-see-um KAR-bon-ayt)
Alka-Mints, Amitone, Antacid Tablets, Apo-Cal ✱, Cal Carb-HD, Calci-Chew, Calciday-667, Calci-Mix, Calcium 600, Cal-Plus, Caltrate ✱, Caltrate 600, Caltrate Jr., Children's Mylanta Upset Stomatch Relief, Chooz, Dicarbosil, Equilet, Extra Strength Antacid, Extra Strength Tums, Florical, Gencalc 600, Maalox Antacid Caplets, Mallamint, Mylanta Lozenges, Nephro-Calci, Os-Cal 500, Os-Cal 500 Chewable, Oysco 500 Chewable, Oyst-Cal 500, Oystercal 500, Oyster Shell Calcium-500, Tums, Tums Ultra, Webber Calcium Carbonate ✱ **(OTC)**
Classification: Calcium salt

See also *Calcium Salts.*
Uses: Mild hypocalcemia, antacid, antihyperphosphatemic.
Special Concerns: Dosage not established in children.
How Supplied: *Capsule:* 500 mg, 600 mg, 900 mg, 1250 mg; *Chew Tablet:* 300 mg, 500 mg, 600 mg, 650 mg; *Lozenge/Troche:* 240 mg; *Suspension:* 500 mg/5 mL; *Tablet*: 10 mg, 250 mg, 375 mg, 420 mg, 500 mg, 600 mg, 625 mg, 650 mg, 750 mg, 1,000 mg, 1,250 mg; *Tablet, Extended Release:* 500 mg

Dosage

- **Chewable Tablets, Tablets, Suspension, Gum, Lozenges, Wafers**

Adults: 0.5–1.5 g, as needed.

- **Capsules, Suspension, Tablets, Chewable Tablets**

Hypocalcemia, nutritional supplement.
Adults: 1.25–1.5 g 1–3 times/day with or after meals.
Antihyperphosphatemic.
Adults: 5–13 g/day in divided doses with meals.
NOTE: The preparation contains 40% elemental calcium and 400 mg elemental calcium/g (20 mEq/g).

- **Florical**

1 capsule or tablet daily (also contains 8.3 mg sodium fluoride per capsule or tablet).

- **Children's Mylanta Upset Stomach Relief Chewable Tablets or Liquid**

Upset stomach in children.
1 tablet or 5 mL for children weighing 24–47 pounds (or those aged 2–5 years) and 2 tablets or 10 mL for children weighing 48–95 pounds (or those aged 6–11).

HEALTH CARE CONSIDERATIONS

See also *Health Care Considerations* for *Calcium Salts.*

Outcome/Evaluate

- Desired serum calcium levels
- ↓ Gastric acidity

Calcium citrate

(KAL-see-um CIH-trayt)
Cal.Citrus ✱, Citracal, Citracal Liquitab **(OTC)**
Classification: Calcium salt

See also *Calcium Salts.*
Additional Uses: Renal osteodystrophy.
Special Concerns: Dosage not established in children.
How Supplied: *Tablet:* 950 mg; *Tablet, Effervescent:* 2376 mg

Dosage

- **Tablets, Effervescent Tablets**

Hypocalcemia.
Adults: 0.9–1.9 g t.i.d.–q.i.d. after meals.
Nutritional supplement.
3.8–7.1 g/day in three to four divided doses.
NOTE: Contains 21.1% elemental calcium and 211 mg calcium/g (10.5 mEq/g).

HEALTH CARE CONSIDERATIONS

See *Health Care Considerations* for *Calcium Salts.*
Outcome/Evaluate: Restoration of serum calcium/electrolyte levels

Calcium glubionate

(KAL-see-um glue-BYE-oh-nayt)

Pregnancy Category: C
Neo-Calglucon, Calcium-Sandoz **(OTC)**
Classification: Calcium salt

See also *Calcium Salts.*
Uses: Hypocalcemia, calcium deficiency, tetany of newborn, hypoparathyroidism, pseudohypoparathyroidism, osteoporosis, rickets, osteomalacia.
How Supplied: *Syrup*

Dosage
- **Syrup**

Dietary supplement.
Adults and children over 4 years: 15 mL t.i.d.–q.i.d. **Pediatric (under 4 years):** 10 mL t.i.d. **Infants:** 5 mL 5 times/day.
Tetany of newborn.
On the basis of laboratory tests, usually 50–150 mg/kg/day in three or more divided doses.
Other calcium deficiencies.
Adults: 15–45 mL 1–3 times/day.
NOTE: The preparation contains 115 mg calcium ion/5 mL.

HEALTH CARE CONSIDERATIONS

See *Health Care Considerations* for *Calcium Salts.*
Outcome/Evaluate
- Desired calcium replacement
- Control of twitching and spasm

Calcium gluconate
(KAL-see-um GLUE-koh-nayt)
Kalcinate (Rx, injection; OTC, tablets)
Classification: Calcium salt

See also *Calcium Salts.*
Uses: Mild hypocalcemia due to neonatal tetany, tetany due to parathyroid deficiency or vitamin D deficiency, and alkalosis. Prophylaxis of hypocalcemia during exchange transfusions. Intestinal malabsorption. Adjunct to treat insect bites or stings to relieve muscle cramping. Depression due to magnesium overdosage. Acute symptoms of lead colic. Rickets, osteomalacia. Reverse symptoms of verapamil overdosage. Decrease capillary permeability in allergic conditions, nonthrombocytopenic purpura, and exudative dermatoses (e.g., dermatitis herpetiformis). Pruritus due to certain drugs. Hyperkalemia to antagonize cardiac toxicity (as long as client is not receiving digitalis).
Contraindications: IM, intramyocardial, or SC use due to severe tissue necrosis, sloughing, and abscess formation.
How Supplied: *Injection:* 100 mg/mL; *Tablet:* 500 mg, 650 mg, 975 mg, 1000 mg

Dosage
- **Chewable Tablets, Tablets**

Treatment of hypocalcemia.
Adults: 8.8–16.5 g/day in divided doses; **pediatric:** 0.5–0.72 g/kg/day in divided doses.
Nutritional supplement.
Adults: 8.8–16.5 g/day in divided doses.
- **IV Only**

Treatment of hypocalcemia.
Adults: 2.3–9.3 mEq (5–20 mL of the 10% solution) as needed (range: 4.65–70 mEq/day). **Children:** 2.3 mEq/kg/day (or 56 mEq/m^2/day) given well diluted and slowly in divided doses. **Infants:** No more than 0.93 mEq (2 mL of the 10% solution).
Emergency elevation of serum calcium.
Adults: 7–14 mEq (15–30.1 mL). **Children:** 1–7 mEq (2.2–15 mL). **Infants:** Less than 1 mEq (2.2 mL). Depending on client response, the dose may be repeated q 1–3 days.
Hypocalcemic tetany.
Children: 0.5–0.7 mEq/kg (1.1–1.5 mL/kg) t.i.d.–q.i.d. until tetany is controlled. **Infants:** 2.4 mEq/kg/day (5.2 mL/kg/day) in divided doses.
Hyperkalemia with cardiac toxicity.
2.25–14 mEq (4.8–30.1 mL) while monitoring the ECG. If needed, the dose can be repeated after 1–2 min.
Magnesium intoxication.
Initial: 4.5–9 mEq (9.7–19.4 mL). Subsequent dosage based on client response.
Exchange transfusion.
Adults: 1.35 mEq (2.9 mL) concurrent with each 100 mL citrated blood. **Neonates:** 0.45 mEq (1 mL)/100 mL citrated blood.
- **IM**

Hypocalcemic tetany.
Adults: 4.5–16 mEq (9.7–34.4 mL) until a therapeutic response is noted.
Magnesium intoxication.
If IV administration is not possible: 2–5 mEq (4.3–10.8 mL) in divided doses as needed.
NOTE: The preparation contains 9% calcium and 90 mg calcium/g (4.5 mEq/g).

HEALTH CARE CONSIDERATIONS

See also *Health Care Considerations* for *Calcium Salts.*
Administration/Storage
1. If a precipitate is noted in the syringe, do not use.
2. If a precipitate is noted in the vials or ampules, heat to 80°C (146°F) in a dry heat oven for 1 hr to dissolve. Shake vigorously and allow to cool to room temperature. Do not use if precipitate remains.

IV 3. IV rate should not exceed 0.5–2 mL/min.
4. Give by intermittent IV infusion at a rate not exceeding 200 mg (19.5 mg calcium ion)/ min. Can also be given by continuous IV infusion.

Outcome/Evaluate
- Restoration of serum calcium levels
- ↓ Magnesium and potassium levels

Calcium lactate

(KAL-see-um LACK-tayt)
(OTC)
Classification: Calcium salt

See also *Calcium Salts*.
Uses: Latent hypocalcemic tetany, hyperphosphatemia.
How Supplied: *Tablet:* 325 mg, 650 mg

Dosage
- **Tablets**

Treatment of hypocalcemia.
Adults: 7.7 g/day in divided doses with meals. **Pediatric:** 0.34–0.5 g/kg/day in divided doses.

NOTE: The preparation contains 13% calcium and 130 mg calcium/g (6.5 mEq/g).

HEALTH CARE CONSIDERATIONS

See *Health Care Considerations* for *Calcium Salts*.
Outcome/Evaluate: Restoration of serum calcium levels

Candesartan cilexetil

(kan-deh-SAR-tan)
Pregnancy Category: C (first trimester), D (second and third trimesters)
Atacand **(Rx)**
Classification: Antihypertensive, angiotensin II receptor blocker

See also *Antihypertensive Drugs*.
Action/Kinetics: Prevents the binding of angiotensin II to the AT_1 receptor, resulting in blockade of the vasoconstrictor and aldosterone-secreting effects of angiotensin II. Is rapidly and completely bioactivated to candesartan by ester hydrolysis during absorption from the GI tract. Food does not affect bioavailability. **t½, elimination:** 9 hr. Candesartan is excreted mainly unchanged in the urine and feces.
Uses: Alone or in combination with other drugs to treat hypertension.
Contraindications: Lactation.
Special Concerns: Fetal and neonatal morbidity and death are possible if given to pregnant women. Safety and efficacy have not been determined in children less than 18 years of age.
Side Effects: *GI:* N&V, abdominal pain, diarrhea, dyspepsia, gastroenteritis. *CNS:* Headache, dizziness, paresthesia, vertigo, anxiety, depression, somnolence. *CV:* Tachycardia, palpitation; rarely, angina pectoris, MI. *Body as a whole:* Fatigue, asthenia, fever, peripheral edema. *Respiratory:* URTI, pharyngitis, rhinitis, bronchitis, coughing, dyspnea, sinusitis, epistaxis. *GU:* Impaired renal function, hematuria. *Dermatologic:* Rash, increased sweating. *Miscellaneous:* Backpain, chest pain, arthralgia, myalgia, angioedema.
Laboratory Test Considerations: ↑ Creatine phosphatase. Albuminuria, hyperglycemia, hypertriglyceridemia, hyperuricemia.
How Supplied: *Tablets:* 4 mg, 8 mg, 16 mg, 32 mg

Dosage
- **Tablets**

Hypertension, monotherapy.
Adults, usual initial: 16 mg once daily in those not volume depleted. Can be given once or twice daily in doses from 8 to 32 mg.

HEALTH CARE CONSIDERATIONS

Administration/Storage
1. Maximum BP reduction is reached within 4 to 6 weeks.
2. Initiate dosage under close supervision in those with possible depletion of intravascular volume. Consider giving a lower dose.
3. Can be given with or without food.
4. If BP is not controlled by candesartan alone, a diuretic may be added.

Assessment
1. Note onset and duration of disease, other agents trialed and the outcome.
2. Assess lytes, renal and LFTs.
3. Ensure adequate hydration, especially with diuretic therapy in renal dysfunction.

Client/Family Teaching
1. Take as directed with or without food.
2. Practice reliable birth control; report if pregnancy suspected.
3. Continue life style modifications, i.e., diet, regular exercise, stress reduction, no smoking, and moderate alcohol intake to ensure desired outcome.

Outcome/Evaluate: ↓ BP

C

Capsaicin

(kap-**SAY**-ih-sin)

Zostrix, Zostrix-HP **(Rx)**

Classification: Topical analgesic

Action/Kinetics: Derived from natural sources from plants of the Solanaceae family. Believed the drug depletes and prevents the reaccumulation of substance P, thought to be the main mediator of pain impulses from the periphery to the CNS.

Uses: Temporary relief of pain due to rheumatoid arthritis and osteoarthritis. Pain following herpes zoster (shingles), painful diabetic neuropathy. *Investigational:* Possible use in psoriasis, vitiligo, intractable pruritus, reflex sympathetic dystrophy, postmastectomy, vulvar vestibulitis, apocrine chromhidrosis, and postamputation and postmastectomy neuroma.

Special Concerns: For external use only.

Side Effects: *Skin:* Transient burning following application, stinging, erythema. *Respiratory:* Cough, respiratory irritation.

How Supplied: *Cream:* 0.025%, 0.075%, 0.25%; *Lotion:* 0.025%, 0.075%

Dosage

- **Cream or Lotion, 0.025% or 0.075%**

Adults and children over 2 years of age: Apply to affected area no more than 3–4 times/day.

HEALTH CARE CONSIDERATIONS

Client/Family Teaching

1. Drug is for external use only. Avoid eyes and broken/irritated skin.Expect transient burning/stinging.
2. Wash hands before and immediately after application.
3. Do not bandage area tightly.
4. Regular use (3–4 times/day) is required for desired response; drug intereferes with substance P (pain neurotransmitter).
5. Report if condition worsens, if symptoms persist > 3 weeks, or if clear then recur within a few days.

Outcome/Evaluate: Relief of pain

Captopril

(**KAP**-toe-prill)

Pregnancy Category: C (first trimester); D (second and third trimesters)

Alti-Captopril ✦, Apo-Capto ✦, Capoten, Gen-Captopril ✦, Med-Captopril ✦, Novo-Captoril ✦, Nu-Capto ✦ **(Rx)**

Classification: Antihypertensive, inhibitor of angiotensin synthesis

See also *Angiotensin-Converting Enzyme Inhibitors*.

Action/Kinetics: Onset: 60–90 min. **Peak serum levels:** 30–90 min; presence of food decreases absorption by 30%–40%. **Plasma protein binding:** 25%–30%. **Time to peak effect:** 60–90 min. **Duration:** 6–12 hr. **t½, normal renal function:** 2 hr; **t½, impaired renal function:** 3.5–32 hr. More than 95% of absorbed dose excreted in urine (40%–50% unchanged). Food decreases bioavailability of captopril by 30%–40%.

Uses: Antihypertensive, alone or in combination with other antihypertensive drugs, especially thiazide diuretics. In combination with diuretics and digitalis in treatment of CHF not responding to conventional therapy. To improve survival following MI in clinically stable clients with LV dysfunction manifested as an ejection fraction of 40% or less. Treatment of diabetic nephropathy (proteinuria > 500 mg/day) in those with type I insulin-dependent diabetes and retinopathy. *Investigational:* Rheumatoid arthritis, hypertensive crisis, neonatal and childhood hypertension, hypertension related to scleroderma renal crisis, diagnosis of anatomic renal artery stenosis, diagnosis of primary aldosteronism, Raynaud's syndrome, diagnosis of renovascular hypertension, enhance sensitivity and specificity of renal scintigraphy, idiopathic edema, and Bartter's syndrome.

Contraindications: Use with a history of angioedema related to previous use of ACE inhibitors.

Special Concerns: Use with caution in cases of impaired renal function and during lactation. Use in children only if other antihypertensive therapy has proven ineffective in controlling BP. May cause a profound drop in BP following the first dose or if used with diuretics.

Side Effects: *Dermatologic:* Rash (usually maculopapular) with pruritus and occasionally fever, eosinophilia, and arthralgia. Alopecia, erythema multiforme, photosensitivity, exfoliative dermatitis, **Stevens-Johnson syndrome,** reversible pemphigoid-like lesions, bullous pemphigus, onycholysis, flushing, pallor, scalded mouth sensation. *GI:* N&V, anorexia, constipation or diarrhea, gastric irritation, abdominal pain, dysgeusia, peptic ulcers, aphthous ulcers, dyspepsia, dry mouth, glossitis, pancreatitis. *Hepatic:* Jaundice, cholestasis, hepatitis. *CNS:* Headache, dizziness, insomnia, malaise, fatigue, paresthesias, confusion, depression, nervousness, ataxia, somnolence. *CV:* Hypotension, angina, ***MI,*** Raynaud's phenomenon, chest pain, palpitations, tachycardia, ***CVA, CHF, cardiac arrest,*** orthostatic hypotension, rhythm disturbances, cerebrovascular insufficiency. *Renal:* Renal insufficiency or failure, proteinuria, urinary frequency, oliguria, polyuria, nephrotic syndrome, interstitial nephritis. *Respiratory:* ***Bronchospasm,*** cough, dyspnea, asthma, ***pulmonary embolism, pulmonary infarction.*** *Hematologic:* Agranulocytosis, neutropenia, thrombocytopenia, pancytopenia, ***aplastic or hemolytic anemia.*** *Other:* Decrease or loss of taste perception with weight loss (reversible), angioedema, asthenia, syncope, fever, myalgia, arthralgia, vasculitis, blurred vision, impotence, hyperkalemia, hyponatremia, myasthenia, gynecomastia, rhinitis, eosinophilic pneumonitis.

Laboratory Test Considerations: False + test for urine acetone.

OD Management of Overdose: *Symptoms:* Hypotension with a systolic BP of <80 mm Hg a possibility. *Treatment:* Volume expansion with NSS (IV) is the treatment of choice to restore BP.

Additional Drug Interactions: Probenecid increases blood levels of captopril due to decreased renal excretion.

How Supplied: *Tablet:* 12.5 mg, 25 mg, 50 mg, 100 mg

Dosage

- **Tablets**

Hypertension.

Adults, initial: 25 mg b.i.d.–t.i.d. If unsatisfactory response after 1–2 weeks, increase to 50 mg b.i.d.–t.i.d.; if still unsatisfactory after another 1–2 weeks, thiazide diuretic should be added (e.g., hydrochlorothiazide, 25 mg/day). Dosage may be increased to 100–150 mg b.i.d.–t.i.d., not to exceed 450 mg/day.

Accelerated or malignant hypertension.

Stop current medication (except for the diuretic) and initiate captopril at a dose of 25 mg b.i.d.–t.i.d. The dose may be increased q 24 hr until a satisfactory response is obtained or the maximum dose reached. Furosemide may be indicated.

Heart failure.

Initial: 25 mg t.i.d.; **then,** if necessary, increase dose to 50 mg t.i.d. and evaluate response; **maintenance:** 50–100 mg t.i.d., not to exceed 450 mg/day.

NOTE: For adults, an initial dose of 6.25–12.5 mg (0.15 mg/kg t.i.d. in children) should be given b.i.d.–t.i.d. to clients who are sodium- and water-depleted due to diuretics, who will continue to be on diuretic therapy, and who have renal impairment.

Left ventricular dysfunction after MI.

Therapy may be started as early as 3 days after the MI. **Initial dose:** 6.25 mg; **then,** begin 12.5 mg t.i.d. and increase to 25 mg t.i.d. over the next several days. The target dose is 50 mg t.i.d. over the next several weeks. Other treatments for MI may be used concomitantly (e.g., aspirin, beta blockers, thrombolytic drugs).

Diabetic nephropathy.

25 mg t.i.d. for chronic use. Other antihypertensive drugs (e.g., beta blockers, centrally-acting drugs, diuretics, vasodilators) may be used with captopril if additional drug therapy is needed to reduce BP.

Hypertensive crisis.

Initial: 25 mg; **then,** 100 mg 90–120 min later, 200–300 mg/day for 2–5 days (then adjust dose). Sublingual captopril, 25 mg, has also been used successfully.

Rheumatoid arthritis.

75–150 mg/day in divided doses.

NOTE: For all uses, doses should be reduced in clients with renal impairment.

Severe childhood hypertension.

Initial: 0.3 mg/kg titrated to 6 mg or less given in 2 to 3 divided doses.

HEALTH CARE CONSIDERATIONS

See also *Health Care Considerations* for *Angiotensin-Converting Enzyme Inhibitors* and *Antihypertensive Agents.*

Administration/Storage

1. Do not discontinue without the provider's consent.
2. Give 1 hr before meals.
3. Discontinue previous antihypertensive medication 1 week before starting captopril, if possible.
4. The tablets can be used to prepare a solution of captopril if desired.

Assessment

1. Obtain baseline hematologic, liver and renal function tests.
2. Determine if diuretics, or nitrates prescribed; may act synergistically and cause a more pronounced response.
3. Record any ACE intolerance.
4. Determine ability to understand and comply with therapy.
5. Note ejection fraction (at or below 40%) in stable, post-MI clients.
6. Usually very effective with heart failure, diabetes, and arthritis.

Interventions

1. Observe for precipitous drop in BP within 3 hr after initial dose if on diuretic therapy and a low-salt diet.
2. If BP falls rapidly, place supine; have saline infusion available.

3. Check for proteinuria monthly and for 9 mo during therapy.
4. Withhold potassium-sparing diuretics; hyperkalemia may result. Hyperkalemia may occur several months after administration of spironolactone and captopril.

Client/Family Teaching

1. Take 1 hr before meals, on an empty stomach; food interferes with drug absorption.
2. Report any fever, skin rash, sore throat, mouth sores, fast or irregular heartbeat, chest pain, or cough.
3. May develop dizziness, fainting, or lightheadedness; usually disappear once the body adjusts to drug. Avoid sudden changes in posture to prevent dizziness/fainting.
4. Loss of taste may be experienced for the first 2–3 months; report if persists/interferes with nutrition.
5. Carry ID and a list of medications currently prescribed.
6. Call with any questions concerning symptoms or effects of drug therapy; do not stop taking abruptly.
7. Insulin-dependent clients may experience hypoglycemia; monitor blood sugar levels closely.
8. Avoid OTC agents without approval.

Outcome/Evaluate

- ↓ BP
- Improvement in symptoms of CHF (↓ preload, ↓ afterload)
- Improved mortality post-MI

Carbamazepine

(kar-bah-**MAYZ**-eh-peen)

Pregnancy Category: C

Apo-Carbamazepine ✦, Atretol, Carbitrol, Epitol, Mazepine ✦, Novo-Carbamaz ✦, Nu-Carbamazepine ✦, PMS-Carbamazepine ✦, Taro-Carbamazepine ✦, Tegretol, Tegretol Chewtabs ✦, Tegretol CR ✦, Tegretol XR **(Rx)**

Classification: Anticonvulsant, miscellaneous

See also *Anticonvulsants*.

Action/Kinetics: Chemically similar to the cyclic antidepressants. It also manifests antimanic, antineuralgic, antidiuretic, anticholinergic, antiarrhythmic, and antipsychotic effects. The anticonvulsant action is not known but may involve depressing activity in the nucleus ventralis anterior of the thalamus, resulting in a reduction of polysynaptic responses and blocking posttetanic potentiation. Due to the potentially serious blood dyscrasias, a benefit-to-risk evaluation should be undertaken before the drug is instituted. **Peak serum levels:** 4–5 hr. **t½** (serum): 12–17 hr with repeated doses. **Therapeutic serum levels:** 4–12 mcg/mL. Metabolized in the liver to an active metabolite (epoxide derivative) with a half-life of 5–8 hr. Metabolites are excreted through the feces and urine.

Uses: Partial seizures with complex symptoms (psychomotor, temporal lobe). Tonic-clonic seizures, diseases with mixed seizure patterns or other partial or generalized seizures. Carbamazepine is often a drug of choice due to its low incidence of side effects. For children with epilepsy who are less than 6 years of age for the treatment of partial seizures, generalized tonic-clonic seizures, and mixed seizure patterns and for treating trigeminal neuralgia. To treat pain associated with tic douloureux (trigeminal neuralgia) and glossopharyngeal neuralgia. *Investigational:* Bipolar disorders, unipolar depression, schizoaffective illness, resistant schizophrenia, dyscontrol syndrome associated with limbic system dysfunction, intermittent explosive disorder, PTSD, atypical psychosis. Management of alcohol, cocaine, and benzodiazepine withdrawal symptoms. Restless leg syndrome, nonneuritic pain syndromes, neurogenic or central diabetes insipidus, hereditary and nonhereditary chorea in children.

Contraindications: History of bone marrow depression. Hypersensitivity to drug or tricyclic antidepressants. Lactation. In clients taking MAO inhibitors, discontinue for 14 days before taking carbamazepine. Use for relief of general aches and pains.

Special Concerns: Safety and effectiveness have not been established in children less than 6 years of age. Use with caution in glaucoma and in hepatic, renal, CV disease, and a history of hematologic reaction. Use with caution in clients with mixed seizure disorder that includes atypical absence seizures (carbamazepine is not effective and may be associated with an increased frequency of generalized convulsions). Use in geriatric clients may cause an increased incidence of confusion, agitation, AV heart block, syndrome of inappropriate antidiuretic hormone, and bradycardia.

Side Effects: *GI:* N&V (common), diarrhea, constipation, gastric distress, abdominal pain, anorexia, glossitis, stomatitis, dryness of mouth and pharynx. *Hematologic:* ***Aplastic anemia,*** leukopenia, eosinophilia, thrombocytopenia, ***agranulocytosis,*** leukocytosis, pancytopenia, ***bone marrow depression.*** *CNS:* Dizziness, drowsiness, disturbances of coordination, headache, fatigue, confusion, speech disturbances, visual hallucinations, depression with agitation, talkativeness, hyperacusis, abnormal involuntary movements, behavioral changes in children. *CV:* CHF, aggravation of hypertension, hypotension, syncope and collapse, edema, recurrence of or primary thrombophlebitis, aggravation of CAD, paralysis and other symptoms of cerebral arterial insufficiency, thromboembolism, ***arrhythmias (including AV block).*** *GU:* Urinary frequency, acute urinary retention, oliguria with hypertension, impotence, renal failure, azotemia, albuminuria, glycosuria, increased BUN, microscopic deposits in urine. *Pulmonary:* Pulmonary hypersensitivity characterized by fever, dyspnea, pneumonitis, or pneumonia. *Dermatologic:* Pruritus, urticaria, photosensitivity, exfoliative dermatitis, erythematous rashes, alterations in pigmentation, alopecia, sweating, purpura, toxic epidermal necrolysis (Lyell's syndrome), ***Stevens-Johnson syndrome,*** aggravation of disseminated lupus erythematosus, alopecia, erythema nodosum or multiforme. *Ophthalmologic:* Nystagmus, double vision, blurred vision, oculomotor disturbances, conjunctivitis; scattered, punctate cortical lens opacities. *Hepatic:* Abnormal liver function tests, cholestatic or hepatocellular jaundice, hepatitis, acute intermittent porphyria. *Other:* Peripheral neuritis, paresthesias, tinnitus, fever, chills, joint and muscle aches and leg cramps, adenopathy or lymphadenopathy, inappropriate ADH secretion syndrome, frank water intoxication with hyponatremia and confusion.

Laboratory Test Considerations: ↓ Calcium, thyroid function tests. Interference with some pregnancy tests.

OD Management of Overdose: *Syptoms:* First appear after 1 to 3 hours. Neuromuscular disturbances are the most common. *Pulmonary:* Irregular breathing, ***respiratory depression.*** *CV:* Tachycardia, hypo- or hypertension, conduction disorders, ***shock.*** *CNS:* Seizures (especially in small children), impaired consciousness (deep coma possible), ***motor restlessness,*** muscle twitching or tremors, athetoid movements, ataxia, drowsiness, dizziness, nystagmus, mydriasis, psychomotor disturbances, hyperreflexia followed by hyporeflexia, opisthotonos, dysmetria, dizziness, EEG may show dysrhythmias. *GI:* N&V. *GU:* Anuria, oliguria, urinary retention. *Treatment:* Stomach should be irrigated completely even if more than 4 hr has elapsed following drug ingestion, especially if alcohol has been ingested. Activated charcoal, 50–100 g initially, using a NGT (dose of 12.5 or more g/hr until client is symptom free). Diazepam or phenobarbital may be used to treat seizures (although they may aggravate respiratory depression, hypotension, and coma). Respiration, ECG, BP, body temperature, pupillary reflexes, and kidney and bladder function should be monitored for several days.

If significant bone marrow depression occurs, the drug should be discontinued and daily CBC, platelet and reticulocyte counts determined. Perform bone marrow aspiration and trephine biopsy immediately and repeat often enough to monitor recovery.

Drug Interactions

Acetaminophen / ↑ Breakdown of acetaminophen → ↓ effect and ↑ risk of hepatotoxicity

Bupropion / ↓ Effect of bupropion due to ↑ breakdown by liver

Charcoal / ↓ Effect of carbamazepine due to ↓ absorption from GI tract

Cimetidine / ↑ Effect of carbamazepine due to ↓ breakdown by liver

Contraceptives, oral / ↓ Effect of contraceptives due to ↑ breakdown by liver

Cyclosporine / ↓ Effect of cyclosporoine due to ↑ breakdown by liver

Danazol / ↑ Effect of carbamazepine due to ↓ breakdown by liver

Diltiazem / ↑ Effect of carbamazepine due to ↓ breakdown by liver

Doxycycline / ↓ Effect of doxycycline due to ↑ breakdown by liver

Erythromycin / ↑ Effect of carbamazepine due to ↓ breakdown by liver

Felbamate / Possible ↓ serum levels of either drug

Felodipine / ↓ Effect of felodipine

Fluoxetine / ↑ Carbamazepine levels → possible toxicity

Fluvoxamine / ↑ Carbamazepine levels → possible toxicity

Haloperidol / ↓ Effect of haloperidol due to ↑ breakdown by liver

Isoniazid / ↑ Effect of carbamazepine due to ↓ breakdown by liver; also, carbamazepine may ↑ risk of isoniazid-induced hepatotoxicity

Lamotrigene / ↓ Effect of lamotrigene; also, ↑ levels of active metabolite of carbamazepine

Lithium / ↑ CNS toxicity

Macrolide antibiotics (e.g., Clarithromycin, Troleandomycin) / Effect of carbamazepine due to breakdown by liver

Muscle relaxants, nondepolarizing / Resistance to or reversal of the neuromuscular blocking effects of these drugs

Phenobarbital / ↓ Effect of carbamazepine due to ↑ breakdown by liver

Phenytoin / ↓ Effect of carbamazepine due to ↑ breakdown by liver; also, phenytoin levels may ↑ or ↓

Primidone / ↓ Effect of carbamazepine due to ↑ breakdown by liver
Propoxyphene / ↑ Effect of carbamazepine due to ↓ breakdown by liver
Ticlopidine / ↑ Effect of carbamazepine due to ↓ breakdown by liver
Tricyclic antidepressants / ↓ Effect of tricyclic antidepressants due to ↑ breakdown by liver; also, ↓ levels of tricyclic antidepressants
Valproic acid / ↓ Effect of valproic acid due to ↑ breakdown by liver; half-life of carbamazepine may be ↑
Vasopressin / ↑ Effect of vasopressin
Verapamil / ↑ Effect of carbamazepine due to ↓ breakdown by liver
Warfarin sodium / ↓ Effect of anticoagulant due to ↑ breakdown by liver

How Supplied: *Capsule, Extended Release:* 200 mg, 300 mg; *Chew Tablet:* 100 mg; *Suspension:* 100 mg/5 mL; *Tablet:* 200 mg; *Tablet, Extended Release:* 100 mg, 200 mg, 400 mg

Dosage

• **Oral Suspension, Extended Release Capsules, Tablets, Chewable Tablets, Extended-Release Tablets**

Anticonvulsant.

Adults and children over 12 years, initial: 200 mg b.i.d. on day 1 (100 mg q.i.d. of suspension). Increase by 200 mg/day or less at weekly intervals until best response is attained. Divide total dose and administer q 6–8 hr; the extended-release tablets may be used for twice-daily dosing instead of dosing 3 or 4 times a day. **Maximum dose, children 12–15 years:** 1,000 mg/day; **adults and children over 15 years:** 1,200 mg/day. **Maintenance:** decrease dose gradually to minimum effective level, usually 800–1,200 mg/day. **Children, 6–12 years: initial,** 100 mg b.i.d. on day 1 (50 mg q.i.d. of suspension); **then,** increase slowly, at weekly intervals, by 100 mg/day or less; dose is divided and given q 6–8 hr. Daily dose should not exceed 1,000 mg. **Maintenance:** 400–800 mg/day. **Children, less than 6 years:** 10–20 mg/kg/day in two to three divided doses (4 times/day with suspension); dose can be increased slowly in weekly increments to maintenance levels of 35 mg/kg/day (not to exceed 400 mg/day).

Trigeminal neuralgia.

Initial: 100 mg b.i.d. on day 1 (50 mg q.i.d. of suspension); increase by no more than 200 mg/day, using increments of 100 mg q 12 hr as needed, up to maximum of 1,200 mg/day. **Maintenance: Usual:** 400–800 mg/day (range: 200–1,200 mg/day). Attempt discontinuation of drug at least 1 time q 3 months.

Manage alcohol withdrawal.

200 mg q.i.d., up to 1,000 mg/day.

Manage cocaine or benzodiazepine withdrawal.

200 mg b.i.d., up to 800 mg/day.

Restless legs syndrome.

100–300 mg at bedtime.

Hereditary or nonhereditary chorea in children.

15–25 mg/kg/day.

Neurogenic or central diabetes.

200 mg b.i.d.–t.i.d.

HEALTH CARE CONSIDERATIONS

See also *Health Care Considerations* for *Anticonvulsants.*

Administration/Storage

1. Do not give for a minimum of 2 weeks after client has received MAO inhibitor drugs.
2. Protect tablets from moisture.
3. Start therapy gradually with the lowest doses of drug to minimize adverse reactions.
4. Add gradually to other anticonvulsant therapy. The other anticonvulsant dosage may be maintained or decreased except for phenytoin, which may need to be increased.
5. If carbamazepine therapy must be discontinued due to side effects, abrupt withdrawal may lead to seizures or status epilepticus.

Assessment

1. Record indications for therapy and pretreatment findings. With seizures, describe type, frequency, and characteristics.
2. Assess for a history of psychosis; drug may activate symptoms.
3. Obtain baseline hematologic, liver, and renal function tests; assess for dysfunction. With high doses, perform weekly CBC for the first 3 mo, then monthly to assess extent of bone marrow depression. At first sign of blood dyscrasia, slowly discontinue drug
4. Review eye exams for evidence of opacities and intraocular pressures.
5. Obtain EEG periodically during therapy. Use seizure precautions with quick withdrawal; may precipitate status epilepticus.
6. During dosage adjustment, monitor I&O and VS for evidence of fluid retention, renal failure, or CV complications.

Client/Family Teaching

1. Take with meals to minimize GI upset. The coating for extended release capsules is not absorbed and may be noticeable in the stool.
2. Withhold drug and report if any of the following symptoms occur:

• Fever, sore throat, mouth ulcers, easy bruising/bleeding; early signs of bone marrow depression.

• Urinary frequency, retention, reduced output, sexual impotence.
• Symptoms of CHF, fainting, collapse, swelling, blood clot, or cyanosis; require immediate attention.
• Loss of symptom control
3. Use caution in operating a car or other dangerous machinery; may interfere with vision and coordination.
4. Report any skin eruptions or pigmentation changes.
5. Avoid excessive sunlight; wear protective clothing and sunscreen.
6. Use nonhormonal birth control.
7. Report for labs to assess for early organ dysfunction.

Outcome/Evaluate
• Control of refractory seizures
• Control of alcohol/drug withdrawal S&S
• ↓ Pain with trigeminal neuralgia
• Therapeutic serum drug levels (4–12 mcg/mL)

Carbenicillin indanyl sodium

(kar-ben-ih-SILL-in)
Pregnancy Category: B
Geocillin **(Rx)**
Classification: Antibiotic, penicillin

See also *Anti-Infectives* and *Penicillins*.
Action/Kinetics: Acid stable drug. **Peak serum levels: PO:** 6.5 mcg/mL after 1 hr. **t½:** 60 min. Rapidly excreted unchanged in urine.
Uses: Upper and lower UTIs or bacteriuria due to *Escherichia coli, Proteus vulgaris and P. mirabilis, Morganella morganii, Providencia rettgeri, Enterobacter, Pseudomonas,* and enterococci. Prostatitis due to *E. coli, Streptococcus faecalis* (enterococci), *P. mirabilis,* and *Enterobacter* species.
Additional Contraindications: Pregnancy.
Special Concerns: Safe use in children not established. Use with caution in clients with impaired renal function.
Additional Side Effects: Neurotoxicity in clients with impaired renal function.
Drug Interactions: Blood levels of carbenicillin may be ↑ with administration of probenecid.
Additional Drug Interactions: When used in combination with gentamicin or tobramycin for *Pseudomonas* infections, effect of carbenicillin may be enhanced.
How Supplied: *Tablet:* 382 mg

Dosage
• **Tablets**
UTIs due to E. coli, Proteus, Enterobacter.
382–764 mg carbenicillin q.i.d.
UTIs due to Pseudomonas and enterococci.
764 mg carbenicillin q.i.d.
Prostatitis due to E. coli, P. mirabilis, Enterobacter, and enterococci.
764 mg carbenicillin q.i.d.

HEALTH CARE CONSIDERATIONS

See also *General Health Care Considerations for All Anti-Infectives* and *Penicillins.*
Administration/Storage
1. Protect from moisture.
2. Store at temperature of 30°C (86°F) or less.

Client/Family Teaching
1. Perform frequent mouth care to minimize nausea and unpleasant aftertaste.
2. Report any neurotoxicity, manifested by hallucinations, impaired sensorium, muscular irritability, and seizures.
3. Hemorrhagic manifestations, such as bruising, discolored skin, and frank bleeding of gums and/or rectum should be reported.

Outcome/Evaluate
• Negative C&S results
• Resolution of infection; symptomatic improvement

Carbidopa

(KAR-bih-doh-pah)
Lodosyn **(Rx)**

COMBINATION DRUG

Carbidopa/Levodopa

(KAR-bih-doh-pah/LEE-voh-doh-pah)
Apo-Levocarb ✤, Endo Levodopa Carbidopa ✤, Nu-Levocarb ✤, Pro-Lecarb ✤, Sinemet CR, Sinemet-10/100, -25/100, or -25/250 **(Rx)**
Classification: Antiparkinson agent

See also *Levodopa*.
Content: Carbidopa/Levodopa: Each 10/100 tablet contains: carbidopa, 10 mg, and levodopa, 100 mg. Each 25/100 tablet contains: carbidopa, 25 mg, and levodopa, 100 mg. Each 25/250 tablet contains: carbidopa, 25 mg, and levodopa, 250 mg. Each sustained-release tablet contains: carbidopa, 50 mg, and levodopa, 200 mg.
Action/Kinetics: Carbidopa inhibits peripheral decarboxylation of levodopa but not central decarboxylation because it does not cross the blood-brain barrier. Since peripheral decarboxylation is inhibited, this allows more levodopa to be available for transport

to the brain, where it will be converted to dopamine, thus relieving the symptoms of parkinsonism. Carbidopa and levodopa are to be given together (e.g., Sinemet). However, *the dosage of levodopa must be reduced by up to 80% when combined with carbidopa*. This decreases the incidence of levodopa-induced side effects. *NOTE:* Pyridoxine will not reverse the action of carbidopa/levodopa. **t½, carbidopa:** 1–2 hr; when given with levodopa, the t½ of levodopa increases from 1 hr to 2 hr (may be as high as 15 hr in some clients). About 30% carbidopa is excreted unchanged in the urine.

Uses: All types of parkinsonism (idiopathic, postencephalitic, following injury to the nervous system due to carbon monoxide and manganese intoxication). Carbidopa alone is used in clients who require individual titration of carbidopa and levodopa. *Investigational:* Postanoxic intention myoclonus. **Warning:** Levodopa must be discontinued at least 8 hr before carbidopa/levodopa therapy is initiated. Also, clients taking carbidopa/levodopa must not take levodopa concomitantly, because the former is a combination of carbidopa and levodopa.

Contraindications: History of melanoma. MAO inhibitors should be stopped 2 weeks before therapy. Lactation.

Special Concerns: Use during pregnancy only if benefits outweigh risks. Safety and efficacy in children less than 18 years of age have not been determined. Lower doses may be necessary in geriatric clients due to aged-related decreases in peripheral dopa decarboxylase.

Side Effects: Because more levodopa reaches the brain, dyskinesias may occur at lower doses with carbidopa/levodopa than with levodopa alone. Clients abruptly withdrawn from levodopa may experience neuroleptic malignant-like syndrome including symptoms of muscular rigidity, hyperthermia, increased serum phosphokinase, and changes in mental status.

Laboratory Test Considerations: ↓ Creatinine, BUN, and uric acid.

Drug Interactions: Use with tricyclic antidepressants may cause hypertension and dyskinesia.

How Supplied: Carbodopa: *Tablet:* 25 mg. Carbidopa/Levodopa: See Content

Dosage

- **Tablets**

Parkinsonism, clients not receiving levodopa.

Initial: 1 tablet of 10 mg carbidopa/100 mg levodopa t.i.d.–q.i.d. or 25 mg carbidopa/100 mg levodopa t.i.d.; **then,** increase by 1 tablet q 1–2 days until a total of 8 tablets/day is taken. If additional levodopa is required, substitute 1 tablet of 25 mg carbidopa/250 mg levodopa t.i.d.–q.i.d.

Parkinsonism, clients receiving levodopa.

Initial: Carbidopa/levodopa dosage should be about 25% of prior levodopa dosage (levodopa dosage is discontinued 8 hr before carbidopa/levodopa is initiated); **then,** adjust dosage as required. Suggested starting dose is 1 tablet of 25 mg carbidopa/250 mg levodopa t.i.d.–q.i.d. for clients taking more than 1500 mg levodopa or 25 mg carbidopa/100 mg levodopa for clients taking less than 1500 mg levodopa.

- **Sustained-Release Tablets**

Parkinsonism, clients not receiving levodopa.

1 tablet b.i.d. at intervals of not less than 6 hr. Depending on the response, dosage may be increased or decreased. Usual dose is 2–8 tablets/day in divided doses at intervals of 4–8 hr during waking hours (if divided doses are not equal, the smaller dose should be given at the end of the day).

Parkinsonism, clients receiving levodopa.

1 tablet b.i.d. Carbidopa is available alone for clients requiring additional carbidopa (i.e., inadequate reduction in N&V); in such clients, carbidopa may be given at a dose of 25 mg with the first daily dose of carbidopa/levodopa. If necessary, additional carbidopa, at doses of 12.5 or 25 mg, may be given with each dose of carbidopa/levodopa.

Clients receiving carbidopa/levodopa who require additional carbidopa.

In clients taking 10 mg carbidopa/100 mg levodopa, 25 mg carbidopa may be given with the first dose each day. Additional doses of 12.5 or 25 mg may be given during the day with each dose. If the client is taking 25 mg carbidopa/250 mg levodopa, a dose of 25 mg carbidopa may be given with any dose, as needed. The maximum daily dose of carbidopa is 200 mg.

HEALTH CARE CONSIDERATIONS

See also *Health Care Considerations* for *Levodopa*.

Administration/Storage

1. Dosage must be individualized.
2. Assess for drug interactions.
3. Do not administer carbidopa/levodopa with levodopa.
4. Administration of the sustained-release form of carbidopa/levodopa with food results in increased availability of levodopa by 50% and increased peak levodopa levels by 25%.

5. Do not crush or chew the sustained-release form of Sinemet but it can be administered as whole or half tablets.
6. Allow a minimum of 3 days to elapse between dosage adjustments of the sustained-release product.
7. When carbidopa is used as a supplement to carbidopa/levodopa, 1 tablet of carbidopa may be added or omitted per day.
8. If general anesthesia is necessary, continue therapy as long as PO fluids and other medication are allowed. Resume therapy when able to take PO medication.

Assessment

1. Assess and record motor function, reflexes, gait, strength of grip, and amount of tremor.
2. Observe extent of tremors, noting muscle weakness, muscle rigidity, difficulty walking, or changing directions. During dosage adjustment period, any involuntary movement may require dosage reduction.
3. Determine usual sleep patterns; assess mental status.
4. Note any history of CV disease, cardiac arrhythmias, or COPD.
5. Elderly clients may require a reduced dosage.
6. Obtain baseline ECG, VS, and respiratory assessment and determine level of bladder function. Monitor BP while supine and standing to detect postural hypotension.
7. Assess need for a drug "holiday" (stopping thedrug for a certain length of time) periodically based on decreased drug response

Client/Family Teaching

1. Report side effects as dose of drug may need to be reduced or temporarily discontinued. May be asked to tolerate certain side effects because of the overall benefits gained with therapy.
2. With improvement, may resume normal activity gradually; with increased activity, other medical conditions must be considered.
3. Do not withdraw abruptly. When changing medication, one drug should be withdrawn slowly and the other started in small doses under supervision. To facilitate adjustment, take the last dose of levodopa at bedtime and start carbidopa/levodopa upon arising. Food may alter availability; do not crush or chew sustained-release form of Sinemet. May take as whole or half tablets.
4. Drug may discolor or darken urine and/or sweat.
5. Muscle/eyelid twitching may indicate toxicity; report immediately.

Outcome/Evaluate: Control of parkinsonian symptoms (e.g., improvement in motor function, reflexes, gait, strength of grip, and amount of tremor)

Carisoprodol

(kar-eye-so-**PROH**-dohl)
Pregnancy Category: C
Soma **(Rx)**
Classification: Skeletal muscle relaxant, centrally acting

See also *Skeletal Muscle Relaxants, Centrally Acting*.

Action/Kinetics: Does not directly relax skeletal muscles. Sedative effects may be responsible for muscle relaxation. **Onset:** 30 min. **Duration:** 4–6 hr. **Peak serum levels:** 4–7 mcg/mL. **t½:** 8 hr. Metabolized in the liver and excreted in the urine.

Uses: As an adjunct to rest, physical therapy, and other measures to treat skeletal muscle disorders including bursitis, low back disorders, contusions, fibrositis, spondylitis, sprains, muscle strains, and cerebral palsy.

Contraindications: Acute intermittent porphyria. Hypersensitivity to carisoprodol or meprobamate. Children under 12 years of age.

Special Concerns: Use with caution during lactation and in impaired liver or kidney function. May cause GI upset and sedation in infants.

Side Effects: *CNS:* Ataxia, dizziness, drowsiness, excitement, tremor, syncope, vertigo, insomnia, irritability, headache, depressive reactions. *GI:* N&V, gastric upset, hiccoughs. *CV:* Flushing of face, postural hypotension, tachycardia. *Allergic reactions:* Pruritus, skin rashes, erythema multiforme, eosinophilia, fever, dizziness, angioneurotic edema, asthmatic symptoms, "smarting" of the eyes, weakness, hypotension, ***anaphylaxis.***

OD **Management of Overdose:** *Symptoms:* Stupor, coma, shock, respiratory depression, and rarely death. *Treatment:* Supportive measures. Diuresis, osmotic diuresis, peritoneal dialysis, hemodialysis. Monitor urinary output to avoid overhydration. Observe client for possible relapse due to incomplete gastric emptying and delayed absorption.

Drug Interactions

Alcohol / Additive CNS depressant effects
Antidepressants, tricyclic / ↑ Effect of carisoprodol
Barbiturates / Possible ↑ effect of carisoprodol, followed by inhibition of carisoprodol
Chlorcyclizine / ↓ Effect of carisoprodol
CNS depressants / Additive CNS depression

MAO inhibitors / ↑ Effect of carisoprodol by ↓ breakdown by liver
Phenobarbital / ↓ Effect of carisoprodol by ↑ breakdown by liver
Phenothiazines / Additive depressant effects
How Supplied: *Tablet:* 350 mg

Dosage

- **Tablets**

Skeletal muscle disorders.

Adults: 350 mg q.i.d. (take last dose at bedtime).

HEALTH CARE CONSIDERATIONS

See also *Health Care Considerations* for *Skeletal Muscle Relaxants, Centrally Acting.*

Assessment

1. Note any hypersensitivity to meprobamate or carisoprodol.
2. Record extent of skeletal muscular disorders noting baseline ROM, stiffness, and level of discomfort.
3. Review drugs prescribed to ensure no interactions.

Client/Family Teaching

1. If unable to swallow tablets, mix with syrup, chocolate, or a jelly mixture.
2. Administer with food if gastric upset occurs.
3. Report side effects of ataxia, or tremors should they occur.
4. Establish a schedule so the last dose is taken at bedtime.
5. Due to the possibility of drug-induced dizziness, drowsiness, and palpitations, use caution when driving or undertaking tasks requiring mental alertness. Report if severe; may necessitate drug withdrawal.
6. Avoid OTC agents and alcohol.
7. Psychologic dependence may occur.

Outcome/Evaluate: Improvement in skeletal muscle pain and spasticity; ↑ ROM

Carteolol hydrochloride

(kar-**TEE**-oh-lohl)
Pregnancy Category: C
Cartrol, Ocupress **(Rx)**
Classification: Beta-adrenergic blocking agent

See also *Beta-Adrenergic Blocking Agents.*
Action/Kinetics: Has both beta-1 and beta-2 receptor blocking activity. It has no membrane-stabilizing activity but does have moderate intrinsic sympathomimetic effects. Low lipid solubility. **t½:** 6 hr. **Duration, ophthalmic use:** 12 hr. Approximately 50%–70% excreted unchanged in the urine.
Uses: PO. Hypertension. *Investigational:* Reduce frequency of anginal attacks. **Ophthalmic.** Chronic open-angle glaucoma and intraocular hypertension alone or in combination with other drugs.
Contraindications: Severe, persistent bradycardia. Bronchial asthma or bronchospasm, including severe COPD.
Special Concerns: Dosage not established in children.
Additional Side Effects: Ophthalmic use. Transient irritation, burning, tearing, conjunctival hyperemia, edema, blurred or cloudy vision, photophobia, decreased night vision, ptosis, blepharoconjunctivitis, abnormal corneal staining, corneal sensitivity.
How Supplied: *Ophthalmic solution:* 1%; *Tablet:* 2.5 mg, 5 mg

Dosage

- **Tablets**

Hypertension.

Initial: 2.5 mg once daily either alone or with a diuretic. If response is inadequate, the dose may be increased gradually to 5 mg and then 10 mg/day as a single dose. **Maintenance:** 2.5–5 mg once daily. Doses greater than 10 mg/day are not likely to increase the beneficial effect and may decrease the response. Increase the dosage interval in clients with renal impairment.

Reduce frequency of anginal attacks.

10 mg/day.

- **Ophthalmic Solution**

Usual: 1 gtt in affected eye b.i.d. If the response is unsatisfactory, concomitant therapy may be initiated.

HEALTH CARE CONSIDERATIONS

See also *Health Care Considerations* for *Beta-Adrenergic Blocking Agents* and *Antihypertensive Agents.*

Assessment

1. Record indications for therapy and note baseline findings.
2. Assess renal function; reduce dose with impairment.

Client/Family Teaching

1. Do not exceed prescribed dose; may alter desired response.
2. May cause increased sensitivity to cold; dress appropriately.
3. Report symptoms of bleeding, infection, dizziness, confusion, depression, SOB, weight gain, or rash.
4. Reinforce diet, exercise, and weight reduction.
5. With ophthalmic solution, report any persistent burning, pain, or visual impairment.

Outcome/Evaluate

- ↓ BP; ↓ anginal attacks
- ↓ Intraocular pressure

C

Carvedilol

(kar-**VAY**-dih-lol)

Pregnancy Category: C

Coreg **(Rx)**

Classification: Alpha/beta-adrenergic blocking agent

Action/Kinetics: Has both alpha- and beta-adrenergic blocking activity. Decreases cardiac output, reduces exercise- or isoproterenol-induced tachycardia, reduces reflex orthostatic hypotension, causes vasodilation, and reduces peripheral vascular resistance. Significant beta-blocking activity occurs within 60 min while alpha-blocking action is observed within 30 min. BP is lowered more in the standing than in the supine position. Significantly lowers plasma renin activity when given for at least 4 weeks. Rapidly absorbed after PO administration, but there is a significant first-pass effect. **Terminal t½:** 7–10 hr. Food delays the rate of absorption. Over 98% is bound to plasma protein. Plasma levels average 50% higher in geriatric compared with younger clients. Extensively metabolized in the liver, with metabolites excreted primarily via the bile into the feces.

Uses: Essential hypertension used either alone or in combination with other antihypertensive drugs, especially thiazide diuretics. Used with digitalis, diuretics, and ACE inhibitors to reduce the progression of mild to moderate CHF of ischemic or cardiomyopathic origin. *Investigational:* Angina pectoris, idiopathic cardiomyopathy.

Contraindications: Clients with New York Heart Association Class IV decompensated cardiac failure, bronchial asthma, or related bronchospastic conditions, second- or third-degree AV block, sick sinus syndrome (unless a permanent pacemaker is in place), cardiogenic shock, severe bradycardia, drug hypersensitivity. Hepatic impairment. Lactation.

Special Concerns: Use with caution in hypertensive clients with CHF controlled with digitalis, diuretics, or an ACE inhibitor. Use with caution in peripheral vascular disease, in surgical procedures using anesthetic agents that depress myocardial function, in diabetics receiving insulin or oral hypoglycemic drugs, in those subject to spontaneous hypoglycemia, or in thyrotoxicosis. Clients with a history of severe anaphylactic reaction to a variety of allergens may be more reactive to repeated challenge while taking beta blockers. Safety and efficacy have not been established in children less than 18 years of age.

Side Effects: *CV:* Bradycardia, postural hypotension, dependent or peripheral edema, AV block, extrasystoles, hypertension, hypotension, palpitations, peripheral ischemia, syncope, angina, ***cardiac failure,*** myocardial ischemia, tachycardia, CV disorder. *CNS:* Dizziness, headache, somnolence, insomnia, ataxia, hypesthesia, paresthesia, vertigo, depression, nervousness, migraine, neuralgia, paresis, amnesia, confusion, sleep disorder, impaired concentration, abnormal thinking, paranoia, emotional lability. *Body as a whole:* Fatigue, viral infection, rash, allergy, asthenia, malaise, pain, injury, fever, infection, somnolence, sweating, ***sudden death.*** *GI:* Diarrhea, abdominal pain, bilirubinemia, N&V, flatulence, dry mouth, anorexia, dyspepsia, melena, periodontitis, increased hepatic enzymes, ***GI hemorrhage***. *Respiratory:* Rhinitis, pharyngitis, sinusitis, bronchitis, dyspnea, ***asthma, bronchospasm,*** pulmonary edema, respiratory alkalosis, dyspnea, respiratory disorder, URTI, coughing. *GU:* UTI, albuminuria, hematuria, frequency of micturition, abnormal renal function, impotence. *Dermatologic:* Pruritus; erythematous, maculopapular, and psoriaform rashes, photosensitivity reaction, exfoliative dermatitis. *Metabolic:* Hypertriglyceridemia, hypercholesterolemia, hyperglycemia, hypovolemia, hyperuricemia, increased weight, gout, dehydration, hypervolemia, glycosuria, hyponatremia, hypokalemia, hyperkalemia, diabetes mellitus. *Hematologic:* Thrombocytopenia, anemia, leukopenia, pancytopenia, purpura, atypical lymphocytes. *Musculoskeletal:* Back pain, arthralgia, myalgia, arthritis. *Otic:* Decreased hearing, tinnitus. *Miscellaneous:* Hot flushes, leg cramps, abnormal vision, ***anaphylactoid reaction.***

Laboratory Test Considerations: ↑ ALT, AST, BUN, NPN, alkaline phosphatase. ↓ HDL.

OD **Management of Overdose:** *Symptoms:* Severe hypotension, bradycardia, cardiac insufficiency, ***cardiogenic shock, cardiac arrest, generalized seizures,*** respiratory problems, bronchospasms, vomiting, lapse of consciousness. *Treatment:* Place the client in a supine position and monitor carefully and treat under intensive care conditions. Treatment should continue for a long enough period of time consistent with the 7- to 10-hr half-life of the drug.

- Gastric lavage or induced emesis shortly after ingestion
- For excessive bradycardia, atropine, 2 mg IV. If the bradycardia is resistant to therapy, perform pacemaker therapy.

• To support cardiovascular function, give glucagon, 5–10 mg IV rapidly over 30 sec, followed by a continuous infusion of 5 mg/hr. Sympathomimetics (dobutamine, isoproterenol, epinephrine) may be given.
• For peripheral vasodilation, give epinephrine or norepinephrine with continuous monitoring of circulatory conditions.
• For bronchospasm, give beta sympathomimetics as aerosol or IV or give aminophylline IV.
• In the event of seizures, give a slow IV injection of diazepam or clonazepam.

Drug Interactions

Antidiabetic agents / The beta-blocking effect may ↑ the hypoglycemic effect of insulin and oral hypoglycemics
Calcium channel blocking agents / ↑ Risk of conduction disturbances
Clonidine / Potentiation of BP and heart rate lowering effects
Digoxin / ↑ Digoxin levels
Rifampin / ↓ Plasma levels of carvedilol

How Supplied: *Tablet:* 3.125 mg, 6.25 mg, 12.5 mg, 25 mg

Dosage

• **Tablets**

Essential hypertension.

Initial: 6.25 mg b.i.d. If this is tolerated, using standing systolic pressure measured about 1 hr after dosing, maintain the dose for 7–14 days. **Then,** increase to 12.5 mg b.i.d., if necessary, based on trough BP, using standing systolic pressure 2 hr after dosing. This dose should be maintained for 7–14 days and can then be adjusted upward to 25 mg b.i.d. if necessary and tolerated. The total daily dose should not exceed 50 mg.

Congestive heart failure.

Initial: 3.125 mg b.i.d. for 2 weeks. If this is tolerated, increase to 6.25 mg b.i.d. Dosing is doubled every 2 weeks to the highest tolerated level, up to a maximum of 25 mg b.i.d. in those weighing less than 85 kg and 50 mg b.i.d. in those weighing over 85 kg.

Angina pectoris.

25–50 mg b.i.d.

Idiopathic cardiomyopathy.

6.25–25 mg b.i.d.

HEALTH CARE CONSIDERATIONS

See also *Health Care Considerations* for *Antihypertensive Agents.*

Administration/Storage

1. The full antihypertensive effect is seen within 7–14 days.
2. Addition of a diuretic can produce additive effects and exaggerate the orthostatic effect.

Assessment

1. Record indications for therapy, type and onset of symptoms, agents trialed, and the outcome.
2. Note any history or evidence of bronchospastic conditions, asthma, advanced AV block, or severe bradycardia as drug is contraindicated.
3. Obtain baseline CBC and liver and renal function studies.

Client/Family Teaching

1. Take as prescribed and with food to slow absorption and decrease incidence of orthostatic effects.
2. Avoid activities that require mental acuity until drug effects realized.
3. Do not stop abruptly due to beta-blocking activity (especially with ischemic heart disease); call provider.
4. To prevent orthostatic hypotension, sit or lie until symptoms subside and rise slowly from a sitting or lying position. Concomitant therapy with a diuretic may aggravate the orthostatic drug effects.
5. Decreased lacrimation may be noted by contact lens wearers.
6. Dosing adjustments will be made every 7–14 days based on standing SBP measured 1 hr after dosing.

Outcome/Evaluate

• Desired reduction of BP
• ↓ Progression of CHF

Cefaclor

(SEF-ah-klor)

Pregnancy Category: B

Apo-Cefaclor ✱, Ceclor, Ceclor CD, PMS-Cefaclor ✱ **(Rx)**

Classification: Cephalosporin, second-generation

See also *Anti-Infectives* and *Cephalosporins.*

Action/Kinetics: Peak serum levels: 5–15 mcg/mL after 1 hr. **t½: PO,** 36–54 min. Well absorbed from GI tract. From 60% to 85% excreted in urine within 8 hr.

Uses: Otitis media due to *Streptococcus pneumoniae, Hemophilus influenzae, Streptococcus pyogenes*, and staphylococci. Upper respiratory tract infections (including pharyngitis and tonsillitis) caused by *S. pyogenes.* Lower respiratory tract infections (including pneumonia) due to *S. pneumoniae, H. influenzae,* and *S. pyogenes.* Skin and skin structure infections due to *Staphylococcus aureus* and *S. pyogenes.* UTIs (including pyelonephritis and cystitis) caused by *Escherichia coli, Proteus mirabilis, Klebsiella,* and coagulase-negative staphylococci.

Extended-release tablets: Acute bacterial exacerbations of chronic bronchitis due to non-β-lactamase-producing strains of *H. influenzae, Moraxella catarrhalis* (including β-lactamase-producing strains), or *S. pneumoniae*. Secondary bacterial infections of acute bronchitis due to *H. influenzae* (non-β-lactamase-producing strains only), *M. catarrhalis* (including β-lactamase-producing strains), or *S. pneumoniae*. Pharyngitis or tonsillitis due to *S. pyogenes*. Uncomplicated skin and skin structure infections due to *S. aureus* (methicillin-susceptible). *Investigational:* Acute uncomplicated UTIs in select populations using a single dose of 2 g.

Special Concerns: Safety for use in infants less than 1 month of age has not been established.

Additional Side Effects: Cholestatic jaundice, lymphocytosis.

How Supplied: *Capsule:* 250 mg, 500 mg; *Powder for Reconstitution:* 125 mg/5 mL, 187 mg/5 mL, 250 mg/5 mL, 375 mg/5 mL; *Tablet, Extended Release:* 375 mg, 500 mg

Dosage

- **Capsules, Oral Suspension**

All uses.

Adults: 250 mg q 8 hr. Dose may be doubled in more severe infections or those caused by less susceptible organisms. Total daily dose should not exceed 4 g. **Children:** 20 mg/kg/day in divided doses q 8 hr. Dose may be doubled in more serious infections, otitis media, or for infections caused by less susceptible organisms. For otitis media and pharyngitis, the total daily dose may be divided and given q 12 hr. Total daily dose should not exceed 2 g.

- **Tablets, Extended Release**

Acute bacterial exacerbations, chronic bronchitis, secondary bacterial infections of acute bronchitis.

500 mg q 12 hr for 7 days.

Pharyngitis, tonsillits.

375 mg q 12 hr for 10 days.

Uncomplicated skin and skin structure infections.

375 mg q 12 hr for 7–10 days.

HEALTH CARE CONSIDERATIONS

See also *General Health Care Considerations for All Anti-Infectives* and *Cephalosporins*.

Administration/Storage

1. Refrigerate suspension after reconstitution; discard after 2 weeks.
2. The extended-release tablet can not be assumed to be equivalent to the capsule or suspension.
3. The total daily dose for otitis media and pharyngitis can be divided and given q 12 hr.

Assessment

1. Record type, onset, duration of symptoms, and agents trialed.
2. Record allergic reactions to penicillin; cross-sensitivity reaction may occur.

Client/Family Teaching

1. Take entire prescription as directed; do not stop when feeling better.
2. Take extended-release tablets with food to enhance absorption. Food does not affect capsule absorption.
3. Report any adverse response or lack of improvement after 48–72 hr.

Outcome/Evaluate: Resolution of infection; symptomatic improvement

Cefadroxil monohydrate

(sef-ah-**DROX**-ill)

Pregnancy Category: B

Duricef **(Rx)**

Classification: Cephalosporin, first-generation

See also *Anti-Infectives* and *Cephalosporins*.

Action/Kinetics: Peak serum levels: PO, 15–33 mcg/mL after 90 min. **t½: PO,** 78–96 min. 90% excreted unchanged in urine within 24 hr.

Uses: UTIs caused by *Escherichia coli, Proteus mirabilis,* and *Klebsiella*. Skin and skin structure infections due to staphylococci or streptococci. Pharyngitis and tonsillitis due to group A beta-hemolytic streptococci.

Special Concerns: Safe use in children not established. C_{CR} determinations must be carried out in clients with renal impairment.

How Supplied: *Capsule:* 500 mg; *Powder for Reconstitution:* 125 mg/5 mL, 250 mg/5 mL, 500 mg/5 mL; *Tablet:* 1 g

Dosage

- **Capsules, Oral Suspension, Tablets**

Pharyngitis, tonsillitis.

Adults: 1 g/day in single or two divided doses for 10 days. **Children:** 30 mg/kg/day in single or two divided doses (for beta-hemolytic streptococcoal infection, dose should be given for 10 or more days).

Skin and skin structure infections.

Adults: 1 g/day in single or two divided doses. **Children:** 30 mg/kg/day in divided doses q 12 hr.

UTIs.

Adults: 1–2 g/day in single or two divided doses for uncomplicated lower UTI (e.g., cystitis). For all other UTIs, the usual dose is

2 g/day in two divided doses. **Children:** 30 mg/kg/day in divided doses q 12 hr.

For clients with C_{CR} rates below 50 mL/min.

Initial: 1 g; **maintenance,** 500 mg at following dosage intervals: q 36 hr for C_{CR} rates of 0–10 mL/min; q 24 hr for C_{CR} rates of 10–25 mL/min; q 12 hr for C_{CR} rates of 25–50 mL/min.

HEALTH CARE CONSIDERATIONS

See also *General Health Care Considerations for All Anti-Infectives* and *Cephalosporins.*

Administration/Storage

1. Give without regard to meals.
2. Shake the suspension well before using.
3. For beta-hemolytic streptococcal infections, continue treatment for 10 days.
4. Refrigerate the reconstituted suspension; discard after 14 days.

Assessment

1. Record indications for therapy, type and onset of symptoms, and pretreatment culture results.
2. Record any penicillin allergy.

Client/Family Teaching

1. Take as directed with or without food.
2. Report adverse side effects or lack of response.

Outcome/Evaluate

- Symptomatic improvement
- Negative culture reports

Cefdinir

(SEF-dih-near)

Pregnancy Category: B

Omnicef **(Rx)**

Classification: Cephalosporin, third generation

See also *Cephalosporins.*

Action/Kinetics: Maximum plasma levels: 2–4 hr. **t½, elimination:** 1.7 hr. Excreted through the urine.

Uses: Adults: (1) Community-acquired pneumonia or acute exacerbations of chronic bronchitis due to *Haemophilus influenzae* (including β-lactamase producing strains), *Haemophilus parainfluenzae* (including β-lactamase producing strains), *Streptococcus pneumoniae* (penicillin-susceptible strains only), and *Moraxella catarrhalis* (including β-lactamase producing strains). (2) Acute maxillary sinusitis due to *Haemophilus influenzae* (including β-lactamase producing strains), *Streptococcius pneumoniae* (penicillin-susceptible strains only), and *Moraxella catarrhalis* (including β-lactamase producing strains). (3) Uncomplicated skin and skin structure infections due to *Staphylococcus aureus* (including β-lactamase producing strains and *Streptococcus pyogenes.)*

Children: (1) Acute bacterial otitis media due to *H. influenzae* (including β-lactamase producing strains), *S. pneumoniae* (penicillin-susceptible strains only), and *M. catarrhalis* (including β-lactamase producing strains). (2) Pharyngitis/tonsillitis due to *S. pyogenes.* (3) Uncomplicated skin and skin structure infections due to *S. aureus* (including β-lactamase producing strains) and *S. pyogenes.*

Contraindications: Allergy to cephalosporins.

Special Concerns: Reduce dose in compromised renal function. Safety and efficacy have not been determined in infants less than 6 months of age.

Side Effects: See Cephalosporins.

Drug Interactions

Antacids, aluminum– or magnesium–containing / ↓ Absorption of cefdinir

Probenecid / ↑ Plasma levels of cefdinir → enhanced effect

How Supplied: *Capsules:* 300 mg; *Oral Suspension:* 125 mg/5mL

Dosage

- **Capsules**

Community-acquired pneumonia, uncomplicated skin and skin structure infections.

Adults and adolescents age 13 and older: 300 mg q 12 hr for 10 days.

Acute exacerbations of chronic bronchitis, acute maxillary sinusitis, or pharyngitis/tonsillitis.

Adults and adolescents age 13 and older: 300 mg q 12 hr or 600 mg q 24 hr for 10 days (5–10 days for pharyngitis/tonsillitis).

- **Oral Suspension**

Acute bacterial otitis media, acute maxillary sinusitis, pharyngitis/tonsillitis.

Children, 6 months through 12 years: 7 mg/kg q 12 hr or 14 mg/kg q 24 hr for 10 days (5–10 days for pharyngitis/tonsillitis).

Uncomplicated skin and skin structure infections.

Children, 6 months through 12 years: 7 mg/kg q 12 hr for 10 days.

HEALTH CARE CONSIDERATIONS

See also *Health Care Considerations* for *Cephalosporins.*

Assessment

1. Determine any cephalosporin or PCN allergy.

2. Record indications for therapy, onset, duration, and characteristics of symptoms.
3. Assess liver and renal function; if C_{CR} < 30 mL/min, reduce dose.

Client/Family Teaching

1. May be taken without regard to food.
2. Iron supplements and multivitamins containing iron interfere with drug absorption as does antacids with aluminum or magnesium; if needed, take either 2 hr before or 2 hr after cefdinir.
3. Oral suspension contains 2.86 grams of sucrose per teaspoon; use capsules with diabetics.
4. May administer suspension in iron fortified infant formula without losing potency.
5. Report if diarrhea is persistent or exceeds 4 episodes/day.
6. Stools may be discolored red; this should subside.

Outcome/Evaluate: Resolution of infection

Cefixime oral

(seh-**FIX**-eem)

Pregnancy Category: B

Suprax **(Rx)**

Classification: Cephalosporin, third-generation

See also *Anti-Infectives* and *Cephalosporins*.

Action/Kinetics: Stable in the presence of beta-lactamase enzymes. **Peak serum levels:** 2–6 hr. **t½:** averages 3–4 hr. About 50% excreted unchanged in the urine and approximately 10% in the bile.

Uses: Uncomplicated UTIs caused by *E. coli* and *P. mirabilis*. Otitis media due to *H. influenzae* (beta-lactamase positive and negative strains), *Moraxella catarrhalis*, and *S. pyogenes*. Pharyngitis and tonsillitis caused by *S. pyogenes*. Acute bronchitis and acute exacerbations of chronic bronchitis caused by *S. pneumoniae* and *H. influenzae* (beta-lactamase positive and negative strains). Uncomplicated cervical or urethral gonorrhea due to *N. gonorrhoeae* (both penicillinase- and non-penicillinase-producing strains).

Special Concerns: Safe use in infants less than 6 months old has not been established.

Additional Side Effects: *GI:* Flatulence. *Hepatic:* Elevated alkaline phosphatase levels. *Renal:* Transient increases in BUN or creatinine.

Additional Laboratory Test Interferences: False + test for ketones using nitroprusside test.

How Supplied: *Powder for Reconstitution:* 100 mg/5 mL; *Tablet:* 200 mg, 400 mg

Dosage

• **Oral Suspension, Tablets**

Adults: Either 400 mg once daily or 200 mg q 12 hr. **Children:** Either 8 mg/kg once daily or 4 mg/kg q 12 hr. Clients on renal dialysis or in whom C_{CR} is 21–60 mL/min, the dose should be 75% of the standard dose (i.e., 300 mg/day). If the C_{CR} is less than 20 mL/min, the dose should be 50% of the standard dose (i.e., 200 mg/day).

Uncomplicated gonorrhea.

One 400-mg tablet daily.

HEALTH CARE CONSIDERATIONS

See also *Health Care Considerations* for *Cephalosporins*.

Administration/Storage

1. Continue therapy for at least 10 days when treating *S. pyogenes*.
2. Give the adult dose to children older than 12 years or weighing more than 50 kg.
3. Treat otitis media using the suspension as higher blood levels are achieved compared with the tablet given at the same dose.
4. Once reconstituted, keep the suspension at room temperature where it maintains potency for 14 days.

Assessment

1. Record any prior sensitivity to cephalosporins or penicillins.
2. Anticipate reduced dose with impaired renal function.
3. Use suspension in children and when treating otitis media.

Client/Family Teaching

1. May cause GI upset; report any bothersome side effects, especially persistent diarrhea.
2. Once-a-day dosing should be taken at the same time each day; prescription cost may be prohibitive.
3. May alter results of urine glucose and ketone testing; do finger sticks for more accurate results.
4. Consult provider if child's condition does not improve or deteriorates after 48–72 hr. Return as scheduled.

Outcome/Evaluate: Resolution of infection; symptomatic improvement

Cefotaxime sodium

(sef-oh-**TAX**-eem)

Pregnancy Category: B

Claforan **(Rx)**

Classification: Cephalosporin, third-generation

See also *Anti-Infectives* and *Cephalosporins*.

Action/Kinetics: t½: 1 hr. **Peak serum levels after 1 g IV:** 42–102 mcg/mL. 60% excreted unchanged in the urine.

Uses: Infections of the GU tract, lower respiratory tract (including pneumonia), skin, skin structures, bones, joints, and CNS (including ventriculitis and meningitis). Intra-abdominal infections (including peritonitis), gynecologic infections (including endometritis, pelvic cellulitis, pelvic inflammatory disease), septicemia, bacteremia, and prophylaxis in surgery. Used with aminoglycosides for gram-positive or gram-negative sepsis where the causative agent has not been identified.

The IV route is preferable for clients with severe or life-threatening infections; for clients after surgery; or for those manifesting malnutrition, trauma, malignancy, heart failure, or diabetes, especially if shock is present or possible.

How Supplied: *Injection:* 1 g/50 mL, 2 g/50 mL; *Powder for injection:* 500 mg, 1 g, 2 g, 10 g

Dosage

- **IV, IM**

Uncomplicated infections.

Adults:1 g q 12 hr.

Moderate to severe infections.

Adults: 1–2 g q 8 hr.

Septicemia.

Adults, IV: 2 g q 6–8 hr, not to exceed 12 g/day.

Life-threatening infections.

Adults, IV: 2 g q 4 hr, not to exceed12 g/day.

Gonorrhea.

Adults, IM: Single dose of 1 g for rectal gonorrhea in males. **IM:** Single dose of 0.5 g for rectal gonorrhea in females or gonococcoal urethritis/cervicitis in males and females.

Preoperative prophylaxis.

Adults: 1 g 30–90 min prior to surgery.

Cesarean section.

IV: 1 g when the umbilical cord is clamped; **then,** give 1 g 6 and 12 hr after the first dose.

Use in children.

Pediatric, 1 month to 12 years, IM, IV: 50–180 mg/kg/day in four to six divided doses; **1–4 weeks, IV:** 50 mg/kg q 8 hr; **0–1 week, IV:** 50 mg/kg q 12 hr. *NOTE:* Use adult dose in children 50 kg or over.

Use in impaired renal function.

If C_{CR} is less than 20 mL/min/1.73m^2, reduce the dose by 50%. If only serum creatinine is available, use the following formulas to calculate C_{CR}:

Males: Weight (kg) x (140-age) / 72 x serum creatinine (mg/dL).
Females: 0.85 x above value.

HEALTH CARE CONSIDERATIONS

See also *Health Care Considerations* for *Cephalosporins.*

Administration/Storage

1. Continue treatment for a minimum of 10 days for group A beta-hemolytic streptococcal infections to minimize the risk of glomerulonephritis or rheumatic fever.
2. For IM use, reconstitute with sterile water for injection or bacteriostatic water for injection. Inject deeply into large muscle. Divide doses of 2 g and administer into different sites.
3. **IV** Discontinue IV administration of other solutions during administration of cefotaxime. Do not mix cefotaxime with aminoglycosides for continuous IV infusion; each should be given separately.
4. Cefotaxime is maximally stable at a pH of 5–7; solutions should not be prepared with diluents having a pH greater than 7.5 (e.g., $NaHCO_3$ injection).
5. Add recommended amount of diluent, shake to dissolve. Do not administer if particles are present or if solution is discolored. The normal color of solution ranges from light yellow to amber.
6. For direct IV administration, mix 1 or 2 g cefotaxime with 10 mL sterile water for injection and administer over 3–5 min. For intermittent administration, dilute in 50–100 mL of solution and infuse over 30 min.
7. After reconstitution, the drug remains stable for 24 hr at room temperature, 5 days refrigerated, and 13 weeks frozen. Thaw frozen samples at room temperature before use. Do not refreeze unused portions.
8. Store dry cefotaxime below 30°C (86°F) and protect from excess heat and light to prevent darkening.

Assessment

1. With joint infections, assess extent of ROM and freedom of movement.
2. With gynecologic infections, determine extent of infection, duration and characteristics of symptoms.
3. Monitor labs and review culture results to determine organism resistance; reduce dose with renal dysfunction.

Client/Family Teaching

1. Review drugs prescribed, side effects, and expected outcomes.
2. Complete course of therapy as prescribed despite feeling better.

3. Review appropriate technique and frequency for administration and proper storage. Inspect injection site for pain and redness; IM may cause thrombophlebitis.
4. Record I&O; report any reduction in urinary output as well as any persistent diarrhea.
5. Avoid alcohol in any form; a disulfiram-type reaction may occur.

Outcome/Evaluate

- Resolution of infection; symptomatic improvement
- Negative culture reports

Cefpodoxime proxetil

(sef-poh-**DOX**-eem)

Pregnancy Category: B

Vantin **(Rx)**

Classification: Cephalosporin, third-generation

See also *Anti-Infectives* and *Cephalosporins*.

Action/Kinetics: t½, after PO: 2–3 hr. From 29% to 33% is excreted unchanged in the urine.

Uses: Acute, community-acquired pneumonia due to *Streptococcus pneumoniae* or *Hemophilus influenzae* (non-β-lactamase-producing strains only). Acute bacterial exacerbation of chronic bronchitis caused by *S. pneumoniae,* non-beta-lactamase-producing *H. influenzae,* or M. catarrhalis. Acute otitis media caused by *S. pneumoniae, H. influenzae* (including beta-lactamase-producing strains), and *Moraxella catarrhalis*. Pharyngitis or tonsillitis due to *Streptococcus pyogenes*. Acute, uncomplicated urethral and cervical gonorrhea caused by *Neisseria gonorrhoeae* (including penicillinase-producing strains). Acute, uncomplicated anorectal infections in women due to *N. gonorrhoeae* (including penicillinase-producing strains). Uncomplicated skin and skin structure infections due to *Staphylococcus aureus* (including penicillinase-producing strains) or *S. pyogenes*. Uncomplicated UTIs (cystitis) due to *Escherichia coli, Klebsiella pneumoniae, Proteus mirabilis,* or *Staphyloccus saprophyticus*.

How Supplied: *Granule for Reconstitution:* 50 mg/5 mL, 100 mg/5 mL; *Tablet:* 100 mg, 200 mg

Dosage

- **Tablets, Suspension**

Acute community-acquired pneumonia.

Adults and children over 13 years: 200 mg q 12 hr for 14 days.

Acute bacterial exacerbations of chronic bronchitis.

Adults and children over 13 years: 200 mg q 12 hr for 10 days. Use the tablets.

Uncomplicated gonorrhea (men and women) and rectal gonococcal infections (women).

Adults and children over 13 years: Single dose of 200 mg.

Skin and skin structure infections.

Adults and children over 13 years: 400 mg q 12 hr for 7–14 days.

Pharyngitis, tonsillitis.

Adults and children over 13 years: 100 mg q 12 hr for 5–10 days. **Children, 5 months–12 years:** 5 mg/kg (maximum of 100 mg/dose) q 12 hr (maximum daily dose: 200 mg) for 5–10 days.

Uncomplicated UTIs.

Adults and children over 13 years: 100 mg q 12 hr for 7 days.

Acute otitis media.

Children, 5 months–12 years: 5 mg/kg (maximum of 200 mg/dose) q 12 hr or 10 mg/kg (maximum of 400 mg/dose) q 24 hr for 10 days.

HEALTH CARE CONSIDERATIONS

See also *General Health Care Considerations for All Anti-Infectives* and *Cephalosporins*.

Administration/Storage

1. In severe renal impairment (C_{CR} < 30 mL/min), increase the dosing interval to q 24 hr. If on hemodialysis, use a dosage frequency of 3 times/week after hemodialysis. Adjustment not required with cirrhosis.
2. May use the following formula to estimate C_{CR} (mL/min): males: weight (kg) × (140 − age)/72 × serum creatinine (mg/100 mL); females: 0.85 × male value.
3. Prepare suspension by adding a total of 58 mL of distilled water to the 50 mg/mL product or 57 mL of distilled water to the 100 mg/5 mL product. Tap the bottle gently to loosen the powder, then add 25 mL of water and shake vigorously for 15 sec to wet the powder. Add the remainder of the water and shake the bottle vigorously for 3 min or until all particles are suspended. Shake well before using.
4. After reconstitution, store suspension in the refrigerator; discard unused portion after 14 days.
5. Give tablets with food to enhance absorption. The oral suspension may be given without regard to food.

Assessment

1. Note any reactions to cephalosporins or penicillins as cross-sensitivity can occur.

2. Document and record source of infection; obtain baseline cultures.
3. Note any renal dysfunction; alter dosage if evident.
4. Obtain serologic test for syphilis with gonorrhea treatment.
5. Monitor VS and I&O; persistent diarrhea should be evaluated for other causes, such as *C. difficile*.
6. Discontinue therapy and report if seizures occur.

Client/Family Teaching
1. Take with food to enhance absorption and to diminish GI upset.
2. Report any persistent N&V or diarrhea as drug or dosage may require adjustment.
3. If receiving treatment for gonorrhea, have partner tested and treated and use barrier contraception to prevent reinfections. Drug is not effective against syphilis; all partners should be tested so that appropriate treatment may be provided.

Outcome/Evaluate
- Resolution of infection
- Symptomatic improvement

Cefprozil

(SEF-proh-zill)
Pregnancy Category: B
Cefzil **(Rx)**
Classification: Cephalosporin, second-generation

See also *Anti-Infectives* and *Cephalosporins*.
Action/Kinetics: t½, after PO: 78 min. Sixty percent is recovered in the urine unchanged.
Uses: Pharyngitis and tonsillitis due to *Streptococcus pyogenes*. Acute bacterial sinusitis due to *Streptococcus pneumoniae, Staphylococcus aureus, Haemophilus influenzae* (including β-lactamase producing strains), and *Morazella catarrhalis* (including β-lactamase producing strains). Otitis media caused by *S. pneumoniae, H. influenzae,* and *M. catarrhalis*. Uncomplicated skin and skin structure infections due to *S. aureus* (including penicillinase-producing strains) and *S. pyogenes*. Secondary bacterial infection of acute bronchitis and acute bacterial exacerbation of chronic bronchitis due to *S. pneumoniae, H. influenzae* (beta-lactamase positive and negative strains), and *M. catarrhalis*.
How Supplied: *Powder for Reconstitution:* 125 mg/5 mL, 250 mg/5 mL; *Tablet:* 250 mg, 500 mg

Dosage
- **Suspension, Tablets**

Pharyngitis, tonsillitis.
Adults and children over 13 years of age: 500 mg q 24 hr for at least 10 days (for *S. pyogenes* infections, give 10 or more days). **Children, 2–12 years of age:** 7.5 mg/kg q 12 hr for at least 10 days (for *S. pyogenes* infections,give 10 or more days).

Acute sinusitis.
Adults and children over 13 years of age: 250 mg q 12 hr or 500 mg q 12 hr for 10 days. Use the higher dose for moderate to severe infections. **Children, 6 months–12 years of age:** 7.5 mg/kg q 12 hr or 15 mg/kg q 12 hr for 10 days. Use the higher dose for moderate to severe infections.

Secondary bacterial infections of acute bronchitis and acute bacterial exacerbation of chronic bronchitis.
Adults and children over 13 years of age: 500 mg q 12 hr for 10 days.

Uncomplicated skin and skin structure infections.
Adults and children over 13 years of age: Either 250 mg q 12 hr, 500 mg q 24 hr, or 500 mg q 12 hr (all for a duration of 10 days). **Children, 2–12 years of age:** 20 mg/kg q 24 hr for 10 days.

Otitis media.
Infants and children 6 months–12 years: 15 mg/kg q 12 hr for 10 days.

HEALTH CARE CONSIDERATIONS

See also *General Health Care Considerations for All Anti-Infectives* and *Cephalosporins*.

Administration/Storage
1. With impaired renal function (C_{CR} of 0–30 mL/min), give 50% of the usual dose at standard intervals.
2. After reconstitution, refrigerate suspension; discard any unused portion after 14 days.

Assessment: Reduce dose with impaired renal function; monitor I&O and VS.

Client/Family Teaching
1. Take exactly as directed. Report lack of response.
2. Refrigerate suspension; discard any unused portion after 14 days.

Outcome/Evaluate
- Symptomatic improvement
- Resolution of infection

Ceftibuten

(sef-TYE-byou-ten)
Pregnancy Category: B
Cedax **(Rx)**
Classification: Cephalosporin, third generation

See also *Cephalosporins.*
Action/Kinetics: Resistant to beta-lactamase. Is well absorbed from the GI tract. Food delays the time to peak serum concentration, lowers the peak cencentration, and decreases the total amount of drug absorbed. **Peak serum levels:** 2 to 3 hours. **t½:** 144 min. 56% excreted in the urine unchanged.
Uses: Acute bacterial exacerbations of chronic bronchitis due to *Haemophilus influenzae* (including β-lactamase-producing strains), *Moraxella catarrhalis* (including β-lactamase-producing strains), and penicillin-susceptible strains of *Streptococcus pneumoniae.* Acute bacterial otitis media due to *H. influenzae* (including β-lactamase-producing strains), *M. catarrhalis* (including β-lactamase-producing strains), and *Staphylococcus pyogenes.* Pharyngitis and tonsillitis due to *S. pyogenes.*
Special Concerns: Although ceftibuten has been approved for pharyngitis or tonsillitis, only penicillin has been shown to be effective in preventing rheumatic fever.
Side Effects: See *Cephalosporins.* Ceftibuten is usually well tolerated. The most common side effect is diarrhea.
How Supplied: *Capsules:* 400 mg; *Oral Suspension*: 90 mg/5mL, 180 mg/5 mL.

Dosage

- **Capsules, Oral Suspension**

All uses.

Adults and children over 12 years of age: 400 mg once daily for 10 days. The maximum daily dose is 400 mg. Adjust the dose in clients with a creatinine clearance (C_{CR}) less than 50 mL/min as follows. If the C_{CR} is between 30 and 49 mL/min, the recommended dose is 4.5 mg/kg or 200 mg once daily. If the C_{CR} is between 5 and 29 mL/min, the recommended dose is 2.25 mg/kg or 100 mg once daily. In clients undergoing hemodialysis 2 or 3 times/week, a single 400-mg dose of ceftibuten capsules or a single dose of 9 mg/kg (maximum of 400 mg) of PO suspension can be given at the end of each hemodialysis session.

Children: pharyngitis, tonsillitis, acute bacterial otitis media.
9 mg/kg, up to a maximum of 400 mg daily, for a total of 10 days. Give children over 45 kg the maximum daily dose of 400 mg.

HEALTH CARE CONSIDERATIONS

See also *Health Care Considerations* for *Cephalosporins.*

Administration/Storage
1. Follow directions for mixing ceftibuten suspension carefully, depending on the final concentration and the bottle size. First, tap bottle to loosen powder; then add the appropriate amount of water in two portions. Shake well after each portion.
2. After mixing, the suspension may be kept for 14 days under refrigeration. Keep the container tightly closed and shake well before each use. Discard any unused drug after 14 days.

Assessment
1. Record type, onset, duration, and characteristics of symptoms.
2. Obtain cultures and renal function studies; reduce dose with impaired function.
3. Review conditions requiring treatment as drug is only approved for chronic bronchitis, bacterial otitis media, and pharyngitis or tonsillitis, with limitations based on the infective organisms.

Client/Family Teaching
1. Suspension must be consumed on an empty stomach, at least 2 hr before or 1 hr after a meal.
2. Complete entire prescription; do not stop despite feeling better.
3. Report persistent diarrhea.
4. Return for F/U (e.g., ear check, throat culture, X-ray).

Outcome/Evaluate
- Resolution of underlying infection
- Symptomatic improvement

Cefuroxime axetil

(sef-your-**OX**-eem)
Pregnancy Category: B
Ceftin **(Rx)**

Cefuroxime sodium

(sef-your-**OX**-eem)
Pregnancy Category: B
Kefurox, Zinacef **(Rx)**
Classification: Cephalosporin, second-generation

See also *Anti-Infectives* and *Cephalosporins.*
Action/Kinetics: Cefuroxime axetil is used PO, whereas cefuroxime sodium is used either IM or IV. **IM, IV: t½,** 80 min. **Peak serum levels after 1.5 g IV:** 100 mcg/mL. 66%–100% is excreted unchanged in the urine. t½ will be prolonged in clients with renal failure.
Uses: PO (axetil). Pharyngitis, tonsillitis, otitis media, acute bacterial maxillary sinusitis, acute bacterial exacerbations of chronic bronchitis and secondary bacterial infections

of acute bronchitis, uncomplicated UTIs, uncomplicated skin and skin structure infections, uncomplicated gonorrhea (urethral and endocervical) caused by non-penicillinase-producing strains of *Neisseria gonorrhoeae*. Early Lyme disease due to *Borrelia burgdorferi*. The suspension is indicated for children from 3 months to 12 years to treat pharyngitis, tonsillitis, acute bacterial otitis media, and impetigo.

IM, IV (sodium). Infections of the urinary tract, lower respiratory tract (including pneumonia), skin and skin structures, bones, and joints. Septicemia, meningitis, uncomplicated and disseminated gonococcal infections due to penicillinase- or non-penicillinase-producing strains of *N. gonorrhoeae* in men and women. Mixed infections in which several organisms have been identified. Prophylaxis of postoperative infections in surgical procedures such as vaginal hysterectomy.

Additional Side Effects: Decrease in H&H.

Additional Laboratory Test Interferences: False – reaction in the ferricyanide test for blood glucose.

How Supplied: Cefuroxime axetil: *Powder for Reconstitution:* 125 mg/5 mL, 250 mg/5 mL; *Tablet:* 125 mg, 250 mg, 500 mg Cefuroxime sodium: *Injection:* 750 mg/50 mL, 1.5 g/50 mL; *Powder for injection:* 750 mg, 1.5 g, 7.5 g

Dosage

CEFUROXIME AXETIL

- **PO (Cefuroxime Axetil)**

Pharyngitis, tonsillits.

Adults and children over 13 years: 250 mg q 12 hr for 10 days. **Children:** 125 mg q 12 hr for 10 days.

Acute bacterial exacerbations of chronic bronchitis and secondary bacterial infections of acute bronchitis, uncomplicated skin and skin structure infections.

Adults and children over 13 years: 250 or 500 mg q 12 hr for 10 days (5 days for secondary bacterial infections of acute bronchitis).

Uncomplicated UTIs.

Adults and children over 13 years: 125 or 250 mg q 12 hr for 7–10 days. **Infants and children less than 12 years:** 125 mg b.i.d.

Acute otitis media.

Children: 250 mg b.i.d. for 10 days.

Uncomplicated gonorrhea.

Adults and children over 13 years: 1,000 mg as a single dose.

Early Lyme disease.

500 mg/day for 20 days.

- **Suspension**

Pharyngitis, tonsillitis.

Children, 3 months to 12 years: 20 mg/kg/day in 2 divided doses, not to exceed 500 mg total dose/day, for 10 days.

Acute otitis media, impetigo.

Children, 3 months to 12 years: 30 mg/kg/day in 2 divided doses, not to exceed 1,000 mg total dose/day, for 10 days.

CEFUROXIME SODIUM

- **IM, IV**

Uncomplicated infections, including urinary tract, uncomplicated pneumonia, disseminated gonococcal, skin and skin structure.

Adults: 750 mg q 8 hr. **Pediatric, over 3 months:** 50–100 mg/kg/day in divided doses q 6–8 hr (not to exceed adult dose for severe infections).

Severe or complicated infections; bone and joint infections.

Adults: 1.5 g q 8 hr. **Pediatric, over 3 months:** *bone and joint infections,* **IV:** 150 mg/kg/day in divided doses q 8 hr (not to exceed adult dose).

Life-threatening infections or those due to less susceptible organisms.

Adults: 1.5 g q 6 hr.

Bacterial meningitis.

Adults: Up to 3 g q 8 hr. **Pediatric, over 3 months, initial, IV:** 200–240 mg/kg/day in divided doses q 6–8 hr; **then,** after clinical improvement, 100 mg/kg/day.

Gonorrhea (uncomplicated).

1.5 g as a single IM dose given at two different sites together with 1 g PO probenecid.

Prophylaxis in surgery.

Adults, IV: 1.5 g 30–60 min before surgery; if procedure is of long duration, **IM, IV,** 0.75 g q 8 hr.

Open heart surgery, prophylaxis.

IV: 1.5 g when anesthesia is initiated; **then,** 1.5 g q 12 hr for a total of 6 g.

Note: Reduce the dose in impaired renal function as follows: C_{CR} over 20 mL/min: 0.75–1.5 g q 8 hr; C_{CR}, 10–20 mL/min: 0.75 g q 12 hr; C_{CR}, less than 10 mL/min: 0.75 g q 24 hr.

HEALTH CARE CONSIDERATIONS

See also *General Health Care Considerations for All Anti-Infectives* and *Cephalosporins.*

Administration/Storage

1. Cefuroxime axetil for PO use is available in tablet and suspension forms. Tablets should be swallowed whole and not crushed, as the crushed tablet has a strong, bitter, persistent taste. The tablets may be taken without regard for food; however, the suspension must be taken with food. Protect tablets from excessive moisture.

2. To reconstitute suspension, loosen the powder by shaking the bottle. Add the appropriate amount of water (depending on bottle size). Invert the bottle and shake vigorously. Shake before each use. Store reconstituted suspension either at room temperature or in the refrigerator. Discard any unused portion after 10 days.
3. Tablet and suspension are not bioequivalent and not substitutable on a milligram-per-milligram basis.
4. For IM use, inject deep into a large muscle mass.
IV 5. Use IV route for severe or life-threatening infections such as septicemia or in poor-risk clients, especially in presence of shock.
6. For direct IV, reconstitute 750 mg with 8 mL sterile water and give over 3–5 min. For intermittent IV, further dilute in 100 mL of dextrose or saline solution and infuse over 30 min.
7. For direct intermittent IV administration, slowly inject drug over 3 to 5 min, or give in tubing of other IV solutions. For intermittent IV infusion with a Y-type administration set, the dose can be given in the tubing through which the client is receiving other medications; however, during drug infusion, discontinue administration of other solutions. For continuous IV infusion, the drug may be added to 0.9% NaCl injection, 5% or 10% dextrose injection, 5% dextrose and 0.45% or 0.9% NaCl, and M/6 sodium lactate injection.
8. Do not add cefuroxime sodium to solutions of aminoglycosides; if both required, give separately.
9. Prior to reconstitution, protect the drug from light. The powder and reconstituted drug may darken without affecting potency.
10. Continue therapy for at least 10 days in infections due to *Streptococcus pyogenes*.

Assessment:

1. Record indications for therapy and note baseline assessments.
2. Assess for any evidence of anemia or renal dysfunction. Reduce dose with impaired renal function.

Client/Family Teaching

1. Take tablets and/or suspension with food to enhance absorption.
2. Report S&S of anemia (SOB, dizziness, pale skin, etc.) immediately.
3. Crushed tablets have a distinctive bitter taste even when hidden in foods. If intolerable, report so alternative drug therapy may be instituted.

Outcome/Evaluate

- Resolution of S&S of infection
- Normal H&H
- Surgical infection prophylaxis

Celecoxib

(sell-ah-KOX-ihb)
Pregnancy Category: C
Celebrex **(Rx)**
Classification: Nonsteroidal anti-inflammatory drug, COX-2 inhibitor

See also *Nonsteroidal Anti-Inflammatory Drugs*.

Action/Kinetics: Inhibits prostaglandin synthesis, primarily by inhibiting cyclooxygenase-2 (COX-2); it does not inhibit the cyclooxygenase-1 (COX-1) isoenzyme. **Peak plasma levels:** 3 hr. About 97% protein bound. **t½, terminal:** 11 hr when fasting; low solubility prolongs absorption. Metabolized in the liver to inactive compounds; excreted in the urine and feces. Blacks show a 40% increase in the total amount absorbed compared with Caucasians.

Uses: Relief of signs and symptoms of rheumatoid arthritis in adults and of osteoarthritis.

Contraindications: Use in severe hepatic impairment, in those who have shown an allergic reaction to sulfonamides, or in those who have experienced asthma, urticaria, or allergic-type reactions after taking aspirin or other NSAIDs. Use in late pregnancy (may cause premature closure of ductus arteriosus). Lactation.

Special Concerns: Use with caution in preexisting asthma, with drugs that are known to inhibit P450 2C9 in the liver, or when initiating the drug in significant dehydration. Use with extreme caution in those with a prior history of ulcer disease or GI bleeding. Safety and efficacy have not been determined in clients less than 18 years of age.

Side Effects: Listed are side effects with a frequency of 0.1% or greater. *GI:* Dyspepsia, diarrhea, abdominal pain, N&V, dry mouth, flatulence, constipation, GI bleeding, diverticulitis, dysphagia, eructation, esophagitis, gastritis, gastroenteritis, gastroesophageal reflux, hemorrhoids, hiatal hernia, melena, stomatitis, tooth disorder, abnormal hepatic function. *CNS:* Headache, dizziness, insomnia, anorexia, anxiety, depression, nervousness, somnolence, hypertonia, hypoesthesia, migraine, neuropathy, paresthesia, vertigo, increased appetite. *CV:* Aggravated hypertension, angina pectoris, coronary artery disorder, ***MI,*** palpitation, tachycardia, thrombocythemia. *Respiratory:* URI, sinusitis, pharyngitis, rhinitis, bronchitis, bronchospasm, coughing, dyspnea, laryngitis, pneumonia. *Dermatologic:* Rash, ecchymosis, alopecia, dermatitis, nail disorder, photosensitivity, pruritus, erythematous rash, maculopapular rash, skin disorder, dry skin, increased sweating, urticara. *Body as a whole:* Accidental injury, back pain, peripheral edema, aggravated allergy, allergic reaction, asthenia, chest pain, fluid retention, generalized edema, fatigue, fever, hot flushes, flu-like symptoms, pain, peripheral pain, weight increase. *Musculoskeletal:* Arthralgia, arthrosis, bone disorder, accidental fracture, myalgia, stiff neck, synovitis, tendinitis. *Infections:* Bacterial, fungal, or viral infection; herpes simplex, herpes zoster, soft tissue infection, moniliasis, genital moniliasis, otitis media. *GU:* Cystitis, dysuria, frequent urination, renal calculus, urinary incontinence, UTI, breast fibroadenosis, breast neoplasm, breast pain, dysmenorrhea, menstrual disorder, vaginal hemorrhage, vaginitis, prostatic disorder. *Ophthalmic:* Glaucoma, blurred vision, cataract, conjunctivitis, eye pain. *Otic:* Deafness, ear abnormality, earache, tinnitus. *Miscellaneous:* Tenesmus, facial edema, leg cramps, diabetes mellitus, epistaxis, anemia, taste perversion.

Laboratory Test Considerations: ↑ ALT, AST, BUN, CPK, NPN, creatinine, alkaline phosphatase. Hypercholesterolemia, hyperglycemia, hypokalemia, albuminuria, hematuria.

Drug Interactions

ACE Inhibitors / ↓ Antihypertensive effect
Antacids, aluminum- and magnesium-containing / ↓ Absorption of celecoxib
Aspirin / ↑ Risk of GI ulceration
Fluconazole / ↑ Plasma levels of celecoxib
Furosemide / ↓ Natriuretic effect of furosemide
Lithium / ↑ Plasma levels of lithium
Thiazide diuretics / ↓ Natriuretic effect of thiazides

How Supplied: *Capsules:* 100 mg, 200 mg

Dosage

- **Capsules**

Osteoarthritis.

Adults: 100 mg b.i.d. or 200 mg as a single dose.

Rheumatoid arthritis.

Adults: 100–200 mg b.i.d.

HEALTH CARE CONSIDERATIONS

See also *Health Care Considerations* for *Nonsteroidal Anti-Inflammatory Drugs.*

Assessment

1. Record indications for therapy, onset and characteristics of disease, ROM, deformity/loss of function, level of pain, other agents trialed and the outcome.
2. Determine any GI bleed or ulcer history, sulfonamide allergy or aspirin or other NSAID-induced asthma, urticaria, or allergic-type reactions.
3. List drugs prescribed to ensure none interact.
4. Assess for liver/renal dysfunction; monitor lytes, renal and LFTs.

Client/Family Teaching

1. Take exactly as directed and generally at the same time each day.
2. Report any unusual or persistent side effects including dyspepsia, abdominal pain, dizziness, and changes in stool or skin color.
3. Avoid therapy during pregnancy.
4. Report weight gain, swelling of ankles, chest pain, or SOB.

Outcome/Evaluate

- Relief of joint pain and inflammation with improved mobility

Cellulose sodium phosphate

(SELL-you-lohs)
Pregnancy Category: C
Calcibind **(Rx)**
Classification: Calcium-binding agent

Action/Kinetics: A synthetic, nonabsorbable compound insoluble in water. The sodium ion exchanges for calcium; the cellulose phospate-bound calcium (from both dietary and endogenous sources) is then excreted in the feces. Urinary calcium is decreased while urinary phosphorus and oxalate are increased.

Uses: Decrease incidence of new renal stone formation in absorptive hypercalciuria Type I. Diagnostic test for causes of hypercalciuria other than hyperabsorption.

Contraindications: Primary or secondary hyperparathyroidism, hypocalcemia, hypomagnesemia, enteric hyperoxaluria, osteoporosis, osteomalacia, osteitis, low intestinal absorption or renal excretion of calcium, when hypercalciuria is due to mobilization from bones. Children under age 16.

Special Concerns: Use with caution in CHF or ascites.

Side Effects: *GI:* Diarrhea, dyspepsia, loose bowel movements. *Other:* Hyperparathyroid bone disease, hyperoxaluria, hypomagnesiuria, loss of copper, zinc, iron. Long-term use may cause hyperoxaluria and hypomagnesiuria.

How Supplied: *Powder*

Dosage

- **Powder**

Urinary calcium greater than 300 mg/day.
5 g with each meal.
Urinary calcium less than 150 mg/day.
2.5 g with breakfast and lunch and 5 g with dinner.

HEALTH CARE CONSIDERATIONS

Administration/Storage

1. Monitor parathyroid hormone levels at least once between 2 weeks and 3 mo after therapy initiated.
2. A moderate calcium intake is recommended.
3. Mix each dose with water, juice, or soft drink, and take within 30 min of the meal.
4. Magnesium gluconate supplements may be given as follows:
- 1.5 g before breakfast and at bedtime if receiving 15 g cellulose/day.
- 1 g, as in the preceding, with 10 g cellulose daily.
- To avoid binding, give magnesium either 1 hr before or 1 hr after cellulose.

5. Stop treatment if urinary oxalate is greater than 55 mg/day with moderate dietary oxalate restriction.
6. Magnesium, iron, and other trace-metal supplements may be ordered.

Assessment: Record indications for therapy; note baseline labs and any history of CHF or ascites.

Client/Family Teaching

1. Take with meals to maximize the uptake of dietary calcium.
2. Avoid calcium-containing foods such as milk, cheese, or ice cream.
3. Avoid eating spinach and dark green vegetables, rhubarb, chocolate, and brewed tea since all of these contain oxalates, which may lead to calcium stone formation.
4. Avoid vitamin C as it is metabolized to oxalate; avoid salt and lightly salted foods.
5. Drink plenty of fluids; the urinary output should be 2 L/day.

Outcome/Evaluate

- ↓ Urinary calcium
- Prophylaxis in new renal stone formation

Cephalexin hydrochloride monohydrate

(sef-ah-**LEX**-in)
Pregnancy Category: B
Keftab **(Rx)**

Cephalexin monohydrate

(sef-ah-**LEX**-in)
Pregnancy Category: B
Apo-Cephalex ✱, Biocef, Dom-Cephalexin ✱, Keflex, Novo–Lexin ✱, Nu-Cephalex ✱, Penta-Cephalexin ✱, PMS-Cephalexin ✱, STCC-Cephalexin ✱ **(Rx)**
Classification: Cephalosporin, first-generation

See also *Anti-Infectives* and *Cephalosporins*.

Action/Kinetics: Peak serum levels: PO, 9–39 mcg/mL after 1 hr. **t½, PO:** 50–80 min. Absorption delayed in children. The HCl monohydrate does not require conversion in the stomach before absorption. Ninety percent of drug excreted unchanged in urine within 8 hr.

Uses: Respiratory tract infections caused by *Streptococcus pneumoniae* and group A β-hemolytic streptococci. Otitis media due to *S. pneumoniae, Hemophilus influenzae, Moraxella catarrhalis* (use monohydrate only), staphylococci, streptococci, and *N. catarrhalis*. GU infections (including acute prostatitis) due to *Escherichia coli, Proteus mirabilis,* or *Klebsiella* species. Bone infections caused by *P. mirabilis* or staphylococci. Skin and skin structure infections due to staphylococci and streptococci.

Special Concerns: Safety and effectiveness of the HCl monohydrate has not been determined in children.

Additional Side Effects: Nephrotoxicity, cholestatic jaundice.

How Supplied: Cephalexin hydrochloride monohydrate: *Tablet:* 500 mg. Cephalexin monohydrate: *Capsule:* 250 mg, 500 mg; *Powder for Reconstitution:* 125 mg/5 mL, 250 mg/5 mL; *Tablet:* 250 mg, 500 mg

Dosage

- **Capsules, Oral Suspension, Tablets**

General infections.

Adults, usual: 250 mg q 6 hr up to 4 g/day. **Pediatric:** *Monohydrate,* 25–50 mg/kg/day in four equally divided doses.

Infections of skin and skin structures, streptococcal pharyngitis, uncomplicated cystitis, over 15 years.

Adults: 500 mg q 12 hr. Large doses may be needed for severe infections or for less susceptible organisms. For streptococcal pharyngitis in children over 1 year and for skin and skin structure infections, the total daily dose should be divided and given q 12 hr. In severe infections, the dose should be doubled.

Otitis media.

Pediatric: 75–100 mg/kg/day in four divided doses.

C

HEALTH CARE CONSIDERATIONS

See also *General Health Care Considerations for All Anti-Infectives* and *Cephalosporins*.

Administration/Storage

1. After reconstitution, refrigerate; discard any unused drug after 14 days.
2. If the total daily dose is more than 4 g, use parenteral therapy.
3. Continue treatment for at least 10 days for beta-hemolytic streptococcal infections.
4. Dosage may have to be reduced with impaired renal function or increased for severe infections. Drug action can be prolonged by concurrently giving probenecid.

Client/Family Teaching

1. Take with meals for GI upset.
2. Consume 2–3 L/day of fluids to prevent dehydration.
3. Report changes in elimination patterns, yellow discoloration of the skin/eyes, or lack of response.

Outcome/Evaluate

- Resolution of infection
- Symptomatic improvement

Cephradine

(SEF-rah-deen)
Pregnancy Category: B
Velosef **(Rx)**
Classification: Cephalosporin, first-generation

See also *Anti-Infectives* and *Cephalosporins*.

Action/Kinetics: Similar to cephalexin. Rapidly absorbed PO or IM (30 min–2 hr); 60%–90% excreted after 6 hr. **Peak serum levels: PO,** 8–24 mcg/mL after 30–60 min; **IM,** 5.6–13.6 mcg/mL after 1–2 hr. **t½:** 42–80 min; 80%–95% excreted in urine unchanged.

Uses: Oral. Respiratory tract infections (tonsillitis, pharyngitis, lobar pneumonia) due to *Streptococcus pneumoniae* and group A β–hemolytic streptococci. Otitis media due to group A β–hemolytic streptococci, *S. pneumoniae, Haemophilus influenzae,* and staphylococci. Skin and skin structure infections due to staphylococci (penicillinase/nonpencilliase–producing) and β–streptococci. UTIs (including prostatitis) due to *Escherichia coli, Proteus mirabilis,* and *Klebsiella* species.

Parenteral. Respiratory tract infections due to *S. pneumoniae, Klebsiella* species, *H. influenzae, S. aureus* (penicillinase/non–penicillinase–producing), and group A β–hemolytic streptococci. UTIs due to *E. coli, P. mirabilis,* and *Klebsiella* species. Skin and skin structure infections due to *S. aureus* and group A β–hemolytic streptococci. Bone infections due to *S. aureus*. Septicemia due to *S. pneumoniae, S. aureus, P. mirabilis,* and *E. coli*. To prevent infections before, during, and after surgery for vaginal hysterectomy and other surgical procedures.

Special Concerns: Safe use during pregnancy, of the parenteral form in infants under 1 month of age, and of the PO form in children less than 9 months of age has not been established.

Additional Laboratory Test Interferences: False + reactions using sulfosalicylic acid for urinary protein tests. High concentrations may interfere with measurement of creatinine by the Jaffe method.

How Supplied: *Capsule:* 250 mg, 500 mg; *Powder for Reconstitution:* 125 mg/5 mL, 250 mg/5 mL

Dosage

- **Capsules, Oral Suspension**

Skin and skin structures, respiratory tract infections (other than lobar pneumonia).

Adults, usual: 250 mg q 6 hr or 500 mg q 12 hr.

Lobar pneumonia.

Adults: 500 mg q 6 hr or 1 g q 12 hr.

Uncomplicated UTIs.

Adults, usual: 500 mg q 12 hr.

More serious UTIs and prostatitis.

500 mg q 6 hr or 1 g q 12 hr (severe, chronic infections may require up to 1 g q 6 hr).

Use in children.

Pediatric, over 9 months: 25–50 mg/kg/day in equally divided doses q 6–12 hr (75–100 mg/kg/day for otitis media). Do not exceed 4 g/day.

- **Deep IM, IV**

General infections.

Adults: 2–4 g/day in equally divided doses q.i.d.

Surgical prophylaxis.

Adults: 1 g 30–90 min before surgery; **then,** 1 g q 4–6 hr for one to two doses (or up to 24 hr postoperatively).

Cesarean section, prophylaxis.

IV: 1 g when the umbilical cord is clamped; **then,** give two additional 1-g doses **IV or IM** 6 and 12 hr after the initial dose.

Use in children.

Pediatric, over 1 year: 50–100 mg/kg/day in equally divided doses q.i.d. Do not exceed adult dose.

Note: For clients not on dialysis, use the following dosage in renal impairment: C_{CR}, over 20 mL/min: 500 mg q 6 hr; C_{CR}, 5–20 mL/min: 250 mg q 6 hr; C_{CR}, less than 5 mL/min: 250 mg q 12 hr. For those on chronic, intermittent hemodialysis, give 250 mg initially; repeat at 12 hr and after 36–48 hr.

HEALTH CARE CONSIDERATIONS

See also *General Health Care Considerations for All Anti-Infectives* and *Cephalosporins.*

Administration/Storage

1. Give oral medication without regard to meals.
2. Do not store the oral suspension above 30°C (86°F) before reconstitution. After reconstitution, suspension retains potency for 7 days at room temperature and 14 days if refrigerated.
3. For IM, reconstitute with sterile or bacteriostatic water for injection.
4. Inject IM into a large muscle; rotate injection sites. Sterile abscesses from accidental SC injection have occurred.

IV 5. For direct IV administration, add 5 mL of diluent to the 250 or 500 mg vials, 10 mL to the 1 g vial, or 20 mL to the 2 g vial. Inject slowly over 3–5 min or give through tubing. Diluents include sterile water for injection, 5% dextrose injection, and NaCl injection.

6. For continuous or intermittent IV infusion, add 10 or 20 mL sterile water for injection (or other diluent—see package insert) to the 1 g vial or 2 g bottle, respectively. Withdraw entire contents and transfer to an IV infusion container.
7. Do not mix cephradine with other antibiotics. Do not mix with lactated Ringer's solution.
8. Use IM or direct IV solutions within 2 hr at room temperature. Solutions refrigerated at 5°C (41°F) retain potency for 24 hr. The IV infusion retains potency for 10 hr at room temperature or 48 hr at 5°C (42°F). Infusion solutions in sterile water for injection, frozen immediately after reconstitution are stable for 6 weeks at –20°C (–4°F).
9. To ensure stability, replace medication infusion solution during prolonged IV administration q 10 hr.

Assessment: Note any previous penicillin reaction; reduce dose with renal dysfunction.

Outcome/Evaluate

- Resolution of S&S of infection
- Infection prophylaxis in surgery
- Negative culture reports

Cerivastatin sodium

(seh-**RIHV**-ah-stat-in)

Pregnancy Category: X

Baycol **(Rx)**

Classification: Antihyperlipidemic, HMG-CoA reductase inhibitor

See also *Antihyperlipidemic Agents—HMG-CoA Reductase Inhibitors.*

Action/Kinetics: Competitive inhibitor of HMG-CoA reductase leading to inhibition of cholesterol synthesis and decrease in plasma cholesterol levels. **Peak plasma levels:** 2.5 hr. **t½, terminal:** 2–3 hr. Food does not affect blood levels. Metabolized in liver and excreted through urine and feces.

Uses: Adjunct to diet to reduce elevated total and LDL cholesterol in clients with primary hypercholesterolemia and mixed dyslipidemia (Types IIA and IIb) when response to diet or other non-pharmacologic approaches have not been adequate.

Contraindications: Use in active liver disease or unexplained elevation of serum transaminases. Pregnancy, lactation.

Special Concerns: Use in women of childbearing age only when pregnancy is unlikely and they have been informed of potential risks. Drug has not been evaluated in rare homozygous familial hypercholesterolemia. Due to interference with cholesterol synthesis and lower cholesterol levels, may be blunting of adrenal or gonadal steroid hormone production. Use with caution in renal or hepatic insufficiency. Safety and efficacy have not been determined in children.

Side Effects: See also *HMG-CoA Reductase Inhibitors. Musculoskeletal:* Rarely, rhabdomyolysis with acute renal failure secondary to myoglobinemia.

Laboratory Test Considerations: ↑ ALT, AST.

Drug Interactions: ↑ Risk of myopathy when used with azole antifungals, cyclosporine, erythromycin, fibric acid derivatives, and lipid-lowering doses of niacin.

How Supplied: *Tablets:* 0.2 mg, 0.3 mg

Dosage

- **Tablets**

Hypercholesterolemia.

Adults: 0.3 mg once daily in evening. Recommended starting dose in those with significant renal impairment (C_{CR} less than 60 mL/min/1.73 m^2) is 0.2 mg once daily in evening.

HEALTH CARE CONSIDERATIONS

See also *Health Care Considerations* for *Antihyperlipidemic Agents—HMG-CoA Reductase Inhibitors.*

C

Administration/Storage
1. Place client on standard cholesterol-lowering diet before giving cerivastatin. Diet should continue during therapy.
2. When given with bile-acid-binding resin (e.g., cholestyramine), give cerivastatin at least 2 hr after resin.

Assessment
1. Record indications for therapy, previous agents/therapies trialed, and outcome.
2. Assess liver and renal function; reduce dose with dysfunction. Monitor LFTs at 6 and 12 weeks initially and with dose increases, then biannually.

Client/Family Teaching
1. Take as directed. May be taken with or without food.
2. Continue regular exercise and low fat, low cholesterol diet during therapy.
3. Report any unexplained muscle pain, weakness, or tenderness, especially if malaise or fever present.
4. Females should avoid pregnancy.
5. Report for F/U labs as scheduled.

Outcome/Evaluate: ↓ Total and LDL cholesterol

Cetirizine hydrochloride

(seh-**TIH**-rah-zeen)
Pregnancy Category: B
Reactine ✱, Zyrtec **(Rx)**
Classification: Antihistamine

See also *Antihistamines*.
Action/Kinetics: A potent H_1-receptor antagonist. A mild bronchodilator that protects against histmine-induced bronchospasm; negligible anticholinergic and sedative activity. Rapidly absorbed after PO administration; however, food delays the time to peak serum levels but does not decrease the total amount of drug absorbed. Poorly penetrates the CNS, but high levels are distributed to the skin. **t½:** 8.3 hr (longer in elderly clients and in those with impaired liver or renal function). Excreted mostly unchanged (95%) in the urine; 10% is excreted in the feces.
Uses: Relief of symptoms associated with seasonal allergic rhinitis due to ragweed, grass, and tree pollens; perennial allergic rhinitis due to allergens such as dust mites, animal dander, and molds. Chronic idiopathic urticaria.
Contraindications: Lactation. In those hypersensitive to hydroxyzine.
Special Concerns: Due to the possibility of sedation, use with caution in situations requiring mental alertness. Safety and efficacy have not been determined in children less than 12 years of age.
Side Effects: See *Antihistamines*. The most common side effects are somnolence, dry mouth, fatigue, pharyngitis, and dizziness.
OD Management of Overdose: *Symptoms*: Somnolence. *Treatment*: Symptomatic and supportive. Dialysis is not effective in removing the drug from the body.
How Supplied: *Syrup:* 1 mg/mL; *Tablets:* 5 mg, 10 mg.

Dosage

- **Tablets, Syrup**

Seasonal or perennial allergic rhinitis, chronic urticaria.

Adults and children over 6 years of age, initial: Depending on the severity of the symptoms, 5 or 10 mg (most common initial dose) once daily. In clients with decreased renal function (C_{CR}: 11–31 mL/min), in hemodialysis clients (C_{CR} less than 7 mL/min), and in those with impaired hepatic function, the dose is 5 mg once daily.

HEALTH CARE CONSIDERATIONS

See also *Health Care Considerations* for *Antihistamines*.

Assessment
1. Record type, onset, and characteristics of symptoms; note triggers.
2. Note any hypersensitivity to hydroxyzine.

Client/Family Teaching
1. May take with or without food; time of administration may be varied depending on client needs.
2. Use caution when performing activities that require mental alertness until drug effects realized; may cause drowsiness.
3. Drug may cause dry mouth and fatigue; report adverse effects that inhibit compliance with therapy.
4. Avoid alcohol or any other CNS depressants.
5. Review allergens that trigger symptoms, e.g., ragweed, dust mites, molds, animal dander, etc., and instruct in how to control and avoid contact.

Outcome/Evaluate
- Symptom relief with seasonal and perennial allergic rhinitis
- ↓ Occurrence, duration, and severity of hives; ↓ pruritus

Chenodiol (Chenodeoxycholic acid)

(kee-noh-**DYE**-ohl)
Pregnancy Category: X
Chenix **(Rx)**
Classification: Naturally occurring human bile acid

Action/Kinetics: By reducing hepatic synthesis of cholesterol and cholic acid, replaces both cholic and deoxycholic acids in the bile acid pool. This helps desaturation of biliary cholesterol and leads to dissolution of radiolucent cholesterol gallstones. Is ineffective on calcified gallstones or on radiolucent bile pigment stones. Fifty percent of clients have stone recurrence within 5 years. Also increases LDLs and inhibits absorption of fluid from the colon. Well absorbed following PO administration. Metabolized by bacteria in the colon to lithocholic acid, most of which is excreted in the feces.
Uses: In radiolucent cholesterol gallstones where surgery is a risk due to age or systemic disease. Ineffective in some. Best results in thin females with a serum cholesterol not higher than 227 mg/dL and who have a small number of radiolucent cholesterol gallstones.
Contraindications: Known hepatic dysfunction or bile ductal abnormalities. Colon cancer. Pregnancy or in those who may become pregnant.
Special Concerns: Safety and efficacy in lactation and in children have not been established.
Side Effects: Hepatotoxicity including increased ALT in one-third of clients, intrahepatic cholestasis. *GI:* Diarrhea (common), anorexia, constipation, dyspepsia, flatulence, heartburn, cramps, epigastric distress, N&V, abdominal pain. *Hematologic:* Decreased white cell count. ***Chenodiol may contribute to colon cancer in susceptible clients.***

Drug Interactions
Antacids, aluminum / ↓ Effect of chenodiol due to ↓ absorption from GI tract
Cholestyramine / See *Antacids*
Clofibrate / ↓ Effect of chenodiol due to ↑ biliary cholesterol secretion
Colestipol / See *Antacids*
Estrogens, oral contraceptives / ↓ Effect of chenodiol due to ↑ biliary cholesterol secretion
How Supplied: *Tablet:* 250 mg

Dosage
- **Tablets**

Radiolucent cholesterol gallstones.
Adults, initial: 250 mg b.i.d. for 2 weeks; **then,** increase by 250 mg/week until maximum tolerated or recommended dose is reached (13–16 mg/kg/day in two divided doses morning and night with milk or food). *NOTE:* Doses less than 10 mg/kg are usually ineffective and may result in increased risk of cholecystectomy.

HEALTH CARE CONSIDERATIONS

Assessment
1. Record type/onset of symptoms, and any previous therapy.
2. List drugs currently prescribed; note any potential interactions.
3. Test for pregnancy.
4. Obtain liver and renal function studies and serum cholesterol; monitor for stone dissolution.

Client/Family Teaching
1. Drug may need to be taken for 24 mo before gallstones are dissolved; gallstones may recur even after successful treatment.
2. Immediately report any severe, sudden upper quadrant pain that radiates to the shoulder, nonspecific abdominal pain, nausea, or vomiting; may indicate gallstone complications.
3. Avoid pregnancy during therapy; report any possibility of conception. Oral contraceptives may decrease the effectiveness of chenodiol; practice alternative birth control.
4. Stress importance of periodic LFTs and cholecystograms or gallbladder ultrasonography to evaluate the effectiveness of the drug therapy.
5. Consult with provider if antacids are needed; most have an aluminum base that absorbs the drug.
6. Report any incidence of diarrhea; this may be drug related and can be relieved by changes in dosage or with antidiarrheal agents.
7. Discuss drug relationship to colon cancer and potential risks.

Outcome/Evaluate: Dissolution of radiolucent cholesterol gallstones

Chloral hydrate
(**KLOH**-ral **HY**-drayt)
Pregnancy Category: C
Aquachloral Supprettes, Novo-Chlorhydrate ✦, PMS-Chloral Hydrate ✦ **(C-IV) (Rx)**
Classification: Nonbenzodiazepine, nonbarbiturate sedative-hypnotic

Action/Kinetics: Metabolized to trichloroethanol, which is the active metabolite causing CNS depression. Produces only slight hangover effects and is said not to affect REM sleep. High doses lead to severe CNS depression, as well as depression of respiratory and vasomotor centers (hypotension). Both psychologic and physical dependence develop. **Onset:** Within 30 min. **Duration:** 4–8 hr. **t½, trichloroethanol:** 7–10 hr. Readily absorbed from the GI tract and distrib-

uted to all tissues; passes the placental barrier and appears in breast milk. Metabolites excreted by kidney.
Uses: Short-term hypnotic. Daytime sedative and sedation prior to EEG procedures. Preoperative sedative and postoperative as adjunct to analgesics. Prevent or reduce symptoms of alcohol withdrawal.
Contraindications: Marked hepatic or renal impairment, severe cardiac disease, lactation. PO use in clients with esophagitis, gastritis, or gastric or duodenal ulcer.
Special Concerns: Use by nursing mothers may cause sedation in the infant. Dose decrease may be necessary in geriatric clients due to age-related decrease in both hepatic and renal function.
Side Effects: *CNS:* Paradoxical paranoid reactions. Sudden withdrawal in dependent clients may result in "chloral delirium." ***Sudden intolerance to the drug following prolonged use may result in respiratory depression, hypotension, cardiac effects, and possibly death.*** *GI:* N&V, diarrhea, bad taste in mouth, gastritis, increased peristalsis. *GU:* Renal damage, decreased urine flow and uric acid excretion. *Miscellaneous:* Skin reactions, hepatic damage, allergic reactions, leukopenia, eosinophilia.

Chronic toxicity is treated by gradual withdrawal and rehabilitative measures such as those used in treatment of the chronic alcoholic. Poisoning by chloral hydrate resembles acute barbiturate intoxication; the same supportive treatment is indicated (see *Barbiturates*).
Laboratory Test Considerations: ↑ 17-Hydroxycorticosteroids. Interference with fluorescence tests for catecholamines and copper sulfate test for glucose.

Drug Interactions

Anticoagulants, oral / ↑ Effect of anticoagulants by ↓ plasma protein binding
CNS depressants / Additive CNS depression; concomitant use may lead to drowsiness, lethargy, stupor, respiratory collapse, coma, or death
Furosemide (IV) / Concomitant use results in diaphoresis, tachycardia, hypertension, flushing
How Supplied: *Capsule:* 500 mg; *Suppository:* 325 mg, 500 mg, 650 mg; *Syrup:* 500 mg/5 mL

Dosage

- **Capsules, Syrup**

Daytime sedative.
Adults: 250 mg t.i.d. after meals.
Preoperative sedative.
Adults: 0.5–1.0 g 30 min before surgery.
Hypnotic.
Adults: 0.5–1 g 15–30 min before bedtime. **Pediatric:** 50 mg/kg (1.5 g/m^2) at bedtime (up to 1 g may be given as a single dose).
Daytime sedative.
Pediatric: 8.3 mg/kg (250 mg/m^2) up to a maximum of 500 mg t.i.d. after meals.
Premedication prior to EEG procedures.
Pediatric: 20–25 mg/kg.

- **Suppositories, Rectal**

Daytime sedative.
Adults: 325 mg t.i.d. **Pediatric:** 8.3 mg/kg (250 mg/m^2) t.i.d.
Hypnotic.
Adults: 0.5–1 g at bedtime. **Pediatric:** 50 mg/kg (1.5 g/m^2) at bedtime (up to 1 g as a single dose).

HEALTH CARE CONSIDERATIONS

See also *Health Care Considerations* for *Pentobarbital Sodium*.

Administration/Storage

1. PO: give capsules after meals with a full glass of water. Give the syrup with half a glass of juice, water, or ginger ale.
2. PO syrups have an unpleasant taste, which can be reduced by chilling the syrup before administration.
3. Have emergency drugs and equipment available should the client require supportive, physiologic treatment of acute poisoning.

Assessment

1. Record indications for therapy and evaluate sleep habits and patterns and life-style.
2. Assess mental status and response to stimuli. Monitor level and pattern of alertness and compare with the premedication history.
3. Observe respiratory and cardiac responses; record evidence of vasomotor depression and dilatation of cutaneous blood vessels.
4. Note any history of cardiac disease, liver or renal dysfunction. Monitor labs for evidence of impairment; drug is metabolized to an alcohol component.
5. Report any psychologic and physical dependence; symptoms resemble those of acute alcoholism, but with more severe gastritis.

Client/Family Teaching

1. Take only as directed.
2. Store away from the bedside.
3. Avoid activities that require mental alertness. Use measures that promote comfort and relaxation. To protect from injury, ambulate with assistance, use side rails, call for help, and use a night light.
4. Drug is for short-term use only; may cause psychologic and physical dependence.

5. Review methods to enhance sleep, i.e., no caffeine, increased exercise, muscle relaxation exercises, no daytime napping.
6. Review drug side effects, note those that require immediate attention.

Outcome/Evaluate

- Desired level of sedation
- ↓ Alcohol withdrawal symptoms
- Improved sleep patterns

Chlorambucil

(klor-**AM**-byou-sill)
Pregnancy Category: D
Leukeran (Abbreviation: CHL) **(Rx)**
Classification: Antineoplastic, alkylating agent

See also *Antineoplastic Agents* and *Alkylating Agents.*

Action/Kinetics: Cell-cycle nonspecific; cytotoxic to nonproliferating cells and has immunosuppressant activity. Forms an unstable ethylenimmonium ion which binds (alkylates) with intracellular substances such as nucleic acids. The cytotoxic effect is due to cross-linking of strands of DNA and RNA and inhibition of protein synthesis. Rapidly absorbed from the GI tract. **Peak plasma levels:** 1 hr. **t½, plasma;:** 1.5 hr. 99% bound to plasma proteins, especially albumin. Extensively metabolized by the liver; at least one metabolite is active. Fifteen to 60% is excreted through the urine 24 hr after drug administration; 40% is bound to tissues, including fat.

Uses: Palliation in chronic lymphocytic leukemia, malignant lymphomas (including lymphosarcoma), giant follicular lymphomas, and Hodgkin's disease. *Investigational:* Uveitis and meningoencephalitis associated with Behcet's disease. With a corticosteroid for idiopathic membranous nephropathy. Rheumatoid arthritis. Possible alternative to MOPP in combination with vinblastine, procarbazine, and prednisone.

Special Concerns: Use during lactation only if benefits outweigh risks. Safety and efficacy have not been established in children. The drug is carcinogenic in humans and may be both mutagenic and teratogenic in humans. It also affects fertility. May be cross-hypersensitivity with other alklyating agents.

Laboratory Test Considerations: ↑ Uric acid levels in serum and urine.

Additional Side Effects: *Hepatic:* Hepatotoxicity with jaundice. *Pulmonary:* ***Pulmonary fibrosis,*** bronchopulmonary dysplasia. *CNS:* Children with nephrotic syndrome have an increased risk of seizures. *Miscellaneous:* Keratitis, drug fever, sterile cystitis, interstitial pneumonia, peripheral neuropathy. Cross-sensitivity (skin rashes) may occur with other alkylating agents.

OD **Management of Overdose:** *Symptoms:* Pancytopenia (reversible), ataxia, agitated behavior, ***clonic-tonic seizures.*** *Treatment:* General supportive measures. Monitor blood profiles carefully; blood transfusions may be required.

How Supplied: *Tablet:* 2 mg

Dosage

- **Tablets**

Leukemia, lymphomas.

Individualized according to response of client. **Adults, children, initial dose:** 0.1–0.2 mg/kg (or 4–10 mg) daily in single or divided doses for 3–6 weeks; **maintenance:** 0.03–0.1 mg/kg/day depending on blood counts.

Alternative for chronic lymphocytic leukemia.

Initial: 0.4 mg/kg; **then,** repeat this dose every 2 weeks increasing by 0.1 mg/kg until either toxicity or control of condition is observed.

Nephrotic syndrome, immunosuppressant.

Adults, children: 0.1–0.2 mg/kg body weight daily for 8–12 weeks.

Uveitis and meningoencephalitis associated with Behcet's disease.

0.1 mg/kg/day.

Idiopathic membranous nephropathy.

0.1–0.2 mg/kg/day every other month, alternating with a corticosteroid for 6 months duration.

Rheumatoid arthritis.

0.1–0.3 mg/kg/day.

HEALTH CARE CONSIDERATIONS

See also *Health Care Considerations* for *Antineoplastic Agents.*

Administration/Storage: Store at 15°C–25°C (59°F–77°F) in a dry place.

Assessment

1. Record indications for therapy, noting pretreatment lab and physical assessment findings.
2. Drug may cause severe granulocyte and lymphocyte suppression. Nadir: 21 days; recovery: 42–56 days.

Client/Family Teaching

1. Take 1 hr before breakfast or 2 hr after the evening meal.
2. Consume 2–3 L/day of fluids to decrease urate crystals.

3. Report side effects; skin rash may result from cross-sensitivity with other alkylating agents.
4. Drug is carcinogenic and may also be mutagenic and teratogenic; practice reliable birth control.

Outcome/Evaluate

- Positive tumor response evidenced by ↓ tumor size/spread; suppression of malignant cell proliferation
- Immunosuppressant activity

Chlordiazepoxide

(klor-dye-**AYZ**-eh-**POX**-eyed)

Pregnancy Category: D

Apo-Chlordiazepoxide ✱, Corax ✱, Libritabs, Librium, Lipoxide, Mitran, Novo-Poxide ✱, Reposans-10 **(C-IV) (Rx)**

Classification: Antianxiety agent, benzodiazepine

See also *Tranquilizers/Antimanic Drugs/Hypnotics.*

Action/Kinetics: Onset: PO, 30–60 min; **IM,** 15–30 min (absorption may be slow and erratic); **IV,** 3–30 min. **Peak plasma levels (PO):** 0.5–4 hr. **Duration: t½:** 5–30 hr. Is metabolized to four active metabolites: desmethylchlordiazepoxide, desmethyldiazepam, oxazepam, and demoxepam. Has less anticonvulsant activity and is less potent than diazepam.

Uses: Anxiety, acute withdrawal symptoms in chronic alcoholics. Sedative-hypnotic. Preoperatively to reduce anxiety and tension. Tension headache. Antitremor agent (PO). Antipanic (parenteral).

Laboratory Test Considerations: ↑ 17-Hydroxycorticosteroids, 17-ketosteroids, alkaline phosphatase, bilirubin, serum transaminase, porphobilinogen. ↓ PT (clients on Coumarin).

Additional Side Effects: Jaundice, acute hepatic necrosis, hepatic dysfunction.

How Supplied: *Capsule:* 5 mg, 10 mg, 25 mg; *Powder for injection:* 100 mg; *Tablet:* 10 mg, 25 mg

Dosage

- **Capsules, Tablets**

Anxiety and tension.

Adults: 5–10 mg t.i.d.–q.i.d. (up to 20–25 mg t.i.d.–q.i.d. in severe cases). Reduce dose to 5 mg b.i.d.–q.i.d. in geriatric or debilitated clients. **Pediatric, over 6 years, initial,** 5 mg b.i.d.–q.i.d. May be increased to 10 mg b.i.d.–q.i.d.

Preoperatively.

Adults: 5–10 mg t.i.d.–q.i.d. on day before surgery.

Alcohol withdrawal/sedative-hypnotic.

Adults: 50–100 mg; may be increased to 300 mg/day; **then,** reduce to maintenance levels.

- **IM, IV (not recommended for children under 12 years)**

Acute/severe agitation, anxiety.

Initial: 50–100 mg; **then,** 25–50 mg t.i.d.–q.i.d.

Preoperatively.

Adults: 50–100 mg IM 1 hr before surgery.

Alcohol withdrawal.

Adults: 50–100 mg IM or IV; repeat in 2–4 hr if necessary. Dosage should not exceed 300 mg/day.

Antipanic.

Adults, initial: 50–100 mg; dose may be repeated in 4–6 hr if needed.

HEALTH CARE CONSIDERATIONS

See also *Health Care Considerations* for *Tranquilizers/Antimanic Drugs/Hypnotics.*

Administration/Storage

1. **IM:** Prepare solution immediately before administration by adding diluent, which is provided, to ampule. Shake until dissolved. Discard any unused solution. Inject slowly into upper, outer quadrant of gluteal muscle.
IV 2. Prepare immediately before administration by diluting with 5 mL of sterile water for injection or sterile 0.9% NaCl solution. Inject directly into vein over 1-min period. Do not add to IV infusion because of instability of drug. Do not use IV solution for IM administration.

Assessment

1. Record indications for therapy and pretreatment symptoms.
2. Maintain a quiet, supervised environment; keep recumbent for 3 hr following parenteral administration.
3. Obtain LFTs to R/O impairment.

Client/Family Teaching

1. Take with food and as directed.
2. Consume extra fluids and bulk to minimize constipating effects.
3. Use caution, may cause dizziness and drowsiness.
4. Avoid all OTC agents, alcohol, and any other CNS depressants.

Outcome/Evaluate

- ↓ Tremors; ↓ anxiety; sedation
- Termination of panic attacks
- ↓ Alcohol withdrawal symptoms

Chloroquine hydrochloride

(**KLOR**-oh-kwin)

Aralen HCl **(Rx)**

Chloroquine phosphate

(KLOR-oh-kwin)

Aralen Phosphate, Novo-Chloroquine ✱ **(Rx)**

Classification: 4-Aminoquinoline, antimalarial, amebicide

Special Concerns: Use during pregnancy only if benefits outweigh risks.

Additional Side Effects: Chloroquine may exacerbate psoriasis and precipitate an acute attack.

Drug Interactions

Cimetidine / ↓ Oral clearance rate and metabolism of chloroquine

Kaolin / ↓ Effect of chloroquine due to ↓ absorption from GI tract

Magnesium trisilicate / ↓ Effect of chloroquine due to ↓ absorption from GI tract

How Supplied: Chloroquine hydrochloride: *Injection:* 50 mg/mL Chloroquine phosphate: *Tablet:* 250 mg, 500 mg

Dosage

CHLOROQUINE HYDROHLORIDE

• **IM**

Acute malarial attack.

Adults, initial: 200–250 mg (160–200 mg base); repeat dosage in 6 hr if necessary. Total daily dose in first 24 hr should not exceed 1 g (800 mg base). Begin PO therapy as soon as possible. **IM, SC. Children and infants:** 6.25 mg/kg (5 mg base/kg) repeated in 6 hr; dose should not exceed 12.5 mg/kg/day (10 mg base/kg/day).

Extraintestinal amebiasis.

Adults: 200–250 mg/day (160–200 mg of the base) for 10–12 days. Begin PO therapy as soon as possible. **Children:** 7.5 mg/kg/day for 10–12 days.

• **IV Infusion**

Acute malarial attack.

Adults, initial: 16.6 mg/kg over 8 hr; **then,** 8.3 mg/kg q 6–8 hr by continuous infusion.

CHLOROQUINE PHOSPHATE

• **Tablets**

Acute malarial attack.

Adults, Day 1: 1 g (600 mg base); **then,** 500 mg (300 mg base) 6 hr later. **Days 2 and 3:** 500 mg/day (300 mg base/day). **Children, Day 1:** 10 mg base/kg; **then,** 5 mg base/kg 6 hr later. **Days 2 and 3:** 5 mg base/kg/day.

Suppression (prophylaxis) of malaria.

Adults: 500 mg/week (300 mg base/week) on same day each week. If therapy has not been initiated 14 days before exposure, an initial loading dose of 1 g (600 mg base) may be given in 500-mg doses 6 hr apart. **Children:** 5 mg base/kg/week, not to exceed the adult dose of 300 mg of the base, given on same day each week. If therapy has not been initiated 14 days before exposure, an initial loading dose of 10 mg/kg of the base may be given in two divided doses 6 hr apart.

Extraintestinal amebiasis.

Adults: 1 g (600 mg base) given as 250 mg q.i.d. for 2 days; **then,** 500 mg (300 mg base) given as 250 mg b.i.d. for 2–3 weeks (combine with an intestinal amebicide). **Children:** 10 mg/kg (not to exceed 500 mg) daily for 3 weeks.

HEALTH CARE CONSIDERATIONS

Assessment

1. Record indications for therapy and onset of symptoms.
2. Determine any history of psoriasis; drug may exacerbate condition and precipitate an acute attack.
3. Note drugs currently prescribed to prevent adverse interactions.

Client/Family Teaching

1. Take only as directed; complete prescribed course of therapy.
2. To minimize GI upset, take with food.
3. Avoid activities that require mental alertness until drug effects realized; drug may cause dizziness.
4. Avoid direct sun exposure; wear protective clothing, sunglasses, and sunscreens.
5. Urine may be discolored dark yellow or reddish brown.
6. Review appropriate methods for protection against mosquitoes, i.e., long pants and long-sleeved shirts, repellents, and netting or screens.
7. Avoid ingestion of alcohol in any form.

Outcome/Evaluate

- Symptomatic improvement
- Negative culture reports
- Malarial prophylaxis

Chlorothiazide

(klor-oh-THIGH-ah-zyd)

Pregnancy Category: C

Diuril **(Rx)**

Chlorothiazide sodium

(klor-oh-THIGH-ah-zyd)

Pregnancy Category: C

Sodium Diuril **(Rx)**

Classification: Diuretic, thiazide type

See also *Diuretics, Thiazides*.

Action/Kinetics: Onset: 2 hr for PO, 15 min for IV; **Peak effect:** 4 hr for PO, 30 min for IV; **Duration:** 6–12 hr. **t½:** 45–120 min. Incompletely absorbed from the GI tract. Pro-

duces a greater diuretic effect if given in divided doses.
Special Concerns: Geriatric clients may be more sensitive to the usual adult dose.
Additional Side Effects: Hypotension, renal failure, renal dysfunction, interstitial nephritis. Following IV use: Alopecia, hematuria, exfoliative dermatitis, toxic epidermal necrolysis, erythema multiforme, ***Stevens-Johnson syndrome.***
How Supplied: Chlorothiazide: *Suspension:* 250 mg/5 mL; *Tablet:* 250 mg, 500 mg. Chlorothiazide sodium: *Powder for injection:* 0.5 g

Dosage

- **Oral Suspension, Tablets, IV**

Diuretic.

Adults: 0.5–2 g 1–2 times/day either PO or IV (reserved for clients unable to take PO medication or in emergencies). Some clients may respond to the drug given 3–5 days each week.

Antihypertensive.

Adults, IV, PO: 0.5–1 g/day in one or more divided doses. **Pediatric, 6 months and older, PO:** 22 mg/kg/day (10 mg/lb/day) in two divided doses; **6 months and younger, PO:** 33 mg/kg/day (15 mg/lb/day) in two divided doses. Thus, children up to 2 years of age may be given 125–375 mg/day in two doses while children 2–12 years of age may be given 375 mg–1 g/day in two doses. IV use in children is not recommended.

HEALTH CARE CONSIDERATIONS

See also *Health Care Considerations* for *Diuretics, Thiazides* and *Antihypertensive Agents.*

Administration/Storage

1. Do not give SC or IM.
2. IV Reserve IV use for adults in emergency situations or those unable to take medication PO.
3. To obtain an isotonic solution for injection, add 18 mL sterile water for injection to 500 mg powder and administer over 5 min.
4. Avoid simultaneous administration of whole blood or derivatives.
5. IV solution is compatible with NaCl or dextrose solutions.
6. Discard unused reconstituted solutions after 24 hr.

Assessment: List drugs currently prescribed; note any sulfa allergy.

Client/Family Teaching

1. May cause orthostatic hypotension; use caution when rising or changing positions.
2. Follow high-potassium diet.
3. Use sun screens (avoid ones with PABA), sunglasses, and protective clothing to diminish photosensitivity.
4. Avoid alcohol and OTC agents.

Outcome/Evaluate

- ↓ BP
- Enhanced diuresis with ↓ edema

Chlorpheniramine maleate

(klor-fen-**EAR**-ah-meen)

Pregnancy Category: B

Syrup, Tablets, Chewable Tablets: Aller-Chlor, Allergy, Chlo-Amine, Chlor-Trimeton Allergy 4 Hour, Chlor-Tripolon ✦ **(OTC), Extended-release Tablets:** Chlor-Trimeton 8 Hour and 12 Hour **(OTC), Injectable:** Chlorpheniramine maleate **(Rx)**

Classification: Antihistamine, alkylamine type

See also *Antihistamines.*
Action/Kinetics: Moderate anticholinergic and low sedative activity. **Onset:** 15–30 min **t½:** 21–27 hr. **Time to peak effect:** 6 hr. **Duration:** 3–6 hr.
Uses: PO: Allergic rhinitis. **IM, SC:** Allergic reactions to blood and plasma and adjunct to anaphylaxis therapy.
Contraindications: IV or intradermal use. Parenteral route for neonates. Use for children under 6 years of age.
Special Concerns: Geriatric clients may be more sensitive to the adult dose.
How Supplied: *Injection:* 10 mg/mL; *Syrup:* 2 mg/5 mL; *Tablet:* 4 mg; *Tablet, Extended Release:* 8 mg, 12 mg

Dosage

- **Syrup, Tablets, Chewable Tablets**

Adults and children over 12 years: 4 mg q 6 hr, not to exceed 24 mg in 24 hr. **Pediatric, 6–12 years:** 2 mg (break 4-mg tablets in half) q 4–6 hr, not to exceed 12 mg in 24 hr. **2–6 years:** 1 mg (¼ of a 4-mg tablet) q 4–6 hr.

- **Extended-Release Tablets**

Adults and children over 12 years: 8 mg q 8–12 hr or 12 mg q 12 hr, not to exceed 24 mg in 24 hr.

- **IM, SC**

Adults and children over 12 years: 5–40 mg for uncomplicated allergic reactions; 10–20 mg for amelioration of allergic reactions to blood or plasma or to treat anaphylaxis. Maximum dose per 24 hr: 40 mg.

HEALTH CARE CONSIDERATIONS

See also *Health Care Considerations* for *Antihistamines.*

Client/Family Teaching

1. Absorption is delayed if given with food.

2. May cause drowsiness; use caution.
3. Avoid alcohol in any form.
4. Anticipate dry mouth and use appropriate remedies.

Outcome/Evaluate: ↓ Nasal congestion and associated allergic manifestations

Chlorpromazine hydrochloride

(klor-**PROH**-mah-zeen)

Pregnancy Category: C

Chlorprom ✱, Chlorpromanyl ✱, Largactil ✱, Novo-Chlorpromazine ✱, Thorazine **(Rx)**

Classification: Antipsychotic, dimethylamino-type phenothiazine

See also *Antipsychotic Agents, Phenothiazines.*

Action/Kinetics: Has significant antiemetic, hypotensive, and sedative effects; moderate anticholinergic and extrapyramidal effects. **Peak plasma levels:** 2–3 hr after both PO and IM administration. **t½** (after IV, IM): **Initial,** 4–5 hr; **final,** 3–40 hr. Extensively metabolized in the intestinal wall and liver; certain of the metabolites are active. **Steady-state plasma levels** (in psychotics): 10–1,300 ng/mL. After 2–3 weeks of therapy, plasma levels decline, possibly because of reduction in drug absorption and/or increase in drug metabolism.

Uses: Acute and chronic psychoses, including schizophrenia; manic phase of manic-depressive illness. Acute intermittent porphyria. Preanesthetic, adjunct to treat tetanus, intractable hiccoughs, severe behavioral problems in children, and N&V. *Investigational:* Treatment of phencyclidine psychosis. IM or IV to treat migraine headaches.

Special Concerns: Use during pregnancy only if benefits outweigh risks. Safety for use during lactation has not been established. PO dosage for psychoses and N&V has not been established in children less than 6 months of age.

Laboratory Test Considerations: Possible ↑ plasma cholesterol.

Additional Drug Interactions

Epinephrine / Chlorpromazine ↓ peripheral vasoconstriction and may reverse action of epinephrine

Norepinephrine / Chlorpromazine ↓ pressor effect and eliminates bradycardia due to norepinephrine

Valproic acid / ↑ Effect of valproic acid due to ↓ clearance

How Supplied: *Capsule, Extended Release:* 30 mg, 75 mg, 150 mg; *Concentrate:* 30 mg/mL, 100 mg/mL; *Injection:* 25 mg/mL; *Rectal Suppository:* 25 mg, 100 mg; *Syrup:* 10 mg/5 mL; *Tablet:* 10 mg, 25 mg, 50 mg, 100 mg, 200 mg

Dosage

• **Tablets, Extended-Release Capsules, Oral Concentrate, Syrup**

Outpatients, general uses.

Adults: 10 mg t.i.d.–q.i.d. or 25 mg b.i.d.–t.i.d. For more serious cases, 25 mg t.i.d. After 1 or 2 days, increase daily dose by 20 to 50 mg semiweekly, until client becomes calm and cooperative. Maximum improvement may not be seen for weeks or months. Continue optimum dosage for 2 weeks; then, reduce gradually to maintenance levels (200 mg/day is usual). Up to 800 mg/day may be needed in discharged mental clients.

Psychotic disorders, less acutely disturbed.

Adults and adolescents: 25 mg t.i.d.; dosage may be increased by 20–50 mg/day q 3–4 days as needed, up to 400 mg/day.

Behavioral disorders in children.

Outpatients: 0.5 mg/kg (0.25 mg/lb) q 4–6 hr, as needed. **Hospitalized:** Start with low doses and increase gradually. For severe conditions: 50–100 mg/day. In older children, 200 mg or more/day may be needed.

N&V.

Adults and adolescents: 10–25 mg (of the base) q 4 hr; dosage may be increased as needed. **Pediatric:** 0.55 mg/kg (15 mg/m^2) q 4–6 hr.

Preoperative sedation.

Adults and adolescents: 25–50 mg 2–3 hr before surgery. **Pediatric:** 0.5 mg/kg (15 mg/m^2) 2–3 hr before surgery.

Hiccoughs or porphyria.

Adults and adolescents: 25–50 mg t.i.d.–q.i.d.

• **IM**

Psychotic disorders, acutely manic or disturbed.

Adults, initial: 25 mg. If necessary, give an additional 25–50 mg in 1 hr. Increase gradually over several days; up to 400 mg q 4–6 hr may be needed in severe cases. Client usually becomes quiet and cooperative within 24–48 hr. Substitute PO dosage and increase until client is calm (usually 500 mg/day). **Pediatric, over 6 months:** 0.5 mg/kg (0.25 mg/lb) q 6–8 hr as needed. Do not exceed 75 mg/day in children 5 to 12 years of age or 40 mg/day in children up to 5 years of age.

Intraoperative to control N&V.

Adults: 12.5 mg; repeat in 30 min if necessary and if no hypotension occurs. **Pediatric:**

0.25 mg/kg (0.125 mg/lb); repeat in 30 min if necessary and if no hypotension occurs.

Preoperative sedative.

Adults: 12.5–25 mg 1–2 hr before surgery. **Pediatric:** 0.5 mg/kg (0.25 mg/lb) 1–2 hr before surgery.

Hiccoughs.

Adults: 25–50 mg (base) t.i.d.–q.i.d.

Acute intermittent porphyria.

Adults: 25 mg q 6–8 hr until client can take PO therapy.

Tetanus.

Adults: 25–50 mg t.i.d.–q.i.d., usually with barbiturates.

- **Suppositories**

Behavioral disorders in children.

1 mg/kg (0.5 mg/lb) q 6–8 hr, as needed.

HEALTH CARE CONSIDERATIONS

See also *Health Care Considerations* for *Antipsychotic Agents, Phenothiazines.*

Administration/Storage

1. The maximum daily PO and parenteral dose for adults and adolescents should be 1 g of the base.
2. Swallow sustained-release capsules whole.
3. The concentrate (to be used in hospitals only) can be mixed with 60 mL or more of fruit or tomato juice, orange or simple syrup, milk, carbonated drinks, coffee, tea, water, or semisolid foods (e.g., soup, pudding).
4. When administering the drug IM, select a large, well-developed muscle mass. Use the dorsogluteal site or rectus femoris in adults and the vastus lateralis in children; rotate injection sites.
5. Solutions may cause contact dermatitis; avoid solution contact with hands or clothing.
6. Slight discoloration of injection or PO solutions will not affect drug action.
7. IV Discard solutions with marked discoloration. Consult with pharmacist if unsure of drug potency.
8. A precipitate or discoloration may occur when chlorpromazine is mixed with morphine, meperidine, or other drugs preserved with cresols.

Assessment

1. Record any seizure disorders; drug may be contraindicated.
2. Obtain baseline CBC, liver and renal function studies.
3. Assess male clients for S&S of prostatic hypertrophy.

Client/Family Teaching

1. Review side effects; report any extrapyramidal symptoms, especially uncontrolled twitching.
2. Urine may become discolored pinkish to brown.
3. Protect self during sun exposure; exposed skin surfaces may develop pigmentation changes.
4. Use caution when performing activities that require mental acuity.
5. Avoid alcohol and any other CNS depressants; may potentiate orthostatic hypotension.
6. Perform frequent toothbrushing and flossing to discourage oral fungal infections.
7. Report unusual bruising/bleeding, fever, sore throat, or malaise.
8. Avoid temperature extremes; drug may impair body's ability to regulate temperature.
9. Therapeutic psychologic effects may require 7–8 weeks of therapy.

Outcome/Evaluate

- ↓ Psychotic/manic manifestations
- Control of N&V
- Cessation of hiccoughs
- Sedation; ↓ muscular twitching

Chlorpropamide

(klor-**PROH**-pah-myd)

Pregnancy Category: C

Apo-Chlorpropamide ✱, Diabinese, Novo-Propamide ✱ **(Rx)**

Classification: Sulfonylurea, first-generation

See also *Antidiabetic Agents: Hypoglycemic Agents* and *Insulin.*

Action/Kinetics: May be effective in clients who do not respond well to other antidiabetic agents. **Onset:** 1 hr. **t½:** 35 hr. **Time to peak levels:** 2–4 hr. **Duration:** Up to 60 hr (due to slow excretion). Eighty percent metabolized in liver; 80%–90% excreted in the urine.

Additional Uses: *Investigational:* Neurogenic diabetes insipidus.

Special Concerns: Monitor frequently in those susceptible to fluid retention or impaired cardiac function.

Additional Side Effects: Side effects are frequent. Severe diarrhea, occasionally accompanied by bleeding in the lower bowel. Relieve severe GI distress by dividing total daily dose in half. In older clients, hypoglycemia may be severe. Inappropriate ADH secretion, leading to hyponatremia, water retention, low serum osmolality, and high urine osmolality.

Additional Drug Interactions

Ammonium chloride / ↑ Effect of chlorpropamide due to ↓ excretion by kidney

Disulfiram / More likely to interact with chlorpropamide than other oral antidiabetics
Probenecid / ↑ Effect of chlorpropamide
Sodium bicarbonate / ↓ Effect of chlorpropamide due to ↑ excretion by kidney
How Supplied: *Tablet:* 100 mg, 250 mg

Dosage

- **Tablets**

Diabetes.

Adults, middle-aged clients, mild to moderate diabetes, initial: 250 mg/day as a single or divided dose; **geriatric, initial:** 100–125 mg/day. **All clients, maintenance:** 100–250 mg/day as single or divided doses. Severe diabetics may require 500 mg/day; doses greater than 750 mg/day are not recommended.

Neurogenic diabetes insipidus.

Adults: 200–500 mg/day.

HEALTH CARE CONSIDERATIONS

Assessment

1. Elderly clients tend to be more sensitive to hypoglycemic agents and exhibit more side effects.
2. Determine if pregnant; drug is contraindicated.
3. Obtain baseline CBC, HbA1C, and LFTs.
4. Assess for cardiac dysfunction or fluid retention. Monitor I&O, serum electrolytes, and urine osmolality.

Client/Family Teaching

1. Record weight and BP.
2. Report any confusion, dizziness, depression, or nausea; may be S&S of inappropriate ADH secretion.
3. Review weight loss, diet, and exercise guidelines.

Outcome/Evaluate: Normalization of serum glucose levels

Chlorthalidone

(klor-THAL-ih-dohn)

Pregnancy Category: B

Apo-Chlorthalidone ✱, Hygroton, Novo-Thalidone ✱, Thalitone, Uridon ✱ **(Rx)**

Classification: Diuretic, thiazide

See also *Diuretics, Thiazides.*

Action/Kinetics: Onset: 2–3 hr. **Peak effect:** 2–6 hr. **Duration:** 24–72 hr. **t½:** 40 hr. Bioavailability may be dose-dependent.

Additional Uses: To potentiate and reduce dosage of other antihypertensive agents.

Special Concerns: Geriatric clients may be more sensitive to the usual adult dose.

Additional Side Effects: Exfoliative dermatitis, toxic epidermal necrolysis.

How Supplied: *Tablet:* 15 mg, 25 mg, 50 mg, 100 mg

Dosage

- **Tablets**

Edema.

Adults, initial: 50–100 mg/day (30–60 mg Thalitone) or 100–200 mg (60 mg Thalitone) on alternate days. Some clients require 150 or 200 mg (90–120 mg Thalitone). **Maximum daily dose:** 200 mg (120 mg Thalitone). **Pediatric:** All uses, 2 mg/kg (60 mg/m^2) 3 times/week.

Hypertension.

Adults, initial: Single dose of 25 mg (15 mg Thalitone); if response is not sufficient, dose may be increased to 50 mg (30 mg Thalitone). For additional control, increase the dose to 100 mg/day (except Thalitone) or a second antihypertensive drug may be added to the regimen. **Maintenance:** Determined by client response. *NOTE:* Doses greater than 25 mg/day are likely to increase potassium excretion but not cause further benefit in sodium excretion or BP reduction.

HEALTH CARE CONSIDERATIONS

See also *Health Care Considerations for Diuretics, Thiazides* and *Antihypertensive Agents.*

Administration/Storage

1. Start with the lowest possible dose. Maintenance doses may be lower than initial doses.
2. Doses higher than 25 mg/day will increase potassium excretion but will not cause further benefit in sodium excretion or reduction of BP.

Assessment

1. Note indications for therapy, other agents trialed, and the outcome.
2. Monitor CBC, electrolytes, glucose, BUN, and creatinine.

Client/Family Teaching: Take in the morning with food.

Outcome/Evaluate

- Enhanced diuresis; ↓ edema
- ↓ BP

Chlorzoxazone

(klor-ZOX-ah-zohn)

Parafon Forte DSC, Remular-S **(Rx)**

Classification: Muscle relaxant, centrally acting

See also *Skeletal Muscle Relaxants, Centrally Acting.*
Action/Kinetics: Inhibits polysynaptic reflexes at both the spinal cord and subcortical areas of the brain. Effects may also be due to sedation. **Onset:** 1 hr. **Time to peak blood levels:** 1–2 hr. **Peak serum levels:** 10–30 mcg/mL (after 750-mg dose). **Duration:** 3–4 hr. **t½:** 1 hr. Metabolized in the liver and inactive metabolites excreted in the urine.
Uses: As adjunct to rest, physical therapy, and other approaches for treatment of acute, painful musculoskeletal conditions (e.g., muscle spasms, sprains, muscle strain).
Special Concerns: Use during pregnancy only if benefits clearly outweigh risks. Use with caution in clients with known allergies or a history of allergic reactions to drugs.
Side Effects: *CNS:* Dizziness, drowsiness, lightheadedness, overstimulation, malaise. *Dermatologic:* Allergic-type skin rashes, petechiae, ecchymoses (rare). *GI:* GI upset, GI bleeding (rare). *Allergic Reactions:* ***Angioneurotic edema, anaphylaxis*** (rare). *Miscellaneous:* Discoloration of urine, liver damage.
OD Management of Overdose: *Symptoms:* N&V, diarrhea, drowsiness, dizziness, lightheadedness, headache, malaise, sluggishness. May be followed by marked loss of muscle tone (voluntary movement may be impossible), decreased or absent deep tendon reflexes, respiratory depression, decreased BP. *Treatment:* Supportive.
How Supplied: *Tablet:* 250 mg, 500 mg

Dosage

- **Tablets**

Skeletal muscle disorders.

Adults: 250–750 mg t.i.d.–q.i.d. with meals and at bedtime; **pediatric:** 125–500 mg t.i.d.–q.i.d. (or 20 mg/kg in three to four divided doses daily).

HEALTH CARE CONSIDERATIONS

See also *Health Care Considerations* for *Skeletal Muscle Relaxants, Centrally Acting.*

Assessment

1. Record indications for therapy; note pretreatment findings.
2. During physical exam test for weakness, stiffness, ROM, reflexes; with low-back pain, perform rectal exam and note sphincter tone.
3. Obtain baseline renal and LFTs; assess for dysfunction.

Client/Family Teaching

1. May take with food if GI upset occurs. May be mixed with food or beverages for children.
2. Do not operate dangerous machinery or drive a car until drug effects evident; causes drowsiness.
3. Drug may cause urine to have an orange or purple-red color when exposed to the air.
4. Review importance of RICE (rest, ice, compression, and elevation) in the setting of an acute injury.
5. Do not overuse extremity during therapy; drug may mask pathology.
6. Return to provider in 3 weeks if no improvement in symptoms.

Outcome/Evaluate: Relief of musculoskeletal spasm and pain

Cholestyramine resin

(koh-less-**TEER**-ah-meen)
Alti-Cholestyramine Light ✦, LoCholest, Novo-Cholaine Light ✦, PMS-Cholestyramine ✦, Prevalite, Questran, Questran Light **(Rx)**
Classification: Hypocholesterolemic agent, bile acid sequestrant

Action/Kinetics: Binds sodium cholate (bile salts) in the intestine; thus, the principal precursor of cholesterol is not absorbed due to formation of an insoluble complex, which is excreted in the feces. Decreases cholesterol and LDL and either has no effect or increases triglycerides, VLDL, and HDL. Also, itching is relieved as a result of removing irritating bile salts. The antidiarrheal effect results from the binding and removal of bile acids. **Onset, to reduce plasma cholesterol:** Within 24–48 hr, but levels may continue to fall for 1 yr; **to relieve pruritus:** 1–3 weeks; **relief of diarrhea associated with bile acids:** 24 hr. Cholesterol levels return to pretreatment levels 2–4 weeks after discontinuance. Fat-soluble vitamins (A, D, K) and possibly folic acid may have to be administered IM during long-term therapy because cholestyramine binds these vitamins in the intestine.
Uses: Adjunct to reduce elevated serum cholesterol in primary hypercholesterolemia in those who do not respond adequately to diet. Pruritus associated with partial biliary obstruction. Diarrhea due to bile acids. *Investigational:* Antibiotic-induced pseudomembranous colitis (i.e., due to toxin produced by *Clostridium difficile*), digitalis toxicity, treatment of chlordecone (Kepone) poisoning, treatment of thyroid hormone overdose.
Contraindications: Complete obstruction or atresia of bile duct.
Special Concerns: Use during pregnancy only if benefits outweigh risks. Use with caution during lactation and in children. Long-term effects and efficacy in decreasing cholesterol levels in pediatric clients are not

known. Geriatric clients may be more likely to manifest GI side effects as well as adverse nutritional effects. Exercise caution in phenylketonurics as Prevalite contains 14.1 mg phenylalanine per 5.5-g dose.

Side Effects: *GI:* Constipation (may be severe), N&V, diarrhea, heartburn, GI bleeding, anorexia, flatulence, belching, abdominal distention, abdominal pain or cramping, loose stools, indigestion, aggravation of hemorrhoids, rectal bleeding or pain, black stools, bleeding duodenal ulcer, peptic ulceration, GI irritation, dysphagia, dental bleeding, hiccoughs, sour taste, pancreatitis, diverticulitis, cholescystitis, cholelithiasis. Fecal impaction in elderly clients. Large doses may cause steatorrhea. *CNS:* Migraine or sinus headaches, dizziness, anxiety, vertigo, insomnia, fatigue, lightheadedness, syncope, drowsiness, femoral nerve pain, paresthesia. *Hypersensitivity:* Urticaria, dermatitis, asthma, wheezing, rash. *Hematologic:* Increased PT, ecchymosis, anemia. *Musculoskeletal:* Muscle or joint pain, backache, arthritis, osteoporosis. *GU:* Hematuria, dysuria, burnt odor to urine, diuresis. *Other:* Bleeding tendencies (due to hypoprothrombinemia). Deficiencies of vitamins A and D. Uveitis, weight loss or gain, osteoporosis, swollen glands, increased libido, weakness, SOB, edema, swelling of hands/feet; hyperchloremic acidosis in children, rash and irritation of the skin, tongue, and perianal area.

Laboratory Test Considerations: Liver function abnormalities.

OD **Management of Overdose:** *Symptoms:* GI tract obstruction.

Drug Interactions

Anticoagulants, PO / ↓ Anticoagulant effect due to ↓ absorption from GI tract
Aspirin / ↓ Absorption of aspirin from GI tract
Clindamycin / ↓ Absorption of clindamycin from GI tract
Clofibrate / ↓ Absorption of clofibrate from GI tract
Digitalis glycosides / ↓ Effect of digitalis due to ↓ absorption from the GI tract
Furosemide / ↓ Absorption of furosemide from GI tract
Gemfibrozil / ↓ Bioavailability of gemfibrozil
Glipizide / ↓ Serum glipizide levels
Hydrocortisone / ↓ Effect of hydrocortisone due to ↓ absorption from GI tract
Imipramine / ↓ Absorption of imipramine from GI tract
Iopanoic acid / Results in abnormal cholecystography
Lovastatin / Effects may be additive
Methyldopa / ↓ Absorption of methyldopa from GI tract
Nicotinic acid / ↓ Absorption of nicotinic acid from GI tract
Penicillin G / ↓ Effect of penicillin G due to ↓ absorption from GI tract
Phenytoin / ↓ Absorption of phenytoin from GI tract
Phosphate supplements / ↓ Absorption of phosphate supplements from GI tract
Piroxicam / ↑ Elimination
Propranolol / ↓ Effect of propranolol due to ↓ absorption from GI tract
Tetracyclines / ↓ Effect of tetracyclines due to ↓ absorption from GI tract
Thiazide diuretics / ↓ Effect of thiazides due to ↓ absorption from GI tract
Thyroid hormones / ↓ Effect of thyroid hormones due to ↓ absorption from GI tract
Tolbutamide / ↓ Absorption of tolbutamide from GI tract
Ursodiol / ↓ Effect of ursodiol due to ↓ absorption from GI tract
Vitamins A, D, E, K / Malabsorption of fat-soluble vitamins

NOTE: These drug interactions may also be observed with colestipol.

How Supplied: *Powder for Reconstitution:* 4 g/5 g, 4 g/5.5 g, 4 g/5.7 g, 4 g/9 g

Dosage

- **Powder**

Adults, initial: 1 g 1–2 times/day. Dose is individualized. For Prevalite, give 1 packet or 1 level scoopful (5.5 g Prevalite: 4 g anhydrous cholestyramine). **Maintenance:** 2–4 packets or scoopfuls/day (8–16 g anhydrous cholestyramine resin) mixed with 60–180 mL water or noncarbonated beverage. The recommended dosing schedule is b.i.d. but it can be given in one to six doses/day. Maximum daily dose: 6 packets or scoopsful (equivalent to 24 g cholestyramine).

HEALTH CARE CONSIDERATIONS

Administration/Storage

1. Always mix powder with 60–180 mL water or noncarbonated beverage before administering; resin may cause esophageal irritation or blockage. Highly liquid soups or pulpy fruits such as applesauce or crushed pineapple may be used.
2. After placing contents of 1 packet of resin on the surface of 4–6 oz of fluid, allow it to stand without stirring for 2 min, occasionally twirling the glass, and then stir slowly (to prevent foaming) to form a suspension.

3. Avoid inhaling the powder while mixing as it may be irritating to mucous membranes.
4. Cholestyramine may interfere with the absorption of other drugs taken orally; thus, take other drug(s) 1 hr before or 4–6 hr after dosing.

Assessment

1. Record type and onset of symptoms, and other agents trialed.
2. Determine onset of pruritus and note bile acid level.
3. Monitor CBC, cholesterol profile, and liver and renal function studies.
4. Vitamins A, D, E, K, and folic acid will need to be administered in a water-miscible form during long-term therapy.
5. Assess skin and eyes for evidence of jaundice or bile deposits.

Client/Family Teaching

1. Other prescribed medications should be taken at least 1 hr before or 4 hr after taking drug. These drugs interfere with the absorption and desired effects of other medications.
2. Review constipating effects of drug and ways to control: daily exercise, fluid intake of 2.5–3 L/day, increased intake of citrus fruits, fruit juices, and high-fiber foods; also, a stool softener may help. If constipation persists, a change in dosage or drug may be indicated.
3. If diarrhea develops, stop constipation measures, record I&O, and weight and report.
4. Clients with high cholesterol levels should follow dietary restrictions of fat and cholesterol as well as smoking cessation, alcohol reduction, and regular exercise.
5. Report tarry stools or abnormal bleeding as supplemental vitamin K (10 mg/week) may be necessary. CBC, PT, and renal function tests should be done routinely.
6. Pruritus may subside 1–3 weeks after taking the drug but may return after the medication is discontinued. Corn starch or oatmeal baths may also assist to alleviate symptoms.

Outcome/Evaluate

- Control of pruritus
- ↓ Serum cholesterol levels
- ↓ Diarrheal stools
- ↓ Bile acid levels

Chorionic gonadotropin (HCG)

(kor-ee-**ON**-ik go-**NAD**-oh-troh-pin)

Pregnancy Category: X

A.P.L., Chorex-5 and -10, Choron 10, Gonic, Pregnyl, Profasi **(Rx)**

Classification: Gonadotropic hormone

Action/Kinetics: The actions of HCG, produced by the trophoblasts of the fertilized ovum and then by the placenta, resemble those of LH. In males, HCG stimulates androgen production by the testes, the development of secondary sex characteristics, and testicular descent when no anatomic impediment is present. In women, HCG stimulates progesterone production by the corpus luteum and completes expulsion of the ovum from a mature follicle. No significant evidence that HCG causes a more attractive or "normal" distribution of fat or that it decreases hunger and discomfort due to calorie-restricted diets.

Uses: Males: Prepubertal cryptorchidism, hypogonadism due to pituitary insufficiency. **Females:** Infertility not due to primary ovarian failure (used with menotropins).

Contraindications: Precocious puberty, prostatic cancer or other androgen-dependent neoplasm, hypersensitivity to drug. Development of precocious puberty is cause for discontinuance of therapy. Pregnancy.

Special Concerns: Since HCG increases androgen production, drug should be used with caution in clients in whom androgen-induced edema may be harmful (epilepsy, migraines, asthma, cardiac or renal diseases). Use with caution during lactation. Safety and efficacy have not been shown in children less than 4 years of age.

Side Effects: *CNS:* Headache, irritability, restlessness, depression, fatigue, aggressive behavior. *GU:* Precocious puberty, ovarian hyperstimulation syndrome, ovarian malignancy (rare), ***enlargement of preexisting ovarian cysts with possible rupture.*** *Miscellaneous:* Edema, gynecomastia, pain at injection site, fluid retention, arterial thromboembolism.

How Supplied: *Powder for injection:* 5,000 U, 10,000 U, 20,000 U

Dosage

- **IM Only**

Prepubertal cryptorchidism, not due to anatomic obstruction.

Various regimens including (1) 4,000 USP units 3 times/week for 3 weeks; (2) 5,000 USP units every other day for 4 injections; (3) 15 injections over a period of 6 weeks of 500–1,000 USP units/injection; (4) 500 USP units 3 times/week for 4–6 weeks; may be repeated after 1 month using 1,000 USP units.

Hypogonadotropic hypogonadism in males.

The following regimens may be used: (1) 500–1,000 USP units 3 times/week for 3 weeks; **then,** same dose twice weekly for 3 weeks; (2) 4,000 USP units 3 times/week for 6–9 months; then, 2,000 USP units 3 times/

week for 3 more months; (3) 1,000–2,000 USP units 3 times/week.

HEALTH CARE CONSIDERATIONS

Administration/Storage

1. Reconstituted solutions are stable for 1–3 months, depending on manufacturer, when stored at 2°C–8°C (35°F–46°F).
2. Have emergency drugs and equipment available in the event of an acute allergic response.

Assessment

1. Record indications for therapy, symptom onset, and clinical presentation.
2. Note any drug sensitivity.
3. Assess prepubescent male for appearance of secondary sex characteristics; drug is contraindicated.

Client/Family Teaching

1. Review indications for therapy and the anticipated results.
2. May cause pain at injection site.
3. Record daily weights and report extent of edema which is common.
4. Delayed menses, excessive menstrual bleeding, pain in the pelvic region, weakness, and fatigue are S&S of ectopic pregnancy; report now.
5. When used with menotropins may experience multiple births .
6. With corpus luteum deficiency, if bleeding occurs after day 15 of therapy, hold drug and report.
7. Report headache, easy fatigue, and restlessness; if increasingly irritable, depressed, and changes in attention to physical appearance occur, may have to stop drug.
8. Gynecomastia may develop in young males. Report the beginning of secondary sex characteristics, as this is an indication of sexual precocity and drug should be withdrawn
9. With cryptorchidism, examine weekly for testicular descent.
10. Return for follow-up visits to monitor drug effectiveness.

Outcome/Evaluate

- Testicular descent
- Functional spermatozoa
- ↑ Progesterone → ovum release
- Sexual maturation

Ciclopirox olamine

(sye-kloh-**PEER**-ox)

Pregnancy Category: B

Loprox **(Rx)**

Classification: Broad-spectrum topical antifungal

Action/Kinetics: At lower concentrations the drug blocks the transport of amino acids into the cell, whereas at higher concentrations the cell membrane of the fungus is altered so that intracellular material leaks out. May also inhibit synthesis of RNA, DNA, and protein in growing fungal cells. A small amount of drug is absorbed through the skin; it also penetrates to the sebaceous glands and dermis as well as into the hair.

Uses: Effective against dermatophytes, yeast, *Malassezia furfur, Trichophyton rubrum, T. mentagrophytes, Epidermophyton floccosum, Microsporum canis,* and *Candida albicans* that cause tinea pedis, tinea corporis, tinea cruris, tinea versicolor, candidiasis.

Contraindications: Use in or around the eyes.

Special Concerns: Safety and efficacy in lactation and in children under 10 years of age not established.

Side Effects: *Dermatologic:* Irritation, redness, burning, pain, skin sensitivity, pruritus at application site.

How Supplied: *Cream:* 1%; *Gel:* 0.77%; *Lotion:* 1%

Dosage

- **Cream, Gel, Lotion**

Massage gently into the affected area and surrounding skin morning and evening. If there is no improvement after 4 weeks, reevaluate diagnosis.

HEALTH CARE CONSIDERATIONS

Assessment

1. Record indications for therapy, onset and duration of symptoms.
2. Describe lesion presentation and obtain scrapings.

Client/Family Teaching

1. Cleanse skin with soap and water and dry thoroughly. Apply cream with a glove; wash hands before and after therapy.
2. Avoid occlusive dressings or wrappings; adult incontinence pads/diapers are occlusive.
3. Even if symptoms have improved, use for the full time.
4. Change shoes and socks at least once daily. Shoes should be well-fitted and ventilated.
5. Report any evidence of blistering, burning, itching, oozing, redness, or swelling.

Outcome/Evaluate

- Resolution of infection; wound healing
- Symptomatic improvement

Cilostazol

(sih-**LESS**-tah-zohl)
Pregnancy Category: C
Pletal **(Rx)**
Classification: Antiplatelet drug

Action/Kinetics: Inhibits cellular phosphodiesterase (PDE), especially PDE III. Cilostazol and several metabolites inhibit cyclic AMP PDE III. Suppression of this isoenzyme causes increased levels of cyclic AMP resulting in vasodilation and inhibition of platelet aggregation. Inhibits platelet aggregation caused by thrombin, ADP, collagen, arachidonic acid, epinephrine, and shear stress. High fat meals significantly increase absorption. Significantly plasma protein bound. Extensively metabolized by the liver with two of the metabolites being active. Primarily excreted through the urine (74%) with the rest in the feces.
Uses: Reduce symptoms of intermittent claudication.
Contraindications: CHF of any severity (may cause a decreased survival rate in clients with class III-IV CHF). Concurrent use of grapefruit juice. Lactation.
Special Concerns: Safety and efficacy have not been determined in children.
Side Effects: *GI:* Abnormal stool, diarrhea, dyspepsia, flatulence, N&V, abdominal pain, anorexia, cholelithiasis, colitis, duodenal ulcer, duodenitis, esophageal hemorrhage, esophagitis, gastritis, gastroenteritis, gum hemorrhage, hematemesis, melena, gastric ulcer, periodontal abscess, rectal hemorrhage, stomach ulcer, tongue edema. *CNS:* Headache, dizziness, vertigo, anxiety, insomnia, neuralgia. *CV:* Palpitation, tachycardia, hypertension, angina pectoris, atrial fibrillation/flutter, cerebral infarct, cerebral ischemia, CHF, ***heart arrest, hemorrhage,*** hypotension, MI, myocardial ischemia, nodal arrhythmia, postural hypotension, supraventricular tachycardia, syncope, varicose veins, vasodilation, ventricular extrasystole or ***ventricular tachycardia*** *Respiratory:* Rhinitis, pharyngitis, increased cough, dyspnea, bronchitis, asthma, epistaxis, hemoptysis, pneumonia, sinusitis. *Musculoskeletal:* Back pain, myalgia, asthenia, leg cramps, arthritis, arthralgia, bone pain, bursitis. *Dermatologic:* Rash, dry skin, furunculosis, skin hypertrophy, urticaria. *GU:* Hematuria, UTI, cystitis, urinary frequency, vaginal hemorrhage, vaginitis. *Hematologic:* Anemia, ecchymosis, iron deficiency anemia, polycythemia, purpura. *Ophthalmic:* Amblyopia, blindness, conjunctivitis, diplopia, eye hemorrhage, retinal hemorrhage. *Miscellaneous:* Infection, peripheral edema, hyperesthesia, paresthesia, flu syndrome, ear pain, tinnitus, chills, facial edema, fever, generalized edema, malaise, neck rigidity, pelvic pain, ***retroperitoneal hemorrhage,*** diabetes mellitus.
Laboratory Test Considerations: ↑ GGT, creatinine. Albuminuria, hyperlipemia, hyperuricemia.
OD **Management of Overdose:** *Symptoms:* Severe headache, diarrhea, hypotension, tachycardia, possible cardiac arrhythmias. *Treatment:* Observe client carefully and provide symptomatic treatment.
Drug Interactions: Diltiazem, erythromycin, grapefruit juice, itraconazole, ketoconazole, macrolide antibiotics, and omeprazole inhibit liver enzymes that breakdown cilostazol, resulting in ↑ plasma levels. Reduce dose of these drugs if used concomitantly.
How Supplied: *Tablets:* 50 mg, 100 mg

Dosage

- **Tablets**

Intermittent claudication.

100 mg b.i.d. taken 30 min or more before or 2 hr after breakfast and dinner. Consider a dose of 50 mg b.i.d. during coadministration of diltiazem, erythromycin, itraconazole, or ketoconazole.

HEALTH CARE CONSIDERATIONS

Administration/Storage: The dosage of cilostazol may be reduced or discontinued without platelet hyperaggregability.

Assessment

1. Determine and record onset and characteristics of symptoms. Measure distance walked before pain elicited.
2. Determine any history or evidence of CHF.
3. Monitor labs for liver or renal dysfunction.
4. Assess extent/amount/duration of nicotine use.

Client/Family Teaching

1. Take 30 minutes before or 2 hr after meals. Avoid consuming grapefruit juice.
2. Read the patient package insert carefully before starting therapy and each time therapy is renewed.
3. May experience headaches, GI upset, dizziness, or runny nose; report if bothersome.
4. Do not smoke; enroll in formal smoking cessation program.
5. Beneficial effects may not be immediate. May see in 2 to 4 weeks, but up to 12 weeks may be needed before a beneficial effect is seen.

Outcome/Evaluate

- Increased walking distance without pain
- ↓ S&S intermittent claudication

Cimetidine

(sye-**MET**-ih-deen)

Pregnancy Category: B

Apo-Cimetidine ✱, Gen-Cimetidine ✱, Novo-Cimetine ✱, Nu-Cimet ✱, Peptol ✱, PMS-Cimetidine ✱, Tagamet **(Rx)**, Tagamet HB **(OTC)**

Classification: Histamine H_2 receptor blocking agent

See also *Histamine H_2 Antagonists.*

Action/Kinetics: Reduces postprandial daytime and nighttime gastric acid secretion by about 50%–80%. May increase gastromucosal defense and healing in acid-related disorders (e.g., stress-induced ulcers) by increasing production of gastric mucus, increasing mucosal secretion of bicarbonate and gastric mucosal blood flow as well as increasing endogenous mucosal synthesis of prostaglandins. It also inhibits cytochrome P-450 and P-448, which will affect metabolism of drugs. Also possesses antiandrogenic activity and will increase prolactin levels following an IV bolus injection. Well absorbed from GI tract. **Peak plasma level, PO:** 45–90 min. **Time to peak effect, after PO:** 1–2 hr. **Peak plasma levels, after PO use:** 0.7–3.2 mcg/mL (after a 300 mg dose; **after IV:** 3.5–7.5 mcg/mL. **Protein binding:** 13%–25%. **Duration, nocturnal:** 6–8 hr; **basal:** 4–5 hr. **t½:** 2 hr, longer in presence of renal impairment. After PO use, most metabolized in liver; after parenteral use, about 75% of drug excreted unchanged in the urine.

Uses: Rx. Treatment and maintenance of active duodenal ulcers. Short-term (6 weeks) treatment of benign gastric ulcers (in rare cases, healing has occurred). As part of multidrug regimen to eradicate *Helicobacter pylori.* Management of gastric acid hypersecretory states (Zollinger-Ellison syndrome, systemic mastocytosis). GERD, including erosive esophagitis. Prophylaxis of UGI bleeding in critically ill hospitalized clients. *Investigational:* Prior to surgery to prevent aspiration pneumonitis, secondary hyperparathyroidism in chronic hemodialysis clients, prophylaxis of stress-induced ulcers, hyperparathyroidism, dyspepsia, herpes virus infections, tinea capitis, hirsute women, chronic idiopathic urticaria, dermatologic anaphylaxis, acetaminophen overdosage, warts, colorectal cancer.

OTC. Relief of symptoms of heartburn, acid indigestion, and sour stomach.

Contraindications: Children under 16, lactation. Cirrhosis, impaired liver and renal function.

Special Concerns: In geriatric clients with impaired renal or hepatic function, confusion is more likely to occur. Not recommended for children less than 16 years of age.

Side Effects: *GI:* Diarrhea, pancreatitis (rare), hepatitis, hepatic fibrosis. *CNS:* Dizziness, sleepiness, headache, confusion, delirium, hallucinations, double vision, dysarthria, ataxia. Severely ill clients may manifest agitation, anxiety, depression, disorientation, hallucinations, mental confusion, and psychosis. *CV:* Hypotension and arrhythmias following rapid IV administration. *Hematologic:* Agranulocytosis, thrombocytopenia, ***hemolytic or aplastic anemia,*** granulocytopenia. *GU:* Impotence (high doses for prolonged periods of time), gynecomastia (long-term treatment). *Dermatologic:* Exfoliative dermatitis, erythroderma, erythema multiforme. *Musculoskeletal:* Arthralgia, reversible worsening of joint symptoms with preexisting arthritis (including gouty arthritis). *Other:* Hypersensitivity reactions, pain at injection site, myalgia, rash, cutaneous vasculitis, peripheral neuropathy, galactorrhea, alopecia, bronchoconstriction.

Drug Interactions

Antacids / ↓ Effect of cimetidine due to ↓ absorption from GI tract
Anticholinergics / ↓ Effect of cimetidine due to ↓ absorption from GI tract
Benzodiazepines / ↑ Effect of benzodiazepines due to ↓ breakdown by liver
Beta-adrenergic blocking drugs / ↑ Effect of beta blockers due to ↓ breakdown by liver
Caffeine / ↑ Effect of caffeine due to ↓ breakdown by liver
Calcium channel blockers / ↑ Effect of calcium channel blockers due to ↓ breakdown by liver
Carbamazepine / ↑ Effect of carbamazepine due to ↓ breakdown by liver
Carmustine / Additive bone marrow depression
Chloroquine / ↑ Effect of chloroquine due to ↓ breakdown by liver
Chlorpromazine / ↓ Effect of chlorpromazine due to ↓ absorption from GI tract
Digoxin / ↓ Serum levels of digoxin
Flecainide / ↑ Effect of flecainide
Fluconazole / ↓ Effect of fluconazole due to ↓ absorption from GI tract
Fluorouracil / ↑ Serum levels of fluorouracil following chronic cimetidine use
Indomethacin / ↓ Effect of indomethacin due to ↓ absorption from GI tract
Iron salts / ↓ Effect of iron due to ↓ absorption from GI tract

Ketoconazole / ↓ Effect of ketoconazole due to ↓ absorption from GI tract
Labetalol / ↑ Effect of labetalol due to ↓ breakdown by liver
Lidocaine / ↑ Effect of lidocaine due to ↓ breakdown by liver
Metoclopramide / ↓ Effect of cimetidine due to ↓ absorption from GI tract
Metoprolol / ↑ Effect of metoprolol due to ↓ breakdown by liver
Metronidazole / ↑ Effect of metronidazole due to ↓ breakdown by liver
Moricizine / ↑ Effect of moricizine due to ↓ breakdown by liver
Narcotics / Possible ↑ toxic effects (respiratory depression) of narcotics
Pentoxifylline / ↑ Effect of pentoxifylline due to ↓ breakdown by liver
Phenytoin / ↑ Effect of phenytoin due to ↓ breakdown by liver
Procainamide / ↑ Effect of procainamide due to ↓ excretion by kidney
Propafenone / ↑ Effect of propafenone due to ↓ breakdown by liver
Propranolol / ↑ Effect of propranolol due to ↓ breakdown by liver
Quinidine / ↑ Effect of quinidine due to ↓ breakdown by liver
Quinine / ↑ Effect of quinine due to ↓ breakdown by liver
Sildenafil / ↑ Effect of sildenafil due to ↓ breakdown by liver
Succinylcholine / ↑ Neuromuscular blockade → respiratory depression and extended apnea
Sulfonylureas / ↑ Effect of sulfonylureas due to ↓ breakdown by liver
Tacrine / ↑ Effect of tacrine due to ↓ breakdown by liver
Tetracyclines / ↓ Effect of tetracyclines due to ↓ absorption from GI tract
Theophyllines / ↑ Effect of theophyllines due to ↓ breakdown by liver
Tocainide / ↓ Effect of tocainide
Triamterene / ↑ Effect of triamterene due to ↓ breakdown by liver
Tricyclic antidepressants / ↑ Effect of tricyclic antidepressants due to ↓ breakdown by liver
Valproic acid / ↑ Effect of valproic acid due to ↓ breakdown by liver
Warfarin / ↑ Effect of anticoagulant due to ↓ breakdown by liver

How Supplied: *Injection:* 150 mg/mL, 300 mg/50 mL; *Solution:* 300 mg/5 mL; *Tablet:* 100 mg (OTC), 200 mg, 300 mg, 400 mg, 800 mg

Dosage

• **Tablets, Oral Solution**

Duodenal ulcers, short-term.

Adults: 800 mg at bedtime. Alternate dosage: 300 mg q.i.d. with meals and at bedtime for 4–6 weeks (administer with antacids, staggering the dose of antacids) or 400 mg b.i.d. (in the morning and evening). **Maintenance:** 400 mg at bedtime.

Active benign gastric ulcers.

Adults: 800 mg at bedtime (preferred regimen) or 300 mg q.i.d. with meals and at bedtime for no more than 8 weeks.

Pathologic hypersecretory conditions.

Adults: 300 mg q.i.d. with meals and at bedtime up to a maximum of 2,400 mg/day for as long as needed.

Erosive gastroesophageal reflux disease.

Adults: 800 mg b.i.d. or 400 mg q.i.d. for 12 weeks. Use beyond 12 weeks has not been determined.

Heartburn, acid indigestion, sour stomach (OTC only).

200 mg with water as symptoms present up to b.i.d.

Dyspepsia.

Adults: 400 mg b.i.d.

Prophylaxis of aspiration pneumonitis.

Adults: 400–600 mg 60–90 min before anesthesia.

Primary hyperparathyroidism, secondary hyperparathyroidism in chronic hemodialysis clients.

Up to 1 g/day.

• **IM, IV, IV Infusion**

Hospitalized clients with pathologic hypersecretory conditions or intractable ulcers or those unable to take PO medication.

Adults: 300 mg IM or IV q 6–8 hr. If an increased dose is necessary, administer 300 mg more frequently than q 6–8 hr, not to exceed 2,400 mg/day.

Prophylaxis of upper GI bleeding.

Adults: 50 mg/hr by continuous IV infusion. If C_{CR} is less than 30 mL/min, use one-half the recommended dose. Treatment beyond 7 days has not been studied.

Prophylaxis of aspiration pneumonitis.

Adults: 300 mg IV 60–90 min before induction of anesthetic.

HEALTH CARE CONSIDERATIONS

See also *Health Care Considerations* for *Histamine H_2 Antagonists.*

Administration/Storage

1. Do not use the OTC product continuously for more than 2 weeks except under medical supervision.
2. If antacids are used, stagger dose with that of cimetidine; antacids (but not food) decrease absorption.

3. Administer PO medication with meals and with a snack at bedtime.
4. In renal dysfunction, a dose of 300 mg PO or IV q 12 hr may be necessary. The dose may be given, with caution, q 8 hr if needed.
5. For IM use, give undiluted.
IV 6. For IV injections, dilute 300 mg in 0.9% NaCl injection (or other compatible solution) to a total volume of 20 mL. Inject over at least 2 min.
7. For intermittent IV infusion, dilute 300 mg in at least 50 mL of dextrose or saline solution and infuse over 15–20 min.
8. For continuous IV infusion, give a loading dose of 150 mg (by intermittent IV infusion); then, administer 37.5 mg/hr (900 mg/day) in 0.9% NaCl injection, 5% or 10% dextrose injection, 5% $NaHCO_3$ injection, RL solution, or as part of TPN. Is stable for 24 hr at room temperature if mixed with these diluents.
9. May be diluted in 100–1,000 mL; if the volume for a 24-hr infusion is less than 250 mL, use a pump.
10. Do *not* introduce drugs or additives to cimetidine solutions in plastic containers.
11. Cimetidine is incompatible with aminophylline and barbiturates in IV solutions and in the same syringe with pentobarbital sodium and a pentobarbital sodium/atropine sulfate combination.
12. Do not expose premixed single-dose product to excessive heat; store at 15°C–30°C (59°F–86°F).

Assessment

1. Note general client condition. Those receiving radiation therapy or myelosuppressive drugs may have additional side effects.
2. List drugs prescribed to ensure none interact unfavorably.
3. Record indications for therapy, type/onset of symptoms, and anticipated length of therapy.
4. Assess location, characteristics, extent of abdominal pain; note blood in emesis, stool, or gastric aspirate. Maintain gastric pH above 5 to enhance mucosal healing.
5. Document radiologic and/or endoscopic findings; check for *H. Pylori.*
6. Monitor CBC, I&O, electrolytes, liver and renal function studies, especially for the elderly, severely ill, or those with renal impairment.

Client/Family Teaching

1. Take with meals and/or a snack at bedtime. Avoid antacids 1 hr before or after dose; establish schedule to assure compliance.
2. Take entire prescription even if symptoms disappear.
3. Review dietary modifications, especially if being treated for GI problems; consult dietitian as needed.
4. Do not perform tasks that require mental alertness until drug effects realized.
5. Report gynecomastia or galactorrhea.
6. Report if abdominal pain, bloody stools, or other S&S of reactivated ulcer are evident.
7. Avoid alcohol, caffeine, spicy foods, and aspirin-containing products; may enhance GI irritation.
8. Do not smoke after the last dose of cimetidine to ensure optimal suppression of nocturnal gastric acid secretion. Attend smoking cessation program if unable to quit.
9. Report any new symptoms of confusion/mood swings; more common among the elderly.
10. Note any increased susceptibility to infections; may develop agranulocytosis, thrombocytopenia, or anemia; obtain periodic CBC.
11. If diarrhea develops, maintain adequate hydration, monitor frequency and severity, and report.
12. Report skin rashes/changes.
13. May alter response to skin tests with allergenic extracts. Provider may stop drug 48–72 hr prior to testing.

Outcome/Evaluate

- ↓ Abdominal pain; ulcer healing
- Control of acid hypersecretion
- Prophylaxis of GI bleeding

Cinoxacin

(sin-**OX**-ah-sin)
Pregnancy Category: B
Cinobac Pulvules **(Rx)**
Classification: Urinary anti-infective

See also *Anti-Infectives.*
Action/Kinetics: Related chemically to nalidixic acid. Acts by inhibiting DNA replication, resulting in a bactericidal action. Rapidly absorbed after PO administration; a 500-mg dose results in a urine concentration of 300 mcg/mL during the first 4-hr period and 100 mcg/mL during the second 4-hr period. Within 24 hr, 97% is excreted in the urine, 60% unchanged. **Mean serum t½:** 1.5 hr. Food decreases peak serum levels by approximately 30% but not the total amount absorbed.
Uses: Initial and recurrent UTIs caused by *Escherichia coli, Proteus mirabilis, P. vulgaris, Klebsiella,* and *Enterobacter* species. Prevents UTIs for up to 5 months in women with a history of UTIs. *NOTE:* Cinoxacin is ineffective against *Pseudomonas,* staphylococci, and enterococci infections. Prophylaxis of UTIs.

Contraindications: Hypersensitivity to cinoxacin or other quinolones. Infants and prepubertal children. Anuric clients. Lactation.
Special Concerns: Use with caution in clients with hepatic or kidney disease. Safety and efficacy in children less than 18 years of age have not been determined.
Side Effects: *GI:* N&V, anorexia, abdominal cramps and pain, diarrhea, altered sensation of taste. *CNS:* Headache, dizziness, insomnia, drowsiness, confusion, nervousness. *Hypersensitivity:* Rash, pruritus, urticaria, edema, angioedema, eosinophilia, ***anaphylaxis (rare),*** toxic epidermal necrolysis (rare), erythema multiforme, ***Stevens-Johnson syndrome***. *Other:* Tingling sensation, photophobia, perineal burning, tinnitus, thrombocytopenia.
Laboratory Test Considerations: ↑ BUN, AST, ALT, serum creatinine, and alkaline phosphatase. ↓ Hematocrit/hemoglobin.
OD **Management of Overdose:** *Symptoms:* Anorexia, N&V, epigastric distress, diarrhea, headache, dizziness, insomnia, photophobia, tinnitus, and a tingling sensation. *Treatment:* Well hydrate the client to prevent crystalluria. Maintain an airway and support ventilation and perfusion. Carefully monitor VS, blood gases, and serum electrolytes. Give activated charcoal to decrease absorption.
Drug Interactions: Probenecid ↓ excretion of cinoxacin → ↓ concentration in the urine.
How Supplied: *Capsule:* 250 mg, 500 mg

Dosage

- **Capsules**

UTIs.

Adults: 1 g/day in two to four divided doses for 7–14 days. *In clients with impaired renal function:* **Initial,** 500 mg; **then,** dosage schedule based on creatinine clearance (see package insert).

Prophylaxis of UTIs in women.

250 mg at bedtime for up to 5 months.

HEALTH CARE CONSIDERATIONS

See also *General Health Care Considerations for All Anti-Infectives.*

Assessment: Obtain baseline liver and renal function studies; hold if anuric.

Client/Family Teaching

1. Take exactly as directed.
2. Consume 2–3 L/day of fluids to ensure adequate hydration.
3. Acidic fluids enhance drug action (cranberry, prune juice); limit intake of alkaline products (milk, bicarb).
4. Avoid sun; use sunscreens, protective clothing, and sunglasses to limit photosensitivity reaction.

Outcome/Evaluate

- ↓ S&S of UTI (dysuria, frequency)
- Recurrent UTI prophylaxis

Ciprofloxacin hydrochloride

(sip-row-**FLOX**-ah-sin)
Pregnancy Category: C
Ciloxan Ophthalmic, Cipro, Cipro Cystitis Pack, Cipro I.V. **(Rx)**
Classification: Fluoroquinolone anti-infective

See also *Fluoroquinolones.*
Action/Kinetics: Effective against both gram-positive and gram-negative organisms. Rapidly and well absorbed following PO administration. Food delays absorption of the drug. **Maximum serum levels:** 2–4 mcg/mL 1–2 hr after dosing. **t½:** 4 hr for PO use and 5–6 hr for IV use. Avoid peak serum levels above 5 mcg/mL. About 40%–50% of a PO dose and 50%–70% of an IV dose is excreted unchanged in the urine.
Uses: Systemic. UTIs caused by *Escherichia coli, Enterobacter cloacae, Citrobacter diversus, Citrobacter freundii, Klebsiella pneumoniae, Proteus mirabilis, Providencia rettgeri, Pseudomonas aeruginosa, Morganella morganii, Serratia marcescens, Serratia epidermidis,* and *Streptococcus faecalis.* Uncomplicated cervical and urethral gonorrhea due to *Neisseria gonorrhoeae.* Chancroid due to *Haemophilus ducreyi*; uncomplicated or disseminated gonococcal infections.

Mild to moderate chronic bacterial prostatitis due to *E. coli* or *P. mirabilis.*

Mild to moderate sinusitis due to *S. pneumoniae, H. influenzae,* or *M. catarrhalis.*

Lower respiratory tract infections caused by *E. coli, E. cloacae, K. pneumoniae, P. mirabilis, P. aeruginosa, Haemophilus influenzae, H. parainfluenzae,* and *Streptococcus pneumoniae.*

Bone and joint infections due to *E. cloacae, P. aeruginosa,* and *S. marcescens.*

Skin and skin structure infections caused by *E. coli, E. cloacae, Citrobacter freundii, M. morganii, K. pneumoniae, P. aeruginosa, P. mirabilis, Proteus vulgaris, Providencia stuartii, Staphylococcus pyogenes, Staphylococcus epidermidis,* and penicillinase- and non-penicillinase-producing strains of *Staphylococcus aureus.*

Infectious diarrhea caused by enterotoxigenic strains of *E. coli.* Also, *Campylobacter jejuni, Shigella flexneri,* and *Shigella sonnei.*

Typhoid fever (enteric fever) due to *Salmonella typhi.* Efficacy in eradicating the chronic typhoid carrier state has not been shown.

IV as empirical therapy in febrile neutropenia.

Investigational: Clients, over 14 years of age, with cystic fibrosis who have pulmonary exacerbations due to susceptible microorganisms. Malignant external otitis. In combination with rifampin and other tuberculostatics for tuberculosis.

Ophthalmic. Superficial ocular infections due to *Staphylococcus* species (including *S. aureus*), *Streptococcus* species (including *S. pneumoniae, S. pyogenes*), *E. coli, H. ducreyi, H. influenzae, H. parainfluenzae, K. pneumoniae, N. gonorrhoeae, Proteus* species, *Klebsiella* species, *Acinetobacter calcoaceticus, Enterobacter aerogenes, P. aeruginosa, S. marcescens, Chlamydia trachomatis, Vibrio* species, and *Providencia* species.

Contraindications: Hypersensitivity to quinolones. Use in children. Lactation. Ophthalmic use in the presence of dendritic keratitis, varicella, vaccinia, and mycobacterial and fungal eye infections and after removal of foreign bodies from the cornea.

Special Concerns: Safety and effectiveness of ophthalmic, PO, or IV use have not been determined in children.

Laboratory Test Considerations: ↑ ALT, AST, alkaline phosphatase, serum bilirubin, LDH, serum creatinine, BUN, serum gamma-glutamyltransferase, serum amylase, uric acid, blood monocytes, potassium, PT, triglycerides, cholesterol. ↓ H&H. Either ↑ or ↓ blood glucose, platelets.

Additional Side Effects

See also *Side Effects* for *Fluoroquinolones.*

GI: N&V, abdominal pain/discomfort, diarrhea, dry/painful mouth, dyspepsia, heartburn, constipation, flatulence, pseudomembranous colitis, oral candidiasis, ***intestinal perforation,*** anorexia, GI bleeding, bad taste in mouth. *CNS:* Headache, dizziness, fatigue, lethargy, malaise, drowsiness, restlessness, insomnia, nightmares, hallucinations, tremor, lightheadedness, irritability, confusion, ataxia, mania, weakness, psychotic reactions, depression, depersonalization, seizures. *GU:* Nephritis, hematuria, cylindruria, renal failure, urinary retention, polyuria, vaginitis, urethral bleeding, acidosis, renal calculi, interstitial nephritis, vaginal candidiasis. *Skin:* Urticaria, photosensitivity, hypersensitivity, flushing, erythema nodosum, cutaneous candidiasis, hyperpigmentation, rash, paresthesia, edema (of lips, neck, face, conjunctivae, hands), angioedema, toxic epidermal necrolysis, exfoliative dermatitis, ***Stevens-Johnson syndrome.*** *Ophthalmic:* Blurred or disturbed vision, double vision, eye pain, nystagmus. *CV:* Hypertension, syncope, angina pectoris, palpitations, atrial flutter, ***MI, cerebral thrombosis,*** ventricular ectopy, ***cardiopulmonary arrest,*** postural hypotension. *Respiratory:* Dyspnea, ***bronchospasm, pulmonary embolism, edema of larynx or lungs,*** hemoptysis, hiccoughs, epistaxis. *Hematologic:* Eosinophilia, pancytopenia, leukopenia, anemia, leukocytosis, ***agranulocytosis,*** bleeding diathesis. *Miscellaneous:* Superinfections; fever; chills; tinnitus; joint pain or stiffness; back, neck, or chest pain; flare-up of gout; flushing; worsening of myasthenia gravis; ***hepatic necrosis;*** cholestatic jaundice; hearing loss, dysphasia.

After ophthalmic use: Irritation, burning, itching, angioneurotic edema, urticaria, maculopapular and vesicular dermatitis, crusting of lid margins, conjunctival hyperemia, bad taste in mouth, corneal staining, keratitis, keratopathy, allergic reactions, photophobia, decreased vision, tearing, lid edema. Also, a white, crystalline precipitate in the superficial part of corneal defect (onset within 1–7 days after initiating therapy; lasts about 2 weeks and does not affect continued use of the medication).

Additional Drug Interactions

Azlocillin / ↓ Excretion of ciprofloxacin → possible ↑ effect
Caffeine / ↓ Excretion of caffeine → ↑ pharmacologic effects
Cyclosporine / ↑ Nephrotoxic effect of cyclosporine
Hydantoins / ↓ Phenytoin serum levels
Theophylline / Should not be taken with ciprofloxacin

How Supplied: *Injection:* 10 mg/mL, 200 mg/100 mL, 400 mg/200 mL; *Ophthalmic solution:* 0.3%; *Ophthalmic ointment:* 0.3%; *Powder for Reconstitution:* 250 mg/5 mL, 500 mg/5 mL; *Tablet:* 100 mg, 250 mg, 500 mg, 750 mg

Dosage

- **Suspension, Tablets**

UTIs.

250 mg (mild to moderate) to 500 mg (severe/complicated) q 12 hr for 7–14 days.

Mild to moderate chronic bacterial prostatitis.

Adults: 500 mg b.i.d. for 28 days.

Mild to moderate sinusitis.

Adults: 500 mg b.i.d. for 10 days.

Urethral or cervical gonococcal infections, uncomplicated.

250 mg in a single dose.

Infectious diarrhea.

500 mg q 12 hr for 5–7 days.

Skin, skin structures, lower respiratory tract, bone and joint infections.

500 mg (mild to moderate) to 750 mg (severe or complicated) q 12 hr for 7–14 days. Treatment may be required for 4–6 weeks in bone and joint infections.

Typhoid fever.

500 mg (mild to moderate) q 12 hr for 10 days.

*Chancroid (*H. ducreyi infection).

500 mg b.i.d. for 3 days.

Disseminated gonococcal infections.

500 mg b.i.d. to complete a full week of therapy after initial treatment with ceftriaxone, 1 g IM or IV q 24 hr for 24–48 hr after improvement begins.

Uncomplicated gonococcal infections.

500 mg in a single dose plus doxycycline.

NOTE: Dose must be reduced with a C_{CR} less than 50 mL/min. The PO dose should be 250–500 mg q 12 hr if the C_{CR} is 30–50 mL/min and 250–500 mg q 18 hr (IV: 200–400 mg q 18–24 hr) if the C_{CR} is 5–29 mL/min. If the client is on hemodialysis or peritoneal dialysis, the PO dose should be 250–500 mg q 24 hr after dialysis.

• **Cipro Cystitis Pack**

Uncomplicated UTI infections.

100 mg b.i.d. for 3 days. The pack contains six 100-mg tablets of ciprofloxacin and is intended to increase compliance.

• **Ophthalmic Solution**

Acute infections.

Initial, 1–2 gtt q 15–30 min; **then,** reduce dosage as infection improves.

Moderate infections.

1–2 gtt 4–6 (or more) times/day.

HEALTH CARE CONSIDERATIONS

See also *Health Care Considerations for All Anti-infectives* and *Fluoroquinolones.*

Administration/Storage

1. Although food delays absorption of the drug, it may be taken with or without meals; recommended dosing time is 2 hr after a meal.
2. Clients on theophylline or probenecid require close observation and potential medication adjustments.
3. Do not administer to children.
4. Following instillation of ophthalmic solution, apply light finger pressure to lacrimal sac for 1 min.

Assessment

1. Note indications for therapy; obtain cultures prior to use.
2. Determine age. Not for use in children under 18 as irreversible collagen destruction has occurred.
3. Note meds currently prescribed. Fatal reactions have been reported with concurrent administration of IV ciprofloxacin and theophylline.

Client/Family Teaching

1. Take 2 hr after meals; food may delay absorption, as will antacids containing magnesium or aluminum.
2. Drink 2–3 L/day of fluids to keep the urine acidic and to minimize the risk of crystalluria.
3. May cause dizziness; use caution in any activity that requires mental alertness or coordination.
4. Report any persistent GI symptoms such as diarrhea, vomiting, or abdominal pain.
5. Review side effects; note those that should be reported immediately.

Outcome/Evaluate

• Symptomatic improvement; ↓ fever, ↓ WBCs, ↑ appetite
• Negative culture reports

Citalopram hydrobromide

(sigh-TAL-oh-pram)

Pregnancy Category: C

Celexa **(Rx)**

Classification: Antidepressant, selective serotonin-reuptake inhibitor

See also *Antidepressants.*

Action/Kinetics: Acts to inhibit reuptake of serotonin into CNS neurons resulting in increased levels of serotonin in synapses. Has minimal effects on reuptake of norepinephrine and dopamine. **Peak blood levels:** 4 hr. **t½, terminal:** 35 hr. Half-life is increased in geriatric clients. **Steady state plasma levels:** About 1 week. Metabolized in the liver and excreted in the urine.

Uses: Treatment of depression in those with DSM-IV category of major depressive disorder.

Contraindications: Use with MAO inhibitors or with alcohol. Lactation.

Special Concerns: Use with caution in severe renal impairment, a history of seizure disorders, or in diseases or conditions that produce altered metabolism or hemodynamic responses. Safety and efficacy have not been determined in children.

Side Effects: *CNS:* Activation of mania/hypomania, dizziness, insomnia, agitation, somnolence, insomnia, anorexia, paresthesia, migraine, hyperkinesia, vertigo, hypertonia, extrapyramidal disorder, neuralgia, dystonia, abnormal gait, hypesthesia, ataxia, aggravated depression, suicide attempt, confusion, aggressive reaction, drug dependence, depersonalization, hallucinations, euphoria, psychotic depression, delusions, paranoid reaction, emotional lability, panic reaction, psychosis. *GI:* N&V, dry mouth, diarrhea, dyspepsia, abdominal pain, increased salivation, flatulence, gastritis, gastroenteritis, stomatitis, eructation, hemorrhoids, dysphagia, teeth grinding, gingivitis, esophagitis. *CV:* Tachycardia, postural hypotension, hypertension, bradycardia, edema of extremities, angina pectoris, extrasystoles, ***cardiac failure, MI, CVA,*** flushing, myocardial ischemia. *Musculoskeletal:* Arthralgia, myalgia, arthritis, muscle weakness, skeletal pain, leg cramps, involuntary muscle contraction. *Hematologic:* Purpura, anemia, leukocytosis, lymphadenopathy. *Metabolic/nutritional:* Decreased or increased weight, thirst. *GU:* Ejaculation disorder, impotence, dysmenorrhea, decreased or increased libido, amenorrhea, galactorrhea, breast pain, breast enlargement, vaginal hemorrhage, polyuria, frequent micturition, urinary incontinence, urinary retention, dysuria. *Respiratory:* Coughing, epistaxis, bronchitis, dyspnea, pneumonia. *Dermatologic:* Rash, pruritus, photosensitivity reaction, urticaria, acne, skin discoloration, eczema, dermatitis, dry skin, psoriasis. *Ophthalmic:* Abnormal accommodation, conjunctivitis, eye pain. *Body as a whole:* Asthenia, fatigue, fever. *Miscellaneous:* Hyponatremia, increased sweating, yawning, hot flushes, rigors, alcohol intolerance, syncope, flu-like symptoms, taste perversion, tinnitus.

Laboratory Test Considerations: ↑ Hepatic enzymes, alkaline phosphatase. Abnormal glucose tolerance.

OD **Management of Overdose:** *Symptoms:* Dizziness, sweating, N&V, tremor, somnolence, sinus tachycardia. Rarely, amnesia, confusion, coma, convulsions, hyperventilation, cyanosis, rhabdomyolysis, ECG changes (including QTc prolongation, nodal rhythm, ventricular arrhythmias). *Treatment:* Establish and maintain an airway. Gastric lavage with use of activated charcoal. Monitor cardiac and vital signs. General symptomatic and supportive care.

Drug Interactions

Azole antifungals / ↑ Citalopram plasma levels

Carbamazepine / ↓ Citalopram plasma levels

Imipramine / ↑ Imipramine metabolite (desimpramine) by 50%

Lithium / Possible ↑ serotonergic effects of citalopram

Macrolide antibiotics / ↑ Citalopram plasma levels

MAO inhibitors / Possible serious and sometimes fatal reactions, including hyperthermia, rigidity, myoclonus, autonomic instability, mental status changes (extreme agitation, delirium, coma)

How Supplied: *Tablets:* 20 mg, 40 mg

Dosage

- **Tablets**

Depression.

Adults, initial: 20 mg once daily in the a.m. or p.m. with or without food. Increase the dose in increments of 20 mg at intervals of no less than 1 week. Doses greater than 40 mg/day are not recommended. For the elderly or those with hepatic impairment, 20 mg/day is recommended; titrate to 40 mg/day only for nonresponders. Initial treatment is continued for 6 or 8 weeks. **Maintenance:** Up to 24 weeks.

HEALTH CARE CONSIDERATIONS

See also *Health Care Considerations* for *Antidepressants.*

Administration/Storage: Allow at least 14 days to elapse between discontinuation of a monoamine oxidase inhibitor and initiation of citalopram or vice versa.

Assessment

1. Record indications for therapy, onset and characteristics of symptoms.
2. Note other drugs prescribed to ensure none interact. Avoid use with MAOs or within 14 days before or after MAO use.
3. Determine any liver or renal dysfunction or seizure disorder.
4. Assess for altered metabolic/hemodynamics; reduce dose with liver or renal dysfunction.

Client/Family Teaching

1. Take as directed, once daily, with or without food.
2. Use caution operating machines or cars until drug effects known.
3. Avoid alcohol or other CNS depressants.
4. Use reliable birth control.
5. May see improvement in 1 to 4 weeks; continue therapy as prescribed.

Outcome/Evaluate: Relief/control of depression

Clarithromycin

(klah-**rith**-roh-**MY**-sin)

Pregnancy Category: C

Biaxin **(Rx)**

Classification: Antibiotic, macrolide

See also *Anti-Infectives.*

C

Action/Kinetics: Macrolide antibiotic that acts by binding to the 50S ribosomal subunit of susceptible organisms, thus interfering with or inhibiting microbial protein synthesis. Rapidly absorbed from the GI tract although food slightly delays the onset of absorption and the formation of the active metabolite but does not affect the extent of the bioavailability. **Peak serum levels:** When fasting, 2 hr for the tablet and 3 hr for the suspension. **Steady-state peak serum levels:** 1 mcg/mL within 2–3 days after 250 mg q 12 hr and 2–3 mcg/mL after 500 mg q 12 hr. Clarithromycin and 14-OH clarithromycin (active metabolite) are readily distributed to body tissues and fluids. **t½, elimination:** 3–7 hr (depending on the dose) for clarithromycin and 5–6 hr for 14-OH clarithromycin. Up to 30% of a dose is excreted unchanged in the urine.

Uses: Mild to moderate infections caused by susceptible strains of the following. **Adults.** Pharyngitis/tonsillitis due to *Streptococcus pyogenes*. Acute maxillary sinusitis or acute bacterial exacerbaton of chronic bronchitis due to *Sreptococcus pneumoniae*, *Haemophilus influenzae*, and *Moraxella catarrhalis*. The active metabolite, 14-OH clarithromycin, has significant activity (twice the parent compound) against *H. influenzae*. Pneumonia due to *Mycoplasma pneumoniae*, *S. pneumoniae*, or *Chlamydia pneumoniae*. Uncomplicated skin and skin structure infections due to *Staphylococcus aureus* or *S. pyogenes*. Treatment of disseminated mycobacterial infections due to *Mycobacterium avium* (commonly seen in AIDS clients) and *M. intracellulare*. Prevention of disseminated *M. avium* complex (MAC) in individuals with advanced HIV.

Used with omeprazole or ranitidine bismuth citrate (Tritec) for the eradication of *Helicobacter pylori* infection in clients with active duodenal ulcers associated with *H. pylori* infection. Also with amoxicillin and lansoprazole for the same purpose.

Children. Pharyngitis or tonsillitis due to *S. pyogenes*. Acute maxillary sinusitis or acute otitis media due to *S. pneumoniae*, *H. influenzae*, and *M. catarrhalis*. Uncomplicated skin and skin structure infections due to *S. aureus* or *S. pyogenes*. Disseminated mycobacterial infections due to *M. avium* or *M. intracellulare*. Prevention of disseminated MAC disease in clients with advanced HIV infection. Community-acquired pneumonia caused by *M. pneumoniae*, *Chlamydia pneumoniae*, and *S. pneumoniae*.

Contraindications: Hypersensitivity to clarithromycin, other macrolide antibiotics, or erythromycin. Clients taking astemizole, terfenadine, cisapride, or pimozide. Use with ranitidine bismuth citrate in those with a history of acute porphyria.

Special Concerns: Use with caution in severe renal impairment with or without concomitant hepatic impairment and during lactation. Safety and effectiveness in children less than 6 months of age have not been determined. Safety has not been determined in MAC clients less than 20 months of age.

Side Effects: *GI:* Diarrhea, nausea, abnormal taste, dyspepsia, abdominal discomfort or pain, pseudomembranous colitis, glossitis, stomatitis, oral moniliasis, vomiting. *CNS:* Headache, dizziness, behavioral changes, confusion, depersonalization, disorientation, hallucinations, insomnia, nightmares, vertigo. *Allergic:* Urticaria, mild skin eruptions and, rarely, ***anaphylaxis and Stevens-Johnson syndrome.*** *Hepatic:* Hepatocellular cholestatic hepatitis with or without jaundice, increased liver enzymes, ***hepatic failure.*** *Miscellaneous:* Hearing loss (usually reversible), alteration of sense of smell (usually with taste perversion).

In children, the most common side effects are diarrhea, vomiting, abdominal pain, rash, and headache.

Laboratory Test Considerations: ↑ ALT, AST, GGT, alkaline phosphatase, LDH, total bilirubin, BUN, serum creatinine, PT. ↓ WBC count.

Drug Interactions

See also *Drug Interactions* for *Erythromycins.*

Anticoagulants / ↑ Anticoagulant effects
Astemizole / ↑ Astemizole levels; side effects, including ventricular arrhythmias, torsades de pointes, cardiac arrest, and death
Benzodiazepines / ↑ Plasma levels of certain benzodizepines → ↑ and prolonged CNS effects
Buspirone / ↑ Plasma levels of buspirone → ↑ risk of side effects
Carbamazepine / ↑ Blood levels of carbamazepine
Cisapride / Possibility of serious cardiac arrhythmias, including ventricular tachycardia, ventricular fibrillation, torsade de pointes, and QT prolongation
Cyclosporine ↑ Levels of cyclosporine → ↑ risk of nephrotoxicity and neurotoxicity
Digoxin / ↑ Plasma levels ofdigoxin due to ↓ metabolism of digoxin by the gut flora
Disopyramide / ↑ Plasma levels → arrhythmias and ↑ QTc intervals
Ergot alkaloids / Acute ergot toxicity, including severe peripheral vasospasm and dysesthesia
Fluconazole / ↑ Blood levels of clarithromycin

HMG–CoA Reductase Inhibitors / ↑ Risk of severe myopathy or rhabdomyolysis
Omeprazole / ↑ Plasma levels of omeprazole, clarithromycin, and 14-OH-clarithromycin
Pimozide / ↑ Risk of sudden death; do not use together
Ranitidine bismuth citrate / ↑ Levels of ranitidine, bismuth citrate, and 14–OH clarithromycin
Rifabutin, Rifampin / ↓ Effect of clarithromycin and ↑ GI side effects
Tacrolimus / ↑ Plasma tacrolimus levels → ↑ risk of toxicity (e.g., nephrotoxicity)
Terfenadine / ↑ Plasma levels of the active acid metabolite of terfenadine; ↑ risk of cardiac arrhythmias, including QT interval prolongation
Theophylline / ↑ Serum levels of theophylline
Triazolam / ↑ Risk of somnolence and confusion
Zidovudine (AZT) / ↓ Steady-state AZT levels in HIV-infected clients; however, peak serum AZT levels may be ↑ or ↓
How Supplied: *Granules for Oral Suspension after Reconstitution:* 125 mg/5 mL, 250 mg/5 mL; *Tablet:* 250 mg, 500 mg

Dosage

- **Tablets, Oral Suspension**

Pharyngitis, tonsillitis.
Adults: 250 mg q 12 hr for 10 days.
Acute exacerbation of chronic bronchitis due to S. pneumoniae *or* M. catarrhalis; *pneumonia due to* S. pneumoniae *or* M. pneumoniae; *uncomplicated skin and skin structure infections.*
Adults: 250 mg q 12 hr for 7–14 days.
Acute maxillary sinusitis, acute exacerbation of chronic bronchitis due to H. influenzae.
Adults: 500 mg q 12 hr for 7–14 days.
Disseminated MAC or prophylaxis of MAC.
Adults: 500 mg b.i.d.; **children:** 7.5 mg/kg b.i.d. up to 500 mg b.i.d.
NOTE: The usual daily dose for children is 15 mg/kg q 12 hr for 10 days.
Community-acquired pneumonia in children.
15 mg/kg/day of the suspension, divided and given q 12 hr for 10 days.
Active duodenal ulcers associated with H. pylori *infection.*
Clarithromycin, 500 mg t.i.d., with omeprazole, 40 mg, each morning for 2 weeks. **Then,** omeprazole is given alone at a dose of 20 mg/day for 2 more weeks. Or, clarithromycin, 500 mg t.i.d., with ranitidine bismuth citrate, 400 mg b.i.d., for 2 weeks. **Then,** ranitidine bismuth citrate is given alone at a dose of 400 mg b.i.d. for 2 more weeks. Or, clarithromycin 500 mg, plus lansoprazole, 30 mg, and amoxicillin, 1 g b.i.d. for 10 days.

C

HEALTH CARE CONSIDERATIONS

Administration/Storage

1. May be given with or without food, and both tablets and suspension can be given with milk. Food delays both the onset of absorption and the formation of 14-OH clarithromycin (the active metabolite).
2. Consider decreased doses or prolonging the dosing interval with severe renal impairment with or without hepatic impairment.
3. Shake the reconstituted suspension well before each use; use within 14 days and do not refrigerate.

Assessment

1. Note any sensitivity to erythromycin or any of the macrolide antibiotics.
2. Record type, severity, onset, and duration of symptoms.
3. List drugs currently prescribed to prevent any interactions.
4. Obtain baseline cultures, CBC, liver and renal function studies.

Client/Family Teaching

1. May take with or without meals; food delays onset of absorption. Drug may cause a bitter taste.
2. Report any persistent diarrhea; an antibiotic-associated colitis may be precipitated by *C. difficile* and require alternative management.
3. Report if no symptom improvement after 48–72 hr.

Outcome/Evaluate

- Symptomatic improvement
- Negative follow-up cultures

Clemastine fumarate

(kleh-**MAS**-teen)
Pregnancy Category: B
Antihist-1 **(OTC)**, Tavist **(Rx)**
Classification: Antihistamine

See also *Antihistamines.*
Action/Kinetics: Moderate sedative effects, high anticholinergic activity, and moderate to high antiemetic effects. **Peak blood levels:** 2–4 hr. **Peak effects:** 5–7 hr. **Duration:** 10–12 hr (up to 24 hr in some clients). Metabolized in the liver and excreted through the urine.

C

Uses: Allergic rhinitis. Urticaria and angioedema.

Contraindications: Use in newborns or premature infants. Lactation. Treatment of lower respiratory tract symptoms, including asthma. Use with monoamine oxidase (MAO) inhibitors.

Special Concerns: Use with caution in clients with narrow angle glaucoma, stenosing peptic ulcer, pyloroduodenal obstruction, symptomatic prostatic hypertrophy, and bladder neck obstruction. Use with caution in clients 60 years of age and older and in those with a history of bronchial asthma, increased intraocular pressure, hyperthyroidism, CV disease, and hypertension. Safety and efficacy have not been determined in children less than 12 years of age.

Side Effects: *CNS:* Drowsiness (common), sedation, sleepiness, dizziness, incoordination, fatigue, confusion, restlessness, excitation, nervousness, tremor, irritability, insomnia, euphoria, paresthesia, blurred vision, diplopia, vertigo, tinnitus, acute labyrinthitis, hysteria, neuritis, ***convulsions.*** *GI:* Epigastric distress, anorexia, N&V, diarrhea, constipation. *CV:* Hypotension, headache, palpitations, tachycardia, extrasystoles. *Respiratory:* Thickening of bronchial secretions, tightness of chest, wheezing, nasal stuffiness. *Hematologic:* Hemolytic anemia, thrombocytopenia, agranulocytosis. *GU:* Urinary frequency, difficulty in urination, urinary retention, early menses.

How Supplied: *Syrup:* 0.5 mg/5 mL; *Tablets:* 1.34 mg, 2.68 mg.

Dosage

- **Syrup, Tablets**

Allergic rhinitis.

Adults and children over 12 years of age, initial: 1.34 mg (1 mg clemastine) b.i.d., up to a maximum dose of 8.04 mg (60 mL of syrup or 6 tablets) daily. **Children, aged 6 to 12 years of age, initial:** 0.67 mg (0.5 mg clemastine) b.i.d., up to a maximum of 4.02 mg (3 mg) daily. Use only the syrup in children.

Urticaria and angioedema.

Adults and children over 12 years of age, initial: 2.68 mg (use tablet) 1–3 times/day, not to exceed 8.04 mg (6 tablets) daily. **Children, aged 6 to 12 years, initial:** 1.34 mg (use syrup only) b.i.d., not to exceed 4.02 mg daily.

HEALTH CARE CONSIDERATIONS

See also *Health Care Considerations* for *Antihistamines.*

Administration/Storage: Store the syrup below 77°F (25°C) in a tight, amber glass bottle. Store tablets at room temperatures between 15°C and 30°C (59°F–86°F) in a tight, light-resistant container.

Assessment

1. Record onset, duration, and characteristics of symptoms; identify triggers.
2. Determine any evidence or history of asthma, BPH, HTN, PUD, or glaucoma.
3. Obtain baseline CBC, VS, ECG, ENT, and CP assessments.

Client/Family Teaching

1. Take as directed; do not exceed prescribed dose.
2. Do not perform activities that require mental alertness until drug effects realized; dizziness and drowsiness may occur.
3. Avoid alcohol and any other CNS depressants.
4. Use sugarless gum and candy or sips of water for dry mouth symptoms. Report any intolerable side effects or loss of symptom control.

Outcome/Evaluate: Relief of allergic manifestations.

Clindamycin hydrochloride

(klin-dah-**MY**-sin)

Pregnancy Category: B

Cleocin, Dalacin C ✱ **(Rx)**

Clindamycin palmitate hydrochloride

(klin-dah-**MY**-sin)

Pregnancy Category: B

Cleocin Pediatric, Dalacin C Palmitate ✱ **(Rx)**

Clindamycin phosphate

(klin-dah-**MY**-sin)

Pregnancy Category: B (vaginal cream, topical gel, lotion, solution)

Cleocin Phosphate, Cleocin T, Cleocin Vaginal Cream, Clinda-Derm, C/T/S, Dalacin C Phosphate ✱, Dalacin T Topical ✱, Dalacin Vaginal Cream ✱ **(Rx)**

Classification: Antibiotic, clindamycin and lincomycin

See also *Anti-Infectives.*

Action/Kinetics: A semisynthetic antibiotic that suppresses protein synthesis by microorganism by binding to ribosomes (50S subunit) and preventing peptide bond formation. Is both bacteriostatic and bactericidal. **Peak serum concentration: PO,** 4 mcg/mL after 300 mg; **IM,** 4.9 mcg/mL after 300 mg; **IV,** 14.7 mcg/mL after 300 mg. **t½:** 2.4–3 hr. In serious infections the rate of IV administration is adjusted to maintain appropriate serum drug concentrations: 4–6 mcg/mL.

Uses: Should not be used for trivial infections. **Systemic.** *Anareobes:* Serious respiratory tract infections (e.g., empyema, lung abscess, anaerobic pneumonitis). Serious skin and soft tissue infections, septicemia, intra-abdominal infections (e.g., peritonitis, intra–abdominal abscess), infections of the female pelvis and genital tract (e.g., PID, endometritis, nongonococcal tubo–ovarian abscess, pelvic cellulitis, postsurgical vaginal cuff infection). *Streptococci/staphylococci:* Serious respiratory tract infections, serious skin and soft tissue infections, septicemia (parenteral use), acute staphylococcal hematogenous osteomyelitis (parenteral use). *Pneumonococcus:* Serious respiratory tract infections. Adjunct to surgery for chronic bone/joint infections. *Investigational:* Alternative to sulfonamides in combination with pyrimethamine in the acute treatment of CNS toxoplasmosis in AIDS clients. In combination with primaquine to treat *Pneumocystis carinii* pneumonia. Chlamydial infections in women. Bacterial vaginosis due to *Gardnerella vaginalis*. **Topical Use.** Used topically for inflammatory acne vulgaris. Vaginally to treat bacterial vaginosis. *Investigational:* Treatment of rosacea (lotion used).

Contraindications: Hypersensitivity to either clindamycin or lincomycin. Use in treating viral and minor bacterial infections or in clients with a history of regional enteritis, nonbacterial infections (e.g., most URIs), ulcerative colitis, meningitis, or antibiotic-associated colitis. Lactation.

Special Concerns: Use with caution in infants up to 1 month of age, in clients with GI disease, liver or renal disease, or a history of allergy or asthma. Safety and efficacy of topical products have not been established in children less than 12 years of age.

Side Effects: *GI:* N&V, diarrhea, ***pseudomembranous colitis*** (more frequent after PO use), abdominal pain, esophagitis, unpleasant or metallic taste (after high IV doses), glossitis, stomatitis. *CV:* Hypotension, ***rarely, cardiopulmonary arrest after too rapid IV use.*** *Allergic:* Morbilliform rash (most common), skin rashes, urticaria, erythema multiforme, ***anaphylaxis, Stevens-Johnson-like syndrome,*** maculopapular rash, angioneurotic edema. *Hematologic:* Leukopenia, neutropenia, thrombocytopenia, transient eosinophilia, ***agranulocytosis, aplastic anemia.*** *Hepatic:* Jaundice, abnormal LFT's. *GU:* Renal dysfunction (azotemia, oliguria, proteinuria), vaginitis. *Miscellaneous:* Superinfection, tinnitus, polyarthritis. Also sore throat, fatigue, urinary frequency, headache.

Following IV use: Thrombophlebitis, erythema, pain, swelling. *Following IM use:* Pain, induration, sterile abscesses.

Following topical use: Erythema, irritation, dryness, peeling, itching, burning, oiliness of skin.

Following vaginal use: Cervicitis, vaginitis, vulvar irritation, urticaria, rash.

NOTE: The injection contains benzyl alcohol, which has been associated with ***fatal "gasping syndrome" in infants.***

Laboratory Test Considerations: ↓ Levels of AST, ALT, NPN, alkaline phosphatase, bilirubin, BSP retention, and ↓ platelet count.

Drug Interactions

Antiperistaltic antidiarrheals (opiates, Lomotil) / ↑ Diarrhea due to ↓ removal of toxins from colon

Ciprofloxacin HCl / Additive antibacterial activity

Erythromycin / Cross-interference → ↓ effect of both drugs

Kaolin/Pectin (e.g., Kaopectate) / ↓ Effect due to ↓ absorption from GI tract

Neuromuscular blocking agents / ↑ Effect of blocking agents

How Supplied: Clindamycin hydrochloride: *Capsule:* 75 mg, 150 mg, 300 mg. Clindamycin palmitate: *Granule for oral solution:* 75 mg/5 mL. Clindamycin phosphate: *Vaginal cream:* 2%; *Gel:* 1%; *Injection:* 150 mg/mL, 300 mg/50 mL, 600 mg/50 mL, 900 mg/50 mL; *Lotion:* 1%; *Solution:* 1%; *Swab:* 1%

Dosage

- **Capsules, Oral Solution**

Serious infections.

Adults: 150–300 mg q 6 hr. **Pediatric, Clindamycin hydrochloride:** 8–16 mg/kg/day divided into three or four equal doses. **Pediatric, clindamycin palmitate hydrochloride:** 8–12 mg/kg/day divided into three or four equal doses.

More severe infections.

Adults: 300–450 mg q 6 hr. **Pediatric, Clindamycin hydrochloride:** 16–20 mg/kg/day divided into three or four equal doses. **Pediatric, clindamycin palmitate hydrochloride:** 13–25 mg/kg/day divided into three or four equal doses. **Children less than 10 kg:** Minimum recommended dose is 37.5 mg t.i.d.

- **IM, IV**

Serious infections due to aerobic gram–positive cocci.

Adults: 600–1,200 mg/day in two to four equal doses. **Pediatric, over 1 month to 16 years:** 350 mg/m²/day.

More severe infections due to B. fragilis, Peptococcus, or Clostridium (other than C.perfringens).

Adults: 1,200–2,700 mg/day in two to four equal doses. May have to be increased in more serious infections. **Pediatric, over 1 month to 16 years:** 450 mg/m²/day.

Life-threatening infections.

Adults: 4.8 g IV. **Pediatric, 1 month to 16 years:** 20–40 mg/kg/day in three to four equal doses depending on severity of infections. **Pediatric, less than 1 month of age:** 15–20 mg/kg/day in three or four equal doses.

Acute pelvic inflammatory disease.

IV: 900 mg q 8 hr plus gentamicin loading dose of 2 mg/kg IV or IM; **then,** gentamicin, 1.5 mg/kg q 8 hr IV or IM. Therapy may be discontinued 24 hr after client improves. After discharge from the hospital, continue with doxycycline PO, 100 mg b.i.d. for 10–14 days. Alternatively, give clindamycin, PO, 450 mg q.i.d. for 14 days.

• **Topical Gel, Lotion, or Solution**

Apply thin film b.i.d. to affected areas. One or more pledgets may also be used.

• **Vaginal Cream (2%)**

Bacterial vaginosis

One applicatorful (containing about 100 mg clindamycin phosphate), preferably at bedtime, for 3 or 7 consecutive days.

HEALTH CARE CONSIDERATIONS

See also *General Health Care Considerations for All Anti-Infectives.*

Administration/Storage

1. For anaerobic infections, use the parenteral form initially; may be followed by PO therapy.
2. For β–hemolytic streptococci infections, continue treatment for at least 10 days.
3. Reduce dosage in severe renal impairment.
4. Single IM injections greater than 600 mg are not advisable. Inject deeply into muscle to prevent induration, pain, and sterile abscesses.
5. Do not refrigerate the reconstituted solution as it may become thickened and difficult to pour.
6. Shake lotion well just before using.

Assessment

1. Record indications for therapy, type and onset of symptoms.
2. Auscultate lungs and note extent of respiratory tract infections.
3. Describe skin and soft tissue infections; note complaints indicative of pelvic inflammatory disease or intra-abdominal infections.
4. Obtain baseline cultures, liver and renal function studies. Note any history of liver or renal disease, allergies, or GI problems.
5. With IV therapy, observe for hypotension; keep in bed for 30 min following infusion. Advise that a bitter taste may be evident.
6. Observe for drug interactions caused by concurrent administration of neuromuscular blocking agents. Be alert to hypotension, bronchospasms, cardiac disturbances, hyperthermia, and respiratory depression.
7. Observe closely for:
   • Skin rash; frequently reported
   • Renal and/or hepatic impairment and newborns for organ dysfunction
   • GI disturbances, such as abdominal pain, diarrhea, anorexia, N&V, bloody or tarry stools, and excessive flatulence.

Client/Family Teaching

1. Take PO medication with a full glass of water to prevent esophageal ulceration. May be taken with or without food.
2. Report any side effects such as persistent vomiting, diarrhea, fever, or abdominal pain and cramping.
3. Pseudomembranous colitis may occur 2–9 days or several weeks after initiation of therapy. Fluids, electrolytes, protein supplements, systemic corticosteroids, and oral antibiotics may be needed. Do not use antiperistaltic agents if diarrhea occurs because these can prolong or aggravate condition. Kaolin will reduce absorption of antibiotic; if prescribed, take 3 hr before drug.
4. The vaginal cream contains mineral oil, which may weaken latex or rubber products, such as condoms or vaginal contraceptive diaphragms; avoid for 72 hr following treatment.
5. Do not engage in intercourse when using the vaginal cream as this may enhance irritation.
6. Do not use any acne or topical mercury preparations containing a peeling agent in affected area; severe irritation may occur.

Outcome/Evaluate

• Resolution of infection
• Symptomatic improvement
• Therapeutic drug levels with IV therapy (4–6 mcg/mL)

Clobetasol propionate

(kloh-**BAY**-tah-sohl)

Pregnancy Category: C

Alti-Clobetasol Propionate ✦, Cormax, Dermasone ✦, Dermovate ✦, Gen-Clobetasol Cream/Ointment ✦, Gen-Clobetasol Scalp Application ✦, Novo-Clobetasol ✦, Temovate **(Rx)**

Classification: Corticosteroid, topical

See also *Corticosteroids.*

Action/Kinetics: Has anti-inflammatory, antipruritic, and vasoconstrictive effects.
Uses: Relief of inflammatory and pruritic dermatoses.
Contraindications: Use in children less than 12 years old, use for more than 2 weeks, to treat rosacea or perioral dermatitis, and use on face, groin, axillae.
Special Concerns: May suppress hypothalamic-pituitary-adrenal (HPA) axis at doses as low as 2 g/day. Use with caution during lactation.
Side Effects: *Dermatologic:* Burning sensation, itching, stinging, irritation, dryness, pruritus, erythema, folliculitis, hypertrichosis, acneform eruptions, hypopigmentation, perioral dermatitis, allergic contact dermatitis, skin maceration, secondary infection, striae, millaria, cracking and fissuring of the skin, skin atrophy, numbness of fingers, telangiectasia. *Miscellaneous:* Cushing's syndrome.
How Supplied: *Cream:* 0.05%; *Foam:* 0.05%; *Gel:* 0.05%; *Ointment:* 0.05%; *Scalp Application:* 0.05%

Dosage

- **Topical cream, foam, gel**

Dermatoses.

Apply thin layer to affected skin b.i.d. once in the morning and once in the evening. Rub in gently and completely. Use no more than 50 g/week.

HEALTH CARE CONSIDERATIONS

Administration/Storage

1. Do not use occlusive dressings.
2. Do not refrigerate.

Assessment

1. Record onset, location, and characteristics of symptoms or photograph area; note other agents trialed and outcome.
2. Drug is a potent corticosteroid for short term use; assess for S&S of HPA axis suppression using ACTH stimulation test, a.m. cortisol, and urinary free cortisol test.

Client/Family Teaching

1. Apply thin layer to affected area and gently rub in. Use only as directed, externally, avoid eye contact.
2. Wash hands before and after application. Do not cover, wrap, or bandage treatment area.
3. Report any failure to heal as this may indicate an allergic contact dermatitis from agent.
4. If skin infections develop, may also need antifungal or antibacterial agent; report if evident.
5. Report any severe burning, stinging, swelling, numbness, or lack of response.

Outcome/Evaluate: Relief of inflammation and pruritic skin manifestations

Clofibrate

(kloh-**FYE**-brayt)

Pregnancy Category: C
Atromid-S, Claripex ✱, Novo-Fibrate ✱ **(Rx)**
Classification: Antihyperlipidemic agent

Action/Kinetics: Decreases triglycerides and VLDL; cholesterol and LDL are decreased less predictably and less effectively. Mechanism may be due to increased catabolism of VLDL to LDL and decreased synthesis of VLDL by the liver. Cholesterol formation is inhibited early in the biosynthetic chain; excretion of neutral streoids is increased. **Peak plasma levels:** 3–6 hr. **t½, plasma:** 15 hr. **Therapeutic effect: Onset,** 2–5 days; **maximum effect:** 3 weeks. Triglycerides return to pretreatment levels 2–3 weeks after therapy is terminated. Hydrolyzed to the active *p*-chlorophenoxyisobutyric acid which is further metabolized and excreted in the urine. Drug may concentrate in fetal blood. LFTs should be performed during therapy.
Uses: Dysbetalipoproteinemia (type III hyperlipidemia) not responding to diet. Hyperlipidemia (types IV and V) with a risk of abdominal pain and pancreatitis not responding to diet.
Contraindications: Impaired hepatic or renal function, primary biliary cirrhosis, lactation, pregnancy, children.
Special Concerns: Use with caution in clients with gout and peptic ulcer. Reduced dosage may be required in geriatric clients due to age-related decreases in renal function.
Side Effects: *GI:* Nausea, dyspepsia, weight gain, gastritis, vomiting, bloating, flatulence, abdominal distress, stomatitis, loose stools, diarrhea, hepatomegaly, cholelithiasis, gallstones. *CNS:* Headaches, dizziness, fatigue, weakness, drowsiness. *CV:* Changes in blood-clotting time, arrhythmias, increased or decreased angina, intermittent claudication, thromboembolic events, thrombophlebitis, swelling and phlebitis at xanthoma site, pulmonary embolism. *Skeletal muscle:* Asthenia, arthralgia, myalgia, weakness, muscle cramps, aches. *GU:* Impotence, dysuria, hematuria, decreased urine output, decreased libido, proteinuria. *Hematologic:* Anemia, leukopenia, eosinophilia. *Dermatologic:* Allergic reactions, including urticaria, skin rash, dry skin, pruritus, dry brittle hair,

alopecia. *Other:* Dyspnea, polyphagia, flu-like symptoms, ***noncardiovascular death.***
Laboratory Test Considerations: ↑ AST, ALT, thymol turbidity, CPK, BSP retention. Proteinuria.

C

Drug Interactions
Anticoagulants / Clofibrate ↑ anticoagulant effect by ↓ plasma protein binding
Antidiabetics (sulfonylureas) / Clofibrate ↑ effect of antidiabetics
Furosemide / Exaggerated diuretic response
Insulin / Clofibrate ↑ effect of insulin
Probenecid / ↑ Therapeutic and toxic effects of clofibrate due to ↓ breakdown by liver and ↓ kidney excretion
Ursodiol / ↑ Risk of gallstone formation
How Supplied: *Capsule:* 500 mg

Dosage

- **Capsules**

Antihyperlipidemic.

Adults: 500 mg q.i.d. Therapeutic response may take several weeks to become apparent. Drug must be administered on a continuous basis because lowered levels of cholesterol and other lipids will return to elevated state within several weeks after administration is stopped. Discontinue after 3 months if response is poor.

HEALTH CARE CONSIDERATIONS

Assessment: Obtain baseline CBC, liver and renal function studies; document cholesterol profile and pregnancy test if appropriate.

Client/Family Teaching

1. If GI upset occurs, take with food. Nausea usually decreases with continued therapy or reduced dose.
2. Anticoagulant dosage is reduced if clofibrate is instituted; report any abnormal bleeding.
3. Report symptoms of hypoglycemia because of possible drug interactions with oral antidiabetic agents.
4. Use contraception during and for several months after drug therapy if pregnancy is planned; drug may be teratogenic.
5. Review potential risks of drug therapy (e.g., gallstones, tumors); report any unusual side effects.
6. Stress importance of adhering to dietary restrictions, daily exercise, and weight loss in the overall management of high cholesterol.

Outcome/Evaluate: Significant ↓ in serum cholesterol and triglyceride levels

Clomiphene citrate

(KLOH-mih-feen)

Clomid, Serophene **(Rx)**
Classification: Ovarian stimulant

Action/Kinetics: Combines with estrogen receptors, thus decreasing the number of available receptor sites. Through negative feedback, the hypothalamus and pituitary are thus stimulated to increase secretion of LH and FSH. Under the influence of increased levels of these hormones, an ovarian follicle develops, followed by ovulation and corpus luteum development. Most women ovulate after the first course of therapy. Further treatment may be inadvisable if pregnancy fails to occur after ovulatory responses. Readily absorbed from the GI tract and excreted in the feces. **t½:** 5–7 days. **Time to peak effect:** 4–10 days after the last day of treatment for ovulation.
Uses: To treat ovulatory failure in women desiring pregnancy and whose partners are fertile and potent. Normal liver function and normal levels of endogenous estrogen are necessary criteria to clomiphene use. Therapy is ineffective in clients with ovarian or pituitary failure. *Investigational:* Male infertility (controversial).
Contraindications: Pregnancy, liver disease or history thereof, abnormal bleeding of undetermined origin. Ovarian cysts or enlargement not due to polycystic ovarian syndrome. Uncontrolled thyroid or adrenal dysfunction, organic intracranial lesion (e.g., pituitary tumor). The absence of neoplastic disease should be established before treatment is initiated.
Special Concerns: Multiple births are possible.
Side Effects: *Ovarian:* Ovarian overstimulation and/or enlargement and subsequent symptoms resembling those of PMS. *Ophthalmologic:* Blurred vision, spots, or flashes, probably due to intensification of after images. Although cause and effect have not been established, the following have been noted in users of clomiphene: posterior capsular cataract, detachment of the posterior vitreous, spasm of retinal arteriole, and thrombosis of temporal arteries of retina. *GI:* Abdominal distention, pain, bloating, or soreness; N&V. *GU:* Abnormal uterine bleeding, breast tenderness, increased urination. *CNS:* Insomnia, nervousness, headache, depression, fatigue, lightheadedness, dizziness. *Other:* Hot flashes, allergic dermatitis, urticaria, weight gain, alopecia (reversible).
Laboratory Test Considerations: ↑ Serum thyroxine, thyroxine-binding globulin, BSP retention.
How Supplied: *Tablet:* 50 mg

Dosage

- **Tablets**

First course.

50 mg/day for 5 days. Therapy may be initiated at any time in clients who have had no recent uterine bleeding.

Second course.

Same dosage if ovulation has occurred. In absence of ovulation, dose may be increased to 100 mg/day for 5 days. This course may be started as early as 30 days after the previous one.

Third course.

Most clients who are going to respond will do so during the first course of therapy. Three courses are an adequate therapeutic trial. If ovulatory menses has not occurred, reevaluate diagnosis.

HEALTH CARE CONSIDERATIONS

Administration/Storage: If the client has had recent uterine bleeding, start the therapy on the fifth day of the cycle.

Assessment

1. Obtain menstrual history and any history of abnormal bleeding of undetermined origin.
2. Note history of hepatic dysfunction; document LFTs and abdominal US.
3. Determine if pregnant.

Client/Family Teaching

1. Take basal temperature and chart on graph to determine if ovulation has occurred; usually 4–10 days after treatment.
2. Take at the same time each day.
3. Discontinue drug and report if pain in the pelvic area or abdominal distention occurs; may indicate ovarian enlargement, presence of an ovarian cyst or rupture.
4. Stop drug if blurred vision or spots or flashes in the eyes occur; the retina may be affected. Report for an ophthalmologic exam.
5. Avoid performing hazardous tasks involving body coordination or mental alertness; drug may cause lightheadedness, dizziness, or visual disturbances.
6. Stop drug and report if pregnancy is suspected; drug may have teratogenic effects.
7. Potential for multiple pregnancy exists.

Outcome/Evaluate

- ↑ Levels of FSH and LH
- Ovulation → pregnancy

Clomipramine hydrochloride

(kloh-**MIP**-rah-meen)

Pregnancy Category: C

Anafranil, Apo-Clomipramine ✦, Gen-Clomipramine ✦, Med-Clomipramine ✦, Novo-Clopamine ✦, Penta-Clomipramine ✦

(Rx)

Classification: Antidepressant, tricyclic

See also *Antidepressants, Tricyclic.*

Action/Kinetics: Significant anticholinergic and sedative effects as well as moderate orthostatic hypotension. Significant serotonin uptake blocking activity and moderate blocking activity for norepinephrine. **t½:** 19–37 hr. **Effective plasma levels:** 80–100 ng/mL. **Time to reach steady state:** 7–14 days. Metabolized to the active desmethylclomipramine.

Uses: Obsessive-compulsive disorder in which the obsessions or compulsions cause marked distress, significantly interfere with social or occupational activities, or are time-consuming. Panic attacks and cataplexy associated with narcolepsy.

Contraindications: To relieve symptoms of depression.

Special Concerns: Safety has not been established for use during lactation or in children less than 10 years of age.

Additional Side Effects: Hyperthermia, especially when used with other drugs. Increased risk of ***seizures.*** Aggressive reactions, asthenia, anemia, eructation, failure to ejaculate, laryngitis, vestibular disorders, muscle weakness.

How Supplied: *Capsule:* 25 mg, 50 mg, 75 mg

Dosage

- **Capsules**

Adult, initial: 25 mg/day; **then,** increase gradually to approximately 100 mg during the first 2 weeks (depending on client tolerance). The dose may then be increased slowly to a maximum of 250 mg/day over the next several weeks. **Adolescents, children, initial:** 25 mg/day; **then,** increase gradually during the first 2 weeks to a maximum of 100 mg or 3 mg/kg, whichever is less. The dose may then be increased to a maximum daily dose of 3 mg/kg or 200 mg, whichever is less. **Maintenance, adults and children:** Adjust the dose to the lowest effective dose with periodic reassessment to determine need for continued therapy.

HEALTH CARE CONSIDERATIONS

See also *Health Care Considerations* for *Antidepressants, Tricyclic.*

Administration/Storage

1. Initially, divide the daily dosage and give with meals to reduce GI side effects.
2. After the optimum dose is determined, the total daily dose can be given at bedtime to minimize daytime sedation.
3. For all ages, adjust to the lowest effective dose and evaluate periodically to determine need for continued treatment.
4. Although efficacy of clomipramine has not been determined after 10 weeks of therapy, clients have successfully used it for up to 1 year without loss of beneficial effects.

Assessment

1. Record indications for therapy and baseline behavorial findings.
2. List drugs currently prescribed, those used previously for this disorder, and the outcome.

Client/Family Teaching

1. Take only as directed. May give with meals to reduce GI side effects.
2. Rise slowly to prevent orthostatic drug effects, i.e., dizziness. May take at bedtime to minimize daytime sedation.
3. Report symptoms of depression.
4. Fluids and lozenges may relieve symptoms of dry mouth.
5. Anticipate 2–3 weeks of therapy before desired effect.

Outcome/Evaluate: Control of obsessive-compulsive behaviors that interfere with normal social or occupational functioning

Clonazepam

(kloh-**NAY**-zeh-pam)

Alti-Clonazepam ✱, Apo-Clonazepam ✱, Clonapam ✱, Dom-Clonazepam ✱, Gen-Clonazepam ✱, Klonopin, Nu-Clonazepam ✱, PMS–Clonazepam ✱, Rivotril ✱ **(C-IV) (Rx)**

Classification: Anticonvulsant, miscellaneous

See also *Anticonvulsants.*

Action/Kinetics: Benzodiazepine derivative which increases presynaptic inhibition and suppresses the spread of seizure activity. **Peak plasma levels:** 1–2 hr. **t½:** 18–60 hr. **Therapeutic serum levels:** 20–80 ng/mL. More than 80% bound to plasma protein; metabolized almost completely in the liver to inactive metabolites, which are excreted in the urine.

Even though a benzodiazepine, clonazepam is used only as an anticonvulsant. However, contraindications, side effects, and so forth are similar to those for diazepam.

Uses: Absence seizures (petit mal) including Lennox-Gastaut syndrome, akinetic and myoclonic seizures. Some effectiveness in clients resistant to succinimide therapy. *Investigational:* Parkinsonian dysarthria, acute manic episodes of bipolar affective disorder, leg movements (periodic) during sleep, adjunct in treating schizophrenia, neuralgias, multifocal tic disorders.

Contraindications: Sensitivity to benzodiazepines. Severe liver disease, acute narrow-angle glaucoma. Pregnancy.

Special Concerns: Effects on lactation not known.

Additional Side Effects: In clients in whom different types of seizure disorders exist, clonazepam may elicit or precipitate ***grand mal seizures.***

Drug Interactions

CNS depressants / Potentiation of CNS depressant effect of clonazepam
Phenobarbital / ↓ Effect of clonazepam due to ↑ breakdown by liver
Phenytoin / ↓ Effect of clonazepam due to ↑ breakdown by liver
Valproic acid / ↑ Chance of absence seizures

How Supplied: *Tablet:* 0.5 mg, 1 mg, 2 mg

Dosage

- **Tablets**

Seizure disorders.

Adults, initial: 0.5 mg t.i.d. Increase by 0.5–1 mg/day q 3 days until seizures are under control or side effects become excessive; **maximum:** 20 mg/day. **Pediatric up to 10 years or 30 kg:** 0.01–0.03 mg/kg/day in two to three divided doses up to a maximum of 0.05 mg/kg/day. Increase by increments of 0.25–0.5 mg q 3 days until seizures are under control or maintenance of 0.1–0.2 mg/kg is attained.

Parkinsonian dysarthria.

Adults: 0.25–0.5 mg/day.

Acute manic episodes of bipolar affective disorder.

Adults: 0.75–16 mg/day.

Periodic leg movements during sleep.

Adults: 0.5–2 mg nightly.

Adjunct to treat schizophrenia.

Adults: 0.5–2 mg/day.

Neuralgias.

Adults: 2–4 mg/day.

Multifocal tic disorders.

Adults: 1.5–12 mg/day.

HEALTH CARE CONSIDERATIONS

See also *Health Care Considerations* for *Tranquilizers/Antimanic Drugs/Hypnotics and Anticonvulsants.*

Administration/Storage

1. Approximately one-third of clients show some loss of anticonvulsant activity within 3 months; dosage adjustment may reestablish effectiveness.

2. Adding clonazepam to existing anticonvulsant therapy may increase the depressant effects.
3. Divide the daily dose into three equal doses; if doses cannot be divided equally, give the largest dose at bedtime.

Assessment

1. Record indications for therapy, onset/cause of symptoms, other agents prescribed, and the outcome.
2. Obtain baseline CBC, liver and renal function studies.

Outcome/Evaluate: ↓ Number and frequency of recurrent seizures

Clonidine hydrochloride

(KLOH-nih-deen)

Pregnancy Category: C

Apo-Clonidine ✱; Catapres; Catapres-TTS-1, -2, and -3; Dixarit ✱; Duraclon, Novo-Clonidine ✱, Nu-Clonidine ✱ **(Rx)**

Classification: Antihypertensive, centrally acting antiadrenergic

See also *Antihypertensive Agents.*

Action/Kinetics: Stimulates alpha-adrenergic receptors of the CNS, which results in inhibition of the sympathetic vasomotor centers and decreased nerve impulses. Thus, bradycardia and a fall in both SBP and DBP occur. Plasma renin levels are decreased, while peripheral venous pressure remains unchanged. Few orthostatic effects. Although NaCl excretion is markedly decreased, potassium excretion remains unchanged. To relieve spasticity, it decreases excitatory amino acids by central presynaptic α–receptor agonism. Tolerance to the drug may develop. **Onset, PO:** 30–60 min; **transdermal:** 2–3 days. **Peak plasma levels, PO:** 3–5 hr; **transdermal:** 2–3 days. **Maximum effect, PO:** 2–4 hr. **Duration, PO:** 12–24 hr; **transdermal:** 7 days (with system in place). **t½:** 12–16 hr. Approximately 50% excreted unchanged in the urine; 20% excreted through the feces.

The transdermal dosage form contains the following levels of drug: Catapres-TTS-1 contains 2.5 mg clonidine (surface area 3.5 cm^2), with 0.1 mg released daily; Catapres-TTS-2 contains 5 mg clonidine (surface area 7 cm^2), with 0.2 mg released daily; and Catapres-TTS-3 contains 7.5 mg clonidine (surface area 10.5 cm^2), with 0.3 mg released daily.

Epidural use causes analgesia at presynaptic and postjunctional alpha-2-adrenergic receptors in the spinal cord due to prevention of pain signal transmission to the brain. **t½, distribution, epidural:** 19 min; **elimination:** 22 hr.

Uses: Oral, Transdermal: Mild to moderate hypertension. A diuretic or other antihypertensive drugs, or both, are often used concomitantly. Treat spasticity. *Investigational:* Alcohol withdrawal, atrial fibrillation, attention deficit hyperactivity disorder, constitutional growth delay in children, cyclosporine-associated nephrotoxicity, diabetic diarrhea, Gilles de la Tourette's syndrome, hyperhidrosis, hypertensive emergencies, mania, menopausal flushing, opiate detoxification, diagnosis of pheochromocytoma, postherpetic neuralgia, psychosis in schizophrenia, reduce allergen-induced inflammatory reactions in extrinsic asthma, restless leg syndrome, facilitate smoking cessation, ulcerative colitis.

Epidural: With opiates for severe pain in cancer clients not relieved by opiate analgesics alone. Most effective for neuropathic pain.

Contraindications: Epidurally: Presence of an injection site infection, clients on anticoagulant therapy, in bleeding diathesis, administration above the C4 dermatome. For obstetric, postpartum, or perioperative pain.

Special Concerns: Use with caution during lactation and in the presence of severe coronary insufficiency, recent MI, cerebrovascular disease, or chronic renal failure. Safe use in children not established. Geriatric clients may be more sensitive to the hypotensive effects; a decreased dosage may also be necessary in these clients due to age-related decreases in renal function. For children, restrict epidural use to severe intractable pain from malignancy that is not responsive to epidural or spinal opiates or other analgesic approaches.

Side Effects: *CNS:* Drowsiness (common), sedation, confusion, dizziness, headache, fatigue, malaise, nightmares, nervousness, restlessness, anxiety, mental depression, increased dreaming, insomnia, hallucinations, delirium, agitation. *GI:* Dry mouth (common), constipation, anorexia, N&V, parotid pain, weight gain, hepatitis, parotitis, ileus, pseudo-obstruction, abdominal pain. *CV:* CHF, severe hypotension, Raynaud's phenomenon, abnormalities in ECG, palpitations, tachycardia and bradycardia, postural hypotension, conduction disturbances, sinus bradycardia, ***CVA***. *Dermatologic:* Urticaria, skin rashes, sweating, ***angioneurotic edema,*** pruritus, thinning of hair, alopecia, skin ulcer. *GU:* Impotence, urinary retention, decreased sexual activity, loss of libido, nocturia, difficulty in urination, UTI. *Respiratory:* Hypoventilation, dyspnea. *Musculoskeletal:* Muscle or joint pain, leg cramps, weakness. *Other:*

Gynecomastia, increase in blood glucose (transient), increased sensitivity to alcohol, chest pain, tinnitus, hyperaesthesia, pain, infection, thrombocytopenia, syncope, blurred vision, withdrawal syndrome, dryness of mucous membranes of nose; itching, burning, dryness of eyes; skin pallor, fever.

Transdermal products: Localized skin reactions, pruritus, erythema, allergic contact sensitization and contact dermatitis, localized vesiculation, hyperpigmentation, edema, excoriation, burning, papules, throbbing, blanching, generalized macular rash.

NOTE: Rebound hypertension may be manifested if clonidine is withdrawn abruptly.

Laboratory Test Considerations: Transient ↑ blood glucose, serum phosphatase, and serum CPK. Weakly + Coombs' test. Alteration of electrolyte balance.

OD **Management of Overdose:** *Symptoms:* Hypotension, bradycardia, respiratory and CNS depression, hypoventilation, hypothermia, apnea, miosis, agitation, irritability, lethargy, ***seizures, cardiac conduction defects, arrhythmias,*** transient hypertension, diarrhea, vomiting. *Treatment:* Maintain respiration; perform gastric lavage followed by activated charcoal. Magnesium sulfate may be used to hasten the rate of transport through the GI tract. IV atropine sulfate (0.6 mg for adults; 0.01 mg/kg for children), epinephrine, tolazoline, or dopamine to treat persistent bradycardia. IV fluids and elevation of the legs are used to reverse hypotension; if unresponsive to these measures, dopamine (2–20 mcg/kg/min) or tolazoline (1 mg/kg IV, up to a maximum of 10 mg/dose) may be used. To treat hypertension, diazoxide, IV furosemide, or an alpha-adrenergic blocking drug may be used.

Drug Interactions

Alcohol / ↑ Depressant effects
Beta-adrenergic blocking agents / Paradoxical hypertension; also, ↑ severity of rebound hypertension following clonidine withdrawal
CNS depressants / ↑ Depressant effect
Levodopa / ↓ Effect of levodopa
Local anesthetics / Epidural clonidine → prolonged duration of epidural local anesthetics
Narcotic analgesics / Potentiation of hypotensive effect of clonidine
Prazosin / ↓ Antihypertensive effect of clonidine
Tolazoline / Blocks antihypertensive effect
Tricyclic antidepressants / Blocks antihypertensive effect
Verapamil / ↑ Risk of AV block and severe hypotension

How Supplied: *Film, Extended Release:* 0.1 mg/24 hrs, 0.2 mg/24 hrs, 0.3 mg/24 hrs; *Injection:* 0.1 mg/mL; *Tablet:* 0.1 mg, 0.2 mg, 0.3 mg

Dosage

- **Tablets**

Hypertension.

Initial: 100 mcg b.i.d.; **then,** increase by 100–200 mcg/day until desired response is attained; **maintenance:** 200–600 mcg/day in divided doses (maximum: 2400 mcg/day). Tolerance necessitates increased dosage or concomitant administration of a diuretic. Gradual increase of dosage after initiation minimizes side effects. **Pediatric:** 50–400 mcg b.i.d.

NOTE: In hypertensive clients unable to take PO medication, clonidine may be administered sublingually at doses of 200–400 mcg/day.

Treat spasticity.

Adults and children: 0.1–0.3 mg/day, given in divided doses.

Alcohol withdrawal.

300–600 mcg q 6 hr.

Atrial fibrillation.

75 mcg 1–2 times/day with or without digoxin.

Attention deficit hyperactivity disorder.

5 mcg/kg/day for 8 weeks.

Constitutional growth delay in children.

37.5–150 mcg/m^2/day.

Diabetic diarrhea.

100–600 mcg q 12 hr.

Gilles de la Tourette syndrome.

150–200 mcg/day.

Hyperhidrosis.

250 mcg 3–5 times/day.

Hypertensive urgency (diastolic > 120 mm Hg).

Initial: 100–200 mcg; **then,** 50– 100 mcg q hr to a maximum of 800 mcg.

Menopausal flushing.

100–400 mcg/day.

Withdrawal from opiate dependence.

15–16 mcg/kg/day.

Diagnosis of pheochromocytoma.

300 mcg.

Postherpetic neuralgia.

200 mcg/day.

Psychosis in schizophrenia.

Less than 900 mcg/day.

Reduce allergen-induced inflammation in extrinsic asthma.

150 mcg for 3 days or 75 mcg/1.5 mL saline by inhalation.

Restless leg syndrome.

100–300 mcg/day, up to 900 mcg/day.

Facilitate cessation of smoking.

150–400 mcg/day.

Ulcerative colitis.
300 mcg t.i.d.

• **Transdermal**

Hypertension.

Initial: Use 0.1-mg system; **then,** if after 1–2 weeks adequate control has not been achieved, can use another 0.1-mg system or a larger system. The antihypertensive effect may not be seen for 2–3 days. The system should be changed q 7 days.

Treat spasticity.

Adults and children: 0.1–0.3 mg; apply patch q 7 days.

Cyclosporine-associated nephrotoxicity.
100–200 mcg/day.

Diabetic diarrhea.
0.3 mg/24 hr patch (1 or 2 patches/week).

Menopausal flushing.
100 mcg/24-hr patch.

Facilitate cessation of smoking.
200 mcg/24-hr patch.

• **Epidural infusion**

Analgesia.

Initial: 30 mcg/hr. Dose may then be titrated up or down, depending on pain relief and side effects.

HEALTH CARE CONSIDERATIONS

See also *Health Care Considerations* for *Antihypertensive Agents.*

Administration/Storage

1. It may take 2–3 days to achieve effective blood levels using the transdermal system. Therefore, reduce any prior drug dosage gradually.
2. Clients with severe hypertension may require other antihypertensive drug therapy in addition to transdermal clonidine.
3. If the drug is to be discontinued, do gradually over a period of 2–4 days.
4. Do not use a preservative when given epidurally.
5. Store the injection at controlled room temperature. Discard any unused portion.

Assessment

1. Record indications for therapy, onset, type of symptoms, and previous treatments.
2. Obtain baseline CBC, liver and renal function studies.
3. Note occupation; drug may interfere with the ability to work.
4. List drugs currently prescribed to prevent any interactions. With propranolol, observe for a paradoxical hypertensive response. With tolazoline or TCA, be aware that these may block the antihypertensive action of clonidine; clonidine dosage may need to be increased
5. Note evidence of alcohol, drug, or nicotine addiction. These agents usually work well for BP control in this group of clients (especially the once-a-week patch).
6. Initially, monitor BP closely. BP decreases occur within 30–60 min after administration and may persist for 8 hr. Note any fluctuations to determine whether to use clonidine alone or concomitantly with a diuretic. A stable BP reduces orthostatic effects with postural changes.

Client/Family Teaching

1. With the transdermal system, apply to a hairless area of skin, such as upper arm or torso. Change the system q 7 days and use a different site with each application.
2. If taken PO, take last dose of the day at bedtime to ensure overnight control of BP.
3. Do not engage in activities that require mental alertness, such as operating machinery or driving a car; may cause drowsiness.
4. Do not change regimen or discontinue drug abruptly. Withdrawal should be gradual to prevent rebound hypertension.
5. Record weight daily, in the morning, in clothing of the same weight, to determine if there is edema caused by sodium retention. Any fluid retention should disappear after 3–4 days.
6. Clonidine may reduce the effect of levodopa; report any increase in the S&S of Parkinson's disease previously controlled with levodopa.
7. Report any depression (may be precipitated by drug), especially with history of mental depression.

Outcome/Evaluate

- ↓ BP; ↓ menopausal S&S
- Control of withdrawal symptoms
- Control of neuropathic pain

Clopidogrel bisulfate

(kloh-**PID**-oh-grel)
Pregnancy Category: B
Plavix **(Rx)**
Classification: Antiplatelet drug

Action/Kinetics: Inhibits platelet aggregation by inhibiting binding of adenosine diphosphate (ADP) to its platelet receptor and subsequent ADP-mediative activation of glycoprotein GPIIb/IIIa complex. Modifies receptor irreversibly; thus, platelets are affected for remainder of their lifespan. Also inhibits platelet aggregation caused by agonists other than ADP by blocking amplification of platelet activation by released ADP. Rapidly absorbed from GI tract; food does not affect bioavailability. **Peak plasma levels:** About 1 hr. Extensively metabolized in liver; about 50% excreted in urine and 46% in feces. **t½, elimination:** 8 hr.

Uses: Reduction of MI, stroke, and vascular death in clients with atherosclerosis documented by recent stroke, MI, or established peripheral arterial disease.

Contraindications: Lactation. Active pathological bleeding such as peptic ulcer or intracranial hemorrhage.

Special Concerns: Use with caution in those at risk of increased bleeding from trauma, surgery, or other pathological conditions. Safety and efficacy have not been determined in children.

Side Effects: *CV:* Edema, hypertension, ***intracranial hemorrhage***. *GI:* Abdominal pain, dyspepsia, diarrhea, nausea, hemorrhage, ulcers (peptic, gastric, duodenal). *CNS:* Headache, dizziness, depression. *Body as a whole:* Chest pain, accidental injury, flu-like symptoms, pain, fatigue. *Respiratory:* URTI, dyspnea, rhinitis, bronchitis, coughing. *Hematologic:* Purpura, epistaxis. *Musculoskeletal:* Arthralgia, back pain. *Dermatologic:* Disorders of skin/appendages, rash, pruritus. *Miscellaneous:* UTI.

Laboratory Test Considerations: Hypercholesterolemia.

Drug Interactions

NSAIDs / ↑ Risk of occult blood loss

Warfarin / Clopidogrel prolongs bleeding time; safety of use with warfarin not established

How Supplied: *Tablets:* 75 mg

Dosage

- **Tablets**

Reduction of atherosclerotic events.

Adults: 75 mg once daily with or without food.

HEALTH CARE CONSIDERATIONS

Administration/Storage: Dosage adjustment not necessary for geriatric clients or with renal disease.

Assessment

1. Record atherosclerotic event (MI, stroke) or established peripheral arterial disease requiring therapy.
2. Assess for any active bleeding as with ulcers or intracranial bleeding.

Client/Family Teaching

1. Take exactly as directed; may take without regard to food.
2. Avoid OTC agents especially aspirin and NSAIDs.
3. Report any unusual bruising or bleeding; advise all providers of prescribed therapy.
4. Drug should be discontinued 7 days prior to elective surgery.

Outcome/Evaluate

- Inhibition of platelet aggregation
- Reduction of atherosclerotic events

Clorazepate dipotassium

(klor-**AYZ**-eh-payt)

Pregnancy Category: D

Apo-Clorazepate ★, Gen-Xene, Novo-Clopate ★, Tranxene-SD, Tranxene-T **(C-IV) (Rx)**

Classification: Antianxiety agent, benzodiazepine type; anticonvulsant

See also *Tranquilizers/Antimanic Drugs/Hypnotics.*

Action/Kinetics: Peak plasma levels: 1–2 hr. **t½:** 30–100 hr. Hydrolyzed in the stomach to desmethyldiazepam, the active metabolite. Oxazepam is also an active metabolite. **t½, desmethyldiazepam:** 30–100 hr; **t½, oxazepam:** 5–15 hr. **Time to peak plasma levels:** 0.5–2 hr. Significantly bound to plasma protein and slowly excreted by the kidneys.

Uses: Anxiety, tension. Acute alcohol withdrawal, as adjunct in treatment of seizures. Adjunct for treating partial seizures.

Additional Contraindications: Depressed clients, nursing mothers.

Special Concerns: Use with caution with impaired renal or hepatic function.

How Supplied: *Tablet:* 3.75 mg, 7.5 mg, 15 mg; *Tablet, Extended Release:* 11.25 mg, 22.5 mg

Dosage

- **Extended-Release Tablets, Tablets**

Anxiety.

Initial: 7.5–15 mg b.i.d.–q.i.d.; **maintenance:** 15–60 mg/day in divided doses. **Elderly or debilitated clients, initial:** 7.5–15 mg/day. **Alternative.** Single daily dosage: **Adult, initial,** 15 mg; **then,** 11.25–22.5 mg once daily.

Acute alcohol withdrawal.

Day 1, initial: 30 mg; **then,** 15 mg b.i.d.–q.i.d. the first day; **day 2:** 45–90 mg in divided doses; **day 3:** 22.5–45 mg in divided doses; **day 4:** 15–30 mg in divided doses. Thereafter, reduce to 7.5/day and discontinue as soon as possible. Maximum daily dose: 90 mg.

Partial seizures.

Adults and children over 12 years, initial: 7.5 mg t.i.d.; increase no more than 7.5 mg/week to maximum of 90 mg/day. **Children (9–12 years), initial:** 7.5 mg b.i.d.; increase by no more than 7.5 mg/week to maximum of 60 mg/day. Not recommended for children under 9 years of age.

HEALTH CARE CONSIDERATIONS

See also *Health Care Considerations* for *Tranquilizers/Antimanic Drugs/Hypnotics*.

Assessment

1. Note any evidence of depression.
2. With excessive alcohol intake, determine time of last drink.

Client/Family Teaching

1. Avoid activities requiring mental alertness until drug effects realized.
2. Avoid alcohol and any other CNS depressants.

Outcome/Evaluate

- ↓ Anxiety and tension
- ↓ S&S of alcohol withdrawal
- Control of seizures

Clotrimazole

(kloh-**TRY**-mah-zohl)

Pregnancy Category: C (systemic use); B (topical/vaginal use)

Canesten ✱, Canestin 1 ✱, Canestin 3 ✱, Clotrimaderm ✱, FemCare, Gyne-Lotrimin, Lotrimin, Lotrimin AF, Mycelex, Mycelex-7, Mycelex-G, Mycelex OTC, Myclo-Derm ✱, Myclo-Gyne ✱, Scheinpharm Clotrimazole ✱, Neo-Zol **(OTC) (Rx)**

Classification: Antifungal

See also *Anti-Infectives*.

Action/Kinetics: Depending on concentration, may be fungistatic or fungicidal. Acts by inhibiting the biosynthesis of sterols, resulting in damage to the cell wall and subsequent loss of essential intracellular elements due to altered permeability. May also inhibit oxidative and peroxidative enzyme activity and inhibit the biosynthesis of triglycerides and phospholipids by fungi. When used for *Candida albicans*, the drug inhibits transformation of blastophores into the invasive mycelial form. Poorly absorbed from the GI tract and metabolized in the liver to inactive compounds that are excreted through the feces. **Duration:** up to 3 hr.

Uses: Broad-spectrum antifungal effective against *Malassezia furfur, Trichophyton rubrum, Trichophyton mentagrophytes, Epidermophyton floccosum, Microsporum canis, C. albicans*. *Oral troche:* Oropharyngeal candidiasis. Reduce incidence of oropharyngeal candidiasis in clients who are immunocompromised due to chemotherapy, radiotherapy, or steroid therapy used for leukemia, solid tumors, or kidney transplant. *Topical OTC products:* Topically to treat tinea pedis, tinea cruris, and tinea corporis. *Topical prescription products:* Same as OTC plus candidiasis and tinea versicolor. *Vaginal products:* Vulvovaginal candidiasis.

Contraindications: Hypersensitivity. First trimester of pregnancy.

Special Concerns: Use with caution during lactation. Safety and effectiveness for PO use in children less than 3 years of age has not been determined.

Side Effects: *Skin:* Irritation including rash, stinging, pruritus, urticaria, erythema, peeling, blistering, edema. *Vaginal:* Lower abdominal cramps; urinary frequency; bloating; vaginal irritation, itching or burning; dyspareunia. *Hepatic:* Abnormal liver function tests. *GI:* N&V following use of troche.

How Supplied: *Kit*; *Lotion:* 1%; *Lozenge/Troche:* 10 mg; *Solution:* 1%; *Topical cream:* 1%; *Vaginal cream:* 1%; *Vaginal tablet:* 100 mg, 500 mg

Dosage

- **Troche**

Treatment of oropharyngeal candidiasis.

One troche (10 mg) 5 times/day for 14 consecutive days.

Prophylaxis of oropharyngeal candidiasis.

One troche t.i.d. for duration of chemotherapy or until maintenance doses of steroids are instituted.

- **Topical Cream, Lotion, Solution (each 1%)**

Massage into affected skin and surrounding areas b.i.d. in morning and evening for 7 consecutive days. Diagnosis should be reevaluated if no improvement occurs in 4 weeks.

- **Vaginal Tablets**

One 100-mg tablet/day at bedtime for 7 days. One 500-mg tablet can be inserted once at bedtime.

- **Vaginal Cream (1%)**

5 g (one full applicator)/day at bedtime for 7 consecutive days.

- **Vaginal Inserts and Clotrimazole, 1%**

Vaginal yeast infections.

Insert daily for 3 consecutive days.

HEALTH CARE CONSIDERATIONS

See also *General Health Care Considerations for All Anti-Infectives*.

Administration/Storage

1. Store Mycelex-G vaginal cream at 2°C–30°C (36°F–86°F). Do not store Mycelex-G 100-mg vaginal tablets above 35°C (95°F); store the 500-mg vaginal tablets below 30°C (86°F).

2. Slowly dissolve the troche in the mouth.
3. Do not allow topical products to come in contact with the eyes.

Client/Family Teaching

1. Review goals of therapy; appropriate method for administration. Wash hands before and after treatments. Unless otherwise directed, apply only after cleaning the affected area.
2. With vaginal infections, do not engage in intercourse; or, to prevent reinfection, have partner wear a condom.
3. To prevent staining of clothes, use a sanitary napkin with vaginal tablets or cream.
4. If exposed to HIV and recurrent vaginal yeast infections occur, seek prompt medical intervention to determine cause of the symptoms.

Outcome/Evaluate

- Eradication of fungal infection
- Symptomatic improvement

Cloxacillin sodium

(klox-ah-**SILL**-in)

Pregnancy Category: B

Apo-Cloxi ✱, Cloxapen, Novo-Cloxin ✱, Nu-Cloxi ✱, Orbenin ✱, Taro-Cloxacillin ✱ **(Rx)**

Classification: Antibiotic, penicillin

See also *Anti-Infectives* and *Penicillins*.

Action/Kinetics: Penicillinase resistant and acid stable. **Peak plasma levels:** 7–15 mcg/mL after 30–60 min. **t½:** 30 min. Protein binding: 95%. Well absorbed from GI tract. Mostly excreted in urine, but some excreted in bile.

Uses: Infections caused by penicillinase-producing staphylococci, including pneumococci, group A beta-hemolytic streptococci, and penicillin G-sensitive and penicillin G-resistant staphylococci.

How Supplied: *Capsule:* 250 mg, 500 mg; *Powder for Reconstitution:* 125 mg/5 mL when reconstituted

Dosage

- **Capsules, Oral Solution**

Skin and soft tissue infections, mild to moderate URTIs.

Adults and children over 20 kg: 250 mg q 6 hr; **pediatric, less than 20 kg:** 50 mg/kg/day in divided doses q 6 hr.

Lower respiratory tract infections or disseminated infections.

Adults and children over 20 kg: 500 mg q 6 hr; **pediatric, less than 20 kg:** 100 mg/kg/day in divided doses q 6 hr. Alternatively, a dose of 50–100 mg/kg/day (up to a maximum of 4 g/day) divided q 6 hr may be used for infants and children.

HEALTH CARE CONSIDERATIONS

See also *Health Care Considerations* for *Penicillins*.

Administration/Storage

1. To reconstitude the oral solutoin, add amount of water stated on label in two portions; shake well after each addition.
2. Shake well before pouring each dose.
3. Refrigerate reconstituted solution and discard unused portion after 14 days.

Assessment: Note any sensitivity to penicillin; obtain baseline CBC, LFTs, and cultures.

Client/Family Teaching

1. Review appropriate guidelines for administration; include frequency and amount. Shake well before using; refrigerate and discard after 14 days.
2. Take as directed, 1 hr before or 2 hr after meals; food interferes with absorption of drug.
3. Complete prescription despite feeling better.

Outcome/Evaluate

- Eradication of infection
- ↓ Fever, ↓ WBCs, ↑ appetite

Clozapine

(**KLOH**-zah-peen)

Pregnancy Category: B

Clozaril **(Rx)**

Classification: Antipsychotic

Action/Kinetics: Interferes with the binding of dopamine to both D-1 and D-2 receptors; more active at limbic than at striatal dopamine receptors. Thus, is relatively free from extrapyramidal side effects and does not induce catalepsy. Also acts as an antagonist at adrenergic, cholinergic, histaminergic, and serotonergic receptors. Increases the amount of time spent in REM sleep. Food does not affect the bioavailability of clozapine. **Peak plasma levels:** 2.5 hr. **Average maximum concentration at steady state:** 122 ng/mL plasma after 100 mg b.i.d. Highly bound to plasma proteins. **t½:** 12 hr. Metabolized in the liver to inactive compounds and excreted through the urine (50%) and feces (30%).

Uses: Severely ill schizophrenic clients who do not respond adequately to conventional antipsychotic therapy, either because of ineffectiveness or intolerable side effects from other drugs. Due to the possibility of development of agranulocytosis and seizures, avoid continued use in clients failing to respond.

Contraindications: Myeloproliferative disorders. Use in those with a history of clozapine–induced agranulocytosis or severe granulocytopenia; use with other agents known to suppress bone marrow function . Severe CNS depression or coma due to any cause. Lactation.

Special Concerns: Use with caution in clients with known CV disease, prostatic hypertrophy, narrow angle glaucoma, hepatic or renal disease.

Side Effects: *Hematologic:* ***Agranulocytosis,*** leukopenia, neutropenia, eosinophilia. *CNS:* ***Seizures*** (appear to be dose dependent), drowsiness or sedation, dizziness, vertigo, headache, tremor, restlessness, nightmares, hypokinesia, akinesia, agitation, akathisia, confusion, rigidity, fatigue, insomnia, hyperkinesia, weakness, lethargy, slurred speech, ataxia, depression, anxiety, epileptiform movements. *CV:* Orthostatic hypotension (especially initially), tachycardia, syncope, hypertension, angina, chest pain, ***cardiac abnormalities,*** changes in ECG. *Neuroleptic malignant syndrome:* ***Hyperpyrexia,*** muscle rigidity, altered mental status, irregular pulse or BP, tachycardia, diaphoresis, cardiac dysrhythmias. *GI:* Constipation, nausea, heartburn, abdominal discomfort, vomiting, diarrhea, anorexia. *GU:* Urinary abnormalities, incontinence, abnormal ejaculation, urinary frequency or urgency, urinary retention. *Musculoskeletal:* Muscle weakness, pain (back, legs, neck), muscle spasm, muscle ache. *Respiratory:* Dyspnea, SOB, throat discomfort, nasal congestion. *Miscellaneous:* Salivation, sweating, visual disturbances, fever (transient), dry mouth, rash, weight gain, numb or sore tongue.

OD **Management of Overdose:** *Symptoms:* Drowsiness, delirium, tachycardia, ***respiratory depression,*** hypotension, hypersalivation, ***seizures, coma.*** *Treatment:* Establish an airway and maintain with adequate oxygenation and ventilation. Give activated charcoal and sorbitol. Monitor cardiac status and VS. General supportive measures.

Drug Interactions

Anticholinergic drugs / Additive anticholinergic effects

Antihypertensive drugs / Additive hypotensive effects

Benzodiazepines / Possible respiratory depression and collapse

Digoxin / ↑ Effect of digoxin due to ↓ binding to plasma protein

Epinephrine / Clozapine may reverse effects if epinephrine is given for hypotension

Warfarin / ↑ Effect of warfarin due to ↓ binding to plasma protein

How Supplied: *Tablet:* 25 mg, 100 mg

Dosage

- **Tablets**

  Schizophrenia.

Adults, initial: 25 mg 1–2 times/day; **then,** if drug is tolerated, the dose can be increased by 25–50 mg/day to a dose of 300–450 mg/day at the end of 2 weeks. Subsequent dosage increments should occur no more often than once or twice a week in increments not to exceed 100 mg. **Usual maintenance dose:** 300–600 mg/day (although doses up to 900 mg/day may be required in some clients). Total daily dose should not exceed 900 mg.

HEALTH CARE CONSIDERATIONS

Administration/Storage

1. Clozapine is available through independent "Clozaril treatment systems" based on a plan developed by physicians and pharmacists to ensure safe use of the drug with respect to weekly blood monitoring, data reporting, and drug dispensing. Prescriptions are limited to 1-week supplies, and the drug may only be dispensed following receipt, by the pharmacist, of weekly WBC test results that fall within the established limits. All weekly blood test results must be reported by participating pharmacists to the Clozaril National Registry.
2. If drug is effective, seek the lowest maintenance doses possible to maintain remission.
3. If termination of therapy is planned, gradually reduce the dose over a 1–2-week period. If cessation of therapy is abrupt due to toxicity, observe client carefully for recurrence of psychotic symptoms.
4. Clozapine therapy may be initiated immediately upon discontinuation of other antipsychotic medication; however, a 24-hr "washout period" is desirable.

Assessment

1. Record indications for therapy; assess behavioral manifestations. List other therapies trialed and the outcome.
2. Note history of seizure disorder.
3. Record baseline VS and ECG; report any irregular pulse, tachycardia, hyperpyrexia, or hypotension.
4. Obtain CBC and LFTs prior to initiating therapy. If WBCs fall below 2,000/mm^3 or granulocyte counts fall below 1,000/mm^3, the drug should be discontinued. Such clients should *not* be restarted on clozapine therapy.
5. Monitor and report WBCs once weekly

for the first six months of therapy, then every 2 weeks if stable.
6. Periodically reassess to determine continued need for therapy.

Client/Family Teaching

1. Take only as directed; do not stop abruptly.
2. Report immediately symptoms of lethargy, weakness, fever, sore throat, malaise, mucous membrane ulceration, or signs of infection.
3. Rinse mouth frequently and perform regular oral care to minimize potential for candidiasis.
4. Avoid driving or other hazardous activity due to possibility of seizures.
5. Because of orthostatic hypotension, especially during initial dosing, use care when rising from a supine or sitting position.
6. Avoid hot showers or baths and hot weather exposure.
7. Report if pregnancy occurs or desires to become pregnant.
8. Do not breast-feed.
9. Do not take any prescription drugs, OTC drugs, or alcohol.
10. Stress importance of weekly WBC test to assess for agranulocytosis. These are reported to a national registry and must be completed before scripts will be issued and filled.

Outcome/Evaluate

- Improved behavior patterns with ↓ agitation, ↓ hyperactivity, ↓ delusions, paranoia, and hallucinations
- Improved coping behaviors and thought patterns

Codeine phosphate

(KOH-deen)
Pregnancy Category: C
Paveral ✱ **(C-II) (Rx)**

Codeine sulfate

(KOH-deen)
Pregnancy Category: C
(C-II) (Rx)
Classification: Narcotic analgesic, morphine type

See also *Narcotic Analgesics.*

Action/Kinetics: Produces less respiratory depression and N&V than morphine. Moderately habit-forming and constipating. Dosages over 60 mg often cause restlessness and excitement and irritate the cough center. In lower doses it is a potent antitussive and is an ingredient in many cough syrups. **Onset:** 10–30 min. **Peak effect:** 30–60 min. **Duration:** 4–6 hr. **t½:** 3–4 hr. Codeine is two-thirds as effective PO as parenterally.

Uses: Relief of mild to moderate pain. Antitussive to relieve chemical or mechanical respiratory tract irritation. In combination with aspirin or acetaminophen to enhance anal-gesia.

Contraindications: Premature infants or during labor when delivery of a premature infant is expected.

Special Concerns: May increase the duration of labor. Use with caution and reduce the initial dose in clients with seizure disorders, acute abdominal conditions, renal or hepatic disease, fever, Addison's disease, hypothyroidism, prostatic hypertrophy, ulcerative colitis, urethral stricture, following recent GI or GU tract surgery, and in the young, geriatric, or debilitated clients.

Additional Drug Interactions: Combination with chlordiazepoxide may induce coma.

How Supplied: Codeine Phosphate: *Injection:* 15 mg/mL, 30 mg/mL, 60 mg/mL; *Solution:* 15 mg/5 mL; *Tablet:* 30 mg, 60 mg. Codeine Sulfate: *Tablet:* 15 mg, 30 mg, 60 mg

Dosage

- **Solution, Tablets, IM, IV, SC**

Analgesia.

Adults: 15–60 mg q 4–6 hr, not to exceed 360 mg/day. **Pediatric, over 1 year:** 0.5 mg/kg q 4–6 hr. IV should not be used in children.

Antitussive.

Adults: 10–20 mg q 4–6 hr, up to maximum of 120 mg/day. **Pediatric, 2–6 years:** 2.5–5 mg PO q 4–6 hr, not to exceed 30 mg/day; **6–12 years:** 5–10 mg q 4–6 hr, not to exceed 60 mg/day.

HEALTH CARE CONSIDERATIONS

See also *Health Care Considerations* for *Narcotic Analgesics.*

Client/Family Teaching

1. Take only as directed. Tylenol or aspirin act synergistically with codeine and are usually given together.
2. Increase intake of fluids, fruits, and fiber to diminish constipation.
3. Drug may cause dizziness and drowsiness.
4. Avoid alcohol/CNS depressants.
5. Report altered mental patterns.
6. If taking codeine syrups to suppress coughs, do not overuse. If productive coughing is suppressed, may cause additional congestion.

Outcome/Evaluate

- Relief of pain
- Control of coughing with improved sleeping patterns

—COMBINATION DRUG—

Codeine phosphate and guaifenesin

(KOH-deen FOS-fayt, gwye-FEN-eh-sin)
Pregnancy Category: C
Brontex **(C-III) (Rx)**
Classification: Antitussive/expectorant

See also *Codeine Phosphate* and *Guaifenesin*.
Content: *Antitussive:* Codeine phosphate, 10 mg/tablet or 20 mL. *Expectorant:* Guaifenesin, 300 mg/tablet or 20 mL.
Uses: Relief of cough due to a cold or inhaled irritants. To loosen mucus and thin bronchial secretions.
Contraindications: Asthma, during labor and delivery. Use of tablets in children less than 12 years of age and use of the liquid in children less than 6 years of age.
Special Concerns: Use with caution in clients with severe CNS depression, respiratory depression, acute alcoholism, chronic pulmonary disease, acute abdominal conditions, seizure disorders, fever, hypothyroidism, Addison's disease, ulcerative colitis, prostatic hypertrophy, following recent GI or urinary tract surgery, and in significant renal or hepatic dysfunction, in the very young and elderly, and during lactation.
Side Effects: *CNS:* CNS depression, lightheadedness, dizziness, sedation, headache, euphoria or dysphoria, transient hallucinations, disorientation, visual disturbances, ***seizures.*** *CV:* Tachycardia, bradycardia, palpitations, syncope, faintness, orthostatic hypotension, circulatory depression. *GI:* N&V, stomach pain, constipation, biliary tract spasm, increased colonic motility in those with ulcerative colitis. *GU:* Oliguria, urinary retention. *Allergic:* Pruritus, urticaria, ***angioneurotic edema, laryngeal edema, anaphylaxis.*** *Miscellaneous:* Flushing of the face, sweating, weakness.
Drug Interactions: Additive CNS depression if used with alcohol, sedatives, antianxiety agents, and MAO inhibitors
How Supplied: See Content

Dosage

- **Oral Solution, Tablets**

Cough/colds, bronchial congestion.
Adults and children over 12 years of age: One tablet q 4 hr or 20 mL (4 teaspoonfuls) q 4 hr. **Children, 6–12 years of age:** 10 mL (2 teaspoonfuls) q 4 hr.

HEALTH CARE CONSIDERATIONS

See also *Health Care Considerations* for *Narcotic Analgesics* and *Guaifenesin*.

Assessment

1. Record indications for therapy, onset and duration of symptoms, other agents used, and the outcome.
2. Note asthma or any conditions that would preclude drug use.

Client/Family Teaching

1. Take as directed with a full glass of water.
2. Report if cough persists; do not increase dose.
3. Do not engage in any activities that require mental or physical alertness until drug effects realized; may cause dizziness and drowsiness.
4. Drug may cause orthostatic hypotension; rise slowly from a sitting or lying position.
5. Avoid alcohol, CNS depressants, sedatives, or antidepressants.
6. Supervise children's activities (i.e., bike riding, games, swings).
7. Drug is for short-term use only; report if symptoms do not subside or get worse after 48 hr.

Outcome/Evaluate: Relief of cough

Colchicine

(KOHL-chih-seen)
Pregnancy Category: C (oral use); D (parenteral use)
(Rx)
Classification: Antigout agent

Action/Kinetics: Colchicine is not uricosuric. It may reduce the crystal-induced inflammation by reducing lactic acid production by leukocytes (resulting in a decreased deposition of sodium urate), by inhibiting leukocyte migration, and by reducing phagocytosis. May also inhibit the synthesis of kinins and leukotrienes. **t½, plasma:** 10–60 min. **Onset, IV:** 6–12 hr; **PO:** 12 hr. **Time to peak levels, PO:** 0.5–2 hr. It concentrates in leukocytes (t½, about 46 hr). Metabolized in the liver and mainly excreted in the feces with 10%–20% excreted unchanged through the urine.
Uses: Prophylaxis and treatment of acute attacks of gout. *Investigational:* To slow progression of chronic progressive multiple sclerosis, to decrease frequency and severity of fever and to prevent amyloidosis in familiar Mediterranean fever, primary biliary cirrhosis, hepatic cirrhosis, adjunct in the treatment of primary amyloidosis, Behcet's disease,

pseudogout due to chondrocalcinosis, refractory idiopathic thrombocytopenic purpura, progressive systemic sclerosis, dermatologic disorders including dermatitis herpetiformis, psoriasis, palmoplantar pustulosis, and pyoderma associated with Crohn's disease.

C

Contraindications: Blood dyscrasias. Serious GI, hepatic, cardiac, or renal disorders.
Special Concerns: Use with caution during lactation. Dosage has not been established for children. Geriatric clients may be at greater risk of developing cumulative toxicity. Use with extreme caution for elderly, debilitated clients, especially in the presence of chronic renal, hepatic, GI, or CV disease. May impair fertility.
Side Effects: The drug is toxic; thus clients must be carefully monitored. *GI:* N&V, diarrhea, abdominal cramping. *Hematologic:* ***Aplastic anemia, agranulocytosis,*** or thrombocytopenia following long-term therapy. *Miscellaneous:* Peripheral neuritis, purpura, myopathy, neuropathy, alopecia, reversible azoospermia, dermatoses, hypersensitivity, thrombophlebitis at injection site (rare), liver dysfunction. If such symptoms appear, discontinue drug at once and wait at least 48 hr before reinstating drug therapy.
Laboratory Test Considerations: Alters liver function tests. ↑ Alkaline phosphatase, AST. False + for hemoglobin or RBCs in urine.
OD **Management of Overdose:** *Symptoms (Acute Intoxication):* Characterized at first by violent GI tract symptoms such as N&V, abdominal pain, and diarrhea. The latter may be profuse, watery, bloody, and associated with severe fluid and electrolyte loss. Also, burning of throat and skin, hematuria and oliguria, rapid and weak pulse, general exhaustion, muscular depression, and CNS involvement. ***Death is usually caused by respiratory paralysis.*** *Treatment (Acute Poisoning):* Gastric lavage, symptomatic support, including atropine and morphine, artificial respiration, hemodialysis, peritoneal dialysis, and treatment of shock.

Drug Interactions

Acidifying agents / Inhibit the action of colchicine
Alkalinizing agents / Potentiate the action of colchicine
CNS depressants / Clients on colchicine may be more sensitive to CNS depressant effect of these drugs
Sympathomimetic agents / Enhanced by colchicine
Vitamin B_{12} / Colchicine may interfere with absorption from the gut

How Supplied: *Injection:* 0.5 mg/ml; *Tablet:* 0.5 mg, 0.6 mg

Dosage

• **Tablets**

Acute attack of gout.
Adults, initial: 1–1.2 mg followed by 0.5–1.2 mg q 1–2 hr until pain is relieved or nausea, vomiting, or diarrhea occurs. **Total amount required:** 4–8 mg.

Prophylaxis for gout.
Adults: 0.5–0.65 mg/day for 3–4 days a week if the client has less than one attack per year or 0.5–0.65 mg/day if the client has more than one attack per year.

Prophylaxis for surgical clients.
Adults: 0.5–0.65 mg t.i.d. for 3 days before and 3 days after surgery.

• **IV Only**

Acute attack of gout.
Adults, initial: 2 mg; **then,** 0.5 mg q 6 hr until pain is relieved; give no more than 4 mg in a 24-hr period. Some physicians recommend a single IV dose of 3 mg while others recommend no more than 1 mg for the initial dose, followed by 0.5 mg once or twice daily, if needed. If pain recurs, 1–2 mg/day may be given for several days; however, colchicine should not be given by any route for at least 7 days after a full course of IV therapy (i.e., 4 mg).

Prophylaxis or maintenance of recurrent or chronic gouty arthritis.
0.5–1 mg 1–2 times/day. However, PO colchicine is preferred (usually with a uricosuric drug).

HEALTH CARE CONSIDERATIONS

Administration/Storage

1. Store in tight, light-resistant containers.
IV 2. Parenterally, give only IV; SC or IM causes severe local irritation.
3. For parenteral administration, give undiluted or may dilute in 10–20 mL of NSS without a bacteriostatic agent or with sterile water. Administer over 2–5 min.
4. Do not use turbid solutions.
5. Not compatible with dextrose-containing solutions.

Assessment

1. Determine symptom onset; any other attacks, frequency, and any preventative therapy prescribed.
2. Note age and general physical condition.
3. Record joint involvement, noting pain, swelling, and degree of mobility; may need to aspirate joint for definitive diagnosis.
4. Monitor CBC, joint X-ray, uric acid levels, and renal and LFTs.

Client/Family Teaching

1. If prescribed for use in acute attacks take at the first S&S of attack to diminish severity. Stop uricosuric agent (if prescribed) during acute attack.
2. Start or increase dosage of colchicine as prescribed; at the first sign of joint pain or other symptom of impending gout attack. The maximum dose is 10 tablets or 10 mg in 24 hr; do not exceed. It usually takes 12–48 hr for relief of symptoms.
3. Acute episodes may be precipitated by aspirin, alcohol, or foods high in purine.
4. Stop drug and report if N&V, or diarrhea develops; signs of toxicity. With severe diarrhea, medication (paregoric) may be needed.
5. Report any evidence of liver dysfunction (yellow discoloration of eyes, skin, or stool). LFTs may be scheduled during long-term use.
6. Females should avoid pregnancy.
7. Consume 3–3.5 L/day of fluids to enhance excretion.
8. NSAIDs may help with pain and inflammation; use as prescribed.

Outcome/Evaluate

- ↓ Joint pain and swelling
- Prophylaxis of acute gout attacks

Colestipol hydrochloride

(koh-**LESS**-tih-poll)

Colestid **(Rx)**

Classification: Hypocholesterolemic, bile acid sequestrant

Action/Kinetics: An anion exchange resin that binds bile acids in the intestine, forming an insoluble complex excreted in the feces. The loss of bile acids results in increased oxidation of cholesterol to bile acids and a decrease in LDL and serum cholesterol. Does not affect (or may increase) triglycerides or HDL and may increase VLDL. Not absorbed from the GI tract. **Onset:** 1–2 days; **maximum effect:** 1 month. Return to pretreatment cholesterol levels after discontinuance of therapy: 1 month.

Uses: As adjunctive therapy in hyperlipoproteinemia (types IIA and IIB) to reduce serum cholesterol in clients who do not respond adequately to diet. *Investigational:* Digitalis toxicity.

Contraindications: Complete obstruction or atresia of bile duct.

Special Concerns: Use during pregnancy only if benefits outweigh risks. Use with caution during lactation and in children. Children may be more likely to develop hyperchloremic acidosis although dosage has not been established. Clients over 60 years of age may be at greater risk of GI side effects and adverse nutritional effects.

Side Effects: *GI:* Constipation (may be severe and accompanied by fecal impaction), N&V, diarrhea, heartburn, GI bleeding, anorexia, flatulence, steatorrhea, abdominal distention/cramping, bloating, loose stools, indigestion, rectal bleeding/pain, black stools, hemorrhoidal bleeding, ***bleeding duodenal ulcer, peptic ulceration,*** ulcer attack, GI irritation, dysphagia, dental bleeding/caries, hiccoughs, sour taste, pancreatitis, diverticulitis, cholecystitis, cholelithiasis. *CV:* Chest pain, angina, tachycardia (rare). *CNS:* Migraine or sinus headache, anxiety, vertigo, dizziness, lightheadedness, insomnia, fatigue, tinnitus, syncope, drowsiness, femoral nerve pain, paresthesia. *Hematologic:* Ecchymosis, anemia, beeding tendencies due to hypoprothrombinemia. *Allergic:* Urticaria, dermatitis, asthma, wheezing, rash. *Musculoskeletal:* Backache, muscle/joint pain, arthritis. *Renal:* Hematuria, burnt odor to urine, dysuria, diuresis. *Miscellaneous:* Uveitis, fatigue, weight loss or gain, increased libido, swollen glands, SOB, edema, weakness, swelling of hands/feet, osteoporosis, calcified material in biliary tree and gall bladder, hyperchloremic acidosis in children.

Drug Interactions

See *Cholestyramine.*

How Supplied: *Granule for Reconstitution:* 5 g/7.5 g, 5 g/packet, 5 g/scoopful; *Tablet:* 1 g

Dosage

- **Oral Granules**

Antihyperlipidemic.

Adults, initial: 5 g 1–2 times/day; **then,** can increase 5 g/day at 1–2-month intervals. **Total dose:** 5–30 g/day given once or in two to three divided doses.

- **Tablets**

Adults, initial: 2 g 1–2 times/day. Dose can be increased by 2 g, once or twice daily, at 1–2-month intervals. **Total dose:** 2–16 g/day given once or in divided doses.

Digitalis toxicity.

10 g followed by 5 g q 6–8 hr.

HEALTH CARE CONSIDERATIONS

See also *Health Care Considerations* for *Cholestyramine.*

Administration/Storage

1. If compliance is good and side effects acceptable but the desired effect is not obtained with 2–16 g/day using tablets, consid-

er combined therapy or alternative treatment.
2. Granules are available in an orange-flavored product.

Client/Family Teaching

1. Take 30 min before meals, preferably with the evening meal, since cholesterol synthesis is increased during the evening hours. Take other drugs 1 hr before or 4 hr after colestipol to reduce interference with their absorption.
2. Never take dose in dry form. Always mix granules with 90 mL or more of fruit juice, milk, water, carbonated beverages, applesauce, soup, cereal, or pulpy fruit before administering to disguise unpalatable taste and to prevent resin from causing esophageal irritation or blockage.
3. Rinse glass with a small amount of additional beverage to ensure the total amount of the drug is taken.
4. Tablets should be swallowed whole (i.e., they should not be cut, crushed, or chewed); may be taken with water or other fluids.
5. Consume adequate amounts of fluids, fruits, and fiber to diminish constipating drug effects.
6. Continue to follow dietary restrictions of fat and cholesterol, regular exercise program, smoking cessation, and weight reduction in the overall goal of cholesterol reduction.
7. Serum cholesterol level will return to pretreatment levels within 1 month if drug is discontinued.

Outcome/Evaluate: ↓ LDL levels

Collagenase

(koh-**LAJ**-eh-nace)
Biozyme-C, Santyl **(Rx)**
Classification: Topical enzyme

Action/Kinetics: Digests collagen, thus, effectively removing tissue debris. Assists in the formation of granulation tissue and subsequent epithelialization of dermal ulcers and severely burned areas. May also reduce the incidence of hypertrophic scarring. Collagen in healthy tissue or newly formed granulation is not affected.
Uses: Reduces pus, odor, necrosis, and inflammation in chronic dermal ulcers and severely burned areas.
Contraindications: Local or systemic hypersensitivity to collagenase.
Side Effects: No allergic sensitivity or toxic reactions have been noted.
Drug Interactions: Detergents, benzalkonium chloride, hexachlorophene, nitrofurazone, tincture of iodine, and certain heavy metal ions used in some antiseptics (e.g., mercury, silver) inhibit the activity of collagenase.
How Supplied: *Ointment:* 250 U/g

Dosage

- **Ointment**

Chronic dermal ulcers, burns.
Apply once daily (more frequently if the dressing becomes soiled).

HEALTH CARE CONSIDERATIONS

Administration/Storage

1. If any of the agents listed under drug interactions have been used, clean the area thoroughly with repeated washings using NSS before collagenase ointment is applied.
2. Before applying, cleanse the site and other material by gently rubbing with a gauze pad saturated with hydrogen peroxide or Dakin's solution followed by sterile NSS.
3. If infection is present, apply a topical antibiotic powder to the lesion before collagenase is applied. If the infection does not respond, discontinue collagenase therapy until the infection is in remission.
4. Apply collagenase to deep lesions using a wooden tongue depressor or spatula; for shallow lesions, a sterile gauze pad may be securely applied to the area.
5. Crosshatching thick eschar with a #10 blade allows more surface area for the collagenase to come in contact with necrotic tissue. Remove as much loosened debris as possible with forceps and scissors.
6. Remove all excess ointment each time the dressing is changed.
7. Terminate therapy when necrotic tissue debridement completed and granulation tissue well established.
8. The action of the enzyme may be stopped by applying Burrow's solution (pH 3.6–4.4) to the lesion.

Assessment: Record underlying cause and assess area to be treated, noting wound size, depth, color, presence of eschar, any evidence of drainage, swelling, or odor and determine wound stage.

Client/Family Teaching

1. Review procedure for tissue preparation and collagenase application.
2. Note importance of frequent position changes, methods to reduce pressure to bony prominences, proper body alignment, proper skin care, adequate nutrition, and clean, dry linens in the overall goal to reduce the size and spread of the disrupted tissue, whether from an ulcer or from a burn.
3. Return for follow-up evaluations to deter-

mine the effectiveness of therapy; report any evidence of infection.

Outcome/Evaluate

- Formation of granulation tissue
- Wound reepithelialization

COMBINATION DRUG

Conjugated estrogens and Medroxyprogesterone acetate

(KON-jyou-gay-ted ES- troh-jens meh-drox-see-proh-JESS-ter- ohn)

Pregnancy Category: X

PremPro **(Rx)**

Classification: Hormones

See also *Conjugated estrogens* and *Medroxyprogesterone acetate.*

Content: Each tablet contains: conjugated estrogens, 0.625 mg, and medroxyprogesterone acetate, 2.5 mg or 5 mg.

Uses: Moderate to severe vasomotor symptoms associated with menopause in women with an intact uterus. Vulvular and vaginal atrophy. Prevention of osteoporosis.

Contraindications: Known or suspected pregnancy, including use for missed abortion or as a diagnostic test for pregnancy. Known or suspected cancer of the breast or estrogen-dependent neoplasia. Undiagnosed abnormal genital bleeding. Active or past history of thrombophlebitis, thromboembolic disease, or stroke. Liver dysfunction or disease. Lactation.

Special Concerns: Estrogens reportedly increase the risk of endometrial carcinoma in postmenopausal women. Use with caution in conditions aggravated by fluid retention, including asthma, epilepsy, migraine, and cardiac or renal dysfunction. Estrogens may cause significant increases in plasma triglycerides that may cause pancreatitis and other complications in clients with familial defects of lipoprotein metabolism.

Side Effects: See individual drug entries.

Drug Interactions: See individual drug entries.

How Supplied: See Content

Dosage

- **Tablets**

Vasomotor symptoms due to menopause, vulvar and vaginal atrophy, prevention of osteoporosis.

Initial: 0.625 mg/2.5 mg estrogen/medroxyprogesterone per day; **then,** increase to 0.625/5 mg estrogen/medroxyprogestrone per day.

HEALTH CARE CONSIDERATIONS

See also *Health Care Considerations* for *Conjugated estrogens* and *Medroxyprogesterone acetate.*

Assessment

1. Record indications for therapy (hormone replacement for menopausal symptoms or osteoporosis prevention), onset and duration of symptoms, and length of therapy.
2. Note any history or experience with replacement therapy.
3. Evaluate for any active or past conditions that may preclude drug therapy: liver dysfunction, thrombophlebitis, thromboembolic disorders, cancer of the breast or estrogen-dependent neoplasia, or any undiagnosed abnormal vaginal bleeding.

Client/Family Teaching

1. Take only as directed; two cards are provided, marked cards 1 and 2.
2. Stress importance of follow-up exams to assess need for continued therapy. When used for treating vasomotor symptoms or vulval and vaginal atrophy, reevaluate every 3–6-mo to assess treatment results.
3. When used to prevent osteoporosis, monitor closely for signs of endometrial cancer. Diagnostic procedures should be undertaken to rule out malignancy in the event of persistent or recurring AVB.

Outcome/Evaluate

- Osteoporosis prophylaxis
- ↓ Menopausal symptoms

Cortisone acetate (Compound E)

(KOR-tih-zohn)

Cortone ✦, Cortone Acetate, Cortone Acetate Sterile Suspension **(Rx)**

Classification: Corticosteroid, glucocorticoid-type

See also *Corticosteroids.*

Action/Kinetics: Possesses both glucocorticoid and mineralocorticoid activity. Short-acting. **t½, plasma:** 30 min; **t½, biologic:** 8–12 hr.

Uses: Replacement therapy in chronic cortical insufficiency. Short-term (due to strong mineralocorticoid effect) for inflammatory or allergic disorders. Sterile suspension: Congenital adrenal hyperplasia in children.

Special Concerns: Use during pregnancy only if benefits outweigh risks.

How Supplied: *Injection:* 50 mg/mL; *Tablet:* 5 mg, 10 mg, 25 mg

Dosage

- **Tablets, Injection**

Initial or during crisis.

25–300 mg/day. Decrease gradually to lowest effective dose.

Anti-inflammatory.

25–150 mg/day, depending on severity of the disease.

Acute rheumatic fever.

200 mg b.i.d. day 1, thereafter, 200 mg/day.

Addison's disease.

Maintenance: 0.5–0.75 mg/kg/day.

HEALTH CARE CONSIDERATIONS

See also *Health Care Considerations* for *Corticosteroids.*

Administration/Storage: Single course of therapy should not exceed 6 weeks. Rest periods of 2–3 weeks are indicated between treatments.

Outcome/Evaluate

- Replacement with insufficiency
- Relief of allergic manifestations
- Normal plasma cortisol levels (138–635 nmol/L at 8 a.m.)

Cromolyn sodium (Sodium cromoglycate)

(CROH-moh-lin)

Pregnancy Category: B

Apo-Cromolyn ✤, Crolom, Gastrocrom, Gen-Cromoglycate Sterinebs ✤, Intal, Nalcrom ✤, Nasalcrom, Novo-Cromolyn ✤, Opticrom ✤, PMS-Sodium Chromoglycate ✤, Rynacrom ✤, Vistacrom ✤ **(OTC) (Rx)**

Classification: Antiasthmatic, antiallergic drug

Action/Kinetics: Acts locally to inhibit the degranulation of sensitized mast cells that occurs after exposure to certain antigens. Prevents the release of histamine, slow-reacting substance of anaphylaxis, and other endogenous substances causing hypersensitivity reactions. When effective, reduces the number and intensity of asthmatic attacks as well as decreasing allergic reactions in the eye. No antihistaminic, anti-inflammatory, or bronchodilator effects and has no role in terminating an acute attack of asthma. After inhalation, some drug is absorbed systemically. **t½:** 81 min; from lungs: 60 min. About 50% excreted unchanged through the urine and 50% through the bile. When used in the eye, approximately 0.03% is absorbed. **Onset, ophthalmic:** Several days. **Onset, nasal:** Less than 1 week. **Time to peak effect, nasal:** Up to 4 weeks.

Uses: Inhalation: Prophylactic and adjunct in the management of severe bronchial asthma in selected clients. Prophylaxis of exercise-induced bronchospasms and bronchospasms due to allergens, cold dry air, or environmental pollutants. **Ophthalmologic:** Conjunctivitis, including vernal keratoconjunctivitis, vernal conjunctivitis, and vernal keratitis. **Nasal, OTC:** Prophylaxis and treatment of allergic rhinitis. **PO:** Mastocytosis (improves symptoms including diarrhea, flushing, headaches, vomiting, urticaria, nausea, abdominal pain, and itching). *Investigational:* PO to treat food allergies.

Contraindications: Hypersensitivity. Acute attacks and status asthmaticus. Due to the presence of benzalkonium chloride in the product, soft contact lenses should not be worn if the drug is used in the eye. For mastocytosis in premature infants.

Special Concerns: Dosage of the ophthalmic product has not been established in children less than 4 years of age; dosage of the nasal product has not been established in children less than 6 years of age. Use with caution for long periods of time, in the presence of renal or hepatic disease, and during lactation.

Side Effects: *Respiratory:* ***Bronchospasm, laryngeal edema (rare),*** cough, eosinophilic pneumonia. *CNS:* Dizziness, drowsiness, headache. *Allergic:* Urticaria, rash, angioedema, serum sickness, ***anaphylaxis.*** *Other:* Nausea, urinary frequency, dysuria, joint swelling and pain, lacrimation, swollen parotid gland.

Following nebulization: Sneezing, wheezing, itching, nose bleeds, burning, nasal congestion. **Following nasal solution:** Burning, stinging, irritation of nose; sneezing, nose bleeds, headache, bad taste in mouth, postnasal drip. **Following ophthalmic use:** Stinging and burning after use. Also, conjunctival injection, watery or itchy eyes, dryness around the eye, puffy eyes, eye irritation, styes.

Following PO use: *GI:* Diarrhea, taste perversion, spasm of esophagus, flatulence, dysphagia, burning of mouth and throat. *CNS:* Headache, dizziness, fatigue, migraine, paresthesia, anxiety, depression, psychosis, behavior changes, insomnia, hallucinations, lethargy, lightheadedness after eating. *Dermatologic:* Flushing, angioedema, urticaria, skin burning, skin erythema. *Musculoskeletal:* Arthralgia, stiffness and weakness in legs. *Miscellaneous:* Altered liver function test, dyspnea, dysuria, polycythemia, neutropenia.

How Supplied: *Oral concentrate:* 100 mg/5 mL; *Metered dose inhaler:* 0.8 mg/inh; *Ophthalmic solution:* 4%; *Solution:* 10 mg/mL; *Nasal spray:* 5.2 mg/inh

Dosage

- **Capsules or Metered Dose Inhaler**

Prophylaxis of bronchial asthma.

Adults: 20 mg q.i.d. at regular intervals. Adjust dosage as required.

Prophylaxis of bronchospasm.

Adults: 20 mg as a single dose just prior to exposure to the precipitating factor. If used chronically, 20 mg q.i.d, up to a maximum of 160 mg/day.

- **Ophthalmic Solution**

Allergic ocular disorders.

Adults and children over 4 years: 1–2 gtt of the 4% solution in each eye 4–6 times/day at regular intervals.

- **Nasal Spray (OTC)**

Allergic rhinitis.

Adults and children over 6 years: 5.2 mg in each nostril 3–4 times/day at regular intervals (e.g., q 4–6 hr). May be used up to 6 times/day.

- **Oral Capsules**

Mastocytosis.

Adults: 200 mg q.i.d. 30 min before meals and at bedtime. **Pediatric, term to 2 years:** 20 mg/kg/day in four divided doses; should be used in this age group only in severe incapacitating disease where benefits outweigh risks. **Pediatric, 2–12 years:** 100 mg q.i.d. 30 min before meals and at bedtime. If relief is not seen within 2–3 weeks, dose may be increased, but should not exceed 40 mg/kg/day for adults and children over 2 years of age and 30 mg/kg/day for children 6 months–2 years.

HEALTH CARE CONSIDERATIONS

Administration/Storage

1. Continue corticosteroid dosage when initiating cromolyn therapy. If improvement occurs, taper the steroid dosage slowly. May have to reinstitute steroids if cromolyn inhalation is impaired, in times of stress, or in adrenocortical insufficiency.
2. One drop of ophthalmic solution contains 1.6 mg cromolyn sodium.
3. Protect ophthalmic solution from direct sunlight and, once opened, discard after 4 weeks.
4. The ophthalmic solution contains benzylkonium chloride; don't wear soft contact lenses during treatment.
5. Keep ophthalmic solution tightly closed and protect from light (store in original carton). Store between 15°C–30°C (59°F–85°F).

Client/Family Teaching

1. Institute only after acute episode is over, when airway is clear and able to inhale adequately.
2. When administered by Spinhaler, use the following guidelines:
   - Puncture and load the capsule into the Spinhaler.
   - Inhale and exhale fully; place the mouthpiece between the lips.
   - Tilt head back and inhale deeply and rapidly through the inhaler; causes propeller to turn rapidly and supply more medication in one breath.
   - Remove inhaler, hold breath a few seconds, and exhale slowly.
   - Repeat until the powder is completely administered.
   - Do not wet powder with breath while exhaling.
   - Taking a sip of water or rinsing the mouth immediately before and after using the Spinhaler will diminish the throat irritation and/or cough.
   - Replace Spinhaler q 6 mo.
3. Continue prescribed medications; may take up to 4 weeks for frequency of asthmatic attacks to decrease.
4. With exposure bronchoconstriction, use inhaler within 10–15 min prior to precipitating agent (i.e., exercise, antigen, environmental pollutants) for best results.
5. Use a peak expiratory flow meter to monitor asthma control; establish level to seek medical assistance.
6. Do not discontinue medication abruptly. Rapid withdrawal of the drug may precipitate an asthmatic attack, and concomitant corticosteroid therapy may require adjustment.
7. When used in the *eye*:
   - Do not wear soft contacts until medically cleared.
   - Drug may sting on application, but this should subside.

Outcome/Evaluate

- ↓ Frequency of asthmatic attacks
- Prevention of exposure-induced bronchoconstriction
- Control of symptoms of mastocytosis (↓ diarrhea, N&V, headache, flushing, and abdominal pain)
- Relief of ocular and/or nasal allergic manifestations

Cyanocobalamin (Vitamin B_{12})

(sye-**an**-oh-koh-**BAL**-ah-min)

Pregnancy Category: C

Nasal gel: Ener-B, Nascobal **(OTC)**., **Parenteral:** Berubigen, Kaybovite-1000, Redisol, Rubramin ✱, Rubramin PC, Scheinpharm B12 ✱ **(OTC) (Rx)**

Cyanocobalamin crystalline

(sye-an-oh-koh-**BAL**-ah-min)
Pregnancy Category: C
Crystamine, Crysti 1000, Cyanoject, Cyomin, Rubesol-1000 **(OTC: Tablets; Rx: Injection)**
Classification: Vitamin $_B$12

Action/Kinetics: Cyanocobalamin (vitamin B_{12}), a cobalt-containing vitamin, can be isolated from liver and is identical to that of the antianemic factor of liver. Required for hematopoiesis, cell reproduction, nucleoprotein and myelin synthesis. Plasma vitamin B_{12} levels: 150–750 pg/mL.

Intrinsic factor is required for adequate absorption of PO vitamin B_{12}, and in pernicious anemia and malabsorption diseases intrinsic factor is administered simultaneously. Rapidly absorbed following IM or SC administration. Following absorption, vitamin B_{12} is carried by plasma proteins to the liver where it is stored until required for various metabolic functions.

Products containing less than 500 mcg vitamin B_{12} are nutritional supplements and are not to be used for the treatment of pernicious anemia. **t½:** 6 days (400 days in the liver). **Time to peak levels, after PO:** 8–12 hr.

Uses: Nutritional vitamin B_{12} deficiency, including cancer of the bowel or pancreas, sprue, total or partial gastrectomy, accompanying folic acid deficiency, GI surgery or pathology, gluten enteropathy, fish tapeworm infestation, bacterial overgrowth of the small intestine. Do not use PO products to treat pernicious anemia. Also, in conditions with an increased need for vitamin B_{12} such as thyrotoxicosis, hemorrhage, malignancy, pregnancy, and in liver and kidney disease. Vitamin B_{12} is particularly suitable for the treatment of clients allergic to liver extract.

Investigational: Diagnosis of vitamin B_{12} deficiency.

NOTE: Folic acid is not a substitute for vitamin B_{12} although concurrent folic acid therapy may be required.

Contraindications: Hypersensitivity to cobalt, Leber's disease.

Special Concerns: Use with caution in clients with gout.

Side Effects: Following parenteral use. *Allergic:* Urticaria, itching, transitory exanthema, ***anaphylaxis, shock, death.*** *CV:* ***Peripheral vascular thrombosis,*** CHF, ***pulmonary edema.*** *Other:* Polycythemia vera, optic nerve atrophy in clients with hereditary optic nerve atrophy, diarrhea, hypokalemia, body feels swollen.

Following intranasal use. *GI:* Glossitis, N&V. *Miscellaneous:* Asthenia, headache, infection (sore throat, common cold), paresthesia, rhinitis.

NOTE: Benzyl alcohol, which is present in certain products, may cause ***fatal "gasping syndrome"*** in premature infants.

Laboratory Test Considerations: Antibiotics, methotrexate, or pyrimethamine invalidate folic acid and vitamin B_{12} diagnostic blood assays.

Drug Interactions
Alcohol / ↓ Vitamin B_{12} absorption
Chloramphenicol / ↓ Response to vitamin B_{12} therapy
Cholestyramine / ↓ Vitamin B_{12} absorption
Cimetidine / ↓ Digestion and release of vitamin B_{12}
Colchicine / ↓ Vitamin B_{12} absorption
Neomycin / ↓ Vitamin B_{12} absorption
PAS / ↓ Vitamin B_{12} absorption
Potassium, timed-release / ↓ Vitamin B_{12} absorption

How Supplied: Cyanocobalamin: *Lozenge:* 100 mcg, 250 mcg, 300 mcg; *Tablet:* 50 mcg, 100 mcg, 250 mcg, 500 mcg, 1,000 mcg, 2,000 mcg 2,500 mcg, 5,000 mcg; *Tablet, Extended Release:* 1,000 mcg, 1,500 mcg. Cyanocobalamin crystalline: *Injection:* 2 mcg/mL, 100 mcg/mL, 1,000 mcg/mL

Dosage

CYANOCOBALAMIN

- **Tablets, Extended-Release Tablets**

Nutritional supplement.

Adults: 1 mcg/day (up to 25 mcg for increased requirements). The RDA is 2 mcg/day. **Pediatric, up to 1 year:** 0.3 mcg/day; **over 1 year:** 1 mcg/day.

Nutritional deficiency.

25–250 mcg/day.

- **Nasal gel**

Nutritional deficiency.

500 mcg/0.1 mL weekly given intranasally.

CYANOCOBALAMIN CRYSTALLINE

- **IM, Deep SC**

Addisonian pernicious anemia.

Adults: 100 mcg/day for 6–7 days; **then,** 100 mcg every other day for seven doses. If improvement is noted along with a reticulocyte response, 100 mcg q 3–4 days for 2–3 weeks; **maintenance, IM:** 100 mcg once a month for life. Give folic acid if necessary.

Vitamin B_{12} deficiency.

Adults: 30 mcg daily for 5–10 days; **then,** 100–200 mcg/month. Doses up to 1,000 mcg have been recommended. **Pediatric, for hematologic signs:** 10–50 mcg/day for 5–10 days followed by 100–250 mcg/dose q 2–4 weeks. **Pediatric, for neurologic signs:** 100 mcg/day for 10–15 days; **then,** 1–2 times/week for several months (can possibly be tapered to 250–1,000 mcg/month by 1 year).

Diagnosis of vitamin B_{12} deficiency. **Adults:** 1 mcg/day IM for 10 days plus low dietary folic acid and vitamin B_{12}. Loading dose for the Schilling test is 1,000 mcg given IM.

HEALTH CARE CONSIDERATIONS

Administration/Storage

1. Protect cyanocobalamin crystalline injection from light. Do not freeze.
2. With pernicious anemia, the drug cannot be administered PO.
3. Clients should be in hematologic remission before use of the nasal gel.

Assessment

1. Record indications for therapy, type and onset of symptoms.
2. Determine if allergic to cobalt.
3. Note if prescribed chloramphenicol; this drug antagonizes the hematopoietic response to vitamin B_{12}.
4. Perform a baseline assessment of peripheral pulses and assess for neuropathy.
5. Monitor CBC, potassium, and B_{12} levels if being treated for megaloblastic anemia.
6. With pernicious anemia and malabsorption syndromes, administer intrinsic factor simultaneously.

Client/Family Teaching

1. With pernicious anemia, *must take* vitamin B_{12} replacement for life.
2. When repository vitamin B_{12} used, it provides drug for 4 weeks.
3. The stinging, burning sensation after injection is transitory.
4. If vitamin B_{12} therapy is the result of dietary deficiency, identify foods (such as meats, especially liver, fermented cheeses, egg yolks, and seafood) high in B_{12} and review diet.
5. Avoid alcohol; interferes with drug absorption.
6. Report any symptoms of urticaria, itching, and evidence of anaphylaxis immediately.
7. If diarrhea occurs, record the frequency, quantity, and consistency of stools; may require a drug change.

Outcome/Evaluate

- Cause of B_{12} deficiency state
- Symptomatic improvement
- Plasma vitamin B_{12} levels of 350–750 pg/mL

Cyclobenzaprine hydrochloride

(sye-kloh-**BENZ**-ah-preen)

Pregnancy Category: B

Alti-Cyclobenzaprine ✱, Apo-Cyclobenzaprine ✱, Flexeril, Novo-Cycloprine ✱, Nu-Cyclobenzaprine ✱, PMS-Cyclobenzaprine ✱ **(Rx)**

Classification: Skeletal muscle relaxant, centrally acting

See also *Skeletal Muscle Relaxants, Centrally Acting.*

Action/Kinetics: Related to the tricyclic antidepressants; possesses both sedative and anticholinergic properties. Thought to inhibit reflexes by reducing tonic somatic motor activity. **Onset:** 1 hr. **Time to peak plasma levels:** 4–6 hr. **Therapeutic plasma levels:** 20–30 ng/mL. **Duration:** 12–24 hr. **t½:** 1–3 days. Highly bound to plasma protein. Inactive metabolites are excreted in the urine.

Uses: Adjunct to rest and physical therapy for relief of muscle spasms associated with acute and/or painful musculoskeletal conditions. Not indicated for the treatment of spastic diseases or for cerebral palsy. *Investigational:* Adjunct in the treatment of fibrositis syndrome.

Contraindications: Hypersensitivity. Arrhythmias, heart block or conduction disturbances, CHF, or during acute recovery phase of MI. Hyperthyroidism. Concomitant use of MAO inhibitors or within 14 days of their discontinuation.

Special Concerns: Safe use during lactation and in children under age 15 has not been established. Due to atropine-like effects, use with caution in situations where cholinergic blockade is not desired (e.g., history of urinary retention, angle-closure glaucoma, increased intraocular pressure). Geriatric clients may be more sensitive to cholinergic blockade.

Side Effects: Since cyclobenzaprine resembles tricyclic antidepressants, side effects to these drugs should also be noted. *GI:* Dry mouth, N&V, constipation, dyspepsia, unpleasant taste, anorexia, diarrhea, GI pain, gastritis, thirst, flatulence, ageusia, paralytic ileus, discoloration of tongue, stomatitis, parotid swelling. *CNS:* Drowsiness, dizziness, fatigue, asthenia, blurred vision, nervousness, headache, ***convulsions,*** ataxia, vertigo, dysarthria, paresthesia, hypertonia, tremors, malaise, abnormal gait, delusions, Bell's palsy, alteration in EEG patterns, extrapyramidal symptoms. Psychiatric symptoms include: confusion, insomnia, disorientation, depressed mood, abnormal sensations, anxiety, agitation, abnormal thinking or dreaming, excitement, hallucinations. *CV:* Tachycardia, syncope, ***arrhythmias,*** vasodilation, palpitations, hypotension, edema, chest pain, hypertension, MI, heart block, stroke. *GU:* Urinary frequency or retention, impaired urination, dilation of urinary tract, impotence, decreased or increased libido, testicular swelling, gynecomastia, breast enlargement, galactorrhea. *Dermatologic:* Sweating, skin rashes, urticaria, pruritus, photosensitivity, alopecia. *Musculoskeletal:* Muscle twitching, weakness, myalgia. *Hematologic:* Purpura, bone marrow depression, leukopenia, eosinophilia, thrombocytopenia. *Hepatic:* Abnormal liver function, hepatitis, jaundice, cholestasis. *Miscellaneous:* Tinnitus, diplopia, peripheral neuropathy, increase and decrease of blood sugar, weight gain or loss, ***edema of the face and tongue,*** inappropriate ADH syndrome, dyspnea.

OD **Management of Overdose:** *Symptoms:* Temporary confusion, disturbed concentration, transient visual hallucinations, agitation, hyperactive reflexes, muscle rigidity, vomiting, ***hyperpyrexia.*** Also, drowsiness, hypothermia, tachycardia, ***cardiac arrhythmias such as bundle branch block, ECG evidence of impaired conduction,*** CHF, dilated pupils, ***seizures, severe hypotension,*** stupor, ***coma,*** paradoxical diaphoresis. *Treatment:* In addition to the treatment outlined in , for physostigmine salicylate, 1–3 mg IV may be used to reverse symptoms of severe cholinergic blockade.

Drug Interactions: *NOTE:* Because of the similarity of cyclobenzaprine to tricyclic antidepressants, the drug interactions for tricyclics should also be consulted.

Anticholinergics / Additive anticholinergic side effects

CNS depressants / Additive depressant effects

Guanethidine / Cyclobenzaprine may block effect

MAO inhibitors / Hypertensive crisis, severe convulsions

Tricyclic antidepressants / Additive side effects

How Supplied: *Tablet:* 10 mg

Dosage

- **Tablets**

  Skeletal muscle disorders.

Adults: 20–40 mg/day in three to four divided doses (usual: 10 mg t.i.d.), up to a maximum of 60 mg/day in divided doses.

HEALTH CARE CONSIDERATIONS

See also *Health Care Considerations* for *Skeletal Muscle Relaxants, Centrally Acting.*

Administration/Storage

1. Use only for 2–3 weeks.
2. If taking an MAO inhibitor, do not administer cyclobenzaprine for at least 2 weeks after discontinuing.

Assessment

1. Record indications for therapy, extent of acute or painful musculoskeletal condition, DTRs, ROM, and evidence of weakness, . Review RICE (rest, ice, compression, and elevation) with acute injury to reduce swelling and recovery time.
2. Note any hypersensitivity or spastic diseases.
3. Check for evidence of cardiac arrhythmias; note history of MI.
4. Obtain ECG, CBC, and LFTs.

Client/Family Teaching

1. Report any unusual fatigue, sore throat, fever, easy bruising/bleeding; S&S of blood dyscrasia.
2. Report nausea or abdominal pain, itchy skin, or evidence of yellow sclera or skin; S&S of hepatic toxicity.
3. Symptoms of dry mouth, blurred vision, dizziness, tachycardia, or urinary retention should be reported.
4. Due to drug-induced drowsiness, dizziness, and/or blurred vision, observe caution if performing activities that require mental alertness.
5. Notify provider if S&S do not improve within 2–3 weeks of therapy.

Outcome/Evaluate: Relief of musculoskeletal spasms/pain; ↑ ROM

Cycloserine

(sye-kloh-**SEE**-reen)

Pregnancy Category: C

Seromycin **(Rx)**

Classification: Antitubercular agent for retreatment regimens

Action/Kinetics: Produced by a strain of *Streptomyces orchidaceus* or *Garyphalus lavendulae.* Acts by inhibiting cell wall synthesis by interfering with the incorporation of the amino acid alanine. Well absorbed from the GI tract and widely distributed in body tissues. **Time to peak plasma levels:** 3–8 hr. CSF levels are similar to those in plasma. **t½:** 10 hr. From 60% to 70% is excreted unchanged in urine.

Uses: With other drugs to treat active pulmonary and extrapulmonary tuberculosis only when primary therapy cannot be used. To treat UTIs when other therapy has failed or if the organism has demonstrated sensitivity.

Contraindications: Hypersensitivity to cycloserine, epilepsy, depression, severe anxiety, psychosis, severe renal insufficiency, and alcoholism. Lactation.

Special Concerns: Safe use during pregnancy and in children has not been established.
Side Effects: *CNS:* Drowsiness, headache, mental confusion, tremors, vertigo, loss of memory, psychoses (possibly with ***suicidal tendencies),*** character changes, hyperirritability, aggression, increased reflexes, ***seizures,*** paresthesias, paresis, coma. Neurotoxic effects depend on blood levels of cycloserine. Hence, frequent determinations of cycloserine blood levels are indicated, especially during the initial period of therapy. *Other:* Sudden development of CHF, skin rashes, increased transaminase.
OD Management of Overdose: *Symptoms:* CNS depression, including drowsiness, mental confusion, headache, vertigo, paresthesias, dysarthrias, hyperirritability, psychosis, paresis, ***seizures,*** and ***coma.*** *Treatment:* Supportive therapy. Charcoal may be more effective than emesis or gastric lavage. Hemodialysis may be used for life-threatening toxicity. Pyridoxine may treat neurotoxic effects.
Drug Interactions
Ethanol / ↑ Risk of epileptic episodes
Isoniazid / ↑ Risk of cycloserine CNS side effects (especially dizziness)
How Supplied: *Capsule:* 25 mg

Dosage
- **Capsules**

Adults, initially: 250 mg q 12 hr for first 2 weeks; **then,** 0.5–1 g/day in divided doses based on blood levels. Dosage should not exceed 1 g/day. **Pediatric:** 10–20 mg/kg/day, not to exceed 0.75–1 g/day. *NOTE:* Pyridoxine, 200–300 mg/day may prevent neurotoxic effects.

HEALTH CARE CONSIDERATIONS

See also *General Health Care Considerations for All Anti-Infectives.*
Assessment
1. Note any evidence of depression, anxiety, seizures, or excessive alcohol use. Report any psychotic or neurologic reactions that may necessitate temporary drug withdrawal.
2. Monitor I&O; observe for any S&S of CHF with high-dose therapy.
3. Monitor liver and renal function studies and cycloserine levels throughout therapy (<25–30 mcg/mL).
Client/Family Teaching
1. May cause drowsiness and dizziness; do not perform tasks that require mental alertness; report if symptoms persist.
2. Consume 2–3 L/day of fluids.
3. Avoid alcohol.
4. Immediately report any SOB, skin rashes, or overt behavioral changes, especially suicide ideations.
Outcome/Evaluate
- Negative sputum cultures for acid-fast bacilli
- Improved CXR and PFTs

Cyclosporine
(sye-kloh-**SPOR**-een)
Pregnancy Category: C
Neoral, Sandimmune, Sandimmune I.V. ✱, Sandimmune Neoral ✱ **(Rx)**
Classification: Immunosuppressant

Action/Kinetics: Thought to act by inhibiting the immunocompetent lymphocytes in the G_0 or G_1 phase of the cell cycle. T-lymphocytes are specifically inhibited; both the T-helper cell and the T-suppressor cell may be affected. Also inhibits interleukin 2 or T-cell growth factor production and release. Absorption from the GI tract is incomplete and variable. Children often require larger PO doses than adults, which may be due to the smaller absorptive surface area of their intestines. **Peak plasma levels:** 3.5 hr. Food may both delay and impair drug absorption. **t½:** Approximately 19 hr for adults and 7 hr in children. Metabolized by the liver; inactive metabolites are excreted mainly through the bile.

Neoral immediately forms a microemulsion in an aqueous environment. This product has better bioequivalency; thus, Sandimmune and Neoral are not bioequivalent and cannot be used interchangeably without medical supervision. **Time to peak blood levels:** 1.5–2 hr. Food decreases the amount of drug absorbed.
Uses: Prophylaxis of rejection in kidney, liver, and heart allogeneic transplants. Sandimmune is always to be taken with adrenal corticosteroids while Neoral has been used in combination with azathioprine and corticosteroids. Neoral microemulsion: Alone or in combination with methotrexate for severe, active rheumatoid arthritis which has not responded to methotrexate alone. Neoral microemulsion: Severe recalcitrant plaque psoriasis. Sandimmune: Treatment of chronic rejection in clients previously treated with other immunosuppressants. Sandimmune has been used in children as young as 6 months with no unusual side effects. *Investigational:* Aplastic anemia, myasthenia gravis, atopic dermatitis, Crohn's disease, Graves ophthalmology, severe psoriasis, multiple sclerosis,

polymyositis, Behcet's disease, biliary cirrhosis, corneal transplantation (or other diseases of the eye which have an autoimmune component), dermatomyositis, insulin-dependent diabetes mellitus, lichen planus, lupus nephritis, nephrotic syndrome, pemphigus and pemphigoid, psoriatic arthritis, pulmonary sarcoidosis, pyoderma gangrenosum, alopecia areata, ulcerative colitis, uveitis.

Contraindications: Hypersensitivity to cyclosporine or polyoxyethylated castor oil. Lactation. Use of potassium-sparing diuretics. Neoral in psoriasis or rheumatoid arthritis with abnormal renal function, uncontrolled hypertension, or malignancies. Neoral together with PUVA or UVB in psoriasis.

Special Concerns: Use with caution in clients with impaired renal or hepatic function. Safety and efficacy have not been established in children. Clients with malabsorption may not achieve therapeutic levels following PO use.

Side Effects: *GI:* N&V, diarrhea, gum hyperplasia, anorexia, gastritis, hiccoughs, peptic ulcer, abdominal discomfort, upper GI bleeding, pancreatitis, constipation, mouth sores, difficulty in swallowing. *Hematologic:* Leukopenia, lymphoma, thrombocytopenia, anemia, microangiopathic hemolytic anemia syndrome. *Allergic:* ***Anaphylaxis (rare).*** *CV:* Hypertension, edema, chest pain, cramps, ***MI*** (rare). *CNS:* Headache, tremor, confusion, fever, ***seizures,*** anxiety, depression, weakness, lethargy, ataxia. *GU:* Renal dysfunction, glomerular capillary thrombosis, nephrotoxicity. *Dermatologic:* Acne, hirsutism, brittle finger nails, hair breaking, pruritus. *Miscellaneous:* Hepatotoxicity, flushing, paresthesia, sinusitis, gynecomastia, conjunctivitis, hearing loss, tinnitus, muscle pain, infections (including fungal, viral), *Pneumocystis carinii* pneumonia, hematuria, blurred vision, weight loss, joint pain, night sweats, tingling, hypomagnesemia in some clients with seizures, infectious complications, increased risk of cancer.

Laboratory Test Considerations: ↑ Serum creatinine, BUN, total bilirubin, alkaline phosphatase, serum potassium. Possibly ↑ cholesterol, LDL, and apolipoprotein B. Hyperglycemia, hyperkalemia, hyperuricemia.

OD **Management of Overdose:** *Symptoms:* Transient hepatotoxicity and nephrotoxicity. *Treatment:* Induction of vomiting (up to 2 hr after ingestion). General supportive measures.

Drug Interactions

Aminoglycosides / ↑ Risk of nephrotoxicity
Amiodarone / ↑ Blood levels of cyclosporine → ↑ risk of nephrotoxicity
Amphotericin B / ↑ Risk of nephrotoxicity
Azathioprine / ↑ Immunosuppression due to suppression of lymphocytes → possible infection and malignancy
Bromocriptine / ↑ Plasma level of cyclosporine due to ↓ breakdown by liver
Calcium channel blockers / / ↑ Plasma levels of cyclosporine due to ↓ breakdown by liver; ↑ risk of toxicity
Carbamazepine / ↓ Plasma level of cyclosporine due to ↑ breakdown by liver
Cimetidine / ↑ Risk of nephrotoxicity
Clarithromycin / ↑ Plasma levels of cyclosporine due to ↓ breakdown by liver; ↑ risk of nephrotoxicity, neurotoxicity
Colchicine / Severe side effects, including GI, hepatic, renal, and neuromuscular toxicity
Corticosteroids / ↑ Immunosuppression due to suppression of lymphocytes → possible infection and malignancy
Cyclophosphamide / ↑ Immunosuppression due to suppression of lymphocytes → possible infection and malignancy
Danazol / ↑ Plasma level of cyclosporine due to ↓ breakdown by liver
Diclofenac / ↑ Risk of nephrotoxicity
Digoxin / ↑ Digoxin levels due to ↓ clearance; also, ↓ volume of distribution of digoxin → toxicity
Diltiazem / ↑ Plasma level of cyclosporine due to ↓ breakdown by liver → possible nephrotoxicity
Erythromycin / ↑ Plasma level of cyclosporine due to ↓ breakdown by liver and ↓ biliary excretion → possible nephrotoxicity
Etoposide / ↓ Etoposide renal clearance → increased toxicity
Fluconazole / ↑ Plasma level of cyclosporine due to ↓ gut and liver metabolism → possible nephrotoxicity
Foscarnet ↑ Risk of renal failure
HIV protease inhibitors / ↑ Plasma levels of cyclosporine due to ↓ breakdown by liver → toxicity
Imipenem-cilastatin / ↑ Blood levelsof cyclosporine → CNS toxicity
Isoniazid / ↓ Plasma level of cyclosporine due to ↑ breakdown by liver
Itraconazole / ↑ Plasma level of cyclosporine due to ↓ breakdown by liver
Ketoconazole / ↑ Plasma level of cyclosporine due to ↓ breakdown by gut and liver metabolism → possible nephrotoxicity
Lovastatin / ↑ Risk of myopathy and rhabdomyolysis
Melphalan / ↑ Risk of nephrotoxicity
Methylprednisolone / ↑ Blood levels of cyclosporine due to ↓ breakdown by liver → toxicity

Metoclopramide / ↑ Plasma level of cyclosporine due to ↓ breakdown by liver → toxicity
Naproxen / ↑ Risk of nephrotoxicity
Nephrotoxic drugs / Additive nephrotoxicity
Nicardipine / ↑ Plasma level of cyclosporine due to ↓ breakdown by liver → possible nephrotoxicity
Nifedipine / ↑ Risk of gingival hyperplasia
Octreotide / ↓ Plasma level of cyclosporine due to ↑ breakdown by liver
Oral contraceptives / ↑ Plasma level of cyclosporine due to ↓ breakdown by liver; possible severe hepatotoxicity
Phenobarbital / ↓ Plasma level of cyclosporine due to ↑ breakdown by liver
Phenytoin / ↓ Plasma level of cyclosporine due to ↑ breakdown by liver
Probucol / ↓ Bioavailability of cyclosporine → ↓ clinical effect
Ranitidine / ↑ Risk of nephrotoxicity
Rifabutin/Rifampin / ↓ Plasma level of cyclosporine due to ↑ breakdown by liver
Sulfamethoxazole and/or trimethoprim / ↑ Risk of nephrotoxicity; also, ↓ serum levels of cyclosporine → possible rejection
Sulindac / ↑ Risk of nephrotoxicity
Tacrolimus / ↑ Risk of nephrotoxicity
Terbenafine / ↓ Serum levels of cyclosporine due to ↑ breakdown by liver
Vancomycin / ↑ Risk of nephrotoxicity
Verapamil / ↑ Immunosuppression

How Supplied: *Capsule:* 25 mg, 100 mg, 250 mg; *Injection:* 50 mg/mL; *Solution:* 100 mg/mL

Dosage

- **Capsules, Oral Solution**

Allogenic transplants.

Adults and children, initial: A single 15 mg/kg dose given 4–12 hr before transplantation; there is a trend to use lower initial doses of 10–14 mg/kg/day. The dose should be continued postoperatively for 1–2 weeks followed by 5% decrease in dose per week to maintenance dose of 5–10 mg/kg/day (some have used a dose of 3 mg/kg/day successfully). Compared with Sandimmune, lower maintenance doses of Neoral may be sufficient.

If converting from Sandimmune to Neoral, start with a 1:1 conversion. Then, adjust the Neoral dose to reach the pre-conversion cyclosporine blood trough levels. Until this level is reached, monitor the cyclosporine trough level q 4–7 days.

Rheumatoid arthritis (Neoral only).

Initial: 1.25 mg/kg b.i.d. PO. Salicylates, NSAIDs, and PO corticosteroids may be continued. If sufficient beneficial effect is not seen and the client is tolerating the medication, the dose may be increased by 0.5–0.75 mg/kg/day after 8 weeks and again after 12 weeks to a maximum dose of 4 mg/kg/day. If no benefit is seen after 16 weeks, discontinue therapy. If Neoral is combined with methotrexate, the same initial dose and dose range of Neoral can be used.

Psoriasis (Neoral only).

Initial: 1.25 mg/kg b.i.d. PO. Maintain this dose for 4 weeks if tolerated. If significant improvement is not seen, increase the dose at 2-week intervals. Based on client response, make dose increases of about 0.5 mg/kg/day to a maximum of 4 mg/kg/day. Discontinue treatment if beneficial effects can not be achieved after 6 weeks at 4 mg/kg/day. Once beneficial effects are seen, decrease the dose (doses less than 2.5 mg/kg/day may be effective). To control side effects, make dose decreases by 25% to 50% at any time.

HEALTH CARE CONSIDERATIONS

Administration/Storage

1. Sandimmune and Neoral are not bioequivalent and should not be used interchangeably without the supervision of someone experienced in immunosuppressive therapy. Conversion from Neoral to Sandimmune using a 1:1 ratio (mg/kg/day) may result in lower cyclosporine blood levels.
2. Sandimmune capsules and oral solution are bioequivalent. Neoral capsules and oral solution are bioequivalent.
3. May dilute the PO solution with milk, chocolate milk, orange or apple juice immediately before administering. Dilute Neoral, preferably, with orange or apple juice; grapefruit juice affects metabolism of cyclosporine and is not to be used. After removal of the protective cover, transfer the solution, using the dosing syringe supplied, and transfer the solution to a glass of diluent. Stir well and drink at once. Do not allow diluted solution to stand beofre drinking. Use a glass container (not plastic). Rinse the glass with more diluent to ensure the total dose is taken. Do not store PO solutions in the refrigerator; contents should be used within 2 months after being opened.
4. At temperatures less than 20°C (68°F), Neoral solution may gel; light flocculation or the formation of a light sediment may also occur. This will not affect product peformance or dosing using the syringe provided. Allow

to warm to room temperature to reverse such changes.
5. Due to variable absorption of the PO solution, monitor blood levels.
6. Clients with malabsorption from the GI tract may not achieve appropriate blood levels.

Assessment

1. Record indications for therapy; note any previous treatments. List drugs prescribed and note any potential interactions. Anticipate concomitant administration of adrenal corticosteroids.
2. Monitor VS, CBC, cyclosporine levels, liver and renal function studies. Drug may increase BP, serum K, lipid, and uric acid levels.
3. Differentiate nephrotoxicity from rejection using criteria provided by the manufacturer.

Client/Family Teaching

1. Review importance of following the written guidelines for medication therapy explicitly. Drug must be taken throughout one's lifetime to prevent transplant rejection.
2. Because this drug is so important in preventing rejection, a written list of all possible drug side effects and those which need to be reported will be provided.
3. Taking the drug with food may reduce nausea and GI upset. If PO form unpalatable, mix with milk or juice in a glass container to minimize container adherence. Measure dose accurately and take immediately after mixing.
4. Do not stop abruptly; must be discontinued gradually.
5. Record BP, I&O, and daily weights. Report any persistent diarrhea and N&V.
6. Avoid crowds and persons with infectious illnesses.
7. Practice reliable birth control.
8. Use nystatin swish and swallow to prevent development of thrush; perform oral care and routine dental exams.
9. May develop acne and hirsutism; report as dermatologic referral may be needed.
10. Yellow discoloration of eyes, skin, or stools; fever; other signs of hepatotoxicity require reporting.
11. Report increased fatigue, malaise, unexplained bleeding or bruising, or hematuria.

Outcome/Evaluate

- Prevention of transplant rejection; improved organ function
- Cyclosporine trough levels (100–200 ng/mL)

Cyproheptadine hydrochloride

(sye-proh-**HEP**-tah-deen)
Pregnancy Category: B
Periactin, PMS-Cyproheptadine ✱ **(Rx)**
Classification: Antihistamine, piperidine-type

See also *Antihistamines*.
Action/Kinetics: Moderate anticholinergic activity and low sedative effects. **Onset:** 15–30 min. **Duration:** 3–6 hr.
Uses: Hypersensitivity reactions: Perennial and seasonal allergic rhinitis, vasomotor rhinitis, allergic conjunctivitis, uncomplicated allergic skin reactions of urticaria and angioedema, allergic reactions to blood or plasma, cold urticaria, adjunct to treat anaphylaxis, dermographism. *Investigational:* Stimulate appetite in anorexia nervosa and for cachexia associated with cancer. Vascular cluster headaches.
Additional Contraindications: Glaucoma, urinary retention.
Special Concerns: Geriatric clients may be more sensitive to the usual adult dose.
Laboratory Test Considerations: ↑ Serum amylase and prolactin if given with thyroid-releasing hormone.
Additional Side Effects: Increased appetite.
How Supplied: *Syrup:* 2 mg/5 mL; *Tablet:* 4 mg

Dosage

- **Syrup, Tablets**

Hypersensitivity reactions.
Adults, initial: 4 mg q 8 hr; **then,** 4–20 mg/day, not to exceed 0.5 mg/kg/day. **Pediatric, 2–6 years:** 2 mg q 8–12 hr, not to exceed 12 mg/day; **6–14 years:** 4 mg q 8–12 hr, not to exceed 16 mg/day.
Appetite stimulant.
Adults: 4 mg t.i.d. with meals. **Pediatric, 6–14 years, initial:** 2 mg t.i.d.–q.i.d. with meals; **then,** reduce dose to 4 mg t.i.d. **Pediatric, 2–6 years, initial:** 2 mg t.i.d. with meals; **then,** dose may be increased to a total of 8 mg/day.

HEALTH CARE CONSIDERATIONS

See also *Health Care Considerations* for *Antihistamines*.
Administration/Storage: Do not give for more than 6 months to adults and 3 months to children for appetite stimulation.

Outcome/Evaluate

- ↓ Allergic manifestations
- Weight gain
- Relief of cluster headaches

Cysteamine bitartrate

(SIS-tee-ah-meen)

Pregnancy Category: C

Cystagon **(Rx)**

Classification: Urinary tract product

Action/Kinetics: Lowers cystine levels of cells in cystinosis, which is an inherited defect of lysosomal transport. In those with cystinosis, cystine transport out of lysosomes is abnormal, resulting in the formation of crystals which damage the kidney. Other tissues are damaged as well, including the retina, muscles, and CNS. Acts within the cell to convert cystine into both cysteine and cysteine-cysteamine mixed disulfide, which can leave the lysosome in those with cystinosis.
Uses: Management of nephropathic cystinosis in adults and children.
Contraindications: Hypersensitivity to cysteamine or penicillamine. Use during lactation.
Side Effects: *CNS:* Lethargy, somnolence, depression, encephalopathy, ***seizures,*** headache, ataxia, confusion, tremor, hyperkinesia, dizziness, jitteriness, nervousness, abnormal thinking, emotional lability, hallucinations, nightmares. *GI:* N&V, anorexia, abdominal pain (may be severe), diarrhea, bad breath, dyspepsia, constipation, gastroenteritis, duodenitis, duodenal ulceration. *Hematologic:* Reversible leukopenia, anemia. *Miscellaneous;* Decreased hearing, fever, rash, dehydration, hypertension, urticaria.
Laboratory Test Considerations: Abnormal LFTs.
OD Management of Overdose: *Symptoms:* Extension of side effects, respiratory symptoms. *Treatment:* Support the cardiovascular and respiratory systems. Hemodialysis may be effective in removing the drug from the body.
How Supplied: *Capsule:* 50 mg, 150 mg

Dosage

- **Capsules**

Nephropathic cystinosis.

Initial: New clients should be started on one-fourth to one-sixth of the maintenance dose. The dose is then raised gradually over 4–6 weeks to avoid intolerance. **Maintenance, children up to age 12 years:** 1.3 g/m²/day (of the free base) given in four divided doses. **Maintenance, children over 12 years and over 110 lb:** 2 g/day in four divided doses.

HEALTH CARE CONSIDERATIONS

Administration/Storage

1. Begin therapy in children and adults promptly after the diagnosis has been confirmed by increased white cell cystine levels.
2. Do not give intact cysteamine capsules to children less than 6 years of age due to the possibility of aspiration. Sprinkle contents of the capsule over food.
3. The goal is to keep leukocyte cystine levels less than 1 nmol/½ cystine/mg protein 5–6 hr following administration of cysteamine. Those with intolerance to cysteamine can still get a beneficial effect if cystine levels are less than 2 nmol/½ cystine/mg protein. To achieve this level, the dose of cysteamine may be increased to a maximum of 1.95 g/m²/day.
4. Cystinotic clients taking cysteamine HCl or phosphocysteamine solutions may be transferred to equimolar doses of cysteamine bitartrate capsules. Clients being transferred should have their white cell cystine levels measured in 2 weeks and every 3 months thereafter.

Assessment: Obtain baseline CBC, liver and renal function tests, C_{CR} and white cell cystine levels; repeat levels 5–6 hr after drug administered.

Client/Family Teaching

1. Take only as directed. May be given with electrolyte and mineral replacements, vitamin D, and thyroid hormone to manage renal tubular Fanconi syndrome.
2. Report rash; provider will withhold drug until cleared and then reinstitute at a lower dose with gradual increases to therapeutic dose. This may also have to be done if CNS or GI side effects occur.
3. Obtain labs to assess for leukocyte cystine levels, abnormal liver function, or reversible leukopenia.

Outcome/Evaluate

- Prevention of organ damage R/T cystine accumulation
- White cell cystine levels of <1 nmol/½ cystine/mg protein

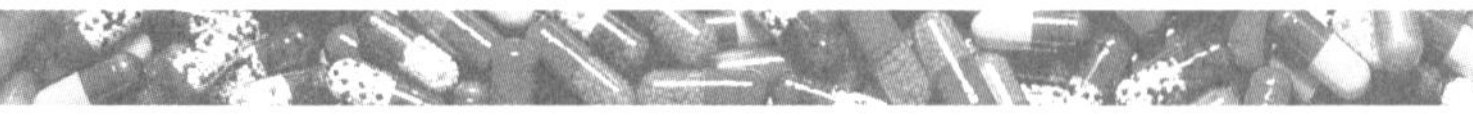

Danazol

(DAN-ah-zohl)

Cyclomen ✱, Danocrine **(Rx)**

Classification: Synthetic androgen (gonadotropin inhibitor)

Action/Kinetics: Inhibits the release of gonadotropins (FSH and LH) by the anterior pituitary; thus, inhibits synthesis of sex steroids and competitively inhibits binding of steroids to their cytoplasmic receptors in target tissues. In women this action arrests ovarian function, induces amenorrhea, and causes atrophy of normal and ectopic endometrial tissue. Has weak androgenic effects. **Onset, fibrocystic disease:** 4 weeks. **Time to peak effect, amenorrhea and anovulation:** 6-8 weeks; **fibrocystic disease:** 2-3 months to eliminate breast pain and tenderness and 4-6 months for elimination of nodules. **t½:** 4.5 hr. **Duration:** Ovulation and cyclic bleeding usually resume 60-90 days after cessation of therapy.

Uses: Endometriosis amenable to hormonal management in clients who cannot tolerate or who have not responded to other drug therapy. Fibrocystic breast disease. Hereditary angioedema in males and females. *Investigational:* Gynecomastia, menorrhagia, precocious puberty, idiopathic immune thrombocytopenia, lupus-associated thrombocytopenia, and autoimmune hemolytic anemia.

Contraindications: Undiagnosed genital bleeding; markedly impaired hepatic, renal, and cardiac function; pregnancy and lactation.

Special Concerns: Use with caution in children treated for hereditary angioedema due to the possibility of virilization in females and precocious sexual development in males. Use with caution in conditions aggravated by fluid retention (e.g., epilepsy, migraine, cardiac, or renal dysfunction). Geriatric clients may have an increased risk of prostatic hypertrophy or prostatic carcinoma.

Side Effects: *Androgenic:* Acne, decrease in breast size, oily hair and skin, weight gain, deepening of voice and hair growth, clitoral hypertrophy, testicular atrophy. *Estrogen deficiency:* Flushing, sweating, vaginitis, nervousness, changes in emotions. *GI:* N&V, constipation, gastroenteritis. *Hepatic:* Jaundice, dysfunction. *CNS:* Fatigue, tremor, headache, dizziness, sleep problems, paresthesia of extremities, anxiety, depression, appetite changes. *Musculoskeletal:* Muscle cramps or spasms, joint swelling or lock-up, pain in back, legs, or neck. *Miscellaneous:* Allergic reactions (skin rashes and rarely nasal congestion), hematuria, increased BP, chills, pelvic pain, carpal tunnel syndrome, hair loss, change in libido.

Drug Interactions

Insulin / Danazol ↑ insulin requirements

Warfarin / Danazol ↑ PT in warfarin-stabilized clients

How Supplied: *Capsule:* 50 mg, 100 mg, 200 mg

Dosage

- **Capsules**

Endometriosis.

400 mg b.i.d. (moderate to severe) or 100-200 mg b.i.d. (mild) for 3-6 months (up to 9 months may be required in some clients). Begin therapy during menses, if possible, to be sure that client is not pregnant.

Fibrocystic breast disease.

50-200 mg b.i.d. beginning on day 2 of menses. Begin therapy during menses to assure client is not pregnant.

Hereditary angioedema.

Initial: 200 mg b.i.d.-t.i.d.; after desired response, decrease dosage by 50% (or less) at 1-3-month intervals. Treat subsequent attacks by giving up to 200 mg/day. No more than 800 mg/day should be given to adults.

HEALTH CARE CONSIDERATIONS

Administration/Storage: Breast pain and tenderness in fibrocystic disease are usually relieved within 30 days and eliminated in 2-3 mo; elimination of nodularity requires 4-6 mo of uninterrupted therapy. Treatment may be reinstituted if symptoms recur (50% have recurring symptoms within 6 mo).

Assessment

1. Note reports of endometrial pain, breast pain, tenderness, and the presence of any nodules.
2. Determine any undiagnosed vaginal bleeding; note onset, frequency, extent, and precipitating factors.
3. Obtain baseline CBC, renal and LFTs; determine if pregnant.
4. Identify factors that trigger angioedema (usually C-1 inhibitor deficiency).

Client/Family Teaching

1. Take with meals to decrease GI upset.
2. Virilization may occur with drug therapy (e.g., abnormal hair growth, acne, reduced breast size, increased skin oiliness, enlarged clitoris, voice deepening); report so dosage

can be adjusted. Hypoestrogenic side effects usually disappear once discontinued; ovulation will resume in 60-90 days.
3. Wear cotton underwear and pay careful attention to hygiene to diminish danazol-induced vaginitis.
4. Practice birth control; continue breast self-exams and report changes
5. Clients with a history of epilepsy, migraines, and cardiac or renal dysfunction may develop fluid retention; stop drug and report.
6. Several months of therapy may be required before improvements.

Outcome/Evaluate

- ↓ Endometrial pain (3-6 mo)
- ↓ Breast pain (2-3 mo)

Dapiprazole hydrochloride

(dah-**PIP**-rah-zol)
Pregnancy Category: B
Rev-Eyes **(Rx)**
Classification: Ophthalmic alpha-adrenergic blocking agent

Action/Kinetics: Produces miosis by blocking the alpha-adrenergic receptors on the dilator muscle of the iris. No significant action on ciliary muscle contraction; thus, there are no changes in the depth of the anterior chamber or the thickness of the lens. Does not alter the IOP either in normal eyes or in eyes with elevated IOP. The rate of pupillary constriction may be slightly slower in clients with brown irides than in clients with blue or green irides.
Uses: To reverse diagnostic mydriasis induced by adrenergic (e.g., phenylephrine) or parasympatholytic (e.g., tropicamide) agents.
Contraindications: Acute iritis or other conditions where miosis is not desirable. To reduce IOP or to treat open-angle glaucoma.
Special Concerns: Use with caution during lactation. Safety and effectiveness have not been determined in children. The drug may cause difficulty in adaptation to dark and may reduce the field of vision.
Side Effects: *Ophthalmic:* Conjunctival injection lasting 20 min, burning on instillation, ptosis, lid erythema, itching, lid edema, chemosis, corneal edema, punctate keratitis, photophobia, tearing and blurring of vision, dryness of eyes. *Miscellaneous:* Headaches, browache.
How Supplied: *Ophthalmic Powder for Reconstitution:* 0.5%

Dosage

- **Ophthalmic Solution**
  Reverse mydriasis.

2 gtt followed in 5 min by 2 more gtt applied to the conjunctiva of the eye after ophthalmic examination.

HEALTH CARE CONSIDERATIONS

Administration/Storage

1. Do not use more frequently than once a week.
2. To prepare the solution, remove and discard aluminum seals and rubber plugs from the drug and diluent vials. Pour the diluent into the drug vial; remove the dropper assembly from its sterile wrapping and attach to the drug vial. Shake container for several minutes to ensure adequate mixing.
3. Store reconstituted eye drops at room temperature for 21 days. Discard solution if not clear and colorless.

Assessment

1. Determine any hypersensitivity to alpha-adrenergic blocking agents.
2. Note eye color. Pupillary constriction may be slightly slower in clients with brown irides as opposed to those with blue or green irides.

Client/Family Teaching: May cause burning on instillation. Use care; may impair adaptation to dark and reduce field of vision.
Outcome/Evaluate: Reversal of drug-induced mydriasis (constriction of pupils)

Dapsone (DDS, Diphenylsulfone)

(**DAP**-sohn)
Pregnancy Category: C
Avlosulfon ✱ **(Rx)**
Classification: Sulfone, leprostatic

Action/Kinetics: Has both bacteriostatic and bactericidal activity, especially against *Mycobacterium leprae* (Hansen's bacillus). Thought to interfere with the metabolism of the infectious organism. Widely distributed throughout the body. **Peak plasma levels:** 4-8 hr. Doses of 200 mg/day for 8 days will lead to a plateau plasma level of 0.1-7 mcg/mL. From 70% to 90% is bound to plasma proteins. **t½:** About 28 hr. Acetylated in the liver and metabolites excreted in the urine. However, excretion is slow and constant blood levels can be maintained with usual dosage.
Uses: Lepromatous and tuberculoid types of leprosy, dermatitis herpetiformis. *Investigational:* Relapsing polychondritis, prophylaxis

of malaria, inflammatory bowel disease, leishmaniasis, *Pneumocystis carinii* pneumonia, rheumatoid arthritis, lupus erythematosus, bites of the brown recluse spider.

Contraindications: Advanced amyloidosis of kidneys. Lactation.

D

Side Effects: *Hematologic:* ***Hemolytic anemia, agranulocytosis,*** methemoglobinemia. *GI:* N&V, anorexia, abdominal discomfort. *CNS:* Headache, insomnia, vertigo, paresthesia, psychoses, peripheral neuropathy. *Dermatologic:* Photosensitivity, lupus-like syndrome. *Hypersensitivity:* Severe skin reactions including exfoliative dermatitis, erythema multiforme, toxic erythema, urticaria, erythema nodosum, toxic erythema, toxic epidermal necrolysis, morbilliform and scarlatiniform reactions. *Sulfone syndrome:* ***Potentially fatal hypersensitivity reaction***, including symptoms of fever, malaise, jaundice with ***hepatic necrosis,*** exfoliative dermatitis, lymphadenopathy, methemoglobinemia, and ***hemolytic anemia.*** *Renal:* Nephrotic syndrome, renal papillary necrosis, albuminuria. *Miscellaneous:* Muscle weakness, blurred vision, tinnitus, male infertility, fever, tachycardia, mononucleosis-type syndrome, pulmonary eosinophilia, pancreatitis.

A leprosy-reactional state may occur in large numbers of clients during therapy with dapsone. Type 1 occurs soon after therapy is initiated. Clients manifest an enhanced delayed hypersensitivity syndrome, leading to swelling of existing nerve and skin lesions with possible neuritis. However, this is not an indication to discontinue therapy. Steroids, analgesics, and surgical decompression of swollen nerve trunks may be used to reduce symptoms. Type 2 occurs in nearly 50% of clients during the first year of therapy. Symptoms include fever, erythematous skin nodules, joint swelling, neuritis, orchitis, malaise, depression, iritis, or epistaxis. Usually therapy is continued with the use of analgesics, steroids, or clofazimine to suppress the reaction.

Laboratory Test Considerations: Altered liver function tests.

OD **Management of Overdose:** *Symptoms:* N&V, hyperexcitability (up to 24 hr after ingestion of an overdose). Methemoglobin-induced depression, ***seizures,*** severe cyanosis, headache, hemolysis. *Treatment:* Gastric lavage. In normal and methemoglobin-reductase deficient clients, give methylene blue, 1-2 mg/kg by slow IV (may need to be repeated if methemoglobin reaccumulates). In nonemergencies, methylene blue may be given PO, 3-5 mg/kg/4-6 hr.

Drug Interactions

Charcoal, activated / ↓ Absorption of dapsone from GI tract

Didanosine / Possible therapeutic failure of dapsone → increased infection

Para-aminobenzoic acid / ↓ Effect of dapsone

Probenecid / ↑ Effect of dapsone due to inhibition of renal excretion

Pyrimethamine / ↑ Risk of hematologic reactions

Rifampin / ↓ Effect of dapsone due to ↑ plasma clearance

Trimethoprim / ↑ Serum levels of both drugs → pharmacologic and toxic effects of both

How Supplied: *Tablet:* 25 mg, 100 mg

Dosage

- **Tablets**

Leprosy.

Adults: 50-100 mg/day. Initiate and continue the full dose without interruption.

Leprosy, bacteriologically negative tuberculoid and indeterminate type.

Adults: 100 mg/day with rifampin, 600 mg/day for 6 months; **then,** continue for a minimum of 3 years.

Leprosy, lepromatous and borderline clients.

100 mg/day for at least 2 years with rifampin, 600 mg/day. A third antileprosy drug may be added such as clofazimine, 50-100 mg/day or ethionamide, 250-500 mg/day. Dapsone is continued for up to 10 years until skin scrapings and biopsies are negative for 1 year.

Dermatitis herpetiformis.

Adults, initial: 50 mg/day; dosage may be increased to 300 mg/day or higher, if necessary. **Maintenance:** Reduce dosage to minimum maintenance dose as soon as possible; maintenance dosage may be reduced or eliminated in clients on a gluten-free diet. Dosage is correspondingly less in children.

HEALTH CARE CONSIDERATIONS

See also *General Health Care Considerations for All Anti-Infectives.*

Administration/Storage

1. For tuberculoid and indeterminate clients, continue dosage for at least 3 years.
2. For lepromatous clients, full dosage may be necessary for life.
3. Carefully evaluate possible resistance to dapsone, especially if lepromatous or borderline lepromatous clients relapse. If no response to therapy within 3-6 mo, confirm dapsone resistance.

Assessment

1. Note indications for therapy; onset of symptoms. Record size, extent, and location of lesions.

2. Observe clients with other concurrent chronic conditions closely; reduce dose of sulfones.
3. Increase dosage slowly during initiation period; determine if client to receive hematinics.
4. Monitor CBC, liver and renal function studies. Assess for anemia; report if WBCs < 4,500/mm³; RBC < 2,500,000/mm³ or if remains low during first 6 weeks of therapy.

Client/Family Teaching
1. Take exactly as ordered.
2. Follow prescribed diet (e.g., gluten-free) and see dietitian as needed for instruction.
3. Lactating mothers should report cyanosis of nursing infant; this indicates high sulfone levels, and drug withdrawal may be indicated.
4. Report any evidence of psychoses, GI disturbances, lepra reaction, headaches, dizziness, lethargy, severe malaise, tinnitus, paresthesias, deep aches, neuralgic pains, and ocular disturbances.
5. Report allergic dermatitis (usually appears before week 10); may develop into fatal exfoliative dermatitis.
6. Lab studies and FU visits are needed to evaluate drug effectiveness.
7. Identify local support groups that may assist client to understand and cope with this chronic disease.

Outcome/Evaluate
- ↓ Size and extent of lesions
- ↓ Inflammation and ulceration of mucous membranes
- Malaria prophylaxis

COMBINATION DRUG

Darvocet-N 50 and Darvocet-N 100

(DAR-voh-set)
(Rx)
Classification: Analgesic

See also *Acetaminophen* and *Propoxyphene.*
Content: *Nonnarcotic analgesic:* Acetaminophen, 325 (Darvocet-N 50) or 650 mg (Darvocet-N 100). *Analgesic:* Propoxyphene napsylate, 50 or 100 mg.
Uses: Mild to moderate pain (may be used if fever is present).
Special Concerns: Use during pregnancy only if benefits outweigh risks. Safety and a suitable dosage regimen have not been established in children. Increased dosing intervals should be considered in geriatric clients.
How Supplied: See Content

Dosage
- **Tablets**

Analgesia.
Two Darvocet-N 50 tablets or 1 Darvocet-N 100 tablet q 4 hr, not to exceed 600 mg/day of propoxyhene napsylate. Reduce total daily dose in impaired hepatic or renal function.

HEALTH CARE CONSIDERATIONS

See *Health Care Considerations* for *Acetaminophen* and *Propoxyphene.*
Assessment: Record indications for therapy, type, duration, and onset of symptoms. Anticipate reduced dose with renal and hepatic dysfunction.
Outcome/Evaluate: ↓ Pain and discomfort

COMBINATION DRUG

Darvon Compound 65

(DAR-von)
(Rx)
Classification: Analgesic

See also *Acetylsalicylic acid* and *Propoxyphene.*
Content: Darvon Compound 65: *Analgesic:* Propoxyphene HCl, 65 mg. *Nonnarcotic analgesic:* Aspirin, 389 mg. *CNS stimulant:* Caffeine, 32.4 mg.
Uses: Mild to moderate pain, with or without accompanying fever.
Special Concerns: Use during pregnancy only if benefits outweigh risks.
How Supplied: See Content

Dosage
- **Capsules**

Analgesia.
One capsule q 4 hr. Total daily dose of propoxyphene HCl should not exceed 390 mg. Decrease total daily dosage in hepatic or renal impairment.

HEALTH CARE CONSIDERATIONS

See also *Health Care Considerations* for *Acetylsalicylic acid* and *Propoxyphene.*
Assessment: Record indications for therapy, onset and type of symptoms; reduce dose with renal or liver dysfunction.

Client/Family Teaching
1. Use caution when performing tasks that require mental alertness; may cause dizziness and sedation.
2. Do *NOT* drink alcohol.
3. Keep out of reach of children.
4. Psychologic and physical dependence may occur.

Outcome/Evaluate: ↓ Pain and discomfort

Delavirdine mesylate

(deh-lah-**VIR**-deen)

Pregnancy Category: C

Rescriptor **(Rx)**

Classification: Antiviral drug, reverse transcriptase inhibitor

D

See also *Antiviral Drugs*.

Action/Kinetics: Non-nucleoside reverse transcriptase inhibitor that binds directly to reverse transcriptase and blocks RNA-dependent and DNA-dependent DNA polymerase activities. Effect is additive if used with other antiviral drugs. Delavirdine may confer cross-resistance to other non-nucleoside reverse transcriptase inhibitors when used alone or in combination. Rapidly absorbed. **Peak plasma levels:** About 1 hr. Extensively bound to plasma albumin. Converted to inactive metabolites which are excreted in urine and feces. It inhibits its own metabolism.

Uses: Treatment of HIV-1 infections in combination with appropriate antiretroviral agents.

Special Concerns: Use with caution in impaired hepatic function. Safety and efficacy in combination with other antiretroviral drugs have not been determined in HIV-1-infected clients less than 16 years of age.

Side Effects: *Body as a whole:* Headache, fatigue, asthenia, allergic reaction, chest pain, chills, general or local edema, fever, flu syndrome, lethargy, malaise, neck rigidity, general or local pain, trauma. *CV:* Bradycardia, migraine, pallor, palpitation, postural hypotension, syncope, tachycardia, vasodilation. *CNS:* Abnormal coordination, agitation, amnesia, anxiety, change in dreams, cognitive impairment, confusion, decreased libido, depression, disorientation, dizziness, emotional lability, hallucinations, hyperesthesia, hyperreflexia, hypesthesia, impaired coordination, insomnia, mania, nervousness, neuropathy, nightmares, paralysis, paranoia, paresthesia, restlessness, somnolence, tingling, tremor, vertigo, weakness. *GI:* N&V, diarrhea, anorexia, aphthous stomatitis, bloody stool, colitis, constipation, appetite decreased or increased, diarrhea, duodenitis, dry mouth, diverticulitis, dyspepsia, dysphagia, fecal incontinence, flatulence, enteritis, esophagitis, gastritis, gagging, gastroesophageal reflux, GI bleeding or disorder, gingivitis, gum hemorrhage, increased saliva, increased thirst, mouth ulcer, abdominal cramps/distention/pain, lip edema, hepatitis (nonspecified), pancreatitis, rectal disorder, sialadenitis, stomatitis, tongue edema, ulceration. *Dermatologic:* Skin rashes, maculopapular rash, pruritus, angioedema, dermal leukocytoblastic vasculitis, dermatitis, desquamation, diaphoresis, dry skin, erythema, erythema multiforme, folliculitis, fungal dermatitis, alopecia, nail disorder, petechial rash, seborrhea, skin disorder, skin nodule, ***Stevens-Johnson syndrome,*** vesiculobullous rash, sebaceous cyst. *GU:* Breast enlargement, kidney calculi, epididymitis, hematuria, hemospermia, impotence, kidney pain, metrorrhagia, nocturia, polyuria, proteinuria, vaginal moniliasis. *Musculoskeletal:* Back pain, neck rigidity, arthritis or arthralgia of single or multiple joints, bone disorder or pain, leg cramps, muscle weakness, myalgia, tendon disorder, tenosynovitis, tetany, muscle cramps. *Respiratory:* Upper respiratory infection, bronchitis, chest congestion, cough, dyspnea, epistaxis, laryngismus, pharyngitis, rhinitis, sinusitis. *Hematologic:* Anemia, bruises, ecchymosis, eosinophilia, granulocytosis, neutropenia, pancytopenia, petechiae, purpura, spleen disorder, thrombocytopenia. *Ophthalmic:* Nystagmus, blepharitis, conjunctivitis, diplopia, dry eyes, photophobia. *Miscellaneous:* Alcohol intolerance, peripheral edema, weight increase or decrease, taste perversion, tinnitus, ear pain.

Laboratory Test Considerations: ↑ ALT, AST, bilirubin, GGT, lipase, serum alkaline phosphatase, serum amylase, serum creatinine phosphatase, serum creatinine. Bilirubinemia, hyperkalemia, hyperuricemia, hypocalcemia, hyponatremia, hypophosphatemia

Drug Interactions

Antacids / ↓ Absorption of delavirdine; separate doses by 1 hr

Anticonvulsants / ↓ Plasma levels of delavirdine due to ↑ hepatic metabolism

Astemizole / Possible serious or life-threatening side effects of astemizole due to ↓ metabolism

Benzodiazpines / Possible serious or life-threatening side effects of benzodiazepines due to ↓ metabolism

Calcium channel blockers, dihydropyridine-type / Possible serious or life-threatening side effects of calcium channel blocker due to ↓ metabolism

Cisapride / Possible serious or life-threatening side effects of cisapride due to ↓ metabolism

Clarithromycin / Significant ↑ in amount absorbed of both drugs; possible serious side effects

Dapsone / Possible serious or life-threatening side effects of dapsone due to ↓ metabolism

Didanosine / ↓ Absorption of both drugs; separate administration by at least 1 hr

Ergot derivatives / Possible serious or life-threatening side effects of ergot due to ↓ metabolism
Fluoxetine / ↑ Trough levels of delavirdine by 50%
Indinavir / ↑ Levels of indinavir due to ↓ metabolism; possible serious side effects
Quinidine / Possible serious or life-threatening side effects of quinidine due to ↓ metabolism
Rifabutin, Rifampin / ↓ Plasma levels of delavirdine due to ↑ hepatic metabolism
Saquinavir / ↑ Levels of saquinavir due to ↓ metabolism; possible serious side effects
Terfenadine / Possible serious or life-threatening side effects of terfenadine due to ↓ metabolism
Warfarin / Possible serious or life-threatening side effects of warfarin due to ↓ metabolism
How Supplied: *Tablets:* 100 mg

Dosage

- **Tablets**

  HIV-1 infection.

400 mg (4-100 mg tablets) t.i.d. in combination with other antiretroviral therapy.

HEALTH CARE CONSIDERATIONS

Administration/Storage

1. Give with or without food.
2. In achlorhydria, take with an acidic beverage (e.g., orange or cranberry juice).

Assessment

1. Record disease onset/exposure times, likelihood of transmission, and disease characteristics such as stage of infection, viral load.
2. List drugs prescribed.
3. Monitor CBC, LFTs, viral load, CD_4 counts.
4. Assess lifestyle and potential to resume risky behaviors.

Client/Family Teaching

1. Take as directed, with or without food. Take antacids 1 hr before or 1 hr after drug ingestion.
2. Tablets may be dispersed with water prior to consumption. To prepare, add 4 tablets to at least 3 ounces of water and allow to stand for a few minutes. Stir until a uniform dispersion occurs and consume promptly. Rinse glass and swallow rinse to ensure entire dose is taken.
3. Always administer with other antiretroviral therapy. Drug is not a cure for HIV; may continue to acquire opportunistic infections.
4. Rash on upper body and arms may necessitate interruption of therapy. Report especially if accompanied by fever, blistering, myalgia, eye or mouth lesions.
5. Avoid OTC agents without approval.
6. Continue barrier contraception; does not reduce risk of transmission.

Outcome/Evaluate: Post-exposure prophylaxis; ↓ viral load

D

Desipramine hydrochloride

(dess-IP-rah-meen)

Alti-Desipramine ✱, Apo-Desipramine ✱, Dom-Desipramine ✱, Norpramin, Novo-Desipramine ✱, Nu-Desipramine ✱, Pertofrane ✱, PMS-Desipramine ✱ **(Rx)**

Classification: Antidepressant, tricyclic

See also *Antidepressants, Tricyclic.*
Action/Kinetics: Slight anticholinergic, sedative, and orthostatic hypotensive effects. **Effective plasma levels:** 125-300 ng/mL. **t½:** 12-24 hr. **Time to reach steady state:** 2-11 days. Response usually seen within the first week.
Uses: Symptoms of depression. Bulimia nervosa. To decrease craving and depression during cocaine withdrawal. To treat severe neurogenic pain. Cataplexy associated with narcolepsy. Attention deficit disorders with or without hyperactivity in children over 6 years of age.
Contraindications: Use in children less than 12 years of age.
Special Concerns: Safe use during pregnancy has not been established. Safety and efficacy have not been established in children.
Additional Side Effects: Bad taste in mouth, hypertension during surgery.
How Supplied: *Tablet:* 10 mg, 25 mg, 50 mg, 75 mg, 100 mg, 150 mg

Dosage

- **Tablets**

  Antidepressant.

Initial: 100-200 mg/day in single or divided doses. **Maximum daily dose:** 300 mg in severely ill clients. **Maintenance:** 50-100 mg/day. **Geriatric clients:** 25-50 mg/day in divided doses up to a maximum of 150 mg/day. **Adolescents and geriatric clients:** 25-50 mg/day in divided doses up to a maximum of 150 mg.

  Cocaine withdrawal.

50-200 mg/day.

HEALTH CARE CONSIDERATIONS

See also *Health Care Considerations* for *Antidepressants, Tricyclic.*

Administration/Storage
1. Initiate in a hospital setting for those requiring 300 mg/day.
2. Give maintenance doses for at least 2 months following a satisfactory response.
3. Give single daily dose or any dosage increases at bedtime to reduce daytime sedation.

Outcome/Evaluate
- ↓ Perceived depression; ↑ self-worth
- Relief of neurogenic pain
- Therapeutic levels (125-300 ng/mL)

Dexamethasone

(dex-ah-**METH**-ah-zohn)
Oral: Decadron, Dexameth, Dexamethasone Intensol, Dexasone ✱, Dexone, Hexadrol **(Rx)**. **Topical:** Aeroseb-Dex, Decaderm **(Rx)**. **Ophthalmic:** Maxidex Ophthalmic **(Rx)**
Classification: Glucocorticoid, synthetic

See also *Corticosteroids*.
Action/Kinetics: Long-acting. Low degree of sodium and water retention. Diuresis may ensue when transferred from other corticosteroids to dexamethasone. **t½:** 110-210 min.
Additional Uses: In acute allergic disorders, PO dexamethasone may be combined with dexamethasone sodium phosphate injection and used for 6 days. To test for adrenal cortical hyperfunction. Cerebral edema due to brain tumor, craniotomy, or head injury. *Investigational:* Diagnosis of depression. Antiemetic in cisplatin-induced vomiting. Prophylaxis or treatment of acute mountain sickness. Decrease hearing loss in bacterial meningitis. Bronchopulmonary dysplasia in preterm infants. Hirsutism.
Contraindications: Use for replacement therapy in adrenal cortical insufficiency.
Special Concerns: Use during pregnancy only if benefits outweigh risks.
Additional Drug Interactions: Ephedrine ↓ effect of dexamethasone due to ↑ breakdown by the liver.
How Supplied: *Aerosol, topical:* 0.01%, 0.04%; *Elixir:* 0.5 mg/5 mL; *Ophthalmic suspension:* 0.1%; *Oral Solution:* 0.5 mg/0.5 mL, 0.5 mg/5 mL; *Tablet:* 0.25 mg, 0.5 mg, 0.75 mg, 1 mg, 1.5 mg, 2 mg, 4 mg, 6 mg

Dosage
- **Oral Concentrate, Tablets, Elixir**

Most uses.
Initial: 0.75-9 mg/day; **maintenance:** gradually reduce to minimum effective dose (0.5-3 mg/day).

Suppression test for Cushing's syndrome.
0.5 mg q 6 hr for 2 days for 24-hr urine collection (or 1 mg at 11 p.m. with blood withdrawn at 8 a.m. for blood cortisol determination).

Suppression test to determine cause of pituitary ACTH excess.
2 mg q 6 hr for 2 days (for 24-hr urine collection).

Acute allergic disorders or acute worsening of chronic allergic disorders.
Day 1: Dexamethasone sodium phosphate injection, 4-8 mg IM. **Days 2 and 3:** Two 0.75-mg dexamethasone tablets b.i.d. **Day 4:** One 0.75-mg dexamethasone tablet b.i.d. **Days 5 and 6:** One 0.75-mg dexamethasone tablet. **Day 7:** No treatment. **Day 8:** Follow-up visit to physician.
- **Topical Aerosol, Cream**

Apply sparingly as a light film to affected area b.i.d.-t.i.d.
- **Ophthalmic Suspension**

1-2 gtt in the conjunctival sac q hr during day and q 2 hr during night until a satisfactory response obtained; **then,** 1 gtt q 4 hr and finally 1 gtt q 6-8 hr.

HEALTH CARE CONSIDERATIONS

See also *Health Care Considerations* for *Corticosteroids*.

Client/Family Teaching
1. Use exactly as directed; do not exceed dose and do not stop abruptly unless ordered.
2. May take with food to decrease GI upset.
3. Report loss of response, worsening of symptoms, excessive thirst and urinary frequency.

Outcome/Evaluate
- Status of adrenal cortical function
- ↓ Symptoms of allergic response
- ↓ Cerebral edema

Dexamethasone acetate

(dex-ah-**METH**-ah-zohn)
Dalalone D.P., Dalalone L.A., Decadron-LA, Decaject-L.A., Dexasone L.A., Dexone LA, Solurex LA **(Rx)**
Classification: Glucocorticoid, synthetic

See also *Corticosteroids*.
Action/Kinetics: Practically insoluble; provides the prolonged activity suitable for repository injections, although it has a prompt onset of action. Not for IV use.
Special Concerns: Use during pregnancy only if benefits outweigh risks.
How Supplied: *Injection:* 8 mg/mL, 16 mg/mL

Dosage
- **Repository Injection, IM**

8-16 mg q 1-3 weeks, if necessary.
- **Intralesional**

0.8-1.6 mg.

- **Soft Tissue and Intra-articular**

4-16 mg repeated at 1-3-week intervals.

HEALTH CARE CONSIDERATIONS

See also *Health Care Considerations* for *Corticosteroids.*

Client/Family Teaching: Do not overuse joint/limb as further injury may occur.

Outcome/Evaluate

- ↓ Inflammation
- Symptomatic improvement

Dexamethasone sodium phosphate

(dex-ah-**METH**-ah-zohn)

Systemic: Dalalone, Decadron Phosphate, Decaject, Dexasone, Dexone, Hexadrol Phosphate, R.O.-Dexone ✦, Solurex **(Rx)**. **Inhaler:** Decadron Phosphate Respihaler **(Rx)**. **Nasal:** Decadron Phosphate Turbinaire **(Rx)**. **Ophthalmic:** AK-Dex, Decadron Phosphate Ophthalmic, Diodex ✦, PMS-Dexamethasone Sodium Phosphate ✦, Spersadex ✦ **(Rx)**. **Otic:** AK-Dex, Decadron, I-Methasone **(Rx)**. **Topical:** Decadron Phosphate **(Rx)**

Classification: Glucocorticoid, synthetic

See also *Corticosteroids.*

Action/Kinetics: Rapid onset and short duration of action.

Additional Uses: For IV or IM use in emergency situations when dexamethasone cannot be given PO. Intranasally for nasal polyps, allergic or inflammatory nasal conditions.

Contraindications: Acute infections, persistent positive sputum cultures of *Candida albicans.* Lactation.

Special Concerns: Use during pregnancy only if benefits outweigh risks.

Side Effects: *Following inhalation:* Nasal and nasopharyngeal irritation, burning, dryness, stinging, headache.

How Supplied: *Metered dose inhaler* 0.1 mg/inh; *Injection:* 4 mg/mL, 10 mg/mL, 24 mg/mL; *Ophthalmic ointment:* 0.05%; *Ophthalmic solution:* 0.1%

Dosage

- **IM, IV**

Most uses.

Range: 0.5-9 mg/day (1/3-1/2 the PO dose q 12 hr).

Cerebral edema.

Adults, initial: 10 mg IV; **then,** 4 mg IM q 6 hr until maximum effect obtained (usually within 12-24 hr). Switch to PO therapy (1-3 mg t.i.d.) as soon as feasible and then slowly withdraw over 5-7 days.

Shock, unresponsive.

Initial: either 1-6 mg/kg IV or 40 mg IV; **then,** repeat IV dose q 2-6 hr as long as necessary.

- **Intralesional, Intra-articular, Soft Tissue Injections**

0.4-6 mg, depending on the site (e.g., small joints: 0.8-1 mg; large joints: 2-4 mg; soft tissue infiltration: 2-6 mg; ganglia: 1-2 mg; bursae: 2-3 mg; tendon sheaths: 0.4-1 mg.

- **Metered Dose Inhaler**

Bronchial asthma.

Adults, initial: 3 inhalations (84 mcg dexamethasone/inhalation) t.i.d.-q.i.d.; **maximum:** 3 inhalations/dose; 12 inhalations/day. **Pediatric: initial,** 2 inhalations t.i.d.-q.i.d.; **maximum:** 2 inhalations/dose; 8 inhalations/day.

- **Intranasal**

Allergies, nasal polyps.

Adults: 2 sprays (total of 168 mcg dexamethasone) in each nostril b.i.d.-t.i.d. (maximum: 12 sprays/day); **pediatric, 6-12 years:** 1-2 sprays (total of 84-168 mcg dexamethasone) in each nostril b.i.d. (maximum: 8 sprays/day).

- **Ophthalmic Ointment**

Instill a small amount of the ointment into the conjunctival sac t.i.d.-q.i.d. As response is obtained, reduce the number of applications.

- **Ophthalmic Solution**

Initial: Instill 1-2 gtt into the conjunctival sac q hr during the day and q 2 hr at night until response obtained. After a favorable response, reduce to 1 gtt q 4 hr and later 1 gtt t.i.d.-q.i.d.

- **Otic Solution**

3-4 gtt into the ear canal b.i.d.-t.i.d.

- **Topical Cream**

Apply sparingly to affected areas and rub in.

HEALTH CARE CONSIDERATIONS

See also *Health Care Considerations* for *Corticosteroids.*

Administration/Storage

1. For intranasal use, some are controlled using 1 spray in each nostril b.i.d.
2. The ophthalmic ointment is useful when an eye pad is used and for situations when prolonged contact of dexamethasone with ocular tissues is required.
3. **IV** For IV administration may give undiluted over 1 min. Do not use preparation containing lidocaine IV.

Client/Family Teaching: Review appropriate method/frequency for administration and use as directed; report loss of response or worsening of symptoms.

Outcome/Evaluate

- Improved airway exchange
- Relief of allergic manifestations
- Suppression of inflammatory response; improved circulation of blood to tissues

D

Dexchlorpheniramine maleate

(dex-klor-fen-EAR-ah-meen)

Pregnancy Category: B

Polaramine **(Rx)**

Classification: Antihistamine, alkylamine type

See also *Antihistamines.*

Action/Kinetics: Minimal sedative and moderate anticholinergic effects. **Duration:** 8 hr.

Contraindications: Use of extended-release tablets in children.

Special Concerns: Geriatric clients may be more sensitive to the usual adult dose.

How Supplied: *Syrup:* 2 mg/5 mL; *Tablet:* 2 mg; *Tablet, Extended Release:* 4 mg, 6 mg

Dosage

- **Syrup, Tablets**

Adults: 2 mg q 4-6 hr. **Pediatric, 5-12 years:** 1 mg q 4-6 hr; **2-5 years:** 0.5 mg q 4-6 hr.

- **Extended-Release Tablets**

Adults and children over 12 years: 4-6 mg at bedtime or q 8-10 hr. **Children, 6-12 years:** 4 mg/day, taken preferably at bedtime.

HEALTH CARE CONSIDERATIONS

See also *Health Care Considerations* for *Antihistamines.*

Client/Family Teaching: Take as directed; report adverse side effects or lack of response.

Outcome/Evaluate: Symptomatic relief; ↓ allergic signs & symptons

Dextroamphetamine sulfate

(dex-troh-am-FET-ah-meen)

Pregnancy Category: C

Dexedrine, Oxydess II, Spancap No. 1 **(C-II) (Rx)**

Classification: Central nervous system stimulant, amphetamine type

See also *Amphetamines and Derivatives.*

Action/Kinetics: Stronger CNS effects and weaker peripheral action than amphetamine; thus, dextroamphetamine manifests fewer undesirable CV effects. After PO, completely absorbed in 3 hr. **Duration: PO,** 4-24 hr; **t½, adults:** 10-12 hr; **children:** 6-8 hr. Excreted in urine. Acidification will increase excretion, while alkalinization will decrease it.

Uses: Attention deficit disorders in children, narcolepsy.

Additional Contraindications: Lactation. Use for obesity.

Special Concerns: Use of extended-release capsules for attention deficit disorders in children less than 6 years of age and the elixir or tablets for attention deficit disorders in children less than 3 years of age is not recommended. Dosage for narcolepsy has not been determined in children less than 6 years of age.

How Supplied: *Capsule, Extended Release:* 5 mg, 10 mg, 15 mg; *Tablet:* 5 mg, 10 mg

Dosage

- **Tablets**

Attention deficit disorders in children.

3-5 years, initial: 2.5 mg/day; increase by 2.5 mg/day at weekly intervals until optimum dose is achieved (usual range 0.1-0.5 mg/kg/dose each morning). **6 years and older, initial:** 5 mg 1-2 times/day; increase in increments of 5 mg/week until optimum dose is achieved (rarely over 40 mg/day).

Narcolepsy.

Adults: 5-60 mg in divided doses daily. **Children over 12 years, initial:** 10 mg/day; increase in increments of 10 mg/day at weekly intervals until optimum dose is reached. **Children, 6-12 years, initial:** 5 mg/day; increase in increments of 5 mg/week until optimum dose is reached (maximum is 60 mg/day).

- **Extended-Release Capsule**

Attention deficit disorders.

Children, 6 years and older: 5-15 mg/day.

Narcolepsy.

Adults: 5-30 mg/day. **Children, 6-12 years:** 5-15 mg/day; **12 years and older:** 10-15 mg/day.

HEALTH CARE CONSIDERATIONS

See also *Health Care Considerations* for *Amphetamines and Derivatives.*

Administration/Storage

1. Long-acting products may be used for once-a-day dosing in attention deficit disorders and narcolepsy.
2. When tablets or elixir are used for ADD or narcolepsy, give first dose upon awakening with one or two additional doses given at intervals of 4-6 hr. Give the last dose 6 hr before bedtime.

3. If receiving an MAO inhibitor, wait 14 days after stopping before initiating dextroamphetamine.

Client/Family Teaching

1. Take last dose at least 6 hr before bedtime to ensure adequate rest.
2. Avoid activities that require alertness until drug effects realized.

Outcome/Evaluate

- Improved attention span and concentration levels
- ↓ Daytime sleeping

Dextromethorphan hydrobromide

(dex-troh-meth-**OR**-fan)

Balminil DM Children ✱, Balminil DM Syrup ✱, Benylin DM, Benylin DM for Children, Children's Hold, Delsym, Drixoral Cough Liquid Caps ✱, Hold DM, Koffex DM Children ✱, Koffex DM Syrup ✱, Novahistex DM ✱, Novahistine DM ✱, Pertussin CS, Pertussin ES, Robitussin Cough Calmers, Robitussin Pediatric, St. Joseph Cough Suppressant, Scot-Tussin DM Cough Chasers, Sucrets Cough Control, Suppress, Triaminic DM ✱, Triaminic DM Long Lasting For Children ✱, Trocal, Vick's Formula 44, Vick's Formula 44 Pediatric Formula **(OTC)**

Classification: Nonnarcotic antitussive

Action/Kinetics: Selectively depresses the cough center in the medulla. Dextromethorphan 15-30 mg is equal to 8-15 mg codeine as an antitussive. Does not produce physical dependence or respiratory depression. Well absorbed from GI tract. **Onset:** 15-30 min. **Duration:** 3-6 hr. The sustained liquid contains dextromethorphan plistirex equivalent to 30 mg dextromethorphan hydrobromide per 5 mL.

Uses: Symptomatic relief of nonproductive cough due to colds or inhaled irritants.

Contraindications: Persistent or chronic cough or when cough is accompanied by excessive secretions. Use during first trimester of pregnancy unless directed otherwise by physician. Use in children less than 2 years of age.

Special Concerns: Use with caution in clients with nausea, vomiting, high fever, rash, or persistent headache.

Side Effects: *CNS:* Dizziness, drowsiness. *GI:* N&V, stomach pain.

OD **Management of Overdose:** *Symptoms:* **Adults:** Dysphoria, slurred speech, ataxia, altered sensory perception. **Children:** Ataxia, ***convulsions, respiratory depression.*** *Treatment:* Treat symptoms and provide support.

Drug Interactions: Use with MAO inhibitors may cause nausea, hypotension, hyperpyrexia, myoclonic leg jerks, and coma. Use with caution with patients taking SSRI's.

How Supplied: *Concentrate:* 40 mg/5 mL; *Liquid:* 3.5 mg/5 mL, 5 mg/5 mL, 7.5 mg/5 mL, 15 mg/5 mL; *Lozenge/troche:* 2.5 mg, 5 mg, 15 mg; *Suspension, Extended Release:* 30 mg/5 mL; *Syrup:* 3.5 mg/5 mL, 5 mg/5 mL, 7.5 mg/5 mL, 10 mg/5 mL, 15 mg/5 mL, 20 mg/15 mL; *Tablet:* 15 mg

Dosage

- **Capsules, Liquid, Lozenges, Syrup, Concentrate, Tablets**

Antitussive.

Adults and children over 12 years: 10-30 mg q 4-8 hr, not to exceed 120 mg/day; **pediatric, 6-12 years:** either 5-10 mg q 4 hr or 15 mg q 6-8 hr, not to exceed 60 mg/day; **pediatric, 2-6 years:** either 2.5-7.5 mg q 4 hr or 7.5 mg q 6-8 hr of the syrup, not to exceed 30 mg/day.

- **Sustained-Release Suspension**

Antitussive.

Adults: 60 mg q 12 hr. **Pediatric, 6-12 years:** 30 mg q 12 hr, not to exceed 60 mg/day; **pediatric, 2-6 years:** 15 mg q 12 hr, not to exceed 30 mg/day.

HEALTH CARE CONSIDERATIONS

Administration/Storage

1. Increasing the dose of dextromethorphan will not increase its effectiveness but will increase the duration of action.
2. Do not give lozenges to children under 6 years of age.

Assessment

1. Record sputum production and characteristics. Note duration of cough. If it persists beyond several weeks, stop dextromethorphan.
2. Determine presence of nausea, vomiting, persistent headaches, or a high fever.
3. If pregnant, determine trimester; contraindicated in first trimester.

Client/Family Teaching

1. Avoid tasks that require mental alertness until drug effects realized.
2. Avoid alcohol in any form.
3. Add humidity to environment.
4. Increase fluids to decrease viscosity of secretions.
5. Cigarette smoke, dust, and chemical fumes are irritants that may aggravate condition.
6. Symptoms that persist for more than a week require medical intervention; record

onset, triggers, characteristics of secretions, medications, and response to therapy.
Outcome/Evaluate: Control of cough with improved sleep patterns

D

Dextrose and electrolytes

(DEX-trohs)
Pedialyte, Rehydralyte, Resol **(Rx)**
Classification: Electrolyte replenisher

Action/Kinetics: PO products that contain varying amounts of sodium, potassium, chloride, citrate, and dextrose (Lytren and Resol contain 20 g/L whereas Pedialyte and Rehydralyte contain 25 g/L). In addition, Resol contains magnesium, calcium, and phosphate. **Time to peak effect:** 8-12 hr.
Uses: Diarrhea. Prophylaxis and treatment of electrolyte depletion in diarrhea or in continuing fluid loss. Maintenance of hydration.
Contraindications: Anuria, oliguria. Severe dehydration including severe diarrhea (IV therapy is necessary for prompt replacement of fluids and electrolytes). Malabsorption of glucose. Severe and sustained vomiting when the client is unable to drink. Intestinal obstruction, perforated bowel, paralytic ileus.
Special Concerns: Use with caution in premature infants.
Side Effects: Overhydration indicated by puffy eyelids. Hypernatremia, vomiting (usually shortly after treatment has started).
How Supplied: *Oral Solution*

Dosage

- **Oral Solution**

Mild dehydration.

Adults and children over 10 years, initial: 50 mL/kg over 4-6 hr; **maintenance:** 100-200 mL/kg over 24 hr until diarrhea stops.

Moderate dehydration.

Adults and children over 10 years, initial: 100 mL/kg over 6 hr; **maintenance:** 15 mL/kg q hr until diarrhea stops.

Moderate to severe dehydration.

Pediatric, 2-10 years, initial: 50 mL/kg over the first 4-6 hr followed by 100 mL/kg over the next 18-24 hr; **less than 2 years, initial:** 75 mL/kg during the first 8 hr and 75 mL/kg during the next 16 hr.

HEALTH CARE CONSIDERATIONS

Administration/Storage

1. Give no more than 1,000 mL/hr to adults and no more than 100 mL/20 min to children.
2. Adjust the amount and rate of solution depending on need, thirst, and response.
3. Assist infants and small children in drinking the solution slowly and frequently in small quantities and, if necessary, feed by a spoon.
4. Do not dilute rehydration solutions with water.

Client/Family Teaching

1. Soft foods such as bananas, cereal, cooked peas, beans, and potatoes should be given to maintain nutrition.
2. Report if fluid output exceeds intake, if there is no weight gain, or if S&S of dehydration persist.
3. If vomiting occurs after PO therapy initiated, continue but give small amounts, frequently and slowly.
4. If dehydration is severe, seek medical attention immediately. IV fluids and electrolytes should be started since the onset of action of PO solution is too slow. Oral solution can be used later for maintenance.

Outcome/Evaluate

- Adequate hydration; no S&S of dehydration
- Prevention of electrolyte depletion

Diazepam

(dye-AYZ-eh-pam)
Pregnancy Category: D
Apo-Diazepam ✦, Diastat, Diazemuls ✦, Diazepam Intensol, Dizac, E Pam ✦, Novo-Dipam ✦, PMS-Diazepam ✦, Valium, Valium Roche ✦, Vivol ✦ **(C-IV) (Rx)**
Classification: Antianxiety agent, anticonvulsant, skeletal muscle relaxant

See also *Tranquilizers/Antimanic Drugs/Hypnotics*.
Action/Kinetics: The skeletal muscle relaxant effect of diazepam may be due to enhancement of GABA-mediated presynaptic inhibition at the spinal level as well as in the brain stem reticular formation. **Onset: PO,** 30-60 min; **IM,** 15-30 min; **IV,** more rapid. **Peak plasma levels: PO,** 0.5-2 hr; **IM,** 0.5-1.5; **IV,** 0.25 hr. **Duration:** 3 hr. **t½:** 20-50 hr. Metabolized in the liver to the active metabolites desmethyldiazepam, oxazepam, and temazepam. Diazepam and metabolites are excreted through the urine. Diazepam is 97%-99% bound to plasma protein.
Uses: Anxiety, tension (more effective than chlordiazepoxide), alcohol withdrawal, muscle relaxant, adjunct to treat seizure disorders, antipanic drug. Use prior to gastroscopy and esophagoscopy, preoperatively and prior to cardioversion. In dentistry to induce sedation. Treatment of status epilepticus. Relief of skeletal muscle spasm due to inflammation of muscles or joints or trauma; spasticity caused by upper motor neuron disorders such as cerebral palsy and paraplegia; athetotis; and stiff-man syndrome. Relieve spasms

of facial muscles in occlusion and temporomandibular joint disorders. **IV:** Status epilepticus, severe recurrent seizures, and tetanus. Rectal gel: Treat epilepsy in those with stable regimens of anticonvulsant drugs who require intermittent diazepam to control increased seizure activity.

Additional Contraindications: Narrow-angle glaucoma, children under 6 months, lactation, and parenterally in children under 12 years.

Special Concerns: When used as an adjunct for seizure disorders, diazepam may increase the frequency or severity of clonic-tonic seizures, for which an increase in the dose of anticonvulsant medication is necessary. Safety and efficacy of parenteral diazepam have not been determined in neonates less than 30 days of age. Prolonged CNS depression has been observed in neonates, probably due to inability to biotransform diazepam into inactive metabolites.

Additional Drug Interactions

Diazepam potentiates antihypertensive effects of thiazides and other diuretics.

Diazepam potentiates muscle relaxant effects of *d*-tubocurarine and gallamine.

Fluoxetine / ↑ half-life of diazepam.

Isoniazid / ↑ half-life of diazepam.

Ranitidine / ↓ GI absorption of diazepam.

How Supplied: *Injection:* 5 mg/mL; *Rectal Gel:* 2.5 mg, 5 mg, 10 mg, 15 mg, 20 mg; *Solution:* 5 mg/5 mL; *Tablet* 2 mg, 5 mg, 10 mg

Dosage

- **Tablets, Oral Solution**

Antianxiety, anticonvulsant, adjunct to skeletal muscle relaxants.

Adults: 2-10 mg b.i.d.-q.i.d. **Elderly, debilitated clients:** 2-2.5 mg 1-2 times/day. May be gradually increased to adult level. **Pediatric, over 6 months, initial:** 1-2.5 mg (0.04-0.2 mg/kg or 1.17-6 mg/m^2) b.i.d.-t.i.d.

Alcohol withdrawal.

Adults: 10 mg t.i.d.-q.i.d. during the first 24 hr; **then,** decrease to 5 mg t.i.d.-q.i.d. as required.

Anticonvulsant.

Adults: 15-30 mg once daily.

- **Rectal Gel**

Anticonvulsant.

Over 12 years: 0.2 mg/kg. **Children, 6-11 years:** 0.3 mg/kg; **2-5 years:** 0.5 mg/kg. If required, a second dose can be given 4 to 12 hr after the first dose. Do not treat more than five episodes per month or more than one episode every 5 days. Adjust dose downward in elderly or debilitated clients to reduce ataxia or oversedation.

- **IM, IV**

Preoperative or diagnostic use.

Adults: 10 mg IM 5-30 min before procedure.

Adjunct to treat skeletal muscle spasm.

Adults, initial: 5-10 mg IM or IV; **then,** repeat in 3-4 hr if needed (larger doses may be required for tetanus).

Moderate anxiety.

Adults: 2-5 mg IM or IV q 3-4 hr if necessary.

Severe anxiety, muscle spasm.

Adults: 5-10 mg IM or IV q 3-4 hr, if necessary.

Acute alcohol withdrawal.

Initial: 10 mg IM or IV; **then,** 5-10 mg q 3-4 hr.

Preoperatively.

Adults: 10 mg IM prior to surgery.

Endoscopy.

IV: 10 mg or less although doses up to 20 mg can be used; **IM:** 5-10 mg 30 min prior to procedure.

Cardioversion.

IV: 5-15 mg 5-10 min prior to procedure.

Tetanus in children.

IM, IV, over 1 month: 1-2 mg, repeated q 3-4 hr as necessary; **5 years and over:** 5-10 mg q 3-4 hr.

- **IV**

Status epilepticus.

Adults, initial: 5-10 mg; **then,** dose may be repeated at 10-15-min intervals up to a maximum dose of 30 mg. Dosage may be repeated after 2-4 hr. **Children, 1 month-5 years:** 0.2-0.5 mg q 2-5 min, up to maximum of 5 mg. Can be repeated in 2-4 hr. **5 years and older:** 1 mg q 2-5 min up to a maximum of 10 mg; dose can be repeated in 2-4 hr, if needed.

NOTE: Elderly or debilitated clients should not receive more than 5 mg parenterally at any one time.

HEALTH CARE CONSIDERATIONS

See also *Health Care Considerations* for *Tranquilizers/Antimanic Drugs/Hypnotics.*

Administration/Storage

1. Mix Intensol solution with beverages such as water, soda, and juices or soft foods such as applesauce or puddings. Use only the calibrated dropper provided to withdraw drug. Once the medication is withdrawn and mixed, use immediately.
2. Except for the deltoid muscle, absorption from IM sites is slow and erratic.
3. **IV** The IV route is preferred in the convulsing client.

4. Dizac, which is an emulsified injection, should only be given IV; it is not to be given IM or SC.
5. Parenteral administration may cause bradycardia, respiratory or cardiac arrest; have emergency equipment and drugs available.
6. Diazepam interacts with plastic; therefore, introducing diazepam into plastic containers or administration sets will decrease drug availability.
7. To reduce reactions at the IV site, give diazepam slowly (5 mg/min); avoid small veins or intra-arterial administration. For pediatric use, give the IV solution slowly over a 3-min period at a dose not exceeding 0.25 mg/kg. The initial dose can be repeated after 15-30 min.
8. Due to the possibility of precipitation and instability, do not infuse diazepam. Do not mix or dilute with other solutions or drugs in the syringe or infusion container.

Assessment

1. Record indications for therapy and time for anticipated results.
2. Determine any depression or drug abuse. Avoid simultaneous use of CNS depressants.
3. Reduce drug gradually to avoid withdrawal symptoms such as anxiety, tremors, anorexia, insomnia, weakness, headache, and N&V.
4. Monitor CBC, renal, and LFTs.
5. Review anxiety level and identify any contributing factors.
6. Elderly clients may experience adverse reactions more quickly than younger clients; use a lower dose in this group.

Client/Family Teaching

1. Drug may cause dizziness and drowsiness. Avoid activities that require mental alertness until drug effects realized.
2. Avoid alcohol and any other CNS depressants.
3. Notify provider if pregnancy suspected.

Outcome/Evaluate

- ↓ Anxiety/tension episodes
- Control alcohol withdrawal
- Control of status epilepticus
- Relief of muscle spasms
- Effective sedation

Diclofenac potassium

(dye-**KLOH**-fen-ack)

Pregnancy Category: B

Cataflam, Voltaren Rapide ✱ **(Rx)**

Diclofenac sodium

(dye-**KLOH**-fen-ack)

Pregnancy Category: B

Apo-Diclo ✱, Apo-Diclo SR ✱, Novo-Difenac ✱, Novo-Difenac SR ✱, Nu-Diclo ✱, Penta-Diclofenac ✱, Taro-Diclofenac ✱, Voltaren, Voltaren Ophtha ✱, Voltaren Ophthalmic, Voltaren-XR **(Rx)**

Classification: Nonsteroidal anti-inflammatory analgesic

See also *Nonsteroidal Anti-Inflammatory Drugs.*

Action/Kinetics: Available as both the potassium (immediate-release) and sodium (delayed-release) salts. *Immediate-release product.* **Onset:** 30 min. **Peak plasma levels:** 1 hr. **Duration:** 8 hr. *Delayed-release product.* **Peak plasma levels:** 2-3 hr. **t½:** 1-2 hr. For all dosage forms, food will affect the rate, but not the amount, absorbed from the GI tract. Metabolized in the liver and excreted by the kidneys.

Uses: PO, Immediate-release: Analgesic, primary dysmenorrhea. **PO, Immediate- or Delayed-release:** Rheumatoid arthritis, osteoarthritis, ankylosing spondylitis. **PO, Delayed-release:** Osteoarthritis, rheumatoid arthritis. *Investigational:* Mild to moderate pain, juvenile rheumatoid arthritis, acute painful shoulder, sunburn. **Ophthalmic:** Postoperative inflammation following cataract or corneal refractive surgery.

Contraindications: Wearers of soft contact lenses.

Special Concerns: Use with caution during lactation. Safety and effectiveness have not been determined in children. When used ophthalmically, may cause increased bleeding of ocular tissues in conjunction with ocular surgery. Healing may be slowed or delayed.

Side Effects: *Following ophthalmic use:* Keratitis, increased intraocular pressure, ocular allergy, N&V, anterior chamber reaction, viral infections, transient burning and stinging on administration. When used with soft contact lenses, may cause ocular irritation, including redness and burning.

How Supplied: Diclofenac potassium: *Tablet:* 50 mg Diclofenac sodium: *Enteric Coated Tablet:* 25 mg, 50 mg, 75 mg; *Ophthalmic solution:* 0.1%; *Tablet, Extended Release:* 100 mg

Dosage

- **Immediate-Release Tablets, Delayed-Release Tablets**

Analgesia, primary dysmenorrhea.

Adults: 50 mg t.i.d. of immediate-release tablets. In some, an initial dose of 100 mg followed by 50-mg doses may achieve better results. After the first day, the total daily dose should not exceed 150 mg.

Rheumatoid arthritis.

Adults: 100-200 mg/day in divided doses (e.g., 50 mg t.i.d. or q.i.d.; 75 mg b.i.d. of the sodium salt). For chronic therapy, use extended-release tablets, 100 mg once or twice daily, not to exceed 225 mg/day.

Osteoarthritis.

Adults: 100-150 mg/day in divided doses (e.g., 50 mg b.i.d. or t.i.d.; 75 mg b.i.d. of the sodium salt). For chronic therapy, use extended-release tablets, 100 mg/day. Doses greater than 200 mg/day have not been evaluated.

Ankylosing spondylitis.

Adults: 25 mg q.i.d. with an extra 25-mg dose at bedtime, if necessary. Doses greater than 125 mg/day have not been evaluated.

• **Ophthalmic Solution, 0.1%**

Following cataract surgery.

1 gtt in the affected eye q.i.d. beginning 24 hr after cataract surgery and for 2 weeks thereafter.

Corneal refractive surgery.

1-2 gtt within 1 hr prior to surgery; then, apply 1-2 gtt within 15 min of surgery and continue q.i.d. for three days or less.

HEALTH CARE CONSIDERATIONS

See also *Health Care Considerations* for *Nonsteroidal Anti-Inflammatory Drugs.*

Administration/Storage: Up to 3 weeks may be required for beneficial effects to be realized when used for rheumatoid arthritis or osteoarthritis.

Assessment

1. Assess for redness, infection, pain, or vision changes with ophthalmic therapy.
2. With arthritis, assess joints for inflammation, ROM, pain, and loss of function.
3. Monitor CBC, liver and renal function studies; perform FOB with long-term therapy.
4. Ensure that drug is administered in high enough doses for anti-inflammatory effect when needed and in low doses for an analgesic effect.

Client/Family Teaching

1. May take with meals, a full glass of water or milk if GI upset occurs.
2. Do not crush or chew delayed-release tablets.
3. Limit intake of sodium, monitor weights, and report any evidence of edema or unusual weight gain.
4. Clients with diabetes should monitor BS levels closely as drug may alter response to antidiabetic agents.
5. Avoid alcohol and OTC products.
6. Maintain fluid intake of 2 L/day.
7. Report any changes in stools.

Outcome/Evaluate

• Relief of joint pain and inflammation with improved mobility
• Control of eye inflammation

COMBINATION DRUG

Diclofenac sodium and Misoprostol

(dye-**KLOH**-fen-ack/my-soh-**PROST**-ohl)

Pregnancy Category: X

Arthrotec 50, Arthrotec 75 **(Rx)**

Classification: Nonsteroidal anti-Inflammatory

See also *Diclofenac sodium* and *Misoprostol.*

Content: Arthrotec 50 contains: *NSAID:* Diclofenac sodium, 50 mg and *Prostaglandin:* Misoprostol, 200 mcg. Arthrotec 75 contains: Diclofenac sodium, 75 mg and Misoprostol, 200 mcg.

Action/Kinetics: Diclofenac is a NSAID with anti-inflammatory and analgesic effects. Misoprostol, a synthetic prostaglandin E1 analog, maintains gastroduodenal integrity and minimizes NSAID-induced gastric and duodenal ulcer formation. See individual drugs.

Uses: Treatment of osteoarthritis and rheumatoid arthritis in those at high risk of developing NSAID-induced gastric and duodenal ulcers.

Contraindications: Use in those with active GI bleeding, gastric and/or duodenal ulceration, porphyria. Pregnancy or in women planning pregnancy. Lactation. Known hypersensitivity to diclofenac, aspirin, other NSAIDs, misoprostol, or other prostaglandins.

Special Concerns: Use in premenopausal women only if effective contraception has been used and they have been advised of the risks of taking the drug if pregnant. Use with caution in renal, cardiac, or hepatic impairment. Safety and efficacy have not been determined in children.

Side Effects: See individual drugs. *GI:* Abdominal pain, diarrhea, nausea, dyspepsia, flatulence, vomiting, gastritis, constipation, eructation, GI bleeding, GI perforation, gastroduodenal ulcerations or erosions. *CNS:* Headache, dizziness. *GU:* Menorrhagia, intermenstrual bleeding, vaginal bleeding, papillary necrosis, interstitial nephritis. *Hematologic:* Decreased platelet aggregation, prolonged bleeding time, anemia. *Miscellaneous:* Skin rashes, allergic reactions, ***anaphylaxis,***fluid retention, edema.

Laboratory Test Considerations: ↑ AST, ALT, alkaline phosphatase, bilirubin.

Drug Interactions
Antacids, magnesium-containing / Worsening of diarrhea
Aspirin / ↓ Effect of diclofenac
Cyclosporine / ↑ Nephrotoxicity
Digoxin / ↑ Plasma digoxin levels
Diuretics / ↓ Effect of diuretics
Diuretics, potassium-sparing / ↑ Serum potassium levels
Lithium / ↑ Plasma lithium levels
Methotrexate / Possible enhanced methotrexate toxicity due to ↑ plasma levels
Warfarin / ↑ Risk of GI bleeding
How Supplied: See Content

Dosage
- **Tablets**

Osteoarthrits.
Adults: 1 Arthrotec 50 tablet with food t.i.d.
Rheumatoid arthritis.
Adults: 1 Arthrotec 50 tablet with food t.i.d. or q.i.d.
Note: For clients who experience intolerance, Arthrotec 75 b.i.d. or Arthrotec 50 b.i.d. can be used, but are less effective in preventing ulcers.

HEALTH CARE CONSIDERATIONS

See also *Health Care Considerations* for *Diclofenac sodium* and *Misoprostol.*
Administration/Storage: Swallow tablets whole; do not chew.
Assessment
1. Assess joints for inflammation, ROM, pain, and loss of function.
2. Note any cardiac, hepatic, or renal impairment; monitor CBC, liver and renal function studies.

Client/Family Teaching
1. Take with food as directed.
2. Drug contains an anti-inflammatory drug with a drug to protect the stomach from ulcers.
3. Report any unusual side effects, bruising or bleeding or loss of effect.
4. Practice reliable birth control.

Outcome/Evaluate: Relief of joint pain and inflammation with improved mobility

Dicloxacillin sodium
(dye-klox-ah-**SILL**-in)
Pregnancy Category: B
Dycill, Dynapen, Pathocil **(Rx)**
Classification: Antibiotic, penicillin

See also *Anti-Infectives* and *Penicillins.*
Action/Kinetics: Penicillinase-resistant and acid-stable. **Peak serum levels: IM, PO,** 4-20 mcg/mL after 1 hr. **t½:** 40 min. 98% bound to plasma proteins. Chiefly excreted in urine.
Uses: Infections due to penicillinase-producing staphylococci. To initiate therapy in any suspected staphylococcal infection. Infections due to *Streptococcus pneumoniae.*
Contraindications: Treatment of meningitis. Use in newborns.
How Supplied: *Capsule:* 250 mg, 500 mg; *Powder for reconstitution:* 62.5 mg/5 mL

Dosage
- **Capsules, Oral Suspension**

Skin and soft tissue infections, mild to moderate URTIs.
Adults and children over 40 kg: 125 mg q 6 hr; **pediatric, less than 40 kg:** 12.5 mg/kg/day in four equal doses given q 6 hr.
More severe lower respiratory tract infections or disseminated infections.
Adults and children over 40 kg: 250 mg q 6 hr, up to a maximum of 4 g/day; **pediatric, less than 40 kg:** 25 mg/kg/day in four equal doses given q 6 hr.

HEALTH CARE CONSIDERATIONS

See also *General Health Care Considerations for All Anti-Infectives* and *Penicillins.*
Administration/Storage
1. To prepare PO suspension, shake container to loosen powder, measure water for reconstitution as indicated on label, add half of the water, and immediately shake vigorously because usual handling may cause lumps. Add the remainder of the water and again shake vigorously.
2. Shake well before pouring each dose.
3. The reconstituted PO solution is stable for 7 days at room temperature, 10 days if refrigerated, and 21 days if frozen.

Assessment: Note indications for therapy, onset and duration of symptoms. Obtain cultures when indicated.
Client/Family Teaching: Preferable to take on an empty stomach 1-2 hr before meals.
Outcome/Evaluate: Symptomatic relief; negative cultures with resolution of infection

Dicyclomine hydrochloride
(dye-**SYE**-kloh-meen)
Pregnancy Category: C
Antispas, A-Spas, Bentyl, Bentylol ✦, Byclomine, Dibent, Di-Cyclonex, Dilomine, Di-Spaz, Formulex ✦, Or-Tyl **(Rx)**
Classification: Cholinergic blocking agent

See also *Cholinergic Blocking Agents.*
Action/Kinetics: t½, initial: 1.8 hr; **secondary:** 9-10 hr.

Uses: Hypermotility and spasms of GI tract associated with irritable colon and spastic colitis, mucous colitis.
Additional Contraindications: Use for peptic ulcer.
Special Concerns: Lower doses may be needed in elderly clients due to confusion, agitation, excitement, or drowsiness.
Additional Side Effects: Brief euphoria, slight dizziness, feeling of abdominal distention. **Use of the syrup in infants less than 3 months of age:** ***Seizures,*** syncope, respiratory symptoms, fluctuations in pulse rate, ***asphyxia,*** muscular hypotonia, ***coma.***
How Supplied: *Capsules:* 10 mg; *Injection:* 10 mg/mL; *Syrup:* 10 mg/1.5 mL; *Tablets:* 20 mg

Dosage

- **Capsules, Syrup, Tablets**

Hypermotility and spasms of GI tract.
Adults: 10-20 mg t.i.d.-q.i.d.; **then,** may increase to total daily dose of 160 mg if side effects do not limit this dosage. **Pediatric, 6 years and older, capsules or tablets:** 10 mg t.i.d.-q.i.d.; adjust dosage to need and incidence of side effects. **Pediatric, 6 months-2 years, syrup:** 5-10 mg t.i.d.-q.i.d.; **2 years and older:** 10 mg t.i.d.-q.i.d. The dose should be adjusted to need and incidence of side effects.

- **IM**

Hypermotility and spasms of GI tract.
Adults: 20 mg q 4-6 hr. **Not for IV use.**

HEALTH CARE CONSIDERATIONS

See also *Health Care Considerations* for *Cholinergic Blocking Agents.*
Administration/Storage: Can be administered to clients with glaucoma.
Assessment
1. Record indications for therapy, onset and duration of symptoms.
2. List other agents trialed and the outcome.
3. Determine any presence of PUD.

Client/Family Teaching: Take as directed and report any loss of response or adverse side effects.
Outcome/Evaluate: Restoration of normal bowel function/GI motility

Didanosine (ddI, dideoxyinosine)

(die-**DAN**-oh-seen)
Pregnancy Category: B
Videx **(Rx)**
Classification: Antiviral

See also *Antiviral Agents.*
Action/Kinetics: A nucleoside analog of deoxyadenosine. After entering the cell, it is converted to the active dideoxyadenosine triphosphate (ddATP) by cellular enzymes. Due to the chemical structure of ddATP, its incorporation into viral DNA leads to chain termination and therefore inhibition of viral replication. ddATP also inhibits viral replication by interfering with the HIV-RNA-dependent DNA polymerase by competing with the natural nucleoside triphosphate for binding to the active site of the enzyme. Didanosine has shown in vitro antiviral activity in a variety of HIV-infected T cell and monocyte/macrophage cell cultures. Is broken down quickly at acidic pH; therefore, PO products contain buffering agents to increase the pH of the stomach. Food decreases the rate of absorption. **t½, elimination:** 1.6 hr for adults and 0.8 hr for children. Metabolized in the liver and excreted mainly through the urine.
Uses: Advanced HIV infection in adult and pediatric (over 6 months of age) clients who are intolerant of AZT therapy or who have demonstrated decreased effectiveness of AZT therapy. Use in adults with HIV infection who have received prolonged AZT therapy. Treatment of HIV infection when antiretroviral therapy is indicated. AZT should be considered as initial therapy for the treatment of advanced HIV infection, unless contraindicated, since this drug prolongs survival and decreases the incidence of opportunistic infections. May be used as monotherapy for the treatment of AIDS.
Contraindications: Lactation.
Special Concerns: Use with caution in renal and hepatic impairment and in those on sodium-restricted diets. Opportunistic infections and other complications of HIV infection may continue to develop; thus, keep clients under close observation.
Side Effects: Commonly pancreatitis and peripheral neuropathy (manifested by distal numbness, tingling, or pain in the feet or hands). Neuropathy occurs more frequently in clients with a history of neuropathy or neurotoxic drug therapy.

In adults. *GI:* Diarrhea, abdominal pain, N&V, anorexia, dry mouth, ileus, colitis, constipation, eructation, flatulence, gastroenteritis, ***GI hemorrhage,*** oral moniliasis, stomatitis, mouth sores, sialadenitis, ***stomach ulcer hemorrhage,*** melena, oral thrush, liver abnormalities. *CNS:* Headache, ***tonic-clonic seizures,*** abnormal thinking, anxiety, nervousness, twitching, confusion, depression, acute brain syndrome, amnesia, aphasia, ataxia, dizziness, hyperesthesia, hypertonia, incoordination, ***intracranial hemorrhage,*** paralysis, paranoid reaction, psychosis, insomnia, sleep disorders, speech disorders, tremor. *Hematologic:* Leukopenia, granulocytopenia, thrombocytopenia, microcytic anemia, ***hemorrhage,*** ecchymosis, petechiae. *Dermatologic:* Rash, pruritus, herpes simplex, skin disorder, sweating, eczema, impetigo, excoriation, erythema. *Musculoskeletal:* Asthenia, myopathy, arthralgia, arthritis, myalgia, muscle atrophy, decreased strength, hemiparesis, neck rigidity, joint disorder, leg cramps. *CV:* Chest pain, hypertension, hypotension, migraine, palpitation, peripheral vascular disorder, syncope, vasodilation, arrhythmias. *Body as a whole:* Chills, fever, infection, allergic reaction, pain, abscess, cellulitis, cyst, dehydration, malaise, flu syndrome, numbness of hands and feet, weight loss, alopecia. *Respiratory:* Pneumonia, dyspnea, asthma, bronchitis, increased cough, rhinitis, rhinorrhea, epistaxis, laryngitis, decreased lung function, pharyngitis, hypoventilation, sinusitis, rhonchi, rales, congestion, interstitial pneumonia, respiratory disorders. *Ophthalmic:* Blurred vision, conjunctivitis, diplopia, dry eye, glaucoma, retinitis, photophobia, strabismus. *Otic:* Ear disorder, otitis (externa and media), ear pain. *GU:* Impotency, kidney calculus, kidney failure, abnormal kidney function, nocturia, urinary frequency, vaginal hemorrhage. *Miscellaneous:* Peripheral edema, sarcoma, hernia, hypokalemia, lymphoma-like reaction.

In children. *GI:* Diarrhea, N&V, liver abnormalities, abdominal pain, stomatitis, mouth sores, pancreatitis, anorexia, increase in appetite, constipation, oral thrush, melena, dry mouth. *CNS:* Headache, nervousness, insomnia, dizziness, poor coordination, lethargy, neurologic symptoms, ***seizures.*** *Hematologic:* Ecchymosis, ***hemorrhage,*** petechiae, leukopenia, granulocytopenia, thrombocytopenia, anemia. *Dermatologic:* Rash, pruritus, skin disorder, eczema, sweating, impetigo, excoriation, erythema. *Musculoskeletal:* Arthritis, myalgia, muscle atrophy, decreased strength. *Body as a whole:* Chills, fever, asthenia, pain, malaise, failure to thrive, weight loss, flu syndrome, alopecia, dehydration. *CV:* Vasodilation, arrhythmia. *Respiratory:* Cough, rhinitis, dyspnea, asthma, rhinorrhea, epistaxis, pharyngitis, hypoventilation, sinusitis, rhonchi, rales, congestion, pneumonia. *Ophthalmic:* Photophobia, strabismus, visual impairment. *Otic:* Ear pain, otitis. *Miscellaneous:* Urinary frequency, diabetes mellitus, diabetes insipidus, liver abnormalities.

Laboratory Test Considerations: ↑ AST, ALT, alkaline phosphatase, bilirubin, uric acid, amylase.

OD Management of Overdose: *Symptoms:* Pancreatitis, peripheral neuropathy, diarrhea, hyperuricemia, hepatic dysfunction. *Treatment:* There are no antidotes; treatment should be symptomatic.

Drug Interactions

Ketoconazole / ↓ Absorption of ketoconazole due to gastric pH change caused by buffering agents in didanosine
Pentamidine (IV) / ↑ Risk of pancreatitis
Quinolone antibiotics / ↓ Plasma levels of quinolone antibiotics
Ranitidine / ↓ Absorption of ranitidine due to gastric pH change caused by buffering agents in didanosine
Tetracyclines / ↓ Absorption of tetracyclines from the stomach due to the buffering agents in didanosine

How Supplied: *Chew Tablet:* 25 mg, 50 mg, 100 mg, 150 mg; *Powder for reconstitution:* 10 mg/mL, 100 mg, 167 mg, 250 mg

Dosage

• **Chewable/Dispersible Buffered Tablets, Buffered Powder for Oral Solution, Powder for Pediatric Oral Solution**

Adults, initial, weight over 60 kg: 200 mg q 12 hr (with 250 mg buffered powder q 12 hr). **Weight less than 60 kg:** 125 mg q 12 hr (with 167 mg buffered powder q 12 hr). **Pediatric, BSA 1.1-1.4 m²:** Two 50-mg tablets q 12 hr or 125 mg of the pediatric powder q 12 hr; **BSA 0.8-1.0 m²:** One 50- and one 25-mg tablet q 12 hr or 94 mg of the pediatric powder q 12 hr. **BSA 0.5-0.7 m²:** Two 25-mg tablets q 12 hr or 62 mg of the pediatric powder q 12 hr. **BSA less than 0.4 m²:** One 25-mg tablet q 12 hr or 31 mg of the pediatric powder q 12 hr.

HEALTH CARE CONSIDERATIONS

See also *Health Care Considerations* for *Antiviral Agents.*

Administration/Storage

1. Give on an empty stomach.
2. Give adult and pediatric clients (over 1 yr) a 2-tablet dose to prevent gastric acid degradation. Give those under 12 months old a 1-tablet dose.
3. To prepare the buffered powder for PO solution, mix with 4 oz of drinking water; do not mix the powder with fruit juice or other acid-containing beverages. Stir the mixture until the powder dissolves completely (about 2-3 min). Take the entire solution immediately.

4. To prepare the powder for pediatric oral solution, mix the dry powder with purified water to an initial concentration of 20 mg/mL. The resulting solution is then mixed with antacid to a final concentration of 10 mg/mL. Shake this admixture thoroughly prior to use. May be stored in a tightly closed container in the refrigerator for up to 30 days.

Assessment

1. Record all previous experience with AZT therapy; list reasons for transfer to didanosine.
2. Monitor CBC, CD_4 counts/viral load, liver and renal function studies.
3. Anticipate reduced dose with liver and renal impairment. Note baseline VS and weight.

Client/Family Teaching

1. Food decreases the rate of drug absorption; take on empty stomach.
2. Do not swallow tablets whole. Tablets may be chewed or crushed thoroughly before taking or dispersed in at least 1 oz of drinking water (stir thoroughly and drink immediately).
3. Report any symptoms of neuropathy (numbness, burning, or tingling in the hands or feet); drug should be discontinued until symptoms subside. May tolerate a reduced dose once these symptoms resolved.
4. Report any abdominal pain and N&V immediately; may be clinical signs of pancreatitis. Stop drug and report; resume only after pancreatitis has been ruled out.
5. With Na-restricted diets, Na content is more in the single-dose packet than the two-tablet dose.
6. Increase fluid intake; report S&S of diarrhea or hyperuricemia.
7. Any changes in vision should be evaluated by an ophthalmologist. Get retinal exams every 6 mo to rule out depigmentation with children.
8. Avoid alcohol and any other drugs that may exacerbate toxicity of didanosine.
9. Drug is not a cure, but alleviates the symptoms of HIV infections; may continue to acquire opportunistic infections.
10. *Does not* reduce the risk of transmission of HIV to others through sexual contact or blood contamination; use appropriate precautions.
11. Identify local support groups that may assist client/family to understand and cope with disease.

Outcome/Evaluate: Control of symptoms of AIDS, ARC, and opportunistic infections in clients with HIV who are intolerant or have clinically deteriorated during AZT therapy

Diethylstilbestrol diphosphate

(dye-eth-ill-still-**BESS**-trohl)

Pregnancy Category: X

Honvol ✱, Stilphostrol (Abbreviation: DES)

(Rx)

Classification: Estrogen, synthetic, nonsteroidal

See also *Estrogens* and *Antineoplastic Agents*.

Action/Kinetics: Synthetic estrogen, which competes with androgen receptors, thereby preventing androgen from inducing further growth of the neoplasm. Also binds to cytoplasmic receptor protein. The estrogen-receptor complex translocates to the nucleus, where metabolic alterations ensue. Metabolized in the liver.

Uses: Palliative treatment of inoperable, progressive prostatic cancer. Postcoital contraceptive (emergency use only).

Contraindications: Known or suspected breast cancer, estrogen-dependent neoplasia, active thrombophlebitis, thromboembolic disease, markedly impaired liver function. **Not to be used during pregnancy because of the possibility of vaginal cancer in female offspring.** The diphosphate is not to be used to treat any disorder in women.

Special Concerns: Use with caution in presence of hypercalcemia, epilepsy, migraine, asthma, cardiac and renal disease. Use with caution in children in whom bone growth is incomplete.

Side Effects: *CV: **Thrombophlebitis, pulmonary embolism, cerebral thrombosis,*** neuro-ocular lesions. *GI:* N&V, anorexia. *CNS:* Headaches, malaise, irritability. *Skin:* Allergic rash, itching. *GU:* Gynecomastia, changes in libido. *Other:* Porphyria, backache, pain and sterile abscess at injection site, postinjection flare.

How Supplied: *Injection:* 250 mg/5 mL

Dosage

- **Tablets**

Palliative treatment of prostatic carcinoma.

50 mg t.i.d. up to 200 mg t.i.d., not to exceed 1 g/day.

- **IV**

Palliative treatment of prostatic carcinoma.

500 mg (in 250 mL 5% dextrose or saline) on day 1 followed by 1 g (in 250-500 mL 5% dextrose or saline) daily for 5 days. **Maintenance, IV:** 250-500 mg 1-2 times/week. Maintenance dose may also be given PO.

D

HEALTH CARE CONSIDERATIONS

See also *Health Care Considerations* for *Antineoplastic Agents* and *Estrogens*.

Administration/Storage

IV 1. Administer slowly by IV drip (20-30 gtt/min for first 10-15 min); then adjust for a total administration period of 1 hr.
2. Solution is stable for 5 days at room temperature if stored away from direct light. Do not use if cloudy or has a precipitate.

Assessment

1. Record indications for therapy and onset of symptoms. Do not use the diphosphate to treat any disorder in women.
2. Note any history of thrombophlebitis, thromboembolic conditions, or impaired liver function.
3. Withhold and report high serum calcium levels; effect of the steroid and osteolytic metastases may result in hypercalcemia. Monitor closely (VS, weights, and I&O) once drug-induced hypercalcemia is corrected. Promote a high fluid intake to minimize hypercalcemia.
4. Assess client with poor cardiac function for edema; monitor ECG.
5. Determine if pregnant; not given during pregnancy because of the high incidence of genital tumors in offspring.
6. May prevent gynecomastia in men by administering low doses of radiation prior to initiating therapy.

Client/Family Teaching

1. Take with solid foods; may relieve nausea.
2. Report any ↑ N&V, lethargy, insomnia, anorexia, visual changes, SOB, or painful swelling of breasts or extremities.
3. With poor cardiac function, record daily weights and and check for edema.
4. Do not smoke.
5. Withdrawal bleeding may occur if drug stopped suddenly in females.
6. May alter amount of antidiabetic agent required.
7. May cause photosensitivity reaction; use sunscreen or protective clothing and/or wide brim hats.

Outcome/Evaluate: Inhibition of malignant cell proliferation

—COMBINATION DRUG—

Difenoxin hydrochloride with Atropine sulfate

(dye-fen-**OX**-in, **AH**-troh-peen)

Pregnancy Category: C

Motofen **(Rx)**

Classification: Antidiarrheal

See also *Cholinergic Blocking Agents*.

Content: Each tablet contains: *Antidiarrheal:* Difenoxin HCl, 1 mg. *Anticholinergic:* Atropine sulfate, 0.025 mg.

Action/Kinetics: Related chemically to meperidine; thus, atropine sulfate is incorporated to prevent deliberate overdosage. Difenoxin is the active metabolite of diphenoxylate and is effective at one-fifth the dosage of diphenoxylate. Slows intestinal motility by a local effect on the GI wall. **Peak plasma levels:** 40-60 min. The drug and its inactive metabolites are excreted through both the urine and feces.

Uses: Management of acute nonspecific diarrhea and acute episodes of chronic functional diarrhea.

Contraindications: Diarrhea caused by *Escherichia coli, Salmonella,* or *Shigella;* pseudomembranous colitis caused by broad-spectrum antibiotics; jaundice; children less than 2 years of age.

Special Concerns: Use with caution in ulcerative colitis, liver and kidney disease, lactation, and in clients receiving dependence-producing drugs or in those who are addiction prone. Safety and effectiveness in children less than 12 years of age have not been determined.

Side Effects: *GI:* N&V, dry mouth, epigastric distress, constipation. *CNS:* Lightheadedness, dizziness, drowsiness, headache, tiredness, nervousness, confusion, insomnia. *Ophthalmic:* Blurred vision, burning eyes.

OD **Management of Overdose:** *Symptoms:* Initially include dry skin and mucous membranes, hyperthermia, flushing, and tachycardia. These are followed by hypotonic reflexes, nystagmus, miosis, lethargy, coma, and ***respiratory depression*** (may occur up to 30 hr after overdose taken). *Treatment:* Naloxone may be used to treat respiratory depression.

Drug Interactions

Antianxiety agents / Potentiation or addition of CNS depressant effects
Barbiturates / Potentiation or addition of CNS depressant effects
Ethanol / Potentiation or addition of CNS depressant effects
MAO inhibitors / Precipitation of hypertensive crisis
Narcotics / Potentiation or addition of CNS depressant effects

How Supplied: See Content

Dosage

• **Tablets**

Adults, initial: 2 tablets (2 mg difenoxin); **then,** 1 tablet (1 mg difenoxin) after each loose stool or 1 tablet q 3-4 hr as needed. Total dose during a 24-hr period should not exceed 8 mg (i.e., 8 tablets).

HEALTH CARE CONSIDERATIONS

Administration/Storage: Treatment beyond 48 hr is usually not necessary for acute diarrhea or acute exacerbation of functional diarrhea and generally not recommended if clinical improvement is not noted.

Assessment

1. Note the onset, characteristics, and frequency of diarrhea; identify precipitating factors, e.g., travel, stress, food, medication regimens.
2. Assess for evidence of dehydration (weakness, weight loss, poor skin turgor, higher temperature, rapid weak pulse, or decreased urinary output) or electrolyte imbalance (weakness, irritability, anorexia, nausea, and dysrhythmias).
3. Send stool for analysis; C&S.
4. Monitor LFTs; may precipitate hepatic coma with dysfunction.
5. Contains atropine sulfate.
6. May precipitate hypertensive crisis with MAO inhibitors.
7. With overdose, hospitalize, since latent (12-30 hr later) respiratory depression may occur.

Client/Family Teaching

1. Do not perform tasks that require mental alertness until drug effects are realized.
2. Take only as directed; do not share.
3. Chew sugarless gum; use sugarless candy or ice chips for dry mouth. Report any swelling of gums or extremity numbness.
4. Keep out of child's reach; may be fatal if ingested.
5. Do *not* take if breast feeding.
6. Avoid alcohol or any other unprescribed CNS depressants.
7. May take 24-36 hr before effects are evident. Record the number, frequency, and characteristics of the stools; report if S&S persist more than 5 days.

Outcome/Evaluate: ↓ Frequency and number of diarrheal stools

Diflunisal

(dye-**FLEW**-nih-sal)

Pregnancy Category: C

Apo-Diflunisal ✱, Dolobid, Novo-Diflunisal ✱, Nu-Diflunisal ✱ **(Rx)**

Classification: Nonsteroidal analgesic, anti-inflammatory, antipyretic

Action/Kinetics: A salicylic acid derivative, although not metabolized to salicylic acid. Mechanism not known; may be an inhibitor of prostaglandin synthetase. **Onset:** 20 min (analgesic, antipyretic). **Peak plasma levels:** 2-3 hr. **Peak effect:** 2-3 hr. **Duration:** 4-6 hr **t½:** 8-12 hr. Ninety-nine percent protein bound. Metabolites excreted in urine.

Uses: Analgesic, rheumatoid arthritis, osteoarthritis, ankylosing spondylitis, psoriatic arthritis, musculoskeletal pain. Prophylaxis and treatment of vascular headaches.

Contraindications: Hypersensitivity to diflunisal, aspirin, or other anti-inflammatory drugs. Acute asthmatic attacks, urticaria, or rhinitis precipitated by aspirin. During lactation and in children less than 12 years of age.

Special Concerns: Use with caution in presence of ulcers or in clients with a history thereof, in clients with hypertension, compromised cardiac function, or in conditions leading to fluid retention. Use with caution in only first two trimesters of pregnancy. Geriatric clients may be at greater risk of GI toxicity.

Side Effects: *GI:* Nausea, dyspepsia, GI pain and bleeding, diarrhea, vomiting, constipation, flatulence, peptic ulcer, eructation, anorexia. *CNS:* Headache, fatigue, fever, malaise, dizziness, somnolence, insomnia, nervousness, vertigo, depression, paresthesias. *Dermatologic:* Rashes, pruritus, sweating, ***Stevens-Johnson syndrome,*** dry mucous membranes, erythema multiforme. *CV:* Palpitations, syncope, edema. *Other:* Tinnitus, asthenia, chest pain, hypersensitivity reactions, ***anaphylaxis,*** dyspnea, dysuria, muscle cramps, thrombocytopenia.

OD **Management of Overdose:** *Symptoms:* Drowsiness, N&V, diarrhea, tachycardia, hyperventilation, stupor, disorientation, diminished urine output, ***coma, cardiorespiratory arrest.*** *Treatment:* Supportive measures. To empty the stomach, induce vomiting, or perform gastric lavage. Hemodialysis may not be effective since the drug is significantly bound to plasma protein.

Drug Interactions

Acetaminophen / ↑ Plasma levels of acetaminophen
Antacids / ↓ Plasma levels of diflunisal
Anticoagulants / ↑ PT
Furosemide / ↓ Hyperuricemic effect of furosemide
Hydrochlorothiazide / ↑ Plasma levels and ↓ hyperuricemic effect of hydrochlorothiazide
Indomethacin / ↓ Renal clearance of indomethacin → ↑ plasma levels
Naproxen / ↓ Urinary excretion of naproxen and metabolite

How Supplied: *Tablet:* 250 mg, 500 mg

Dosage

- **Tablets**

Mild to moderate pain.

Adults, initial: 1,000 mg; **then,** 250-500 mg q 8-12 hr.

Rheumatoid arthritis, osteoarthritis.

Adults: 250-500 mg b.i.d. Doses in excess of 1,500 mg/day are not recommended. For some, an initial dose of 500 mg followed by 250 mg q 8-12 hr may be effective. Reduce dosage with impaired renal function.

D

HEALTH CARE CONSIDERATIONS

Administration/Storage: Maximum relief occurs in 2-3 weeks when used for the pain and swelling of arthritis. Serum salicylate levels are not used as a guide to dosage or toxicity because the drug is not hydrolyzed to salicylic acid.

Assessment

1. Note any hypersensitivity to salicylates or other NSAIDs.
2. Determine any history of PUD, HTN, or compromised cardiac function.
3. Check for pregnancy; avoid drug or use with extreme caution during the first two trimesters.
4. Give in high enough doses for anti-inflammatory effects when needed and use the lower dose for analgesic effects.
5. With long-term therapy, monitor CBC, liver and renal function studies.

Client/Family Teaching

1. May be given with water, milk, or meals to reduce gastric irritation. Do not crush or chew tablets.
2. Report unusual bruising or bleeding; may inhibit platelet aggregation which is reversible with drug discontinuation. Do not give with acetaminophen or aspirin.
3. May cause dizziness or drowsiness; use care when operating machinery or driving.
4. Report stool color changes or diarrhea; can cause an electrolyte imbalance or GI bleed.
5. Must take on a regular basis to sustain the anti-inflammatory effect.
6. Report for medical follow-up; drug needs to be adjusted according to age, condition, and changes in disease activity.

Outcome/Evaluate

- ↓ Pain and inflammation; ↑ joint mobility
- Prevention of vascular headaches

Digitoxin

(dih-jih-TOX-in)

Pregnancy Category: C

Digitaline ✱ **(Rx)**

Classification: Cardiac glycoside

Action/Kinetics: Most potent of the digitalis glycosides. Slow onset makes it unsuitable for emergency use. Almost completely absorbed from GI tract. **Onset: PO,** 1-4 hr; maximum effect: 8-12 hr. **t½:** 5-9 days; **Duration:** 2 weeks. Significant protein binding (over 90%). Metabolized by the liver and excreted as inactive metabolites through the urine. **Therapeutic serum levels:** 14-26 ng/mL. Withhold drug and check with provider if serum level exceeds 35 ng/mL, indicating toxicity.

Uses: Maintenance in CHF.

Special Concerns: Digitalis tablets may not be suitable for small children; thus, other digitalis products should be considered.

Additional Drug Interactions

Aminoglutethimide / ↓ Effect of digitoxin due to ↑ breakdown by liver
Barbiturates / ↓ Effect of digitoxin due to ↑ breakdown by liver
Diltiazem / May ↑ serum levels of digitoxin
Phenylbutazone / ↓ Effect of digitoxin due to ↑ breakdown by liver
Phenytoin / ↓ Effect of digitoxin due to ↑ breakdown by liver
Quinidine / May ↑ serum levels of digitoxin
Rifampin / ↓ Effect of digitoxin due to ↑ breakdown by liver
Verapamil / May ↑ serum levels of digitoxin

How Supplied: *Tablets:* 0.1 mg

Dosage

- **Tablets**

Digitalizing (loading) dose: Rapid.

Adults: 0.6 mg followed by 0.4 mg in 4-6 hr; **then,** 0.2 mg q 4-6 hr until therapeutic effect achieved.

Digitalizing (loading) dose: Slow.

Adults: 0.2 mg b.i.d. for 4 days.

Digitalizing (loading) dose: children.

After the neonatal period, the doses are as follows: **Under one year:** 0.045 mg/kg/day divided into three, four, or more doses with 6 hr between doses; **one to two years:** 0.04 mg/kg/day divided into three, four, or more doses with 6 hr between doses; **over two years:** 0.03 mg/kg/day (0.75 mg/m²) divided into three, four, or more doses with 6 hr between doses.

Maintenance dose: PO.

Adults: 0.05-0.3 mg/day (**usual:** 0.15 mg/day). **Children:** Give one-tenth of the digitalizing dose.

HEALTH CARE CONSIDERATIONS

Administration/Storage

1. Incompatible with acids/alkali.

2. Protect from light.
3. Premature/immature infants are especially sensitive to digitoxin; carefully determine lowered dose.

Outcome/Evaluate

- Control of S&S of CHF
- Digitoxin level (14-26 ng/mL)

Digoxin

(dih-**JOX**-in)

Pregnancy Category: A

Lanoxicaps, Lanoxin, Novo-Digoxin ✱ **(Rx)**

Classification: Cardiac glycoside

Action/Kinetics: Action prompter and shorter than that of digitoxin. **Onset: PO,** 0.5-2 hr; **time to peak effect:** 2-6 hr. **Duration:** Over 24 hr. **Onset, IV:** 5-30 min; **time to peak effect:** 1-4 hr. **Duration:** 6 days. **t½:** 30-40 hr. **Therapeutic serum level:** 0.5-2.0 ng/mL. From 20% to 25% is protein bound. Serum levels above 2.5 ng/mL indicate toxicity. Fifty percent to 70% is excreted unchanged by the kidneys. Bioavailability depends on the dosage form: tablets (60%-80%), capsules (90%-100%), and elixir (70%-85%). Thus, changing dosage forms may require dosage adjustments.

Uses: May be drug of choice for CHF because of rapid onset, relatively short duration, and ability to be administered PO or IV.

OD **Management of Overdose:** *Treatment:* See Digoxin immune Fab.

Additional Drug Interactions

1. The following drugs increase serum digoxin levels, leading to possible toxicity: Aminoglycosides, amiodarone, anticholinergics, benzodiazepines, captopril, diltiazem, erythromycin, esmolol, flecainide, hydroxychloroquine, ibuprofen, indomethacin, nifedipine, quinidine, quinine, tetracyclines, tolbutamide, verapamil.
2. Disopyramide may alter the pharmacologic effect of digoxin.
3. Penicillamine decreases serum digoxin levels.

How Supplied: *Capsule:* 0.05 mg, 0.1 mg, 0.2 mg; *Elixir:* 0.05 mg/mL; *Injection:* 0.1 mg/mL, 0.25 mg/mL; *Tablet:* 0.125 mg, 0.25 mg, 0.5 mg

Dosage

- **Capsules**

Digitalization: Rapid.

Adults: 0.4-0.6 mg initially followed by 0.1-0.3 mg q 6-8 hr until desired effect achieved.

Digitalization: Slow.

Adults: A total of 0.05-0.35 mg/day divided in two doses for a period of 7-22 days to reach steady-state serum levels. **Pediatric.** Digitalizing dosage is divided into three or more doses with the initial dose being about one-half the total dose; doses are given q 4-8 hr. **Children, 10 years and older:** 0.008-0.012 mg/kg. **5-10 years:** 0.015-0.03 mg/kg. **2-5 years:** 0.025-0.035 mg/kg. **1 month-2 years:** 0.03-0.05 mg/kg. **Neonates, full-term:** 0.02-0.03 mg/kg. **Neonates, premature:** 0.015-0.025 mg/kg.

Maintenance.

Adults: 0.05-0.35 mg once or twice daily. **Premature neonates:** 20%-30% of total digitalizing dose divided and given in two to three daily doses. **Neonates to 10 years:** 25%-35% of the total digitalizing dose divided and given in two to three daily doses.

- **Elixir, Tablets**

Digitalization: Rapid.

Adults: A total of 0.75-1.25 mg divided into two or more doses each given at 6-8-hr intervals.

Digitalization: Slow.

Adults: 0.125-0.5 mg/day for 7 days. **Pediatric.** (Digitalizing dose is divided into two or more doses and given at 6-8-hr intervals.) **Children, 10 years and older, rapid or slow:** Same as adult dose. **5-10 years:** 0.02-0.035 mg/kg. **2-5 years:** 0.03-0.05 mg/kg. **1 month-2 years:** 0.035-0.06 mg/kg. **Premature and newborn infants to 1 month:** 0.02-0.035 mg/kg.

Maintenance.

Adults: 0.125-0.5 mg/day. **Pediatric:** One-fifth to one-third the total digitalizing dose daily. *NOTE:* An alternate regimen (referred to as the “small-dose” method) is 0.017 mg/kg/day. This dose causes less toxicity.

- **IV**

Digitalization.

Adults: Same as tablets. **Maintenance:** 0.125-0.5 mg/day in divided doses or as a single dose. **Pediatric:** Same as tablets.

HEALTH CARE CONSIDERATIONS

Administration/Storage

1. Lanoxicaps gelatin capsules are more bioavailable than tablets. Thus, the 0.05-mg capsule is equivalent to the 0.0625-mg tablet; the 0.1-mg capsule is equivalent to the 0.125-mg tablet, and the 0.2-mg capsule is equivalent to the 0.25-mg tablet.
2. Differences in bioavailability have been noted between products; monitor clients when changing from one product to another.

3. Protect from light.

IV 4. Give IV injections over 5 min (or longer) either undiluted or diluted fourfold or greater with sterile water for injection, 0.9% NaCl injection, RL injection, or D5W.

Client/Family Teaching

1. Check when to hold digoxin, (i.e., HR < 50-60 or > 120.
2. Report S&S of digoxin toxicity: abdominal pain, N&V, visual disturbances, irregular heart beat.
3. Continue Na-restricted, low-fat diet.

Outcome/Evaluate

- Control of S&S of CHF (↑ CO, ↓ HR, ↓ SOB)
- Serum level (0.5-2.0 ng/mL)

Dihydroergotamine mesylate

(dye-hy-droh-er-**GOT**-ah-meen)

Pregnancy Category: X

D.H.E. 45, Dihydroergotamine (DHE) Sandoz ✱, Migranal Nasal Spray **(Rx)**

Classification: Alpha-adrenergic blocking agent

Action/Kinetics: Manifests alpha-adrenergic receptor blocking activity as well as a direct stimulatory action on vascular smooth muscle of peripheral and cranial blood vessels, resulting in vasoconstriction, thus preventing the onset of a migraine attack. Manifests greater adrenergic blocking activity, less pronounced vasoconstriction, less N&V, and less oxytocic properties than does ergotamine. More effective when given early in the course of a migraine attack. **Onset: IM,** 15-30 min; **IV,**< 5 min. **Duration: IM,** 3-4 hr. **t½: initial,**1.4 hr; **final,**18-22 hr. Metabolized in liver and excreted in feces with less than 10% excreted through the urine.

Uses: IM, IV. To prevent or abort migraine, migraine variant, histaminic cephalalgia (cluster headaches). Especially useful when rapid effect is desired or when other routes of administration are not possible. **Nasal Spray.** Acute treatment of migraine headaches with or without aura.

Contraindications: Lactation. Pregnancy. Peripheral vascular disease, coronary heart disease, hypertension, impaired hepatic or renal function, sepsis, hypersensitivity, malnutrition, severe pruritus, presence of infection.

Special Concerns: Safety and efficacy have not been determined in children. Geriatric clients may be more affected by peripheral vasoconstriction that results in hypothermia. Prolonged administration may cause ergotism and gangrene.

Side Effects: *CV:* Precordial pain, transient tachycardia or bradycardia. Large doses may cause increased BP, vasoconstriction of coronary arteries, and bradycardia. *GI:* N&V, diarrhea. *Other:* Numbness and tingling of fingers and toes, muscle pain in extremities, weakness in legs, localized edema, and itching. *Prolonged use:* Gangrene, ergotism.

OD **Management of Overdose:** *Symptoms:* N&V, pain in limb muscles, tachycardia or bradycardia, precordial pain, numbness and tingling of fingers and toes, weakness of the legs, hypertension or hypotension, localized edema, S&S of ischemia due to vasoconstriction of peripheral arteries and arterioles. Symptoms of ischemia include the feet and hands becoming cold, pale, and numb; muscle pain, gangrene. Occasionally confusion, depression, drowsiness, and ***seizures.*** *Treatment:* Maintain adequate circulation. IV nitroglycerin and nitroprusside to treat vasospasm. IV heparin and low molecular weight dextran to minimize thrombosis.

Drug Interactions

Beta-adrenergic blockers / ↑ Peripheral ischemia resulting in cold extremities and possibly peripheral gangrene

Macrolide antibiotics / Acute ergotism resulting in peripheral ischemia

Nitrates / ↑ Bioavailability of hydroergotamine and ↓ anginal effects of nitrates

How Supplied: *Injection:* 1 mg/mL; *Nasal Spray:* 0.5 mg/inh

Dosage

- **IM**

Suppress vascular headache.

Adults, initial: 1 mg at first sign of headache; repeat q hr for a total of 3 mg (not to exceed 6 mg/week).

- **IV**

Suppress vascular headache.

Similar to IM but to a maximum of 2 mg/attack or 6 mg/week.

- **Nasal spray**

Acute migraine headaches.

Single treatment of 0.5 mg spray in each nostril followed in 15 min by a second 0.5 mg spray in each nostil (i.e., total of 2 mg).

HEALTH CARE CONSIDERATIONS

Administration/Storage: Adjust dosage if client complains of severe headaches; use this dose when subsequent headaches begin.

Assessment

1. Obtain a thorough medical, diet, and drug history; note any contributing factors (i.e., cigarette smoking, alcohol ingestion, OTC agents, stress).
2. Do not take with nitrates or if any sensitivity to ergotamine.
3. Determine severity and characteristics of headaches and what relieved them.

4. Assess for pregnancy; has an oxytocic effect.
5. Note any liver or renal dysfunction, HTN, PVD, or CAD.

Client/Family Teaching
1. Take at the onset of migraine; most effective when administered early in an attack.
2. Seek bed rest in a darkened room for 1-2 hr after drug ingestion.
3. Practice alternative methods for dealing with stress, such as relaxation.
4. Report evidence of cold extremities and numbness or tingling; to avoid gangrene.
5. Take only as directed and do not stop abruptly.
6. Keep a headache diary; list foods, events, activities surrounding onset.

Outcome/Evaluate: Relief of migraine headaches

Diltiazem hydrochloride

(dill-**TIE**-ah-zem)

Pregnancy Category: C

Alti-Diltiazem ✱, Alti-Diltiazem CD ✱, Apo-Diltiaz ✱, Apo-Diltiaz CD ✱, Cardizem, Cardizem CD, Cardizem Injectable, Cardizem Lyo-Ject, Cardizem-SR, Dilacor XR, Diltiazem HCl Extended Release, Gen-Diltiazem ✱, Med Diltiazem ✱, Novo-Diltazem ✱, Novo-Diltazem SR ✱, Nu-Diltiaz ✱, Taro-Diltiazem ✱, Tiamate, Tiazac **(Rx)**

Classification: Calcium channel blocking agent (antianginal, antihypertensive)

See also *Calcium Channel Blocking Agents.*

Action/Kinetics: Decreases SA and AV conduction and prolongs AV node effective and functional refractory periods. Also decreases myocardial contractility and peripheral vascular resistance. **Tablets: Onset,** 30-60 min; **time to peak plasma levels:** 2-3 hr; **t½, first phase:** 20-30 min; **second phase:** about 3-4.5 hr (5-8 hr with high and repetitive doses); **duration:** 4-8 hr. **Extended-Release Capsules: Onset,** 2-3 hr; **time to peak plasma levels:** 6-11 hr; **t½:** 5-7 hr; **duration:** 12 hr. **Therapeutic serum levels:** 0.05-0.2 mcg/mL. Metabolized to desacetyldiltiazem, which manifests 25%-50% of the activity of diltiazem. Excreted through both the bile and urine.

Uses: Tablets: Vasospastic angina (Prinzmetal's variant). Chronic stable angina (classic effort-associated angina), especially in clients who cannot use beta-adrenergic blockers or nitrates or who remain symptomatic after clinical doses of these agents. **Sustained-Release Capsules:** Essential hypertension, angina. **Parenteral:** Atrial fibrillation or flutter. Paroxysmal SVT. Cardizem Lyo-Ject is used on an emergency basis for atrial fibrillation or atrial flutter. Cardizem Monovial is used to maintain control of HR for up to 24 hr in atrial fibrillation or flutter. *Investigational:* Prophylaxis of reinfarction of nonQ wave MI; tardive dyskinesia, Raynaud's syndrome.

Contraindications: Hypotension. Second- or third-degree AV block and sick sinus syndrome except in presence of a functioning ventricular pacemaker. Acute MI, pulmonary congestion. Lactation.

Special Concerns: Safety and effectiveness in children have not been determined. The half-life may be increased in geriatric clients. Use with caution in hepatic disease and in CHF. Abrupt withdrawal may cause an increase in the frequency and duration of chest pain. Use with beta blockers or digitalis is usually well tolerated, although the effects of coadministration cannot be predicted (especially in clients with left ventricular dysfunction or cardiac conduction abnormalities).

Side Effects: *CV:* AV block, bradycardia, CHF, hypotension, syncope, palpitations, peripheral edema, ***arrhythmias,*** angina, tachycardia, ***abnormal ECG, ventricular extrasystoles.*** *GI:* N&V, diarrhea, constipation, anorexia, abdominal discomfort, cramps, dry mouth, dysgeusia. *CNS:* Weakness, nervousness, dizziness, lightheadedness, headache, depression, psychoses, hallucinations, disturbances in sleep, somnolence, insomnia, amnesia, abnormal dreams. *Dermatologic:* Rashes, dermatitis, pruritus, urticaria, erythema multiforme, ***Stevens-Johnson syndrome.*** *Other:* Photosensitivity, joint pain or stiffness, flushing, nasal or chest congestion, dyspnea, SOB, nocturia/polyuria, sexual difficulties, weight gain, paresthesia, tinnitus, tremor, asthenia, gynecomastia, gingival hyperplasia, petechiae, ecchymosis, purpura, bruising, hematoma, leukopenia, double vision, epistaxis, eye irritation, thirst, alopecia, ***bundle branch block,*** abnormal gait, hyperglycemia.

Laboratory Test Considerations: ↑ Alkaline phosphatase, CPK, LDH, AST, ALT.

Additional Drug Interactions

Anesthetics / ↑ Risk of depression of cardiac contractility, conductivity, and automaticity as well as vascular dilation

Carbamazepine / ↑ Effect of diltiazem due to ↓ breakdown by liver

Cimetidine / ↑ Bioavailability of diltiazem

Cyclosporine / ↑ Effect of cyclosporine possibly leading to renal toxicity

Digoxin / ↑ Serum digoxin levels are possible

Lithium / ↑ Risk of neurotoxicity
Ranitidine / ↑ Bioavailability of diltiazem
Theophyllines / ↑ Risk of pharmacologic and toxicologic effects of theophyllines
How Supplied: *Capsule, Extended Release:* 60 mg, 90 mg, 120 mg, 180 mg, 240 mg, 300 mg, 360 mg; *Injection:* 5 mg/mL; *Monovial:* 100 mg freeze-dried diltiazem; *Powder for Injection:* 10 mg, 25 mg; *Tablet:* 30 mg, 60 mg, 90 mg, 120 mg; *Tablet, Extended Release:* 120 mg, 180 mg, 240 mg

Dosage

• **Tablets**

Angina.

Adults, initial: 30 mg q.i.d. before meals and at bedtime; **then,** increase gradually to total daily dose of 180-360 mg (given in three to four divided doses). Increments may be made q 1-2 days until the optimum response is attained.

• **Capsules, Sustained-Release**

Angina.

Cardizem CD: Adults, initial: 120 or 180 mg once daily. Up to 480 mg/day may be required. Dosage adjustments should be carried out over a 7-14-day period.

Dilacor XR: Adults, initial: 120 mg once daily; **then,** dose may be titrated, depending on the needs of the client, up to 480 mg once daily. Titration may be carried out over a 7-14-day period.

Hypertension.

Cardizem CD: Adults, initial: 180-240 mg once daily. Maximum antihypertensive effect usually reached within 14 days. Usual range is 240-360 mg once daily.

Cardizem SR: Adults, initial: 60-120 mg b.i.d.; **then,** when maximum antihypertensive effect is reached (approximately 14 days), adjust dosage to a range of 240-360 mg/day.

Dilacor XR: Adults, initial: 180-240 mg once daily. Usual range is 180-480 mg once daily. The dose may be increased to 540 mg/day with little or no increased risk of side effects.

Tiazac: Adults, initial: 120-240 mg once daily. Usual range is 120-360 mg once daily, although doses up to 540 mg once daily have been used.

• **IV Bolus**

Atrial fibrillation/flutter; paroxysmal SVT.

Adults, initial: 0.25 mg/kg (average 20 mg) given over 2 min; **then,** if response is inadequate, a second dose may be given after 15 min. The second bolus dose is 0.35 mg/kg (average 25 mg) given over 2 min. Subsequent doses should be individualized. Some clients may respond to an initial dose of 0.15 mg/kg (duration of action may be shorter).

• **IV Infusion**

Atrial fibrillation/flutter.

Adults: 10 mg/hr following IV bolus dose(s) of 0.25 mg/kg or 0.35 mg/kg. Some clients may require 5 mg/hr while others may require 15 mg/hr. Infusion may be maintained for 24 hr.

• **Cardizem Lyo-Ject**

Atrial fibrillation/atrial flutter.

Delivery system consists of a dual-chamber, prefilled, calibrated syringe containing 25 mg of diltiazem hydrochloride in one chamber and 5 mL of diluent in the other chamber.

HEALTH CARE CONSIDERATIONS

See also *Health Care Considerations* for *Calcium Channel Blocking Agents.*

Administration/Storage

1. Sublingual nitroglycerin may be taken concomitantly for acute angina. Diltiazem may also be taken together with long-acting nitrates.
2. Clients taking other forms of diltiazem can be safely switched to Dilacor XR at the nearest equivalent total daily dose. Titration to larger or smaller doses may be necessary.
3. Use with beta blockers or digitalis is usually well tolerated, but the combined effects cannot be predicted, especially with cardiac conduction abnormalities or LV dysfunction.

Assessment

1. Record indications for therapy, symptom onset, and any previous treatments.
2. Note any edema or CHF; review ECG for evidence of AV block.
3. Monitor renal and LFTs; reduce dose with impaired function.
4. The drug half-life may be prolonged in the elderly; monitor closely.

Client/Family Teaching

1. Take the sustained-release capsules on an empty stomach. Do not open, chew, or crush; should be swallowed whole.
2. May cause drowsiness or dizziness.
3. Rise slowly from a lying to a sitting and standing position; may cause postural hypotension.
4. Report persistent and bothersome side effects including constipation, unusual tiredness, or weakness.
5. Continue carrying short-acting nitrites (nitroglycerin) at all times and use as directed.
6. Continue diet (low fat and low Na), regular exercise, and decreased intake of caffeine, tobacco, and alcohol.

Outcome/Evaluate

• ↓ Frequency and intensity of vasospastic anginal attacks
• ↓ BP; stable cardiac rhythm

Dimenhydrinate

(dye-men-**HY**-drih-nayt)

Pregnancy Category: B

Oral Liquid, Syrup, Tablets, Chewable Tablets: Apo-Dimenhydrinate ✦, Calm-X, Dimentabs, Dramamine, Gravol ✦, Marmine, Motion-Aid, PMS-Dimenhydrinate ✦, Travamine, Travel Tabs ✦, Traveltabs ✦, Triptone **(OTC)**. **Injection:** Dimenhydrinate Injection ✦, Dinate, Dramanate, Dramilin, Dymenate, Gravol ✦, Hydrate, Marmine, Reidamine **(Rx)**

Classification: Antihistamine, antiemetic

See also *Antihistamines* and *Antiemetics.*

Action/Kinetics: Contains both diphenhydramine and chlorotheophylline. Antiemetic mechanism not known, but it does depress labyrinthine and vestibular function. May mask ototoxicity due to aminoglycosides. Possesses anticholinergic activity. **Duration:** 3-6 hr.

Uses: Motion sickness, especially to relieve nausea, vomiting, or dizziness. Treat vertigo.

Special Concerns: Use of the injectable form is not recommended in neonates. Geriatric clients may be more sensitive to the usual adult dose.

How Supplied: *Chew Tablet:* 50 mg; *Injection:* 50 mg/mL; *Liquid:* 12.5 mg/4 mL, 12.5 mg/5 mL; *Tablet:* 25 mg, 50 mg

Dosage

- **Elixir, Syrup, Tablets, Chewable Tablets**

Motion sickness.

Adults: 50-100 mg q 4 hr, not to exceed 400 mg/day. **Pediatric, 6-12 years:** 25-50 mg q 6-8 hr, not to exceed 150 mg/day; **2-6 years:** 12.5-25 mg q 6-8 hr, not to exceed 75 mg/day.

- **IM, IV**

Adults: 50 mg as required. **Pediatric, over 2 years:** 1.25 mg/kg (37.5 mg/m^2) q.i.d., not to exceed 300 mg/day.

- **IV**

Adults: 50 mg in 10 mL sodium chloride injection given over 2 min; may be repeated q 4 hr as needed. **Pediatric:** 1.25 mg/kg (37.5 mg/m^2) in 10 mL of 0.9% sodium chloride injection given slowly over 2 min; may be repeated q 6 hr, not to exceed 300 mg/day.

HEALTH CARE CONSIDERATIONS

See also *Health Care Considerations* for *Antihistamines* and *Antiemetics.*

Assessment: Record indications for therapy and symptom onset; assess for vestibular damage when administered with antihistamines.

Client/Family Teaching

1. Avoid activities that require mental alertness until effects realized.
2. May alter skin testing results.

Outcome/Evaluate: Prevention of N&V; control of vertigo

D

Diphenhydramine hydrochloride

(dye-fen-**HY**-drah-meen)

Pregnancy Category: B

Allerdryl ✦, AllerMax, AllerMax Allergy & Cough Formula, Banophen Caplets, Benadryl, Benadryl Allergy, Benadryl Allergy Ultratabs, Benadryl Dye-Free Allergy, Benadryl Dye-Free Allergy Liqui Gels, Diphen AF, Diphen Cough, Diphenhist, Genahist, Hyrexin-50, Nytol ✦, Nytol Extra Strength ✦, PMS-Diphenhydramine ✦, Scheinpharm Diphenhydramine ✦, Scot-Tussin DM, Siladryl, Tusstat**(OTC and Rx).**, **Sleep-Aids:** Dormin, Miles Nervine, Nighttime Sleep Aid, Nytol, Sleep-eze 3, Sleep-Eze D ✦, Sleepwell 2-nite, Sominex **(OTC)**

Classification: Antihistamine, ethanolamine-type; antiemetic

See also *Antihistamines*, *Antiemetics*, and *Antiparkinson Drugs.*

Action/Kinetics: High sedative, anticholinergic, and antiemetic effects.

Uses: Hypersensitivity reactions, motion sickness (PO only), parkinsonism, nighttime sleep aid (PO only), antitussive (syrup only).

Contraindications: Topically to treat chickenpox, poison ivy, or sunburn. Topically on large areas of the body or on blistered or oozing skin.

How Supplied: *Balm:* 2%; *Capsule:* 25 mg, 50 mg; *Chew Tablet:* 12.5 mg; *Cream:* 2%; *Elixir:* 12.5 mg/5 mL; *Injection:* 10 mg/mL, 50 mg/mL; *Liquid:* 6.25 mg/5 mL, 12.5 mg/5 mL, 50 mg/15 mL; *Lotion:* 0.5%; *Spray:* 1%, 2%; *Syrup:* 12.5 mg/5 mL; *Tablet:* 25 mg, 50 mg

Dosage

- **Capsules, Chewable Tablets, Elixir, Liquid, Syrup, Tablets**

Antihistamine, antiemetic, antimotion sickness, parkinsonism.

Adults: 25-50 mg t.i.d.-q.i.d.; **pediatric, over 10 kg:** 12.5-25 mg t.i.d.-q.i.d. (or 5 mg/kg/day not to exceed 300 mg/day or 150 mg/m^2/day).

Sleep aid.

Adults and children over 12 years: 50 mg at bedtime.

Antitussive (syrup only).

Adults: 25 mg q 4 hr, not to exceed 100 mg/day; **pediatric, 6-12 years:** 12.5-25 mg q 4 hr, not to exceed 50 mg/day; **pediatric, 2-6 years:** 6.25 mg q 4 hr, not to exceed 25 mg/day.

• **IV, Deep IM**

Parkinsonism.

Adults: 10-50 mg up to 100 mg if needed (not to exceed 400 mg/day); **pediatric:** 1.25 mg/kg (or 37.5 mg/m²) q.i.d., not to exceed a total of 300 mg/day.

HEALTH CARE CONSIDERATIONS

See also *Health Care Considerations* for *Antihistamines*, *Antiemetics*, and *Antiparkinson Drugs*.

Administration/Storage

1. With motion sickness, give the full prophylactic dose 30 min prior to travel and 1-2 hr before exposures that precipitate sickness.
2. Take similar doses with meals and at bedtime.
3. Do not use more than 2 weeks to treat insomnia.

IV 4. For IV, may give undiluted; each 25 mg over at least 1 min.

Client/Family Teaching

1. May cause drowsiness; use caution until drug effects realized.
2. Use protection; may cause photosensitivity reaction.
3. Use sugarless gum/candy to diminish dry mouth effects.
4. Avoid alcohol and any other CNS depressants unless prescribed.

Outcome/Evaluate

- ↓ Allergic manifestations
- Relief of nausea
- Promotion of sleep
- Relief of dyskinesias/extrapyramidal symptoms with parkinsonism

COMBINATION DRUG

Diphenoxylate hydrochloride with Atropine sulfate

(dye-fen-**OX**-ih-layt, **AH**-troh-peen)

Pregnancy Category: C

Lofene, Logen, Lomanate, Lomodix, Lomotil, Lonox, Low-Quel **(C-V) (Rx)**

Classification: Antidiarrheal agent, systemic

See also *Cholinergic Blocking Agents*.

Content: Each tablet or 5 mL of liquid contains: *Antidiarrheal:* Diphenoxylate HCl, 2.5 mg. *Anticholinergic:* Atropine sulfate, 0.025 mg.

Action/Kinetics: Chemically related to the narcotic analgesic drug meperidine but without the analgesic properties. Inhibits GI motility and has a constipating effect. May aggravate diarrhea due to organisms that penetrate the intestinal mucosa (e.g., *Escherichia coli, Salmonella, Shigella)* or in antibiotic-induced pseudomembranous colitis. High doses over prolonged periods may cause euphoria and physical dependence. The product also contains small amounts of atropine sulfate which will prevent abuse by deliberate overdosage. **Onset:** 45-60 min. **t½, diphenoxylate:** 2.5 hr; **diphenoxylic acid:** 12-24 hr. **Duration:** 2-4 hr. Metabolized in the liver to the active diphenoxylic acid and excreted through the urine.

Uses: Symptomatic treatment of chronic and functional diarrhea. Also, diarrhea associated with gastroenteritis, irritable bowel, regional enteritis, malabsorption syndrome, ulcerative colitis, acute infections, food poisoning, postgastrectomy, and drug-induced diarrhea. Therapeutic results for control of acute diarrhea are inconsistent. Also used in the control of intestinal passage time in clients with ileostomies and colostomies.

Contraindications: Obstructive jaundice, liver disease, diarrhea associated with pseudomembranous enterocolitis after antibiotic therapy or enterotoxin-producing bacteria, children under the age of 2.

Special Concerns: Use with caution during lactation, when anticholinergics may be contraindicated, and in advanced hepatic-renal disease or abnormal renal functions. Children (especially those with Down syndrome) are susceptible to atropine toxicity. Children and geriatric clients may be more sensitive to the respiratory depressant effects of diphenoxylate. Dehydration, especially in young children, may cause a delayed diphenoxylate toxicity.

Side Effects: *GI:* N&V, anorexia, abdominal discomfort, paralytic ileus, megacolon. *Allergic:* Pruritus, ***angioneurotic edema,*** swelling of gums. *CNS:* Dizziness, drowsiness, malaise, restlessness, headache, depression, numbness of extremities, ***respiratory depression, coma.*** *Topical:* Dry skin and mucous membranes, flushing. *Other:* Tachycardia, urinary retention, hyperthermia.

OD **Management of Overdose:** *Symptoms:* Dry skin and mucous membranes, flushing, ***hyperthermia,*** mydriasis, restlessness, tachycardia followed by miosis, lethargy, hypotonic reflexes, nystagmus, ***coma, severe (and possibly fatal) respiratory depression.*** *Treatment:* Gastric lavage, induce vomiting, establish a patent airway, and assist respiration. Activated charcoal (100 g) given as a slurry. IV administration of a narcotic antagonist. Administration may be repeated after

10-15 min. Observe client and readminister antagonist if respiratory depression returns.

Drug Interactions

Alcohol / Additive CNS depression

Antianxiety agents / Additive CNS depression

Barbiturates / Additive CNS depression

MAO inhibitors / ↑ Chance of hypertensive crisis

Narcotics / ↑ Effect of narcotics

How Supplied: See Content

Dosage

- **Oral Solution, Tablets**

Adults, initial: 2.5-5 mg (of diphenoxylate) t.i.d.-q.i.d.; **maintenance:** 2.5 mg b.i.d.-t.i.d. **Pediatric, 2-12 years:** 0.3-0.4 mg/kg/day (of diphenoxylate) in divided doses.

HEALTH CARE CONSIDERATIONS

See also *Health Care Considerations* for *Difenoxin hydrochloride with Atropine sulfate.*

Administration/Storage

1. For liquid preparations, use only the plastic dropper supplied by the manufacturer to measure dosage.
2. If clinical improvement is not evident after 10 days with a maximum dose of 20 mg/day, further use will not likely control symptoms.

Assessment

1. Record indications for therapy, onset, duration of symptoms, and other agents trialed.
2. Determine fluid and electrolyte status. Dehydration in young children may cause delayed toxicity.
3. Review culture reports to determine if drug is appropriate if not effective after 24-36 hr.
4. Note any hepatic or renal dysfunction.
5. Assess for abdominal distension and toxic megacolon.

Pediatric / Dose

2-3 years / 0.75-1.5 mg q.i.d.

3-4 years / 1-1.5 mg q.i.d.

4-5 years / 1-2 mg q.i.d.

5-6 years / 1.25-2.25 mg q.i.d.

6-9 years / 1.25-2.5 mg q.i.d.

9-12 years / 1.75-2.5 mg q.i.d.

Based on 4 mL/tsp or 2 mg of diphenoxylate. Each tablet or 5 mL of liquid preparation contains 2.5 mg diphenoxylate hydrochloride and 25 mcg of atropine sulfate. Dosage should be maintained at initial levels until symptoms are under control; then reduce to maintenance levels.

Client/Family Teaching: Take only as prescribed; do not exceed dosage, report lack of response. May cause drowsiness; use caution.

Outcome/Evaluate: Relief of diarrhea

Dipyridamole

(dye-peer-**ID**-ah-mohl))

Pregnancy Category: B

Apo-Dipyridamole FC ✱, Apo-Dipyridamole SC ✱, Novo-Dipiradol ✱, Persantine **(Rx)**

Classification: Platelet adhesion inhibitor

Action/Kinetics: In higher doses may act by several mechanisms, including inhibition of red blood cell uptake of adenosine, itself an inhibitor of platelet reactivity; inhibition of platelet phosphodiesterase, which leads to accumulation of cAMP within platelets; direct stimulation of release of prostacyclin or prostaglandin D_2; and/or inhibition of thromboxane A_2 formation. Dipyridamole prolongs platelet survival time in clients with valvular heart disease and has maintained platelet count in open heart surgery. Also causes coronary vasodilation which may be due to inhibition of adenosine deaminase in the blood, thus allowing accumulation of adenosine which is a potent vasodilator. Vasodilation may also be caused by delaying the hydrolysis of cyclic 3', 5'-adenosine monophosphate as a result of inhibition of the enzyme phosphodiesterase. Incompletely absorbed from the GI tract. **Peak plasma levels, after PO:** 45-150 min. **$t^1/_2$, after PO: initial,** 40-80 min; **terminal,** 10-12 hr. Metabolized in the liver and mainly excreted in the bile.

Uses: PO. As an adjunct to coumarin anticoagulants in preventing post-operative thromboembolic complications of cardiac valve replacement. **IV.** As an alternative to exercise in thallium myocardial perfusion imaging for the evaluation of CAD in those who cannot exercise adequately. *Investigational:* Alone or as an adjunct to treat angina, to prevent graft occlusion in those undergoing arterial reconstructive bypass surgery, intralingual bypass grafts, and to prevent deterioration of coronary vessel patency after percutaneous transluminal angioplasty. Use with aspirin for preventing migraine headaches, MI, to reduce platelet aggregation at the carotid endarterectomy, to slow progression of peripheral occlusive arterial disease, to reduce incidence of DVT, to reduce the number of platelets deposited on dacron aortofemoral artery grafts, and TIAs.

NOTE: Not effective for the treatment of

acute episodes of angina and is not a substitute for the treatment of angina pectoris.

Special Concerns: Use with caution in hypotension and during lactation. Safety and efficacy have not been determined in children less than 12 years of age.

Side Effects: After PO use. *GI:* GI intolerance, N&V, diarrhea. *CNS:* Dizziness, headache, syncope. *CV:* Peripheral vasodilation, flushing. Rarely, angina pectoris or aggravation of angina pectoris (usually at the beginning of therapy). *Miscellaneous:* Weakness, rash, pruritus.

After IV use. Most common side effects (1% or greater) are listed. *GI:* Nausea, dyspepsia. *CNS:* Headache, dizziness, paresthesia, fatigue. *CV:* Chest pain, angina pectoris, ECG abnormalities (ST-T changes, extrasystoles, tachycardia), precipitation of acute myocardial ischemia in clients with CAD, hypotension, flushing, blood pressure lability, hypertension. *Miscellaneous:* Dyspnea, unspecified pain.

OD **Management of Overdose:** *Symptoms:* Hypotension of short duration. *Treatment:* Use of a vasopressor may be beneficial. Due to the high percentage of protein binding of dipyridamole, dialysis is not likely to be beneficial.

How Supplied: *Injection:* 5 mg/mL; *Tablets:* 25 mg, 50 mg, 75 mg.

Dosage

- **Tablets**

Adjunct in prophylaxis of thromboembolism after cardiac valve replacement.

Adults: 75-100 mg q.i.d. as an adjunct to warfarin therapy.

Prevention of thromboembolic complications in other thromboembolic disorders.

Adults: 150-400 mg/day in combination with another platelet-aggregation inhibitor (e.g., aspirin) or an anticoagulant.

- **IV**

Adjunct to thallium myocardial perfusion imaging.

Adjust the dose according to body weight. Recommended dose is 0.142 mg/kg/min infused over 4 min. Total dose should not exceed 60 mg.

HEALTH CARE CONSIDERATIONS

Administration/Storage

IV 1. When used IV, to prevent irritation, dilute the injection in at least a 1:2 ratio with 0.45% NaCl injection, 0.9% NaCl injection, or D5W. The total volume should be 20 to 50 mL.

2. With imaging, give thallium-201 within 5 min after the IV injection.

3. Do not mix with other drugs in the same syringe or infusion container.

Assessment

1. Record indications for therapy, type, onset, duration, and characteristics of symptoms.

2. List all drugs currently prescribed to ensure none interact unfavorably.

3. Record mental status, skin color, and cardiopulmonary findings.

4. Monitor VS, ECG, CBC, PT, PTT, and INR.

Client/Family Teaching

1. Drug helps prevent clots by inhibiting platelet stickiness.

2. Avoid alcohol and tobacco due to hypotensive vasoconstrictive effects; and any other unprescribed drugs including aspirin without approval.

3. Drug may cause dizziness and lightheadedness; change positions slowly.

4. Try small frequent meals if nausea or gastric distress is experienced.

5. Report any increased chest pain, skin rash, fainting or severe headaches.

Outcome/Evaluate

- CAD evaluation with imaging
- Prevention of thromboembolism

COMBINATION DRUG

Dipyridamole and Aspirin

(dye-peh-**RID**-ah-mohl, **ASS**-per-in)

Pregnancy Category: Dipyridamole: B; aspirin: D

Aggrenox **(Rx)**

Classification: Antiplatelet agent

Action/Kinetics: An antithrombotic action resulting from additive antiplatelet effects. See monographs for dipyridamole and aspirin (acetylsalicylic acid). **t½:** Dipyridamole, 13.6 hr; aspirin, 1.71 hr. **Peak:** Dipyridamole, 2 hr; aspirin: 0.63 hr.

Uses: Reduce risk of stroke in patients who have had transient ischemia of the brain or ischemic stroke due to thrombosis.

Contraindications: Hypersensitivity to dipyridamole, aspirin, or any component; allergy to NSAIDs; patients with asthma, rhinitis, and nasal polyps; bleeding disorders (factors VII or IX deficiencies); children <16 years of age with viral infections; pregnancy (especially 3rd trimester).

Special Concerns: Patients who drink >3 alcoholic drinks per day are at risk of bleeding. Caution should be used in patients with inherited or acquired bleeding disorders including those of liver disease or vitamin K deficiency. Use should be avoided in persons with active peptic ulcer disease. Avoid use in patients with severe renal failure.

OD **Management of Overdose:** Dipyridamole overdose might predominate due to the low dosage of aspirin and the high ratio of dipyridamole to aspirin. *Symptoms:* Major symptoms include hypotension and peripheral vasodilation. *Treatment:* IV fluids and possibly vasopressors, careful medical monitoring and management.

Drug Interactions: Adenosine, angiotensin-converting enzyme inhibitors, acetoazolamide, anticoagulants, cholinesterase inhibitors, diuretics, methotrexate, NSAIDs, phenytoin, probenecid, sulfinpyrazone, valproic acid, and verapamil.

Laboratory Test Interferences: Monitor CBC, INR, PT.

How Supplied: Capsule: Dipyridamole (extended-release) 200 mg and aspirin 25 mg

Dosage

- **Capsules**

  Reduce risk of stroke

Adults: 1 capsule (200 mg dipyridamole, 25 mg aspirin) orally twice daily.

HEALTH CARE CONSIDERATIONS

Administration/Storage: Do not crush capsules.

Assessment

1. Record indications for therapy.
2. List all drugs currently prescribed to ensure none interact unfavorably.
3. Record mental status, skin color, and cardiopulmonary findings.
4. Monitor VS, CBC, ECG, PT, PTT, and INR.

Interventions

1. Watch for signs and symtoms of GI ulcers and bleeding.
2. Monitor for dizziness, tinnitus, or impaired hearing.
3. Use may be discontinued. Notify medical provider.

Client/Family Teaching

1. Swallow whole, do not crush or chew.
2. Drug helps prevent clots by inhibiting platelet stickiness.
3. Avoid alcohol and tobacco (cause hypotensive vasoconstrictive effects) and any other unprescribed medications including OTCs without medical provider approval.
4. Report any signs or symptoms of bleeding, i.e. bloody or tarry stools.
5. Report any dizziness, tinnitus, or impaired hearing while taking this medication. Change positions slowly.
6. Try small frequent meals if nausea or gastric distress occurs.
7. Report any chest pain, skin rash, fainting or severe headaches.

Outcome/Evaluate: CAD evaluation with imaging. Prevention of thromboembolism.

Dirithromycin

(die-**rih**-throw-**MY**- sin)

Pregnancy Category: C

Dynabac **(Rx)**

Classification: Antibiotic, macrolide

Action/Kinetics: Rapidly absorbed and converted during intestinal absorption to the active erythromycylamine. Distributed throughout the body, including the lungs, GI tract, skin, soft tissues, and GU tract. Erythromycylamine acts by binding to the 50S ribosomal subunits of microorganisms, resulting in inhibition of protein synthesis. **t½:** 2-36 hr. From 81% to 97% of erythromycylamine is excreted in the feces via the bile.

Uses: Acute bacterial exacerbations of chronic bronchitis due to *Haemophilus influenzae, Moraxella catarrhalis* or *Streptococcus pneumoniae.* Secondary bacterial infections of acute bronchitis due to *M. catarrhalis* or *S. pneumoniae.* Community-acquired pneumonia due to *Legionella pneumophila, Mycoplasma pneumoniae,* or *S. pneumoniae.* Pharyngitis or tonsillitis due to *Streptococcus pyogenes.* Uncomplicated infections of the skin and skin structures due to *Staphylococcus aureus* or *S. pyogenes.*

Contraindications: Hypersensitivity to erythromycin or any other macrolide antibiotic. Use in children less than 12 years of age. Use in clients with known, suspected, or potential bacteremias since serum levels of the drug are not high enough in the serum to be effective. Use for the empiric treatment of acute bacterial exacerbations of chronic or secondary bacterial infections of acute bronchitis or for empiric treatment of uncomplicated skin and skin structure infections.

Special Concerns: Although dirithromycin eradicates *S. pyogenes* from the nasopharynx, data are lacking as to its effectiveness in preventing rheumatic fever. Use with caution during lactation. Safety and efficacy have not been determined in children less than 12 years of age.

Side Effects: *GI:* ***Pseudomembranous colitis,*** abdominal pain, nausea, diarrhea, vomiting, dyspepsia, GI disorder, flatulence, abnormal stools, constipation, dry mouth, gastritis, gastroenteritis, mouth ulceration, taste perversion, thirst, dysphagia. *CNS:* Headache, dizziness, vertigo, insomnia, anxiety, depression, nervousness, paresthesia, somnolence. *CV:* Palpitation, vasodilation, syncope. *GU:* Dysmenorrhea, urinary frequency, vaginal moniliasis, vaginitis. *Dermatologic:* Rash, pruritus, urticaria, sweating. *Respiratory:* Increased cough, dyspnea, hyperventilation. *Miscellaneous:* Nonspecific pain, asthenia, anorexia, dehydration, edema, epistaxis, eye disorder, fever, flu syndrome, hemoptysis, malaise, peripheral edema, ***allergic reaction,*** amblyopia, myalgia, neck pain, tinnitus, tremor, thirst.

Laboratory Test Considerations: ↑ ALT, AST, alkaline phosphatase, potassium, serum CPK, bands, segs, basophils, eosinophils, platelet count, total bilirubin, creatinine, GGT, leukocyte count, lymphocytes, monocytes, phosphorus, uric acid, Ca, hematocrit, hemoglobin. ↓ Platelet count, albumin, chloride, hematocrit, hemoblobin, lymphocytes, segmented neutrophils, phosphorus, serum alkaline phosphatase, serum uric acid, total protein.

OD **Management of Overdose:** *Symptoms:* N&V, epigastric distress, diarrhea. *Treatment:* Treat symptoms.

Drug Interactions

Antacids / Slightly ↑ absorption of dirithromycin

H_2-Antagonists / Slightly ↑ absorption of dirithromycin

Pimozide / Not to be used together due to possible sudden death

How Supplied: *Enteric-coated tablet:* 250 mg

Dosage

- **Tablets, Enteric-Coated**

Acute bacterial exacerbations of chronic bronchitis. Secondary bacterial infection of acute bronchitis.

Adults and children over 12 years of age: 500 mg once a day for 7 days.

Community-acquired pneumonia.

Adults and children over 12 years of age: 500 mg once a day for 14 days.

Pharyngitis or tonsillitis.

Adults and children over 12 years of age: 500 mg once a day for 10 days.

Uncomplicated skin and skin structure infections.

Adults and children over 12 years of age: 500 mg once a day for 5-7 days.

HEALTH CARE CONSIDERATIONS

See also *General Health Care Considerations for All Anti-infectives.*

Assessment

1. Record indications for therapy, type, onset, and duration of symptoms.
2. Obtain cultures for C&S initially; assess for any superinfections.
3. Does not appear to cause CV problems.

Client/Family Teaching

1. Take as prescribed with food or within 1 hr of eating.
2. Do not crush, cut, or chew enteric-coated tablets.
3. Report new diarrhea; drug alters normal colon flora, permitting clostridia overgrowth; requires drug withdrawal and symptom management.

Outcome/Evaluate

- Resolution of infection
- Negative culture reports

Disopyramide phosphate

(dye-so-**PEER**-ah-myd)

Pregnancy Category: C

Norpace, Norpace CR, Rythmodan-LA ✱

(Rx)

Classification: Antiarrhythmic, class IA

Action/Kinetics: Decreases the rate of diastolic depolarization (phase 4), decreases the upstroke velocity (phase 0), increases the action potential duration (of normal cardiac cells), and prolongs the refractory period (phases 2 and 3). Weak anticholinergic effects; fewer side effects than quinidine. Does not affect BP significantly; can be used in digitalized and nondigitalized clients. **Onset:** 30 min. **Peak plasma levels:** 2 hr. **Duration:** average of 6 hr (range 1.5-8 hr). **t½:** 4-10 hr. **Therapeutic serum levels:** 2-4 mcg/mL. Do not use serum levels to adjust the dose because of variance in protein binding and potential toxicity of unbound drug. **Protein binding:** 40%-60%. Bioavailability of the controlled-release capsules appears to be similar to that of the immediate-release capsules. Both unchanged drug (50%) and metabolites (30%) are excreted through the urine. Approximately 15% is excreted through the bile.

Uses: Life-threatening ventricular arrhythmias (e.g., sustained ventricular tachycardia). Not been shown to improve survival in clients with ventricular arrhythmias. *Investigational:* Paroxysmal SVT.

Contraindications: Hypersensitivity to drug. Cardiogenic shock, heart failure, heart block (especially preexisting second- and third-degree AV block if no pacemaker is present), congenital QT prolongation, asymptomatic ventricular premature contractions, sick sinus syndrome, glaucoma, urinary retention, myasthenia gravis. Use of controlled-release capsules in clients with severe renal insufficiency. Lactation.

Special Concerns: Safe use during childhood, labor, and delivery has not been established. Use with caution in Wolff-Parkinson-White syndrome or bundle branch block. Decrease dosage in impaired hepatic function. Geriatric clients may be more sensitive to the anticholinergic effects of this drug. The drug may be ineffective in hypokalemia and toxic in hyperkalemia.

Side Effects: ***Increased risk of death when used in clients with non-life-threatening cardiac arrhythmias.*** *CV:* Hypotension, CHF, ***worsening of arrhythmias,*** edema, weight gain, cardiac conduction disturbances, SOB, syncope, chest pain, AV block, ***severe myocardial depression (with hypotension and increased venous pressure).*** *Anticholinergic:* Dry mouth, urinary retention, constipation, blurred vision, dry nose, eyes, and throat. *GU:* Urinary frequency and urgency, urinary retention, impotence, dysuria. *GI:* Nausea, pain, flatulence, anorexia, diarrhea, vomiting, severe epigastric pain. *CNS:* Headache, nervousness, dizziness, fatigue, depression, insomnia, psychoses. *Dermatologic:* Rash, dermatoses, itching. *Other:* Fever, respiratory problems, gynecomastia, ***anaphylaxis,*** malaise, muscle weakness, numbness, tingling, angle-closure glaucoma, hypoglycemia, reversible cholestatic jaundice, symptoms of lupus erythematosus (usually in clients switched to disopyramide from procainamide).

Laboratory Test Considerations: ↑ Creatinine, BUN, cholesterol, triglycerides, and liver enzymes.

OD Management of Overdose: *Symptoms:* Apnea, loss of consciousness, ***cardiac arrhythmias*** (widening of QRS complex and QT interval, conduction disturbances), hypotension, bradycardia, anticholinergic symptoms, ***loss of spontaneous respiration, death.*** *Treatment:* Induction of vomiting, gastric lavage, or a cathartic followed by activated charcoal. Monitor ECG. IV isoproterenol, IV dopamine, cardiac glycosides, diuretics, intra-aortic balloon counterpulsation, artificial respiration, hemodialysis. Use endocardial pacing to treat AV block and neostigmine to treat anticholinergic symptoms.

Drug Interactions

Anticoagulants / ↓ PT after discontinuing disopyramide

Beta-adrenergic blockers / Possible ↓ clearance of disopyramide; sinus bradycardia, hypotension

Digoxin / ↑ Serum digoxin levels (may be beneficial)

Erythromycin / ↑ Disopyramide levels → arrhythmias and ↑ QTc intervals

Phenytoin / ↓ Effect due to ↑ breakdown by liver; ↑ anticholinergic effects

Quinidine / ↑ Disopyramide serum levels or ↓ quinidine levels

Rifampin / ↓ Effect due to ↑ breakdown by liver

How Supplied: *Capsule:* 100 mg, 150 mg; *Capsule, Extended Release:* 100 mg, 150 mg

Dosage

- **Immediate-Release Capsules**

Antiarrhythmic.

Adults, initial loading dose: 300 mg of immediate-release capsule (200 mg if client weighs less than 50 kg); **maintenance:** 400-800 mg/day in four divided doses (usual: 150 mg q 6 hr). **For clients less than 50 kg, maintenance:** 100 mg q 6 hr. **Children, less than 1 year:** 10-30 mg/kg/day in divided doses q 6 hr; **1-4 years of age:** 10-20 mg/kg/day in divided doses q 6 hr; **4-12 years of age:** 10-15 mg/kg/day in divided doses q 6 hr; **12-18 years of age:** 6-15 mg/kg/day in divided doses q 6 hr.

Severe refractory tachycardia.

Up to 400 mg q 6 hr may be required.

Cardiomyopathy.

Do not administer a loading dose; give 100 mg q 6 hr of immediate-release or 200 mg q 12 hr for controlled-release.

- **Extended-Release Capsules**

Antiarrhythmic, maintenance only.

Adults: 300 mg q 12 hr (200 mg q 12 hr for body weight less than 50 kg).

NOTE: For all uses, decrease dosage in clients with renal or hepatic insufficiency.

Moderate renal failure or hepatic failure.

100 mg q 6 hr (or 200 mg/12 hr of sustained-release form).

Severe renal failure.

100 mg q 8-24 hr depending on severity (with or without an initial loading dose of 150 mg).

HEALTH CARE CONSIDERATIONS

See also *Health Care Considerations* for *Antiarrhythmic Agents.*

Administration/Storage

1. Administer drug only after ECG assessment has been done.
2. Use with other antiarrhythmics (e.g., class IA or propranolol) should be reserved for life-threatening arrhythmias unresponsive to a single agent.
3. Do not use the controlled-release capsule for initial dosage. These are intended for maintenance therapy.
4. When being transferred from the regular PO capsule, give the first controlled-release capsule 6 hr after the last regular dose.
5. For children, a 1-10-mg/mL suspension may be made; add contents of the immediate-release capsule (do NOT use the controlled-release capsule) to cherry syrup. Syrup is

stable for 1 month if refrigerated; shake thoroughly before use and dispense in an amber bottle.

Assessment

1. Record indications for therapy, type and onset of symptoms.
2. If taking other antiarrhythmic agents, identify/record response.
3. Assess for drug hypersensitivity.
4. Note any urine dribbling, frequency, or sensation of bladder fullness; may worsen with disopyramide. Important in men with BPH and in elderly clients who have had prior urinary tract problems; palpate bladder if hesitancy is severe.
5. Obtain ECG, liver and renal function studies; check serum potassium levels and correct if low.
6. Monitor for hypotensive effect; clients with poor LV function are more likely to develop hypotension.
7. If receiving drug in the hospital, monitor ECG for QRS widening, QT prolongation, or first-degree heart block. Hold drug and report if evident.

Client/Family Teaching

1. Take at the same time each day.
2. Increase intake of fruit juices and bulk foods to prevent constipation.
3. For dry mouth, use mouth rinses, sugarless gum/hard candy.
4. Avoid alcohol in any form.
5. Report symptoms of CHF (edema, cough, weight gain, ↑ SOB).
6. Change positions slowly; avoid hot showers, temperature extremes, sun exposure, or prolonged standing.
7. Report any mental status changes or confusion.

Outcome/Evaluate: Control of ventricular arrhythmias; stable cardiac rhythm

Disulfiram

(dye-**SUL**-fih-ram)
Antabuse **(Rx)**
Classification: Treatment of alcoholism

Action/Kinetics: Produces severe hypersensitivity to alcohol. Inhibits liver enzymes that participate in the normal degradation of alcohol. This results in accumulation of acetaldehyde in the blood. High levels of acetaldehyde produce a series of symptoms referred to as the disulfiram-alcohol reaction or syndrome. The specific symptoms are listed under *Side Effects*. The symptoms vary individually, are dose-dependent with respect to both alcohol and disulfiram, and persist for periods ranging from 30 min to several hours. A single dose of disulfiram may be effective for 1-2 weeks. **Onset:** May be delayed up to 12 hr because disulfiram is initially localized in fat stores.

Uses: To prevent further ingestion of alcohol in chronic alcoholics. Should be given only to cooperating clients fully aware of the consequences of alcohol ingestion.

Contraindications: Alcohol intoxication. Severe myocardial or occlusive coronary disease. Use of paraldehyde or alcohol-containing products such as cough syrups. If client is exposed to ethylene dibromide.

Special Concerns: Use in pregnancy only if benefits outweigh risks. Use with caution in narcotic addicts or clients with diabetes, goiter, epilepsy, psychosis, hypothyroidism, hepatic cirrhosis, or nephritis.

Side Effects: In the absence of alcohol, the following symptoms have been reported: Drowsiness (most common), headache, restlessness, fatigue, psychoses, peripheral neuropathy, dermatoses, hepatotoxicity, metallic or garlic taste, arthropathy, impotence. **In the presence of alcohol,** the following symptoms may be manifested. *CV:* Flushing, chest pain, palpitations, tachycardia, hypotension, syncope, arrhythmias, ***CV collapse, MI, acute CHF.*** *CNS:* Throbbing headaches, vertigo, weak-ness, uneasiness, confusion, unconsciousness, ***seizures, death.*** *GI:* Nausea, severe vomiting, thirst. *Respiratory:* Respiratory difficulties, dyspnea, hyperventilation, ***respiratory depression.*** *Other:* Throbbing in head and neck, sweating. In the event of an Antabuse-alcohol interaction, measures should be undertaken to maintain BP and treat shock. Oxygen, antihistamines, ephedrine, and/or vitamin C may also be used.

Drug Interactions

Anticoagulants, oral / ↑ Effect of anticoagulants by ↑ hypoprothrombinemia
Barbiturates / ↑ Effect of barbiturates due to ↓ breakdown by liver
Chlordiazepoxide, diazepam / ↑ Effect of chlordiazepoxide or diazepam due to ↓ plasma clearance
Isoniazid / ↑ Side effects of isoniazid (especially CNS)
Metronidazole / Acute toxic psychosis or confusional state
Paraldehyde / Concomitant use produces Antabuse-like effect
Phenytoin / ↑ Effect of phenytoin due to ↓ breakdown by liver
Tricyclic antidepressants / Acute organic brain syndrome

How Supplied: *Tablet:* 250 mg, 500 mg

Dosage

- **Tablets**

  Alcoholism.

Adults, initial (after alcohol-free interval of 12-48 hr): 500 mg/day for 1-2 weeks; **maintenance: usual,** 250 mg/day (range: 120-500 mg/day). Do not exceed 500 mg/day.

HEALTH CARE CONSIDERATIONS

Client/Family Teaching

1. Tablets can be crushed or mixed with liquid.
2. Never give without client's knowledge. Ingesting 30 mL of 100-proof alcohol (e.g., one shot) may cause severe symptoms (within 15 min; lasting several hours) and possibly death. Avoid alcohol in any form, in foods, sauces, or other meds, such as cough syrups or tonics; avoid vinegar, paregoric, skin products, linaments, or lotions containing alcohol. Read all labels before consuming.
3. CNS side effects should lessen with continued therapy.
4. May feel tired, experience drowsiness and headaches, and develop a metallic or garlic-like taste; should subside after 2 weeks of therapy.
5. May have occasional impotence, usually transient; report.
6. Report if skin eruptions occur; an antihistamine may be prescribed.
7. Carry card stating "taking disulfiram" and describing symptoms and treatment if a disulfiram reaction occurs. Include provider and phone number. (Cards may be obtained from the Wyeth-Ayerst Laboratories, P.O. Box 8299, Philadelphia, PA 19101-1245; attention: Professional Services.)
8. Attend local support group meetings, e.g., Alcoholics Anonymous (AA) and Al-Anon, to gain the support, structure, referral, and encouragement to obtain an alcohol-free life.

Outcome/Evaluate: Freedom from alcohol and its effects; sobriety

Divalproex sodium

(dye-**VAL**-proh-ex)
Depakote, Epival ✱ **(Rx)**

See *Valproic Acid.*
How Supplied: *Enteric Coated Capsule:* 125 mg; *Enteric Coated Tablet:* 125 mg, 250 mg, 500 mg

Docusate calcium (Dioctyl calcium sulfosuccinate)

(**DEW**-kyou-sayt)
Pregnancy Category: C
Albert Docusate ✱, DC Softgels, PMS Docusate Calcium ✱, Pro-Cal-Sof, Soflax C ✱, Sulfalax Calcium, Surfak ✱, Surfak Liquigels **(OTC)**

Docusate potassium (Dioctyl potassium sulfosuccinate)

(**DEW**-kyou-sayt)
Pregnancy Category: C
Dialose, Diocto-K **(OTC)**

Docusate sodium (Dioctyl sodium sulfosuccinate)

(**DEW**-kyou-sayt)
Pregnancy Category: C
Colace, Diocto, Dioeze, Disonate, DOK, DOS Softgel, D-S-S, Modane Soft, PMS-Docusate Sodium ✱, Regulax SS, Selax ✱ **(OTC)**
Classification: Laxative, emollient

See also *Laxatives.*
Action/Kinetics: Acts by lowering the surface tension of the feces and promoting penetration by water and fat, thus increasing the softness of the fecal mass. Not absorbed systemically and does not seem to interfere with the absorption of nutrients. A microenema formulation is available for clients aged 3 and older. **Onset:** 24-72 hr.; **onset, microenema formulation:** 15 min.
Uses: To lessen strain of defecation in persons with hernia or CV diseases or other diseases in which straining at stool should be avoided. Megacolon or bedridden clients. Constipation associated with dry, hard stools. The microemulsion formulation is indicated for relief of occasional constipation in children over the age of 3 years.
Contraindications: Nausea, vomiting, abdominal pain, and intestinal obstruction.
Drug Interactions: Docusate may ↑ absorption of mineral oil from the GI tract.
How Supplied: Docusate calcium: *Capsule:* 240 mg. Docusate potassium: *Capsule:* 100 mg, 240 mg Docusate sodium: *Capsule:* 50 mg, 100 mg, 240 mg, 250 mg; *Oral Liquid:* 200 mg/5 mL, 150 mg/15 mL; *Powder for Reconstitution:* 283 mg; *Solution:* 100 mg/15 mL; *Syrup:* 50 mg/15 mL, 60 mg/15 mL; *Tablet:* 100 mg

Dosage

DOCUSATE CALCIUM

- **Capsules**

Adults: 240 mg/day until bowel movements are normal; **pediatric, over 6 years:** 50-150 mg/day.

DOCUSATE POTASSIUM

- **Capsules**

Adults: 100-300 mg/day; **pediatric, over 6 years:** 100 mg at bedtime.

DOCUSATE SODIUM

- **Capsules, Oral Liquid, Syrup, Tablets**

Adults and children over 12 years: 50-500 mg; **pediatric, under 3 years:** 10-40 mg; **3-6 years:** 20-60 mg; **6-12 years:** 40-120 mg.

- **Rectal Solution**

Flushing or retention enema.

Adults: 50-100 mg.

HEALTH CARE CONSIDERATIONS

See also *Health Care Considerations* for *Laxatives*.

Client/Family Teaching

1. May give PO solutions with milk or juices to help mask bitter taste.
2. Drink a glass of water with each PO dose.
3. When used in enemas, add 50-100 mg (5-10 mL) to a retention or flushing enema.
4. Because docusate salts are minimally absorbed, it may require 1-3 days to soften fecal matter.

Outcome/Evaluate: Elimination of a soft, formed stool; ↓ straining

Dofetilide

(doh-**FET**-ih-lyd)

Pregnancy Category: C

Tikosyn **(Rx)**

Classification: Antiarrhythmic drug

See also *Antiarrhythmic Drugs*.

Action/Kinetics: Acts by blocking the cardiac ion channel carrying the rapid component of the delayed rectifier potassium currents. Blocks only I_{Kr} with no significant block of other repolarizing potassium currents (e.g., I_{Ks}, I_{K1}). No effect on sodium channels or adrenergic receptors. Dofetilide increases the monophasic action potential duration due to delayed repolarization. **Maximum plasma levels:** 2-3 hr during fasting. Steady state plasma levels reached in 2-3 days. Metabolized in the liver and excreted in the urine. **t½, terminal:** About 10 hr. Women have lower oral clearances than men.

Uses: Conversion of atrial fibrillation or atrial flutter to normal sinus rhythm. Maintenance of normal sinus rhythm in clients witih atrial fibrillation/atrial flutter of more than 1 week duration and who have been converted to normal sinus rhythm. Reserve for those in whom atrial fibrillation/atrial flutter is highly symptomatic due to life-threatening ventricular arrhythmias. *NOTE:* Available only to hospitals and prescribers who receive dosing and treatment initiation education through the *Tikosyn* education program.

Contraindications: Congenital or acquired long QT syndromes, in those with a baseline QT interval greater than 440 msec (500 msec in clients with ventricular conduction abnormalities), severe renal impairment (C_{CR} less than 20 mL/min). Concomitant use of verapamil, cimetidine, trimethoprim (alone or with sulfamethoxazole), ketoconazole, prochlorperazine, megestrol. Lactation.

Special Concerns: There is a greater risk of dofetilide-induced TdP (type of ventricular tachycardia) in female clients than in male clients. Use with caution in severe hepatic impairment. Use with drugs that prolong the QT interval has not been studied with dofetilide use; therefore, do not use bepridil, certain macrolide antibiotics, phenothiazines, or TCAs with dofetilide. Safety and efficacy have not been determined in children less than 18 years of age.

Side Effects: *CV:* Ventricular arrhythmias (especially TdP type ventricular tachycardia), ***torsades de pointes,*** angina pectoris, atrial fibrillation, hypertension, palpitation, supraventricular tachycardia, ventricular tachycardia, bradycardia, cerebral ischemia, ***CVA, MI, heart arrest, ventricular fibrillation,*** AV block, bundle branch block, heart block. *CNS:* Headache, dizziness, insomnia, anxiety, paresthesia. *GI:* Nausea, diarrhea, abdominal pain. *Respiratory:* Respiratory tract infection, dyspnea, increased cough. *Miscellaneous:* Chest pain, flu syndrome, accidental injury, back pain, rash, arthralgia, asthenia, pain, peripheral edema, sweating, UTI, angioedema, edema, facial paralysis, flaccid paralysis, liver damage, paralysis, ***sudden death,*** syncope.

OD **Management of Overdose:** *Symptoms:* Excessive prolongation of QT interval. *Treatment:* Symptomatic and supportive. Initiate cardiac monitoring. Can use charcoal slur but is effective only when given within 15 min of dofetilide. To treat TdP or overdose, may give isoproterenol infusion, with or without cardiac pacing. IV magnesium sulfate may be useful to manage TdP. Monitor until QT interval returns to normal.

Drug Interactions

Amiloride / Possible ↑ dofetilide levels
Amiodarone / Possible ↑ dofetilide levels
Cannabinoids / Possible ↑ dofetilide levels
Cimetidine / ↑ Risk of arrhythmia (TdP) R/T ↓ liver metabolism of dofetilide
Digoxin / ↑ Risk of torsades de pointes
Diltiazem / Possible ↑ dofetilide levels

Grapefruit juice / Possible ↑ dofetilide levels
Ketoconazole / ↑ Risk of arrhythmia (TdP) R/T ↓ liver metabolism of dofetilide
Macrolide antibiotics / Possible ↑ dofetilide levels
Megestrol / Possible ↑ dofetilide levels
Metformin / Possible ↑ dofetilide levels
Nefazadone / Possible ↑ dofetilide levels
Norfloxacin / Possible ↑ dofetilide levels
Potassium-depleting diuretics / Hypokalemia or hypomagnesemia may occur, → ↑ potential for torsades de pointes
Prochlorperazine / Possible ↑ dofetilide levels
Quinine / Possible ↑ dofetilide levels
Triamterene / Possible ↑ dofetilide levels
Trimethoprim or Trimethoprim/Sulfamethoxazole / ↑ Risk of arrhythmia (TdP) R/T ↓ liver metabolism of dofetilide
Verapamil / Possible ↑ dofetilide levels
Zafirlukast / Possible ↑ dofetilide levels

How Supplied: *Capsules:* 125 mcg, 250 mcg, 500 mcg

Dosage

- **Capsules**

Conversion of atrial fibrillation/flutter; maintenance of normal sinus rhythm.

The dosing for dofetilide must be undertaken using the following steps:

1. Before giving the first dose, determine the QTc using an average of 5-10 beats. If the QTc is greater than 440 msec (500 msec in those with ventricular conduction abnormalities), dofetilide is contraindicated. Also, do not use if the heart rate is less than 60 bpm.
2. Before giving the first dose, calculate the C_{CR} using the following formulas:
Males: Weight (kg) x (140 - age)/72 x serum creatinine (mg/dL)
Females: 0.84 x above value
3. Determine the starting dose of dofetilide as follows: **C_{CR}, greater than 60 mL/min:** 500 mcg b.i.d.; **C_{CR}, 40-60 mL/min:** 250 mcg b.i.d.; **C_{CR}, 20-less than 40 mL/min:** 125 mcg b.i.d.; **C_{CR}, less than 20 mL/min:** DO NOT USE DOFETILIDE; CONTRAINDICATED IN THESE CLIENTS. The maximum daily dose is 500 mcg b.i.d.
4. Give the adjusted dose based on C_{CR} and begin continuous ECG monitoring.
5. At 2-3 hr after giving the first dofetilide dose, determine the QTc. If the QTc has increased by more than 15% compared with the baseline established in Step 1 or if the QTc is 500 msec (550 msec in those with ventricular conduction abnormalities), adjust subsequent dosing as follows: If the starting dose based on C_{CR} is 500 mcg b.i.d., the adjusted dose (for QTc prolongation) is 250 mcg b.i.d. If the starting dose is 250 mcg b.i.d., the adjusted dose (for QTc prolongation) is 125 mcg b.i.d. If the starting dose is 125 mcg b.i.d., the adjusted dose (for QTc prolongation) is 125 mcg once daily.
6. At 2-3 hr after each subsequent dose of dofetilide, determine QTc for in-hospital doses 2 through 5. No further down titration of dofetilide based on QTc is recommended. Discontinue if at any time after the second dose of dofetilide, the QTc is greater than 500 msec (550 msec in those with ventricular conduction abnormalities).
7. Continuously monitor by ECG for a minimum of 3 days or for a minimum of 12 hr after electrical or pharmacological conversion to normal sinus rhythm, whichever time is greater.

HEALTH CARE CONSIDERATIONS

See also *Health Care Considerations* for *Antiarrhythmic Drugs.*

Administration/Storage

1. Therapy must be started (and, if necessary, reinitiated) in a setting where continuous ECG monitoring and personnel trained in the management of serious ventricular arrhythmias are available for a minimum of 3 days.
2. Do not discharge clients within 12 hr of electrical or pharmacological conversion to normal sinus rhythm.
3. Prior to electrical or pharmacological cardioversion, anticoagulate clients with atrial fibrillation according to usual medical practices. Anticoagulants may be continued after cardioversion. Correct hypokalemia before starting dofetilide therapy.
4. Re-evaluate renal function q 3 months or as warranted. Discontinue dofetilide if the QTc is greater than 500 msec (550 msec in those with ventricular conduction abnormalities) and monitor carefully until QTc returns to baseline levels. If renal function decreases, adjust the dose as described under Dosage.
5. The highest dose of 500 mcg b.i.d. is the most effective. However, the risk of torsades de pointes is increased. Thus, a lower dose may be used. If at any time the lower dose is increased, the client must be hospitalized for 3 days. Previous tolerance of higher doses does not eliminate the need for hospitalization.

6. Do not consider electrical conversion if the client does not convert to normal sinus rhythm within 24 hr after starting dofetilide.
7. Withdraw previous antiarrhythmic drug therapy before starting dofetilide therapy; during withdrawal, carefully monitor for a minimum of 3 plasma half-lives. Do not initiate dofetilide following amiodarone therapy until amiodarone plasma levels are less than 0.3 mcg/mL or until amiodarone has been withdrawn for 3 or more months.
8. Protect from moisture and humidity. Dispense in tight containers.

Assessment

1. Identify arrhythmia and duration. Note any S&S associated with arrhythmia.
2. Note drugs prescribed to ensure none interact. Avoid use of drugs that prolong the QT interval.
3. Monitor renal and LFTs; avoid use with dysfunction.
4. Drug is available only through the Tikosyn Dosing Program with provider education.

Client/Family Teaching

1. Take exactly as prescribed; avoid grapefruit juice.
2. Do not double the next dose if a dose is missed. Take next dose at usual time.
3. Report any change in prescriptions or OTC/supplement use. Inform all providers especially if hospitalized or prescribed a new medication for any condition.
4. Read the package insert prior to use. Drug adherance is imperative with this therapy. Must report as scheduled for ECG evaluation and report any side effects to ensure no serious drug related complications.

Outcome/Evaluate: Conversion of atrial fibrillation/flutter to NSR; maintenance of NSR once converted

Dolasetron mesylate

(dohl-**AH**-seh-tron)
Pregnancy Category: B
Anzemet **(Rx)**
Classification: Antinauseant/antiemetic, serotonin 5-HT_3 antagonist

Action/Kinetics: Selective serotonin 5-HT_3 antagonist that prevents N&V by inhibiting released serotonin from combining with receptors on vagal efferents that initiate vomiting reflex. May also cause acute, usually reversible, PR and QT_c prolongation and QRS widening, perhaps due to blockade of sodium channels by active metabolite of dolasetron. Well absorbed from GI tract. Metabolized to active hydrodolasetron: **peak plasma levels:** 1 hr; **t½:** 8.1 hr. Food does not affect bioavailability. Hydrodolasetron is excreted through urine and feces. Is eliminated more quickly in children than in adults.

Uses: Prevention of N&V associated with moderately-emetogenic cancer chemotherapy (initially and repeat courses). Prevention of postoperative N&V.

Special Concerns: Use with caution during lactation and in those who have or may develop prolongation of cardiac conduction intervals, including QT_c. These include clients with hypokalemia or hypomagnesemia, those taking diuretics with potential for electrolyte abnormalities, in congenital QT syndrome, those taking anti-arrhythmic drugs or other drugs which lead to QT prolongation, and cumulative high dose anthracycline therapy. Safety and efficacy in children less than 2 years of age have not been determined.

Side Effects: Chemotherapy clients. Headache, fatigue, diarrhea, bradycardia, dizziness, pain, tachycardia, dyspepsia, chills, shivering. **Postoperative clients.** Headache, hypotension, dizziness, fever, pruritus, oliguria, hypertension, tachycardia. **Chemotherapy or postoperative clients.** *CV:* Hypotension, edema, peripheral edema, peripheral ischemia, thrombophlebitis, phlebitis. *GI:* Constipation, dyspepsia, abdominal pain, anorexia, pancreatitis, taste perversion. *CNS:* Flushing, vertigo, paresthesia, tremor, ataxia, twitching, agitation, sleep disorder, depersonalization, confusion, anxiety, abnormal dreaming. *Dermatologic:* Rash, increased sweating. *Hematologic:* Hematuria, epistaxis, anemia, purpura, hematoma, thrombocytopenia. *Hypersensitivity:* Rarely, ***anaphylaxis,*** facial edema, urticaria. *Musculoskeletal:* Myalgia, arthralgia. *Respiratory:* Dyspnea, bronchospasm. *GU:* Dysuria, polyuria, acute renal failure. *Ophthalmic:* Abnormal vision, photophobia. *Miscellaneous:* Tinnitus.

Laboratory Test Considerations: ↑ PTT, AST, ALT, alkaline phosphatase. Prolonged prothrombin time.

Drug Interactions: There is the potential for dolasetron to interact with other drugs that prolong the QT_c interval.

How Supplied: *Injection:* 20 mg/mL; *Tablet:* 50 mg, 100 mg

Dosage

- **Tablets**

Prevention of N&V during chemotherapy.
Adults: 100 mg within 1 hr before chemotherapy. **Children, 2 to 16 years:** 1.8 mg/kg within 1 hr before chemotherapy, up to a maximum of 100 mg.

Prevention of postoperative N&V.

Adults: 100 mg within 2 hr before surgery. **Children, 2 to 16 years:** 1.2 mg/kg within 2 hr before surgery, up to a maximum of 100 mg.

HEALTH CARE CONSIDERATIONS

Assessment

1. Record indications for therapy.
2. List drugs prescribed to ensure none interact unfavorably.
3. Monitor CBC, electrolytes, Mg and ECG.
4. Give 1 hr before chemo or 2 hrs before surgery to gain desired effect.
5. With children, calculate appropriate dose (cancer chemo or postop N&V); may administer orally with apple or apple-grape juice.

Outcome/Evaluate: Inhibition of chemotherapy induced/postop N&V

Donepezil hydrochloride

(dohn-**EP**-eh-zil)

Pregnancy Category: C

Aricept **(Rx)**

Classification: Psychotherapeutic drug for Alzheimer's disease

Action/Kinetics: A decrease in cholinergic function may be the cause of Alzheimer's disease. Donepezil is a cholinesterase inhibitor and exerts its effect by enhancing cholinergic function by increasing levels of acetylcholine. No evidence that the drug alters the course of the underlying dementing process. Well absorbed from the GI tract. **Peak plasma levels:** 3-4 hr. Food does not affect the rate or extent of absorption. Metabolized in the liver, and both unchanged drug and metabolites are excreted in the urine and feces.
Uses: Treatment of mild to moderate dementia of the Alzheimer's type.
Contraindications: Hypersensitivity to piperidine derivatives.
Special Concerns: Use with caution in clients with a history of asthma or obstructive pulmonary disease. Safety and efficacy have not been determined for use in children.
Side Effects: *NOTE:* Side effects with an incidence of 1% or greater are listed. *GI:* N&V, diarrhea, anorexia, fecal incontinence, GI bleeding, bloating, epigastric pain. *CNS:* Insomnia, dizziness, depression, abnormal dreams, somnolence. *CV:* Hypertension, vasodilation, atrial fibrillation, hot flashes, hypotension, bradycardia. *Body as a whole:* Headache, pain (in various locations), accident, fatigue, influenza, chest pain, toothache. *Musculoskeletal:* Muscle cramps, arthritis, bone fracture. *Dermatologic:* Diaphoresis, urticaria, pruritus. *GU:* Urinary incontinence, nocturia, frequent urination. *Respiratory:* Dyspnea, sore throat, bronchitis. *Ophthalmic:* Cataract, eye irritation, blurred vision. *Miscellaneous:* Dehydration, syncope, ecchymosis, weight loss.
OD **Management of Overdose:** *Symptoms:* Cholinergic crisis characterized by severe N&V, salivation, sweating, bradycardia, hypotension, respiratory depression, collapse, con-vulsions, increased muscle weakness (may cause death if respiratory muscles are involved). *Treatment:* Atropine sulfate at an initial dose of 1-2 mg IV with subsequent doses based on the response. General supportive measures.

Drug Interactions

Anticholinergic drugs / The cholinesterase inhibitor activitiy of donepezil interferes with the activity of anticholinergics
Bethanechol / Synergistic effect
NSAIDs / ↑ Gastric acid secretion → ↑ risk of active or occult GI bleeding
Succinylcholine / ↑ Muscle relaxant effect

How Supplied: *Tablet:* 5 mg, 10 mg

Dosage

- **Tablets**

Alzheimer's disease.

Initial: 5 mg. Use of a 10-mg dose did not provide a clinical effect greater than the 5-mg dose; however, in some clients, 10 mg daily may be superior. Do not increase the dose to 10 mg until clients have been on a daily dose of 5 mg for 4 to 6 weeks.

HEALTH CARE CONSIDERATIONS

Administration/Storage: Store at controlled room temperatures from 15°C to 30°C (59°F to 86°F).

Assessment

1. Record onset/duration, other agents trialed, and the outcome.
2. Describe clinical presentation.
3. Note any history of asthma or COPD.
4. Obtain ECG and labs.

Client/Family Teaching

1. Take in the evening, just prior to bedtime.
2. May take with or without food.
3. Report any irregular pulse or dizzy spells, lack of response or worsening of symptoms.

Outcome/Evaluate: Improved cognitive functioning with Alzheimer's.

COMBINATION DRUG

Donnatal Capsules, Elixir, Tablets

(DON-nah-tal)
Pregnancy Category: C
(Rx)
Classification: Anticholinergic

D

Content: Each tablet, capsule, or 5 mL elixir contains: *Anticholinergic:* Atropine sulfate, 0.0194 mg. *Anticholinergic:* Hyoscyamine sulfate, 0.1037 mg. *Anticholinergic:* Scopolamine hydrobromide, 0.0065 mg. *Sedative:* Phenobarbital, 16.2 mg. *NOTE:* The Extentabs contain three times the amount of drugs found in tablets.
Uses: Possibly effective as an adjunct in the treatment of irritable colon, spastic colon, mucous colitis, and acute enterocolitis. Has also been used in the treatment of duodenal ulcer.
Special Concerns: It is not known with certainty whether or not anticholinergic drugs aid in the healing in duodenal ulcer or decrease the rate of recurrence or prevent complications.
How Supplied: See Content

Dosage

- **Tablets, Capsules, Extentabs, Elixir**

Adults, usual: 1-2 tablets or capsules t.i.d.-q.i.d. (or one Extentab q 12 hr). If the elixir is used, **adult, usual:** 5-10 mL t.i.d.-q.i.d. **Pediatric:** Use elixir as follows: **4.5-9.0 kg:** 0.5 mL q 4 hr or 0.75 mL q 6 hr; **9.1-13.5 kg:** 1.0 mL q 4 hr or 1.5 mL q 6 hr; **13.6-22.6 kg:** 1.5 mL q 4 hr or 2.0 mL q 6 hr; **22.7-33.9 kg:** 2.5 mL q 4 hr or 3.75 mL q 6 hr. **34.0-45.3 kg:** 3.75 mL q 4 hr or 5 mL q 6 hr; **45.4 kg:** 5 mL q 4 hr or 7.5 mL q 6 hr.

HEALTH CARE CONSIDERATIONS

See also *Health Care Considerations* for *Cholinergic Blocking Agents.*
Client/Family Teaching: Take as directed; report lack of response or adverse side effects.
Outcome/Evaluate: Relief of abdominal pain; improved bowel motility

Dorzolamide hydrochloride ophthalmic solution

(dor-ZOH-lah-myd)
Pregnancy Category: C
Trusopt (Rx)
Classification: Carbonic anhydrase inhibitor

Action/Kinetics: Decreases aqueous humor secretion in the ciliary processes of the eye by inhibiting carbonic anhydrase. Occurs by decreasing the formation of bicarbonate ions with a reduction in sodium and fluid transport and a subsequent decrease in intraocular pressure. The drug may reach the systemic circulation, where it and the metabolite are excreted through the urine. The drug and metabolite also accumulate in RBCs.
Uses: Elevated intraocular pressure (IOP) in those with ocular hypertension or open-angle glaucoma.
Contraindications: Use with severe renal impairment (C_{CR} < 30 mL/min) or in soft contact lens wearers as the preservative (benzalkonium chloride) may be absorbed by the lenses. Lactation.
Special Concerns: Dorzolamide is a sulfonamide and, as such, may cause similar systemic reactions, including side effects and allergic reactions, as sulfonamides. Use with caution in hepatic impairment. Due to additive effects, concurrent use of dorzolamide with systemic carbonic anhydrase inhibitors is not recommended. Safety and efficacy have not been determined in children. It is possible geriatric clients may show greater sensitivity to the drug.
Side Effects: *Ophthalmic:* Conjunctivitis, lid reactions, bacterial keratitis (due to contamination by concurrent corneal disease). Ocular burning, stinging, or discomfort immediately following administration. Also, superficial punctate keratitis, ocular allergic reaction, blurred vision, tearing, dryness, photophobia, iridocyclitis (rare). *Miscellaneous:* Acid-base and electrolyte disturbances (i.e., similar to systemic use of carbonic anhydrase inhibitors). Also, bitter taste following instillation, headache, nausea, asthenia, fatigue. Rarely, skin rashes, urolithiasis.
How Supplied: *Solution:* 2%

Dosage

- **Ophthalmic Solution**

Increased intraocular pressure.
Adults: 1 gtt in the affected eye(s) t.i.d.

HEALTH CARE CONSIDERATIONS

Administration/Storage: Protect from light and store at 15°C-30°C (59°F-86°F).
Assessment: Record visual symptoms and baseline IOP. Note any sensitivity to sulfonamides or impaired renal function.
Client/Family Teaching
1. Do not let dispenser tip come in contact with eye or surrounding structures; contamination may result.
2. Use only as prescribed. Report any evidence of conjunctivitis or eye or lid reaction.

Burning or stinging may accompany administration; a bitter taste may also be noted.
3. May be used with other topical ophthalmic drugs. If more than one is being used, give them at least 10 min apart.
4. Do not administer drops while wearing contact lenses as they may absorb solution preservative.
Outcome/Evaluate: ↓ IOP

COMBINATION DRUG

Dorzolamide hydrochloride and Timolol maleate

(dor-**ZOH**-lah-myd/**TIE**-moh-lohl)
Pregnancy Category: C
Cosopt **(Rx)**
Classification: Topical carbonic anhydrase inhibitor and a topical beta-adrenergic blocking agent

See also *Dorzolamide hydrochloride* and *Timolol maleate.*
Content: *Ophthalmic Solution:* Dorzolamide 2%, Timolol 0.5%
Action/Kinetics: Both drugs decrease elevated IOP by reducing aqueous humor production. Inhibition of carbonic anhydrase by dorzolamide decreases aqueous humor secretion by slowing formation of bicarbonate ions with subsequent reduction in sodium and fluid transport. Timolol is a nonspecific beta-receptor blocking agent.
Uses: To reduce elevated IOP in open-angle glaucoma or ocular hypertension in those inadequately controlled with beta-blockers.
Contraindications: Use in bronchial asthma or history thereof, severe COPD, sinus bradycardia, second or third degree AV block, overt cardiac failure, cardiogenic shock. Lactation.
Special Concerns: Use beta-blockers with caution in diabetics receiving insulin or oral hypoglycemic drugs or in those subject to spontaneous hypoglycemia. Timolol may mask signs and symptoms of hypoglycemia or hyperthyroidism. Safety and efficacy have not been determined in children.
Side Effects: See individual drugs. *Ophthalmic:* Conjunctival hyperemia, ocular burning and/or stinging, blurred vision, superficial punctate keratitis, eye itching, blepharitis, cloudy vision, conjunctival discharge, conjunctival edema, conjunctival follicles, conjunctival injections, corneal erosion, corneal staining, cortical lens opacity, dryness of eyes, eye debris, eye discharge, eye pain, eye tearing, eyelid edema, eyelid erythema, eyelid exudate/scales, eyelid pain or discomfort, foreign body sensation, glaucomatous cupping, lens nucleus coloration, lens opacity, nuclear lens opacity, postsubcapsular cataract, visual field defect, vitreous detachment. *GI:* Taste perversion (bitter, sour, or unusual taste), abdominal pain, dyspepsia, nausea. *Respiratory:* Bronchitis, cough, pharyngitis, sinusitis, URI. *Miscellaneous:* Back pain, dizziness, headache, hypertension, influenza, UTI.
Drug Interactions: See individual drugs.
How Supplied: See Content

Dosage

- **Ophthalmic Solution**

  Elevated IOP.

Adults: 1 gtt of Cosopt in the affected eye(s) b.i.d.

HEALTH CARE CONSIDERATIONS

See also *Health Care Considerations* for *Dorzolamide hydrochloride* and *Timolol maleate.*
Administration/Storage: Store at 15°C-25°C (59°F-77°F). Protect from light.
Assessment
1. Avoid contaminating tip or product by improper handling or container contact with the eye or surrounding tissues. Serious eye damage or loss of vision may occur from contaminated solutions.
2. Wait 10 min between drops if more than one eye drug prescribed.
3. The product contains benzalkonium chloride which may be absorbed by soft contact lenses. Remove lenses prior to instillation and wait 15 min before reinsertion.
4. Stop drug and report if eye lid reactions or redness of the eye is observed.
Outcome/Evaluate: ↓ IOP

Doxazosin mesylate

(dox-**AYZ**-oh-sin)
Pregnancy Category: B
Cardura, Cardura-1, -2, -4 ✱ **(Rx)**
Classification: Antihypertensive

Action/Kinetics: Blocks the alpha-1 (postjunctional) adrenergic receptors resulting in a decrease in systemic vascular resistance and a corresponding decrease in BP. **Peak plasma levels:** 2-3 hr. **Peak effect:** 2-6 hr. Significantly bound (98%) to plasma proteins. Metabolized in the liver to active and inactive metabolites, which are excreted through the feces and urine. **t½:** 22 hr.
Uses: Alone or in combination with diuretics, calcium channel blockers, or beta blockers to treat hypertension. Treatment of BPH.

Contraindications: Clients allergic to prazosin or terazosin.
Special Concerns: Use with caution during lactation, in impaired hepatic function, or in those taking drugs known to influence hepatic metabolism. Safety and effectiveness have not been demonstrated in children. Due to the possibility of severe hypotension, do not use the 2-, 4-, and 8-mg tablets for initial therapy.
Side Effects: *CV:* Dizziness (most frequent), syncope, vertigo, lightheadedness, edema, palpitation, arrhythmia, postural hypotension, tachycardia, peripheral ischemia. *CNS:* Fatigue, headache, paresthesia, kinetic disorders, ataxia, somnolence, nervousness, depression, insomnia. *Musculoskeletal:* Arthralgia, arthritis, muscle weakness, muscle cramps, myalgia, hypertonia. *GU:* Polyuria, sexual dysfunction, urinary incontinence, urinary frequency. *GI:* Nausea, diarrhea, dry mouth, constipation, dyspepsia, flatulence, abdominal pain, vomiting. *Respiratory:* Fatigue or malaise, rhinitis, epistaxis, dyspnea. *Miscellaneous:* Rash, pruritus, flushing, abnormal vision, conjunctivitis, eye pain, tinnitus, chest pain, asthenia, facial edema, generalized pain, slight weight gain.
OD **Management of Overdose:** *Symptoms:* Hypotension. *Treatment:* IV fluids.
How Supplied: *Tablet:* 1 mg, 2 mg, 4 mg, 8 mg

Dosage

- **Tablets**

Hypertension.

Adults: initial, 1 mg once daily at bedtime; **then,** depending on the response (client's standing BP both 2-6 hr and 24 hr after a dose), the dose may be increased to 2 mg/day. A maximum of 16 mg/day may be required to control BP.

Benign prostatic hyperplasia.

Initial: 1 mg once daily. **Maintenance:** Depending on the urodynamics and symptoms, dose may be increased to 2 mg daily and then 4-8 mg once daily (maximum recommended dose). The recommended titration interval is 1-2 weeks.

HEALTH CARE CONSIDERATIONS

Administration/Storage

1. To minimize the possibility of severe hypotension, limit initial dosage to 1 mg/day.
2. Increasing the dose higher than 4 mg/day increases the possibility of severe syncope, postural dizziness, vertigo, and postural hypotension.

Assessment

1. Note any allergy to prazosin or terazosin; drug is a quinazoline derivative.
2. Assess liver function and BP.
3. When used for BPH, numerically score severity.

Client/Family Teaching

1. Take once daily; do not stop abruptly.
2. Record BP/weight; check for edema.
3. Rise slowly to a sitting position before attempting to stand to prevent postural hypotension. Postural effects may occur 2-6 hr after a dose.
4. Driving and hazardous tasks should be avoided for 24 hr after first dose until effects are evident.
5. Report if S&S do not improve after several weeks of therapy as drug dosage may need adjustment.

Outcome/Evaluate

- ↓ BP
- ↓ Nocturnal dysuria

Doxepin hydrochloride

(DOX-eh-pin)
Alti-Doxepin ✱, Apo-Doxepin ✱, Novo-Doxepin ✱, Rho-Doxepin ✱, Sinequan, Triadapin ✱, Zonalon ✱ **(Rx)**
Classification: Antidepressant, tricyclic

See also *Antidepressants, Tricyclic.*
Action/Kinetics: Metabolized to the active metabolite, desmethyldoxepin. Moderate anticholinergic effects and orthostatic hypotension; high sedative effects. **Therapeutic plasma levels of both doxepin and desmethyldoxepin:** 100-200 ng/mL. **Time to reach steady state:** 2-8 days. **t½:** 8-24 hr.
Uses: Psychoneurotic clients with depression or anxiety. Depression or anxiety due to organic disease or alcoholism. Psychotic depressive disorders with associated anxiety, including involutional depression and manic-depressive disorders. Chronic, severe neurogenic pain. PUD. Dermatologic disorders including chronic urticaria, angioedema, and nocturnal pruritus due to atopic eczema.
Contraindications: Use in children less than 12 years of age. Glaucoma or a tendency for urinary retention.
Special Concerns: Safety has not been determined in pregnancy.
Additional Side Effects: Doxepin has a high incidence of side effects, including a high degree of sedation, decreased libido, extrapyramidal symptoms, dermatitis, pruritus, fatigue, weight gain, edema, paresthesia, breast engorgement, insomnia, tremor, chills, tinnitus, and photophobia.
How Supplied: *Capsule:* 10 mg, 25 mg, 50 mg, 75 mg, 100 mg, 150 mg; *Concentrate:* 10 mg/mL; *Cream:* 5%

Dosage

- **Capsules, Oral Concentrate**

Antidepressant, mild to moderate anxiety or depression.

Adults: 25 mg t.i.d. (or up to 150 mg can be given at bedtime); **then,** adjust dosage to individual response (usual optimum dosage: 75-150 mg/day). **Geriatric clients, initially:** 25-50 mg/day; dose can be increased as needed and tolerated.

Severe symptoms.

Initial: 50 mg t.i.d.; **then,** gradually increase to 300 mg/day.

Emotional symptoms with organic disease.

25-50 mg/day.

Antipruritic.

10-30 mg at bedtime.

- **Cream 5%**

Apply a thin film q.i.d. with at least a 3-4 hr interval between applications.

HEALTH CARE CONSIDERATIONS

See also *Health Care Considerations* for *Antidepressants, Tricyclic.*

Administration/Storage

1. Oral concentrate is to be diluted with 4 oz water, milk, or orange, grapefruit, tomato, prune, or pineapple juice just before ingestion. Do not mix the concentrate with carbonated beverages or grape juice.
2. The antianxiety effect is manifested rapidly; however, it may take 2 to 3 weeks to observe the optimum antidepressant effect.

Assessment

1. Record type, onset and characteristics of symptoms.
2. List any other prescribed therapy for this problem and the outcome.
3. Record clinical presentation and attempt to identify any factors contributing to this disorder.

Client/Family Teaching

1. Beneficial antidepressant effects may take up to 3 weeks, whereas antianxiety effects occur rapidly.
2. Do not perform activities that require mental alertness until drug effects realized.
3. Avoid alcohol and any other CNS depressants.

Outcome/Evaluate

- ↓ Symptoms of anxiety and depression
- Improved sleeping patterns
- Control of neurogenic pain
- Relief of nocturnal pruritus

Doxycycline calcium

(dox-ih-**SYE**-kleen)

Pregnancy Category: D

Vibramycin **(Rx)**

Doxycycline hyclate

(dox-ih-**SYE**-kleen)

Pregnancy Category: D

Alti-Doxycycline ✱, Apo-Doxy ✱, Apo-Doxy-Tabs ✱, Doryx, Doxy 100 and 200, Doxy-Caps, Doxycin ✱, Doxychel Hyclate, Doxytec ✱, Novo-Doxylin ✱, Nu-Doxycycline ✱, Rho-Doxycyline ✱, Vibramycin, Vibramycin IV, Vibra-Tabs, Vibra-Tabs C-Pak ✱, Vivox **(Rx)**

Doxycycline monohydrate

(dox-ih-**SYE**-kleen)

Pregnancy Category: D

Monodox, Vibramycin **(Rx)**

Classification: Antibiotic, tetracycline

See also *Anti-Infectives* and *Tetracyclines.*

Action/Kinetics: More slowly absorbed, and thus more persistent, than other tetracyclines. Preferred for clients with impaired renal function for treating infections outside the urinary tract. From 80% to 95% is bound to serum proteins. **t½:** 14.5-22 hr; 30%-40% excreted unchanged in urine.

Additional Uses: Orally for uncomplicated gonococcal infections in adults (except anorectal infections in males); acute epididymo-orchitis caused by *Neisseria gonorrhoeae* and *Chlamydia trachomatis;* gonococcal arthritis-dermatitis syndrome; nongonococcal urethritis caused by *C. trachomatis* and *Ureaplasma urealyticum.* Prophylaxis of malaria due to *Plasmodium falciparum* in short-term travelers (< 4 months) to areas with chloroquine- or pyrime-thamine-sulfadoxine-resistant strains.

Contraindications: Prophylaxis of malaria in pregnant individuals and in children less than 8 years old. Use during the last half of pregnancy and in children up to 8 years of age (tetracycline may cause permanent discoloration of the teeth). Lactation.

Special Concerns: Safety for IV use in children less than 8 years of age has not been established.

Additional Drug Interactions: Carbamazepine, phenytoin, and barbiturates ↓ effect of doxycycline by ↑ breakdown of doxycycline by the liver.

How Supplied: Doxycycline calcium: *Syrup:* 50 mg/5 mL. Doxycyline hyclate: *Capsule:* 50 mg, 100 mg; *Enteric Coated Capsule:* 100 mg; *Powder for injection:* 100 mg; *Tablet:* 100 mg. Doxycycline monohydrate: *Cap-*

sule: 50 mg, 100 mg; *Powder for Reconstitution:* 25 mg/5 mL

Dosage

• **Capsules, Delayed-Release Capsules, Oral Suspension, Syrup, Tablets, IV**

Infections.

Adult: First day, 100 mg q 12 hr; **maintenance:** 100-200 mg/day, depending on severity of infection. **Children, over 8 years (45 kg or less): First day,** 4.4 mg/kg in 1-2 doses; **then,** 2.2-4.4 mg/kg/day in divided doses depending on severity of infection. Children over 45 kg should receive the adult dose.

Acute gonorrhea.

200 mg at once given PO; **then,** 100 mg at bedtime on first day, followed by 100 mg b.i.d. for 3 days. Alternatively, 300 mg immediately followed in 1 hr with 300 mg.

Syphilis (primary/secondary).

300 mg/day in divided PO doses for 10 days.

C. trachomatis infections.

100 mg b.i.d. PO for minimum of 7 days.

Prophylaxis of "traveler's diarrhea."

100 mg/day given PO.

Prophylaxis of malaria.

Adults: 100 mg PO once daily; **children, over 8 years of age:** 2 mg/kg/day up to 100 mg/day.

• **IV**

Endometritis, parametritis, peritonitis, salpingitis.

100 mg b.i.d. with 2 g cefoxitin, IV, q.i.d. continued for at least 4 days or 2 days after improvement observed. This is followed by doxycycline, PO, 100 mg b.i.d. for 10-14 days of total therapy.

NOTE: The Centers for Disease Control and Prevention (CDC) have established treatment schedules for STDs.

HEALTH CARE CONSIDERATIONS

See also *General Health Care Considerations for All Anti-Infectives* and *Tetracyclines.*

Administration/Storage

1. Prophylaxis for malaria can begin 1-2 days before travel begins, during travel, and for 4 weeks after leaving the malarious area.
2. The powder for suspension expires 12 months from date of issue.
3. Solution is stable for 2 weeks when stored in refrigerator.

Client/Family Teaching

1. May take with food; take with a full glass of water to prevent esophageal ulceration.
2. Avoid direct exposure to sunlight and wear protective clothing and sunscreens when exposed .
3. With STDs advise that partner be tested and treated. Use condoms until medically cleared.
4. Take entire prescription; do not stop if symptoms subside.

Outcome/Evaluate

- Resolution of infection
- Symptomatic improvement

Dronabinol (Delta-9-tetrahydro-cannabinol)

(droh-**NAB**-ih-nohl)

Pregnancy Category: C

Marinol **(C-II) (Rx)**

Classification: Antinauseant

Action/Kinetics: As the active component in marijuana, significant psychoactive effects may occur. (See *Side Effects.*) In therapeutic doses, the drug also causes conjunctival injection and an increased HR. Antiemetic effect may be due to inhibition of the vomiting center in the medulla. **Peak plasma levels:** 2-3 hr. Significant first-pass effect. The 11-hydroxytetrahydrocannabinol metabolite is active. **t½, biphasic:** 4 hr and 25-36 hr. **t½, 11-hydroxy-THC:** 15-18 hr. Metabolized in the liver and mainly excreted in the feces. Cumulative toxicity using clinical doses may occur. Highly bound to plasma proteins and may thus displace other protein-bound drugs.

Uses: Nausea and vomiting associated with cancer chemotherapy, especially in clients who have not responded to other antiemetic treatment. To stimulate appetite and prevent weight loss in AIDS clients.

Contraindications: Nausea and vomiting from any cause other than cancer chemotherapy. Lactation. Hypersensitivity to sesame oil.

Special Concerns: Monitor pediatric and geriatric clients carefully due to an increased risk of psychoactive effects. Use with caution in clients with hypertension, occasional hypotension, syncope, tachycardia; those with a history of substance abuse, including alcohol abuse or dependence; clients with mania, depression, or schizophrenia (the drug may exacerbate these illnesses); clients receiving sedatives, hypnotics, or other psychoactive drugs (due to the potential for additive or synergistic CNS effects).

Side Effects: *CNS:* Side effects are due mainly to the psychoactive effects of the drug and, in addition to those listed in the preceding, include dizziness, muddled thinking, coordination difficulties, irritability, weakness, headache, ataxia, cannabinoid "high," paresthesia, hallucinations, visual distortions, depersonalization, confusion, nightmares, disorientation, and confusion. *CV:* Palpitations, tachycardia, vasodilation, facial flush, hypotension. *GI:* Abdominal pain, N&V, diarrhea, dry mouth, fecal incontinence, anorexia. *Respiratory:* Cough, rhinitis, sinusitis. *Other:* Asthenia, conjunctivitis, myalgias, tinnitus, speech difficulty, vision difficulties, chills, headache, malaise, sweating, elevated hepatic enzymes.

Symptoms of Abstinence Syndrome: An abstinence syndrome has been reported following discontinuation of doses greater than 210 mg/day for 12-16 days. Symptoms include irritability, insomnia, and restlessness within 12 hr; within 24 hr, symptoms include "hot flashes," sweating, rhinorrhea, loose stools, hiccoughs, and anorexia. Disturbed sleep may occur for several weeks.

OD **Management of Overdose:** *Symptoms:* Extension of the pharmacologic effects. Symptoms of mild overdose include: drowsiness, euphoria, heightened sensory awareness, altered time perception, reddened conjunctiva, dry mouth, and tachycardia. Symptoms of moderate toxicity include impaired memory, depersonalization, mood alteration, urinary retention, and reduced bowel motility. Severe intoxication includes decreased motor coordination, lethargy, slurred speech, and postural hypotension. Seizures may occur in clients with existing seizure disorders. Hallucinations, psychotic episodes, ***respiratory depression,*** and ***coma*** have been reported. *Treatment:* Clients with depressive, hallucinatory, or psychotic reactions should be placed in a quiet environment and provided supportive treatment, including reassurance. Diazepam (5-10 mg PO) may be used for extreme agitation. Hypotension usually responds to IV fluids and Trendelenburg position. In unconscious clients with a secure airway, administer activated charcoal (30-100 g in adults and 1-2 g/kg in children); this may be followed by a saline cathartic.

Drug Interactions

Amphetamine / Additive hypertension, tachycardia, possibly cardiotoxicity

Anticholinergics / Additive or super-additive tachycardia; drowsiness

CNS depressants / Additive CNS depressant effects

Cocaine / See *Amphetamine*

Antidepressants, tricyclic / Additive tachycardia, hypertension, drowsiness

Ethanol / During subchronic dronabinol use, lower and delayed peak alcohol blood levels

Sympathomimetics / See *Amphetamine*

Theophylline / Possible increased metabolism of theophylline

How Supplied: *Capsule:* 2.5 mg, 5 mg, 10 mg

Dosage

- **Capsules**

Antiemetic.

Adults and children, initial: 5 mg/m² 1-3 hr before chemotherapy; **then,** 5 mg/m² q 2-4 hr for a total of four to six doses/day. If ineffective, this dose may be increased by 2.5 mg/m² to a maximum of 15 mg/m²/dose. However, the incidence of serious psychoactive side effects increases dramatically at these higher dose levels.

Appetite stimulation.

Initial: 2.5 mg b.i.d. before lunch and dinner. If unable to tolerate 5 mg/day, reduce the dose to 2.5 mg/day as a single evening or bedtime dose. If side effects are absent or minimal and an increased effect is desired, the dose may be increased to 2.5 mg before lunch and 5 mg before dinner (or 5 mg at lunch and 5 mg after dinner). The dose may be increased to 20 mg/day in divided doses. The incidence of side effects increases at higher doses.

HEALTH CARE CONSIDERATIONS

Administration/Storage

1. Due to its CNS effects, use only when client closely supervised.
2. Due to abuse potential, limit prescriptions to one course of chemotherapy (i.e., several days) and reorder PRN.

Assessment

1. Note any allergy to sesame oil or seeds.
2. Record onset of symptoms; assess if N&V may be caused by anything other than chemotherapy.
3. List other agents trialed.
4. Assess for symptoms of abstinence syndrome which may be seen following withdrawal of doses greater than 210 mg/day for 12-16 days.

Client/Family Teaching

1. Take 1-3 hr before chemotherapy.
2. Avoid sudden position changes; dizziness may occur.
3. Do not drive or perform hazardous tasks requiring mental acuity.
4. Potential for psychoactive symptoms, visual distortions, and mental confusion; these may be minimized by a quiet, supportive environment.
5. Keep out of child's reach; do not share regardless of symptoms.

Outcome/Evaluate

- Relief of chemotherapy-induced N&V
- ↑ Appetite; ↓ weight loss

Droperidol

(droh-PER-ih-dol)

Pregnancy Category: C

Inapsine **(Rx)**

Classification: Antipsychotic, butyrophenone; antianxiety agent

D

Action/Kinetics: Causes sedation, alpha-adrenergic blockade, peripheral vascular dilation; has antiemetic properties. For other details, see *Haloperidol*, and *Phenothiazines*. **Onset** (after IM, IV): 3-10 min. **Peak effect:** 30 min. **Duration:** 2-4 hr, although alteration of consciousness may last up to 12 hr. **t½:** 2.2 hr. Metabolized in the liver and excreted in both the feces and urine.

Uses: Preoperatively; induction and maintenance of anesthesia. To relieve N&V and reduce anxiety in diagnostic procedures or surgery. Neuroleptic analgesia. Antiemetic in cancer chemotherapy (used IV).

Special Concerns: Use with caution during lactation; in the elderly, debilitated, or poor risk client; and in renal or hepatic impairment. Safety for use during labor has not been established. Safety and efficacy have not been established in children less than 2 years of age.

Side Effects: *CNS:* Postoperative drowsiness (common), restlessness, hyperactivity, anxiety, dizziness, postoperative hallucinations; extrapyramidal symptoms (e.g., akathisia, dystonia, oculogyric crisis). *CV:* Hypotension and tachycardia (common), increase in BP (when combined with fentanyl or other parenteral analgesics). *Respiratory:* ***Respiratory depression (when combined with fentanyl), laryngospasm, bronchospasm.*** *Miscellaneous:* Chills, shivering.

Drug Interactions

Anesthetics, conduction (e.g., spinal) / Peripheral vasodilation and hypotension

CNS depressants / Additive or potentiating effects

Narcotic analgesics / ↑ Respiratory depressant effects

How Supplied: *Injection:* 2.5 mg/mL

Dosage

- **IM**

Preoperatively.

Adults: 2.5-10 mg 30-60 min before surgery (modify dosage in elderly, debilitated); **pediatric, 2-12 years,** 88-165 mcg/kg.

Diagnostic procedures.

Adults: 2.5-10 mg 30-60 min before procedure; **then,** if necessary, **IV,** 1.25-2.5 mg.

- **IV**

Adjunct to general anesthesia.

Adults: 0.28 mg/kg with analgesic or anesthetic; **maintenance:** 1.25-2.5 mg (total dose).

- **IV (Slow) or IM**

Adjunct to regional anesthesia.

Adults: 2.5-5 mg.

HEALTH CARE CONSIDERATIONS

See also *Health Care Considerations* for *Antipsychotic Agents, Phenothiazines.*

Administration/Storage

IV 1. May be administered by direct IV slowly over 1 min; may also be reconstituted in 250 mL of D5W or NSS and administered slowly via infusion control device.

2. At a concentration of 1 mg/50 mL, droperidol is stable for 7-10 days in glass bottles with D5W, RL injection, and 0.9% NaCl injection. Droperidol is stable for 7 days in PVC bags containing D5W or 0.9% NaCl injection.

3. If used with Innovar injection (fentanyl plus droperidol), consider the dose of droperidol in the injection.

4. Droperidol is compatible at a concentration of 2.5 mg/mL for 15 min when combined in a syringe with the following: atropine sulfate, butorphanol tartrate, chlorpromazine hydrochloride, diphenhydramine hydrochloride, fentanyl citrate, glycopyrrolate, hydroxyzine hydrochloride, meperidine hydrochloride, morphine sulfate, perphenazine, promazine hydrochloride, promethazine hydrochloride, and scopolamine hydrobromide.

5. A precipitate will form if droperidol is mixed with barbiturates.

Interventions

1. Keep on bedrest; supervise activities and ambulation until VS stable. Drug causes orthostatic hypotension and drowsiness

2. Assess for extrapyramidal S&S; may use anticholinergics as needed.

Outcome/Evaluate

- ↓ Procedure anxiety
- Control of N&V

E 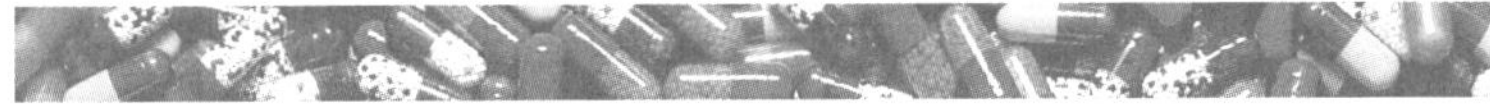

Econazole nitrate

(ee-**KON**-ah-zohl)
Pregnancy Category: C
Ecostatin ✦, Spectazole **(Rx)**
Classification: Antifungal, topical

Action/Kinetics: Fungistatic or fungicidal, depending on concentration. Inhibits the synthesis of sterols that damages the cell membrane and increases the permeability, resulting in a loss of essential intracellular elements. May also inhibit biosynthesis of triglycerides and phospholipids and inhibit oxidative and peroxidative enzyme activity. Effective concentrations are found in the stratum corneum, epidermis, and the dermis. Systemic absorption is low.
Uses: Broad-spectrum fungicide effective against *Microsporum audouinii, M. canis, M. gypseum, Epidermophyton floccosum, Trichophyton mentagrophytes, T. rubrum, T. tonsurans, Candida albicans, Malassezia furfur,* and some gram-positive bacteria. Used to treat tinea cruris, tinea corporis, tinea pedis, tinea versicolor, cutaneous candidiasis.
Contraindications: Hypersensitivity. Ophthalmic use.
Special Concerns: Use with caution in pregnancy and lactation.
Side Effects: *Topical:* Burning, erythema, itching, stinging.
How Supplied: *Cream:* 1%

Dosage

- **Topical Cream (1%)**

Tinea cruris, tinea corporis, tinea pedis, tinea versicolor.
Apply sufficient cream to cover the affected areas once daily.
Cutaneous candidiasis.
Apply b.i.d. in the morning and evening. If no improvement is noted after recommended treatment period, reevaluate diagnosis.

HEALTH CARE CONSIDERATIONS

See also *General Health Care Considerations for All Anti-Infectives.*
Client/Family Teaching
1. Wash hands before and after therapy. Clean area with soap and water; dry thoroughly; apply cream.
2. For athlete's foot, the shoes and socks should be changed at least once daily; wear well-fitted, ventilated shoes.
3. To reduce chance of reinfection, treat tinea pedis for 1 month; treat tinea cruris, tinea corporis, and candidal infections for 2 weeks.
4. Use for the full prescribed time even if symptoms have improved.
5. Report if condition worsens or symptoms of burning, itching, redness, and stinging occur.

Outcome/Evaluate
- Resolution of fungal infection
- Symptomatic improvement

Edrophonium chloride

(ed-roh-**FOH**-nee-um)
Pregnancy Category: C
Enlon, Reversol, Tensilon **(Rx)**

COMBINATION DRUG

Edrophonium chloride and Atropine sulfate

(ed-roh-**FOH**-nee-um)
Pregnancy Category: C
Enlon-Plus **(Rx)**
Classification: Cholinesterase inhibitor, indirectly-acting

See also *Neostigmine* and *Atropine sulfate.*
Action/Kinetics: By increasing the duration of action at the motor end plate, edrophonium causes a transient increase in muscle strength in myasthenia gravis clients and either no change or a slight weakness in muscle strength in clients with other disorders. Atropine counteracts the muscarinic side effects that will occur due to edrophonium (e.g., increased secretions, bradycardia, bronchoconstriction). **Onset: IM,** 2-10 min; **IV,** <1 min. **Duration: IM,** 5-30 min; **IV,** 10 min. Eliminated through the kidneys.
Uses: Edrophonium: Differential diagnosis of myasthenia gravis. Adjunct to evaluate requirements for treating myasthenia gravis. Adjunct to treat respiratory depression due to curare and similar nondepolarizing agents such as gallamine, pancuronium, and tubocurarine.

Edrophonium and Atropine: To antagonize or reverse nondepolarizing neuromuscular blocking agents. Adjunct to treat respiratory depression caused by overdosage of curare.
Contraindications: Edrophonium combined with atropine in the differential diagnosis of myasthenia gravis.

Special Concerns: Edrophonium combined with atropine is not effective against depolarizing neuromuscular blocking agents.
How Supplied: Edrophonium chloride: *Injection:* 10 mg/mL. Edrophonium chloride and Atropine sulfate: *Injection:* 10 mg-0.14 mg/mL

Dosage

- **Edrophonium, IV**

Differential diagnosis of myasthenia gravis.
IV, Adults: 2 mg initially over 15-30 sec; with needle in place, wait 45 sec; if no response occurs after 45 sec inject an additional 8 mg. If a cholinergic reaction is obtained following 2 mg (muscarinic side effects, skeletal muscle fasciculations, increased muscle weakness), test is discontinued and atropine, 0.4-0.5 mg, is given IV. The test may be repeated in 30 min. **Pediatric, up to 34 kg, IV:** 1 mg; if no response after 45 sec, can give up to 5 mg. **Pediatric, over 34 kg, IV:** 2 mg; if no response after 45 sec, can give up to 10 mg in 1-mg increments q 30-45 sec. **Infants:** 0.5 mg. If IV injection is not feasible, IM can be used.

To evaluate treatment needs in myasthenic clients.
1 hr after PO administration of drug used to treat myasthenia, give edrophonium IV, 1-2 mg. (*NOTE:* Response will be myasthenic in undertreated clients, adequate in controlled clients, and cholinergic in overtreated clients.)

Curare antagonist.
Slow IV: 10 mg over 30-45 sec to detect onset of cholinergic reaction; repeat if necessary to maximum of 40 mg. Should not be given before use of curare, gallamine, or tubocurarine.

- **Edrophonium, IM**

Differential diagnosis of myasthenia gravis.
Adults: 10 mg; if hyperreactivity occurs, retest after 30 min with 2 mg IM to rule out false negative. **Pediatric, up to 34 kg:** 2 mg; **more than 34 kg:** 5 mg. (There is a 2-10-min delay in reaction with IM route.)

- **Edrophonium and Atropine, IV**

Adults: 0.5-1 mg/kg edrophonium and 0.007-0.014 mg/kg atropine.

HEALTH CARE CONSIDERATIONS

See also *Health Care Considerations* for *Neostigmine* and *Atropine Sulfate*.

Administration/Storage

IV 1. Do not give edrophonium before curare or curare-like drugs.
2. Have IV atropine sulfate available to use as an antagonist.
3. When atropine is combined with edrophonium, monitor carefully; assisted or controlled ventilation should be undertaken.
4. Recurarization has not been noted following satisfactory reversal with edrophonium and atropine.

Assessment

1. Record therapy indications.
2. List drugs currently prescribed.
3. Note any history of asthma, seizures, CAD, or hyperthyroidism.

Interventions

1. Monitor closely during administration; effects last up to 30 min.
2. Monitor VS and I&O at least q 4 hr.
3. Record any increased salivation, bronchial spasm, bradycardia, and cardiac arrhythmia; especially important with the elderly.
4. When administered as an antidote for curare, assess for each dose effect; do not administer the next dose unless prior effects have been observed. Larger doses may potentiate effects.
5. Evaluate respiratory effort and provide assisted ventilation prn.
6. During cholinergic crisis, monitor state of consciousness closely.

Outcome/Evaluate

- With myasthenia gravis (transient ↑ muscle strength, improved gait)
- Curare antagonist
- Reversal of respiratory depression
- Differentiation of myasthenic from cholinergic crisis

Efavirenz

(eh-**FAH**-vih-rehnz)
Pregnancy Category: C
Sustiva **(Rx)**
Classification: Antiviral drug

See also *Antiviral Agents.*
Action/Kinetics: A non-nucleoside reverse transcriptase inhibitor of HIV-1. Action is mainly by non-competitive inhibition of HIV-1. **Peak plasma levels:** 3-5 hr. **Steady-state plasma levels:** 6-10 days. Highly protein bound. Metabolized by the cytochrome P450 system to inactive metabolites which are excreted in the urine and feces. Will induce its own metabolism. **t½, terminal:** 52-76 hr after a single dose and 40-55 hr after multiple doses.
Uses: In combination with other antiretroviral drugs to treat HIV-1 infection.
Contraindications: Use as a single agent to treat HIV or added on as a sole agent to a failing regimen.
Special Concerns: HIV-infected mothers should not breastfeed to avoid risking post-

natal transmission of HIV infection. Use with caution in impaired hepatic function.

Side Effects: *CNS:* Delusions, inappropriate behavior (especially in those with a history of mental illness or substance abuse), severe acute depression with suicidal ideation/attempts, dizziness, impaired con-centration, somnolence, abnormal dreams, insomnia, fatigue, headache, hypoesthesia, depression, anorexia, nervousness, ataxia, confusion, convulsions, impaired coordination, migraine headaches, neuralgia, paresthesia, peripheral neuropathy, speech disorder, tremor, vertigo, aggravated depression, agitation, amnesia, anxiety, apathy, emotional lability, euphoria, hallucinations, psychosis. *Dermatologic:* Skin rash, including moist or dry desquamation, ulceration, erythema, pruritus, diffuse maculopapular rash, vesiculation, erythema multiforme. Increased sweating, alopecia, eczema, folliculitis, urticaria. Rarely, ***Stevens-Johnson syndrome, toxic epidermal necrolysis,*** necrosis requiring surgery, exfoliative dermatitis. *GI:* N&V, diarrhea, dyspepsia, abdominal pain, flatulence, dry mouth, pancreatitis. *GU:* Hematuria, renal calculus. *CV:* Flushing, palpitations, tachycardia, thrombophlebitis. *Musculoskeletal:* Arthralgia, myalgia. *Ophthalmic:* Abnormal vision, diplopia. *Miscellaneous:* Parosmia, taste perversion, alcohol intolerance, allergic reaction, asthenia, fever, hot flushes, malasie, pain, peripheral edema, syncope, tinnitus, hepatitis, asthma.

Laboratory Test Considerations: ↑ AST, ALT, total cholesterol, serum triglycerides.

OD **Management of Overdose:** *Symptoms:* Increased nervous system symptoms. *Treatment:* General supportive measures, including monitoring of vital signs.

Drug Interactions

Astemizole / Inhibition of the metabolism of astemizole → possible cardiac arrhythmias, prolonged sedation, or respiratory depression

Cisapride / Inhibition of the metabolism of cisapride → possible cardiac arrhythmias, prolonged sedation, or respiratory depression

Clarithromycin / ↓ Clarithromycin plasma levels and ↑ levels of metabolite; use alternative therapy such as azithromycin

CNS depressants / Additive CNS depression

Ergot derivatives / Inhibition of the metabolism of ergot derivatives → possible cardiac arrhythmias, prolonged sedation, or respiratory depression

Midazolam / Inhibition of the metabolism of midazolam → possible cardiac arrhythmias, prolonged sedation, or respiratory depression

Ritonavir / Higher frequency of dizziness, nausea, paresthesia, and elevated liver enzymes

Triazolam / Inhibition of the metabolism of triazolam → possible cardiac arrhythmias, prolonged sedation, or respiratory depression

How Supplied: *Capsules:* 50 mg, 100 mg, 200 mg

Dosage

- **Capsules**

  HIV-1 infections.

Adults: 600 mg once daily in combination with a protease inhibitor or nucleoside analog reverse transcriptase inhibitors. **Children, 3 years and older. 10-< 15 kg:** 200 mg once daily; **15-< 20 kg:** 250 mg once daily; **20-< 25 kg:** 300 mg once daily; **25-< 32.5 kg:** 350 mg once daily; **32.5-< 40 kg:** 400 mg once daily; **40 kg or more:** 600 mg once daily.

HEALTH CARE CONSIDERATIONS

See also *Health Care Considerations* for *Antiviral Agents.*

Administration/Storage

1. Always initiate therapy with 1 or more other new antiretroviral drugs to which the client has not been previously exposed.
2. May be taken with or without food; however, high-fat meals may increase the absorption and are to be avoided.
3. Use bedtime dosing during the first 2 to 4 weeks to improve tolerability of nervous system side effects.

Assessment

1. Note indications for therapy and other agents trialed.
2. May cause false-positive cannabinoid urine test.

Client/Family Teaching

1. Take as directed and with other antiretroviral agents.
2. May take with food but avoid high fat meals as these may increase drug absorption.
3. Drug does not cure disease but works to reduce viral load.
4. Practice reliable barrier contraception with additional form of birth control; do not breast feed.
5. May cause dizziness, drowsiness, delusions, and impaired concentration. Take at bedtime to increase tolerability and avoid tasks requiring concentration and dexterity until effects realized.

E

6. Most will experience a rash. This should resolve after several weeks; report if persistent or extensive.
7. Avoid alcohol and any OTC agents.

Outcome/Evaluate: ↓ HIV-RNA levels; ↑ CD4 cell counts

Emedastine difumarate
(em-eh-**DAS**-teen)

Pregnancy Category: B

Emadine **(Rx)**

Classification: Antihistamine, ophthalmic

See also *Antihistamines*.

Action/Kinetics: Selective H_1 antagonist which inhibits histamine-stimulated vascular permeability in the conjunctiva. Very little reaches the systemic circulation.

Uses: Relieve signs and symptoms of allergic conjunctivitis.

Contraindications: Parenteral or oral use. Use to treat contact lens-related irritation.

Special Concerns: Use with caution during lactation. Safety and efficacy have not been established in children less than 3 years of age.

Side Effects: *Ophthalmic:* Blurred vision, burning or stinging, corneal infiltrates, corneal staining, dry eyes, foreign body sensation, hyperemia, keratitis, tearing. *CNS:* Headache, abnormal dreams. *Respiratory:* Pruritus, rhinitis, sinusitis. *Miscellaneous:* Asthenia, bad taste, dermatitis, discomfort.

How Supplied: *Solution:* 0.05%

Dosage

- **Solution**

  Allergic conjunctivitis.

One drop in the affected eye(s) up to q.i.d.

HEALTH CARE CONSIDERATIONS

See also *Health Care Considerations* for *Antihistamines*.

Administration/Storage: Store at 4°C-30°C (39°F-86°F).

Assessment: Note time of year and events/triggers that surround symptoms.

Client/Family Teaching

1. Use as directed; avoid triggers that precipitate symptoms.
2. To prevent contamination, do not allow the dropper tip to touch the eyelids or surrounding areas.
3. Keep bottle tightly closed; do not use if the solution becomes discolored.
4. Avoid contact lens if eye irritated or red. Do not insert soft contact lens for 15 min after instilling drops; the preservative, benzalkonium chloride, may be absorbed.

Outcome/Evaluate

- Relief of S&S of allergic conjunctivitis
- ↓ Ocular itching

Enalapril maleate
(en-**AL**-ah-prill)

Pregnancy Category: D

Vasotec, Vasotec I.V. **(Rx)**

Classification: Angiotensin-converting enzyme inhibitor

See also *Angiotensin-Converting Enzyme Inhibitors*.

Action/Kinetics: Converted in the liver by hydrolysis to the active metabolite, enalaprilat. The parenteral product is enalaprilat injection. **Onset, PO:** 1 hr; **IV,** 15 min. **Time to peak action, PO:** 4-6 hr; **IV,** 1-4 hr. **Duration, PO:** 24 hr; **IV,** About 6 hr. Approximately 50%-60% is protein bound. **t½, enalapril, PO:** 1.3 hr; **IV,** 15 min. **t½, enalaprilat, PO:** 11 hr. Excreted through the urine (half unchanged) and feces; over 90% of enalaprilat is excreted through the urine.

Uses: Alone or in combination with a thiazide diuretic for the treatment of hypertension (step I therapy). As adjunct with digitalis and diuretic in acute and chronic CHF. *Investigational:* Hypertension in children, hypertension related to scleroderma renal crisis, diabetic nephropathy, asymptomatic left ventricular dysfunction following MI. Enalaprilat may be used for hypertensive emergencies (effect is variable).

Special Concerns: Use with caution during lactation. Safety and effectiveness have not been determined in children.

Side Effects: *CV:* Palpitations, hypotension, chest pain, angina, ***CVA, MI,*** orthostatic hypotension, disturbances in rhythm, tachycardia, ***cardiac arrest,*** orthostatic effects, atrial fibrillation, tachycardia, bradycardia, Raynaud's phenomenon. *GI:* N&V, diarrhea, abdominal pain, alterations in taste, anorexia, dry mouth, constipation, dyspepsia, glossitis, ileus, melena, stomatitis. *CNS:* Insomnia, headache, fatigue, dizziness, paresthesias, nervousness, sleepiness, ataxia, confusion, depression, vertigo, abnormal dreams. *Hepatic:* Hepatitis, hepatocellular or cholestatic jaundice, pancreatitis, elevated liver enzymes, hepatic failure. *Respiratory:* Bronchitis, cough, dyspnea, bronchospasm, URI, pneumonia, pulmonary infiltrates, asthma, ***pulmonary embolism and infarction, pulmonary edema.*** *Renal:* Renal dysfunction, oliguria, UTI, transient increases in creatinine and BUN. *Hematologic:* Rarely, neutropenia, thrombocytopenia, bone marrow depression, decreased H&H in hypertensive or CHF clients. Hemolytic anemia, including hemolysis, in clients with G6PD deficiency. *Dermatologic:* Rash, pruritus, alopecia, flushing, erythema multiforme, exfoliative dermatitis, photosensitivity, urticaria, increased sweating, pemphigus, ***Stevens-Johnson syndrome,*** herpes zoster, toxic epidermal necrolysis. *Other:* Angioedema, asthenia, impotence, blurred vision, fever, arthralgia, arthritis, vasculitis, eosinophilia, tinnitus, syncope, myalgia, muscle cramps, rhinorrhea, sore throat, hoarseness, conjunctivitis, tearing, dry eyes, loss of sense of smell, hearing loss, peripheral neuropathy, anosmia, myositis, flank pain, gynecomastia.

Additional Drug Interactions: Rifampin may ↓ the effects of enalapril. Do not discontinue without first reporting to the provider.

How Supplied: *Tablet:* 2.5 mg, 5 mg, 10 mg, 20 mg; *Injection:* 1.25 mg/mL

Dosage

- **Tablets (Enalapril)**

Antihypertensive in clients not taking diuretics.

Initial: 5 mg/day; **then,** adjust dosage according to response (range: 10-40 mg/day in one to two doses).

Antihypertensive in clients taking diuretics.

Initial: 2.5 mg. Since hypotension may occur following the initiation of enalapril, the diuretic should be discontinued, if possible, for 2-3 days before initiating enalapril. If BP is not maintained with enalapril alone, diuretic therapy may be resumed.

Adjunct with diuretics and digitalis in heart failure.

Initial: 2.5 mg 1-2 times/day; **then,** depending on the response, 5-20 mg/day in two divided doses. Dose should not exceed 40 mg/day. Dosage must be adjusted in clients with renal impairment or hyponatremia.

In clients with impaired renal function.

Initial: 5 mg/day if C_{CR} ranges between 30 and 80 mL/min and serum creatinine is less than 3 mg/dL; 2.5 mg/day if C_{CR} is less than 30 mL/min and serum creatinine is more than 3 mg/dL and in dialysis clients on dialysis days.

Renal impairment or hyponatremia.

Initial: 2.5 mg/day if serum sodium is less than 130 mEq/L and serum creatinine is more than 1.6 mg/dL. The dose may be increased to 2.5 mg b.i.d. and then 5 mg b.i.d. or higher if required; dose is given at intervals of 4 or more days. Maximum daily dose is 40 mg.

Asymptomatic LV dysfunction following MI.

2.5-20 mg/day beginning 72 hr or longer after onset of MI. Therapy is continued for 1 year or longer.

NOTE: Dosage should be decreased in clients with a C_{CR} less than 30 mL/min and a serum creatinine level greater than 3 mg/dL.

- **IV (Enalaprilat)**

Hypertension.

1.25 mg over a 5-min period; repeat q 6 hr.

Antihypertensive in clients taking diuretics.

Initial: 0.625 mg over 5 min; if an adequate response is seen after 1 hr, administer another 0.625-mg dose. Thereafter, 1.25 mg q 6 hr.

Clients with impaired renal function.

Give enalaprit, 1.25 mg q 6 hr for clients with a C_{CR} more than 30 mL/min and an initial dose of 0.625 mg for clients with a C_{CR} less than 30 mL/min. If there is an adequate response, an additional 0.625 mg may be given after 1 hr; thereafter, additional 1.25-mg doses can be given q 6 hr. For dialysis clients, the initial dose is 0.625 mg q 6 hr.

HEALTH CARE CONSIDERATIONS

See also *Health Care Considerations* for *Angiotensin-Converting Enzyme Inhibitors* and *Antihypertensive Agents.*

Administration/Storage

1. To convert from IV to PO therapy in clients on a diuretic, begin with 2.5 mg/day for clients responding to a 0.625-mg IV dose. Thereafter, 2.5 mg/day may be given.
2. Use lower dose if receiving diuretics or with impaired renal function.
3. **IV** To convert from PO to IV therapy in clients not on a diuretic, use the recommended IV dose (i.e., 1.25 mg/6 hr). To convert from IV to PO therapy, begin with 5 mg/day.
4. Following IV administration, first dose peak effect may take 4 hr (whether or not on a diuretic). For subsequent doses, the peak effect is usually within 15 min.
5. Give enalaprilat as a slow IV infusion (over 5 min) either alone or diluted up to 50 mL with an appropriate diluent. Any of the following can be used: D5W, D5/RL, Isolyte E, 0.9% NaCl, D5/0.9% NaCl.
6. When used initially for heart failure, observe for at least 2 hr after the initial dose and until BP has stabilized for an additional hour. If possible, reduce dose of diuretic.

Assessment

1. Record indications for therapy, presenting symptoms, other agents trialed, and the outcome.
2. Record ECG, VS, and weight.

3. Monitor CBC, electrolytes, liver and renal function studies. Reduce dose with impaired renal function.

Client/Family Teaching

1. Use caution, may cause orthostatic effects and dizziness.
2. Maintain a healthy diet; limit intake of caffeine; avoid alcohol, salt substitutes, or high-Na and high-K foods.
3. Report any weight loss that may result from the loss of taste or rapid weight gain that may result from fluid overload.
4. Any flu-like symptoms should be reported immediately.

Outcome/Evaluate

- ↓ BP
- ↓ Preload and afterload with CHF

COMBINATION DRUG

Enalapril maleate and Hydrochlorothiazide

(en-**AL**-ah-prill, **high**-droh-**KLOR**oh-**THIGH**-ah-zyd)

Pregnancy Category: D

Vaseretic **(Rx)**

Classification: Antihypertensive

See also *Enalapril maleate* and *Hydrochlorothiazide*.

Content: *ACE inhibitor:* Enalapril, 5 mg or 10 mg. *Diuretic:* Hydrochlorothiazide, 12.5 mg or 25 mg.

Uses: Combination therapy for hypertension.

Contraindications: Use for initial therapy of hypertension. Anuria or severe renal dysfunction. History of angioedema related to use of ACE inhibitors. Lactation.

Special Concerns: Excessive hypotension may be observed in clients with severe salt or volume depletion such as those treated with diuretics or on dialysis. Significant hypotension may also be seen with severe CHF, with or without associated renal insufficiency. A significant fall in BP may result in MI or CVA in clients with ischemic heart or cerebrovascular disease. Safety and effectiveness have not been established in children.

How Supplied: See Content

Dosage

- **Tablets**

Adults: 1-2 tablets once daily.

HEALTH CARE CONSIDERATIONS

See also *Health Care Considerations* for *Antihypertensive Agents* and individual agents.

Administration/Storage

1. Individualize the dose determined by the titration of the individual components. Once successfully titrated with the individual components, Vaseretic (1 or 2 of the 10-25 tablets) may be given once daily if titrated doses are the same as those in the fixed combination.
2. Do not exceed 2 tablets/day.
3. If being treated with hydrochlorothiazide, hypotension may occur following the initial dose of enalapril. Thus, if possible, discontinue the diuretic 2-3 days before beginning therapy with enalapril. If diuretic cannot be discontinued, use an initial dose of 2.5 mg enalapril under close medical supervision for at least 2 hr and until BP has stabilized for another 1 hr.
4. The usual dose of Vaseretic is recommended with a C_{CR} > 30 mL/min.

Assessment

1. Monitor BP, CBC, electrolytes, liver and renal function.
2. Note any evidence of heart failure, cerebrovascular disease, angioedema, gout, elevated cholesterol levels, or diabetes.

Client/Family Teaching

1. Take as directed and do not stop abruptly.
2. Avoid activities that require mental alertness until drug effects realized.
3. Avoid alcohol, xanthines, potassium supplements or salt substitutes, potassium-sparing drugs, and OTC agents without approval.

Outcome/Evaluate: Control of hypertension

Enoxacin

(ee-**NOX**-ah-sin)

Pregnancy Category: C

Penetrex **(Rx)**

Classification: Antibacterial, fluoroquinolone derivative

See also *Fluoroquinolones*.

Action/Kinetics: Inhibits certain isozymes of the cytochrome P-450 hepatic microsomal enzyme system, resulting in alterations of metabolism of some drugs. **Peak plasma levels:** 0.83 mcg/mL 1-3 hr after a 200-mg dose and 2 mcg/mL 1-3 hr after a 400-mg dose. Mean peak plasma levels are 50% higher in geriatric clients than in young adults. Diffuses into the cervix, fallopian tubes, and myometrium at levels 1-2 times those seen in plasma and into kidney and prostate at levels 2-4 times those seen in plasma. **t½:** 3-6 hr. More than 40% excreted unchanged through the urine.

Uses: To treat uncomplicated urethral or cervical gonorrhea due to *Neisseria gonorrhoeae*. To treat uncomplicated UTIs due *Escherichia coli, Staphylococcus epidermidis,* or *S. saprophyticus;* for complicated UTIs due to *E. coli, Klebsiella pneumoniae, Proteus mirabilis, Pseudomonas aeruginosa, S. epidermidis,* or *Enterobacter cloacae*. Not effective for syphilis.
Contraindications: Lactation.
Special Concerns: Safety and efficacy have not been determined in children less than 18 years of age. Dosage adjustment is not required in elderly clients with normal renal function. Not efficiently removed by hemodialysis or peritoneal dialysis.
Laboratory Test Considerations: ↑ ALT, AST, alkaline phosphatase, bilirubin. Proteinuria, albuminuria.
Additional Side Effects: *GI:* Anorexia, bloody stools, gastritis, stomatitis. *CNS:* Confusion, nervousness, anxiety, tremor, agitation, myoclonus, depersonalization, hypertonia. *Dermatologic:* Toxic epidermal necrolysis, ***Stevens-Johnson syndrome,*** urticaria, hyperhidrosis, mycotic infection, erythema multiforme. *CV:* Palpitations, tachycardia, vasodilation. *Respiratory:* Dyspnea, cough, epistaxis. *GU:* Vaginal moniliasis, urinary incontinence, renal failure. *Hematologic:* Eosinophilia, leukopenia, increased or decreased platelets, decreased hemoglobin, leukocytosis. *Miscellaneous:* Glucosuria, pyuria, increased or decreased potassium, asthenia, back or chest pain, myalgia, arthralgia, purpura, vertigo, unusual taste, tinnitus, conjunctivitis.
Additional Drug Interactions
Bismuth subsalicylate / Bioavailability of enoxacin is ↓ when bismuth subsalicylate is given within 1 hr; should not use together
Digoxin / ↓ Serum digoxin levels
How Supplied: *Tablet:* 200 mg, 400 mg

Dosage
- **Tablets**

Uncomplicated gonorrhea.
Adults: 400 mg for one dose.
Uncomplicated UTIs, cystitis.
Adults: 200 mg q 12 hr for 7 days.
Complicated UTIs.
Adults: 400 mg q 12 hr for 14 days.

HEALTH CARE CONSIDERATIONS

See also *General Health Care Considerations for All Anti-Infectives* and *Fluoroquinolones.*

Administration/Storage: Adjust the dose if C_{CR} is 30 mL (or less)/min/1.73 m^2. After a normal initial dose, use a 12-hr interval and one-half the recommended dose.
Assessment
1. Note any sensitivity to quinolones.
2. Identify source of infection; obtain cultures.
3. Obtain CBC, liver and renal function studies; reduce dose with renal dysfunction.
Client/Family Teaching
1. Take only as directed; 1 hr before or 2 hr after meals.
2. Increase fluid intake to prevent crystallization within the kidney which may result in damage to the kidneys.
3. Avoid high intake of alkaline foods (dairy products) and drugs (antacids).
4. With STDs, inform partners so thay can receive treatment, to prevent reinfections.
Outcome/Evaluate
- Resolution of infection
- Relief of pain and burning R/T UTI

Entacapone

(en-**TAH**-kah-pohn)
Pregnancy Category: C
Comtan **(Rx)**
Classification: Antiparkinson drug

Action/Kinetics: A selective and reversible catechol-O-methyltransferase (COMT) inhibitor. COMT eliminates catechols (e.g., dopa, dopamine, norepinephrine, epinephrine) and in the presence of a decarboxylase inhibitor (e.g., carbidopa), COMT becomes the major metabolizing enzyme for dopa. Thus, in the presence of a COMT inhibitior, levels of dopa and dopamine increase. When entacapone is given with levodopa and carbidopa, plasma levels of levodopa are greater and more sustained than after levodopa/carbidopa alone. This leads to more constant dopaminergic stimulation in the brain resulting in improvement of the signs and symptoms of Parkinson's disease. Rapidly absorbed. High plasma protein binding (98%). Almost completely metabolized in the liver with most excreted in the feces. **$t^1/_2$, elimination:** Biphasic 0.4-0.7 hr and 2.4 hr.
Uses: As an adjunct to levodopa/carbidopa to treat idiopathic Parkinsonism clients who experience signs and symptoms of end-of-dose "wearing-off."
Contraindications: Concomitant use with a nonselective MAO inhibitor (e.g., phenelzine, tranylcypromine).
Special Concerns: Use with caution during lactation and in clients with biliary obstruction.

At the present, there is no potential use in children. Use with caution with drugs known to be metabolized by COMT (e.g., apomorphine, bitolterol, dobutamine, dopamine, epinephrine, isoetharine, isoproterenol, methyldopa, norepinephrine) due to the possibility of increased HRs, arrhythmias, and excessive changes in BP.

E

Side Effects: *CNS:* Dyskinesia, hyperkinesia, hypokinesia, dizziness, anxiety, somnolence, agitation, hallucinations. *GI:* Nausea, diarrhea, abdominal pain, constipation, vomiting, dry mouth, dyspepsia, flatulence, gastritis, GI disorder. *Body as a whole:* Fatigue, asthenia, increased sweating, bacterial infection. *Miscellaneous:* Urine discoloration, back pain, dsypnea, purpura, taste perversion, rhabdomyolysis.

OD **Management of Overdose:** *Symptoms:* Abdominal pain, loose stools. *Treatment:* Symptomatic with supportive care. Consider hospitalization. Monitor respiratory and circulatory systems. Review for possible drug interactions.

Drug Interactions

Ampicillin / ↓ Biliary excretion of entacapone
Apomorphine / Possible ↑ HR, arrhythmias, and excessive changes in BP
Bitolterol / Possible ↑ HR, arrhythmias, and excessive changes in BP
Chloramphenicol / ↓ Biliary excretion of entacapone
Cholestyramine / ↓ Biliary excretion of entacapone
Dobutamine / Possible ↑ HR, arrhythmias, and excessive changes in BP
Dopamine / Possible ↑ HR, arrhythmias, and excessive changes in BP
Epinephrine / Possible ↑ HR, arrhythmias, and excessive changes in BP
Erythromycin / ↓ Biliary excretion of entacapone
Isoetharine / Possible ↑ HR, arrhythmias, and excessive changes in BP
Isoproterenol / Possible ↑ HR, arrhythmias, and excessive changes in BP
MAO inhibitors (phenylzine, tranylcypromine) / Significant ↑ levels of catecholamines
Methyldopa / Possible ↑ HR, arrhythmias, and excessive changes in BP
Norepinephrine / Possible ↑ HR, arrhythmias, and excessive changes in BP
Probenecid / ↓ Biliary excretion of entacapone
Rifamipicin / ↓ Biliary excretion of entacapone

How Supplied: *Tablets:* 200 mg

Dosage

- **Tablets**

Parkinsonism.

200 mg given concomitantly with each levodopa/carbidopa dose up to a maximum of 8 times/day (i.e., 1,600 mg/day).

HEALTH CARE CONSIDERATIONS

Administration/Storage

1. Always give entacapone in combination with levodopa/carbidopa; entacapone has no antiparkinson effect by itself.
2. Most clients required a decreased daily levodopa dose (about 25%) if their daily levodopa dose was 800 mg or more, or if they had moderate or severe dyskinesias prior to entacapone treatment.
3. Entacapone can be given with either immediate- or sustained-release levodopa/carbidopa formulations.
4. Rapid withdrawal or abrupt reduction in the entacapone dose can lead to emergence of S&S of Parkinsonism and could lead to a complex resembling neuroleptic malignant syndrome (hyperpyrexia and confusion).
5. If necessary to discontinue treatment, withdraw clients slowly from entacapone.

Assessment

1. Note onset of Parkinson''s disease, levodopa/carbidopa dosage, and when symtoms occur in dosage cycle.
2. Determine any evidence of liver or bilary dysfunction.
3. List drugs prescribed to ensure none interact.

Client/Family Teaching

1. Take as directed with levodopa/carbidopa.
2. Drug is used to prevent end-of-dose "wearing off" effects of Sinemet; alone it has no antiparkinson effect.
3. Report any high fever or rigidity immediately.
4. Do not perform activities that require mental or physical alertness until drug effects realized.
5. May experience syncope, nausea, diarrhea, hallucinations, increase in dyskinesia, altered pulmonary or kidney function. Report if bothersome or persistent.
6. Urine may appear brownish-orange in color.
7. Rise slowly from a sitting or lying position to prevent postural hypotension or syncope.
8. Drug is not for use during pregnancy or breastfeeding. Report if pregnancy suspected or desired.

Outcome/Evaluate: Improved control of "end of dose" S&S of Parkinson''s disease i.e.; ↓ stiffness, tremor and shuffling; ↑ coordination

Ephedrine sulfate

(eh-**FED**-rin)

Pregnancy Category: C

Nasal decongestants: Kondon's Nasal, Pretz-D, Vatronol Nose Drops **(OTC)**. **Systemic:** Ephed II (**Rx:** Injection; **OTC:** Oral dosage forms)

Classification: Adrenergic agent, direct- and indirect-acting

See also *Sympathomimetic Drugs*.

Action/Kinetics: Releases norepinephrine from synaptic storage sites. Has direct effects on alpha, beta-1, and beta-2 receptors, causing increased BP due to arteriolar constriction and cardiac stimulation, bronchodilation, relaxation of GI tract smooth muscle, nasal decongestion, mydriasis, and increased tone of the bladder trigone and vesicle sphincter. It may also increase skeletal muscle strength, especially in myasthenia clients. Significant CNS effects include stimulation of the cerebral cortex and subcortical centers. Hepatic glycogenolysis is increased, but not as much as with epinephrine. More stable and longer-lasting than epinephrine. Rapidly and completely absorbed following parenteral use. **Onset, IM:** 10-20 min; **PO:** 15-60 min; **SC:** < 20 min. **Duration, IM, SC:** 30-60 min; **PO:** 3-5 hr. **t½, elimination:** About 3 hr when urine is at a pH of 5 and about 6 hr when urinary pH is 6.3. Excreted mostly unchanged through the urine (rate dependent on urinary pH—increased in acid urine).

Uses: Bronchial asthma and reversible bronchospasms associated with obstructive pulmonary diseases. Nasal congestion in vasomotor rhinitis, acute sinusitis, hay fever, and acute coryza. Parenterally to treat narcolepsy and depression and as a vasopressor to treat shock. In acute hypotension states, especially that associated with spinal anesthesia and Stokes-Adams syndrome with complete heart block.

Additional Contraindications: Angle closure glaucoma, anesthesia with cyclopropane or halothane, thyrotoxicosis, diabetes, obstetrics where maternal BP is greater than 130/80. Lactation.

Special Concerns: Geriatric clients may be at higher risk to develop prostatic hypertrophy. May cause hypertension resulting in intracranial hemorrhage or anginal pain in clients with coronary insufficiency or ischemic heart disease.

Additional Side Effects: *CNS:* Nervousness, shakiness, confusion, delirium, hallucinations. Anxiety and nervousness following prolonged use. *CV:* Precordial pain, ***excessive doses may cause hypertension sufficient to result in cerebral hemorrhage***. *GU:* Difficult and painful urination, urinary retention in males with prostatism, decrease in urine formation. *Miscellaneous:* Pallor, respiratory difficulty, hypersensitivity reactions. *Abuse:* Prolonged abuse can cause an anxiety state, including symptoms of paranoid schizophrenia, tachycardia, poor nutrition and hygiene, dilated pupils, cold sweat, and fever.

Additional Drug Interactions

Dexamethasone / Ephedrine ↓ effect of dexamethasone

Diuretics / Diuretics ↓ response to sympathomimetics

Furazolidone / ↑ Pressor effect → possible hypertensive crisis and intracranial hemorrhage

Guanethidine / ↓ Effect of guanethidine by displacement from its site of action

Halothane / Serious arrhythmias due to sensitization of the myocardium to sympathomimetics by halothane

MAO Inhibitors / ↑ Pressor effect → possible hypertensive crisis and intracranial hemorrhage

Methyldopa / Effect of ephedrine ↓ in methyldopa-treated clients

Oxytocic drugs / Severe persistent hypertension

How Supplied: *Capsule:* 24.3 mg, 25 mg, 50 mg; *Injection:* 50 mg/mL; *Spray:* 0.25%

Dosage

- **Capsules**

Bronchodilator, systemic nasal decongestant, CNS stimulant.

Adults: 25-50 mg q 3-4 hr. **Pediatric:** 3 mg/kg (100 mg/m²) daily in four to six divided doses.

- **SC, IM, Slow IV**

Bronchodilator.

Adults: 12.5-25 mg; subsequent doses determined by client response. **Pediatric:** 3 mg/kg (100 mg/m²) daily divided into four to six doses SC or IV.

Vasopressor.

Adults: 25-50 mg (IM or SC) or 5-25 mg (by slow IV push) repeated at 5- to 10-min intervals, if necessary. Absorption following IM is more rapid than following SC use. **Pediatric (IM):** 16.7 mg/m² q 4-6 hr.

- **Topical (0.25% Spray)**

Nasal decongestant.

Adults and children over 6 years: 2-3 gtt of solution or small amount of jelly in each nostril q 4 hr. Do not use topically for more than 3 or 4 consecutive days. Do not use in children under 6 years of age unless ordered by provider.

HEALTH CARE CONSIDERATIONS

See also *Health Care Considerations* for *Sympathomimetic Drugs.*

Administration/Storage

1. Tolerance may develop; however, temporary cessation of therapy restores the original drug response.

IV 2. May administer 10 mg IV undiluted over at least 1 min.

3. Use only clear solutions and discard any unused solution with IV therapy. Protect against exposure to light; drug is subject to oxidation.

Assessment

1. Record indications for therapy, type and onset of symptoms.

2. Assess mental status and pulmonary function; monitor ECG and VS. If administered for hypotension, monitor BP until stabilized.

3. If used for prolonged periods, assess for drug resistance. Rest without medication for 3-4 days, then resume to regain response.

Client/Family Teaching

1. Notify provider if SOB is unrelieved by medication and accompanied by chest pain, dizziness, or palpitations. Report any elevated or irregular pulse.

2. With males, report any difficulty or pain with voiding; may be drug-induced urinary retention.

3. Report any signs of depression, lack of interest in personal appearance, or complaints of insomnia or anorexia.

4. Avoid OTC drugs and alcohol.

Outcome/Evaluate

- Improved airway exchange
- ↓ Nasal congestion/mucus
- ↑ BP
- Control of narcolepsy

Epinephrine

(ep-ih-**NEF**-rin)

Pregnancy Category: C

Adrenalin Chloride Solution, Bronkaid Mist, Bronkaid Mistometer ✱, Epi E-Z Pen, Epi E-Z Pen Jr., Epipen, Epipen Jr., Primatene Mist Solution, Sus-Phrine (Both Rx and OTC)

Epinephrine bitartrate

(ep-ih-**NEF**-rin)

Pregnancy Category: C

Asthmahaler Mist, Bronitin Mist, Bronkaid Mist Suspension, Epitrate, Primatene Mist Suspension **(OTC)**

Epinephrine borate

(ep-ih-**NEF**-rin)

Pregnancy Category: C

Epinal Ophthalmic Solution **(Rx)**

Epinephrine hydrochloride

(ep-ih-**NEF**-rin)

Pregnancy Category: C

Adrenalin Chloride, AsthmaNefrin, Epifrin, Glaucon, microNefrin, Nephron, S-2 Inhalant, Vaponefrin (Both Rx and OTC)

Classification: Adrenergic agent, direct-acting

See also *Sympathomimetic Drugs.*

Action/Kinetics: Causes marked stimulation of alpha, beta-1, and beta-2 receptors, causing sympathomimetic stimulation, pressor effects, cardiac stimulation, bronchodilation, and decongestion. It crosses the placenta but not the blood-brain barrier. **Extreme caution must be taken never to inject 1:100 solution intended for inhalation—injection of this concentration has caused death. SC: Onset,** 6-15 min; **duration:** <1-4 hr. **Inhalation: Onset,** 1-5 min; **duration:** 1-3 hr. **IM, Onset:** variable; duration: <1-4 hr. Ineffective when given PO.

Uses: Cardiac arrest, Stokes-Adams syndrome, low CO following ECB. To prolong the action of local anesthetics. As a hemostatic during ocular surgery; treatment of conjunctival congestion during surgery; to induce mydriasis during surgery; treat ocular hypertension during surgery. Topically to control bleeding. Acute bronchial asthma, bronchospasms due to emphysema, chronic bronchitis, or other pulmonary diseases. Treatment of anaphylaxis, angioedema, anaphylactic shock, drug-induced allergic reactions, transfusion reactions, insect bites or stings. As an adjunct in the treatment of open-angle glaucoma (may be used with miotics, beta blockers, hyperosmotic agents, or carbonic anhydrase inhibitors). To produce mydriasis; to treat conjunctivitis. *NOTE:* Autoinjectors are available for emergency self-administration of first aid for anaphylactic reactions due to insect stings or bites, foods, drugs, and other allergens as well as idiopathic or exercise-induced anaphylaxis.

Additional Contraindications: Narrow-angle glaucoma. Use when wearing soft contact lenses (may discolor lenses). Aphakia. Lactation.

Special Concerns: May cause anoxia in the fetus. Safety and efficacy of ophthalmic products have not been determined in children; administer parenteral epinephrine to children with caution. Syncope may occur if epinephrine is given to asthmatic children. Administration of the SC injection by the IV route may cause severe or fatal hypertension or cerebrovascular hemorrhage. Epinephrine may temporarily increase the rigidity and tremor of parkinsonism. Use with caution and in small quantities in the toes, fingers, nose, ears, and genitals or in the presence of peripheral vascular disease as vasoconstriction-induced tissue sloughing may occur.

Laboratory Test Considerations: False + or ↑ BUN, fasting glucose, lactic acid, urinary catecholamines, glucose (Benedict's). ↓ Coagulation time. The drug may affect electrolyte balance.

Additional Side Effects: *CV:* ***Fatal ventricular fibrillation, cerebral or subarachnoid hemorrhage,*** obstruction of central retinal artery. ***Rapid and large increase in BP may cause aortic rupture, cerebral hemorrhage, or angina pectoris.*** *GU:* Decreased urine formation, urinary retention, painful urination. *CNS:* Anxiety, fear, pallor. Parenteral use may cause or aggravate disorientation, memory impairment, psychomotor agitation, panic, hallucinations, ***suicidal or homicidal tendencies,*** schizophrenic-type behavior. *Miscellaneous:* Prolonged use or overdose may cause elevated serum lactic acid with severe metabolic acidosis. *At injection site:* Bleeding, urticaria, wheal formation, pain. Repeated injections at the same site may cause necrosis from vascular constriction. *Ophthalmic:* Transient stinging or burning when administered, conjunctival hyperemia, brow ache, headache, blurred vision, photophobia, allergic lid reaction, ocular hypersensitivity, poor night vision, eye ache, eye pain. Prolonged ophthalmic use may cause deposits of pigment in the cornea, lids, or conjunctiva. When used for glaucoma in aphakic clients, reversible cystoid macular edema.

Additional Drug Interactions

Beta-adrenergic blocking agents / Initial effectiveness in treating glaucoma of this combination may ↓ over time

Chymotrypsin / Epinephrine, 1:100, will inactivate chymotrypsin in 60 min

How Supplied: Epinephrine: *Metered dose inhaler:* 0.22 mg/inh; *Injection:* 1 mg/mL, 5 mg/mL; *Kit:* 0.5 mg/mL, 1 mg/mL; Epinephrine bitartrate: *Metered dose inhaler:* 0.3 mg/inh; Epinephrine hydrochloride: *Injection:* 0.1 mg/mL, 1 mg/mL; *Solution:* 1:100, 1:1000; *Ophthalmic solution:* 0.5%, 1%, 2%

Dosage

- **Metered Dose Inhaler**

  Bronchodilation.

Adults and children over 4 years of age: 0.2-0.275 mg (1 inhalation) of the aerosol or 0.16 mg (1 inhalation) of the bitartrate aerosol; may be repeated after 1-2 min if needed. At least 3 hr should elapse before subsequent doses. Dosage not established in children less than 4 years of age.

- **Inhalation Solution**

  Bronchodilation.

Adults and children over 6 years of age: 1 inhalation of the 1% solution (of the base); may be repeated after 1-2 min.

- **IM, IV, SC**

  Bronchodilation using the solution (1:1,000).

Adults: 0.3-0.5 mg SC or IM repeated q 20 min-4 hr as needed; dose may be increased to 1 mg/dose. **Infants and children (except premature infants and full-term newborns):** 0.01 mg/kg (0.3 mg/m^2) SC up to a maximum of 0.5 mg/dose; may be repeated q 15 min for two doses and then q 4 hr as needed.

Bronchodilation using the sterile suspension (1:200).

Adults: 0.5-1.5 mg SC. **Infants and children, 1 month-12 years:** 0.025 mg/kg SC; **children less than 30 kg:** 0.75 mg as a single dose.

Anaphylaxis.

Adults: 0.2-0.5 mg SC q 10-15 min as needed, up to a maximum of 1 mg/dose if needed. **Pediatric:** 0.01 mg/kg (0.3 mg/m^2) up to a maximum of 0.5 mg/dose; may be repeated q 15 min for two doses and then q 4 hr as needed.

- **Autoinjector, IM**

  First aid for anaphylaxis.

The autoinjectors deliver a single dose of either 0.3 mg or 0.15 mg (for children) of epinephrine. In cases of a severe reaction, repeat injections may be necessary.

Vasopressor.

Adults, IM or SC, initial: 0.5 mg repeated q 5 min if needed; **then,** give 0.025-0.050 mg IV q 5-15 min as needed. **Adults, IV, initial:** 0.1-0.25 mg given slowly. May be repeated q 5-15 min as needed. Or, use IV infusion beginning with 0.001 mg/min and increasing the dose to 0.004 mg/min if needed. **Pediatric, IM, SC:** 0.01 mg/kg, up to a maximum of 0.3 mg repeated q 5 min if needed. **Pediatric, IV:** 0.01 mg/kg/5-15 min if an inadequate response to IM or SC administration is observed.

Cardiac stimulant.

Adults, intracardiac or IV: 0.1-1 mg repeated q 5 min if needed. **Pediatric, intracardiac or IV:** 0.005-0.01 mg/kg (0.15-0.3

mg/m^2) repeated q 5 min if needed; this may be followed by IV infusion beginning at 0.0001 mg/kg/min and increased in increments of 0.0001 mg/kg/min up to a maximum of 0.0015 mg/kg/min.

Adjunct to local anesthesia.

Adults and children: 0.1-0.2 mg in a 1:200,000-1:20,000 solution.

Adjunct with intraspinal anesthetics.

Adults: 0.2-0.4 mg added to the anesthetic spinal fluid.

- **Solution**

Antihemorrhagic, mydriatic.

Adults and children, intracameral or subconjunctival: 0.01%-0.1% solution.

Topical antihemorrhagic.

Adults and children: 0.002%-0.1% solution.

Nasal decongestant.

Adults and children over 6 years of age: Apply 0.1% solution as drops or spray or with a sterile swab as needed.

- **Borate Ophthalmic Solution, Hydrochloride Ophthalmic Solution**

Glaucoma.

Adults: 1-2 gtt into affected eye(s) 1-2 times/day. Determine frequency of use by tonometry. Dosage has not been established in children.

HEALTH CARE CONSIDERATIONS

See also *Health Care Considerations* for *Sympathomimetic Drugs.*

Administration/Storage

1. Briskly massage site of SC or IM injection to hasten drug action. Do not expose to heat, light, or air, as this causes deterioration of the drug.
2. Discard solution if reddish brown and after expiration date.
3. With sodium bisulfite as a preservative in the topical preparation, there may be slight stinging after administration.
4. Do not use the topical preparation in children under 6 years of age.
5. Ophthalmic use may result in discomfort, which decreases over time.
6. The ophthalmic preparation is not for injection or intraocular use.
7. If ophthalmic glaucoma product used with a miotic, instill miotic first.
8. Keep the ophthalmic product tightly sealed and protected from light. Store at 2°C-4°C (36°F-75°F). Discard the solution if it becomes discolored or contains a precipitate.

IV 9. *Never administer* 1:100 solution IV. Use 1:1,000 solution for IV administration.

10. Use a tuberculin syringe to measure; parenteral doses are small and drug is potent, errors in measurement may be disastrous.
11. For direct IV administration to adults, the drug must be well diluted as a 1:1,000 solution; inject quantities of 0.05-0.1 mL of solution cautiously taking about 1 min for each injection; note response (BP and pulse). Dose may be repeated several times if necessary. May be further diluted in D5W or NSS.

Assessment

1. Note history of sulfite sensitivity.
2. Record indications for therapy; describe type and onset of symptoms and anticipated results.
3. Assess cardiopulmonary function.
4. During IV therapy, continuously monitor ECG, BP, and pulse until desired effect achieved. Then take VS every 2-5 min until condition has stabilized; once stable, monitor BP q 15-30 min.
5. Note any symptoms of shock such as cold, clammy skin, cyanosis, and loss of consciousness.

Client/Family Teaching

1. Review method for administration carefully. When prescribed for anaphylaxis, administer autoinjector immediately and then seek further medical care.
2. Report any increased restlessness, chest pain, or insomnia as dosage adjustment may be necessary.
3. Limit intake of caffeine, as with colas, coffee, tea, and chocolate; avoid OTC drugs without approval.
4. Rinse mouth after MDI use.
5. Ophthalmic solution may burn on administration; this should subside. May stain contact lens.
6. Use caution when performing activities that require careful vision; ophthalmic solution may diminish visual fields, cause double vision, and alter night vision.

Outcome/Evaluate

- Restoration of cardiac activity
- Improved CO with EC bypass
- ↓ IOP
- Reversal of S&S of anaphylaxis
- Improved airway exchange
- Hemostasis with ocular surgery

Epoprostenol sodium

(eh-poh-**PROST**-en-ohl)

Pregnancy Category: B

Flolan **(Rx)**

Classification: Antihypertensive, miscellaneous

See also *Antihypertensive Agents.*

Action/Kinetics: Acts by direct vasodilation of pulmonary and systemic arterial vascular beds and by inhibition of platelet aggregation. IV infusion in clients with pulmonary hypertension results in increases in cardiac index and SV and decreases in pulmonary vascular resistance, total pulmonary resistance, and mean systemic arterial pressure. Is rapidly hydrolyzed at the neutral pH of the blood as well as by enzymatic degradation. Metabolites are less active than the parent compound. **t½:** 6 min.

Uses: Long-term IV treatment of primary pulmonary hypertension in New York Heart Association Class III and Class IV clients.

Contraindications: Chronic use in those with CHF due to severe LV systolic dysfunction and in those who develop pulmonary edema during dose ranging.

Special Concerns: Abrupt withdrawal or sudden large decreases in the dose may cause rebound pulmonary hypertension. Use caution in dose selection in the elderly due to the greater frequency of decreased hepatic, renal, or cardiac function, as well as concomitant disease or other drug therapy. Use with caution during lactation. Safety and efficacy have not been determined in children.

Side Effects: Side effects have been classified as those occurring during acute dose ranging, those as a result of the drug delivery system, and those occurring during chronic dosing.

Those occurring during acute dose ranging. *CV:* Flushing, hypotension, bradycardia, tachycardia. *GI:* N&V, abdominal pain, dyspepsia. *CNS:* Headache, anxiety, nervousness, agitation, dizziness, hypesthesia, paresthesia. *Miscellaneous:* Chest pain, musculoskeletal pain, dyspnea, back pain, sweating.

Those occurring as a result of the drug delivery system. *Due to the chronic indwelling catheter:* Local infection, pain at the injection site, sepsis, infections.

Those occurring during chronic dosing. *CV:* Flushing, tachycardia. *GI:* N&V, diarrhea. *CNS:* Headache, anxiety, nervousness, tremor, dizziness, hypesthesia, hyperesthesia, paresthesia. *Musculoskeletal:* Jaw pain, myalgia, nonspecific musculoskeletal pain. *Miscellaneous:* Flu-like symptoms, chills, fever, sepsis.

OD **Management of Overdose:** *Symptoms:* Flushing, headache, hypotension, tachycardia, nausea, vomiting, diarrhea. *Treatment:* Reduce dose of epoprostenol.

Drug Interactions

Anticoagulants / Possible ↑ risk of bleeding

Antiplatelet drugs / Possible ↑ risk of bleeding

Diuretics / Additional ↓ in BP

Vasodilators / Additional ↓ in BP

How Supplied: *Powder for injection:* 0.5 mg, 1.5 mg

Dosage

- **Chronic IV Infusion**

Pulmonary hypertension.

Acute dose ranging: The initial chronic infusion rate is first determined. The mean maximum dose that did not elicit dose-limiting pharmacologic effects was 8.6 ng/kg/min. **Continuous chronic infusion, initial:** 4 ng/kg/min less than the maximum-tolerated infusion rate determined during acute dose ranging. If the maximum-tolerated infusion rate is less than 5 ng/kg/min, start the chronic infusion at one-half the maximum-tolerated infusion rate. **Dosage adjustments:** Changes in the chronic infusion rate are based on persistence, recurrence, or worsening of the symptoms of primary pulmonary hypertension. If symptoms require an increase in infusion rate, increase by 1-2 ng/kg/min at intervals (at least 15 min) sufficient to allow assessment of the clinical response. If a decrease in infusion rate is necessary, gradually make 2-ng/kg/min decrements every 15 min or longer until the dose-limiting effects resolve. Avoid abrupt withdrawal or sudden large reductions in infusion rates.

HEALTH CARE CONSIDERATIONS

See also *Health Care Considerations* for *Antihypertensive Agents.*

Administration/Storage

IV 1. Chronic administration is delivered continuously by a permanent indwelling central venous catheter and an ambulatory infusion pump (see package insert for requirements for the infusion pump). Unless contraindicated, give anticoagulant therapy to decrease the risk of pulmonary thromboembolism or systemic embolism.

2. Do not dilute reconstituted solutions or administer with other parenteral solutions or medications.

3. Check package insert carefully to make 100 mL of a solution with the appropriate final concentration of drug and for infusion delivery rates for doses equal to or less than 16 ng/kg/min based on client weight, drug delivery rate, and concentration of solution to be used.

4. Protect unopened vials from light and store at 15°C-25°C (59°F-77°F). Protect reconstituted solutions from light and refrigerate at 2°C-8°C (36°F-46°F) for no more than 40 hr.
5. Do not freeze reconstituted solutions; discard any solution refrigerated for more than 48 hr.
6. A single reservoir of reconstituted solution can be given at room temperature for 8 hr; alternatively, it can be used with a cold pouch and given for up to 24 hr. Do not expose solution to sunlight.

Assessment
1. Perform a full cardiopulmonary assessment. Based on symptoms, determine New York Heart Association functional class (III or IV). Note other agents used and outcome.
2. Determine mental status and ability to handle medication preparation and IV administration; or identify someone in the home that can and is willing to perform this function on a regular basis and/or initiate home infusion referral.
3. Determine that a permanent indwelling central venous catheter is available for continuous ambulatory delivery once dose ranging completed.
4. Assess central venous access site for any evidence of infection, discharge, odor, erythema, or swelling.
5. Consult manufacturer's guidelines for dosage and delivery rate based on client weight for acute dose ranging.

Client/Family Teaching
1. Drug helps reduce RV and LV afterload and increases CO and SV, thereby improving symptoms of SOB, fatigue, and exercise intolerance.
2. Administered continously through an indwelling catheter to the heart by a portable external infusion pump; may be needed for years to help control symptoms.
3. Proper site care and pump maintenance as well as appropriate reconstitution for desired drug concentration, proper storage, protection from light, pouch filling, pump settings, and accessing VAD are imperative to safe therapy.
4. Review written guidelines for drug preparation, infusion, dose reduction, storage, and administration and site inspection and care; pump maintenance, programming, trouble shooting, and care.
5. When drug is reconstituted and administered at room temperature, the pump must be programmed to administer pouch contents in 8 hr, whereas if drug is reconstituted and refrigerated at 2°C-8°C (36°F-46°F) it may be administered over 24 hr.
6. Side effects that indicate excessive dosing and require a reduction in dosage and reporting include tachycardia, headache, N&V, diarrhea, hypotension.
7. Brief interruptions in therapy may cause rapid deterioration in condition.

Outcome/Evaluate: Improvement in exercise capacity; ↓ dyspnea and fatigue

Eprosartan mesylate

(eh-proh-**SAR**-tan)
Pregnancy Category: C (first trimester), D (second and third trimesters)
Teveten **(Rx)**
Classification: Antihypertensive, angiotensin II receptor antagonist

Action/Kinetics: Acts by blocking the vasoconstrictor and aldosterone-secreting effects of angiotensin II by blocking selectively the binding of angiotensin II to angiotensin II receptors located in the vascular smooth muscle and adrenal gland. **Peak plasma levels:** 1-2 hr. Food delays absorption. **t½, terminal:** 5-9 hr. Significantly bound (98%) to plasma protein. Excreted mostly unchanged in both the feces and urine.

Uses: Used alone or with other antihypertensives (diuretics, calcium channel blockers) to treat hypertension.

Special Concerns: Drugs that act on the renin-angiotensin system directly during the second and third trimesters of pregnancy may cause fetal and neonatal injury. Symptomatic hypotension may be seen in clients who are volume- and/or salt-depleted (e.g., those taking diuretics). Safety and efficacy have not been determined in children.

Side Effects: *GI:* Abdominal pain, diarrhea, dyspepsia, anorexia, constipation, dry mouth, esophagitis, flatulence, gastritis, gastroenteritis, gingivitis, nausea, peridontitis, toothache, vomiting. *CNS:* Depression, headache, dizziness, anxiety, ataxia, insomnia, migraine, neuritis, nervousness, paresthesia, somnolence, tremor, vertigo. *CV:* Angina pectoris, bradycardia, abnormal ECG, extrasystoles, atrial fibrillation, hypotension, tachycardia, palpitations, peripheral ischemia. *Respiratory:* URTI, sinusitis, bronchitis, chest pain, rhinitis, pharyngitis, coughing, asthma, epistaxis. *Musculoskeletal:* Arthralgia, myalgia, arthritis, aggravated arthritis, arthrosis, skeletal pain, tendonitis, back pain. *GU:* UTI, albuminuria, cystitis, hematuria, frequent micturition, polyuria, renal calculus, urinary incontinence. *Metabolic:* Diabetes mellitus, gout. *Body as a whole:* Viral infection, injury, fatigue, alcohol intolerance, asthenia, substernal chest pain, peripheral edema, depen-

dent edema, fatigue, fever, hot flushes, flu-like symptoms, malasie, rigors, pain, leg cramps, herpes simplex. *Hematologic:* Anemia, purpura, leukopenia, neutropenia, thrombocytopenia. *Dermatologic:* Eczema, furunculosis, pruritus, rash, maculopapular rash, increased sweating. *Ophthalmic:* Conjunctivitis, abnormal vision, xerophthalmia. *Otic:* Otitis externa, otitis media, tinnitus.
Laboratory Test Considerations: ↑ ALT, AST, creatine phosphokinase, BUN, creatinine, alkaline phosphatase. ↓ Hemoglobin. Glycosuria, hypercholesterolemia, hyperglycemia, hyperkalemia, hypokalemia, hyponatremia.
How Supplied: *Tablets:* 400 mg, 600 mg

Dosage

- **Tablets**

Hypertension.
Adults, initial: 600 mg once daily as monotherapy in clients who are not volume-depleted. Can be given once or twice daily with total daily doses ranging from 400-800 mg.

HEALTH CARE CONSIDERATIONS

See also *Health Care Considerations* for *Antihypertensive Agents.*
Administration/Storage
1. If the antihypertensive effect using once daily dosing is inadequate, a twice-a-day regimen at the same total daily dose or an increase in dose may be more effective.
2. Maximum BP reduction may not occur for 2-3 weeks.
3. May be used in combination with thiazide diuretics or calcium channel blockers if additional BP lowering effect is needed.
4. Discontinuing treatment does not lead to a rapid rebound increase in BP.

Assessment
1. Record/document disease onset, symptoms, and other agents trialed.
2. Monitor CBC, K^+, renal, and LFTs.

Client/Family Teaching
1. Take as directed once or twice daily with or without food.
2. Continue life style modifications such as regular exercise, weight loss, smoking/alcohol cessation, low fat, low salt diet in the overall goal of BP control.
3. Practice reliable birth control. Report if pregnancy suspected or desired.
4. Keep a record of BP readings and bring to F/U visits.

Outcome/Evaluate: ↓ BP; control of HTN

COMBINATION DRUG

Equagesic

(eh-kwah-**JEE**-sik)
(Rx)
Classification: Analgesic

See also *Acetylsalicylic acid* and *Meprobamate.*
Content: *Nonnarcotic Analgesic:* Aspirin, 325 mg. *Antianxiety agent:* Meprobamate, 200 mg. See also information on individual components.
Uses: Short-term treatment of pain due to musculoskeletal disease accompanied by anxiety and tension.
Additional Contraindications: Pregnancy. Children under 12 years of age. Use for longer than 4 months.
How Supplied: See Content

Dosage

- **Tablets**

Pain due to musculoskeletal disease.
Adults: 1-2 tablets t.i.d.-q.i.d.

HEALTH CARE CONSIDERATIONS

See also *Health Care Considerations* for *Acetylsalicylic acid* and *Meprobamate.*
Outcome/Evaluate: Relief of pain; ↓ anxiety and tension

Erythromycin base

(eh-**rih**-throw-**MY**-sin)
Pregnancy Category: B (A/T/S, Erymax, Staticin, and T-Stat are C)
Capsules/Tablets: Alti-Erythromycin ★, Apo-Erythro Base ★, Apo-Erythro-EC ★, Diomycin ★, E-Base, E-Mycin, Erybid ★, Eryc, Ery-Tab, Erythro-Base ★, Erythromid ★, Erythromycin Base Film-Tabs, Novo-Rythro EnCap ★, PCE Dispertab, PMS-Erythromycin ★, **Gel, topical:**A/T/S, Erygel. **Ointment, topical:** Aknemycin. **Ointment, ophthalmic:** Ilotycin Ophthalmic, **Pledgets:** Erycette, T-Stat. **Solution:**, Del-Mycin, Eryderm 2%, Erymax, Erythra-Derm, Staticin, Theramycin Z, T-Stat **(Rx)**
Classification: Antibiotic, erythromycin

See also *Anti-Infective Agents.*
Action/Kinetics: Erythromycins are macrolide antibiotics. They inhibit protein synthesis of microorganisms by binding reversibly to a ribosomal subunit (50S), thus interfering with the transmission of genetic information and inhibiting protein synthesis. The drugs are effective only against rapidly multiplying organisms. Absorbed from the upper part of the small intestine. Those for PO use are manu-

factured in enteric-coated or film-coated forms to prevent destruction by gastric acid. Erythromycin is approximately 70% bound to plasma proteins and achieves concentrations in body tissues about 40% of those in the plasma. Diffuses into body tissues; peritoneal, pleural, ascitic, and amniotic fluids; saliva; through the placental circulation; and across the mucous membrane of the tracheobronchial tree. Diffuses poorly into spinal fluid, although penetration is increased in meningitis. Alkalinization of the urine (to pH 8.5) increases the gram-negative antibacterial action. **Peak serum levels: PO,** 1-4 hr. **t½:** 1.5-2 hr, *but prolonged in clients with renal impairment.* Partially metabolized by the liver and primarily excreted in bile. Also excreted in breast milk.

Uses

1. Mild to moderate upper respiratory tract infections due to *Streptococcus pyogenes* (group a beta-hemolytic streptococci), *Streptococcus pneumoniae,* and *Haemophilus influenzae* (combined with sulfonamides).
2. Mild to moderate lower respiratory tract infections due to *S. pyogenes* (group a beta-hemolytic streptococci) and *S. pneumoniae.* Respiratory tract infections due to *Mycoplasma pneumoniae.*
3. Pertussis (whooping cough) caused by *Bordetella pertussis;* may also be used as prophylaxis of pertussis in exposed individuals.
4. Mild to moderate skin and skin structure infections due to *S. pyogenes* and *Staphylococcus aureus.*
5. As an adjunct to antitoxin in diphtheria (caused by *Corynebacterium diphtheriae*), to prevent carriers, and to eradicate the organism in carriers.
6. Intestinal amebiasis due to *Entamoeba histolytica* (PO erythromycin only).
7. Acute pelvic inflammatory disease due to *Neisseria gonorrhoeae.*
8. Erythrasma due to *Corynebacterium minutissimum.*
9. *Chlamydia trachomatis* infections causing urogenital infections during pregnancy, conjunctivitis in the newborn, or pneumonia during infancy. Also, uncomplicated chlamydial infections of the urethra, endocervix, or rectum in adults (when tetracyclines are contraindicated or not tolerated).
10. Nongonococcal urethritis caused by *Ureaplasma urealyticum* when tetracyclines are contraindicated or not tolerated.
11. Legionnaires' disease due to *Legionella pneumophilia.*
12. PO as an alternative to penicillin (in penicillin-sensitive clients) to treat primary syphilis caused by *Treponema pallidum.*
13. Prophylaxis of initial or recurrent attacks of rheumatic fever in clients allergic to penicillin or sulfonamides.
14. Infections due to *Listeria monocytogenes.*
15. Bacterial endocarditis due to alpha-hemolytic streptococci, Viridans group, in clients allergic to penicillins.

Investigational: Severe or prolonged diarrhea due to *Campylobacter jejuni.* Genital, inguinal, or anorectal infections due to *Lymphogranuloma venereum.* Chancroid due to *Haemophilus ducreyi.* Primary, secondary, or early latent syphilis due to *T. pallidum.* Erythromycin base used with PO neomycin prior to elective colorectal surgery to reduce wound complications. As an alternative to penicillin to treat anthrax, Vincent's gingivitis, erysipeloid, actinomycosis, tetanus, with a sulfonamide to treat *Nocardia* infections, infections due to *Eikenella corrodens,* and *Borrelia* infections (including early Lyme disease).

Ophthalmic solution: Treatment of ocular infections (along with PO therapy) due to *Streptococcus pneumoniae, Staphylococcus aureus, S. pyogenes, Corynebacterium* species, *Haemophilus influenzae,* and *Bacteroides* infections. Also prophylaxis of ocular infections due to *Neisseria gonorrhoeae* and *Chlamydia trachomatis.* **Topical solution:** Acne vulgaris. **Topical ointment:** Prophylaxis of infection in minor skin abrasions; treatment of superficial infections of the skin. Acne vulgaris.

Contraindications: Hypersensitivity to erythromycin; in utero syphilis. Use of topical preparations in the eye or near the nose, mouth, or any mucous membrane. Ophthalmic use in dendritic keratitis, vaccinia, varicella, myobacterial infections of the eye, fungal diseases of the eye. Use with steroid combinations following uncomplicated removal of a corneal foreign body.

Special Concerns: Use with caution in liver disease and during lactation. Use may result in bacterial and fungal overgrowth (i.e., superinfection). Use of other drugs for acne may result in a cumulative irritant effect.

Side Effects: *GI:* Abdominal discomort or pain, anorexia, diarrhea or loose stools, dyspepsia, flatulence, GI disorder, N&V, pseudomembranous colitis, hepatotoxicity. *CV:* Ventricular arrhythmias, including ***ventricular tachycardia and torsades de pointes in clients with prolonged QT intervals.*** *Dermatologic:* Pruritus, rash, urticaria, bullous eruptions, eczema, erythema multiforme, ***Stevens-Johnson syndrome, toxic epidermal necrolysis.*** *CNS:* Dizziness, headche, insomnia. *Miscellane-*

ous: Asthenia, dyspnea, increased cough, non-specific pain, vaginitis, allergic reaction, ***anaphylaxis.*** Reversible hearing loss in those with renal or hepatic insufficiency, in the elderly, and after doses greater than 4 g/day.

Following IV use: Venous irritation, thrombophlebitis. *Following IM use:* Pain at the injection site, with development of necrosis or sterile abscesses. *Following topical use:* Itching, burning, irritation, stinging of skin; dry, scaly skin. *When used topically:* Erythema, desquamation, burning sensation, eye irritation, tenderness, dryness, pruritus, oily skin, generalized urticaria.

Laboratory Test Considerations: Interference with fluorometric assay for urinary catecholamines. ↑ Bicarbonate, eosinophils, platelet count, segmented neutrophils, serum CPK.

OD **Management of Overdose:** *Symptoms:* N&V, diarrhea, epigastric distress, acute pancreatitis (mild), hearing loss (with or without tinnitus and vertigo). *Treatment:* Induce vomiting. General supportive measures. Allergic reactions should be controlled with conventional therapy.

Drug Interactions

Alfentanil / ↓ Excretion of alfentanil → ↑ effect

Anticoagulants / ↑ Anticoagulant effect → possible hemorrhage

Astemizole / Serious CV side effects, including torsades de pointes and other ventricular arrhythmias (including QT interval prolongation), cardiac arrest, and death

Antacids / Slight ↓ in elimination rate of erythromycin

Benzodiazepines (Alprazolam, Diazepam, Midazolam, Triazolam) / ↑ Plasma levels of benzodiazepine → ↑ CNS depressant effects

Bromocriptine / ↑ Serum levels of bromocriptine → ↑ pharmacologic and toxic effects

Buspirone / ↑ Plasma levels of buspirone → ↑ pharmacologic and toxic effects

Carbamazepine / ↑ Effect (and toxicity requiring hospitalization and resuscitation) of carbamazepine due to ↓ breakdown by liver

Clindamycin / Antagonism of effect if used together topically

Cisapride / Possible serious cardiac arrhythmias, including ventricular tachycardia, ventricular fibrillation, torsades de pointes, and prolonged QT interval

Cyclosporine / ↑ Effect of cyclosporine due to ↓ excretion (possibly with renal toxicity)

Digoxin / ↑ Serum digoxin levels due to effect on gut flora

Disopyramide / ↑ Plasma levels of disopyramide → arrhythmias and ↑ QTc intervals

Ergot alkaloids / Acute ergotism manifested by peripheral ischemia and dysesthesia

Felodipine / ↑ Plasma levels of felodipine → ↑ pharmacologic and toxic effects

Grepafloxacin / ↑ Risk of life-threatening cardiac arrhythmias, including torsades de pointes

HMG-CoA Reductase inhibitors / ↑ Risk of myopathy or rhabdomyolysis

Lincosamides / Drugs may each other

Methylprednisolone / ↑ Effect of methylprednisolone due to ↓ breakdown by liver

Penicillin / Erythromycins either ↓ or ↑ effect of penicillins

Pimozide / Possibility of sudden death; do not use together

Rifabutin, Rifambin / ↓ Effect of erythromycin; ↑ risk of GI side effects

Sodium bicarbonate / ↑ Effect of erythromycin in urine due to alkalinization

Sparfloxacin / ↑ Risk of life-threatening cardiac arrhythmias, including torsades de pointes

Tacrolimus / ↑ Serum levels of tacrolimus → ↑ risk of nephrotoxicity

Terfenadine / Serious CV side effects, including torsades de pointes and other ventricular arrhythmias (including QT interval prolongation), cardiac arrest, and death

Theophyllines / ↑ Effect of theophylline due to ↓ breakdown in liver; ↓ erythromycin levels may also occur

Vinblastine / ↑ Risk of vinblastine toxicity (constipation, myalgia, neutropenia)

How Supplied: *Enteric Coated Capsule:* 250 mg; *Enteric Coated Tablet:* 250 mg, 333 mg, 500 mg; *Gel/Jelly:* 2%; *Ointment:* 2%; *Ophthalmic ointment:* 5 mg/g; *Pad:* 2%; *Solution:* 1.5%, 2%; *Swab:* 2%; *Tablet:* 250 mg, 500 mg; *Tablet, Coated Particles:* 333 mg, 500 mg

Dosage

Note: Doses are listed as erythromycin base.

• **Delayed-Release Capsules, Enteric-Coated Tablets, Delayed-Release Tablets, Film-Coated Tablets, Suspension**

Respiratory tract infections due to Mycoplasma pneumoniae.

500 mg q 6 hr for 5-10 days (up to 3 weeks for severe infections).

Upper respiratory tract infections (mild to moderate) due to S. pyogenes and S. pneumoniae.

Adults: 250-500 mg q.i.d. for 10 days. **Children:** 20-50 mg/kg/day in divided doses, not to exceed the adult dose, for 10 days.

URTIs due to H. influenzae.
Erythromycin ethylsuccinate, 50 mg/kg/day for children, plus sulfisoxazole, 150 mg/kg/day, given together for 10 days.

Lower respiratory tract infections (mild to moderate) due to S. pyogenes and S. pneumoniae.
250-500 mg q.i.d. (or 20-50 mg/kg/day in divided doses) for 10 days.

Intestinal amebiasis due to Entamoeba histolytica.
Adults: 250 mg q.i.d. for 10-14 days; **pediatric:** 30-50 mg/kg/day in divided doses for 10 days.

Legionnaire's disease.
1-4 g/day in divided doses for 10-14 days.

Bordetella pertussis.
500 mg q.i.d. for 10 days (or for children, 40-50 mg/kg/day in divided doses for 5-14 days).

Infections due to Corynebacterium diphtheriae.
500 mg q 6 hr for 10 days.

Primary syphilis.
20-40 g in divided doses over 10 days.

Conjunctivitis of the newborn, pneumonia of infancy, urogenital infections during pregnancy due to Chlamydia trachomatis.
Infants: 50 mg/kg/day in four divided doses for 14 (conjunctivitis) to 21 (pneumonia) days; **adults:** 500 mg q.i.d. for 7 days or 250 mg q.i.d. for 14 days for urogenital infections.

Mild to moderate skin and skin structure infections due to S. pyogenes *and* S. aureus.
250-500 mg q 6 hr (or 20-50 mg/kg/day for children, in divided doses—to a maximum of 4 g/day) for 10 days.

Listeria monocytogenes *infections.*
Adults: 500 mg q 12 hr (or 250 mg q 6 hr), up to maximum of 4 g/day.

Pelvic inflammatory disease, acute N. gonorrhoeae.
Erythromycin lactobionate, 500 mg IV q 6 hr for 3 days; **then,** 250 mg erythromycin base 250 mg PO q 6 hr for 7 days. Alternatively for pelvic inflammatory disease, 500 mg PO q.i.d. for 10-14 days.

Prophylaxis of initial or recurrent rheumatic fever.
250 mg b.i.d.

Bacterial endocarditis due to alpha-hemolytic streptococcus.
Adults: 1 g 1-2 hr prior to the procedure; **then,** 500 mg 6 hr after the initial dose. **Pediatric,** 20 mg/kg 2 hr prior to the procedure; **then,** 10 mg/kg 6 hr after the initial dose.

Uncomplicated urethral, endocervicial, or rectal infections due to C. trachomatis.
500 mg q.i.d. for 7 days (or 250 mg q.i.d. for 14 days).

Nongonococcal urethritis due to Ureaplasma urealyticum.
500 mg q.i.d. for at least 7 days or 250 mg q.i.d. for 14 days if client can not tolerate high doses of erythromycin.

Erythrasma due to Corynebacterium minutissimum.
250 mg t.i.d. for 21 days.

• **Ophthalmic Ointment**

Mild to moderate infections.
0.5-in. ribbon b.i.d.-t.i.d.

Acute infections.
0.5 in. q 3-4 hr until improvement is noted.

Prophylaxis of neonatal gonococcal or chlamydial conjunctivitis.
0.2-0.4 in. into each conjunctival sac.

• **Topical Gel (2%), Ointment (2%), Solution (2%)**

Clean the affected area and apply, using fingertips or applicator, morning and evening, to affected areas. If no improvement is seen after 6 to 8 weeks, discontinue therapy.

• **Investigational Uses.**

Diarrhea due to Campylobacter enteritis or enterocolitis. Chancroid due to Haemophilus ducreyi.
500 mg q.i.d. for 7 days.

Genital, inguinal, or anorectal Lymphogranuloma venereum.

Early syphilis due to Treponema pallidium.
500 mg q.i.d. for 14 days.

Tetanus due to Clostridium tetani.
500 mg q 6 hr for 10 days.

Granuloma inguinale due to Calymmatobacterium granulomatis.
500 mg PO q.i.d. for 21 or more days.

HEALTH CARE CONSIDERATIONS

See also *General Health Care Considerations for All Anti-Infectives.*

Administration/Storage: Topical gel is prepared by adding 3 mL of ethyl alcohol to the vial and immediately shaking to dissolve erythromycin. This solution is added to the gel and stirred until it appears homogenous (1-1.5 min). Refrigerate gel.

Assessment

1. Identify allergy to any antibiotics; note allergens. Assess for sensitivity reactions.
2. Record type, onset, and characteristics of symptoms, other agents used, and outcome.
3. Obtain cultures, CBC, wound documentation, and appropriate diagnostic studies.

4. Avoid if also prescribed astemizole, seldane, digoxin, and theophyllines, because erythromycins can inhibit cytochrome P-450 and enhance effects of these drugs or cause lethal arrhythmias.

Client/Family Teaching

1. Take on an empty stomach; the delayed-release forms of the base can be taken without regard for meals. Do not administer with or immediately prior to ingestion of fruit juice or other acidic drinks; acidity may decrease drug activity. Consume up to 8 oz of water with each dose and a fluid intake of 2.5 L/day.
2. May take with food to decrease GI upset; food decreases absorption of most erythromycins. Take only as directed and complete entire prescription despite feeling better.
3. If tablets are not coated, take them 2 hr after meals. Stomach acid destroys the erythromycin base thus it must be administered with an enteric coating.
4. Doses should be evenly spaced over 24 hr. Report any unusual or intolerable side effects or lack of response.
5. If nausea intolerable, report so the prescription can be changed to coated tablets that can be taken with meals.
6. Report symptoms of superinfection, i.e., furry tongue, vaginal itching, rectal itching, or diarrhea.
7. Any rash, yellow discoloration of skin or eyes, or irritation of the mouth or tongue should be reported.
8. Drug may increase GI motility with diabetic gastric paresis.
9. With topical use, clean affected area before applying ointment; wash hands before and after therapy.
10. A sterile bandage may be used with the topical ointment.
11. Instill ear solutions at room temperature. Pull ear lobe down and back for children under 3 years of age; pull ear lobe up and back when over 3 years of age.
12. Report any evidence of hearing loss, which is usually temporary.
13. Do not wash ophthalmic ointment from the eyes.
14. The topical and ophthalmic products are for external use only.

Outcome/Evaluate

- Resolution of infection (negative culture reports, ↓ temperature, wound healing, ↓ WBCs, improved appetite)
- Desired infection prophylaxis (pre-vention of recurrence)

Erythromycin estolate

(eh-**rih**-throw-**MY**-sin)

Pregnancy Category: B

Ilosone, Novo-Rythro Estolate ✱ **(Rx)**

Classification: Antibiotic, erythromycin

See also *Erythromycin Base.*

Action/Kinetics: Most active form of erythromycin, with relatively long-lasting activity.

Uses: See Erythromycin Base.

Additional Contraindications: Cholestatic jaundice or preexisting liver dysfunction. Treatment of chronic disorders such as acne, furunculosis, or prophylaxis of rheumatic fever.

How Supplied: *Capsule:* 250 mg; *Suspension:* 125 mg/5 mL, 250 mg/5 mL; *Tablet:* 500 mg

Dosage

- **Capsules, Suspension, Tablets**

See *Erythromycin base.* Similar blood levels are achieved using erythromycin base, estolate, or stearate.

HEALTH CARE CONSIDERATIONS

See also *Health Care Considerations* for *Erythromycin Base.*

Assessment

1. Record indications for therapy, duration and onset of symptoms.
2. Note evidence of liver failure.

Client/Family Teaching

1. Shake suspension well before using; do not store for more than 2 weeks at room temperature.
2. Chew or crush chewable tablets.
3. Take without regard to meals.

Outcome/Evaluate: Resolution of infection

Erythromycin ethylsuccinate

(eh-**rih**-throw-**MY**-sin)

Pregnancy Category: B

Apo-Erythro-ES, E.E.S. 200 and 400, E.E.S. Granules, EryPed, EryPed 200, EryPed 400, EryPed Drops, Erythro-ES ✱, Novo-Rythro Ethylsuccinate ✱ **(Rx)**

Classification: Antibiotic, erythromycin

See also *Erythromycin Base.*

Uses: See Erythromycin Base.

Additional Contraindications: Preexisting liver disease.

How Supplied: *Chew Tablet:* 200 mg; *Granule for Reconstitution:* 100 mg/2.5 mL, 200 mg/5 mL, 400 mg/5 mL; *Suspension:* 200 mg/5 mL, 400 mg/5 mL; *Tablet:* 400 mg

Dosage

- **Oral Suspension, Tablets, Chewable Tablets**

See *Erythromycin base. NOTE:* 400 mg of erythromycin ethylsuccinate will achieve the same blood levels of erythromycin as 250 mg of the base, estolate, or stearate forms.

Hemophilus influenzae infections.

Erythromycin ethylsuccinate, 50 mg/kg/day with sulfisoxazole, 150 mg/kg/day, both for a total of 10 days.

HEALTH CARE CONSIDERATIONS

See also *Health Care Considerations* for *Erythromycin Base.*

Client/Family Teaching

1. Take without regard to meals.
2. Chew or crush chewable tablets.
3. Refrigerate oral suspension; store for 1 week maximum.

Outcome/Evaluate: Resolution of infection

Erythromycin lactobionate

(eh-rih-throw-MY-sin)

Pregnancy Category: B

Erythrocin I.V. ✱, Erythrocin **(Rx)**

Classification: Antibiotic, erythromycin

See also *Erythromycin Base.*

Uses: See Erythromycin Base.

Additional Drug Interactions: Do not add drugs to IV solutions of erythromycin lactobionate.

How Supplied: *Powder for injection:* 500 mg, 1 g

Dosage

- **IV**

Adults and children: 15-20 mg/kg/day up to 4 g/day in severe infections.

Acute pelvic inflammatory disease caused by gonorrhea.

500 mg q 6 hr for 3 days followed by 250 mg erythromycin stearate, **PO,** q 6 hr for 7 days.

Legionnaire's disease.

1-4 g/day in divided doses. Change to PO therapy as soon as possible.

HEALTH CARE CONSIDERATIONS

See also *Health Care Considerations* for *Erythromycin Base.*

Administration/Storage

IV 1. Sterile water for injection is the preferred diluent. However, D5W or D5/RL may also be used if buffered with 4% $NaHCO_3$ injection.

2. For intermittent IV administration, may be further diluted in 100 to 250 mL of D5W or NSS and infused over 20-60 min.

3. The initial reconstituted solution is stable for 2 weeks if refrigerated or for 24 hr at room temperature and if final diluted solution used within 8 hr. Use the reconstituted piggyback vial within 24 hr if stored in the refrigerator or 8 hr if stored at room temperature.

4. If reconstituted solution is frozen, it can be stored for 30 days. Once thawed, use within 8 hr. Do not refreeze thawed solutions.

Assessment

1. Obtain CBC and cultures.
2. Assess for hearing deficits.

Outcome/Evaluate: Resolution of infection; negative cultures

Erythromycin stearate

(eh-rih-throw-MY-sin)

Pregnancy Category: B

Apo-Erythro-S ✱, Erythro ✱, Erythrocin Stearate, Novo-Rythro Stearate ✱, Nu-Erythromycin-S ✱ **(Rx)**

Classification: Antibiotic, erythromycin

See also *Erythromycin Base.*

Uses: See *Erythromycins Base.*

Additional Side Effects: Causes more allergic reactions (e.g., skin rash and urticaria) than other erythromycins.

How Supplied: *Tablet:* 250 mg, 500 mg

Dosage

- **Tablets, Film Coated**

See *Erythromycin base.* Similar blood levels are achieved using erythromycin base, estolate, or stearate forms.

HEALTH CARE CONSIDERATIONS

See also *Health Care Considerations* for *Erythromycin Base.*

Client/Family Teaching

1. Take on an empty stomach; food decreases absorption.
2. Report lack of effect or evidence of allergic reaction, i.e., rash or itching.

Outcome/Evaluate: Resolution of infection

Estazolam

(es-TAYZ-oh-lam)

Pregnancy Category: X

ProSom **(C-IV) (Rx)**

Classification: Hypnotic, benzodiazepine

See also *Tranquilizers, Antimanic Drugs, and Hypnotics.*

Action/Kinetics: Peak plasma levels: 2 hr. **t½:** 10-24 hr. The clearance is increased in smokers compared with nonsmokers. Metabolized in the liver and excreted mainly in the urine. Two metabolites—4'-hydroxy estazolam and 1-oxo-estazolam—have minimal

pharmacologic activity although at the levels present they do not contribute significantly to the hypnotic effect.
Uses: Short-term use for insomnia characterized by difficulty in falling asleep, frequent awakenings, and/or early morning awakenings.
Contraindications: Pregnancy. Use during labor and delivery and during lactation.
Special Concerns: Use with caution in geriatric or debilitated clients, in those with impaired renal or hepatic function, in those with compromised respiratory function, and in those with depression or who show suicidal tendencies. Safety and efficacy have not been determined in children less than 18 years of age.
How Supplied: *Tablet:* 1 mg, 2 mg

Dosage
- **Tablets**

Adults: 1 mg at bedtime (although some clients may require 2 mg). The initial dose in small or debilitated geriatric clients is 0.5 mg. Prolonged use is not recommended or necessary.

HEALTH CARE CONSIDERATIONS

See also *Health Care Considerations* for *Tranquilizers, Antimanic Drugs, and Hypnotics.*

Assessment
1. Note history of depression, suicidal tendencies, or respiratory problems.
2. Monitor liver and renal function studies; reduce dose in geriatric and debilitated clients and those with impaired renal and hepatic function.
3. Identify underlying cause(s) for insomnia; investigate alternative nonpharmacologic methods for sleep inducement.
4. Drug may enhance the duration and quality of sleep for up to 12 weeks; assess need to continue.

Client/Family Teaching
1. Identify symptoms that require immediate reporting.
2. Practice contraception; discontinue drug before becoming pregnant.
3. Do not perform tasks that require mental alertness until drug effects realized; ability to drive or operate machinery may be impaired.
4. Avoid alcohol and OTC drugs; smoking may alter drug absorption.
5. Take only as directed; may cause psychologic/physical dependence.
6. Do not stop abruptly; after prolonged treatment, withdraw slowly.
7. Identify any causative/contributing factors; review alternative methods for sleep induction.

Outcome/Evaluate: Enhanced duration and quality of sleep

Esterified estrogens

(es-**TER**-ih-fyd **ES**-troh-jens)
Pregnancy Category: X
Estratab, Menest, Neo-Estrone ✱ **(Rx)**
Classification: Estrogen, natural

See also *Estrogens.*
Action/Kinetics: This product is a mixture of sodium salts of sulfate esters of natural estrogenic substances: 75%-85% estrone sodium sulfate and 6%-15% equilin sodium sulfate. Less potent than estrone.
Uses: Replacement therapy in primary ovarian failure, following castration, or hypogonadism. Inoperable, progressing prostatic or breast carcinoma (in postmenopausal women and selected men). Moderate to severe vasomotor symptoms, atrophic vaginitis, and kraurosis vulvae due to menopause. Prophylaxis of osteoporosis (0.3 mg tablet).
How Supplied: *Tablet:* 0.3 mg, 0.625 mg, 1.25 mg, 2.5 mg

Dosage
- **Tablets**

Moderate to severe vasomotor symptoms, atrophic vaginitis, or kraurosis vulvae due to menopause.
0.3-1.25 mg/day given cyclically for short-term use. Adjust dose to the lowest effective level and discontinue as soon as possible.

Hypogonadism.
2.5-7.5 mg/day in divided doses for 20 days, followed by a 10-day rest period. If menses does not occur by the end of this period of time, repeat dosage schedule. The number of courses of estrogen required to produce bleeding varies, depending on the responsiveness of the endometrium. If bleeding occurs before the end of the 10-day period, a 20-day estrogen-progestin cycle should be started with 2.5-7.5 mg/day of estrogen with a progestin added the last 5 days. If bleeding occurs before the end of this regimen, discontinue therapy and resume on day 5 of bleeding.

Primary ovarian failure, castration.
1.25 mg/day given cyclically.

Prostatic carcinoma, inoperable and progressing.

1.25-2.5 mg t.i.d. Effectiveness can be determined using phosphatase determinations and symptomatic improvement.

Breast carcinoma, inoperable and progressing, in selected men and postmenopausal women.

10 mg t.i.d. for at least 3 months.

Prophylaxis of osteoporosis.

0.3 mg daily.

E

HEALTH CARE CONSIDERATIONS

See *Health Care Considerations* for *Estrogens.*

Assessment: Record indications for therapy; note type, onset, and characteristics of symptoms.

Outcome/Evaluate

- Stimulation of menses
- Relief of postmenopausal S&S
- Suppression of tumor growth/spread
- Osteoporosis prophylaxis

Estradiol hemihydrate

(ess-trah-**DYE**-ohl)

Pregnancy Category: X

Vagifem **(Rx)**

Classification: Estrogen

See also *Estrogens.*

Uses: Treatment of atrophic vaginitis.

How Supplied: *Tablets, Vaginal:* 25 mcg

Dosage

- **Vaginal Tablets**

Atrophic vaginitis.

Initial: 1 tablet, inserted vaginally, once daily for 2 weeks; **maintenance:** 1 tablet, inserted vaginally, twice a week.

HEALTH CARE CONSIDERATIONS

See also *Health Care Considerations* for *Estrogens.*

Administration/Storage: Attempt to discontinue or taper the drug at 3- to 6-month intervals.

Assessment: Note indications for therapy, age at onset and characteristics of symptoms.

Client/Family Teaching

1. Gently insert the vaginal tablet into the vagina as far as it can comfortably go without force. Use the supplied applicator.
2. Insert the tablet at the same time each day.
3. Report any pain, odor, or increased discharge.

Outcome/Evaluate: Relief of S&S atrophic vaginitis

Estradiol transdermal system

(ess-trah-**DYE**-ohl)

Pregnancy Category: X

Alora, Climara, Esclim, Estraderm, FemPatch, Vivelle **(Rx)**

Classification: Estrogen

See also *Estrogens.*

Action/Kinetics: This transdermal system allows a constant low dose of estradiol to directly reach the systemic circulation. The system overcomes certain problems associated with PO use, including first-pass hepatic metabolism, GI upset, and induction of liver enzymes. The system is available in various surface areas, release rates, and total estradiol content (the package insert should be carefully consulted). The patches are made either with a reservoir and a rate-controlling membrane or using a matrix where estradiol is embedded in the adhesive, allowing for a translucent, small, thin patch.

Uses: Vasomotor symptoms due to menopause, including hot flashes, night sweats, and vaginal burning, itching, and dryness. Female hypogonadism or castration; atrophic vaginitis or kraurosis vulvae due to deficient endogenous estrogen production; primary ovarian failure; prevention of osteoporosis. Abnormal uterine bleeding due to hormonal imbalance in the absence of organic pathology and only when associated with a hypoplastic or atrophic endometrium.

Side Effects: Skin irritation, URTI, headache, breast tenderness.

How Supplied: *Film, Extended Release:* 0.025 mg/24 hr, 0.0375 mg/24 hr, 0.05 mg/24 hr, 0.075 mg/24 hr, 0.1 mg/24 hr; *Insert, Controlled Release:* 0.0075 mg/24 hr

Dosage

- **Dermal System**

Menopausal symptoms.

Initial: Lowest dose needed to control symptoms: One 0.025- or 0.05-mg system applied to the skin twice weekly (if using Alora, Estraderm, Esclim, or Vivelle) or once a week (if using Climara or FemPatch). Adjust dose as necessary to control symptoms. Taper or discontinue dose at 3- to 6-month intervals. Alora is available in strengths to release 0.05-, 0.075-, and 0.1-mg/24 hr. Climara and Estraderm are available in strengths to release 0.05- or 0.1-mg/24 hr. Esclim is available in strengths to release 0.025-, 0.0375-, 0.05-, 0.075-, or 0.1-mg/24 hr. FemPatch is available to release 0.025-mg/24 hr. Vivelle is available in strengths to release 0.0375-, 0.05-, 0.075-, or 0.1-mg/24 hr.

Prevention of osteoporosis.

Initial: 0.05 mg/day as soon as possible after menopause. Adjust dosage to control concurrent menopausal symptoms.

HEALTH CARE CONSIDERATIONS

See also *Health Care Considerations* for *Estrogens.*

Client/Family Teaching

1. If taking oral estrogens, stop pills and wait 1 week before applying the system.
2. Without a hysterectomy, the system is usually used for 3 weeks, followed by 1 week of rest. May be used continuously in those without an intact uterus.
3. Place the system on a clean, dry area of the skin on the trunk of the body (preferably the abdomen). Avoid using areas with excessive amounts of hair. Also may use on the hip or buttock. Do not apply to the breasts or the waistline.
4. Rotate application site; date patch. Allow at least a 1-week interval between reapplication to a particular site.
5. Apply system immediately after the pouch is opened and the protective liner is removed. Firmly press in place with the palm for approximately 10 sec. Ensure good contact, especially around the edges. If system falls, reapply the same system or place a new one and follow the same schedule.
6. Weight gain may occur; report if marked or if edema develops.
7. Stop smoking; smoking increases risk of thromboembolic problems.
8. Addition of a progestin for 7 or more days may reduce the incidence of endometrial hyperplasia.

Outcome/Evaluate

- Relief of menopausal symptoms
- Therapeutic estrogen levels

Estramustine phosphate sodium

(es-trah-**MUS**-teen)
Emcyt **(Rx)**
Classification: Antineoplastic, hormonal agent, alkylating agent

See also *Antineoplastic Agents.*

Action/Kinetics: Water-soluble drug that combines estradiol and mechlorethamine (a nitrogen mustard). Estradiol facilitates uptake into cells containing the estrogen receptor while the nitrogen mustard acts as an alkylating agent. Chronic estramustine administration results in plasma levels and effects of estradiol similar to those of conventional estradiol therapy. Well absorbed from the GI tract and dephosphorylated before reaching the general circulation. Metabolites include estromustine, estrone, and estradiol. **t½:** 20 hr. Major route of excretion is in the feces.

Uses: Palliative treatment of metastatic and/or progressive prostatic carcinoma.

Contraindications: Active thrombophlebitis or thromboembolic disease unless the tumor mass is causing the thromboembolic disorder. Allergy to nitrogen mustard or estrogen.

Special Concerns: Use with caution in presence of cerebrovascular disease, CAD, diabetes, hypertension, CHF, impaired liver or kidney function, and metabolic bone diseases associated with hypercalcemia.

Laboratory Test Considerations: ↑ Bilirubin, AST, LDH. ↓ Glucose tolerance. Abnormal hematologic tests for leukopenia and thrombocytopenia.

Additional Side Effects: *CV:* ***MI, CVA,*** thrombosis, CHF, increased BP, thrombophlebitis, leg cramps, edema. *Respiratory:* ***Pulmonary embolism,*** dyspnea, upper respiratory discharge, hoarseness. *GI:* Flatulence, burning sensation of throat, thirst. *CNS:* Emotional lability, insomnia, anxiety, lethargy, headache. *Dermatologic:* Easy bruising, flushing, peeling of skin or fingertips. *Miscellaneous:* Chest pain, tearing of eyes, leg cramps, breast tenderness or enlargement, decreased glucose tolerance.

OD Management of Overdose: *Symptoms:* Extensions of the side effects. *Treatment:* Gastric lavage; treat symptoms. Monitor blood counts and liver profiles for at least 6 weeks.

Drug Interactions: Drugs or food containing calcium may ↓ absorption of estramustine phosphate sodium.

How Supplied: *Capsule:* 140 mg

Dosage

- **Capsules**

14 mg/kg/day in three to four divided doses (range: 10-16 mg/kg/day) or 600 mg (base)/m^2 daily in three divided doses. One 140-mg capsule is taken for each 10 kg or 22 lb of body weight. Treat for 30-90 days before assessing beneficial effects; continue therapy as long as the drug is effective. Some clients have taken doses from 10 to 16 mg/kg/day for more than 3 years.

HEALTH CARE CONSIDERATIONS

See also *Health Care Considerations* for *Antineoplastic Agents.*

Administration/Storage: Store capsules in the refrigerator at 2°C-8°C (36°F-46°F), although they may be kept at room temperature up to 48 hr without affecting potency.

Assessment

1. Note any allergy to nitrogen mustard or estrogen.
2. Assess diabetics for hyperglycemia, increased fatigue, weakness; glucose tolerance may be decreased.
3. Monitor CBC, electrolytes, liver and renal function studies.
4. Assess for symptoms of hypercalcemia: insomnia, lethargy, anorexia, N&V, coma, and vascular collapse.
5. Assess serum calcium levels (normal: 4.5-5.5 mEq/L). The effect of the steroid and osteolytic metastases may result in hypercalcemia.

Client/Family Teaching

1. Take capsules with water 1 hr before or 2 hr after meals. Do not take milk, milk products, calcium-rich foods and drugs simultaneously with estramustine.
2. Check BP and record; elevations may occur.
3. Consume 2-3 L/day of fluids to minimize hypercalcemia.
4. Report symptoms of hypercalcemia (chest pain, SOB, swelling or redness and pain in an extremity).
5. Impotence resulting from previous estrogen therapy may be reversed.
6. Drug may cause genetic mutation; consider sperm/egg harvesting; practice contraceptive measures to prevent teratogenesis.

Outcome/Evaluate: ↓ Size and spread of prostatic carcinoma

Estrogens conjugated, oral (conjugated estrogenic substances)

(ES-troh-jens)

Pregnancy Category: X

C.E.S. ✦, Congest ✦, Conjugated Estrogens C.S.D. ✦, Premarin **(Rx)**

Estrogens conjugated, parenteral

Pregnancy Category: X

(ES-troh-jens)

Premarin IV **(Rx)**

Estrogens conjugated, synthetic

(ES-troh-jens)

Pregnancy Category: X

Cenestin **(Rx)**

Estrogens conjugated, vaginal

(ES-troh-jens)

Pregnancy Category: X

Premarin Vaginal Cream **(Rx)**

Classification: Estrogen, natural

See also *Estrogens* and *Esterified Estrogens*.

Action/Kinetics: These products contain a blend of various estrogenic substances.

Uses: PO: Moderate to severe vasomotor symptoms due to menopause, atrophic vaginitis, kraurosis vulvae, female hypogonadism, primary ovarian failure, female castration. Palliation in mammary cancer in men or postmenopausal women; prostatic carcinoma (inoperable and progressive). Prophylaxis of osteoporosis.

Parenteral: Abnormal bleeding due to imbalance of hormones and in the absence of disease.

Vaginal: Atrophic vaginitis and kraurosis vulvae associated with menopause.

Special Concerns: Use of estrogen replacement therapy for prolonged periods of time may increase the risk of fatal ovarian cancer, an increased risk of endometrial cancer, and possibly a higher risk of breast cancer.

How Supplied: Estrogens conjugated, oral: *Tablet:* 0.3 mg, 0.625 mg, 0.9 mg, 1.25 mg, 2.5 mg. Estrogens conjugated, parenteral: *Powder for injection:* 25 mg. Estrogens conjugated, synthetic: *Tablet:* 0.625 mg, 0.9 mg. Estrogens conjugated, vaginal: *Cream:* 0.625 mg/g

Dosage

- **Tablets, Estrogens, Conjugated Oral**

Moderate to severe vasomotor symptoms due to menopause.

1.25 mg/day given cyclically. If the client has not menstruated in 2 or more months, begin therapy on any day; if, however, the client is menstruating, begin therapy on day 5 of bleeding.

Primary ovarian failure, female castration.

1.25 mg/day given cyclically (3 weeks on, 1 week off). Adjust dose to lowest effective level.

Atrophic vaginitis or kraurosis vulvae associated with menopause.

0.3-1.25 mg/day (higher doses may be necessary, depending on the response) given cyclically (3 weeks on, 1 week off).

Hypogonadism in females.

2.5-7.5 mg/day in divided doses for 20 days, followed by a 10-day rest period. If menses does not occur by the end of this period of time, repeat the dosage schedule. The number of courses of estrogen required to produce bleeding varies, depending on the responsiveness of the endometrium. If bleeding occurs before the end of the 10-day period, start a 20-day estrogen-progestin cycle with 2.5-7.5 mg/day of estrogen with a progestin added the last 5 days. If bleeding occurs before the end of this regimen, discontinue therapy and resume on day 5 of bleeding.

Palliation of mammary carcinoma in men or postmenopausal women.
10 mg t.i.d. for at least 90 days.

Palliation of prostatic carcinoma.
1.25-2.5 mg t.i.d. Effectiveness can be measured by phosphatase determinations and symptomatic improvement.

Prophylaxis of osteoporosis.
0.625 mg/day given cyclically (3 weeks on, 1 week off). Mainstays of therapy include calcium; exercise and nutrition may be important adjuncts.

• **Tablets, Estrogens, Conjugated Synthetic**

Moderate-to-severe vasomotor symptoms due to menopause.
Initial: 0.625 mg daily; **then,** titrate up to 1.25 mg daily. Discontinue as soon as possible. Attempt to discontinue or taper dosage at 3- to 6-month intervals.

• **IM, IV**

Abnormal bleeding.
25 mg; repeat after 6-12 hr if necessary.

• **Vaginal Cream**

½-2 g daily given for 3 weeks on and 1 week off. Repeat as needed. Attempt to taper the dose or discontinue the medication at 3- to 6-month intervals.

HEALTH CARE CONSIDERATIONS

See also *Health Care Considerations* for *Estrogens.*

Administration/Storage

1. For all uses, except palliation of mammary and prostatic carcinoma and prevention of postpartum breast engorgement, oral conjugated estrogens are best administered cyclically—3 weeks on and 1 week off.
2. When used vaginally, insert the cream high into the vagina (two-thirds the length of the applicator).
IV 3. Administer IV Premarin slowly to prevent flushing.
4. Parenteral solutions of conjugated estrogens are compatible with NSS, invert sugar solutions, and dextrose solutions.
5. Parenteral solutions are incompatible with acid solutions, ascorbic acid solutions, and protein hydrolysates.
6. Use reconstituted parenteral solutions within a few hours after mixing if kept at room temperatures. Put the date and time of reconstitution on the solution label.
7. IV use is preferred over IM as it induces a more rapid response.
8. Use the reconstituted solution within a few hours. If refrigerated, the reconstituted solution is stable for 60 days. Do not use if solution is dark or has a precipitate.

Assessment

1. Record indications for therapy, type, onset, and duration of symptoms.
2. Review potential risks R/T to the development of breast and fatal ovarian cancers with prolonged therapy.
3. Monitor serum phosphatase levels with prostatic cancer.

Client/Family Teaching

1. Take cyclically as directed i.e., 3 weeks on, 1 week off.
2. Cenestin is the only plant derived form of estrogen.
3. Review potential risks of prolonged therapy i.e., endometrial cancer, abnormal blood clotting, gallbladder disease and breast cancer.
4. If no hysterectomy has been performed remember to add progesterone to prevent cancer.

Outcome/Evaluate

• Control of abnormal uterine bleeding
• Osteoporosis prophylaxis
• Relief of menopausal symptoms
• Treatment of urogenital S&S R/T post-menopausal atrophy of vagina and lower urinary tract.

Estropipate (Piperazine estrone sulfate)

(es-troh-**PIE**-payt)
Pregnancy Category: X
Ogen, Ogen Vaginal Cream, Ortho-Est **(Rx)**
Classification: Estrogen, semisynthetic

See also *Estrogens.*

Action/Kinetics: Contains solubilized crystalline estrone stabilized with piperazine.

Uses: PO: Moderate to severe vasomotor symptoms associated with menopause. Vulval and vaginal atrophy. Primary ovarian failure, female castration, female hypogonadism. Prevention of osteoporosis.

Vaginal: Atrophic vaginitis and kraurosis vulvae associated with menopause.

Contraindications: Use during pregnancy.

How Supplied: *Vaginal cream:* 1.5 mg/g; *Tablet:* 0.75 mg, 1.5 mg, 3 mg

Dosage

- **Tablets**

Moderate to severe vasomotor symptoms; atrophic vaginitis or kraurosis vulvae due to menopause.

0.75-6 mg/day for short-term therapy (give cyclically). May also be used continuously. The lowest dose that will control symptoms should be selected. Attempt to discontinue or taper the dose at 3- to 6-month intervals.

Hypogonadism, primary ovarian failure, castration.

1.5-9 mg/day (calculated as 0.625 to 5 mg estrone sulfate) for first 3 weeks; **then,** rest period of 8-10 days. A PO progestin can be given during the third week if withdrawal bleeding does not occur.

Prevention of osteoporosis.

0.625 mg/day for 25 days of a 31-day cycle per month. Mainstays of therapy include calcium; exercise and nutrition may be important adjuncts.

- **Vaginal Cream**

2-4 g (containing 3-6 mg estropipate) daily (depending on severity of condition) for 3 weeks followed by a 1-week rest period. Attempt to taper the dose or discontinue the medication at 3- to 6-month intervals.

HEALTH CARE CONSIDERATIONS

See also *Health Care Considerations* for *Estrogens*.

Administration/Storage

1. Administration should be cyclic—3 weeks on the medication and 1 week off.
2. When used to relieve vasomotor symptoms, cyclic administration is initiated on day 5 of bleeding if menstruating. If the client has not menstruated within the last 2 months (or more), cyclic administration may be initiated at any time.

Client/Family Teaching

1. Take medications at the same time each day.
2. Relieve nausea during PO therapy by consuming solid foods.
3. Report any evidence of thromboembolic S&S (headache, blurred vision, pain, swelling or tenderness in the extremities); fluid retention (weight gain, swelling of extremities); hepatic dysfunction (yellowing of skin or eyes, itching, dark urine, clay-colored stools); changes in mental status or any unusual bleeding.
4. With vaginal preparations, administer at bedtime, remaining recumbent for 30 min; protect clothing and bed linens by using a sanitary pad. To deliver cream, the end of the applicator (after the appropriate amount is introduced) should be inserted into the vagina and the plunger pushed all the way down.
5. Between uses the plunger of the applicator should be pulled out of the barrel and washed in warm, soapy water. Do not put in hot or boiling water.
6. Do not smoke.
7. Drug may cause increased pigmentation of skin. Wear protective clothing and sunscreens and avoid prolonged sun exposures.
8. Stop drug and report if pregnant.

Outcome/Evaluate

- Relief of menopausal symptoms
- Stimulation of menses
- Restoration of hormonal balance

Etanercept

(eh-TAN-er-sept)

Pregnancy Category: B

Enbrel **(Rx)**

Classification: Antiarthritic drug

Action/Kinetics: Binds specifically to tumor necrosis factor (TNF) and blocks its interaction with cell surface TNF receptors. TNF is a cytokine that is involved in normal inflammatory and immune responses. Thus, the drug renders TNF biologically inactive. It is possible for etanercept to affect host defenses against infections and malignancies since TNF mediates inflammation and modulates cellular immune responses. **t½:** 115 hr. Individual clients may undergo a two- to five-fold increase in serum levels with repeated dosing.

Uses: Reduce signs and symptoms of moderately to severely active rheumatoid arthritis in those who have had an inadequate response to one or more antirheumatic drugs. May be used in combination with methotrexate in those who do not respond adequately to methotrexate alone.

Contraindications: Use in clients with sepsis. Administration of live vaccines given concurrently with etanercept. Lactation.

Special Concerns: Safety and efficacy have not been determined in those with immunosuppression or chronic infections or in children less than 4 years of age.

Side Effects: *Injection site reactions:* Erythema and/or itching, pain, swelling. *GI:* Abdominal pain, dyspepsia, cholecystitis, pancreatitis, ***GI hemorrhage***. *CNS:* Headache, dizziness, depression. *CV:* ***Heart failure, MI,*** myocardial ischemia, cerebral ischemia, hypertension, hypotension. *Respiratory:* URI, sinusitis, rhinitis, pharyngitis, cough, respiratory disorder, dyspnea. *Miscellaneous:* Formation of autoimmune antibodies, non-URI, rash, asthenia, bursitis.

How Supplied: *Single-Use Vial:* 25 mg

Dosage

- **SC**

Treat rheumatoid arthritis.

Adults: 25 mg twice weekly SC.

HEALTH CARE CONSIDERATIONS

Administration/Storage

1. Methotrexate, glucocorticoids, salicylates, NSAIDs, or analgesics may be continued during treatment with etanercept.
2. The needle cover of the diluent syringe contains latex; do not handle if sensitive to latex.
3. Reconstitute aseptically with 1 mL of the supplied sterile water for injection. Do not use other diluents. Slowly inject the diluent into the vial. Some foaming will occur. To avoid excessive foaming, do not shake or vigorously agitate. Swirl contents gently during dissolution, which takes less than 5 min. The reconstituted solution should be clear and colorless.
4. Before administration, visually inspect for particulate matter and discoloration. Do not use if discolored, cloudy, or if particulate matter remains after reconstitution.
5. Withdraw the solution into the syringe, removing as much liquid as possible from the vial. The final volume in the syringe will be about 1 mL.
6. Do not add other medications to solutions containing etanercept.
7. Do not filter reconstituted solution during preparation or administration.
8. Refrigerate etanercept sterile powder (do not freeze). Give reconstituted solutions as soon as possible. If not given immediately after reconstitution, solution may be stored in the vial at 2°C-8°C (36°F-46°F) for up to 6 hr.

Assessment

1. Note indications for therapy, joints affected, presenting characteristics, and other agents trialed/failed.
2. Observe client perform first injection after instruction.
3. Discontinue if client develops a serious infection.

Client/Family Teaching

1. Each tray contains all materials needed for administration.
2. Review procedures for storage, reconstitution, inspection, withdraw, administration, site rotation and disposal of syringes.
3. If self-administering etanercept, the first injection will be performed by the client under the supervision of a qualified health care professional.
4. Always rotate sites for self-injection which include the thigh, abdomen, or upper arm. Give new injections at least one inch from the old site and never into areas where the skin is tender, bruised, red, or hard.
5. Report any abdominal pain, S&S of infection, dizziness, SOB, and chest pain.
6. Avoid immunizations with live vaccines.

Outcome/Evaluate: ↓ Joint pain/swelling with RA

E

Ethambutol hydrochloride

(eh-**THAM**-byou-tohl)

Etibi ✦, Myambutol **(Rx)**

Classification: Primary antitubercular agent

Action/Kinetics: Inhibits the synthesis of metabolites resulting in impairment of cell metabolism, arrest of multiplication, and ultimately cell death. Is active against *Mycobacterium tuberculosis,* but not against fungi, other bacteria, or viruses. Readily absorbed after PO administration. Widely distributed in body tissues except CSF. **Peak plasma concentration:** 2-5 mcg/mL after 2-4 hr. **t½:** 3-4 hr. About 65% of metabolized and unchanged drug excreted in urine and 20%-25% unchanged drug excreted in feces. Drug accumulates in clients with renal insufficiency.

Uses: Pulmonary tuberculosis in combination with other tuberculostatic drugs. Use only in conjunction with at least one other antituberculostatic.

Contraindications: Hypersensitivity to ethambutol, preexisting optic neuritis, and in children under 13 years of age.

Special Concerns: Use with caution and in reduced dosage in clients with gout and impaired renal function and in pregnant women.

Side Effects: *Ophthalmologic:* Optic neuritis, decreased visual acuity, loss of color (green) discrimination, temporary loss of vision or blurred vision. *GI:* N&V, anorexia, abdominal pain. *CNS:* Fever, headache, dizziness, confusion, disorientation, malaise, hallucinations. *Allergic:* Pruritus, dermatitis, ***anaphylaxis.*** *Miscellaneous:* Peripheral neuropathy (numbness, tingling), precipitation of gout, thrombocytopenia, joint pain, toxic epidermal necrolysis. Renal damage. Also ***anaphylactic shock,*** peripheral neuritis (rare), hyperuricemia, and decreased liver function. Adverse symptoms usually appear during the early months of therapy and disappear thereafter. Periodic renal and hepatic function tests as well as uric acid determinations are recommended.

Drug Interactions: Aluminum may delay and decrease the absorption of ethambutol.
How Supplied: *Tablet:* 100 mg, 400 mg

Dosage

- **Tablets**

Adults, initial treatment: 15 mg/kg/day until maximal improvement noted; **for retreatment:** 25 mg/kg/day as a single dose with at least one other tuberculostatic drug; **after 60 days:** 15 mg/kg/day.

E

HEALTH CARE CONSIDERATIONS

See also *General Health Care Considerations for All Anti-Infectives.*

Assessment

1. Note indications for therapy, onset and duration of symptoms, other treatments, and outcomes.
2. Obtain a visual acuity test before ethambutol therapy. Document no preexisting visual problems (especially if dose exceeds 15 mg/kg/day).
3. Monitor CBC, cultures, liver and renal function studies.
4. With positive AFB cultures, report contacts and advise treatment.

Client/Family Teaching

1. Take as prescribed to prevent any relapses or complications.
2. Consume 2-3 L/day of fluids to ensure adequate hydration.
3. Avoid aluminum-based antacids; may interfere with drug absorption.
4. Obtain periodic vision testing during therapy (q 1-2 months); report any vision changes that may indicate optic neuritis. Ocular side effects generally disappear within weeks to months after therapy completed.
5. Practice reliable birth control; stop drug and report if pregnancy is suspected.

Outcome/Evaluate

- Negative sputum cultures
- Resolution of infection (↓ fever, WBC, sputum; improved CXR)

Ethosuximide

(eth-oh-**SUCKS**-ih-myd)
Zarontin **(Rx)**
Classification: Anticonvulsant, succinimide type

See also *Anticonvulsants* and *Succinimides.*
Action/Kinetics: Peak serum levels: 3-7 hr. **t½, adults:** 40-60 hr; **t½, children:** 30 hr. Steady serum levels reached in 7-10 days. **Therapeutic serum levels:** 40-100 mcg/mL. Not bound to plasma protein. Metabolized in the liver. Both inactive metabolites and unchanged drug are excreted in the urine.
Uses: Absence (petit mal) seizures.
Additional Drug Interactions: Both isoniazid and valproic acid may ↑ the effects of ethosuximide.
How Supplied: *Capsule:* 250 mg; *Syrup:* 250 mg/5 mL

Dosage

- **Capsules, Syrup**

Absence seizures.

Adults and children over 6 years, initial: 250 mg b.i.d.; the dose may be increased by 250 mg/day at 4-7-day intervals until seizures are controlled or until total daily dose reaches 1.5 g. **Children under 6 years, initial:** 250 mg/day; dosage may be increased by 250 mg/day every 4-7 days until control is established or total daily dose reaches 1 g.

HEALTH CARE CONSIDERATIONS

See also *Health Care Considerations* for *Anticonvulsants* and *Succinimides.*
Administration/Storage: May be given with other anticonvulsants when other forms of epilepsy are present.

Client/Family Teaching

1. Take with meals to minimize GI upset.
2. Do not engage in hazardous activities while on drug therapy.
3. Do not stop abruptly; may precipitate withdrawal seizures.
4. Report loss of seizure control.
5. Need lab studies q 3 mo to assess uric acid levels, hematologic, liver, and renal function.

Outcome/Evaluate

- Control of petit mal seizures
- Therapeutic serum drug levels (40-100 mcg/mL)

Etidronate disodium (oral)

(eh-tih-**DROH**-nayt)
Pregnancy Category: B
Didronel **(Rx)**

Etidronate disodium (parenteral)

(eh-tih-**DROH**-nayt)
Pregnancy Category: C
Didronel IV **(Rx)**
Classification: Bone growth regulator, antihypercalcemic

Action/Kinetics: Slows bone metabolism, thereby decreasing bone resorption, bone turnover, and new bone formation; it also reduces bone vascularization. Renal tubular reabsorption of calcium is not affected. **Absorption:** Dose-dependent; after 24 hr, one-half of absorbed drug is excreted unchanged. Absorption is affected by food or preparations containing divalent ions. **Onset:** 1 month for Paget's disease and within 24 hr for hypercalcemia. The drug remaining in the body is adsorbed to bone, where therapeutic effects for Paget's disease persist 3-12 months after discontinuation of the drug. **Plasma t½:** 6 hr; **bone t½:** Over 90 days. Approximately 50% excreted unchanged in the urine; unabsorbed drug is excreted through the feces.

Uses: PO: Paget's disease (osteitis deformans), especially of the polyostotic type accompanied by pain and increased urine levels of hydroxyproline and serum alkaline phosphatase. Heterotopic ossification due to spinal cord injury or total hip replacement. **Parenteral:** Hypercalcemia of malignancy inadequately managed by dietary modification or oral hydration or which persists after adequate hydration is restored. *Investigational:* Postmenopausal osteoporosis and prevention of bone loss in early menopause.

Contraindications: Enterocolitis, fracture of long bones, hypercalcemia of hyperparathyroidism. Serum creatinine greater than 5 mg/dL.

Special Concerns: Use with caution in the presence of renal dysfunction, in active UGI problems, and during lactation. Safety and efficacy have not been established in children.

Side Effects: *GI:* Nausea, diarrhea, constipation, ulcerative stomatitis. *Bones:* Increased incidence of bone fractures and increased or recurrent bone pain. Drug should be discontinued if fracture occurs and not restarted until healing takes place. *Allergy:* Angioedema, rash, pruritus, urticaria. *Electrolytes:* Hypophosphatemia, hypomagnesemia. *Miscellaneous:* Metallic taste, chest pain, abnormal hepatic function, fever, fluid overload, dyspnea, convulsions. Symptoms of rachitic syndrome have been reported in children receiving 10 mg or more/kg daily for long periods (up to 1 year) to treat heterotopic ossification or soft tissue calcification.

Laboratory Test Considerations: Hypomagnesemia, hypophosphatemia.

OD **Management of Overdose:** *Symptoms:* Following PO ingestion, hypocalcemia may occur. Rapid IV administration may cause renal insufficiency. *Treatment:* Gastric lavage following PO ingestion. Treat hypocalcemia by giving calcium IV.

Drug Interactions: Products containing calcium or other multivalent cations ↓ absorption of etidronate

How Supplied: Etidronate disodium (oral): *Tablet:* 200 mg, 400 mg. Etidronate disodium (parenteral): *Injection:* 50 mg /mL

Dosage

- **Tablets**

Paget's disease.

Adults, initial: 5-10 mg/kg/day for 6 months or less; or, 11-20 mg/kg for a maximum of 3 months. Reserve doses above 10 mg/kg when lower doses are ineffective, when there is a need for suppression of increased bone turnover, or when a prompt decrease in CO is needed. Do not exceed doses of 20 mg/kg/day. Another course of therapy may be instituted after rest period of 3 months if there is evidence of active disease process. Monitor every 3 to 6 months.

Heterotopic ossification due to spinal cord injury.

Adults: 20 mg/kg/day for 2 weeks; **then** 10 mg/kg/day for 10 weeks. Treatment should be initiated as soon as possible after the injury, preferably before evidence of heterotopic ossification.

Heterotopic ossification complicating total hip replacement.

Adults: 20 mg/kg/day for 30 days preoperatively; **then,** 20 mg/kg/day for 90 days postoperatively.

- **IV Infusion**

Hypercalcemia due to malignancy.

7.5 mg/kg/day for 3 successive days. If necessary, a second course of treatment may be instituted after a 7-day rest period. The safety and effectiveness of more than two courses of therapy has not been determined. Reduce the dose in those with renal impairment. Etidronate tablets may be started the day after the last infusion at a dose of 20 mg/kg/day for 30 days (treatment may be extended to 90 days if serum calcium levels are normal). Use for more than 90 days is not recommended.

HEALTH CARE CONSIDERATIONS

Administration/Storage

1. Administer PO as a single dose (if GI upset occurs, divide dose) with juice or water 2 hr before meals.
2. There are no indications to date that etidronate will affect mature heterotopic bone.
3. IV Dilute IV dose in at least 250 mL of sterile NSS and administer over a 2-hr period.

4. May experience a metallic taste during IV administration.
5. The diluted solution shows no loss of drug for 48 hr if stored between 15°C and 30°C (59°F and 86°F).

Assessment
1. Note indications for therapy.
2. Assess for evidence of renal dysfunction. Monitor uric acid, alkaline phosphatase, urinary hydroxyproline excretion, electrolytes, magnesium, phosphate, calcium, and renal function studies.
3. Determine if pregnant.

Client/Family Teaching
1. Maintain a well-balanced diet with adequate intake of calcium and vitamin D; see dietitian prn.
2. Do not eat for 2 hr after taking medication. Foods high in calcium (e.g., milk, milk products) and vitamins with mineral supplements (e.g., aluminum, calcium, iron, or magnesium) may decrease absorption. If GI upset with single dose, may divide dose.
3. Report any S&S of hypercalcemia, i.e., lethargy, N&V, anorexia, tremors, and bone pain.
4. Obtain lab studies as scheduled: with Paget's disease, levels of urinary hydroxyproline excretion and serum alkaline phosphatase reductions indicate a beneficial therapeutic response. Levels usually decrease 1-3 months after initiation of therapy.
5. With hypercalcemia, serum calcium levels show drug response and need for continued therapy. Reduction usually occurs in 2-8 days in hypercalcemia R/T bone metastasis. Therapy may be repeated only after 7 days of rest; risk for hypocalcemia greatest 3 days after IV therapy.

Outcome/Evaluate
- Suppression of bone resorption
- ↓ Serum calcium levels
- ↓ Pain with Paget's disease

Etodolac

(ee-toh-**DOH**-lack)
Pregnancy Category: C
Lodine **(Rx)**, Lodine XL
Classification: Nonsteroidal anti-inflammatory drug

See also *Nonsteroidal Anti-Inflammatory Drugs.*

Action/Kinetics: Etodolac is a NSAID in a class called the pyranocarboxylic acids. **Time to peak levels:** 1-2 hr. **Onset of analgesic action:** 30 min; **duration:** 4-12 hr. **t½:** 7.3 hr. The drug is metabolized by the liver and metabolites are excreted through the kidneys.

Uses: Acute and chronic treatment of osteoarthritis and rheumatoid arthritis. Mild to moderate pain.

Contraindications: Clients in whom etodolac, aspirin, or other NSAIDs have caused asthma, rhinitis, urticaria, or other allergic reactions. Use during lactation, during labor and delivery, and in children.

Special Concerns: Use with caution in impaired renal or hepatic function, heart failure, those on diuretics, and in geriatric clients. Safety and effectiveness have not been determined in children.

Laboratory Test Considerations: False + reaction for urinary bilirubin and for urinary ketones (using the dip-stick method). ↑ Liver enzymes, serum creatinine. ↑ Bleeding time.

Additional Side Effects: *GI:* Diarrhea, gastritis, thirst, ulcerative stomatitis, anorexia. *CNS:* Nervousness, depression. *CV:* Syncope. *Respiratory:* Asthma. *Dermatologic:* Angioedema, vesiculobullous rash, cutaneous vasculitis with purpura, hyperpigmentation. *Miscellaneous:* Jaundice, hepatitis.

OD Management of Overdose: *Symptoms:* N&V, drowsiness, lethargy, epigastric pain, ***anaphylaxis.*** Rarely, hypertension, acute renal failure, respiratory depression. *Treatment:* Since there are no antidotes, treatment is supportive and symptomatic. If discovered within 4 hr, emesis followed by activated charcoal and an osmotic cathartic may be tried.

Additional Drug Interactions
Cyclosporine / ↑ Serum levels of cyclosporine due to ↓ renal excretion; ↑ risk of cyclosporine-induced nephrotoxicity
Digoxin / ↑ Serum levels of digoxin due to ↓ renal excretion
Lithium / ↑ Serum levels of lithium due to ↓ renal excretion
Methotrexate / ↑ Serum levels of methotrexate due to ↓ renal excretion

How Supplied: *Capsule:* 200 mg, 300 mg; *Tablet:* 400 mg, 500 mg; *Tablet, Extended Release:* 400 mg, 500 mg, 600 mg

Dosage

- **Capsules, Tablets, Extended Release Tablets**

Osteoarthritis, rheumatoid arthritis.

Adults, initial: 300 mg b.i.d. or t.i.d. or 400 mg b.i.d. or 500 mg b.i.d. using capsules or tablets. Dose my be adjusted up or down during long-term use, depending on the clinical response. Extended-release tablets: 400-1,000 mg given once daily. Doses above 1,000 mg/day have not been evaluated adequately.

Acute pain.

Adults: 200-400 mg q 6-8 hr, up to 1,000 mg. Use capsules or tablets.

HEALTH CARE CONSIDERATIONS

See also *Health Care Considerations* for *Nonsteroidal Anti-Inflammatory Drugs*.

Administration/Storage: The capsules should be protected from moisture.

Assessment

1. Note any previous experience with NSAIDs or acetylsalicylic acid and the results.
2. Record indications for therapy (i.e., analgesic or anti-inflammatory), include onset and characteristics of symptoms and status of ROM.
3. With long-term therapy, monitor CBC chemistry, liver and renal function studies periodically.
4. Determine any history of heart disease or cardiac failure.
5. Note age and weight of client and if currently prescribed diuretics.

Client/Family Teaching

1. Take with food to decrease GI upset.
2. Report any unusual bruising/bleeding, rash, or yellow skin discoloration,

Outcome/Evaluate: Control of pain and inflammation with improved joint mobility

F

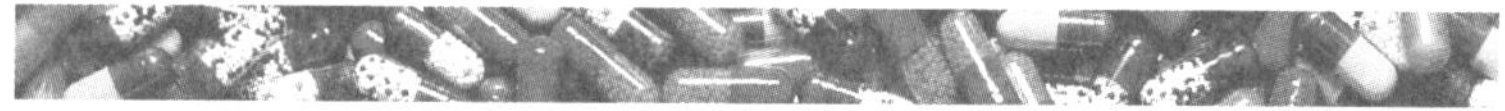

Famciclovir

(fam-**SY**-kloh-veer)

Pregnancy Category: B

Famvir **(Rx)**

Classification: Antiviral agent

See also *Antiviral Agents*.

Action/Kinetics: Undergoes rapid biotransformation to the active compound penciclovir. Inhibits viral DNA synthesis and therefore replication in HSV types 1 (HSV-1) and 2 (HSV-2) and varicella-zoster virus. Penciclovir is further metabolized to inactive compounds that are excreted through the urine. **t½, plasma:** 2 hr following IV administration of penciclovir and 2.3 hr following PO use of famciclovir. Half-life increased in renal insufficiency.

Uses: Management of acute herpes zoster (shingles). Treatment of recurrent herpes simplex (genital herpes and cold sores), including those infected with HIV. To prevent outbreaks of recurrent genital herpes.

Contraindications: Use during lactation.

Special Concerns: The dose should be adjusted in clients with C_{CR} less than 60 mL/min. Safety and efficacy have not been determined in children less than 18 years of age.

Side Effects: *GI:* N&V, diarrhea, constipation, anorexia, abdominal pain, dyspepsia, flatulence. *CNS:* Headache, dizziness, paresthesia, somnolence, insomnia. *Body as a whole:* Fatigue, fever, pain, rigors. *Musculoskeletal:* Back pain, arthralgia. *Respiratory:* Pharyngitis, sinusitis, upper respiratory infection. *Dermatologic:* Pruritus; signs, symptoms, and complications of zoster and genital herpes.

Drug Interactions

Digoxin / ↑ Levels of digoxin

Probenecid / Probenecid ↑ plasma levels of penciclovir

Theophylline / ↑ Levels of penciclovir

How Supplied: *Tablet:* 125 mg, 250 mg, 500 mg

Dosage

- **Tablets**

Herpes zoster infections.

500 mg q 8 hr for 7 days. Dosage reduction is recommended in clients with impaired renal function: for C_{CR} of 40–59 mL/min, the dose should be 500 mg q 12 hr; for C_{CR} of 20–39 mL/min, the dose should be 500 mg q 24 hr; for C_{CR} less than 20 mL/min, the dose should be 250 mg q 48 hr. For hemodialysis clients, the recommended dose is 250 mg given after each dialysis treatment.

Recurrent genital herpes.

125 mg b.i.d. for 5 days. Should be taken within 6 hr of symptoms or lesion onset. Dosage reduction is as follows for those with impaired renal function: for C_{CR} of 40 mL/min or greater, use the recommended dose of 125 mg b.i.d.; for C_{CR} of 20–39 mL/min, the dose should be 125 mg q 24 hr; for C_{CR} less than 20 mL/min, the dose should be 125 mg q 48 hr. For hemodialysis clients, the recommended dose is 125 mg given after each dialysis treatment.

Recurrent orolabial or genital herpes infection in HIV-infected clients.

500 mg b.i.d. for 7 days.

Prevent outbreaks of genital herpes.
250 mg b.i.d.

HEALTH CARE CONSIDERATIONS

See also *Health Care Considerations* for *Antiviral Agents.*

Administration/Storage

1. Start therapy as soon as herpes zoster is diagnosed and at the first symptoms of genital herpes.
2. Therapy is most useful if started within first 48 hr of rash appearance.
3. Effect greatest in those over 50 years of age.
4. May be taken without regard for meals.

Assessment

1. Record onset of symptoms, location, extent of lesions; note duration and frequency of recurrence.
2. Start drug as soon as diagnosis is confirmed.
3. Monitor CBC and renal function studies. Anticipate reduced dosage with renal dysfunction; follow dosing guidelines.

Client/Family Teaching

1. Review frequency, amount of drug to consume, and duration of therapy.
2. Side effects frequently associated with therapy include diarrhea, nausea, headaches, and fatigue;report if intolerable.
3. When lesions are open and draining, carrier is extremely contagious and should avoid any exposure or outside contact unless confirmed that the person(s) have had the chickenpox and are not pregnant.

Outcome/Evaluate

- Resolution of herpetic lesions
- ↓ Duration of neuralgia

Famotidine

(fah-**MOH**-tih-deen)

Pregnancy Category: B

Apo-Famotidine ✱, Gen-Famotidine ✱, Novo-Famotidine ✱, Nu-Famotidine ✱, Pepcid, Pepcid AC Acid Controller, Pepcid IV, Pepcid RPD **(Rx)** (Pepcid AC is OTC)

Classification: Histamine H_2 receptor antagonist

See also *Histamine H_2 Antagonists.*

Action/Kinetics: Competitive inhibitor of histamine H_2 receptors leading to inhibition of gastric acid secretion. Both basal and nocturnal gastric acid secretion and secretion stimulated by food or pentagastrin are inhibited. **Peak plasma levels:** 1–3 hr. **t½:** 2.5–3.5 hr. **Onset:** 1 hr. **Duration:** 10–12 hr. Does not inhibit the cytochrome P-450 system in the liver; thus, drug interactions due to inhibition of liver metabolism are not expected to occur. From 25% to 30% of a PO dose is eliminated through the kidney unchanged; from 65% to 70% of an IV dose is excreted through the kidney unchanged.

Uses: Rx: Treatment of active duodenal ulcers. Maintenance therapy for duodenal ulcer, at reduced dosage, after active ulcer has healed. Pathologic hypersecretory conditions such as Zollinger-Ellison syndrome or multiple endocrine adenomas. GERD, including erosive esophagitis. Treatment of benign gastric ulcer. *Investigational:* Prevent aspiration pneumonitis, for prophylaxis of stress ulcers, prevent acute upper GI bleeding, as part of multidrug therapy to eradicate *Helicobacter pylori.*

OTC: Relief of and prevention of the symptoms of heartburn, acid indigestion, and sour stomach.

Contraindications: Cirrhosis of the liver, impaired renal or hepatic function, lactation.

Special Concerns: Safety and efficacy in children have not been established.

Side Effects: *GI:* Constipation, diarrhea, N&V, anorexia, dry mouth, abdominal discomfort. *CNS:* Dizziness, headache, paresthesias, depression, anxiety, confusion, hallucinations, insomnia, fatigue, sleepiness, agitation, ***grand mal seizure,*** psychic disturbances. *Skin:* Rash, acne, pruritus, alopecia, urticaria, dry skin, flushing. *CV:* Palpitations. *Musculoskeletal:* Arthralgia, asthenia, musculoskeletal pain. *Hematologic:* Thrombocytopenia. *Other:* Fever, orbital edema, conjunctival injection, bronchospasm, tinnitus, taste disorders, decreased libido, impotence, pain at injection site (transient).

Drug Interactions

Antacids / ↓ Absorption of famotidine from the GI tract
Diazepam / ↓ Absorption of diazepam from the GI tract

How Supplied: *Injection:* 10 mg/mL; *Powder for Reconstitution:* 40 mg/5 mL; *Tablet:* 10 mg, 20 mg, 40 mg; *Sublingual Tablet*

Dosage

- **Oral Suspension, Tablets**

Duodenal ulcer, acute therapy.

Adults: 40 mg once daily at bedtime or 20 mg b.i.d. Most ulcers heal within 4 weeks and it is rarely necessary to use the full dosage for 6–8 weeks.

Duodenal ulcer, maintenance therapy.

Adults: 20 mg once daily at bedtime.

Benign gastric ulcers, acute therapy.

Adults: 40 mg at bedtime.

Hypersecretory conditions.

Adults, individualized, initial: 20 mg q 6 hr; **then,** adjust dose to response, although doses of up to 160 mg q 6 hr may be required for severe cases.

Gastroesophageal reflux disease.
Adults: 20 mg b.i.d. for 6 weeks. For esophagitis with erosions and ulcerations, give 20 or 40 mg b.i.d. for up to 12 weeks.
Prophylaxis of upper GI bleeding.
Adults: 20 mg b.i.d.
Prophylaxis of stress ulcers.
Adults: 40 mg/day.
Relief of and prevention of heartburn, acid indigestion, and sour stomach (OTC).
Adults and children over 12 years of age, for relief: 10 mg (1 tablet) with water. **For prevention:** 10 mg 1 hr before eating a meal that may cause symptoms. **Maximum dose:** 20 mg/24 hr. Not to be used continuously for more than 2 weeks unless medically prescribed.
- **IM, IV, IV Infusion**

Hospitalized clients with hypersecretory conditions, duodenal ulcers, gastric ulcers; clients unable to take PO medication.
Adults: 20 mg IV q 12 hr.
Before anesthesia to prevent aspiration of gastric acid.
Adults: 40 mg IM or PO.

HEALTH CARE CONSIDERATIONS

See also *Health Care Considerations* for *Histamine H_2 Antagonists.*

Administration/Storage
1. Use antacids at the same time if needed.
2. If C_{CR} < 10 mL/min, can reduce the dose to 20 mg at bedtime or increase the interval between doses to 36–48 hr.
IV 3. For IV injection, dilute 2 mL (containing 10 mg/mL) with 0.9% NaCl injection to a total volume of 5–10 mL; give over at least a 2-min period.
4. For IV infusion, dilute 2 mL (20 mg) with 100 mL of D5W and infuse over 15–30 min.
5. A solution is stable for 48 hr at room temperature when added to or diluted with water for injection, 0.9% NaCl injection, 5% or 10% dextrose injection, RL injection, or 5% $NaHCO_3$ injection.
6. Stable when mixed with various TPN solutions. Length of stability depends on the solution.

Assessment
1. Record reasons for therapy, type, onset, and duration of symptoms.
2. Note location, extent, and characteristics of abdominal pain.
3. Review UGI findings; note modifications trialed with GERD.
4. Assess mental status.
5. Check for occult blood in stools/GI secretions; note presence of *H. pylori* antibodies.
6. Assess for history of seizures.
7. If pregnant, list benefits versus risks.
8. Note hepatic/renal dysfunction; review CBC, assess for bleeding.

Client/Family Teaching
1. Drug may cause dizziness, headaches, and anxiety; use caution and report if symptoms persist.
2. Increasing lack of concern for personal appearance, depression, or sleeplessness should be reported.
3. Report any diarrhea, constipation, appetite loss, easy bruising, or fatigue.
4. Avoid alcohol, aspirin-containing products, OTC cough and cold products, smoking, and foods that increase GI irritation (i.e., caffeine, black pepper, harsh spices).
5. Report a reduction in urinary output; may need a change in dosage.

Outcome/Evaluate
- ↓ Abdominal pain
- Prophylaxis of stress ulcers
- Control of hypersecretion of acid
- Duodenal ulcer healing
- Control of symptoms of GERD

Felbamate

(FELL-bah-mayt)
Pregnancy Category: C
Felbatol **(Rx)**
Classification: Anticonvulsant, miscellaneous (second-line therapy)

See also *Anticonvulsants.*

NOTE: In August 1994 it was recommended that felbamate treatment be discontinued for epilepsy clients due to several cases of aplastic anemia. Revised labeling states, "...Felbatol should only be used in patients whose epilepsy is so severe that the risk of aplastic anemia is deemed acceptable in light of the benefits conferred by its use..."
Action/Kinetics: Mechanism not known. Felbamate may reduce seizure spread and increase seizure threshold. Has weak inhibitory effects on both GABA and benzodiazepine receptor binding. Well absorbed after PO use. **Terminal t½:** 20–23 hr. Trough blood levels are dose dependent. From 40% to 50% excreted unchanged in the urine.
Uses: Alone or as part of adjunctive therapy for the treatment of partial seizures with and without generalization in adults with epilepsy. As an adjunct in the treatment of partial and generalized seizures associated with Lennox-Gastaut syndrome in children. The

drug should be used only as second-line therapy.

Contraindications: History of hepatic dysfunction or blood dyscrasia. Hypersensitivity to carbamates.

Special Concerns: Aplastic anemia and acute liver failure have been observed in a few clients. Use with caution during lactation. Safety and efficacy have not been established in children other than those with Lennox-Gastaut syndrome.

F

Side Effects: May differ depending on whether the drug is used as monotherapy or adjunctive therapy in adults or for Lennox-Gastaut syndrome in children. *CNS:* Insomnia, headache, anxiety, somnolence, dizziness, nervousness, tremor, abnormal gait, depression, paresthesia, ataxia, stupor, abnormal thinking, emotional lability, agitation, psychologic disturbance, aggressive reaction, hallucinations, euphoria, ***suicide attempt,*** migraine. *GI:* Dyspepsia, vomiting, constipation, diarrhea, dry mouth, nausea, anorexia, abdominal pain, hiccoughs, esophagitis, increased appetite. *Respiratory:* Upper respiratory tract infection, rhinitis, sinusitis, pharyngitis, coughing. *CV:* Palpitation, tachycardia, SVT. *Body as a whole:* Fatigue, weight decrease or increase, facial edema, fever, chest pain, pain, asthenia, malaise, flu-like symptoms, ***anaphylaxis.*** *Ophthalmologic:* Miosis, diplopia, abnormal vision. *GU:* Urinary incontinence, intramenstrual bleeding, UTI. *Hematologic:* ***Aplastic anemia,*** purpura, leukopenia, lymphadenopathy, leukocytosis, thrombocytopenia, granulocytopenia, positive antinuclear factor test, ***agranulocytosis,*** qualitative platelet disorder. *Dermatologic:* Acne, rash, pruritus, urticaria, bullous eruption, buccal mucous membrane swelling, ***Stevens-Johnson syndrome.*** *Miscellaneous:* Otitis media, ***acute liver failure,*** taste perversion, hypophosphatemia, myalgia, photosensitivity, substernal chest pain, dystonia, allergic reaction.

Laboratory Test Considerations: ↑ ALT, AST, gamma-glutamyl transpeptidase, LDH, alkaline phosphatase, CPK. Hypophosphatemia, hypokalemia, hyponatremia.

Drug Interactions

Carbamazepine / Felbamate ↓ steady-state carbamazepine levels and ↑ steady-state carbamazepine epoxide (metabolite) levels. Also, carbamazepine → 50% ↑ in felbamate clearance

Methsuximide / ↑ Normethsuxide levels; decrease methsuximide dose

Phenobarbital / ↑ Phenobarbital plasma levels and a ↓ in felbamate levels

Phenytoin / Felbamate ↑ steady-state phenytoin levels necessitating a 40% decrease in phenytoin dose. Also, phenytoin ↑ felbamate clearance

Valproic acid / Felbamate ↑ steady-state valproic acid levels

How Supplied: *Suspension:* 600 mg/5 mL; *Tablet:* 400 mg, 600 mg

Dosage

- **Suspension, Tablets**

Monotherapy, initial therapy.

Adults over 14 years of age, initial: 1,200 mg/day in divided doses t.i.d.–q.i.d. The dose may be increased in 600-mg increments q 2 weeks to 2,400 mg/day based on clinical response and thereafter to 3,600 mg/day, if needed.

Conversion to monotherapy.

Adults: Initiate at 1,200 mg/day in divided doses t.i.d.–q.i.d. Reduce the dose of present antiepileptic drugs by ⅓ at initiation of felbamate therapy. At week 2, the felbamate dose should be increased to 2,400 mg/day while reducing the dose of other antiepileptic drugs up to another ⅓ of the original dose. At week 3, increase the felbamate dose to 3,600 mg/day and continue to decrease the dose of other antiepileptic drugs as indicated by response.

Adjunctive therapy.

Adults: Add felbamate at a dose of 1,200 mg/day in divided doses t.i.d.–q.i.d. while reducing current antiepileptic drugs by 20%. Further decreases of other antiepileptic drugs may be needed to minimize side effects due to drug interactions. The dose of felbamate can be increased by 1,200-mg/day increments at weekly intervals to 3,600 mg/day.

Lennox-Gastaut syndrome in children, aged 2–14 years.

As an adjunct, add felbamate at a dose of 15 mg/kg/day in divided doses t.i.d.–q.i.d. while decreasing present antiepileptic drugs by 20%. Further decreases in antiepileptic drug dosage may be needed to minimize side effects due to drug interactions. The dose of felbamate may be increased by 15-mg/kg/day increments at weekly intervals to 45 mg/kg/day.

HEALTH CARE CONSIDERATIONS

See also *Health Care Considerations* for *Anticonvulsants.*

Administration/Storage

1. Shake suspension well before use.
2. Store in a tightly closed container at room temperature away from heat, direct sunlight, or moisture and away from children.
3. Most side effects seen during adjunctive therapy are resolved as the dose of other antiepileptic drugs is decreased.

4. For geriatric clients, start at the low end of the dosage range.

Assessment

1. Document type, location, duration, and characteristics of seizures.
2. Determine if monotherapy or adjunctive therapy is needed.
3. List drugs prescribed to ensure none interact unfavorably and to determine need for dosage change.
4. Inform of potentially lethal side effects R/T aplastic anemia.
5. Monitor CBC, renal and LFTs.

Client/Family Teaching

1. Take only as prescribed; store appropriately to prevent loss of effectiveness.
2. Avoid activities that require mental alertness until drug effects realized.
3. Side effects include anorexia, vomiting, insomnia, nausea, and headaches; report if persistent.
4. Report any changes in mental status or loss of seizure control; dosage is determined by clinical response.
5. Do not stop taking due to possibility of increasing seizure frequency.
6. Seizure control benefit should far outweigh the potential for development of aplastic anemia; assess risk.

Outcome/Evaluate: Control of seizures

Felodipine

(feh-**LOHD**-ih-peen)
Pregnancy Category: C
Plendil, Renedil ✱ **(Rx)**
Classification: Calcium channel blocking agent

See also *Calcium Channel Blocking Agents.*
Action/Kinetics: Onset after PO: 120–300 min. **Peak plasma levels:** 2.5–5 hr. Over 99% bound to plasma protein. **t½, elimination:** 11–16 hr. Metabolized in the liver.
Uses: Treatment of mild to moderate hypertension, alone or with other antihypertensives.
Contraindications: Lactation.
Special Concerns: Use with caution in clients with CHF or compromised ventricular function, especially in combination with a beta-adrenergic blocking agent. Use with caution in impaired hepatic function or reduced hepatic blood flow. May cause a greater hypotensive effect in geriatric clients. Safety and effectiveness have not been determined in children.
Side Effects: *CV:* Significant hypotension, syncope, angina pectoris, peripheral edema, palpitations, AV block, ***MI, arrhythmias,*** tachycardia. *CNS:* Dizziness, lightheadedness, headache, nervousness, sleepiness, irritability, anxiety, insomnia, paresthesia, depression, amnesia, paranoia, psychosis, hallucinations. *Body as a whole:* Asthenia, flushing, muscle cramps, pain, inflammation, warm feeling, influenza. *GI:* Nausea, abdominal discomfort, cramps, dyspepsia, diarrhea, constipation, vomiting, dry mouth, flatulence. *Dermatologic:* Rash, dermatitis, urticaria, pruritus. *Respiratory:* Rhinitis, rhinorrhea, pharyngitis, sinusitis, nasal and chest congestion, SOB, wheezing, dyspnea, cough, bronchitis, sneezing, respiratory infection. *Miscellaneous:* Anemia, gingival hyperplasia, sexual difficulties, epistaxis, back pain, facial edema, erythema, urinary frequency or urgency, dysuria.

Additional Drug Interactions

Cimetidine / ↑ Bioavailability of felodipine
Digoxin / ↑ Peak plasma levels of digoxin
Fentanyl / Possible severe hypotension or ↑ fluid volume
Ranitidine / ↑ Bioavailability of felodipine

How Supplied: *Tablet, Extended Release:* 2.5 mg, 5 mg, 10 mg

Dosage

- **Tablets, Extended Release**

  Hypertension.

Initial: 5 mg once daily (2.5 mg in clients over 65 years of age and in those with impaired liver function); **then:** adjust dose according to response, usually at 2-week intervals with the usual dosage range being 2.5–10 mg once daily. Doses greater than 10 mg increase the rate of peripheral edema and other vasodilatory side effects.

HEALTH CARE CONSIDERATIONS

See also *Health Care Considerations* for *Calcium Channel Blocking Agents.*
Administration/Storage: Bioavailability is not affected by food. It is increased more than twofold when taken with doubly concentrated grapefruit juice when compared with water or orange juice.

Assessment

1. Record onset of symptoms, other agents used, and outcome.
2. Note history of heart failure or compromised ventricular function.
3. List drugs currently prescribed; note any potential interactions.
4. During dosage adjustments, monitor BP closely in clients over 65 or with impaired hepatic function.

F

Client/Family Teaching
1. Swallow tablets whole; do not chew or crush.
2. Do not stop abruptly; abrupt withdrawal may increase frequency and duration of chest pain.
3. Avoid activities that require mental alertness until effects are realized.
4. Rise slowly from a lying position and dangle feet before standing to minimize postural effects.
5. Practice frequent careful oral hygiene to minimize the incidence and severity of drug-induced gingival hyperplasia.

Outcome/Evaluate: Control of hypertension

F

Fenofibrate

(fee-noh-FY-brayt)
Pregnancy Category: C
TRICOR **(Rx)**
Classification: Antihyperlipidemic drug

Action/Kinetics: Is converted to the active fenofibric acid, which lowers plasma triglycerides. Probable mechanism is to inhibit triglyceride synthesis, resulting in a reduction of VLDL released into the circulation, and by stimulating catabolism of triglyceride-rich lipoprotein. Also increases urinary excretion of uric acid. Well absorbed; absorption is increased when given with food. **Peak plasma levels:** 6–8 hr; **steady-state plasma levels:** within 5 days. Highly bound to plasma proteins. **t½:** 20 hr with once daily dosing. Fenofibric acid and an inactive metabolite are excreted through the urine.
Uses: Adjunct to diet to treat Types IV and V hyperlipidemia in adults who are at risk of pancreatitis and who do not respond to diet alone.
Contraindications: Hepatic or severe renal dysfunction (including primary biliary cirrhosis), those with unexplained, persistent abnormal liver function, and preexisting gallbladder disease. Lactation.
Special Concerns: Due to similarity to clofibrate and gemfibrozil, side effects, including death, are possible. Safety and efficacy have not been determined in children.
Side Effects: *GI:* Pancreatitis, cholelithiasis, dyspepsia, N&V, diarrhea, abdominal pain, constipation, flatulence, eructation, hepatitis, cholecystitis, hepatomegaly. *CNS:* Decreased libido, dizziness, increased appetite, insomnia, paresthesia. *Respiratory:* Rhinitis, cough, sinusitis, allergic pulmonary alveolitis. *GU:* Polyuria, vaginitis. *Musculoskeletal:* Myopathy, myositis, arthralgia, myalgia, myasthenia, rhabdomyolysis. *Hypersensitivity:* Severe skin rashes, urticaria. *Ophthalmic:* Eye irritation, blurred vision, conjunctivitis, eye floaters. *Miscellaneous:* Infections, pain, headache, asthenia, fatigue, flu syndrome, arrhythmia, photosensitivity, eczema.
Laboratory Test Considerations: ↑ AST, ALT, creatinine, blood urea. ↓ Hemoglobin, uric acid.

Drug Interactions
Anticoagulants / Prolongation of PT
Bile acid sequestrants / ↓ Absorption of fenofibrate due to binding
Cyclosporine / ↑ Risk of nephrotoxicity
HMG-CoA reductase inhibitors / Possibility of rhabdomyolysis, myopathy, and acute renal failure

How Supplied: *Capsules:* 67 mg

Dosage
- **Capsules**

Hypertriglyceridemia.
Initial: 67 mg/day given with meals to optimize bioavailability. Then, individualize based on client response. Increase, if necessary, at 4– 8–week intervals. **Maximuim daily dose:** 201 mg/day (i.e., 3 capsules). If C_{CR} is less than 50 mL/min, start with 67 mg/day; increase dose only after evaluation of effects on renal function and triglyceride levels. In the elderly, limit the initial dose to 67 mg/day.

HEALTH CARE CONSIDERATIONS

Administration/Storage
1. Place clients on an appropriate triglyceride-lowering diet before starting fenofibrate and continue during treatment.
2. Withdraw therapy after 2 months if response is not adequate with the maximum daily dose.

Assessment
1. Note indications for therapy, other agents trialed, and cardiac risk factors.
2. Assess BS, renal and LFTs; avoid drug with severe dysfunction.
3. Monitor lipids, CBC, renal and LFTs; if ALT or AST > 3 times normal, discontinue therapy. Reduce dosage with C_{CR} < 50 mL/min.

Client/Family Teaching
1. Take as directed with meals.
2. Continue to follow diet prescribed for triglyceride reduction as well as a regular exercise program.
3. Report skin rash, GI upset, persistent abdominal pain, or muscle pain, tenderness, or weakness.
4. Avoid therapy with pregnancy and breastfeeding.
5. Report as scheduled for regular liver function tests and triglyceride levels.

Outcome/Evaluate: ↓ Triglyceride levels

Fenoprofen calcium

(fen-oh-**PROH**-fen)
Pregnancy Category: B
Nalfon **(Rx)**
Classification: Nonsteroidal anti-inflammatory analgesic

See also *Nonsteroidal Anti-Inflammatory Drugs.*
Action/Kinetics: Peak serum levels: 1–2 hr. **Peak effect:** 2–3 hr. **Duration:** 4–6 hr. **t½:** 2–3 hr. **Onset, as antiarthritic:** Within 2 days; **maximum effect:** 2–3 weeks. Ninety-nine percent protein bound. Food (but not antacids) delays absorption and decreases the total amount absorbed.
Uses: Rheumatoid arthritis, osteoarthritis, mild to moderate pain. *Investigational:* Juvenile rheumatoid arthritis, prophylaxis of migraine, migraine due to menses, sunburn.
Contraindications: Use in pregnancy and children less than 12 years of age. Renal dysfunction.
Special Concerns: Safety and efficacy in children have not been established.
Additional Side Effects: *GU:* Dysuria, hematuria, cystitis, interstitial nephritis, nephrotic syndrome. Overdosage has caused tachycardia and hypotension.
How Supplied: *Capsule:* 200 mg, 300 mg; *Tablet:* 600 mg

Dosage

- **Capsules, Tablets**

Rheumatoid and osteoarthritis.
Adults: 300–600 mg t.i.d.–q.i.d. Adjust dose according to response of client.
Mild to moderate pain.
Adults: 200 mg q 4–6 hr. Maximum daily dose for all uses: 3,200 mg.

HEALTH CARE CONSIDERATIONS

See also *Health Care Considerations* for *Nonsteroidal Anti-Inflammatory Drugs.*
Administration/Storage: Those over 70 years of age generally require half the usual adult dose.
Assessment
1. Record indications for therapy, type, onset, and duration of symptoms.
2. Perform periodic ophthalmic and auditory tests with chronic therapy.
3. Monitor CBC, PT/PTT, liver and renal function during chronic therapy.

Client/Family Teaching
1. Take 30 min before or 2 hr after meals; food decreases absorption.
2. With swallowing difficulty, the tablets can be crushed and the contents mixed with applesauce or other similar foods.
3. Avoid aspirin and OTC agents.
4. If vomiting or diarrhea occurs, monitor appetite, and weight; report if persistent.
5. Report any unusual bruising/bleeding, blood oozing from gums/nose, sore throat, or fever.
6. Report increased headaches, sleepiness, dizziness, nervousness, weakness, or fatigue.
7. Report evidence of liver toxicity, such as jaundice, RUQ pain, or a change in the color/consistency of stools.

Outcome/Evaluate: ↓ Joint pain and inflammation with ↑ mobility

Fentanyl Transdermal System

(**FEN**-tah-nil)
Pregnancy Category: C
Duragesic-25, -50, -75, and -100 **(C-II) (Rx)**
Classification: Narcotic analgesic, morphine type

See also *Narcotic Analgesics.*
Action/Kinetics: The system provides continuous delivery of fentanyl for up to 72 hr. The amount of fentanyl released from each system each hour depends on the surface area (25 mcg/hr is released from each 10 cm^2). Each system also contains 0.1 mL of alcohol/10 cm^2; the alcohol enhances the rate of drug flux through the copolymer membrane and also increases the permeability of the skin to fentanyl. Following application of the system, the skin under the system absorbs fentanyl, resulting in a depot of the drug in the upper skin layers, which is then available to the general circulation. After the system is removed, the residual drug in the skin continues to be absorbed so that serum levels fall 50% in about 17 hr. Metabolized in the liver and excreted mainly in the urine.
Uses: Restrict use for the management of severe chronic pain that cannot be managed with less powerful drugs. Only use on clients already on and tolerant to narcotic analgesics and who require continuous narcotic administration.
Contraindications: Use for acute or postoperative pain (including out-patient surgeries). To manage mild or intermittent pain that can be managed by acetaminophen-

F

opioid combinations, NSAIDs, or short-acting opioids. Hypersensitivity to fentanyl or adhesives. ICP, impaired consciousness, coma, medical conditions causing hypoventilation. Use during labor and delivery. Use of initial doses exceeding 25 mcg/hr, use in children less than 12 years of age and clients under 18 years of age who weigh less than 50 kg. Lactation.

Special Concerns: Use with caution in clients with brain tumors and bradyarrhythmias, as well as in elderly, cachectic, or debilitated individuals. Safety and efficacy have not been determined in children.

Additional Side Effects: Sustained hypoventilation.

How Supplied: *Film, Extended Release:* 25 mcg/hr, 50 mcg/hr, 75 mcg/hr, 100 mcg/hr

Dosage

- **Transdermal System**

  Analgesia.

Adults, usual initial: 25 mcg/hr unless the client is tolerant to opioids (Duragesic-50, -75, and -100 are intended for use only in clients tolerant to opioids). Initial dose should be based on (1) the daily dose, potency, and characteristics (i.e., pure agonist, mixed agonist/antagonist) of the drug the client has been taking; (2) the reliability of the relative potency estimates used to calculate the dose as estimates vary depending on the route of administration; (3) the degree, if any, of tolerance to narcotics; and (4) the general condition and status of the client.

To convert clients from PO or parenteral opioids to the transdermal system, the following method should be used: (1) the previous 24-hr analgesic requirement should be calculated; (2) convert this amount to the equianalgesic PO morphine dose; (3) find the calculated 24-hr morphine dose and the corresponding transdermal fentanyl dose using the table provided with the product; and (4) initiate treatment using the recommended fentanyl dose. The dose may be increased no more frequently than 3 days after the initial dose or q 6 days thereafter. The ratio of 90 mg/24 hr of PO morphine to 25 mcg/hr increase in transdermal fentanyl dose should be used to base appropriate dosage increments on the daily dose of supplementary opioids.

If the dose of the fentanyl transdermal system exceeds 300 mcg/hr, it may be necessary to change clients to another narcotic analgesic. In such cases, the transdermal system should be removed and treatment initiated with one-half the equianalgesic dose of the new opioid 12–18 hr later. The dose of the new analgesic should be titrated based on the level of pain reported by the client.

HEALTH CARE CONSIDERATIONS

See also *Health Care Considerations* for *Narcotic Analgesics.*

Administration/Storage

1. Multiple systems may be used if the delivery rate needs to exceed 100 mcg/hr.
2. Do not undertake initial evaluation of the maximum analgesic effect until 24 hr after system applied.
3. If required, a short-acting analgesic may be used for the first 24 hr (i.e., until analgesic efficacy reached with transdermal system).
4. Clients may continue to require periodic supplemental doses of a short-acting analgesic to treat breakthrough pain.
5. If opioid therapy is to be discontinued, a gradual decrease in dose is recommended to minimize S&S of abrupt narcotic withdrawal.

Assessment

1. Record indications for therapy, previous agents used, and outcome.
2. Rate pain level at various times throughout the day to ensure adequate dosing. Determine that dose required is based on conversion guidelines provided by manufacturer.
3. Note ↑ ICP or brain tumors.

Client/Family Teaching

1. Apply system to a nonirritated and nonirradiated fatty, flat surface of the skin, preferably on the upper torso. If needed, clip hair (not shaved) from site prior to application.
2. Use only clear water, if needed, to cleanse the site prior to application. Do not use soaps, oils, lotions, alcohol, or other agents that might irritate the skin. Allow the skin to dry completely prior to applying the system. If liquid comes in contact with the skin, use clear water only to remove.
3. Remove the system from the sealed package and apply immediately by pressing firmly in place (for 10–20 sec) with the palm of the hand. *Never cut or open the system.* Ensure complete contact of system, especially around the edges. Date and time patches and tape securely to avoid confusion or dislodgement.
4. Keep each system in place for 72 hr; if additional analgesia is required, a new system can be applied to a different skin site after removal of the previous system.
5. Fold systems removed from a skin site so that the adhesive side adheres to itself; flush down the toilet immediately after removal. Keep systems out of the reach of children.
6. Dispose of any unused systems as soon as they are no longer needed by removing them from their package and flushing down the toilet.

7. Note time and frequency of short-acting analgesic use for breakthrough pain. Report if use exceeds expected needs; transdermal dosage may require adjustment.
8. Use only as prescribed; do not stop suddenly.

Outcome/Evaluate: Desired pain control

Ferrous fumarate

(FAIR-us FYOU-mar-ayt)

Femiron, Feostat, Feostat Drops and Suspension, Hemocyte, Ircon, Nephro-Fer, Scheinpharm Ferrous Fumarate ✦ **(OTC)**

Classification: Antianemic, iron

Action/Kinetics: Better tolerated than ferrous gluconate or ferrous sulfate. Contains 33% elemental iron.

How Supplied: *Chew Tablet:* 100 mg; *Liquid:* 45 mg/0.6 mL; *Suspension:* 100 mg/5 mL; *Tablet:* 63 mg, 200 mg, 324 mg, 325 mg, 350 mg; *Extended Release Capsules* 100–150 mg, 300 mg

Dosage

- **Extended-Release Capsules**

Prophylaxis.

Adults: 325 mg/day.

Anemia.

Adults: 325 mg b.i.d. Capsules are not recommended for use in children.

- **Oral Solution, Oral Suspension, Tablets, Chewable Tablets**

Prophylaxis.

Adults: 200 mg/day. **Pediatric:** 3 g/kg/day.

Anemia.

Adults: 200 mg t.i.d.–q.i.d. **Pediatric:** 3 mg/kg t.i.d., up to 6 mg/kg/day, if needed.

HEALTH CARE CONSIDERATIONS

See *Health Care Considerations* for *Antianemic Drugs*.

Outcome/Evaluate: Restoration of serum iron stores

Ferrous gluconate

(FAIR-us GLUE-kon-ayt)

Apo-Ferrous Gluconate ✦, Fergon **(OTC)**

Classification: Antianemic, iron

Action/Kinetics: Contains about 11% elemental iron.

Uses: Particularly indicated for clients who cannot tolerate ferrous sulfate because of gastric irritation.

How Supplied: *Capsule:* 225 mg and 324 mg; *Extended Release Capsule:* 150 mg, 159 mg, 250 mg; *Drops:* 75 mg/0.6 mL, 25 mg/mL; *Elixir:* 220 mg/5 mL, 300 mg/5 mL; *Oral Liquid/Solution:* 300 mg/5 mL; *Tablet:* 200 mg, 300 mg, 324 mg, 325 mg; *Enteric-Coated Tablet:* 200 mg, 325 mg

Dosage

- **Capsules, Tablets**

Prophylaxis.

Adults: 325 mg/day. **Pediatric, 2 years and older:** 8 mg/kg/day.

Anemia.

Adults: 325 mg q.i.d. Can be increased to 650 mg q.i.d. if needed and tolerated. **Pediatric, 2 years and older:** 16 mg/kg t.i.d.

- **Elixir, Syrup**

Prophylaxis.

Adults: 300 mg/day. **Pediatric, 2 years and older:** 8 mg/kg/day.

Anemia.

Adults: 300 mg q.i.d. Can be increased to 600 mg q.i.d. as needed and tolerated. **Pediatric, 2 years and older:** 16 mg/kg t.i.d. The provider must determine dosage for children less than 2 years of age.

HEALTH CARE CONSIDERATIONS

Outcome/Evaluate:

- Restoration of serum iron stores
- H&H within desired range

Ferrous sulfate

(FAIR-us SUL-fayt)

Apo-Ferrous Sulfate ✦, Feosol, Fer-gen-sol, Fer-in-Sol, Fer-Iron, Ferrodan ✦, Fero-Grad ✦, PMS Ferrous Sulfate ✦ **(OTC)**

Ferrous sulfate, dried

(FAIR-us SUL-fayt)

Fe50, Feosol, Feratab, Slow FE **(OTC)**

Classification: Antianemic, iron

Action/Kinetics: Least expensive, most effective iron salt for PO therapy. Ferrous sulfate products contain 20% elemental iron, whereas ferrous sulfate dried products contain 30% elemental iron. The exsiccated form is more stable in air.

How Supplied: Ferrous sulfate: *Capsule:* 250 mg, 324 mg; *Capsule, Extended Release:* 250 mg; *Elixir:* 220 mg/5 mL; *Enteric Coated Tablet:* 325 mg; *Liquid:* 25 mg/mL, 75 mg/0.6 mL, 300 mg/5 mL; *Solution:* 300 mg/5 mL; *Syrup:* 90 mg/5 mL; *Tablet:* 195 mg, 300 mg, 324 mg, 325 mg; *Tablet, Extended Release:* 250 mg, 525 mg Ferrous sulfate, dried: *Capsule, Extended Release:* 150 mg, 159 mg; *Enteric Coated Tablet:* 200 mg; *Tablet:* 200 mg;

Tablet, Extended Release: 152 mg, 159 mg, 160 mg

Dosage

FERROUS SULFATE

• **Extended-Release Capsules**

Adults: 150–250 mg 1–2 times/day. This dosage form is not recommended for children.

• **Elixir, Oral Solution, Tablets, Enteric-coated Tablets**

Prophylaxis.

Adults: 300 mg/day. **Pediatric:** 5 mg/kg/day.

Anemia.

Adults: 300 mg b.i.d. increased to 300 mg q.i.d. as needed and tolerated. **Pediatric:** 10 mg/kg t.i.d. The enteric-coated tablets are not recommended for use in children.

• **Extended-Release Tablets**

Adults: 525 mg 1–2 times/day. This dosage form is not recommended for use in children.

FERROUS SULFATE, DRIED

• **Capsules**

Prophylaxis.

Adults: 300 mg/day. **Pediatric:** 5 mg/kg/day.

Anemia.

Adults: 300 mg b.i.d. up to 300 mg q.i.d. as needed and tolerated. **Pediatric:** 10 mg/kg t.i.d.

• **Tablets**

Prophylaxis.

Adults: 200 mg/day. **Pediatric:** 5 mg/kg/day.

Anemia.

Adults: 200 mg t.i.d. up to 200 mg q.i.d. as needed and tolerated. **Pediatric:** 10 mg/kg t.i.d.

• **Extended-Release Tablets**

Adults: 160 mg 1–2 times/day. This dosage form is not recommended for use in children.

HEALTH CARE CONSIDERATIONS

Outcome/Evaluate

- Restoration of serum iron levels
- Resolution of S&S of anemia

Fexofenadine hydrochloride

(fex-oh-**FEN**-ah-deen)

Pregnancy Category: C

Allegra **(Rx)**

Classification: Antihistamine

See also *Antihistamines.*

Action/Kinetics: Fexofenadine, a metabolite of terfenadine, is an H_1-histamine receptor blocker. Low to no sedative or anticholinergic effects. **Onset:** Rapid. **Peak plasma levels:** 2.6 hr. **t½, terminal:** 14.4 hr. Approximately 90% of the drug is excreted through the feces (80%) and urine (10%) unchanged.

Uses: Seasonal allergic rhinitis, including sneezing; rhinorrhea; itchy nose, throat, or palate; and itchy, watery, and red eyes in adults and children 12 years of age and older.

Special Concerns: Use with care during lactation. Safety and efficacy have not been determined in children less than 12 years of age.

Side Effects: *CNS:* Drowsiness, fatigue, headache. *GI:* Nausea, dyspepsia. *Respiratory:* Sinusitis, throat irritation, pharyngitis. *Miscellaneous:* Viral infection (flu, colds), dysmenorrhea.

Drug Interactions: No differences in side effects or the QTc interval were observed when fexofenadine was given with either erythromycin or ketoconazole.

How Supplied: *Capsule:* 60 mg

Dosage

• **Capsules**

Seasonal allergic rhinitis.

Adults and children over 12 years of age: 60 mg b.i.d. In clients with decreased renal function, the initial dose should be 60 mg once daily.

HEALTH CARE CONSIDERATIONS

See also *Health Care Considerations* for *Antihistamines.*

Assessment

1. Record onset, duration, and characteristics of symptoms; identify triggers if known.
2. Note other agents trialed, length of use, and outcome.
3. Assess for renal dysfunction; reduce dose if evident.

Client/Family Teaching

1. Take exactly as directed; do not exceed prescribed dosage.
2. May experience headaches, sore throat, nausea, and dysmenorrhea.
3. Report if symptoms intensify or don't improve after 48 hr.
4. Identify and avoid triggers.

Outcome/Evaluate: Control of symptoms of seasonal allergic rhinitis

Finasteride

(fin-**AS**-teh-ride)

Pregnancy Category: X

Propecia, Proscar **(Rx)**

Classification: Androgen hormone inhibitor

Action/Kinetics: Is a specific in-hibitor of 5-α-reductase, the enzyme that converts testosterone to the active 5-α-dihydrotestosterone (DHT). Thus, there are significant decreases in serum and tissue DHT levels, resulting in rapid regression of prostate tissue and an increase in urine flow and symptomatic improvement. Is also a decrease in scalp DHT levels. Well absorbed after PO administration. **Elimination t½:** 6 hr in clients 45–60 years of age and 8 hr in clients over 70 years of age. Slow accumulation after multiple dosing. Metabolized in the liver and excreted through both the urine and feces.

Uses: Treatment of symptomatic benign prostatic hyperplasia. Male pattern baldness (vertex and anterior midscalp). *Investigational:* Adjuvant monotherapy following radical prostatectomy, prevention of the progression of first-stage prostate cancer, acne, and hirsutism.

Contraindications: Hypersensitivity to finasteride or any excipient in the product. Use in women and in children. Lactation.

Special Concerns: Use with caution in clients with impaired liver function.

Side Effects: *GU:* Impotence, decreased libido, decreased volume of ejaculate. *Miscellaneous:* Breast tenderness and enlargement, hypersensitivity reactions (including skin rash and swelling of the lips).

Laboratory Test Considerations: ↓ Serum PSA levels.

How Supplied: *Tablet:* 1 mg, 5 mg

Dosage

- **Tablets**

Benign prostatic hyperplasia.

5 mg/day, with or without meals.

Androgenetic alopecia.

Males: 1 mg once a day with or without meals.

HEALTH CARE CONSIDERATIONS

Administration/Storage

1. At least 6–12 months of therapy may be required in some to determine whether a beneficial response has been achieved for benign prostatic hyperplasia.
2. Daily use for three months or longer is necessary to observe beneficial effects.
3. Continued use is required to sustain beneficial effects for hair growth. Withdrawal leads to reversal of effects within 12 months.
4. Women who are pregnant or may become pregnant should not handle crushed finasteride tablets as there is potential for drug absorption and subsequent potential risk to the male fetus. Also, when the male's sexual partner is or may become pregnant, exposure of semen to his partner should be avoided or drug use discontinued.
5. Do not adjust dosage in the elderly or in those with impaired renal function.

Assessment

1. Record indications for therapy, include onset, characteristics of clinical presentation, and any associated family history.
2. Review urologic exam to rule out other conditions similar to BPH (e.g., prostate cancer, infection, stricture, hypotonic bladder, neurogenic disorders).
3. Monitor LFTs and PSA. May cause a decrease in PSA levels (prostate-specific antigen: a blood screening study to detect prostate cancer) even in the presence of prostate cancer.
4. Schedule regular digital rectal exams to assess prostate gland.
5. Not for use in females.
6. With liver impairment monitor closely; drug is metabolized by the liver.
7. Not all clients show a response to finasteride. With a large residual urinary volume or severely diminished urinary flow assess for obstructive uropathy; may not be a finasteride candidate.
8. May obtain pre-treatment scalp photos to assess/gauge response.
9. Ensure that history and physical exam completed.

Client/Family Teaching

1. The following symptoms of BPH should show improvement with continued drug therapy: hesitancy, feelings of incomplete bladder emptying, interruption of urinary stream, impairment of size and force of urinary stream, and terminal urinary dribbling. May take 6–12 months of continued therapy before a beneficial effect is evident
2. If partner is pregnant or may become pregnant, avoid exposure to semen. Drug may cause damage to male fetus; stop drug or use a condom to prevent exposure.
3. Take once a day with or without meals as directed. More than prescribed dose will not increase hair growth but may cause adverse symptoms. May take 3 mg or more before any response noted.
4. Decreased volume of ejaculate may occur but does not interfere with sexual function. Impotence and decreased libido may also occur.
5. Keep F/U lab, checkup, and prostate exams. Report any unusual side effects.
6. Interruption of therapy will reverse effects within 12 mo and BPH symptoms will return.

Outcome/Evaluate
- ↓ Size of enlarged prostate gland
- Symptomatic improvement
- Regrowth of hair with male pattern baldness

——COMBINATION DRUG——

Fiorinal
(fee-OR-in-al)
(Rx)

Fiorinal with Codeine
(fee-OR-in-al, KOH-deen)
Pregnancy Category: C
(C-III) (Rx)
Classification: Analgesic

See also *Narcotic Analgesics*, *Acetylsalicylic acid*, and *Barbiturates*.

Content: Each Fiorinal capsule or tablet contains:

Nonnarcotic analgesic: Aspirin, 325 mg.
Sedative barbiturate: Butalbital, 50 mg.
CNS stimulant: Caffeine, 40 mg.

In addition to the above, Fiorinal with Codeine capsules contain codeine phosphate, 7.5 mg (No. 1), 15 mg (No. 2), or 30 mg (No. 3).

Uses: Fiorinal: Treat tension headaches. Fiorinal with Codeine: Analgesic for all types of pain.

How Supplied: Fiorinal: See Content. Fiorinal with Codeine: See Content

Dosage
- **Capsules, Tablets**

FIORINAL
1–2 tablets or capsules q 4 hr, not to exceed 6 tablets or capsules/day.

FIORINAL WITH CODEINE
Initial: 1–2 capsules; **then,** dose may be repeated, if necessary, up to maximum of 6 capsules/day.

HEALTH CARE CONSIDERATIONS

See *Health Care Considerations* for *Acetylsalicylic acid* and *Narcotic Analgesics.*

Assessment
1. Record pain level, onset, location, and duration of symptoms.
2. List agents previously used and the outcome.

Outcome/Evaluate
- Control of pain
- Relief of tension headaches

Flavoxate hydrochloride
(flay-VOX-ayt)
Pregnancy Category: B
Urispas **(Rx)**
Classification: Urinary tract antispasmodic

Action/Kinetics: Relieves muscle spasms of the urinary tract by relaxing the detrusor muscle by cholinergic blockade and also by a direct effect. Also has local anesthetic and analgesic effects. Well absorbed from GI tract; 10%–30% is excreted in urine.

Uses: Symptomatic relief of urinary tract irritation, dysuria, urgency, nocturia, suprapubic pain, incontinence associated with cystitis, prostatitis, urethritis, urethrocystitis, and other urinary tract disorders. Compatible for use with urinary tract germicides.

Contraindications: Obstructive disorders of urinary tract, including pyloric or duodenal obstructions, obstructive intestinal lesions, ileus, achalasia, obstructive uropathies of the lower urinary tract, and GI hemorrhage.

Special Concerns: Use with caution in glaucoma and during lactation. Confusion is more likely to occur in geriatric clients. Safety and effectiveness have not been determined in children less than 12 years of age.

Side Effects: *GI:* N&V, xerostomia. *CNS:* Drowsiness, headache, vertigo, nervousness, mental confusion (especially in the elderly). *CV:* Tachycardia, palpitations. *Hematologic:* Eosinophilia, leukopenia. *Ophthalmologic:* Blurred vision, increased ocular tension, accommodation disturbances. *Other:* Urticaria and other dermatoses, fever, dysuria.

How Supplied: *Tablet:* 100 mg

Dosage
- **Tablets**

Adults and children over 12 years: 100 or 200 mg t.i.d.–q.i.d. Reduce dose when symptoms improve.

HEALTH CARE CONSIDERATIONS

See also *Health Care Considerations* for *Cholinergic Blocking Agents.*

Client/Family Teaching
1. Do not drive a car or operate hazardous machinery; may cause drowsiness and blurred vision.
2. Practice good oral hygiene. Relieve dryness of mouth with ice chips or hard candy. Ensure adequate hydration.
3. Avoid strenuous exercise; body's heat-regulating mechanism may be altered and sweating inhibited.
4. Report improvement of symptoms as well as any persistent, bothersome, or new symptoms.

Outcome/Evaluate
- Relief of urinary tract discomfort
- Normal elimination patterns

Flecainide acetate

(fleh-**KAY**-nyd)
Pregnancy Category: C
Tambocor **(Rx)**
Classification: Antiarrhythmic, class IC

See also *Antiarrhythmic Agents.*
Action/Kinetics: The antiarrhythmic effect is due to a local anesthetic action, especially on the His-Purkinje system in the ventricle. Drug decreases single and multiple PVCs and reduces the incidence of ventricular tachycardia. **Peak plasma levels:** 3 hr.; **steady state levels:** 3–5 days. **Effective plasma levels:** 0.2–1 mcg/mL (trough levels). **t½:** 20 hr (12–27 hr). Forty percent is bound to plasma protein. Approximately 30% is excreted in urine unchanged. Impaired renal function decreases rate of elimination of unchanged drug. Food or antacids do not affect absorption.
Uses: Life-threatening arrhythmias manifested as sustained ventricular tachycardia. Prevention of paroxysmal supraventricular tachycardias (PSVT) and paroxysmal atrial fibrillation or flutter (PAF) associated with disabling symptoms but not structural heart disease. Antiarrhythmic drugs have not been shown to improve survival in clients with ventricular arrhythmias.
Contraindications: Cardiogenic shock, preexisting second- or third-degree AV block, right bundle branch block when associated with bifascicular block (unless pacemaker is present to maintain cardiac rhythm). Recent MI. Cardiogenic shock. Chronic atrial fibrillation. Frequent premature ventricular complexes and symptomatic nonsustained ventricular arrhythmias. Lactation.
Special Concerns: Use with caution in sick sinus syndrome, in clients with a history of CHF or MI, in disturbances of potassium levels, in clients with permanent pacemakers or temporary pacing electrodes, renal and liver impairment. Safety and efficacy in children less than 18 years of age are not established. The incidence of proarrhythmic effects may be increased in geriatric clients.
Side Effects: *CV: **New or worsened ventricular arrhythmias, increased risk of death in clients with non-life-threatening cardiac arrhythmias,*** new or worsened CHF, palpitations, chest pain, sinus bradycardia, sinus pause, sinus arrest, ***ventricular fibrillation, ventricular tachycardia that cannot be resuscitated,*** second- or third-degree AV block, tachycardia, hypertension, hypotension, bradycardia, angina pectoris. *CNS:* Dizziness, faintness, syncope, lightheadedness, neuropathy, unsteadiness, headache, fatigue, paresthesia, paresis, hypoesthesia, insomnia, anxiety, malaise, vertigo, depression, ***seizures,*** euphoria, confusion, depersonalization, apathy, morbid dreams, speech disorders, stupor, amnesia, weakness, somnolence. *GI:* Nausea, constipation, abdominal pain, vomiting, anorexia, dyspepsia, dry mouth, diarrhea, flatulence, change in taste. *Ophthalmic:* Blurred vision, difficulty in focusing, spots before eyes, diplopia, photophobia, eye pain, nystagmus, eye irritation, photophobia. *Hematologic:* Leukopenia, thrombocytopenia. *GU:* Decreased libido, impotence, urinary retention, polyuria. *Musculoskeletal:* Asthenia, tremor, ataxia, arthralgia, myalgia. *Dermatologic:* Skin rashes, urticaria, exfoliative dermatitis, pruritus, alopecia. *Other:* Edema, dyspnea, fever, ***bronchospasm,*** flushing, sweating, tinnitus, swollen mouth, lips, and tongue.

F

OD **Management of Overdose:** *Symptoms:* Lengthening of PR interval; increase in QRS duration, QT interval, and amplitude of T wave; decrease in HR and contractility; conduction disturbances; hypotension; ***respiratory failure*** or ***asystole.*** *Treatment:* Charcoal will remove unabsorbed drug up to 90 min after drug ingestion. Administration of dopamine, dobutamine, or isoproterenol. Artificial respiration. Intra-aortic balloon pumping, transvenous pacing (to correct conduction block). Acidification of the urine may be beneficial, especially in those with an alkaline urine. Due to the long duration of action of the drug, treatment measures may have to be continued for a prolonged period of time.

Drug Interactions

Acidifying agents / ↑ Renal excretion of flecainide
Alkalinizing agents / ↓ Renal excretion of flecainide
Amiodarone / ↑ Plasma levels of flecainide
Cimetidine / ↑ Bioavailability and renal excretion of flecainide
Digoxin / ↑ Digoxin plasma levels
Disopyramide / Additive negative inotropic effects
Propranolol / Additive negative inotropic effects; also, ↑ plasma levels of both drugs
Smoking (Tobacco) / ↑ Plasma clearance of flecainide
Verapamil / Additive negative inotropic effects

How Supplied: *Tablet:* 50 mg, 100 mg, 150 mg

Dosage

- **Tablets**

  Sustained ventricular tachycardia.

Initial: 100 mg q 12 hr; **then,** increase by 50 mg b.i.d. q 4 days until effective dose reached. **Usual effective dose:** 150 mg q 12 hr, not to exceed 400 mg/day.

PSVT, PAF.

Initial: 50 mg q 12 hr; **then,** dose may be increased in increments of 50 mg b.i.d. q 4 days until effective dose reached. Maximum recommended dose: 300 mg/day. *NOTE:* For PAF clients, increasing the dose from 50 to 100 mg b.i.d. may increase efficacy without a significant increase in side effects.

NOTE: For clients with a C_{CR} less than 35 mL/min/1.73 m^2, the starting dose is 100 mg once daily (or 50 mg b.i.d.). For less severe renal disease, the initial dose may be 100 mg q 12 hr.

HEALTH CARE CONSIDERATIONS

See also *Health Care Considerations* for *Antiarrhythmic Agents.*

Administration/Storage

1. For most situations, start therapy in a hospital setting (especially in clients with symptomatic CHF, sustained ventricular arrhythmias, compensated clients with significant myocardial dysfunction, or sinus node dysfunction).
2. In renal impairment, increase the dose at intervals greater than 4 days. Monitor for adverse toxic effects.
3. The chance of toxic effects increases if the trough plasma levels exceed 1 mcg/mL.
4. If being transferred to flecainide from another antiarrhythmic, allow at least two to four plasma half-lives to elapse for the drug being discontinued before initiating flecainide therapy.
5. Dosing at 8-hr intervals may benefit some.
6. To minimize toxicity, reduce dose once arrhythmia controlled.

Assessment

1. Record physical assessment findings. Review history, echocardiograms, and ECGs for evidence of CHF, ventricular arrhythmias, sinus node dysfunction, or abnormal EF.
2. Monitor VS, ECG, CXR, electrolytes, liver and renal function studies. Assess ECG for increased arrhythmias or AV block. Preexisting hypo- or hyperkalemia may alter drug effects; should be corrected. Monitor for labile BP.
3. Administration with disopyramide, propranolol, or verapamil will promote negative inotropic effects.
4. Check pacing thresholds of clients with pacemakers; adjust before and 1 week following drug therapy.

Client/Family Teaching

1. Take at the dose and prescribed frequency. Report changes in elimination.
2. Report any bruising or increased bleeding tendencies, dyspnea, edema, or chest pain.
3. Keep appointments so that drug effectiveness can be monitored carefully.
4. Report adverse CNS effects, such as dizziness, visual disturbances, headaches, nausea, or depression.
5. Obtain urinary pH to detect alkalinity or acidity. Alkalinity of the urine decreases renal excretion and acidity increases renal excretion, which affects rate of drug elimination.

Outcome/Evaluate

- Termination of lethal ventricular arrhythmias; stable cardiac rhythm
- Therapeutic serum (trough) drug levels (0.2–1.0 mcg/mL)

Fluconazole

(flew-**KON**-ah-zohl)

Pregnancy Category: C

Diflucan, Difulcan-150 ✱ **(Rx)**

Classification: Antifungal agent

Action/Kinetics: Inhibits the enzyme cytochrome P-450 in the organism, which results in a decrease in cell wall integrity and extrusion of intracellular material, leading to death. Apparently does not affect the cytochrome P-450 enzyme in animals or humans. **Peak plasma levels:** 1–2 hr. **t½:** 30 hr, which allows for once daily dosing. Penetrates all body fluids at steady state. Bioavailability is not affected by agents that increase gastric pH. Eighty percent of the drug is excreted unchanged by the kidneys.

Uses: Oropharyngeal and esophageal candidiasis. Serious systemic candidal infection (including UTIs, peritonitis, and pneumonia). Cryptococcal meningitis. Maintenance therapy to prevent cryptococcal meningitis in AIDS clients. Vaginal candidiasis. To decrease the incidence of candidiasis in clients undergoing a bone marrow transplant who receive cytotoxic chemotherapy or radiation therapy. Treatment of cryptococcal meningitis and candidal infections in children.

Contraindications: Hypersensitivity to fluconazole.

Special Concerns: Use with caution during lactation and if client shows hypersensitivity to other azoles. Efficacy has not been adequately assessed in children.

Side Effects: Following single doses. *GI:* Nausea, abdominal pain, diarrhea, dyspepsia, taste perversion. *CNS:* Headache, dizziness. *Other:* Angioedema, ***anaphylaxis (rare).***

Following multiple doses. Side effects are more frequently reported in HIV-infected clients than in non-HIV-infected clients. *GI:* N&V, abdominal pain, diarrhea, ***serious hepatic reactions***. *CNS:* Headache, ***seizures.*** *Dermatologic:* Skin rash, exfoliative skin disorders (including ***Stevens-Johnson syndrome,*** and toxic epidermal necrolysis), alopecia. *Hematologic:* Leukopenia, thrombocytopenia. *Other:* Hypercholesterolemia, hypertriglyceridemia, hypokalemia.

Laboratory Test Considerations: ↑ AST, serum transaminase (especially if used with isoniazid, oral hypoglycemic agents, phenytoin, rifampin, valproic acid).

Drug Interactions

Cimetidine / ↓ Plasma levels of fluconazole
Cisapride / ↑ Risk of serious cardiac arrhythmias
Cyclosporine / Fluconazole may ↑ cyclosporine levels in renal transplant clients with or without impaired renal function
Hydrochlorothiazide / ↑ Plasma levels of fluconazole due to ↓ renal clearance
Glipizide / ↑ Plasma levels of glipizide due to ↓ breakdown by the liver
Glyburide / ↑ Plasma levels of glyburide due to ↓ breakdown by the liver
Phenytoin / Fluconazole ↑ plasma levels of phenytoin
Rifampin / ↓ Plasma levels of fluconazole due to ↑ breakdown by the liver
Theophylline / ↑ Plasma levels of theophylline
Tolbutamide / ↑ Plasma levels of tolbutamide due to ↓ breakdown by the liver
Warfarin / ↑ PT
Zidovudine / ↑ Plasma levels of AZT

How Supplied: *Injection:* 2 mg/mL, 200 mg/100 mL, 400 mg/200 mL; *Powder for Reconstitution:* 50 mg/5mL, 200 mg/5mL; *Tablet:* 50 mg, 100 mg, 150 mg, 200 mg

Dosage

- **Tablets, Oral Suspension, IV**

Vaginal candidiasis.

150 mg as a single oral dose.

Oropharyngeal or esophageal candidiasis.

Adults, first day: 200 mg; **then,** 100 mg/day for a minimum of 14 days (for oropharyngeal candidiasis) or 21 days (for esophageal candidiasis). Up to 400 mg/day may be required for esophageal candidiasis. **Children, first day:** 6 mg/kg; **then,** 3 mg/kg once daily for a minimum of 14 days (for oropharyngeal candidiasis) or 21 days (for esophageal candidiasis).

Candidal UTI and peritonitis.

50–200 mg/day.

Systemic candidiasis (e.g., candidemia, disseminated candidiasis, and pneumonia).

Optimal dosage and duration in adults have not been determined although doses up to 400 mg/day have been used. **Children:** 6–12 mg/kg/day.

Acute cryptococcal meningitis.

Adults, first day: 400 mg; **then,** 200 mg/day (up to 400 mg may be required) for 10 to 12 weeks after CSF culture is negative. **Children, first day:** 12 mg/kg; **then,** 6 mg/kg once daily for 10 to 12 weeks after CSF culture is negative.

Maintenance to prevent relapse of cryptococcal meningitis in AIDS clients.

Adults: 200 mg once daily. **Pediatric:** 6 mg/kg once daily.

Prevention of candidiasis in bone marrow transplant.

400 mg once daily. In clients expected to have severe granulocytopenia (less than 500 neutrophils/mm^3), start fluconazole several days before the anticipated onset of neutropenia and continue for 7 days after the neutrophil count rises about 1,000 cells/mm^3. In clients with renal impairment, an initial loading dose of 50–400 mg can be given; daily dose is based then on C_{CR}.

HEALTH CARE CONSIDERATIONS

See also *General Health Care Considerations for All Anti-Infectives.*

Administration/Storage

1. The daily dose is the same for PO and IV administration.
2. Usually, a loading dose of twice the daily dose is recommended for the first day of therapy in order to obtain plasma levels close to the steady state by the second day of therapy.
3. Due to a long half-life, once daily dosing (either IV or PO) is possible.
4. To prevent relapse, maintenance therapy is usually required in clients with AIDS, cryptococcal meningitis, or recurrent oropharyngeal candidiasis.
5. Shake the oral suspension well before using. Store the reconstituted suspension at 5°C–30°C (4° F–86°F). Discard any unused drug after 2 weeks. Do not freeze suspension.
6. **IV** Do not use the IV solution if cloudy or precipitated or if seal not intact.
7. Do not exceed a continuous IV infusion rate of 200 mg/hr.
8. Do not add supplementary medication to the IV bag.

Assessment

1. Note any sensitivity to azoles or similar drugs.
2. Determine if HIV infected; may place client at increased risk for side effects.
3. Obtain baseline cultures, liver and renal function studies. If abnormal LFTs occur, monitor closely for the development of more serious liver toxicity.

Client/Family Teaching

1. Review goals of therapy and appropriate method and schedule for medication administration and lab studies. Take as directed.
2. Report any rash or persistent side effects (especially if immunocompromised); drug may need to be discontinued.

Outcome/Evaluate

- Elimination of pathogenic fungi
- Candida prophylaxis in transplant recipients

Flucytosine

(flew-**SYE**-toe-seen)
Pregnancy Category: C
Ancobon **(Rx)**
Classification: Antibiotic, antifungal

Action/Kinetics: Appears to penetrate the fungal cell membrane and, after metabolism, acts as an antimetabolite interfering with nucleic acid and protein synthesis. Less toxic than amphotericin B. Well absorbed from the GI tract and distributed to the joints, aqueous humor, peritoneal and other body fluids and tissues. **Peak plasma concentration:** 2–6 hr. **Therapeutic serum concentration:** 20–25 mcg/mL. **t½:** 2–5 hr, higher in presence of impaired renal function. Eighty percent to 90% of the drug is excreted unchanged in urine.

Uses: Serious systemic fungal infections by susceptible strains of *Candida* (e.g., endocarditis, septicemia, UTIs) or *Cryptococcus* (pulmonary or UTIs, meningitis, septicemia).

Contraindications: Hypersensitivity to drug. Lactation.

Special Concerns: Safety and effectiveness have not been determined in children. Use with extreme caution in clients with kidney disease or history of bone marrow depression. The bone marrow depressant effects may cause an increased incidence of microbial infection, gingival bleeding, and delayed healing.

Side Effects: *GI:* N&V, diarrhea, abdominal pain, dry mouth, anorexia, duodenal ulcer, GI hemorrhage, ulcerative colitis. *Hematologic:* Anemia, leukopenia, thrombocytopenia, ***aplastic anemia, agranulocytosis,*** pancytopenia, eosinophilia. *CNS:* Headache, vertigo, confusion, sedation, hallucinations, paresthesia, parkinsonism, psychosis, pyrexia. *Hepatic:* Hepatic dysfunction, jaundice, elevation of hepatic enzymes, increase in bilirubin. *GU:* Increase in BUN and creatinine, azotemia, crystalluria, renal failure. *Respiratory:* Chest pain, dyspnea, ***respiratory arrest.*** *Dermatologic:* Pruritus, rash, urticaria, photosensitivity. *Other:* Ataxia, hearing loss, peripheral neuropathy, weakness, hypoglycemia, fatigue, ***cardiac arrest,*** hypokalemia.

OD Management of Overdose: *Symptoms (serum levels > 100 mcg/mL):* N&V, diarrhea, leukopenia, thrombocytopenia, hepatitis. *Treatment:* Prompt induction of vomiting or gastric lavage. Adequate fluid intake (by IV if necessary). Monitor blood, liver, and kidney parameters frequently. Hemodialysis will quickly decrease serum levels.

Drug Interactions

Amphotericin B / ↑ Effect and toxicity of flucytosine due to kidney impairment
Cytosine / Inactivates antifungal effect of flucytosine

How Supplied: *Capsule:* 250 mg, 500 mg

Dosage

- **Capsules**

Adult and children: 50–150 mg/kg/day in four divided doses. Use lower doses in renal impairment.

HEALTH CARE CONSIDERATIONS

See also *General Health Care Considerations for All Anti-Infectives.*

Assessment

1. Obtain cultures, CBC, liver and renal function studies; reduce dose with impaired renal function
2. Describe clinical presentation.

Client/Family Teaching

1. Reduce or avoid nausea by administering capsules a few at a time over a 15-min period.
2. Report for weekly cultures to determine that strains have not become resistant. A strain is considered resistant if the MIC is > 100.
3. Report any volume reduction, blood, sediment, or cloudiness in the urine.
4. Side effects that interfere with dosing should be reported.

Outcome/Evaluate

- Resolution of fungal infection
- Therapeutic drug levels (20–25 mcg/mL)

Fludrocortisone acetate

(flew-droh-**KOR**-tih-sohn)
Pregnancy Category: C

Florinef **(Rx)**
Classification: Mineralocorticoid

See also *Corticosteroids.*
Action/Kinetics: Produces marked sodium retention and inhibits excess adrenocortical secretion. Supplementary potassium may be indicated.
Uses: Addison's disease and adrenal hyperplasia.
Contraindications: Use systemically as an anti-inflammatory.
How Supplied: *Tablet:* 0.1 mg

Dosage
- **Tablets**

Addison's disease.
0.1–0.2 mg/day to 0.1 mg 3 times/week, usually in conjunction with hydrocortisone or cortisone.
Salt-losing adrenogenital syndrome.
0.1–0.2 mg/day.

HEALTH CARE CONSIDERATIONS

See *Health Care Considerations* for *Corticosteroids.*
Assessment
1. Record clinical presentation and onset of symptoms.
2. Obtain baseline cortisol test, Na and K levels.
Client/Family Teaching
1. Addison's disease will require lifetime replacement therapy. Do not stop abruptly; may precipitate crisis.
2. Review dietary recommendations of high-potassium, low-sodium diet.
Outcome/Evaluate: Control of symptoms during adrenal cortical hypofunction

Flunisolide

(flew-**NISS**-oh-lyd)
Pregnancy Category: C
Inhalation: AeroBid, Bronalide Aerosol ✤ **(Rx)**, **Intranasal:** Nasalide, Nasarel, Rhinalar ✤ **(Rx)**
Classification: Corticosteroid

See also *Corticosteroids.*
Action/Kinetics: Minimal systemic effects with intranasal use. Significant first-pass after inhalation; rapidly metabolized. Several days may be required for full beneficial effects. **t½:** 1.8 hr.
Uses: Inhalation: Prophylaxis and treatment of bronchial asthma in combination with other therapy. Not used when asthma can be relieved by other drugs, in clients where systemic corticosteroid treatment is infrequent, and in nonasthmatic bronchitis. **Intranasal:** Seasonal or perennial rhinitis, especially if other treatment has proven unsatisfactory.
Contraindications: Active or quiescent TB, especially of the respiratory tract. Untreated fungal, bacterial, systemic viral infections. Ocular herpes simplex. Use until healing occurs following recent ulceration of nasal septum, nasal surgery, or trauma. Lactation.
Special Concerns: Safety and effectiveness in children less than 6 years of age have not been determined.
Additional Side Effects: *Respiratory:* Hoarseness, coughing, throat irritation; *Candida* infections of nose, larynx, and pharynx. *After intranasal use:* Nasopharyngeal irritation, stinging, burning, dryness, headache. *GI:* Dry mouth. Systemic corticosteroid effects, especially if recommended dose is exceeded.
How Supplied: *Metered Dose Inhaler:* 0.25 mg/inh; *Nasal Spray:* 0.025 mg/inh

Dosage
- **Inhalation**

Bronchial asthma.
Adults: 2 inhalations (total of 500 mcg flunisolide) in a.m. and p.m., not to exceed 4 inhalations b.i.d. (i.e., total daily dose of 2,000 mcg). **Pediatric, 6–15 years:** 2 inhalations in the morning and evening, with total daily dose not to exceed 1,000 mcg.
- **Intranasal**

Rhinitis.
Adults, initial: 50 mcg (2 sprays) in each nostril b.i.d.; may be increased to 2 sprays t.i.d. up to maximum daily dose of 400 mcg (i.e., 8 sprays in each nostril). **Pediatric, 6–14 years, initial:** 25 mcg (1 spray) in each nostril t.i.d. or 50 mcg (2 sprays) in each nostril b.i.d., up to maximum daily dose of 200 mcg (i.e., 4 sprays in each nostril). **Maintenance, adults, children:** Smallest dose necessary to control symptoms. Some clients (approximately 15%) are controlled on 1 spray in each nostril daily.

HEALTH CARE CONSIDERATIONS

See also *Health Care Considerations* for *Corticosteroids.*
Administration/Storage
1. When starting the inhalant in clients receiving systemic corticosteroids, use aerosol together with the systemic steroid for 1 week. Then, slowly withdraw the systemic corticosteroid over several weeks.
2. If nasal congestion present, use a decon-

F

gestant before administration to ensure drug reaches site of action.

3. If beneficial effects do not occur within 3 weeks, discontinue therapy. Improvement of symptoms usually is evident within a few days.

Client/Family Teaching

1. Use a demonstrator and instruct client and family how to administer nasal spray or inhalant.

2. Gargle and rinse mouth with water after inhalation to prevent alterations in taste and to maintain adequate oral hygiene. Report any symptoms of fungal infections.

3. Mild nasal bleeding may occur; this is usually transient.

Outcome/Evaluate

- Improved airway exchange
- ↓ Allergic manifestations

Fluoxetine hydrochloride

(flew-**OX**-eh-teen)

Pregnancy Category: B

Apo-Fluoxetine ✱, Dom-Fluoxetine ✱, Novo-Fluoxetine ✱, Nu-Fluoxetine ✱, PMS-Fluoxetine ✱, Prozac, Sarafem, STCC-Fluoxetine ✱ **(Rx)**

Classification: Antidepressant, miscellaneous

Action/Kinetics: Not related chemically to tricyclic, tetracyclic, or other antidepressants. Effect thought to be due to inhibition of uptake of serotonin into CNS neurons. Slight to no anticholinergic, sedative, or orthostatic hypotensive effects. Also binds to muscarinic, histaminergic, and alpha-1-adrenergic receptors, accounting for many of the side effects. Metabolized in the liver to norfluoxetine, a metabolite with equal potency to fluoxetine. Norfluoxetine is further metabolized by the liver to inactive metabolites that are excreted by the kidneys. **Time to peak plasma levels:** 6–8 hr. **Peak plasma concentrations:** 15–55 ng/mL. **t½, fluoxetine:** 1–6 days; **t½, norfluoxetine:** 4–16 days. **Time to steady state:** 2–4 weeks. Active drug maintained in the body for weeks after withdrawal.

Uses: Depression, obsessive-compulsive disorders (as defined in the current edition of DSM), bulimia nervosa. *Investigational:* Many (see *Dosage*).

Contraindications: Use with or within 14 days of discontinuing an MAO inhibitor.

Special Concerns: Use with caution during lactation and in clients with impaired liver or kidney function. Safety and efficacy have not been determined in children. A lower initial dose may be necessary in geriatric clients. Use in hospitalized clients, use for longer than 5–6 weeks for depression, or use for more than 13 weeks for obsessive-compulsive disorder has not been studied adequately.

Side Effects: A large number of side effects have been reported for this drug. Listed are those with a reported frequency of greater than 1%. *CNS:* Headache (most common), activation of mania or hypomania, insomnia, anxiety, nervousness, dizziness, fatigue, sedation, decreased libido, drowsiness, lightheadedness, decreased ability to concentrate, tremor, disturbances in sensation, agitation, abnormal dreams. Although less frequent than 1%, ***some clients may experience seizures or attempt suicide.*** *GI:* Nausea (most common), diarrhea, vomiting, constipation, dry mouth, dyspepsia, anorexia, abdominal pain, flatulence, alteration in taste, gastroenteritis, increased appetite. *CV:* Hot flashes, palpitations. *GU:* Sexual dysfunction, impotence, anorgasmia, frequent urination, UTI, dysmenorrhea. *Respiratory:* URTI, pharyngitis, cough, dyspnea, rhinitis, bronchitis, nasal congestion, sinusitis, sinus headache, yawn. *Skin:* Rash, pruritus, excessive sweating. *Musculoskeletal:* Muscle, joint, or back pain. *Miscellaneous:* Flu-like symptoms, asthenia, fever, chest pain, allergy, visual disturbances, blurred vision, weight loss, bacterial or viral infection, limb pain, chills.

Drug Interactions

Alprazolam / ↑ Alprazolam levels and ↓ psychomotor performance

Buspirone / ↓ Effects of buspirone; worsening of obsessive-compulsive disorder

Carbamazepine / ↑ Serum levels of carbamazepine → toxicity

Clozapine / ↑ Serum clozapine levels

Dextromethorphan / Possibility of hallucinations

Diazepam / Fluoxetine ↑ half-life of diazepam → excessive sedation or impaired psychomotor skills

Haloperidol / ↑ Serum levels of haloperidol

Lithium / ↑ Serum levels of lithium → possible neurotoxicity

MAO inhibitors / MAO inhibitors should be discontinued 14 days before initiation of fluoxetine therapy due to the possibility of symptoms resembling a neuroleptic malignant syndrome or fatal reactions

Phenytoin / Fluoxetine may ↑ phenytoin levels

Tricyclic antidepressants / ↑ Pharmacologic and toxicologic effects of tricyclics due to ↓ breakdown by liver

Tryptophan / Symptoms of CNS toxicity (headache, sweating, dizziness, agitation, aggressiveness) or peripheral toxicity (N&V)

Warfarin / ↑ Bleeding diathesis with unaltered PT

How Supplied: *Capsule:* 10 mg, 20 mg; *Solution:* 20 mg/5 mL

Dosage

- **Capsules, Liquid**

Antidepressant.

Adults, initial: 20 mg/day in the morning. If clinical improvement is not observed after several weeks, the dose may be increased to a maximum of 80 mg/day in two equally divided doses.

Obsessive-compulsive disorder.

Initial: 20 mg/day in the morning. If improvement is not significant after several weeks, the dose may be increased. **Usual dosage range:** 20–60 mg/day; the total daily dosage should not exceed 80 mg.

Treatment of bulimia nervosa.

60 mg/day given in the morning. May be necessary to titrate up to this dose over several days.

Alcoholism.

40–80 mg/day.

Anorexia nervosa, bipolar II affective disorder, trichotillomania.

20–80 mg/day.

Attention deficit hyperactivity disorder, obesity, schizophrenia.

20–60 mg/day.

Borderline personality disorder.

5–80 mg/day.

Cataplexy and narcolepsy, Tourette's syndrome.

20–40 mg/day.

Kleptomania.

60–80 mg/day.

Migraine, chronic daily headaches, tension headaches.

20 mg every other day to 40 mg/day.

Posttraumatic stress disorder.

10–80 mg/day.

Premenstrual syndrome, recurrent syncope.

20 mg/day.

Levodopa-induced dyskinesia.

40 mg/day.

Social phobia.

10–60 mg/day.

HEALTH CARE CONSIDERATIONS

Administration/Storage

1. Divide doses greater than 20 mg/day and give in the morning and at noon.
2. If doses lower than 20 mg are necessary, the drug may be emptied from the capsule into cranberry, orange, or apple juice; this should not be refrigerated (is stable for 2 weeks). *NOTE:* A liquid preparation (20 mg/5 mL) is also available.
3. The maximum therapeutic effect may not be observed until 4 weeks after beginning therapy.
4. Elderly clients, clients taking multiple medications, and those with liver or kidney dysfunction should take lower or less frequent doses.
5. When used for obsessive-compulsive disorders, therapy has been continued for over 6 months. However, reassess periodically to determine if continued drug therapy is needed.

Assessment

1. Record indications for therapy, type and onset of symptoms.
2. Review drugs currently prescribed; note any that may interact unfavorably.
3. Determine if pregnant or lactating.
4. Obtain baseline liver and renal function studies; anticipate reduced dose with hepatic and/or renal insufficiency.
5. Periodically reassess client to determine need for continued therapy.

Client/Family Teaching

1. Use caution when driving or performing tasks that require mental alertness; drug may cause drowsiness and/or dizziness.
2. Report any side effects, especially rashes, hives, increased anxiety, and loss of appetite.
3. Take medication at the specific times designated as nervousness and insomnia may occur.
4. It usually takes 1 month to note any significant benefits from therapy. Do not become discouraged and discontinue the medication before benefits are attained.
5. Avoid alcohol; do not take any OTC medications without approval.
6. Any thoughts of suicide or evidence of increased suicide ideations should be reported immediately.
7. Use reliable birth control during therapy.

Outcome/Evaluate

- ↓ Symptoms of depression, as evidenced by improved sleeping and eating patterns, ↓ fatigue, and ↑ social involvement and activity
- Control of repetitive behavioral manifestations

Fluphenazine decanoate

(flew-**FEN**-ah-zeen)

Modecate Concentrate ✦, Modecate Decanoate ✦, PMS-Fluphenazine ✦, Prolixin Decanoate, Rho-Fluphenazine Decanoate ✦ **(Rx)**

Fluphenazine enanthate

(flew-FEN-ah-zeen)

Moditen Enanthate ✦, Prolixin Enanthate **(Rx)**

Fluphenazine hydrochloride

(flew-FEN-ah-zeen)

Apo-Fluphenazine ✦, Permitil, Prolixin, Moditen HCl ✦, PMS-Fluphenazine ✦ **(Rx)**

Classification: Antipsychotic, piperazine-type phenothiazine

F

See also *Antipsychotic Agents, Phenothiazines.*

Action/Kinetics: High incidence of extrapyramidal symptoms and a low incidence of sedation, anticholinergic effects, antiemetic effects, and orthostatic hypotension. The enanthate and decanoate esters dramatically increase the duration of action. *Decanoate:* **Onset,** 24–72 hr; **peak plasma levels,** 24–48 hr; **t½** (approximate), 14 days; **duration,** up to 4 weeks. *Enanthate:* **Onset,** 24–72 hr; **peak plasma levels,** 48–72 hr; **t½** (approximate), 3.6 days; **duration,** 1–3 weeks.

Fluphenazine hydrochloride can be cautiously administered to clients with known hypersensitivity to other phenothiazines.

Fluphenazine enanthate may replace fluphenazine hydrochloride if desired response occurs with hypersensitivity reaction to fluphenazine.

Uses: Psychotic disorders. Adjunct to tricyclic antidepressants for chronic pain states (e.g., diabetic neuropathy, and clients trying to withdraw from narcotics).

How Supplied: Fluphenazine decanoate: *Injection:* 25 mg/mL Fluphenazine enanthate: *Injection:* 25 mg/mL Fluphenazine hydrochloride: *Concentrate:* 5 mg/mL; *Elixir:* 2.5 mg/5 mL; *Injection:* 2.5 mg/mL; *Tablet:* 1 mg, 2.5 mg, 5 mg, 10 mg

Dosage

Fluphenazine hydrochloride is administered **PO and IM.** Fluphenazine enanthate or decanoate are administered **SC and IM.**

Hydrochloride.

- **Elixir, Oral Solution, Tablets**

Psychotic disorders.

Adults and adolescents, initial: 0.5–10 mg/day in divided doses q 6–8 hr; **then,** reduce gradually to maintenance dose of 1–5 mg/day (usually given as a single dose, not to exceed 20 mg/day). **Geriatric, emaciated, debilitated clients, initial:** 1–2.5 mg/day; **then,** dosage determined by response. **Pediatric:** 0.25–0.75 mg 1–4 times/day.

Hydrochloride.

- **IM**

Psychotic disorders.

Adults and adolescents: 1.25–2.5 mg q 6–8 hr as needed. Maximum daily dose: 10 mg. Elderly, debilitated, or emaciated clients should start with 1–2.5 mg/day.

Decanoate.

- **IM, SC**

Psychotic disorders.

Adults, initial: 12.5–25 mg; **then,** the dose may be repeated or increased q 1–3 weeks. The usual maintenance dose is 50 mg/1–4 weeks. Maximum adult dose: 100 mg/dose. **Pediatric, 12 years and older:** 6.25–18.75 mg/week; the dose can be increased to 12.5–25 mg given q 1–3 weeks. **Pediatric, 5–12 years:** 3.125–12.5 mg with this dose being repeated q 1–3 weeks.

Enanthate.

- **IM, SC**

Psychotic disorders.

Adults and adolescents: 12.5–25 mg; dose can be repeated or increased q 1–3 weeks. For doses greater than 50 mg, increases should be made in increments of 12.5 mg. Maximum adult dose: 100 mg.

HEALTH CARE CONSIDERATIONS

See also *Health Care Considerations* for *Antipsychotic Agents, Phenothiazines.*

Administration/Storage

1. Protect all forms of medication from light.
2. Store at room temperature and avoid freezing the elixir.
3. Color of parenteral solution may vary from colorless to light amber. Do not use solutions that are darker than light amber.
4. Do not mix the hydrochloride concentrate with any beverage containing caffeine, tannates (e.g., tea), or pectins (e.g., apple juice) due to a physical incompatibility.
5. Give the short-acting form when beginning phenothiazine therapy. Consider the decanoate and enanthate forms after the response to the drug has been evaluated and for those who demonstrate compliance problems.

Assessment

1. Record indications for therapy, onset and duration of symptoms, other treatments utilized, and the outcome.
2. Note age, mental status, and physical condition. Elderly and debilitated clients are at increased risk for acute extrapyramidal symptoms.

Client/Family Teaching

1. Review administration techniques; determine if client able to assume responsibility for self-medication.
2. Review written guidelines concerning side effects that should be reported and

when to return for follow-up. Stress importance of regular psychotherapy.

Outcome/Evaluate

- Improved behavior patterns with ↓ agitation, ↓ paranoia and withdrawal
- Control of tics

Flurazepam hydrochloride

(flur-**AYZ**-eh-pam)

Apo-Flurazepam ✱, Dalmane, Durapam, Novo-Flupam ✱, PMS-Flurazepam ✱, Somnol ✱, Som Pam ✱ **(C-IV) (Rx)**

Classification: Benzodiazepine sedative-hypnotic

See also *Tranquilizers, Antimanic Drugs, and Hypnotics.*

Action/Kinetics: Combines with benzodiazepine receptors, which are part of the benzodiazepine-GABA receptor-chloride ionophore complex. Results in enhanced inhibitory action of GABA leading to interference of transmission of nerve impulses in the reticular activating system. **Onset:** 17 min. The major active metabolite, *N*-desalkylflurazepam, is active and has a **t½** of 47–100 hr. **Time to peak plasma levels, flurazepam:** 0.5–1 hr; **active metabolite:** 1–3 hr. **Duration:** 7–8 hr. **Maximum effectiveness:** 2–3 days (due to slow accumulation of active metabolite). Significantly bound to plasma protein. Elimination is slow because metabolites remain in the blood for several days. Exceeding the recommended dose may result in development of tolerance and dependence.

Uses: Insomnia (all types). Is increasingly effective on the second or third night of consecutive use and for one or two nights after the drug is discontinued.

Contraindications: Hypersensitivity. Pregnancy or in women wishing to become pregnant. Depression, renal or hepatic disease, chronic pulmonary insufficiency, children under 15 years.

Special Concerns: Use during the last few weeks of pregnancy may result in CNS depression of the neonate. Use during lactation may cause sedation and feeding problems in the infant. Geriatric clients may be more sensitive to the effects of flurazepam.

Side Effects: *CNS:* Ataxia, dizziness, drowsiness/sedation, headache, disorientation. Symptoms of stimulation including nervousness, apprehension, irritability, and talkativeness. *GI:* N&V, diarrhea, gastric upset or pain, heartburn, constipation. *Miscellaneous:* Arthralgia, chest pains, or palpitations. Rarely, symptoms of allergy, SOB, jaundice, anorexia, blurred vision.

Laboratory Test Considerations: ↑ Alkaline phosphatase, bilirubin, serum transaminases.

Drug Interactions

Cimetidine / ↑ Effect of flurazepam due to ↓ breakdown by liver

CNS depressants / Addition or potentiation of CNS depressant effects—drowsiness, lethargy, stupor, respiratory depression or collapse, coma, and possible death

Disulfiram / ↑ Effect of flurazepam due to ↓ breakdown by liver

Ethanol / Additive depressant effects up to the day following flurazepam administration

Isoniazid / ↑ Effect of flurazepam due to ↓ breakdown by liver

Oral contraceptives / Either ↑ or ↓ effect of benzodiazepines due to effect on breakdown by liver

Rifampin / ↓ Effect of benzodiazepines due to ↑ breakdown by liver

How Supplied: *Capsule:* 15 mg, 30 mg

Dosage

- **Capsules**

Adults: 15–30 mg at bedtime; 15 mg for geriatric and/or debilitated clients.

HEALTH CARE CONSIDERATIONS

See also *Health Care Considerations* for *Tranquilizers, Antimanic Drugs, and Hypnotics.*

Assessment

1. Record indications for therapy, symptom onset, other agents prescribed, and the results.
2. Anticipate short-term therapy. Attempt to identify and address causative factors.

Client/Family Teaching

1. Use caution in driving or operating machinery until daytime sedative effects are evaluated. Report persistent morning "hangover."
2. With simple insomnia, try warm baths, warm drinks, soft music, white noise simulator, and other relaxation methods to induce sleep.
3. Avoid ingestion of alcohol.
4. Report tolerance and any symptoms of psychologic and/or physical dependence. Drug is for short-term therapy; continued use causes a tolerance and a decrease in drug responsiveness.
5. Keep a diary of foods, activities, and events for at least 5 days to determine if there are any relationships to insomnia condition.

Outcome/Evaluate: Improved sleeping patterns and less frequent awakenings

Flurbiprofen

(flur-**BIH**-proh-fen)

Pregnancy Category: B

Alti-Flurbiprofen ✱, Ansaid, Apo-Flurbiprofen ✱, Froben ✱, Froben SR ✱, Novo-Flurprofen ✱, Nu-Flurbiprofen ✱ **(Rx)**

F

Flurbiprofen sodium

(flur-**BIH**-proh-fen)

Pregnancy Category: C

Flurbiprofen Sodium Ophthalmic, Ocufen **(Rx)**

Classification: Nonsteroidal anti-inflammatory drug, ophthalmic and systemic use.

See also *Nonsteroidal Anti-Inflammatory Drugs*.

Action/Kinetics: By inhibiting prostaglandin synthesis, flurbiprofen reverses prostaglandin-induced vasodilation, leukocytosis, increased vascular permeability, and increased intraocular pressure. Also inhibits miosis occurring during cataract surgery. **PO form, time to peak levels:** 1.5 hr; **t½:** 5.7 hr.

Uses: Ophthalmic: Prevention of intraoperative miosis. **PO:** Rheumatoid arthritis, osteoarthritis. *Investigational:* Inflammation following cataract surgery, uveitis syndromes. Topically to treat cystoid macular edema. Primary dysmenorrhea, sunburn, mild to moderate pain.

Contraindications: Dendritic keratitis.

Special Concerns: Use with caution in clients hypersensitive to aspirin or other NSAIDs and during lactation. Wound healing may be delayed with use of the ophthalmic product. Acetylcholine chloride and carbachol may be ineffective when used with ophthalmic flurbiprofen. Safety and efficacy in children have not been established.

Additional Side Effects: *Ophthalmic:* Ocular irritation, transient stinging or burning following use, delay in wound healing. Increased bleeding of ocular tissues in conjunction with ocular surgery.

How Supplied: Flurbiprofen: *Tablet:* 50 mg, 100 mg Flurbiprofen sodium: *Ophthalmic solution:* 0.03%

Dosage

- **Ophthalmic Drops**

Beginning 2 hr before surgery, instill 1 gtt q 30 min (i.e., total of 4 gtt of 0.03% solution).

- **Tablets**

Rheumatoid arthritis, osteoarthritis.

Adults, initial: 200–300 mg/day in divided doses b.i.d.–q.i.d.; **then,** adjust dose to client response. Doses greater than 300 mg/day are not recommended.

Dysmenorrhea.

50 mg q.i.d.

HEALTH CARE CONSIDERATIONS

See also *Health Care Considerations* for *Nonsteroidal Anti-Inflammatory Drugs.*

Administration/Storage: Use a dose of 300 mg only for initiating therapy or for treating acute exacerbations of the disease.

Assessment

1. Record indications for therapy.
2. Assess ROM of involved extremity, noting any discoloration, swelling, crepitus, or warmth.
3. Prior to eye surgery, carefully follow the prescribed dosing intervals.

Client/Family Teaching

1. May take tablets with food to decrease GI upset.
2. Review appropriate method of administering eye medication. Avoid rubbing eyes after medication administered; report any stinging, burning, or irritation immediately.
3. Report delays in wound healing.
4. Muscle-strengthening exercises should be performed daily.

Outcome/Evaluate

- ↓ Pain and inflammation with ↑ joint mobility
- ↓ Optic inflammation
- ↓ Abnormal pupillary contractions

Flutamide

(**FLOO**-tah-myd)

Pregnancy Category: D

Euflex ✱, Novo-Flutamide ✱, PMS-Flutamide ✱, Eulexin **(Rx)**

Classification: Antineoplastic, hormonal agent

See also *Antineoplastic Agents.*

Action/Kinetics: Acts either to inhibit uptake of androgen or to inhibit nuclear binding of androgen in target tissues. Thus, the effect of androgen is decreased in androgen-sensitive tissues. Rapidly metabolized to active (α-hydroxylated derivative) and inactive metabolites in the liver and mainly excreted in the urine. **t½ of active metabolite:** 6 hr (8 hr in geriatric clients). Ninety-four percent to 96% is bound to plasma proteins.

Uses: In combination with leuprolide acetate (i.e., a LHRH agonist) to treat stage D_2 metastatic prostatic carcinoma as well as locally confined stage B_2-C prostate cancer. In combination with goserelin acetate depots (Zolad-

ex) to treat locally confined stage B_2-C prostate cancer.
Contraindications: Use during pregnancy.
Side Effects: Side effects are listed for treatment of flutamide with LHRH agonist. *GU:* Loss of libido, impotence. *CV:* Hot flashes, hypertension. *GI:* N&V, diarrhea, GI disturbances, anorexia. *CNS:* Confusion, depression, drowsiness, anxiety, nervousness. *Hematologic:* Anemia, leukopenia, thrombocytopenia, ***hemolytic anemia,*** macrocytic anemia, methemoglobinemia. *Hepatic:* Hepatitis, cholestatic jaundice, hepatic encephalopathy, ***hepatic necrosis.*** *Dermatologic:* Rash, injection site irritation, erythema, ulceration, bullous eruptions, ***epidermal necrolysis.*** *Miscellaneous:* Gynecomastia, edema, neuromuscular symptoms, pulmonary symptoms, GU symptoms, malignant breast tumors.
Laboratory Test Considerations: ↑ AST, ALT, serum creatinine, SGGT, BUN, bilirubin.
OD Management of Overdose: *Symptoms:* Breast tenderness, gynecomastia, increases in AST. Also possible are ataxia, anorexia, vomiting, decreased respiration, lacrimation, sedation, hypoactivity, and piloerection. *Treatment:* Induce vomiting if client is alert. Frequently monitor VS and observe closely.
How Supplied: *Capsule:* 125 mg

Dosage

- **Capsules**

  Locally confined stage B_2-C and stage D_2 metastatic cancer of the prostate.

  250 mg (2 capsules) t.i.d. q 8 hr for a total daily dose of 750 mg.

HEALTH CARE CONSIDERATIONS

See also *Health Care Considerations* for *Antineoplastic Agents.*

Administration/Storage

1. For stage B_2-C prostatic cancer, start flutamide and the LHRH agonist 8 weeks prior to initiating radiation therapy and continue during radiation therapy.
2. For maximum benefit in stage D_2 metastatic prostatic cancer, start flutamide and the LHRH agonist together and continue until disease progression.

Assessment

1. Record indications for therapy, agents previously used, and the outcome.
2. Administer with an LHRH agonist (such as leuprolide acetate).
3. Monitor CBC and LFTs during long-term therapy.

Client/Family Teaching

1. Take flutamide and the LHRH agonist (leuprolide) at the same time.
2. Drug therapy should not be interrupted or discontinued without consulting the provider.
3. Hot flashes, impotence, and diarrhea are all potential side effects of drug therapy; report if persistent or bothersome.
4. Male sexual problems may be drug induced (impotence, decreased libido, gynecomastia). Counseling may be indicated.
5. Compliance may be a problem if diarrhea experienced. Manage diarrhea by cutting down on dairy products, drinking plenty of fluids, not using laxatives, using antidiarrheal products, and eating smaller, more frequent meals high in dietary fibers.

Outcome/Evaluate

- ↓ Production of testosterone
- Control of metastatic processes

Fluticasone propionate

(flu-**TIH**-kah-sohn)
Pregnancy Category: C
Flonase, Flovent **(Rx)**
Classification: Corticosteroid

See also *Corticosteroids.*
Action/Kinetics: Following intranasal use, a small amount is absorbed into the general circulation. **Onset:** Approximately 12 hr. **Maximum effect:** May take several days. Absorbed drug is metabolized in the liver and excreted in the urine.
Uses: Preventive and maintenance treatment of asthma in adults and children over four years of age. To manage seasonal and perennial allergic rhinitis in adults and children over four years of age.
Contraindications: Use for nonallergic rhinitis. Use following nasal septal ulcers, nasal surgery, or nasal trauma until healing has occurred.
Special Concerns: Clients on immunosuppressant drugs, such as corticosteroids, are more susceptible to infections. Use with caution, if at all, in active or quiescent tuberculosis infections; untreated fungal, bacterial, or systemic viral infections; or ocular herpes simplex. Use with caution during lactation.
Side Effects: *Allergic:* Rarely, immediate hypersensitivity reactions or contact dermatitis. *Respiratory:* Epistaxis, nasal burning, blood in nasal mucus, pharyngitis, irritation of nasal mucous membranes, sneezing, runny nose, nasal dryness, sinusitis, nasal congestion, bronchitis, nasal ulcer, nasal septum excoriation. *CNS:* Headache, dizziness. *Ophthalmologic:* Eye disorder, cataracts, glaucoma, increased intraocular pressure. *GI:* N&V, xe-

rostomia. *Miscellaneous:* Unpleasant taste, urticaria. High doses have resulted in hypercorticism and adrenal suppression.

How Supplied: *Cream:* 0.05%; *Metered Dose Inhaler:* 0.11 mg/inh, 0.22 mg/inh, 0.44 mg/inh; *Nasal spray:* 0.05 mg/inh; *Powder for Inhalation:* 0.044/inh, 0.088/inh, 0.22/inh; *Ointment:* 0.005%; *Rotadisk:* 50 mcg, 100 mcg, 250 mcg

Dosage

- **Metered Dose Inhaler**

  Treatment of asthma.

Adults and children over 4 years of age, initial: 100 mcg b.i.d. For oral steroid sparing, the recommended dose is 1,000 mcg b.i.d.

- **Rotadisk Inhaler**

  Prevention of asthma.

Children over 4 years of age: 50–100 mcg. b.i.d.

- **Nasal Spray**

  Allergic rhinitis.

Adults and children over 4 years of age, initial: One 50-mcg spray in each nostril once a day, for a total daily dose of 100 mcg/day. Maximum dose is two sprays (200 mcg) in each nostril once a day.

- **Ointment, Cream**

Apply sparingly to affected area 2–4 times daily.

HEALTH CARE CONSIDERATIONS

See also *Health Care Considerations* for *Corticosteroids.*

Administration/Storage

1. Effectiveness depends on regular use.
2. Store the spray at 4°C–30°C (39°F–86°F).

Assessment

1. Record indications for therapy, note onset, duration of symptoms, and other agents trialed.
2. Examine for evidence of nasal septal ulcers; note turbinate findings.
3. Determine if immunocompromised or actively infected.

Client/Family Teaching

1. Review technique for administration.
2. Take at regular intervals to ensure effectiveness; do not exceed prescribed dose, it may take several days to achieve full benefits.
3. Do not interrupt therapy if side effects evident; notify provider as drug may require slow withdrawal. The dosage should also be slowly reduced if S&S of hypercorticism or adrenal suppression occur such as depression, lassitude, joint and muscle pain; report if evident, especially when replacing systemic corticosteroids with topical.
4. Use adequate humidity, especially during winter months when dry heat may aggravate mucosa. Patients with mold/mildew allergies should be taught to clean humidifiers daily to prevent the growth of these allergens and thus increasing the symptoms.
5. Avoid persons with active infections. Report exposure to chicken pox or measles. (If not immunized or previously infected with the disease, Varicella or Immune Globulin prophylaxis may be given to high-risk clients on long-term therapy).
6. Height and weight will be monitored periodically in adolescents to detect any growth suppression.
7. Identify triggers that aggravate asthma (dust, pollen, smoke, chemicals, pets). Use peak flow meter to help manage asthma.

Outcome/Evaluate

- Control of asthma
- ↓ Symptoms of allergic rhinitis

Fluvastatin sodium

(flu-vah-**STAH**-tin)

Pregnancy Category: X

Lescol **(Rx)**

Classification: Antihyperlipidemic agent

See also *Antihyperlipidemic Agents—HMG-CoA Reductase Inhibitors.*

Action/Kinetics: **t½:** 1.2 hr. Undergoes extensive first-pass metabolism. Significantly bound (greater than 98%) to plasma protein. Metabolized in the liver with 90% excreted through the feces and 5% through the urine.

Uses: Adjunct to diet for the reduction of elevated total and LDL cholesterol levels in clients with primary hypercholesterolemia. The lipid-lowering effects of fluvastatin are enhanced when it is combined with a bile-acid binding resin or with niacin. To slow the progression of coronary atherosclerosis in coronary heart disease.

Contraindications: Lactation.

Special Concerns: Use with caution in clients with severe renal impairment.

Side Effects: Side effects listed are those most common with fluvastatin. A complete list of possible side effects is provided under *Antihyperlipidemic Agents—HMG-CoA Reductase Inhibitors. GI:* N&V, diarrhea, abdominal pain or cramps, constipation, flatulence, dyspepsia, tooth disorder. *Musculoskeletal:* Myalgia, back pain, arthralgia, arthritis. *CNS:* Headache, dizziness, insomnia. *Respira-tory:* URI, rhinitis, cough, pharyngitis, sinusitis. *Miscellaneous:* Rash, pruritus, fatigue, influenza, allergy, accidental trauma.

Laboratory Test Considerations: ↑ Serum transaminases.

Drug Interactions
Alcohol / ↑ Fluvastatin absorbed
Digoxin / ↓ Bioavailability of fluvastatin
Rifampin / ↓ Fluvastatin clearance
How Supplied: *Capsule:* 20 mg, 40 mg

Dosage

- **Capsules**

Treat primary hypercholesterolemia. Antihyperlipidemic to slow progression of coronary atherosclerosis.
Adults: 20 mg once daily at bedtime. **Dose range:** 20–40 mg/day as a single dose in the evening. Splitting the 40-mg dose into a twice-daily regimen results in a modest improvement in LDL cholesterol.

HEALTH CARE CONSIDERATIONS

See also *Health Care Considerations* for *Antihyperlipidemic Agents—HMG-CoA Reductase Inhibitors.*

Administration/Storage
1. Maximum reductions of LDL cholesterol are usually seen within 4 weeks; order periodic lipid determinations during this time, with dosage adjusted accordingly.
2. To avoid fluvastatin binding to a bile-acid binding resin (if given together), give the fluvastatin at bedtime and the resin at least 2 hr before.

Assessment
1. Monitor LFTs and total cholesterol profile every 3 to 6 months.
2. Evaluate on a standard cholesterol-lowering diet before giving fluvastatin. Continue diet during treatment.

Client/Family Teaching
1. May be taken with or without food but is usually consumed with the evening meal.
2. Drugs are used to lower blood cholesterol and fat levels, which have been proven to promote CAD.
3. Must continue dietary restrictions of saturated fat and cholesterol and regular exercise programs in addition to drug therapy in the overall goal of lowering cholesterol levels.

Outcome/Evaluate: ↓ Triglycerides, LDL, and total cholesterol levels

Fluvoxamine maleate

(flu-**VOX**-ah-meen)
Pregnancy Category: C
Alti-Fluvoxamine ✱, Apo-Fluvoxamine ✱, Luvox **(Rx)**
Classification: Selective serotonin-uptake inhibitor

Action/Kinetics: Mechanism in obsessive-compulsive disorders is likely due to inhibition of serotonin reuptake in the CNS. Produces few if any anticholinergic, sedative, or orthostatic hypotensive effects. **Maximum plasma levels:** 3–8 hr. About 80% if bound to plasma proteins. **t½:** 15.6 hr. **Peak plasma concentration:** 88–546 ng/mL. **Time to reach steady state:** About 7 days. Elderly clients manifest higher mean plasma levels and a decreased clearance. Metabolized in the liver and excreted through the urine.

Uses: Obsessive-compulsive disorder (as defined in DSM-III-R) for adults, adolescents, and children. *Investigational:* Treatment of depression.

Contraindications: Concomitant use with astemizole or terfenadine. Alcohol ingestion. Use with MAO inhibitors or within 14 days of discontinuing treatment with a MAO inhibitor. Lactation.

Special Concerns: Use with caution in clients with a history of mania, seizure disorders, and liver dysfunction and in those with diseases that could affect hemodynamic responses or metabolism. Safety and efficacy have not been determined in children less than 18 years of age.

Side Effects: Side effects listed occur at an incidence of 0.1% or greater. *CNS:* Somnolence, insomnia, nervousness, dizziness, tremor, anxiety, hypertonia, agitation, decreased libido, depression, CNS stimulation, amnesia, apathy, hyperkinesia, hypokinesia, manic reaction, myoclonus, psychoses, fatigue, malaise, agoraphobia, akathisia, ataxia, ***convulsion,*** delirium, delusion, depersonalization, drug dependence, dyskinesia, dystonia, emotional lability, euphoria, extrapyramidal syndrome, unsteady gait, hallucinations, hemiplegia, hostility, hypersomnia, hypochondriasis, hypotonia, hysteria, incoordination, increased libido, neuralgia, paralysis, paranoia, phobia, sleep disorders, stupor, twitching, vertigo. *GI:* Nausea, dry mouth, diarrhea, constipation, dyspepsia, anorexia, vomiting, flatulence, toothache, tooth caries, dysphagia, colitis, eructation, esophagitis, gastritis, gastroenteritis, ***GI hemorrhage,*** GI ulcer, gingivitis, glossitis, hemorrhoids, melena, rectal hemorrhage, stomatitis. *CV:* Palpitations, hypertension, postural hypotension, vasodilation, syncope, tachycardia, angina pectoris, bradycardia, ***cardiomyopathy,*** CV disease, cold extremities, conduction delay, ***heart failure, MI,*** pallor, irregular pulse, ST segment changes. *Respiratory:* URI, dyspnea, yawn, increased cough, sinusitis, asthma, bronchitis, epistaxis, hoarseness, hyperventilation. *Body as a whole:* Headache, asthenia, flu syndrome, chills, malaise, edema, weight gain or loss, dehydration, hypercholesterolemia, allergic reaction, neck pain, neck rigidity, photosensitivity, ***suicide attempt.*** *Dermatologic:* Excessive sweating, acne, alopecia, dry skin, eczema, exfoliative dermatitis, furunculosis, seborrhea, skin discoloration, urticaria. *Musculoskeletal:* Arthralgia, arthritis, bursitis, generalized muscle spasm, myasthenia, tendinous contracture, tenosynovitis. *GU:* Delayed ejaculation, urinary frequency, impotence, anorgasmia, urinary retention, anuria, breast pain, cystitis, delayed menstruation, dysuria, female lactation, hematuria, menopause, menorrhagia, metrorrhagia, nocturia, polyuria, PMS, urinary incontinence, UTI, urinary urgency, impaired urination, ***vaginal hemorrhage,*** vaginitis. *Hematologic:* Anemia, ecchymosis, leukocytosis, lymphadenopathy, thrombocytopenia. *Ophthalmic:* Amblyopia, abnormal accommodation, conjunctivitis, diplopia, dry eyes, eye pain, mydriasis, photophobia, visual field defect. *Otic:* Deafness, ear pain, otitis media. *Miscellaneous:* Taste perversion or loss, parosmia, hypothyroidism, hypercholesterolemia, dehydration.

OD **Management of Overdose:** *Treatment:* Establish an airway and maintain respiration as needed. Monitor VS and ECG. Activated charcoal may be as effective as emesis or lavage in removing the drug from the GI tract. Since absorption in overdose may be delayed, measures to reduce absorption may be required for up to 24 hr.

Drug Interactions

Astemisole / ↑ Risk of severe cardiovascular effects, including QT prolongation, ventricular tachycardia, and torsades de pointes (may be fatal)
Beta-adrenergic blockers / Possible ↑ effects on BP and HR
Carbamazepine / ↑ Risk of carbamazepine toxicity
Cloxapine / ↑ Risk of orthostatic hypotension and seizures
Diazepam / ↑ Effect of diazepam due to ↓ clearance
Diltiazem / ↑ Risk of bradycardia
Haloperidol / ↑ Serum levels of haloperidol
Lithium / ↑ Risk of seizures
MAO inhibitors / Serious and possibly fatal reactions, including hyperthermia, rigidity, myoclonus, rapid fluctuations of VS, changes in mental status (agitation, delirium, coma)
Methadone / ↑ Risk of methadone toxicity
Midazolam / ↑ Effect of midazolam due to ↓ clearance
Sumatriptan / ↑ Risk of weakness, hyperreflexia, incoordination
Terfenadine / ↑ Risk of severe cardiovascular effects, including QT prolongation, ventricular tachycardia, and torsades de pointes (may be fatal)
Theophylline / ↑ Risk of theophylline toxicity (decrease dose by one-third the usual daily maintenance dose)
Triazolam / ↑ Effect of triazolam due to ↓ clearance
Tricyclic antidepressants / Significant ↑ in plasma levels of tricyclic antidepressants
Tryptophan / ↑ Risk of central toxicity (headache, sweating, dizziness, agitation, aggressiveness, worsening of obsessive-compulsive disorder) or peripheral toxicity (N&V)
Warfarin / ↑ Plasma levels of warfarin

How Supplied: *Tablet:* 25 mg, 50 mg, 100 mg

Dosage

- **Tablets**

Obsessive-compulsive disorder.

Adults, initial: 50 mg at bedtime; **then,** increase the dose in 50-mg increments q 4–7 days, as tolerated, until a maximum benefit is reached, not to exceed 300 mg/day. **Children and adolescents, 8 to 17 years:** 25 mg at bedtime; **then,** increase the dose in 25-mg increments q 4–7 days until a maximum benefit is reached, not to exceed 200 mg/day.

HEALTH CARE CONSIDERATIONS

Administration/Storage

1. If total daily dose exceeds 100 mg for adults or 50 mg in children, give in two divided doses. If the doses are unequal, give the larger dose at bedtime.
2. Starting and incremental doses may need to be lower in geriatric clients.
3. Use lowest effective dose; assess periodically to determine need for continued treatment.
4. Use for more than 10 weeks has not been evaluated.

Assessment

1. Record indications for therapy and presenting or described behaviorial manifestations.
2. List agents currently prescribed to ensure none interact unfavorably.
3. Note history of mania, seizure disorders, or liver dysfunction.
4. Monitor ECG, CBC, and liver and renal function studies.

Client/Family Teaching

1. Take only as directed, usually at bedtime, do not exceed dosage.
2. May cause dizziness and drowsiness. Do not perform activities that require mental or physical alertness until drug effects realized.

3. Report any rash, hives, or unusual itching; increased depression or suicide ideations
4. Avoid alcohol and any other drugs without approval.
5. Practice reliable birth control.
6. Report for scheduled appointments so response to therapy, dosage, and need for continued therapy can be determined.

Outcome/Evaluate

- Reduction in excessive, repetitive behaviors
- Control of persistent, recurrent thoughts, ideas, impulses, or images

Folic acid

(FOH-lik AH-sid)

Pregnancy Category: A

Apo-Folic ✤, Folvite, Novo-Folacid ✤ **(Rx) (OTC)**

Classification: Vitamin B complex

Action/Kinetics: Folic acid (which is converted to tetrahydrofolic acid) is necessary for normal production of RBCs and for synthesis of nucleoproteins. Tetrahydrofolic acid is a cofactor in the biosynthesis of purines and thymidylates of nucleic acids. Megaloblastic and macrocytic anemias in folic acid deficiency are believed to be due to impairment of thymidylate synthesis. Natural sources of folic acid include liver, dried beans, peas, lentils, whole-wheat products, asparagus, beets, broccoli, brussels sprouts, spinach, and oranges. Synthetic folic acid is absorbed from the GI tract even if the client suffers from malabsorption syndrome. **Peak plasma levels after an oral dose:** 1 hr. It is stored in the liver.

Uses: Treatment of megaloblastic anemias due to folic acid deficiency (e.g., tropical and nontropical sprue, pregnancy, infancy or childhood, nutritional causes). Diagnosis of folate deficiency.

Contraindications: Use in aplastic, normocytic, or pernicious anemias (is ineffective). Folic acid injection that contains benzyl alcohol should not be used in neonates or immature infants.

Special Concerns: Daily folic acid doses of 0.1 mg or greater may obscure pernicious anemia. Prolonged folic acid therapy may cause decreased vitamin B_{12} levels.

Side Effects: *Allergic:* Skin rash, itching, erythema, general malaise, respiratory difficulty due to bronchospasm. *GI:* Nausea, anorexia, abdominal distention, flatulence, bitter or bad taste (in those taking 15 mg/day for 1 month). *CNS:* In doses of 15 mg daily, altered sleep patterns, irritability, excitement, difficulty in concentration, overactivity, depression, impaired judgment, confusion.

Drug Interactions

Aminosalicylic acid / ↓ Serum folate levels
Corticosteroids (chronic use) / ↑ Folic acid requirements
Methotrexate / Is a folic acid antagonist
Oral contraceptives / ↑ Risk of folate deficiency
Phenytoin / Folic acid ↑ seizure frequency; also, phenytoin ↓ serum folic acid levels.
Pyrimethamine / Folic acid ↓ effect of pyrimethamine in toxoplasmosis; also, pyrimethamine is a folic acid antagonist
Sulfonamides / ↓ Absorption of folic acid
Triamterene / ↓ Utilization of folic acid as it is a folic acid antagonist
Trimethoprim / ↓ Utilization of folic acid as it is a folic acid antagonist

How Supplied: *Injection:* 5 mg/mL; *Tablet:* 0.4 mg, 0.8 mg, 1 mg

Dosage

- **Tablets**

Dietary supplement.

Adults and children: 100 mcg/day (up to 1 mg in pregnancy); may be increased to 500–1,000 mcg if requirements increase.

Treatment of deficiency.

Adults, initial: 250–1,000 mcg/day until a hematologic response occurs; **maintenance:** 400 mcg/day (800 mcg during pregnancy and lactation). **Pediatric, initial:** 250–1,000 mcg/day until a hematologic response occurs. **Maintenance, infants:** 100 mcg/day; **children up to 4 years:** 300 mcg/day; **children 4 years and older:** 400 mcg/day.

- **IM, IV, Deep SC**

Treatment of deficiency.

Adults and children: 250–1,000 mcg/day until a hematologic response occurs.

Diagnosis of folate deficiency.

Adults, IM: 100–200 mcg/day for 10 days plus low dietary folic acid and vitamin B_{12}.

HEALTH CARE CONSIDERATIONS

Administration/Storage

1. Given PO; if there is severe malabsorption, give either IV or SC.
2. Regardless of age, the dosage should never be less than 0.1 mg/day.

IV 3. Folic acid will remain stable in solution if the pH is kept above 5.

4. May be administered IM, by direct IV push or added to infusions. When given IV, the rate should not exceed 5 mcg/min.

5. When parenteral forms are used, have drugs and equipment available to treat anaphylactic reactions.

Assessment

1. Record baseline CBC, reticulocytes, MCV, and serum folate and B_{12} levels.
2. Review drugs prescribed; oral contraceptives, trimethoprim, hydantoins, and alcohol may cause increased body loss of folic acid.

Client/Family Teaching

1. Take only as directed.
2. Dietary sources of folic acid include dark green leafy vegetables, beans, fortified breads, and cereals. Prolonged cooking destroys folate in vegetables.
3. Drug may discolor urine a deep yellow.
4. U.S. Public Health Service recommends that all women of childbearing age consume 0.4 mg of folic acid to reduce the risk of neural tube birth defects. Folic acid may prevent the development of spina bifida or anencephaly, which occur during the first month of pregnancy.

Outcome/Evaluate

- Desired hematologic response
- Reversal in symptoms of folic acid deficiency and megaloblastic anemia
- Prophylaxis of newborn neural tube defects

Fosfomycin tromethamine

(fos-foh-**MY**-sin)

Pregnancy Category: B

Monurol **(Rx)**

Classification: Anti-infective, antibiotic

See also *Anti-Infective Agents.*

Action/Kinetics: Bactericidal drug that inactivates enzyme enolpyruvyl transferase, irreversibly blocking condensation of uridine diphosphate-N-acetylglucosamine with p-enolpyruvate. This is one of first steps in bacterial wall synthesis. Also reduces adherence of bacteria to uroepithelial cells. Rapidly absorbed from GI tract and converted to fosfomycin. **Maximum serum levels:** 2 hr. **t½, elimination:** 5.7 hr. Excreted unchanged in both urine and feces.

Uses: Treatment of uncomplicated urinary tract infections (acute cystitis) in women due to *Escherichia coli* and Enterococcus faecalis.

Contraindications: Lactation.

Special Concerns: Safety and efficacy have not been determined in children 12 years and younger.

Side Effects: *GI:* Diarrhea, nausea, dyspepsia, abdominal pain, abnormal stools, anorexia, constipation, dry mouth, flatulence, vomiting. *CNS:* Headache, dizziness, insomnia, migraine, nervousness, paresthesia, somnolence. *GU:* Vaginitis, dysmenorrhea, dysuria, hematuria, menstrual disorder. *Respiratory:* Rhinitis, pharyngitis. *Miscellaneous:* Asthenia, back pain, pain, rash, ear disorder, fever, flu syndrome, infection, lymphadenopathy, myalgia, pruritus, skin disorder.

Laboratory Test Considerations: ↑ ALT, AST, eosinophil count, bilirubin, alkaline phosphatase. ↓ Hematocrit, hemoglobin. ↑ or ↓ WBC, platelet count.

Drug Interactions

Metoclopramide / ↓ serum levels and urinary excretion of fosfomycin.

How Supplied: *Granules for Reconstitution:* 3 g

Dosage

- **Sachet**

  Acute cystitis.

Women, 18 years and older: One sachet of fosfomycin mixed with water before ingesting.

HEALTH CARE CONSIDERATIONS

See also *Health Care Considerations* for *Anti-Infective Agents.*

Administration/Storage: Store at controlled room temperature.

Assessment

1. Note onset, duration, frequency of occurrence, and symptoms.
2. Assess urine cultures.

Client/Family Teaching

1. Pour entire contents of single-dose sachet into 3 to 4 oz water and stir to dissolve. Do not take dry. Do not use hot water. Take immediately after dissolving in water.
2. May be taken with or without food.
3. Use only one single dose to treat each episode of acute cystitis. Each packet contains 3 g of fosfomycin.
4. Symptoms should improve within 2 to 3 days; if not improved, contact health care provider.

Outcome/Evaluate: Resolution of UTI; symptomatic improvement

Fosinopril sodium

(foh-**SIN**-oh-prill)

Pregnancy Category: D

Monopril **(Rx)**

Classification: Angiotensin-converting enzyme inhibitor

See also *Angiotensin-Converting Enzyme Inhibitors.*

Action/Kinetics: Onset: 1 hr. **Time to peak serum levels:** About 3 hr. Metabolized in the liver to the active fosinoprilat.

Peak effect: 2–6 hr. Over 99% bound to plasma proteins. **t½:** 12 hr for fosinoprilat (prolonged in impaired renal function) following IV administration. **Duration:** 24 hr. Approximately 50% excreted through the urine and 50% in the feces. Food decreases the rate, but not the extent, of absorption of fosinopril.
Uses: Alone or in combination with other antihypertensive agents (especially thiazide diuretics) for the treatment of hypertension. Adjunct in treating CHF in clients not responding adequately to diuretics and digitalis. Diabetic hypertensive clients show a reduction in major CV events.
Contraindications: Use during lactation.
Side Effects: *CV:* Orthostatic hypotension, chest pain, hypotension, palpitations, angina pectoris, ***CVA, MI,*** rhythm disturbances, TIA, tachycardia, ***hypertensive crisis,*** claudication, bradycardia, hypertension, conduction disorder, ***sudden death, cardiorespiratory arrest, shock***. *CNS:* Headache, dizziness, fatigue, confusion, memory disturbance, depression, behavior change, tremors, drowsiness, mood change, insomnia, vertigo, sleep disturbances. *GI:* N&V, diarrhea, abdominal pain, constipation, dry mouth, dysphagia, taste disturbance, abdominal distention, flatulence, heartburn, appetite changes, weight changes. *Hepatic:* Hepatitis, pancreatitis, hepatomegaly, ***hepatic failure.*** *Respiratory:* Cough, sinusitis, dyspnea, URI, ***bronchospasm,*** asthma, pharyngitis, laryngitis, tracheobronchitis, abnormal breathing, sinus abnormalities. *Hematologic:* Leukopenia, eosinophilia, decreases in hemoglobin (mean of 0.1 g/dL) or hematocrit, neutropenia. *Dermatologic:* Diaphoresis, photosensitivity, flushing, exfoliative dermatitis, pruritus, rash, urticaria. *Body as a whole:* Angioedema, muscle cramps, fever, syncope, influenza, cold sensation, pain, myalgia, arthralgia, arthritis, edema, weakness, musculoskeletal pain. *GU:* Decreased libido, sexual dysfunction, renal insufficiency, urinary frequency, abnormal urination, kidney pain. *Miscellaneous:* Paresthesias, tinnitus, gout, lymphade-nopathy, rhinitis, epistaxis, vision disturbances, eye irritation, swelling/weakness of extremities, abnormal vo-calization, pneumonia, muscle ache.
Laboratory Test Considerations: ↑ Serum potassium. Transient ↓ H&H. False low measurement of serum digoxin levels with DigiTab RIA Kit for Digoxin.
How Supplied: *Tablet:* 10 mg, 20 mg, 40 mg

Dosage

- **Tablets**

Hypertension.

Initial: 10 mg once daily; **then,** adjust dose depending on BP response at peak (2–6 hr after dosing) and trough (24 hr after dosing) blood levels. **Maintenance:** Usually 20–40 mg/day, although some clients manifest beneficial effects at doses up to 80 mg.

In clients taking diuretics.

Discontinue diuretic 2–3 days before starting fosinopril. If diuretic cannot be discontinued, use an initial dose of 10 mg fosinopril.

Congestive heart failure.

Initial: 10 mg once daily; **then,** following initial dose, observe the client for at least 2 hr for the presence of hypotension or orthostasis (if either is present, monitor until BP stabilizes). An initial dose of 5 mg is recommended in heart failure with moderate to severe renal failure or in those who have had significant diuresis. The dose is increased over several weeks, not to exceed a maximum of 40 mg daily (usual effective range is 20–40 mg once daily).

HEALTH CARE CONSIDERATIONS

See also *Health Care Considerations* for *Angiotensin-Converting Enzyme Inhibitors* and *Antihypertensive Agents.*

Administration/Storage

1. If antihypertensive effect decreases at the end of the dosing interval with once-daily dosing, consider b.i.d. administration.
2. If also taking a diuretic, discontinue the diuretic 2–3 days prior to beginning fosinopril therapy. If BP is not controlled, reinstitute the diuretic. If the diuretic cannot be discontinued, give an initial dose of fosinopril of 10 mg.
3. Do not adjust the dose of fosinopril in renal insufficiency except as noted in Dosage.

Outcome/Evaluate

- ↓ BP
- Control of symptoms of CHF

Furosemide

(fur-**OH**-seh-myd)
Pregnancy Category: C
Apo-Furosemide ✦, Furoside ✦, Lasix, Lasix Special ✦, Myrosemide, Novo-Semide ✦ **(Rx)**
Classification: Loop diuretic

See also *Diuretics, Loop.*
Action/Kinetics: Inhibits the reabsorption of sodium and chloride in the proximal and distal tubules as well as the ascending loop

of Henle; this results in the excretion of sodium, chloride, and, to a lesser degree, potassium and bicarbonate ions. The resulting urine is more acid. Diuretic action is independent of changes in clients' acid-base balance. Has a slight antihypertensive effect. **Onset: PO, IM:** 30–60 min; **IV:** 5 min. **Peak: PO, IM:** 1–2 hr; **IV:** 20–60 min. **t½:** About 2 hr after PO use. **Duration: PO, IM:** 6–8 hr; **IV:** 2 hr. Metabolized in the liver and excreted through the urine. May be effective for clients resistant to thiazides and for those with reduced GFRs.

F

Uses: Edema associated with CHF, nephrotic syndrome, hepatic cirrhosis, and ascites. IV for acute pulmonary edema. PO to treat hypertension in conjunction with spironolactone, triamterene, and other diuretics *except* ethacrynic acid. *Investigational:* Hypercalcemia.

Contraindications: Never use with ethacrynic acid. Anuria, hypersensitivity to drug, severe renal disease associated with azotemia and oliguria, hepatic coma associated with electrolyte depletion. Lactation.

Special Concerns: Use with caution in premature infants and neonates due to prolonged half-life in these clients (dosing interval must be extended). Geriatric clients may be more sensitive to the usual adult dose. Allergic reactions may be seen in clients who show hypersensitivity to sulfonamides.

Side Effects: *Electrolyte and fluid effects:* Fluid and electrolyte depletion leading to dehydration, hypovolemia, thromboembolism. Hypokalemia and hypochloremia may cause metabolic alkalosis. Hyperuricemia, azotemia, hyponatremia. *GI:* Nausea, oral and gastric irritation, vomiting, anorexia, diarrhea (especially in children) or constipation, cramps, pancreatitis, jaundice, ischemic hepatitis. *Otic:* Tinnitus, hearing impairment (may be reversible or permanent), reversible deafness. Usually following rapid IV or IM administration of high doses. *CNS:* Vertigo, headache, dizziness, blurred vision, restlessness, paresthesias, xanthopsia. *CV:* Orthostatic hypotension, thrombophlebitis, chronic aortitis. *Hematologic:* Anemia, thrombocytopenia, neutropenia, leukopenia, ***agranulocytosis,*** purpura. ***Rarely, aplastic anemia.*** *Allergic:* Rashes, pruritus, urticaria, photosensitivity, exfoliative dermatitis, vasculitis, erythema multiforme. *Miscellaneous:* Interstitial nephritis, fever, weakness, hyperglycemia, glycosuria, exacerbation of, aggravation of or worsening of SLE, increased perspiration, muscle spasms, urinary bladder spasm, urinary frequency.

Following IV use: Thrombophlebitis, ***cardiac arrest.*** *Following IM use:* Pain and irritation at injection site, ***cardiac arrest.***

Because this drug is resistant to the effects of pressor amines and potentiates the effects of muscle relaxants, it is recommended that the PO drug be discontinued 1 week before surgery and the IV drug 2 days before surgery.

OD Management of Overdose: *Symptoms:* Profound water loss, electrolyte depletion (manifested by weakness, anorexia, vomiting, lethargy, cramps, mental confusion, dizziness), decreased blood volume, ***circulatory collapse (possibly vascular thrombosis and embolism).*** *Treatment:* Replace fluid and electrolytes. Monitor urine electrolyte output and serum electrolytes. Induce emesis or perform gastric lavage. Oxygen or artificial respiration may be needed. Treat symptoms.

Additional Drug Interactions

Charcoal / ↓ Absorption of furosemide from the GI tract
Clofibrate / Enhanced diuretic effect
Hydantoins / Hydantoins ↓ the diuretic effect of furosemide
Propranolol / Furosemide may cause ↑ plasma levels of propranolol

How Supplied: *Injection:* 10 mg/mL; *Solution:* 10 mg/ mL, 40 mg/5 mL; *Tablet:* 20 mg, 40 mg, 80 mg

Dosage

- **Oral Solution, Tablets**

Edema.

Adults, initial: 20–80 mg/day as a single dose. For resistant cases, dosage can be increased by 20–40 mg q 6–8 hr until desired diuretic response is attained. Maximum daily dose should not exceed 600 mg. **Pediatric, initial:** 2 mg/kg as a single dose; **then,** dose can be increased by 1–2 mg/kg q 6–8 hr until desired response is attained (up to 5 mg/kg may be required in children with nephrotic syndrome; maximum dose should not exceed 6 mg/kg). A dose range of 0.5–2 mg/kg b.i.d. has also been recommended.

Hypertension.

Adults, initial: 40 mg b.i.d. Adjust dosage depending on response.

CHF and chronic renal failure.

Adults: 2–2.5 g/day.

Antihypercalcemic.

Adults: 120 mg/day in one to three doses.

- **IV, IM**

Edema.

Adults, initial: 20–40 mg; if response inadequate after 2 hr, increase dose in 20-mg increments. **Pediatric, initial:** 1 mg/kg given slowly; if response inadequate after 2 hr, increase dose by 1 mg/kg. Doses greater than 6 mg/kg should not be given.

Antihypercalcemic.

Adults: 80–100 mg for severe cases; dose may be repeated q 1–2 hr if needed.

• **IV**

Acute pulmonary edema.

Adults: 40 mg slowly over 1–2 min; if response inadequate after 1 hr, give 80 mg slowly over 1–2 min. Concomitant oxygen and digitalis may be used.

CHF, chronic renal failure.

Adults: 2–2.5 g/day. For IV bolus injections, the maximum should not exceed 1 g/day given over 30 min.

Hypertensive crisis, normal renal function.

Adults: 40–80 mg.

Hypertensive crisis with pulmonary edema or acute renal failure.

Adults: 100–200 mg.

HEALTH CARE CONSIDERATIONS

See also *Health Care Considerations* for *Diuretics, Loop.*

Administration/Storage

1. Give 2–4 days/week.
2. Food decreases the bioavailability of furosemide and ultimately the degree of diuresis.
3. Slight discoloration resulting from light does not affect potency. However, do not dispense discolored tablets or injection.
4. If used with other antihypertensives, reduce the dose of other agents by at least 50% when furosemide is added in order to prevent an excessive drop in BP.
5. Store in light-resistant containers at room temperature (15°C–30°C, or 59°F–86°F).
6. In CHF or chronic renal failure, oral and parenteral doses of 2–2.5 g/day (or higher) are well tolerated.

IV 7. Give IV injections slowly over 1–2 min.

8. If used IV, do not mix with solutions with a pH below 5.5. After pH adjustment, furosemide can be mixed with NaCl injection, RL injection, and D5W and infused at a rate not to exceed 4 mg/min, to prevent ototoxicity.
9. A precipitate may form if mixed with gentamicin, netilmicin, or milrinone in either D5W or NSS.

Assessment

1. When more than 40 mg/day is required, give in divided doses, i.e., 40 mg PO b.i.d.
2. With renal impairment or if receiving other ototoxic drugs, observe for ototoxicity.
3. Assess closely for signs of vascular thrombosis and embolism, particularly in the elderly.
4. Monitor electrolytes; observe for S&S of hypokalemia.
5. With rapid diuresis, observe for dehydration and circulatory collapse; monitor BP and pulse.
6. With chronic use, assess for thiamine deficiency.

Client/Family Teaching

1. Take in the morning on an empty stomach to enhance absorption and to avoid interruption of sleep. Time administration to participate in social activities and not have to get up during the night to void frequently.
2. Immediately report any muscle weakness, dizziness, numbness, or tingling.
3. Drug may cause orthostatic hypotension.
4. Sorbitol in the solution vehicle may result in diarrhea, especially in children.
5. Monitor weights; report any gains of > 3 lb/day or > 10 lb/week.
6. Consult provider before taking aspirin for any reason. Salicylate intoxication occurs at lower levels than normal because of competition at the renal excretory sites.
7. Use sunscreens and protective clothing when sun exposed to minimize the effects of drug-induced photosensitivity.
8. Supplement diet with vegetables and fruits high in potassium if oral supplements are not prescribed. Those on a salt-restricted diet should not increase salt intake; NSAIDs and alpha blockers may also cause sodium retention with resultant edema.

Outcome/Evaluate

- Enhanced diuresis
- Resolution of pulmonary edema
- ↓ Dependent edema
- ↓ Serum calcium levels

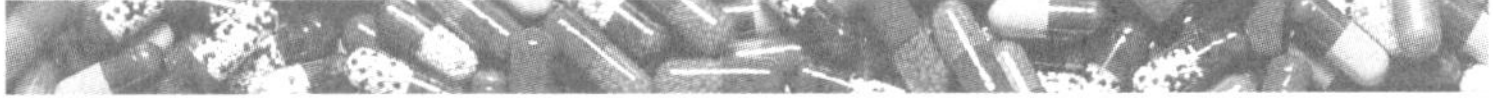

Gabapentin

(gab-ah-PEN-tin)

Pregnancy Category: C

Neurontin **(Rx)**

Classification: Anticonvulsant

See also *Anticonvulsants.*

Action/Kinetics: Anticonvulsant mechanism is not known. Food has no effect on the rate and extent of absorption; however, as the dose increases, the bioavailability decreases.

t½: 5–7 hr. Excreted unchanged through the urine.
Uses: In adults as an adjunct in the treatment of partial seizures with and without secondary generalization.
Special Concerns: Use during lactation only if benefits outweigh risks. Plasma clearance is reduced in geriatric clients and in those with impaired renal function. Safety and efficacy have not been determined in children less than 12 years of age.
Side Effects: Side effects listed are those with an incidence of 0.1% or greater.

CNS: Most commonly: somnolence, ataxia, dizziness, and fatigue. Also, nystagmus, tremor, nervousness, dysarthria, amnesia, depression, abnormal thinking, twitching, abnormal coordination, headache, ***convulsions (including the possibility of precipitation of status epilepticus),*** confusion, insomnia, emotional lability, vertigo, hyperkinesia, paresthesia, decreased/increased/absent reflexes, anxiety, hostility, CNS tumors, syncope, abnormal dreaming, aphasia, hypesthesia, ***intracranial hemorrhage,*** hypotonia, dysesthesia, paresis, dystonia, hemiplegia, facial paralysis, stupor, cerebellar dysfunction, positive Babinski sign, decreased position sense, subdural hematoma, apathy, hallucinations, decreased or loss of libido, agitation depersonalization, euphoria, "doped-up" sensation, ***suicidal tendencies,*** psychoses. *GI:* Most commonly: N&V. Also, dyspepsia, dry mouth and throat, constipation, dental abnormalities, increased appetite, abdominal pain, diarrhea, anorexia, flatulence, gingivitis, glossitis, gum hemorrhage, thirst, stomatitis, taste loss, unusual taste, increased salivation, gastroenteritis, hemorrhoids, bloody stools, fecal incontinence, hepatomegaly. *CV:* Hypertension, vasodilation, hypotension, angina pectoris, peripheral vascular disorder, palpitation, tachycardia, migraine, murmur. *Musculoskeletal:* Myalgia, fracture, tendinitis, arthritis, joint stiffness or swelling, positive Romberg test. *Respiratory:* Rhinitis, pharyngitis, coughing, pneumonia, epistaxis, dyspnea, apnea. *Dermatologic:* Pruritus, abrasion, rash, acne, alopecia, eczema, dry skin, increased sweating, urticaria, hirsutism, seborrhea, cyst, herpes simplex. *Body as a whole:* Weight increase, back pain, peripheral edema, asthenia, facial edema, allergy, weight decrease, chills. *GU:* Hematuria, dysuria, frequent urination, cystitis, urinary retention, urinary incontinence, vaginal hemorrhage, amenorrhea, dysmenorrhea, menorrhagia, breast cancer, inability to climax, abnormal ejaculation, impotence. *Hematologic:* Leukopenia, decreased WBCs, purpura, anemia, thrombocytopenia, lymphadenopathy. *Ophthalmologic:* Diplopia, amblyopia, abnormal vision, cataract, conjunctivitis, dry eyes, eye pain, visual field defect, photophobia, bilateral or unilateral ptosis, eye hemorrhage, hordeolum, eye twitching. *Otic:* Hearing loss, earache, tinnitus, inner ear infection, otitis, ear fullness.
Laboratory Test Considerations: False + reading with Ames N-Multistix SG dipstick test for urinary protein.
OD Management of Overdose: *Symptoms:* Double vision, slurred speech, drowsiness, lethargy, diarrhea. *Treatment:* Hemodialysis.
Drug Interactions
Antacids / Antacids ↓ bioavailability of gabapentin
Cimetidine / Cimetidine ↓ renal excretion of gabapentin
How Supplied: *Capsule:* 100 mg, 300 mg, 400 mg

Dosage

- **Capsules**

Anticonvulsant.

Adults: Dose range of 900–1,800 mg/day in three divided doses. Titration to an effective dose can begin on day 1 with 300 mg followed by 300 mg b.i.d. on day 2 and 300 mg t.i.d. on day 3. If necessary, the dose may be increased to 300–400 mg t.i.d., up to 1,800 mg/day. In clients with a C_{CR} of 30–60 mL/min, the dose is 300 mg b.i.d.; if the C_{CR} is 15–30 mL/min, the dose is 300 mg/day; if the C_{CR} is less than 15 mL/min, the dose is 300 mg every other day.

HEALTH CARE CONSIDERATIONS

See also *Health Care Considerations* for *Anticonvulsants*.

Administration/Storage

1. Do not exceed 12 hr between doses using the t.i.d. daily regimen.
2. If gabapentin is discontinued or an alternate anticonvulsant is added to the regimen, do gradually over a 1-week period.
3. The first dose on day 1 may be taken at bedtime to minimize somnolence, dizziness, fatigue, and ataxia.

Assessment

1. Record type and onset of symptoms, any other agents prescribed, and the outcome.
2. List other drugs prescribed to ensure that none interact unfavorably.
3. Obtain baseline renal function studies; reduce dose in the elderly and with impaired renal function.
4. When drug therapy is discontinued or supplemental therapy is added, do so gradually over at least 1 week.

Client/Family Teaching
1. May be taken with or without food. Do not stop abruptly.
2. Avoid antacids 1 hr before or 2 hr after taking drug.
3. Drug may cause dizziness, fatigue, drowsiness, ataxia, and nystagmus. Do not perform any activities that require mental alertness until full drug effects are realized.
4. Report any new/unusual S&S.

Outcome/Evaluate
- Control of seizure activity
- Chronic pain control

Ganciclovir sodium (DHPG)

(gan-**SYE**-kloh-veer)
Pregnancy Category: C
Cytovene, Vitrasert **(Rx)**
Classification: Antiviral

See also *Antiviral Agents.*
Action/Kinetics: Upon entry into viral cells infected by CMV, ganciclovir is converted to ganciclovir triphosphate by the CMV. Ganciclovir triphosphate inhibits viral DNA synthesis by competitive inhibition of viral DNA polymerases and direct incorporation into viral DNA; this results in eventual termination of viral DNA elongation. Ganciclovir is active against CMV, herpes simplex virus-1 and -2, Epstein-Barr virus, and varicella zoster virus. Use of the intraocular implant causes a significantly slower disease progression than did those treated with IV ganciclovir. **t½:** Approximately 2.9 hr. Believed to cross the blood-brain barrier. Most excreted unchanged through the urine. Renal impairment increases the t½ of the drug; make dosage adjustments based on C_{CR}.
Uses: IV: Immunocompromised clients with CMV retinitis, including AIDS clients. Diagnosis may be confirmed by culture of CMV from the blood, urine, or throat; note that a negative CMV culture does not rule out CMV retinitis. Prevention of CMV disease in transplant clients at risk; duration of treatment depends on duration and degree of immunosuppression. *Investigational:* Treatment of CMV infections (e.g., gastroenteritis, hepatitis, pneumonitis) in immunocompromised clients.

PO: Alternative to IV for maintenance treatment of CMV retinitis in immunocompromised (including AIDS) clients. Prevention of CMV disease in clients with advanced HIV infection at risk for developing CMV disease.

Intraocular implant: CMV retinitis in those with AIDS.

Contraindications: Hypersensitivity to acyclovir or ganciclovir. Lactation. Use when the absolute neutrophil count is less than 500/mm^3 or the platelet count is less than 25,000/mm^3.
Special Concerns: Safety and effectiveness of ganciclovir have not been established for nonimmunocompromised clients, treatment of other CMV infections such as pneumonitis or colitis, or congenital or neonatal CMV disease. Use with caution in impaired renal function, in elderly clients, or with preexisting cytopenias or with a history of cytopenic reactions to other drugs, chemicals, or irradiation. Use in children only if potential benefits outweigh potential risks, including carcinogenicity and reproductive toxicity. Not a cure for CMV retinitis and progression of the disease may continue in immunocompromised clients. Treatment with zidovudine and ganciclovir (e.g., in AIDS clients) will likely not be tolerated and lead to severe granulocytopenia.
Side Effects: *Hematologic:* Granulocytopenia, thrombocytopenia, neutropenia (may be irreversible), eosinophilia, leukopenia, anemia, hypochromic anemia, bone marrow depression, pancytopenia, ***leukemia, lymphoma***. *CNS:* Ataxia, ***coma,*** neuropathy, confusion, abnormal dreams or thoughts, dizziness, headache, paresthesia, psychosis, nervousness, somnolence, tremor, agitation, amnesia, anxiety, depression, euphoria, hypertonia, hypesthesia, insomnia, manic reaction, ***seizures,*** trismus, emotional lability. *GI:* N&V, aphthous stomatitis, diarrhea, anorexia, dry mouth, ***GI hemorrhage, pancreatitis,*** abdominal pain, flatulence, dyspepsia, constipation, dysphagia, esophagitis, eructation, fecal incontinence, melena, mouth ulceration, tongue disorder, hepatitis, weight loss. *CV:* Hypertension or hypotension, arrhythmias, phlebitis, deep thrombophlebitis, ***cardiac arrest, intracranial hypertension, MI, stroke,*** pericarditis, vasodilation, migraine. *Body as a whole:* Fever (most common), chills, edema, infections, malaise, ***sepsis, multiple organ failure,*** asthenia, enlarged abdomen, abscess, back pain, cellulitis, chest pain, facial edema, neck pain or rigidity. *Dermatologic:* Rash (most common), alopecia, pruritus, urticaria, sweating, acne, dry skin, fixed eruption, herpes simplex, maculopapular rash, skin discoloration, vesiculobullous rash, photosensitivity, phototoxicity. *GU:* Hematuria, breast pain, kidney failure, abnormal kidney function, urinary frequency, UTI. *At injection site:* Catheter infection, catheter sepsis, inflammation or pain, abscess, edema, hemorrhage, phle-

bitis. *Musculoskeletal:* Arthralgia, bone pain, leg cramps, myalgia, myasthenia. *Ophthalmologic:* Abnormal vision, amblyopia, blindness, conjunctivitis, eye pain, glaucoma, retinitis, photophobia, cataracts, vitreous disorder. *Respiratory:* Dyspnea, increased cough, pneumonia. *Hepatic:* Cholestasis, cholangitis. *Miscellaneous:* Abnormal gait, decreased libido, deafness, ***anaphylaxis,*** taste perversion, tinnitus, acidosis, congenital anomaly, encephalopathy, impotence, transverse myelitis, infertility, splenomegaly, ***Stevens-Johnson syndrome, unexplained death,*** retinal detachment in CMV retinitis clients.

G

Laboratory Test Considerations: ↑ or ↓ Serum creatinine. ↑ BUN, alkaline phosphatase, CPK, LDH, AST, ALT. ↓ Blood glucose. Abnormal LFT. Hypokalemia, hyponatremia.

OD **Management of Overdose:** *Symptoms:* Neutropenia. Possibility of hypersalivation, anorexia, vomiting, bloody diarrhea, inactivity, cytopenia, testicular atrophy, increased BUN and LFT results. *Treatment:* Hydration, hemodialysis.

Drug Interactions

Adriamycin / Additive cytotoxicity in rapidly dividing cells
Amphotericin B / Additive cytotoxicity in rapidly dividing cells; also, ↑ serum creatinine levels
Cyclosporine / ↑ Serum creatinine levels
Dapsone / Additive cytotoxicity in rapidly dividing cells
Flucytosine / Additive cytotoxicity in rapidly dividing cells
Imipenem/Cilastatin combination / Possibility of seizures
Pentamidine / Additive cytotoxicity in rapidly dividing cells
Probenecid / ↑ Effect of ganciclovir due to ↓ renal excretion
Sulfamethoxazole/Trimethoprim combinations / Additive cytotoxicity in rapidly dividing cells
Vinblastine / Additive cytotoxicity in rapidly dividing cells
Vincristine / Additive cytotoxicity in rapidly dividing cells
Zidovudine (AZT) / ↑ Risk of granulocytopenia and anemia

How Supplied: *Powder for injection:* 500 mg; *Capsules:* 250 mg, 500 mg; *Implant:* 4.5 mg

Dosage

- **IV Infusion, Capsules**

CMV retinitis.

Induction treatment: 5 mg/kg over 1 hr q 12 hr for 14–21 days in clients with normal renal function. Do not use PO treatment for induction. **Maintenance, IV:** 5 mg/kg over 1 hr by IV infusion daily for 7 days or 6 mg/kg/day for 5 days each week. Dosage must be reduced in clients with renal impairment. **Maintenance, PO:** 1,000 mg t.i.d. with food. Or, 500 mg 6 times/day q 3 hr with food during waking hours.

Prevention of CMV retinitis in those with advanced HIV infection and normal renal function.

1,000 mg t.i.d. with food.

Prophylaxis of CMV disease in transplant clients.

Initial dose, IV: 5 mg/kg over 1 hr q 12 hr for 7–14 days. **Maintenance:** 5 mg/kg/day on 7 days each week (or 6 mg/kg/day on 5 days each week).

HEALTH CARE CONSIDERATIONS

See also *Health Care Considerations* for *Antiviral Agents.*

Administration/Storage

1. Use capsules only for whom the risk of a more rapid progression of the disease is offset by the benefit of avoiding daily IV infusions.

Assessment

1. Record onset, duration of symptoms, and any treatments.
2. Determine CMV retinitis by indirect opthalmoscopy.
3. Assess orientation and mentation levels.
4. Monitor CBC and renal function studies; reduce dose with impaired renal function. Granulocytopenia and thrombocytopenia are side effects of drug therapy; do not administer if neutrophil count drops below 500 cells/mm^3 or the platelet count falls below 25,000/mm^3. Concomitant therapy with zidovudine may increase neutropenia.
5. Monitor I&O. Ensure adequate hydration before and during IV therapy.
6. May experience pain and/or phlebitis at infusion site because pH of *diluted* solution is high (pH 9–11). Follow administration guidelines carefully.
7. Review list of drug interactions as some may induce renal failure and have additive toxicity if given during ganciclovir therapy.

Client/Family Teaching

1. Drug is not a cure; is used to control symptoms.
2. Drug therapy should not be interrupted unless deemed necessary by provider; a relapse may occur.
3. Take PO ganciclovir with food to increase bioavailability.
4. Report any dizziness, confusion, and/or seizures immediately.
5. Use protection (sunglasses, clothing/hat,

sunscreen) with sun exposure to prevent photosensitivity reaction.
6. Report for scheduled labs; results may require adjustment of dose or discontinuation of therapy.
7. Have regular ophthalmologic examinations because retinitis may progress to blindness (retinal detachment). With intraocular implant identify side effects that require immediate reporting.
8. May impair fertility; determine if candidate for sperm/egg harvesting.
9. During and for 90 days following drug therapy, women of childbearing age should use safe contraception and men should practice barrier contraception.
10. Report any unusual behavior or altered thought processes.

Outcome/Evaluate

- CMV prophylaxis in transplant and at-risk clients
- ↓ Progression of CMV retinitis
- Prevention of CMV retinitis in those with advanced HIV infection

Ganirelix acetate

(gan-ih-REL-icks)
Pregnancy Category: X
Antagon **(Rx)**
Classification: Infertility drug

Action/Kinetics: Synthetic decapeptide that antagonizes gonadotropin-releasing hormone (GnRH). Acts by competitively blocking GnRH receptors in the pituitary gland leading to a rapid, reversible suppression of gonadotropin secretion. When discontinued, pituitary LH and FSH levels fully recover within 48 hr. **Steady state:** Within 3 days. Metabolized to peptides. Excreted in both the feces and urine. **t½, elimination:** 16.2 hr after multiple doses.

Uses: Infertility treatment to inhibit premature LH surges in women undergoing controlled ovarian stimulation.

Contraindications: Hypersensitivity to ganirelix or any of its components, hypersensitivity to GnRH or GnRH analogs, known or suspected pregnancy. Lactation.

Special Concerns: Use with caution in hypersensitivity to GnRH. Packaging of the product contains natural rubber latex, which may cause allergic reactions.

Side Effects: Abdominal pain (gynecological), fetal death, headache, ovarian hyperstimulation syndrome, vaginal bleeding, injection site reaction, nausea, abdominal pain (GI).

Laboratory Test Considerations: ↑ Neutrophils. ↓ Hematocrit, total bilirubin.

Drug Interactions: Because ganirelix suppresses secretion of pituitary gonadotropins, dosage adjustments of exogenous gonadotropins may be necessary when used during controlled ovarian hyperstimulation.

How Supplied: *Injection:* 250 mcg/0.5 mL

Dosage

- **Injection**

Infertility treatment.

Initiate FSH therapy on day 2 or 3 of the cycle (may reduce exogenous FSH requirement). Give ganirelix, 250 mcg, SC once daily during the early to mid follicular phase. Continue ganirelix treatment daily until the day of chorionic gonadotropion (HCG) treatment. When a sufficient number of follicles of adequate size are present (assess by ultrasound), give HCG to finalize maturation of follicles.

HEALTH CARE CONSIDERATIONS

Administration/Storage

1. The most convenient sites for SC administration are in the upper thigh or in the abdomen around the navel.
2. Swab the injection site with disinfectant. Clean about 2 inches around the point where the needle will be inserted. Let the disinfectant dry a minute or more before proceeding.
3. Pinch up a large area of skin between the finger and thumb. Insert the needle at the base of the pinched-up skin at a 45–90° angle to the skin surface.
4. When the needle is positioned correctly, it will be difficult to draw back on the plunger. If the needle tip penetrates a vein (if blood is drawn into the syringe), withdraw the needle slightly and reposition the needle without removing it from the skin. Alternatively, remove the needle and use a new, sterile, prefilled syringe.
5. Once the needle is positioned correctly, depress the plunger slowly and steadily so the solution is correctly injected and the skin is not damaged.
6. Pull the syringe out quickly and apply pressure to the site with a swab containing disinfectant; the site should stop bleeding within 1 or 2 min.
7. Use the sterile, prefilled syringe only once and dispose of it correctly.
8. Store the syringes at 25°C (77°F). Protect from light.

Assessment
1. Record indications for therapy, other medical conditions and duration of infertility.
2. Use cautiously in gonadotropin-releasing hormone (GnRH) hypersensitivity.
3. Ensure not pregnant.
4. Product packaging contains latex.

Client/Family Teaching
1. Therapy requires SC administration daily during early to mid follicular phases after initial FSH therapy or day 2 or 3 of cycle. It must be continued until day of HCG administration.
2. Follows guidelines for administration under administration/storage and/or review package insert for proper administration procedure.
3. An ultrasound is used to check for sufficient number and size of follicles.
4. May experience abdominal pain, fetal death, headache, ovarian hyperstimulation syndrome, vaginal bleeding, nausea and injection site pain.
5. Not for use in pregnancy as may cause fetal loss.
6. Therapy requires a long term committment for F/U and medical visits from user.

Outcome/Evaluate: Inhibition of premature LH surges during controlled ovarian stimulation; desired pregnancy

G

Gatifloxacin

(gat-ih-FLOX-ah-sin)
Pregnancy Category: C
Tequin **(Rx)**
Classification: Antibiotic, quinolone

See also *Anti-Infective Drugs*.

Action/Kinetics: Well absorbed after PO use. **Peak plasma levels:** 1–2 hr after PO. The PO and IV routes are interchangeable. Steady-state levels are reached by the third daily PO or IV dose. **Mean steady-state peak and trough plasma levels after 400 mg once daily:** About 4.2 mcg/mL and 0.4 mcg/mL, respectively after PO and 4.6 mcg/mL and 0.4 mcg/mL, respectively, after IV. Widely distributed throughout the body. **t½, PO:** 7.1 hr after multiple doses of 400 mg; **t½, IV:** 13.9 hr after multiple doses of 400 mg. Excreted primarily unchanged by the kidneys.

Uses: (1) Acute bacterial exacerbation of chronic bronchitis due to *Streptococcus pneumoniae, Haemophilus influenzae, Haemophilus parainfluenzae, Moraxella catarrhalis,* or *Staphylococcus aureus*. (2) Acute sinusitis due to *S. pneumoniae* or *H. influenzae*. (3) Community-acquired pneumonia due to *S. pneumoniae, H. influenze, H. parainfluenzae, M. catarrhalis, S. aureus, Mycoplasma pneumoniae, Chlamydia pneumoniae,* or *Legionella pneumoniae*. (4) Uncomplicated UTIs (cystitis) or complicated UTIs due to *Escherichia coli, Klebsiella pneumoniae,* or *Proteus mirabilis*. (5) Pyelonephritis due to *E. coli*. (6) Uncomplicated urethral and cervical gonorrhea due to *Neisseria gonorrhoeae*. (7) Acute, uncomplicated rectal infections due to *N. gonorrhoeae*.

Contraindications: Use with drugs that prolong the QTc interval, in clients with uncorrected hypokalemia, and in those receiving Class IA (e.g., quinidine, procainamide) or Class III (e.g., amiodarone, sotalol) antiarrhythmics.

Special Concerns: Reduce dosage in clients with a C_{CR} less than 40 mL/min, including those requiring hemodialysis or continuous ambulatory peritoneal dialysis. Use with caution with antidepressants, antipsychotics, cisapride, or erythromycin or in those with bradycardia or acute myocardial ischemia. Safety and efficacy in children, adolescents (less than 18 years of age), pregnant women, and lactating women have not been established.

Side Effects: *CNS:* Tremors, restlessness, lightheadedness, confusion, hallucinations, paranoia, depression, nightmares, insomnia, paresthesia, vertigo. *GI:* Abdominal pain, constipation, dyspepsia, glossitis, oral moniliaisis, stomatitis, mouth ulcer, vomiting, pseudomembranous colitis, hepatitis, jaundice, ***acute hepatic necrosis or failure.*** *Body as a whole:* Fever, chills, back pain, chest pain. *CV:* Vasculitis, palpitation, vasodilation. *Respiratory:* Dyspnea, pharyngitis, allergic pneumonitis. *Hypersensitivity:* ***Anaphylaxis, CV collapse, angioedema, acute respiratory distress, bronchospasm, shock,*** hypotension, seizure, loss of consciousness, tingling, shortness of breath, dyspnea, urticaria, itching, serious skin reactions. *Hematologic:* Hemolytic or aplastic anemia, thrombotic thrombocytopenic purpura, leukopenia, agranulocytosis, pancytopenia. *Dermatologic:* Rash, sweating, ***toxic epidermal necrolysis, Stevens-Johnson syndrome.*** *Musculoskeletal:* Arthralgia, myalgia. *GU:* Dysuria, hematuria, interstitial nephritis, acute renal insufficiency or failure. *Miscellaneous:* Serum sickness, peripheral edema, abnormal vision, taste perversion, tinnitus.

Laboratory Test Considerations: Hyper- or hypoglycemia, especially in diabetics receiving an oral hypoglycemic or insulin.

Drug Interactions
Aluminum- or magnesium-containing antacids / ↓ Absorption of gatifloxacin
Digoxin / ↑ Risk of digoxin toxicity

Ferrous sulfate / ↓ Bioavailability of gatifloxacin
NSAIDs / ↑ Risk of CNS stimulation and convulsions
Probenecid / ↓ Bioavailability of gatifloxacin
How Supplied: *IV Solution:* 10 mg/mL; *IV Solution, Premix Bags:* 2 mg/mL; *Tablets:* 200 mg, 400 mg

Dosage

- **IV infusion, Tablets**

Acute bacterial exacerbation of chronic bronchitis, complicated UTIs, acute pyelonephritis.
Adults: 400 mg once daily for 7–10 days.
Acute sinusitis.
Adults: 400 mg once daily for 10 days.
Community-acquired pneumonia.
Adults: 400 mg once daily for 7–14 days.
Uncomplicated UTIs (cystitis).
Adults: 400 mg as a single dose or 200 mg daily for 3 days.
Uncomplicated urethral gonorrhea in men, endocervical and rectal gonorrhea in women.
Single dose of 400 mg.

Adjust dosage as follows in clients with impaired renal function. **C_{CR} less than 40 mL/min: Initial,** 400 mg; **then,** 200 mg every day. **Hemodialysis: Initial,** 400 mg; **then,** 200 mg every day. **Continuous peritoneal dialysis: Initial,** 400 mg; **then,** 200 mg every day.

HEALTH CARE CONSIDERATIONS

See also *Health Care Considerations* for *Anti-Infective Drugs.*

Administration/Storage

IV 1. Give by IV infusion over 60 min. Not to be given IM, IP, SC, or intrathecally.
2. No dosage adjustment is needed when switching from IV to PO.

Assessment

1. Note indications for therapy, onset and characteristics of symptoms.
2. Assess for sensitivity to quinolones.
3. Note any congenital prolongation of the QTc interval.
4. Determine if prescribed therapy for heart rhythm disturbance.
5. Assess electrolytes; avoid with hypokalemia and report if taking diuretics.

Client/Family Teaching

1. Take as directed once daily at the same time each day.
2. Can take without regard for food, including milk and calcium-containing dietary supplements.
3. Take at least 4 hr before the administration of ferrous sulfate; dietary supplements containing zinc, magnesium, or iron; aluminum/magnesium-containing antacids; or didanosine buffered tablets, buffered solution, or buffered powder for oral suspension.
4. Complete prescription despite feeling better; report if S&S do not improve with therapy.
5. Avoid activities that require mental alertness until drug effects realized.
6. May cause GI upset, dizziness, and headaches.
7. Report any heart palpitations or fainting spells immediately.
8. Use reliable birth control.
9. Store away from children in a tightly sealed container at room temperature.

Outcome/Evaluate: Resolution of infection; symptomatic improvement

Gemfibrozil

(jem-**FIH**-broh-zill)
Pregnancy Category: B
Apo-Gemfibrozil ✦, Gen-Fibro ✦, Gemcor, Lopid, Novo-Gemfibrozil ✦, Nu-Gemfibrozil ✦, PMS-Gemfibrozil ✦ **(Rx)**
Classification: Antihyperlipidemic

Action/Kinetics: Gemfibrozil, which resembles clofibrate, decreases triglycerides, cholesterol, and VLDL and increases HDL; LDL levels either decrease or do not change. Also, decreases hepatic triglyceride production by inhibiting peripheral lipolysis and decreasing extraction of free fatty acids by the liver. Also, gemfibrozil decreases VLDL synthesis by inhibiting synthesis of VLDL carrier apolipoprotein B as well as inhibits peripheral lipolysis and decreases hepatic extraction of free fatty acids (thus decreasing hepatic triglyceride production). May be beneficial in inhibiting development of atherosclerosis. **Onset:** 2–5 days. **Peak plasma levels:** 1–2 hr; **t½:** 1.5 hr. Nearly 70% is excreted unchanged.
Uses: Hypertriglyceridemia (type IV and type V hyperlipidemia) unresponsive to dietary control or in clients who are at risk of pancreatitis and abdominal pain. Reduce risk of coronary heart disease in clients with type IIb hyperlipidemia who have not responded to diet, weight loss, exercise, and other drug therapy.
Contraindications: Gallbladder disease, primary biliary cirrhosis, hepatic or renal dysfunction.

Special Concerns: Use with caution during lactation. Safety and efficacy have not been established in children. The dose may have to be reduced in geriatric clients due to age-related decreases in renal function.

Side Effects: *GI:* Cholelithiasis, abdominal or epigastric pain, N&V, diarrhea, dyspepsia, constipation, acute appendicitis, colitis, pancreatitis, cholestatic jaundice, hepatoma. *CNS:* Dizziness, headache, fatigue, vertigo, somnolence, paresthesia, hypesthesia, depression, confusion, syncope, ***seizures.*** *CV:* Atrial fibrillation, extrasystole, peripheral vascular disease, ***intracerebral hemorrhage.*** *Hematopoietic:* Anemia, leukopenia, eosinophilia, thrombocytopenia, bone marrow hypoplasia. *Musculoskeletal:* Painful extremities, arthralgia, myalgia, myopathy, myasthenia, rhabdomyolysis, synovitis. *Allergic:* Urticaria, lupus-like syndrome, angioedema, ***laryngeal edema,*** vasculitis, ***anaphylaxis.*** *Dermatologic:* Eczema, dermatitis, pruritus, skin rashes, exfoliative dermatitis, alopecia. *Ophthalmic:* Blurred vision, retinal edema, cataracts. *Miscellaneous:* Increased chance of viral and bacterial infections, taste perversion, impotence, decreased male fertility, weight loss.

Laboratory Test Considerations: ↑ AST, ALT, LDH, CPK, alkaline phosphatase, bilirubin. Hypokalemia. Positive antinuclear antibody. ↓ Hemoglobin, WBCs, hematocrit.

Drug Interactions

Anticoagulants, oral / ↑ Effect of anticoagulants; dosage adjustment necessary
Lovastatin / Possible rhabdomyolysis
Simvastatin / Possible rhabdomyolysis

How Supplied: *Tablet:* 600 mg

Dosage

- **Tablets**

Adults: 600 mg b.i.d. 30 min before the morning and evening meal. Dosage has not been established in children. Discontinue if significant improvement not observed within 3 months.

HEALTH CARE CONSIDERATIONS

See also *Health Care Considerations* for *Clofibrate.*

Assessment

1. Record serum levels and note any previous therapy utilized. (Drug usually reserved until triglycerides greater than 500 mg/dL.)
2. Assess compliance with therapeutic regimens and life-style changes including restriction of fat in diet, weight reduction, regular exercise, and avoidance of alcohol.

Client/Family Teaching

1. Take 30 min before meals.
2. Take as directed; continue to follow prescribed dietary guidelines and regular exercise program.
3. Use caution when driving or performing other dangerous tasks until drug effects realized; may experience dizziness or blurred vision.
4. Report any unusual bruising or bleeding. If also on anticoagulant therapy, a reduction in anticoagulant is indicated with this therapy.
5. Limit intake of alcohol.
6. Report any RUQ abdominal pain or change in stool color or consistency.
7. Report any S&S of gallstones, such as abdominal pain and vomiting.

Outcome/Evaluate: ↓ Serum cholesterol and triglyceride levels

Gentamicin sulfate

(jen-tah-**MY**-sin)

Pregnancy Category: C

Alcomicin ✦, Cidomycin ✦, Diogent ✦, Garamycin, Garamycin Cream or Ointment, Garamycin IV Piggyback, Garamycin Ophthalmic Ointment, Garamycin Ophthalmic Solution, Garatec ✦, Genoptic Ophthalmic Liquifilm, Genoptic S.O.P. Ophthalmic, Gentacidin Ophthalmic, Gentafair, Gentak Ophthalmic, Gentamicin, Gentamicin Ophthalmic, Gentamicin Sulfate IV Piggyback, Gentrasul Ophthalmic, G-myticin Cream or Ointment, Minims Gentamcin ✦, Ocugram ✦, Ophtagram ✦, Pediatric Gentamicin Sulfate, PMS-Gentamicin Sulfate ✦, Sckeinpharm Gentamicin ✦ **(Rx)**

Classification: Antibiotic, aminoglycoside

See also *Aminoglycosides.*

Action/Kinetics: Therapeutic serum levels: IM, 4–8 mcg/mL. **Toxic serum levels:** >12 mcg/mL (peak) and >2 mcg/mL (trough). Prolonged serum levels above 12 mcg/mL should be avoided. **t½:** 2 hr. Can be used with carbenicillin to treat serious *Pseudomonas* infections; do not mix these drugs in the same flask as carbenicillin will inactivate gentamicin.

Uses: Systemic: Serious infections caused by *Pseudomonas aeruginosa, Proteus, Klebsiella, Enterobacter, Serratia, Citrobacter,* and *Staphylococcus.* Infections include bacterial neonatal sepsis, bacterial septicemia, and serious infections of the skin, bone, soft tissue (including burns), urinary tract, GI tract (including peritonitis), and CNS (including meningitis). Should be considered as initial therapy in suspected or confirmed gram-negative infections. In combination with carbenicillin for treating life-threatening infections due to *P. aeruginosa*. In combination with penicillin for treating endocarditis caused by group D streptococci. In combination with penicillin for treating suspected bacterial sepsis or staphylococcal pneumonia in the neonate. Intrathecal administration is used in combination with systemic gentamicin for treating meningitis, ventriculitis, or other serious CNS infections due to *Pseudomonas*. *Investigational:* Pelvic inflammatory disease.

Ophthalmic: Ophthalmic infections due to *Staphylococcus, S. aureus, Streptococcus pneumoniae,* beta-hemolytic streptococci, *Corynebacterium* species, *Streptococcus pyogenes, Escherichia coli, Haemophilus influenzae, H. aegyptius, H. ducreyi, Klebsiella pneumoniae, Neisseria gonorrhoeae, Proteus* species, *Acinetobacter calcoaceticus, Enterobacter aerogenes, P. aeruginosa, Serratia marcescens, Moraxella lacunata.*

Topical: Prevention of infections following minor cuts, wounds, burns, and skin abrasions. Treatment of primary or secondary skin infections. Treatment of infected skin cysts and other skin abscesses when preceded by incision and drainage to permit adequate contact between the drug and the infecting bacteria, infected stasis and other skin ulcers, infected superficial burns, paronychia, infected insect bites and stings, infected lacerations and abrasions and wounds from minor surgery.

Contraindications: Ophthalmic use to treat dendritic keratitis, vaccinia, varicella, mycobacterial infections of the eye, fungal diseases of the eye, use with steroids after uncomplicated removal of a corneal foreign body.

Special Concerns: Use with caution in premature infants and neonates. Ophthalmic ointments may retard corneal epithelial healing.

Additional Side Effects: Muscle twitching, numbness, ***seizures,*** increased BP, alopecia, purpura, pseudotumor cerebri. Photosensitivity when used topically. *After ophthalmic use:* Transient irritation, burning, stinging, itching, inflammation, angioneurotic edema, urticaria, vesicular and maculopapular dermatitis, mydriasis, conjunctival paresthesia, conjunctival hyperemia, nonspecific conjunctivitis, conjunctival epithelial defects, lid itching and swelling, bacterial/fungal corneal ulcers.

Additional Drug Interactions: With carbenicillin or ticarcillin, gentamicin may result in increased effect when used for *Pseudomonas* infections.

How Supplied: *Cream:* 0.1%; *Injection:* 10 mg/mL, 40 mg/mL; *Ointment:* 1%; *Ophthalmic ointment:* 3 mg/g; *Ophthalmic Solution:* 3 mg/mL

Dosage

- **IM (usual), IV**

Adults with normal renal function.

Infections.

1 mg/kg q 8 hr, up to 5 mg/kg/day in life-threatening infections; **children:** 2–2.5 mg/kg q 8 hr; **infants and neonates:** 2.5 mg/kg q 8 hr; **premature infants or neonates less than 1 week of age:** 2.5 mg/kg q 12 hr. Therapy may be required for 7–10 days.

Prevention of bacterial endocarditis, dental or respiratory tract procedures.

Adults: 1.5 mg/kg gentamicin (not to exceed 80 mg) plus 1 g ampicillin, each IM or IV, 30–60 min before the procedure; one additional dose of each can be given 8 hr later (alternative: penicillin V, 1 g PO, 6 hr after initial dose).

Prophylaxis of bacterial endocarditis in GI or GU tract procedures or surgery.

Adults: 1.5 mg/kg gentamicin (not to exceed 80 mg) plus 2 g ampicillin, each IM or IV, 30–60 min before procedure; dose should be repeated 8 hr later. **Children:** 2 mg/kg gentamicin plus penicillin G, 30,000 units/kg, or ampicillin, 50 mg/kg in same dosage interval as for adults. Pediatric dosage should not exceed single or 24-hr adult doses.

NOTE: In clients allergic to penicillin, vancomycin, 1 g IV given slowly over 1 hr, may be substituted; the dose of vancomycin should be repeated 8–12 hr later. **Adults with impaired renal function:** To calculate interval (hr) between doses, multiply serum creatinine level (mg/100 mL) by 8.

- **IV**

Septicemia.

Initially: 1–2 mg/kg infused over 30–60 min; **then,** maintenance doses may be administered.

- **Intrathecal**

Meningitis.

Use only the intrathecal preparation. Adults, usual: 4–8 mg/day; **children and infants 3 months and older:** 1–2 mg/day

Pelvic inflammatory disease.

Initial: 2 mg/kg IV; **then,** 1.5 mg/kg t.i.d. plus clindamycin, 500 mg IV q.i.d. Continue for at least 4 days and at least 48 hr after client improves. Continue clindamycin, 450 mg PO q.i.d. for 10–14 days.

- **Ophthalmic Solution (0.3%)**

Acute infections.

Initially: 1–2 gtt in conjunctival sac q 15–30 min; **then,** as infection improves, reduce frequency.

Moderate infections.

1–2 gtt in conjunctival sac 4–6 times/day.

Trachoma.

2 gtt in each eye b.i.d.–q.i.d.; treatment should be continued for up to 1–2 months.

• **Ophthalmic Ointment (0.3%)**

Depending on the severity of infection, ½-in. ribbon from q 3–4 hr to 2–3 times/day.

• **Topical Cream/Ointment (0.1%)**

Apply 3–4 times/day to affected area. The area may be covered with a sterile bandage.

G

HEALTH CARE CONSIDERATIONS

See also *Health Care Considerations* for *Aminoglycosides.*

Administration/Storage

1. When used intrathecally, the usual site is the lumbar area.

IV 2. For intermittent IV administration, dilute adult dose in 50–200 mL of NSS or D5W and administer over a 30–120-min period; use less volume for infants and children.

3. Do not mix with other drugs for parenteral use.

4. For parenteral use, the duration of treatment is 7–10 days; a longer course may be required for severe or complicated infections.

Assessment

1. Record type, duration, and onset of symptoms.

2. Obtain renal function studies and appropriate specimen for culture.

3. With eye disorders, note baseline ophthalmologic assessments.

4. Assess for tinnitus, vertigo, or hearing losses during therapy. Persistently increased gentamycin levels have been associated with 8th CN dysfunction.

Client/Family Teaching

1. Review the appropriate method and frequency for administration. Wash hands before and after treatment; prepare site and apply as directed.

2. With topical administration:

• Remove crusts of impetigo contagiosa before applying the cream or ointment to permit maximum contact between antibiotic and infection.

• Apply cream or ointment gently and cover with gauze dressing if desirable or as ordered.

• Avoid direct exposure to sunlight as photosensitivity reaction may occur.

• Avoid further contamination of infected skin.

3. Identify symptoms and wound changes that require medical attention; i.e., pain, redness, swelling, increased drainage or odor.

4. Report any evidence of visual impairment, vertigo, dizziness, hearing impairment, or worsening of symptoms.

5. Avoid vaccinia during treatment.

Outcome/Evaluate

• Resolution of infection

• Therapeutic serum drug levels 4–8 mcg/mL; (peak 5–10 mcg/mL trough 1–2 mcg/mL)

Glatiramer acetate

(glah-TER-ah-mer)

Pregnancy Category: B

Copaxone **(Rx)**

Classification: Drug for multiple sclerosis

Action/Kinetics: May act by modifying immune processes responsible for pathology of multiple sclerosis. Some of drug enters lymphatic circulation reaching regional lymph nodes.

Uses: Reduce frequency of relapsing-remitting multiple sclerosis.

Contraindications: Hypersensitivity to glatiramer or mannitol.

Special Concerns: Use with caution during lactation. Safety and efficacy have not been determined in children less than 18 years of age. May interfere with useful immune function.

Side Effects: Side effects listed are those with incidence of 1% or more. *Immediate-post injection reaction:* Flushing, chest pain, palpitations, anxiety, dyspnea, laryngeal constriction, urticaria. *CNS:* Anxiety, hypertonia, tremor, vertigo, agitation, foot drop, nervousness, nystagmus, speech disorder, confusion, abnormal dreams, emotional lability, stupor, migraine. *GI:* Nausea, diarrhea, anorexia, vomiting, GI disorder, abdominal pain, gastroenteritis, bowel urgency, oral moniliasis, salivary gland enlargement, tooth caries, ulcerative stomatitis. *CV:* Vasodilation, palpitations, tachycardia, syncope, hypertension. *Body as a whole:* Infection, asthenia, pain, transient chest pain, flu syndrome, back pain, fever, neck pain, face edema, bacterial infection, chills, cyst, headache, injection site ecchymosis, accidental injury, neck rigidity, malaise, injection site edema or atrophy, abscess, peripheral edema, edema, weight gain. *Dermatologic:* Rash, pruritus, sweating, herpes simplex, erythema, urticaria, skin nodule, eczema, herpes zoster, pustular rash, skin atrophy and warts. *GU:* Urinary urgency, vaginal monoliasis, dysmenorrhea, amenorrhea, hematuria, impotence, menorrhagia, suspicious Pap smear, vaginal hemorrhage. *Hematologic:* Ecchymosis, lymphadenopathy. *Respiratory:* Dyspnea, allergic rhinitis, bronchitis, laryngismus, hyperventilation. *At injection site:* Pain, erythema, inflammation,

pruritus, mass, induration, welt, hemorrhage, urticaria. *Miscellaneous:* Ear pain, eye disorder, arthralgia.
How Supplied: *Powder for Injection:* 20 mg

Dosage
• **SC**
Multiple sclerosis.
Adults: 20 mg/day SC.

HEALTH CARE CONSIDERATIONS

Administration/Storage
1. SC sites include arms, abdomen, hips, and thighs.
2. Reconstitute with diluent provided (sterile water for injection). Gently swirl vial after diluent is added. Let stand at room temperature until solid material is dissolved.
3. Use reconstituted drug immediately as it contains no preservative. Before reconstitution store at 2°C–8°C (36°F–46°F).
Assessment
1. Record age at onset, frequency of exacerbations, degree of physical disability, and other treatments.
2. RRMS is characterized by recurrent attacks of neurologic dysfunction followed by complete or incomplete recovery; assess frequency.
Client/Family Teaching
1. Use exactly as directed, do not stop without consulting provider.
2. Reconstitute with diluent provided and gently swirl vial. Let stand at room temperature until solid material is dissolved. Administer SC into arms, abdomen, hips or thighs, rotating sites.
3. Patient Information booklet is enclosed with drug for review of self–injection procedure.
4. Drug is used to slow accumulation of physical disablilty and to decrease frequency of clinical exacerbations with MS.
5. May experience pain, itching, swelling, and hardening of skin at injection site.
6. Chest tightness, flushing, SOB, and anxiety may occur within minutes of injection and last up to 30 min.
7. Practice reliable contraception.
Outcome/Evaluate: ↓ Frequency and severity of MS exacerbations

Glimepiride

(GLYE-meh-pye-ride)
Pregnancy Category: C
Amaryl **(Rx)**
Classification: Antidiabetic agent, sulfonylurea

Action/Kinetics: Lowers blood glucose by stimulating the release of insulin from functioning pancreatic beta cells and by increasing the sensitivity of peripheral tissues to insulin. Completely absorbed from the GI tract within 1 hr. **Time to maximum effect:** 2–3 hr. Completely metabolized in the liver and metabolites are excreted through both the urine and feces.
Uses: As an adjunct to diet and exercise to lower blood glucose in non-insulin-dependent diabetes mellitus (Type II diabetes mellitus). In combination with insulin to decrease blood glucose in those whose hyperglycemia cannot be controlled by diet and exercise in combination with an oral hypoglycemic drug.
Contraindications: Diabetic ketoacidosis with or without coma. Use during lactation.
Special Concerns: The use of oral hypoglycemic drugs has been associated with increased CV mortality compared with treatment with diet alone or diet plus insulin. Safety and efficacy have not been determined in children.
Side Effects: The most common side effect is hypoglycemia. *GI:* N&V, GI pain, diarrhea, cholestatic jaundice (rare). *CNS:* Dizziness, headache. *Dermatologic:* Pruritus, erythema, urticaria, morbilliform or maculopapular eruptions. *Hematologic:* Leukopenia, agranulocytosis, thrombocytopenia, hemolytic anemia, aplastic anemia, pancytopenia. *Miscellaneous:* Hyponatremia, increased release of ADH, changes in accommodation and/or blurred vision.
Drug Interactions: See *Hypoglycemic Agents.*
How Supplied: *Tablet:* 1 mg, 2 mg, 4 mg

Dosage
• **Tablets**
Non-insulin-dependent diabetes mellitus (Type II diabetes).
Adults, initial: 1–2 mg once daily, given with breakfast or the first main meal. The initial dose should be 1 mg in those sensitive to hypoglycemic drugs, in those with impaired renal or hepatic function, and in elderly, debilitated, or malnourished clients. The maximum initial dose is 2 mg or less daily. **Maintenance:** 1–4 mg once daily up to a maximum of 8 mg once daily. After a dose of 2 mg is reached, increase the dose in increments of 2 mg or less at 1- to 2-week intervals (determined by the blood glucose response). **When combined with insulin therapy:** 8 mg once daily with the first main meal with low-dose insulin. The fasting glucose level for beginning combination thera-

G

py is greater than 150 mg/dL glucose in the plasma or serum.

Type II diabetes—transfer from other hypoglycemic agents
When transferring clients to glimipiride, no transition period is required. However, observe clients closely for 1 to 2 weeks for hypoglycemia when being transferred from longer half-life sulfonylureas (e.g., chlorpropamide) to glimepiride.

HEALTH CARE CONSIDERATIONS

G

Administration/Storage
1. Dispense tablets in well-closed containers with safety caps.
2. Store tablets at 15°C–30°C (59°F–86°F).

Assessment
1. Note indications for therapy, if newly diagnosed or transferred therapy; onset and duration of disease.
2. List drugs currently taking to ensure none interact unfavorably.
3. Obtain baseline labs, including electrolytes, HbA1c, Ca, Mg, urinalysis, liver and renal function studies.

Client/Family Teaching
1. Review dose and frequency for administration.
2. Monitor finger sticks.
3. Continue regular exercise and dietary restrictions in addition to drug therapy.
4. Report as scheduled for teaching reinforcement, follow-up labs, foot exams, and medication evaluation.

Outcome/Evaluate: Blood sugar and HbA1c within desired range

Glipizide
(GLIP-ih-zyd)
Pregnancy Category: C
Glucotrol, Glucotrol XL **(Rx)**
Classification: Sulfonylurea (anti-diabetic), second-generation

See also *Antidiabetic Agents.*
Action/Kinetics: Also has mild diuretic effects. **Onset:** 1–1.5 hr. **t½:** 2–4 hr. **Time to peak levels:** 1–3 hr. **Duration:** 10–16 hr. Metabolized in liver to inactive metabolites, which are excreted through the kidneys.
Uses: Adjunct to diet for control of hyperglycemia in clients with non-insulin-dependent diabetes.
Additional Drug Interactions: Cimetidine may ↑ effect of glipizide due to ↓ breakdown by liver.
How Supplied: *Tablet:* 5 mg, 10 mg; *Tablet, Extended Release:* 5 mg, 10 mg

Dosage
- **Tablets, Extended Release Tablets**
  Diabetes.

Adults, initial: 5 mg 30 min before breakfast; **then,** adjust dosage by 2.5–5 mg every few days, depending on the blood glucose response, until adequate control is achieved. **Maintenance:** 15–40 mg/day. Older clients should begin with 2.5 mg. The Extended Release Tablets are taken once daily (usually at breakfast) in doses of either 5 or 10 mg.

HEALTH CARE CONSIDERATIONS

See also *Health Care Considerations* for *Antidiabetic Agents.*

Administration/Storage
1. Some clients are better controlled on once daily dosing while others are better controlled with divided dosing.
2. Divide maintenance doses greater than 15 mg/day; give before the morning and evening meals. Total daily doses of 30 mg or more may be given safely on twice daily dosing.
3. Assess life-style to ensure that maximal changes in the areas of diet and exercise have been taken before increasing dosage. Once maximum dosage attained, if renal function is normal, consider adding Metformin to decrease production and absorption of gluocose if hyperglycemia is not controlled.

Client/Family Teaching
1. For greatest effect, take 30 min before meals.
2. Report any CNS side effects such as drowsiness or headache; differentiate from hypoglycemia.
3. May experience anorexia, constipation or diarrhea, vomiting, and gastralgia. If severe, record weight, I&O and report.
4. Skin reactions may occur and should be reported. Avoid sun exposure; use sunscreen, sunglasses and protective clothing when out.
5. Avoid alcohol in any form.
6. Practice barrier contraception.
7. Continue prescribed diet and regular exercise program. Monitor fingersticks; report loss of control.

Outcome/Evaluate: BS and HbA1c within desired range

Glucagon
(GLOO-kah-gon)
Pregnancy Category: B
(Rx)
Classification: Insulin antagonist

Action/Kinetics: Produced by the alpha islet cells of the pancreas, glucacon accelerates liver glycogenolysis by stimulating synthesis of cyclic AMP and increasing phosphorylase kinase activity. Increased blood glucose levels result from increased breakdown of glycogen to glucose and inhibition of glycogen synthetase. Glucagon stimulates hepatic gluconeogenesis by increasing the uptake of amino acids and converting them to glucose precursors. Also, lipolysis is increased, resulting in free fatty acids and glycerol for gluconeogenesis. Effective in overcoming hypoglycemia only if the liver has a glycogen reserve. Also relaxes smooth muscle of the GI tract and decreases gastric and pancreatic secretions; increases myocardial contractility. **Onset, hypoglycemia:** 5–20 min. **Maximum effect:** 30 min. **Duration:** 1–2 hr. **t½, plasma:** 3–6 min. Metabolized in the liver, kidney, plasma membrane receptor sites, and plasma.

Uses: Used to terminate insulin-induced shock in diabetic or psychiatric clients. Client usually regains consciousness 5–20 min after the parenteral administration of glucagon. The drug should only be used under medical supervision or in accordance with strict instructions received from the physician. Failure to respond may be an indication for IV administration of glucose—especially true in juvenile diabetics. As a diagnostic aid in radiologic examination of the GI tract when a hypotonic state is desirable. *Investigational:* Treatment of propranolol overdose and cardiovascular emergencies.

Special Concerns: Use with caution during lactation, in clients with renal or hepatic disease, in those who are undernourished and emaciated, and in clients with a history of pheochromocytoma or insulinoma.

Side Effects: *GI:* N&V. *Allergy:* Respiratory distress, urticaria, hypotension. ***Stevens-Johnson syndrome when used as diagnostic aid.***

OD **Management of Overdose:** *Symptoms:* N&V, hypokalemia. *Treatment:* Symptomatic.

Drug Interactions

Anticoagulants, oral / ↑ Effect of anticoagulants by ↑ hypoprothrombinemia

Antidiabetic agents / Hyperglycemic effect of glucagon antagonizes hypoglycemic effect of antidiabetics

Corticosteroids, Epinephrine, Estrogens, Phenytoin / Additive hyperglycemic effect of drugs listed

How Supplied: *Powder for injection:* 1 mg

Dosage

- **IM, IV, SC**

Hypoglycemia.

Children < 20 kg: 0.5 mg; **Adults and children > 20 kg:** 1 mg; one to two additional doses may be given at 20-min intervals, if necessary.

Insulin shock therapy.

IM, IV, SC: 0.5–1 mg after 1 hr of coma; the client will usually awaken in 10–25 min. The dose may be repeated if there is no response.

Diagnostic aid for GI tract.

Dose dependent on desired onset of action and duration of effect necessary for the examination. **IV:** 0.25–0.5 mg (onset: 1 min; duration: 9–17 min); 2 mg (onset: 1 min; duration 22–25 min). **IM:** 1 mg (onset: 8–10 min; duration: 12–27 min); 2 mg (onset: 4–7 min; duration: 21–32 min).

For colon examination.

IM: 2 mg 10 min prior to procedure.

Treatment of toxicity of beta-adrenergic blocking agents.

Adults, IV, initial: 2–3 mg given over 30 sec; may be repeated at the rate of 5 mg/hr until client is stabilized.

HEALTH CARE CONSIDERATIONS

Administration/Storage

1. Once client with hypoglycemia responds, give supplemental carbohydrates to prevent secondary hypoglycemia.

IV 2. Before reconstituting, store powder at room temperature.

3. Following reconstitution, use the solution immediately. If necessary, the solution may be stored at 5°C (41°F) for up to 2 days.

4. Reconstitute doses higher than 2 mg with sterile water for injection and use immediately.

5. With direct IV administration, inject at a rate not exceeding 1 mg/min.

6. Administer with dextrose solutions. A precipitate may form if saline solutions are used.

Client/Family Teaching

1. Instruct family in the administration of glucagon SC or IM in the event of hypoglycemic reaction, loss of consciousness, or inability to swallow.

2. Following administration of glucagon, keep client on their side and administer a CHO once awake.

3. Have rapidly available sugar, such as orange juice and Karo syrup in water (or life savers) to administer. If the shock was caused by a long-acting medication, administer slowly di-

gestible carbohydrates, such as bread with honey.
4. Do not try to administer fluids by mouth if client has a reaction and is not fully conscious; could aspirate fluids into lungs.
5. Record time of day and activity and report all hypoglycemic reactions so that insulin dosage can be adjusted.

Outcome/Evaluate
- Reversal of S&S of hypoglycemia
- Termination of insulin-induced shock
- Inhibition of bowel peristalsis with small muscle relaxation during radiologic imaging of the GI tract

G

Glyburide

(GLYE-byou-ryd)
Pregnancy Category: B
Albert Glyburide ✦, Apo-Glyburide ✦, Diabeta, Euglucon ✦, Gen-Glybe ✦, Glynase PresTab, Med-Glybe ✦, Micronase, Novo-Glyburide ✦, Nu-Glyburide ✦, Penta-Glyburide ✦ **(Rx)**
Classification: Sulfonylurea (anti-diabetic), second-generation

See also *Antidiabetic Agents.*
Action/Kinetics: Has a mild diuretic effect. **Onset, nonmicronized:** 2–4 hr; **micronized:** 1 hr. **t½, nonmicronized:** 10 hr; **micronized:** Approximately 4 hr. **Time to peak levels:** 4 hr. **Duration, both forms:** 24 hr. Metabolized in liver to weakly active metabolites. Excreted in bile (50%) and through the kidneys (50%).
How Supplied: *Tablet:* 1.25 mg, 1.5 mg, 2.5 mg, 3 mg, 5 mg, 6 mg

Dosage
- **Tablets, Nonmicronized (DiaBeta/Micronase)**

Diabetes.
Adults, initial: 2.5–5 mg/day given with breakfast (or the first main meal); **then,** increase by 2.5 mg at weekly intervals to achieve the desired response. **Maintenance:** 1.25–20 mg/day. Clients sensitive to sulfonylureas should start with 1.25 mg/day.
- **Tablets, Micronized (Glynase)**

Diabetes.
Adults, initial: 1.5–3 mg/day given with breakfast (or the first main meal); **then,** increase by no more than 1.5 mg at weekly intervals to achieve the desired response. **Maintenance:** 0.75–12 mg/day.

HEALTH CARE CONSIDERATIONS

See also *Health Care Considerations* for *Antidiabetic Agents* and *Glipizide.*

Administration/Storage
1. For best results, administer just prior to meals.
2. Do not exceed 20 mg/day of the nonmicronized product and 12 mg/day of the micronized product.
3. If daily dosage of the nonmicronized product exceeds 15 mg or the micronized product exceeds 6 mg, divide the dose and give before the morning and evening meals.

Client/Family Teaching
1. Review dose and frequency for administration.
2. Monitor finger sticks.
3. Continue regular exercise and dietary restrictions in addition to drug therapy.
4. Report as scheduled for teaching reinforcement, follow-up labs, foot exams, and medication evaluation.

Outcome/Evaluate: BS and HbA1c within desired range

Gold sodium thiomalate (Sodium aurothiomalate)

(gold SO-dee-um thigh-oh-MAH-layt)
Pregnancy Category: C
Myochrysine ✦ **(Rx)**
Classification: Antirheumatic

Action/Kinetics: Exact mechanism not known. May inhibit lysosomal enzyme activity in macrophages and decrease macrophage phagocytic activity. Other mechanisms may include alteration of the immune response and alteration of biosynthesis of collagen. Gold salts suppress, but do not cure, arthritis and synovitis. Beneficial effects may not be seen for 3–12 months. Most experience transient side effects, although serious effects may be manifested in some. **Peak blood levels (IM):** 4–6 hr. **Steady-state plasma levels:** 1–5 mcg/mL. **t½:** increases with continued therapy. Gold may accumulate in tissues and persist for years. Significantly bound to plasma proteins. Eliminated slowly through both the urine (70%) and feces (30%). This preparation contains 50% gold.
Uses: Adjunct to the treatment of active, early rheumatoid arthritis in children and adults who have insufficient response to or are intolerant of full doses of one or more NSAIDs.
Contraindications: Hepatic disease, CV problems such as hypertension or CHF, severe diabetes, debilitated clients, renal disease, blood dyscrasias, agranulocytosis, hemorrhagic diathesis, clients receiving radiation treatments, colitis, lupus erythematosus, pregnancy, lactation, children under 6 years of age. Clients with eczema or urticaria.

Side Effects: *Skin:* Dermatitis (most common), pruritus, erythema, dermatoses, gray to blue pigmentation of tissues, alopecia, loss of nails. *GI:* Stomatitis (second most common), metallic taste, gastritis, colitis, gingivitis, glossitis, N&V, diarrhea (may be persistent), colic, anorexia, cramps, enterocolitis. *Hematologic:* Anemia, thrombocytopenia, granulocytopenia, leukopenia, eosinophilia, hemorrhagic diathesis. *Allergic:* Flushing, fainting, sweating, dizziness, ***anaphylaxis,*** syncope, bradycardia, angioneurotic edema, respiratory difficulties. *Other:* Interstitial pneumonitis, pulmonary fibrosis, nephrotic syndrome, glomerulitis (with hematuria), proteinuria, hepatitis, fever, headache, arthralgia, ophthalmologic problems including corneal ulcers, iritis, gold deposits, EEG abnormalities, peripheral neuritis. Corticosteroids may be used to treat symptoms such as stomatitis, dermatitis, GI, renal, hematologic, or pulmonary problems. Also, if symptoms are severe and do not respond to corticosteroids, a chelating agent such as dimercaprol may be used. Clients should be monitored carefully.

Laboratory Test Considerations: Alters LFTs. Urinary protein and RBCs, altered blood counts (indicative of toxic effect of drug).

OD **Management of Overdose:** *Symptoms:* Hematuria, proteinuria, thrombocytopenia, granulocytopenia, N&V, diarrhea, fever, papulovesicular lesions, urticaria, exfoliative dermatitis, severe pruritus. *Treatment:* Discontinue use of the drug immediately. Give dimercaprol. Provide supportive treatment for hematologic or renal complications.

Drug Interactions: Concomitant use contraindicated with drugs known to cause blood dyscrasias (e.g., antimalarials, cytotoxic drugs, pyrazolone derivatives, immunosuppressive drugs).

How Supplied: *Injection:* 50 mg/mL

Dosage

- **IM**

Rheumatoid arthritis.

Adults: *week 1:* 10 mg as a single injection; *week 2:* 25 mg as a single dose. Then, 25–50 mg/week until 0.8–1 g total has been given. Thereafter according to individual response. *Usual maintenance:* 25–50 mg every other week for up to 20 weeks. If condition remains stable, the dose can be given every third or fourth week indefinitely. **Pediatric, initial:** *week 1,* 10 mg; **then,** usual dose is 1 mg/kg, not to exceed 50 mg/injection using the same spacing of doses as for adults.

HEALTH CARE CONSIDERATIONS

Administration/Storage

1. Shake vial well to ensure uniformity of suspension before withdrawing medication. Do not use if contents have darkened (color should not exceed pale yellow).
2. Inject into gluteus maximus.
3. May reinstitute therapy following mild toxic symptoms but not after severe symptoms.
4. Geriatric clients manifest a lower tolerance to gold.

Assessment

1. Record indications for therapy, previous treatments utilized, and the outcome.
2. Assess ROM; describe all areas of limitation and pain as well as active synovitis.
3. Monitor urinalysis, CBC, liver and renal function tests every 2 weeks.
4. Have client remain in a recumbent position for at least 20 min after injection to prevent falls resulting from transient vertigo or giddiness. Observe for flushing, dizziness, sweating, and hypotension (nitritoid reaction).
5. Monitor I&O and electrolytes if prolonged diarrhea occurs.

Client/Family Teaching

1. Close medical supervision is required during gold therapy.
2. Do not become discouraged. Beneficial effects are slow to appear; therapy may be continued for up to 12 months in anticipation of relief.
3. Report any unusual bruising or bleeding, skin or mucous membrane lesions, or blood in urine or stools.
4. May rinse with dilute hydrogen peroxide for mild stomatitis; floss daily, use a soft bristle toothbrush, and rinse mouth frequently.
5. Avoid acidic or hot, spicy foods.
6. Practice reliable contraception.
7. Avoid direct sun exposure as a photosensitivity reaction may occur. Wear sunscreen, protective clothing, sunglasses and a hat if exposed.
8. Continue anti-inflammatory doses of NSAIDs for several more weeks.

Outcome/Evaluate: ↓ Joint pain, swelling, and stiffness with ↑ ROM and mobility

Goserelin acetate

(GO-seh-rel-in)

Pregnancy Category: X (when used for endometriosis); D (when used for breast cancer)

Zoladex, Zoladex LA ✱ **(Rx)**
Classification: Antineoplastic, hormonal agent

See also *Antineoplastic Agents.*

Action/Kinetics: Goserelin acetate is a synthetic decapeptide analog of LHRH (or GnRH) which is a potent inhibitor of gonadotropin secretion from the pituitary gland. Initially, there is actually an increase in serum luteinizing hormone and FSH. This is followed by a long-term suppression of pituitary gonadotropins with serum levels of testosterone decreasing to those seen in surgically castrated males. When used for endometriosis, the drug controls the secretion of hormones required for the ovary to synthesize estrogen resulting in plasma estrogen levels seen in menopause. **Peak serum levels after SC implantation of 3.6 mg:** 12–15 days. **Mean peak serum levels:** Approximately 2.5 ng/mL. Available as an implant in a preloaded syringe. For the first 8 days of the treatment cycle, the rate of absorption of the 3.6 mg implant is slower than for the remainder of the period. For the 10.8 mg depot, mean levels increase to a peak within the first 24 hr and then decline rapidly until day 4; thereafter, mean levels remain constant until the end of the treatment period. **t½, elimination:** 4.2 hr for normal renal function and 12.1 hr for C_{CR} less than 20 mL/min. Rapidly cleared by a combination of hepatic metabolism and urinary excretion.

Uses: Implant, 3.6 mg or 10.8 mg: Palliative treatment of advanced prostatic carcinoma as an alternative to orchiectomy or estrogen administration when these are either unacceptable to the client or not indicated. With flutamide (Eulexin) prior to (start 8 weeks before) and during radiation therapy to treat Stage B2-C prostatic carcinoma. **Implant, 3.6 mg only:** Endometriosis, including pain relief and reduction of endometriotic lesions. Palliative treatment of advanced breast cancer in premenopausal and postmenopausal women. For endometrial thinning prior to ablation for dysfunctional uterine bleeding.

Contraindications: Pregnancy, lactation, nondiagnosed vaginal bleeding, hypersensitivity to LHRH or LHRH agonist analogs. Use of the 10.8-mg implant in women.

Special Concerns: Safety and effectiveness have not been determined in clients less than 18 years of age. There may be transient worsening of symptoms during the first few weeks of therapy. Use with caution in males who are at particular risk of developing ureteral obstruction or spinal cord compression.

Side Effects: In males. *GU:* Sexual dysfunction, decreased erections, lower urinary tract symptoms, gynecomastia, renal insufficiency, urinary obstruction, UTI, bladder neoplasm, hematuria, impotence, urinary frequency, incontinence, urinary tract disorder, impaired urination. *CV:* CHF, ***CVA, MI, heart failure, pulmonary embolus,*** arrhythmia, hypertension, peripheral vascular disorder, chest pain, angina pectoris, cerebral ischemia, varicose veins. *CNS:* Lethargy, dizziness, insomnia, asthenia, anxiety, depression, headache, paresthesia. *GI:* N&V, diarrhea, constipation, ulcer, anorexia, hematemesis. *Respiratory:* URI, COPD, increased cough, dyspnea, pneumonia. *Metabolic:* Gout, hypercalcemia, weight increase, diabetes mellitus. *Miscellaneous:* Pelvic or bone pain, anemia, chills, fever, breast pain, breast swelling or tenderness, abdominal or back pain, flu syndrome, sepsis, aggravation reaction, herpes simplex, pruritus, peripheral edema, injection site reaction, hot flashes, rash, sweating, complications of surgery, hypersensitivity, pain, edema.

In females. *GU:* Vaginitis, decreased or increased libido, pelvic symptoms, dyspareunia, dysmenorrhea, urinary frequency, UTI, vaginal bleeding (during the first 2 months) of varying duration and intensity. *CV:* ***Hemorrhage,*** hypertension, palpitations, migraine, tachycardia. *CNS:* Emotional lability, depression, headache, insomnia, dizziness, nervousness, anxiety, paresthesia, somnolence, abnormal thinking, malaise, fatigue, lethargy. *GI:* N&V, abdominal pain, increased appetite, anorexia, constipation, diarrhea, dry mouth, dyspepsia, flatulence. *Musculoskeletal:* Asthenia, back pain, myalgia, hypertonia, arthralgia, joint disorder, decrease of vertebral trabecular bone mineral density. *Dermatologic:* Sweating, acne, seborrhea, hirsutism, pruritus, alopecia, dry skin, ecchymosis, rash, skin discoloration, hair disorders. *Respiratory:* Pharyngitis, bronchitis, increased cough, epistaxis, rhinitis, sinusitis. *Ophthalmic:* Amblyopia, dry eyes. *Miscellaneous:* Hot flashes, breast atrophy or enlargement, breast pain, tumor flare, pain, infection, application site reaction, flu syndrome, voice alterations, weight gain, allergic reaction, chest pain, fever, peripheral edema, hypercalcemia, osteoporosis, hypersensitivity.

Laboratory Test Considerations: ↑ LDL and HDL cholesterol, triglycerides, AST, ALT. Misleading results of pituitary-gonadotropic and gonadal function tests that are conducted during treatment.

How Supplied: *Implant:* 3.6 mg, 10.8 mg

Dosage

- **SC Implant, 3.6 mg**

Prostatic carcinoma, endometriosis, advanced breast cancer, thinning prior to endometrial ablation for dysfunctional uterine bleeding.
3.6 mg q 28 days into the upper abdominal wall using sterile technique under the direction of a physician.

- **SC Implant, 10.8 mg**

Advanced prostatic carcinoma.
10.8 mg q 12 weeks into the upper abdominal wall using sterile technique under the direction of a physician.

With flutamide to treat Stage B2-C prostatic carcinoma.
One goserelin 3.6 mg depot followed in 28 days by one 10.8 mg depot.

HEALTH CARE CONSIDERATIONS

See also *Health Care Considerations* for *Antineoplastic Agents.*

Administration/Storage

1. Do not remove the sterile syringe containing the drug until immediately before use. Examine syringe for damage and to ensure drug is visible in the translucent chamber.
2. Administer drug under the supervision of a physician.
3. Clean the area with an alcohol swab; a topical (i.e., ethyl chloride) or a local anesthetic may be used prior to the injection.
4. To administer, stretch the skin with one hand and grip the needle with the fingers around the barrel of the syringe. Insert the needle into the SC fat; do not aspirate. If a large vessel is penetrated, blood will be seen immediately in the syringe; withdraw the needle and make the injection elsewhere with a new syringe.
5. The direction of the needle is changed so it parallels the abdominal wall. The needle is then pushed in until the barrel hub touches the skin and then withdrawn approximately 1 cm to create a space to inject the drug. The plunger is depressed to deliver the drug. The needle is then withdrawn and the area bandaged.
6. To confirm the drug has been delivered, ensure that the tip of the plunger is visible within the tip of the needle.
7. If there is need to remove goserelin surgically, it can be located by ultrasound.
8. Adhere to the 28-day and 12-week schedules as closely as possible.
9. Store at room temperatures not exceeding 25°C (77°F).
10. There is no evidence the drug accumulates with either hepatic and/or renal dysfunction.
11. Duration of treatment for endometriosis is 6 months.
12. Males with ureteral obstruction or spinal cord compression should have appropriate treatment prior to initiating goserelin therapy.

Client/Family Teaching

1. The most common side effects (especially hot flashes, decreased erections, and sexual dysfunction) are due to decreased testosterone levels.
2. There may be initial worsening of symptoms; results of transient increases of testosterone.
3. May experience an increase in bone pain and develop spinal cord compression or ureteral obstruction; these symptoms are usually only temporary but must be reported promptly so that appropriate treatment may be initiated. Report any unusual or adverse side effects.
4. Goserelin should not be used in women who are likely to become pregnant or who are pregnant. Drug may harm fetus and may impair fertility. Identify appropriate individuals for sperm or egg harvesting.
5. Advise clients with prostate cancer that if they decided against surgery (orchiectomy), for medication therapy, they must come in regularly for abdominal implants for the rest of their lives.
6. Identify appropriate resources and support groups.

Outcome/Evaluate

- Symptom control; ↑ comfort
- ↓ Tumor size and spread
- ↓ Testosterone levels

Granisetron hydrochloride

(gran-**ISS**-eh-tron)
Pregnancy Category: B
Kytril **(Rx)**
Classification: Antinauseant and antiemetic

Action/Kinetics: Selective 5-HT_3 (serotonin) receptor antagonist with little or no affinity for other 5-HT, beta-adrenergic, dopamine, or histamine receptors. During chemotherapy-induced vomiting, mucosal enterochromaffin cells release serotonin, which stimulates 5-HT_3 receptors. The stimulation of 5-HT_3 receptors by serotonin causes vagal discharge resulting in vomiting. Granisetron blocks serotonin stimulation and subsequent vomiting. In adult cancer clients undergoing chemotherapy, infusion of a single 40-mcg/kg dose over 5 min produced the following data. **Peak plasma level:** 63.8 ng/mL. **Plasma t½, terminal:** 8.95 hr. Metabolized in the liver with unchanged drug (12%) and metabolites excreted through both the urine and feces.

Uses: Prevention of N&V associated with initial and repeat cancer chemotherapy, including high-dose cisplatin. *Investigational:* Acute N&V following surgery.

Contraindications: Known hypersensitivity to the drug.

G

Special Concerns: Use with caution during lactation. Safety and efficacy in children less than 2 years of age have not been established.

Side Effects: After IV use. *CNS:* Headache, somnolence, agitation, anxiety, CNS stimulation, insomnia, extrapyramidal syndrome. *GI:* Diarrhea, constipation, taste disorder. *CV:* Hypertension, hypotension, arrhythmias (e.g., sinus bradycardia, atrial fibrillation, ***AV block,*** ventricular ectopy including nonsustained tachycardia, ECG abnormalities). *Allergic:* ***Hypersensitivity reactions (anaphylaxis),*** skin rashes. *Miscellaneous:* Asthenia, fever.

After PO use. *CNS:* Headache, dizziness, insomnia, anxiety, somnolence. *GI:* N&V, diarrhea, constipation, abdominal pain. *CV:* Hypertension, hypotension, angina, atrial fibrillation, syncope (rare). *Hypersensitivity:* Rarely, hypersensitivity reactions; ***severe anaphylaxis,*** shortness of breath, hypotension, urticaria. *Miscellaneous:* Fever, leukopenia, decreased appetite, anemia, alopecia, thrombocytopenia.

Laboratory Test Considerations: ↑ AST, ALT.

Drug Interactions: Because granisetron is metabolized by hepatic cytochrome P-450 drug-metabolizing enzymes, agents that induce or inhibit these enzymes may alter the clearance (and thus the half-life) of granisetron.

How Supplied: *Injection:* 1 mg/mL; *Tablet:* 1 mg

Dosage

- **IV**

Antiemetic during cancer chemotherapy.

Adults and children over 2 years of age: 10 mcg/kg infused over 5 min beginning 30 min before initiation of chemotherapy.

Antiemetic following surgery.

1–3 mg.

- **Tablets**

Protection from chemotherapy-induced nausea and vomiting.

Adults: 1 mg b.i.d. with the first 1 mg-tablet given 1 hr before chemotherapy and the second 1-mg tablet given 12 hr after the first tablet only on days chemotherapy is given. Alternatively, 2 mg once daily taken 1 hr before chemotherapy. Data are not available for PO use in children.

HEALTH CARE CONSIDERATIONS

Administration/Storage

1. Give drug only on the day chemotherapy is given.
2. Dosage adjustment is not necessary for geriatric clients or with impaired renal or hepatic function.

Assessment

1. Note indications for therapy; chemotherapy or postop N&V.
2. Anticipate administration 30 min before the start of emetogenic cancer chemotherapy.

Client/Family Teaching: Review the appropriate method and frequency of dosing to ensure protection from chemotherapy-induced nausea and vomiting.

Outcome/Evaluate

- Prevention of N&V
- Protection from chemotherapy-induced nausea and vomiting

Griseofulvin microsize

(griz-ee-oh-**FULL**-vin)

Pregnancy Category: C

Fulvicin-U/F, Grifulvin V, Grisactin 250, Grisactin 500, Grisovin-FP ★ **(Rx)**

Griseofulvin ultramicrosize

(griz-ee-oh-**FULL**-vin)

Pregnancy Category: C

Fulvicin-P/G, Grisactin Ultra, Gris-PEG **(Rx)**

Classification: Antibiotic, antifungal

See also *Anti-Infectives.*

Action/Kinetics: Derived from a species of *Penicillium.* Believed to interfere with cell division (metaphase) or DNA replication. When taken systemically, the drug is deposited in the newly formed skin and nails, which are then resistant to reinfection by the tinea. Absorbed from the duodenum. **Peak plasma concentration:** 0.5–2 mcg/mL after 4 hr. **t½:** 9–24 hr. Levels may be increased by giving the drug with a high-fat diet. GI absorption of the ultramicrosize products is about 1.5 times that of the microsize products; is no evidence this causes any difference in the safety and effectiveness of the drug compared with the microsize form.

Uses: Tinea (ringworm) infections of skin (including athlete's foot), scalp, groin, and nails. Effective against tinea corporis, tinea pedis, tinea barbae, tinea unguium, tinea cruris, tinea capitis due to *Trichophyton* species, *Microsporum audouinii, M. canis, M. gypseum,* and *Epidermophyton floccosum.* It is the only PO drug effective against dermatophytid (tinea ringworm) infections. Not effective against *Candida.* Establish susceptibility of the infectious agent before treatment is begun.

Contraindications: Pregnancy. Porphyria or history thereof, hepatocellular failure, and hypersensitivity to drug. Exposure to artificial light or sunlight. Use for infections due to bacteria, candidiasis, actinomycosis, sporotrichosis, tinea versicolor, histoplasmosis, chromoblastomycosis, coccidioidomycosis, cryptococcosis, and North American blastomycosis.

Special Concerns: Cross sensitivity with penicillin is possible.

Side Effects: *Hypersensitivity:* Rashes, urticaria, ***angioneurotic edema,*** allergic reactions. *GI:* N&V, diarrhea, epigastric pain, ***GI bleeding.*** *CNS:* Dizziness, headache, confusion, mental fatigue, insomnia. *Miscellaneous:* Oral thrush, acute intermittent porphyria, paresthesias of extremities after long-term therapy, proteinuria, leukopenia, photosensitivity, worsening of lupus erythematosus, menstrual irregularities, hepatic toxicity, granulocytopenia.

Laboratory Test Considerations: ↑ ALT, AST, alkaline phosphatase, BUN, and creatinine level values.

Drug Interactions

Alcohol, ethyl / Tachycardia and flushing
Anticoagulants, oral / ↓ Effect of anticoagulants due to ↑ breakdown in liver
Barbiturates / ↓ Effect of griseofulvin due to ↓ absorption from GI tract
Cyclosporine / ↓ Plasma levels of cyclosporine → ↓ pharmacologic effect
Oral contraceptives / ↓ Effect of contraceptives → breakthrough bleeding, pregnancy, or amenorrhea
Salicylates / ↓ Serum salicylate levels

How Supplied: Griseofulvin microsize: *Capsule:* 250 mg; *Suspension:* 125 mg/5 mL; *Tablet:* 250 mg, 500 mg. Griseofulvin ultramicrosize: *Tablet:* 125 mg; 165 mg; 250 mg; 330 mg

Dosage

- **Capsules, Oral Suspension, Tablets**

Tinea corporis, cruris, or capitis.

Adults: 0.5 g griseofulvin microsize daily in a single dose or divided dose (or 330–375 mg ultramicrosize).

Tinea pedis or unguium.

Adults: 0.75–1 g/day of griseofulvin microsize (or 660–750 mg ultramicrosize). After response, decrease dose of microsize to 0.5 g/day. **Pediatric, 13.6–22.7 kg:** 125–250 mg griseofulvin microsize daily (or 82.5–165 mg ultramicrosize); **pediatric, over 22.7 kg:** 250–500 mg microsize daily (or 165–330 mg ultramicrosize). *NOTE:* Dose has not been determined in children less than 2 years of age.

HEALTH CARE CONSIDERATIONS

See also *General Health Care Considerations for All Anti-Infectives.*

Administration/Storage

1. Assure sufficient length of treatment; i.e., treatment for tinea capitis: 4 to 6 weeks; 2 to 4 weeks for tinea corporis; 4 to 8 weeks for tinea pedis; and 4 to 6 months (fingernails) and 6 to 18 months (toe nails) for tinea unguium.
2. With prolonged therapy, evaluate liver, renal, and hematologic function.
3. May not be the drug of choice with CAD and hyperlipidemia due to the high-fat consumption necessary to enhance absorption.

Assessment

1. Record location, size, and characteristics of skin infection.
2. Obtain baseline CBC, liver and renal function studies. Obtain cultures and scrapings as needed.

Client/Family Teaching

1. Eat high-fat food with drug (i.e., ice cream, bread and butter, gravy, fried chicken); fat enhances absorption of griseofulvin from the intestines.
2. Take all medication as prescribed to prevent any recurrence of infection. If the course of therapy is interrupted or not completed, therapy may have to be started all over again.
3. Practice appropriate hygiene to prevent reinfection.
4. Avoid exposure to intense natural and artificial light because photosensitivity reactions may occur. Wear protective clothing, sunglasses, and a sunscreen if exposure is necessary.
5. Report any fever, sore throat, and malaise, (all symptoms of leukopenia).
6. Use a nonhormonal form of birth control.
7. To be considered cured, repeated cultures and scrapings of affected sites must be negative.
8. Persistent N&V and diarrhea and any mental confusion should be immediately reported.
9. Avoid alcohol during therapy.
10. Anticipate long-term therapy, i.e., 2

G

weeks to 18 months depending on location of infection.

Outcome/Evaluate

- Improvement in symptoms
- Clearing of rash
- Negative cultures and scraping

Guaifenesin (Glyceryl guaiacolate)

(gwye-**FEN**-eh-sin)

Pregnancy Category: C

Allfen, Anti-Tuss, Balminil Expectorant ✱, Benylin-E ✱, Breonesin, Fenesin, Gee-Gee, Genatuss, GG-Cen, Glyate, Glycotuss, Glytuss, Guiatuss, Halotussin, Humibid L.A., Humibid Sprinkle, Hytuss, Hytuss-2X, Mytussin, Naldecon Senior EX, Robitussin, Scot-tussin, Sinumist-SR Capsulets, Touro EX, Uni-tussin **(OTC)**

Classification: Expectorant

Action/Kinetics: May increase the output of fluid of the respiratory tract by reducing the viscosity and surface tension of respiratory secretions, thereby facilitating their expectoration. Data on efficacy are lacking.

Uses: Dry, nonproductive cough due to colds and minor upper respiratory tract infections when there is mucus in the respiratory tract.

Contraindications: Chronic cough (e.g., due to smoking, asthma, or emphysema), cough accompanied by excess secretions. Use in children under age 12 for persistent or chronic cough due to asthma or cough accompanied by excessive mucus (unless prescribed by a provider).

Special Concerns: Persistent cough may indicate a serious infection; thus, the provider should be consulted if cough lasts for more than 1 week, is recurring, or is accompanied by high fever, rash, or persistent headache.

Side Effects: *GI:* N&V, GI upset. *CNS:* Dizziness, headache. *Dermatologic:* Rash, urticaria.

Laboratory Test Considerations: False + urinary 5-hydroxyindoleacetic acid. Color interference with determination of urinary vanillylmandelic acid.

OD Management of Overdose: *Symptoms:* N&V. *Treatment:* Treat symptomatically.

Drug Interactions: Inhibition of platelet adhesiveness by guaifenesin may result in bleeding tendencies.

How Supplied: *Capsule:* 200 mg; *Capsule, Extended Release:* 300 mg; *Liquid:* 100 mg/5 mL, 200 mg/5 mL; *Syrup:* 50 mg/5 mL, 100 mg/5 mL; *Tablet:* 100 mg, 200 mg; *Tablet, Extended Release:* 575 mg, 600 mg, 800 mg, 1000 mg, 1200 mg

Dosage

- **Capsules, Tablets, Oral Liquid, Syrup**

  Expectorant.

Adults and children over 12 years: 100–400 mg q 4 hr, not to exceed 2.4 g/day; **pediatric, 6–12 years:** 100–200 mg q 4 hr, not to exceed 1.2 g/day; **pediatric, 2–6 years:** 50–100 mg q 4 hr, not to exceed 600 mg/day. If less than 2 years of age, individualize the dosage.

- **Sustained-Release Capsules, Sustained-Release Tablets**

  Expectorant.

Adults and children over 12 years: 600–1,200 mg q 12 hr, not to exceed 2.4 g/day; **pediatric, 6–12 years:** 600 mg q 12 hr, not to exceed 1.2 g/day; **pediatric, 2–6 years:** 300 mg q 12 hr, not to exceed 600 mg/day. *NOTE:* The liquid dosage forms may be more suitable for children less than 6 years of age.

HEALTH CARE CONSIDERATIONS

Assessment

1. Record/document pulmonary assessment findings.
2. Note type, frequency, duration, and characteristics of cough and sputum production.
3. Assess for fever/chills, loss of appetite, or increased fatigue.

Client/Family Teaching

1. Take only as directed and do not exceed prescribed dose.
2. If symptoms persist more than 1 week, recur, or are accompanied by a persistent headache, fever, or rash, notify provider.
3. Report any evidence of increased bruising/bleeding or lack or response.
4. Do not perform activities that require mental alertness; may cause drowsiness.
5. Increase fluids to 2.5 L/day to decrease secretion viscosity.
6. Avoid triggers: dust, chemicals, cigarette smoke, pollutants, and perfumes.

Outcome/Evaluate

- Control of coughing episodes
- Mobilization of mucus

Guanabenz acetate

(**GWON**-ah-benz)

Pregnancy Category: C

Wytensin **(Rx)**

Classification: Antihypertensive, centrally acting antiadrenergic

See also *Antihypertensive Agents.*

Action/Kinetics: Stimulates alpha-2-adrenergic receptors in the CNS, resulting in a decrease in sympathetic impulses and in sympathetic tone. It also decreases the pulse rate, but postural hypotension has not been manifested. **Onset:** 60 min. **Peak effect:** 2–4 hr. **Peak plasma levels:** 2–5 hr. **t½:** 6 hr. **Duration:** 8–12 hr.

Uses: Hypertension, alone or as adjunct with thiazide diuretics.

Contraindications: Lactation, children under 12 years of age.

Special Concerns: Use with caution in severe coronary insufficiency, cerebrovascular disease, recent MI, hepatic or renal disease. Geriatric clients may be more sensitive to the hypotensive and sedative effects; dose reduction may be necessary due to age-related decreases in renal function. Sudden cessation may result in an increase in catecholamines and, rarely, "overshoot" hypertension.

Side Effects: *CNS:* Drowsiness and sedation (common), dizziness, weakness, headache, ataxia, depression, disturbances in sleep, excitement. *GI:* Dry mouth (common), N&V, diarrhea, constipation, abdominal discomfort, epigastric pain. *CV:* Palpitations, chest pain, arrhythmias, AV dysfunction or block. *Dermatologic:* Rash, pruritus. *Miscellaneous:* Edema, blurred vision, muscle aches, dyspnea, nasal congestion, urinary frequency, gynecomastia, disturbances of sexual function, taste disorders, aches in extremities.

OD **Management of Overdose:** *Symptoms:* Hypotension, sleepiness, irritability, miosis, lethargy, bradycardia. *Treatment:* Supportive treatment. VS and fluid balance should be monitored. Syrup of ipecac or gastric lavage followed by activated charcoal; administration of fluids, pressor agents, and atropine. Maintain an adequate airway; artificial respiration may be required.

Drug Interactions: Use with CNS depressants may result in additive sedation.

How Supplied: *Tablet:* 4 mg, 8 mg

Dosage

- **Tablets**

  Hypertension.

Adults, initial: 4 mg b.i.d. alone or with a thiazide diuretic; **then,** increase by 4–8 mg/day q 1–2 weeks until control achieved. Maximum recommended dose: 32 mg b.i.d.

HEALTH CARE CONSIDERATIONS

See also *Health Care Considerations* for *Antihypertensive Agents.*

Administration/Storage: The drug should be kept tightly closed and protected from light.

Client/Family Teaching

1. Do not drive or operate machinery until the drug's sedative effect assessed.
2. Report sleep disturbances; may indicate a depressive episode.
3. Avoid tobacco, alcohol, and other CNS depressants.
4. Continue prescribed dietary and exercise recommendations.

Outcome/Evaluate: ↓ BP

G

Guanadrel sulfate

(GWON-ah-drell)

Pregnancy Category: B

Hylorel **(Rx)**

Classification: Antihypertensive, peripherally acting antiadrenergic

See also *Antihypertensive Agents.*

Action/Kinetics: Similar to that of guanethidine. Inhibits vasoconstriction by blocking efferent, peripheral sympathetic pathways by depleting norepinephrine reserves and inhibiting norepinephrine release. Causes increased sensitivity to norepinephrine. **Onset:** 2 hr. **Peak plasma levels:** 1.5–2 hr. **Peak effect:** 4–6 hr. **t½:** Approximately 10 hr. **Duration:** 4–14 hr. Excreted through the urine as unchanged drug (40%) and metabolites.

Uses: Hypertension in those not responding to a thiazide diuretic.

Contraindications: Pheochromocytoma, CHF, within 1 week of MAO drug use, within 2–3 days of elective surgery, lactation.

Special Concerns: Use with caution in bronchial asthma and peptic ulcer. Safety and efficacy not established in children. Geriatric clients may be more sensitive to the hypotensive effects.

Side Effects: *CNS:* Fainting, fatigue, headache, drowsiness, paresthesias, confusion, psychological problems, depression, syncope, sleep disorders, visual disturbances. *CV:* Chest pain, orthostatic hypotension, palpitations, peripheral edema. *Respiratory:* Exertional or resting SOB, coughing. *GI:* Increase in number of bowel movements, constipation, anorexia, indigestion, flatus, glossitis, N&V, dry mouth and throat, abdominal distress or pain. *GU:* Difficulty in ejaculation, impotence, nocturia, hematuria, urinary urgency or frequency. *Miscellaneous:* Leg cramps during both the day and night, excessive weight gain or loss, backache, neckache, joint pain or inflammation, aching limbs.

OD **Management of Overdose:** *Symptoms:* Postural hypotension, syncope, dizziness, blurred vision. *Treatment:* Administration of a vasoconstrictor (e.g., phenylephrine) if hypotension persists. If used, monitor carefully as client may be hypersensitive.

Drug Interactions

Beta-adrenergic blocking agents / Excessive hypotension, bradycardia

Phenothiazines / Reverses effect of guanadrel

Phenylpropanolamine / ↓ Effect of guanadrel

Reserpine / Excessive hypotension, bradycardia

Sympathomimetics / Hypotensive effect of guanadrel may be reversed; also, guanadrel may ↑ the effects of directly acting sympathomimetics

Tricyclic antidepressants / Reverses effect of guanadrel

Vasodilators / ↑ Risk of orthostatic hypotension

How Supplied: *Tablet:* 10 mg

Dosage

- **Tablets**

Hypertension.

Individualized. Initial: 5 mg b.i.d.; **then,** increase dosage to maintenance level of 20–75 mg/day in two to four divided doses. With a C_{CR} of 30–60 mL/min, use an initial dose of 5 mg q 24 hr. If the C_{CR} is less than 30 mL/min, increase the dosing interval to q 48 hr. Make dose changes carefully q 7 or more days for moderate renal insufficiency and q 14 or more days for severe insufficiency.

HEALTH CARE CONSIDERATIONS

See also *Health Care Considerations* for *Antihypertensive Agents.*

Administration/Storage

1. Tolerance may occur with long-term therapy, necessitating a dosage increase.
2. While adjusting dosage, monitor both supine and standing BP.

Client/Family Teaching

1. May develop a dry mouth and become drowsy. Do not perform tasks that require mental alertness, such as driving, until drug effects realized.
2. Diarrhea may occur; if persistent, report as a severe electrolyte imbalance may occur (particularly with the elderly).

Outcome/Evaluate: Control of hypertension

Guanethidine monosulfate

(gwon-**ETH**-ih-deen)

Pregnancy Category: C

Ismelin Sulfate **(Rx)**

Classification: Antihypertensive, peripherally acting antiadrenergic

See also *Antihypertensive Agents.*

Action/Kinetics: Produces selective adrenergic blockade of efferent, peripheral sympathetic pathways by depleting norepinephrine reserve and inhibiting norepinephrine release. Induces a gradual, prolonged drop in both SBP and DBP, usually associated with bradycardia, decreased pulse pressure, a decrease in peripheral resistance, and small changes in CO. Is not a ganglionic blocking agent and does not produce central or parasympathetic blockade. With depleted catecholamines, guanethidine can directly depress the myocardium and can cause an increase in the sensitivity of tissues to catecholamines. Incompletely and variably absorbed from the GI tract (3%–30%) but is relatively constant for any given client. **Peak effect:** 6–8 hr. **Duration:** 24–48 hr. **Maximum effect:** 1–3 weeks. **Duration:** 7–10 days after discontinuation. **t½:** 4–8 days. From 25% to 50% excreted through the kidneys unchanged. Slowly excreted due to extensive tissue binding.

Uses: Moderate to severe hypertension—used alone or in combination. *NOTE:* The use of a thiazide diuretic may increase the effectiveness of guanethidine and reduce the incidence of edema. Also used for renal hypertension, including that secondary to pyelonephritis, renal artery stenosis, and renal amyloidosis.

Contraindications: Mild, labile hypertension; pheochromocytoma, CHF not due to hypertension, use of MAO inhibitors, lactation.

Special Concerns: Administer with caution and at a reduced rate to clients with impaired renal function, coronary disease, CV disease especially when associated with encephalopathy, or severe cardiac failure or to those who have suffered a recent MI. Use with caution in hypertensive clients with renal disease and nitrogen retention or increasing BUN levels. Fever decreases dosage requirements. During prolonged therapy, cardiac, renal, and blood tests should be performed. Used with caution in peptic ulcer. Geriatric clients may be more sensitive to the hypotensive effects of guanethidine; also, it may be necessary to decrease the dose in these clients due to age-related decreases in renal function. Safety and efficacy have not been determined in children.

Side Effects: *CNS:* Dizziness, weakness, lassitude. Rarely, fatigue, psychic depression. *CV:* Syncope due to exertional or postural hypotension, bradycardia, fluid retention and edema with possible CHF. Less commonly, angina. *Respiratory:* Dyspnea, nasal congestion, asthma in susceptible individuals. *GI:* Persistent diarrhea (may be severe enough to cause discontinuation of use), increased frequency of bowel movements. N&V, dry mouth, and parotid tenderness are less common. *GU:* Inhibition of ejaculation, nocturia, urinary incontinence, priapism, impotence. *Hematologic:* Anemia, thrombocytopenia, leukopenia (rare). *Miscellaneous:* Dermatitis, scalp hair loss, blurred vision, myalgia, muscle tremors, chest paresthesia, weight gain, ptosis of the lids.

Laboratory Test Considerations: ↑ BUN, AST, and ALT. ↓ PT, serum glucose, and urine catecholamines. Alteration of electrolyte balance.

OD **Management of Overdose:** *Symptoms:* Bradycardia, postural hypotension, diarrhea (may be severe). *Treatment:* If the client was previously normotensive, keep in a supine position (symptoms usually subside within 72 hr). If the client was previously hypertensive (especially with impaired cardiac reserve or other CV problems or renal disease), intensive treatment may be needed. Vasopressors may be required. Treat severe diarrhea.

Drug Interactions

Alcohol, ethyl / Additive orthostatic hypotension
Amphetamines / ↓ Effect of guanethidine by ↓ uptake of the drug to its site of action
Anesthetics, general / Additive hypotension
Antidepressants, tricyclic / ↓ Effect of guanethidine by ↓ uptake of the drug to its site of action
Antidiabetic drugs / Additive effect ↓ in blood glucose
Cocaine / ↓ Effect of guanethidine by ↓ uptake of the drug at its site of action
Digitalis / Additive slowing of HR
Ephedrine / ↓ Effect of guanethidine by ↓ uptake of the drug at its site of action
Epinephrine / Guanethidine ↑ effect of epinephrine
Haloperidol / ↓ Effect of guanethidine by ↓ uptake of the drug at its site of action
Levarterenol / See *Norepinephrine*
MAO inhibitors / Reverse effect of guanethidine
Metaraminol / Guanethidine ↑ effect of metaraminol
Methotrimeprazine / Additive hypotensive effect
Methoxamine / Guanethidine ↑ effect of methoxamine
Methylphenidate / ↓ Effect of guanethidine
Minoxidil / Profound drop in BP
Norepinephrine / ↑ Effect of norepinephrine probably due to ↑ sensitivity of norepinephrine receptor and ↓ uptake of norepinephrine by the neuron
Oral contraceptives / ↓ Effect of guanethidine by ↓ uptake of the drug to its site of action
Phenothiazines / ↓ Effect of guanethidine by ↓ uptake of the drug to its site of action
Phenylephrine / ↑ Response to phenylephrine in guanethidine-treated clients
Procainamide / Additive hypotensive effect
Procarbazine / Additive hypotensive effect
Propranolol / Additive hypotensive effect
Pseudoephedrine / ↓ Effect of guanethidine by ↓ uptake of the drug at its site of action
Quinidine / Additive hypotensive effect
Reserpine / Excessive bradycardia, postural hypotension, and mental depression
Sympathomimetics / ↓ Effect of guanethidine; also, guanethidine potentiates the effects of directly acting sympathomimetics
Thiazide diuretics / Additive hypotensive effect
Thioxanthenes / ↓ Effect of guanethidine by ↓ uptake of the drug at its site of action
Tricyclic antidepressants / Inhibition of the effects of guanethidine
Vasodilator drugs, peripheral / Additive hypotensive effect
Vasopressor drugs / ↑ Effect of vasopressor agents probably due to ↑ sensitivity of norepinephrine receptor and ↓ uptake of vasopressor agent by the neuron

How Supplied: *Tablet:* 10 mg, 25 mg

Dosage

- **Tablets**

Ambulatory clients.

Initial: 10–12.5 mg/day; increase in 10–12.5-mg increments q 5–7 days; **maintenance:** 25–50 mg/day.

Hospitalized clients.

Initial: 25–50 mg; increase by 25 or 50 mg/day or every other day; **maintenance:** approximately one-seventh of loading dose. **Pediatric, initial:** 0.2 mg/kg/day (6 mg/m²) given in one dose; **then,** dose may be increased by 0.2 mg/kg/day q 7–10 days to maximum of 3 mg/kg/day.

G

HEALTH CARE CONSIDERATIONS

See also *Health Care Considerations* for *Antihypertensive Agents.*

Administration/Storage

1. For severe hypertension, give the loading dose t.i.d. at 6-hr intervals with no nighttime dose.
2. Effects are cumulative; use small initial doses, increase gradually in small increments.
3. Often used with thiazide diuretics to reduce severity of sodium and water retention caused by guanethidine. When used together, reduce the dose of guanethidine.
4. When control is achieved, reduce dose to the minimal required to maintain lowest possible BP.
5. Discontinue or decrease dosage at least 2 weeks before surgery; discontinue MAO inhibitors at least 1 week before starting guanethidine.

Assessment

1. Obtain baseline hepatic and renal function studies.
2. List drugs currently prescribed to ensure none interact unfavorably.
3. Assess VS; report bradycardia. An anticholinergic drug, i.e., atropine, may be indicated if severe.
4. Assess life-style and emotional state.

Client/Family Teaching

1. Limit alcohol intake; may precipitate orthostatic hypotension. Postural hypotension more prevalent in the morning; may be worsened by hot weather, alcohol, or exercise.
2. Avoid any sudden or prolonged standing or exercise.
3. Report any persistent nausea, vomiting, or diarrhea; severe electrolyte imbalances may occur.
4. Perform daily weights. Report any sudden increases in weight, ↑ SOB, reduction in urine volume or edema.

Outcome/Evaluate: ↓ BP

Guanfacine hydrochloride

(GWON-fah-seen)

Pregnancy Category: B

Tenex **(Rx)**

Classification: Antihypertensive, centrally acting

See also *Antihypertensive Agents.*

Action/Kinetics: Thought to act by central stimulation of alpha-2 receptors. Causes a decrease in peripheral sympathetic output and HR resulting in a decrease in BP. May also manifest a direct peripheral alpha-2 receptor stimulant action. **Onset:** 2 hr. **Peak plasma levels:** 1–4 hr. **Peak effect:** 6–12 hr. **t½:** 12–23 hr. **Duration:** 24 hr. Approximately 50% excreted through the kidneys unchanged.

Uses: Hypertension alone or with a thiazide diuretic. *Investigational:* Withdrawal from heroin use, to reduce the frequency of migraine headaches.

Contraindications: Hypersensitivity to guanfacine. Acute hypertension associated with toxemia. Children less than 12 years of age.

Special Concerns: Use with caution during lactation and in clients with recent MI, cerebrovascular disease, chronic renal or hepatic failure, or severe coronary insufficiency. Geriatric clients may be more sensitive to the hypotensive and sedative effects. Safety and efficacy in children less than 12 years of age have not been determined.

Side Effects: *GI:* Dry mouth, constipation, nausea, abdominal pain, diarrhea, dyspepsia, dysphagia, taste perversion or alterations in taste. *CNS:* Sedation, weakness, dizziness, headache, fatigue, insomnia, amnesia, confusion, depression, vertigo, agitation, anxiety, malaise, nervousness, tremor. *CV:* Bradycardia, substernal pain, palpitations, syncope, chest pain, tachycarida, cardiac fibrillation, CHF, heart block, MI (rare), cardiovascular accident (rare). *Ophthalmic:* Visual disturbances, conjunctivitis, iritis, blurred vision. *Dermatologic:* Pruritus, dermatitis, purpura, sweating, skin rash with exfoliation, alopecia, rash. *GU:* Decreased libido, impotence, urinary incontinence or frequency, testicular disorder, nocturia, acute renal failure. *Musculoskeletal:* Leg cramps, hypokinesia, arthralgia, leg pain, myalgia. *Other:* Rhinitis, tinnitus, dyspnea, paresthesias, paresis, asthenia, edema, abnormal LFTs.

OD Management of Overdose: *Symptoms:* Drowsiness, bradycardia, lethargy, hypotension. *Treatment:* Gastric lavage. Supportive therapy, as needed. The drug is not dialyzable.

Drug Interactions: Additive sedative effects when used concomitantly with CNS depressants.

How Supplied: *Tablet:* 1 mg, 2 mg

Dosage

- **Tablets**

  Hypertension.

Initial: 1 mg/day alone or with other antihypertensives; if satisfactory results are not obtained in 3–4 weeks, dosage may be increased by 1 mg at 1–2-week intervals up to a maximum of 3 mg/day in one to two divided doses.

Heroin withdrawal.
0.03–1.5 mg/day.

Reduce frequency of migraine headaches.
1 mg/day for 12 weeks.

HEALTH CARE CONSIDERATIONS

See also *Health Care Considerations* for *Antihypertensive Agents.*

Administration/Storage

1. Divide the daily dose if a decrease in BP is not maintained for over 24 hr; however, the incidence of side effects increases.
2. Adverse effects increase significantly when dose exceeds 3 mg/day.
3. Initiate antihypertensive therapy in clients already taking a thiazide diuretic.
4. Abrupt cessation may result in increases in plasma and urinary catecholamines, symptoms of nervousness and anxiety, and BPs greater than those prior to therapy.

Assessment

1. Record indications for therapy, onset of symptoms, and any previous agents used and the outcome.
2. Determine the extent of CAD, and note any evidence of renal or liver dysfunction.

Client/Family Teaching

1. To minimize daytime drowsiness, take at bedtime. Do not perform activities that require mental alertness until drug effects realized.
2. Do not stop drug abruptly; may experience rebound effect.
3. May cause skin rash; report if persistent or severe.
4. Avoid OTC cough/cold remedies.

Outcome/Evaluate

- ↓ BP
- ↓ S&S of heroin withdrawal
- ↓ Migraine headaches

H

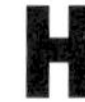

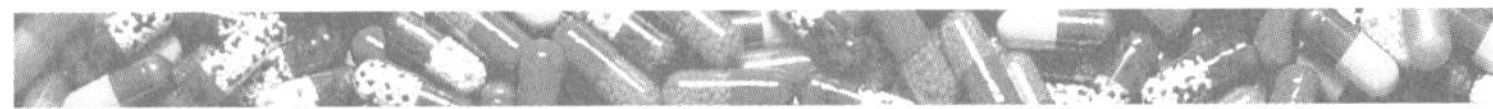

Haloperidol

(hah-low-**PAIR**-ih-dohl)

Pregnancy Category: C

Apo-Haloperidol ✦, Haldol, Novo-Peridol ✦, Peridol ✦, PMS Haloperidol ✦, PMS Haloperidol LA ✦ **(Rx)**

Haloperidol decanoate

(hah-low-**PAIR**-ih-dohl)

Pregnancy Category: C (decanoate form)

Haldol Decanoate 50 and 100, Haldol LA ✦, Rho-Haloperidol Decanoate ✦ **(Rx)**

Haloperidol lactate

(hah-low-**PAIR**-ih-dohl)

Pregnancy Category: C

Haldol Lactate **(Rx)**

Classification: Antipsychotic, butyrophenone

Action/Kinetics: Precise mechanism not known. Competitively blocks dopamine receptors in the tuberoinfundibular system to cause sedation. Also causes alpha-adrenergic blockade, decreases release of growth hormone, and increases prolactin release by the pituitary. Causes significant extrapyramidal effects, as well as a low incidence of sedation, anticholinergic effects, and orthostatic hypotension. Narrow margin between the therapeutically effective dose and that causing extrapyramidal symptoms. Also has antiemetic effects. **Peak plasma levels: PO,** 3–5 hr; **IM,** 20 min; **IM, decanoate:** approximately 6 days. **Therapeutic serum levels:** 3–10 ng/mL. **t½, PO:** 12–38 hr; **IM:** 13–36 hr; **IM, decanoate:** 3 weeks; **IV:** approximately 14 hr. **Plasma protein binding:** 90%. Metabolized in liver, slowly excreted in urine and bile.

Uses: Psychotic disorders including manic states, drug-induced psychoses, and schizophrenia. Severe behavior problems in children (those with combative, explosive hyperexcitability not accounted for by immediate provocation). Short-term treatment of hyperactive children who show excessive motor activity with accompanying conduct consisting of impulsivity, poor attention, aggression, mood lability, or poor frustration tolerance. Control of tics and vocal utterances associated with Gilles de la Tourette's syndrome in adults and children. The decanoate is used for prolonged therapy in chronic schizophrenia.

Investigational: Antiemetic for cancer chemotherapy, phencyclidine psychosis, intractable hiccoughs, infantile autism. IV for acute psychiatric conditions.

Contraindications: Use with extreme caution, or not at all, in clients with parkinsonism. Lactation.

Special Concerns: PO dosage has not been determined in children less than 3 years of age; IM dosage is not recommended in children. Geriatric clients are more likely to exhibit orthostatic hypotension, anticholinergic effects, sedation, and extrapyramidal side effects (such as parkinsonism and tardive dyskinesia).

Side Effects: Extrapyramidal symptoms, especially akathisia and dystonias, occur more frequently than with the phenothiazines. Overdosage is characterized by severe extrapyramidal reactions, hypotension, or sedation. The drug does not elicit photosensitivity reactions like those of the phenothiazines.

Laboratory Test Considerations: ↑ Alkaline phosphatase, bilirubin, serum transaminase; ↓ PT (clients on coumarin), serum cholesterol.

OD **Management of Overdose:** *Symptoms:* CNS depression, hypertension or hypotension, extrapyramidal symptoms, agitation, restlessness, fever, hypothermia, hyperthermia, ***seizures, cardiac arrhythmias,*** changes in the ECG, autonomic reactions, ***coma.*** *Treatment:* Treat symptomatically. Antiparkinson drugs, diphenhydramine, or barbiturates can be used to treat extrapyramidal symptoms. Fluid replacement and vasoconstrictors (either norepinephrine or phenylephrine) can be used to treat hypotension. Ventricular arrhythmias can be treated with phenytoin. To treat seizures, use pentobarbital or diazepam. A saline cathartic can be used to hasten the excretion of sustained-release products.

Drug Interactions

Amphetamine / ↓ Effect of amphetamine by ↓ uptake of drug at its site of action

Anticholinergics / ↓ Effect of haloperidol

Antidepressants, tricyclic / ↑ Effect of antidepressants due to ↓ breakdown by liver

Barbiturates / ↓ Effect of haloperidol due to ↑ breakdown by liver

Guanethidine / ↓ Effect of guanethidine by ↓ uptake of drug at site of action

Lithium / ↑ Toxicity of haloperidol

Methyldopa / ↑ Toxicity of haloperidol

Phenytoin / ↓ Effect of haloperidol due to ↑ breakdown by liver

How Supplied: Haloperidol: *Tablet:* 0.5 mg, 1 mg, 2 mg, 5 mg, 10 mg, 20 mg. Haloperidol decanoate: *Injection:* 50 mg/mL, 100 mg/mL. Haloperidol lactate: *Concentrate:* 2 mg/mL; *Injection:* 5 mg/mL; *Solution:* 1 mg/mL

Dosage

- **Oral Solution, Tablets**

Psychoses.

Adults: 0.5–2 mg b.i.d.–t.i.d. up to 3–5 mg b.i.d.–t.i.d. for severe symptoms; **maintenance:** reduce dosage to lowest effective level. Up to 100 mg/day may be required in some. **Geriatric or debilitated clients:** 0.5–2 mg b.i.d.–t.i.d. **Pediatric, 3–12 years or 15–40 kg:** 0.5 mg/day in two to three divided doses; if necessary the daily dose may be increased by 0.5-mg increments q 5–7 days for a total of 0.15 mg/kg/day for psychotic disorders.

Tourette's syndrome.

Adults, initial: 0.5–1.5 mg t.i.d., up to 10 mg daily. Adjust dose carefully to obtain the optimum response. **Children, 3 to 12 years:** 0.05–0.075 mg/kg/day. Higher doses may be needed for those severely disturbed.

Behavioral disorders/hyperactivity in children.

Children, 3 to 12 years: 0.05–0.075 mg/kg/day. Higher doses may be needed for those severely disturbed.

Intractable hiccoughs (investigational).

1.5 mg t.i.d.

Infantile autism (investigational).

0.5–4 mg/day.

- **IM, Lactate**

Acute psychoses.

Adults and adolescents, initial: 2–5 mg to control acute agitation; may be repeated if necessary q 4–8 hr to a total of 100 mg/day. Switch to **PO** therapy as soon as possible.

- **IM, Decanoate**

Chronic therapy.

Adults, initial dose: 10–15 times the daily PO dose, not to exceed 100 mg initially, regardless of the previous oral antipsychotic dose; **then,** repeat q 4 weeks (decanoate is not to be given IV).

HEALTH CARE CONSIDERATIONS

See also *Health Care Considerations* for *Antipsychotic Agents, Phenothiazines.*

Administration/Storage

1. Give the decanoate by deep IM injection using a 21-gauge needle. Do not exceed a volume of 3 mL/site.
2. Do not give decanoate IV.

Assessment

1. Record type, onset, and duration of symptoms.
2. Use with caution in the elderly; they tend to exhibit toxicity more frequently; may also benefit from a periodic "drug holiday."
3. Record evidence of new onset of extrapyramidal symptoms; may be drug induced.

Outcome/Evaluate

- Improved behavior patterns: ↓ agitation, ↓ hostility, ↓ psychosis, ↓ delusions
- Control of tics/vocal utterances
- ↓ Hyperactive behaviors

Heparin calcium

(HEP-ah-rin)

Pregnancy Category: C

Heparin sodium and sodium chloride

(HEP ah-rin)

Pregnancy Category: C

Heparin Sodium and 0.45% Sodium Chloride, Heparin Sodium and 0.9% Sodium Chloride **(Rx)**

Heparin sodium injection

(HEP-ah-rin)

Pregnancy Category: C

Hepalean ✱, Hepalean-Lok ✱, Heparin Leo ✱ **(Rx)**

Heparin sodium lock flush solution

(HEP-ah-rin)

Pregnancy Category: C

Heparin lock flush, Hep-Lock, Hep-Lock U/P **(Rx)**

Classification: Anticoagulant

Action/Kinetics: Heparin potentiates the inhibitory action of antithrombin III on various coagulation factors including factors IIa, IXa, Xa, XIa, and XIIa. This occurs due to the formation of a complex with and causing a conformational change in the antithrombin III molecule. Inhibition of factor Xa results in interference with thrombin generation; thus, the action of thrombin in coagulation is inhibited. Heparin also increases the rate of formation of antithrombin III–thrombin complex causing inactivation of thrombin and preventing the conversion of fibrinogen to fibrin. By inhibiting the activation of fibrin-stabilizing factor by thrombin, heparin also prevents formation of a stable fibrin clot. Therapeutic doses of heparin prolong thrombin time, whole blood clotting time, activated clotting time, and PTT. Heparin also decreases the levels of triglycerides by releasing lipoprotein lipase from tissues; the resultant hydrolysis of triglycerides causes increased blood levels of free fatty acids. **Onset: IV,** immediate; **deep SC:** 20–60 min. **Peak plasma levels, after SC:** 2–4 hr. **t½:** 30–180 min in healthy persons. t½ increases with dose, severe renal disease, and cirrhosis and in anephric clients and decreases with pulmonary embolism and liver impairment other than cirrhosis. *Metabolism:* Probably by reticuloendothelial system although up to 50% is excreted unchanged in the urine. Clotting time returns to normal within 2–6 hr.

Uses: Pulmonary embolism, peripheral arterial embolism, prophylaxis, and treatment of venous thrombosis and its extension. Atrial fibrillation with embolization. Diagnosis and treatment of disseminated intravascular coagulation. Low doses to prevent deep venous thrombosis and pulmonary embolism in pregnant clients with a history of thromboembolism, urology clients over 40 years of age, clients with stroke or heart failure, AMI or pulmonary infection, high-risk surgery clients, moderate and high-risk gynecologic clients with no malignancy, neurology clients with extracranial problems, and clients with severe musculoskeletal trauma. Prophylaxis of clotting in blood transfusions, extracorporeal circulation, dialysis procedures, blood samples for lab tests, and arterial and heart surgery. *Investigational:* Prophylaxis of post-MI, CVAs, and LV thrombi. By continuous infusion to treat myocardial ischemia in unstable angina refractory to usual treatment. Adjunct to treat coronary occlusion with AMI. Prophylaxis of cerebral thrombosis in evolving stroke.

Heparin lock flush solution: Dilute solutions are used to maintain patency of indwelling catheters used for IV therapy or blood sampling. Not to be used therapeutically.

Contraindications: Active bleeding, blood dyscrasias (or other disorders characterized by bleeding tendencies such as hemophilia), purpura, thrombocytopenia, liver disease with hypoprothrombinemia, suspected intracranial hemorrhage, suppurative thrombophlebitis, inaccessible ulcerative lesions (especially of the GI tract), open wounds, extensive denudation of the skin, and increased capillary permeability (as in ascorbic acid deficiency). IM use.

Do not administer during surgery of the eye, brain, or spinal cord or during continuous tube drainage of the stomach or small intestine. Use is also contraindicated in subacute endocarditis, shock, advanced kidney disease, threatened abortion, severe hypertension, or hypersensitivity to drug. Premature neonates due to the possibility of a fatal "gasping syndrome."

Special Concerns: NaCl, 0.9%, is effective in maintaining patency of peripheral (noncentral) intermittent infusion devices and in reducing added medical costs. The following procedure has been recommended:

- Determine patency by aspirating lock.
- Flush with 2 mL NSS.
- Administer medication therapy. (Flush between drugs.)
- Flush with 2 mL NSS.

• Frequency of flushing to maintain patency when not actively in use varies from every 8 hr to every 24–48 hr.
• This does *NOT* apply to any central venous access devices.

Side Effects: *CV:* ***Hemorrhage ranging from minor local ecchymoses to major hemorrhagic complications from any organ or tissue.*** Higher incidence is seen in women over 60 years of age. Hemorrhagic reactions are more likely to occur in prophylactic administration during surgery than in the treatment of thromboembolic disease. White clot syndrome. *Hematologic:* Thrombocytopenia (both early and late). *Hypersensitivity:* Chills, fever, urticaria are the most common. Rarely, asthma, lacrimation, headache, N&V, rhinitis, ***shock, anaphylaxis.*** Allergic vasospastic reaction within 6–10 days after initiation of therapy (lasts 4–6 hr) including painful, ischemic, cyanotic limbs. Use a test dose of 1,000 units in clients with a history of asthma or allergic disease. *Miscellaneous:* Hyperkalemia, cutaneous necrosis, osteoporosis (after long-term high doses), delayed transient alopecia, priapism, suppressed aldosterone synthesis. Discontinuance of heparin has resulted in rebound hyperlipemia. *Following IM (usual), SC:* Local irritation, erythema, mild pain, ulceration, hematoma, and tissue sloughing.

Laboratory Test Considerations: ↑ AST and ALT.

OD **Management of Overdose:** *Symptoms:* Nosebleeds, hematuria, tarry stools, petechiae, and easy bruising may be the first signs. *Treatment:* Drug withdrawal is usually sufficient to correct heparin overdosage. Protamine sulfate (1%) solution; each mg of protamine neutralizes about 100 USP heparin units.

Drug Interactions
Alteplase, recombinant / ↑ Risk of bleeding, especially at arterial puncture sites
Anticoagulants, oral / Additive ↑ PT
Antihistamines / ↓ Effect of heparin
Aspirin / Additive ↑ PT
Cephalosporins / ↑ Risk of bleeding due to additive effect
Dextran / Additive ↑ PT
Digitalis / ↓ Effect of heparin
Dipyridamole / Additive ↑ PT
Hydroxychloroquine / Additive ↑ PT
Ibuprofen / Additive ↑ PT
Indomethacin / Additive ↑ PT
Insulin / Heparin antagonizes effect of insulin
Nicotine / ↓ Effect of heparin
Nitroglycerin / ↓ Effect of heparin
NSAIDs / Additive ↑ PT
Penicillins / ↑ Risk of bleeding due to possible additive effects
Salicylates / ↑ Risk of bleeding
Streptokinase / Relative resistance to effects of heparin
Tetracyclines / ↓ Effect of heparin
Ticlopidine / Additive ↑ PT

How Supplied: Heparin sodium injection: *Injection:* 1,000 U/mL, 2,000 U/mL, 2,500 U/mL, 5,000 U/mL, 7,500 U/mL, 10,000 U/mL, 20,000 U/mL. Heparin sodium and sodium chloride: *Injection:* 200 U/100 mL-0.9%, 5,000 U/100 mL-0.45%, 10,000 U/100 mL-0.45%; *Pack:* 10U/mL-0.9%, 100 U/mL-0.9%. Heparin sodium lock flush solution: *Kit:* 10 U/mL, 100 U/mL

Dosage

NOTE: Adjusted for each client on the basis of laboratory tests.

• **Deep SC**

General heparin dosage.

Initial loading dose: 10,000–20,000 units; **maintenance:** 8,000–10,000 units q 8 hr or 15,000–20,000 units q 12 hr. *Use concentrated solution.*

Prophylaxis of postoperative thromboembolism.

5,000 units of concentrated solution 2 hr before surgery and 5,000 units q 8–12 hr thereafter for 7 days or until client is ambulatory.

• **Intermittent IV**

General heparin dosage.

Initial loading dose: 10,000 units undiluted or in 50–100 mL saline; **then,** 5,000–10,000 units q 4–6 hr undiluted or in 50–100 mL saline.

• **Continuous IV Infusion**

General heparin dosage.

Initial loading dose: 20,000–40,000 units/day in 1,000 mL saline (preceded initially by 5,000 units IV).

• **Special Uses**

Surgery of heart and blood vessels.

Initial, 150–400 units/kg to clients undergoing total body perfusion for open heart surgery. *NOTE:* 300 units/kg may be used for procedures less than 60 min while 400 units/kg is used for procedures lasting more than 60 min. To prevent clotting in the tube system, add heparin to fluids in pump oxygenator.

Extracorporeal renal dialysis.

See instructions on equipment.

Blood transfusion.

400–600 units/100 mL whole blood. 7,500 units should be added to 100 mL 0.9% sodium chloride injection; from this dilution, add 6–8 mL/100 mL whole blood.

Laboratory samples.

70–150 units/10- to 20-mL sample to prevent coagulation.

Heparin lock sets.

To prevent clot formation in a heparin lock set, inject 10–100 units/mL heparin solution through the injection hub in a sufficient quantity to fill the entire set to the needle tip.

HEALTH CARE CONSIDERATIONS

Administration/Storage

1. Do *not* administer IM.
2. Administer by deep SC injection to minimize local irritation, hematoma, and tissue sloughing and to prolong action of drug.
• Z-track method: Use any fat roll, but abdominal fat rolls are preferred. Use a ½-in. or ⅝-in., 25- or 27-gauge needle. Grasp the skin layer of the fat roll and lift it up. Insert the needle at about a 45° angle to the skin's fat layer and then administer the medication. It is not necessary to aspirate to check if needle is in a blood vessel. Rapidly withdraw the needle while releasing the skin.
• "Bunch technique" method: Grasp tissue around the injection site, creating a tissue roll of about ½ in. in diameter. Insert needle into the tissue roll at a 90° angle to the skin surface and inject the medication. Again, it is not necessary to aspirate. Withdraw the needle rapidly when the skin is released.
• Do not administer within 2 in. of the umbilicus; due to increased vascularity of area.
3. Do not massage site.
4. Rotate sites of administration.
5. Slight discoloration does not affect potency.
IV 6. Hospitalize for IV therapy.
7. May be diluted in dextrose, NSS, or Ringer's solution and administered over 4–24 hr with an infusion pump.
8. Protect solutions from freezing.
9. Have protamine sulfate, a heparin antagonist, available should excessive bleeding occur.

Assessment

1. Identify any bleeding incidents, i.e., bleeding tendencies, family history, or any other incidents of unexplained or active bleeding.
2. Note history of PUD; may be a potential site of bleeding.
3. Perform test dose (1,000 units SC) to clients with multiple allergies or asthma history.
4. Note any evidence of intracranial hemorrhage.
5. If receiving drugs that interact with anticoagulants, anticipate heparin dosage adjustment.
6. Monitor CBC, PT, PTT, and liver and renal function studies.

Interventions: for *Heparin Lock Flush Solution*.

1. Aspirate lock to determine patency. Maintain patency: inject 1 mL of flush solution into device diaphragm after each use (maintains catheter patency for up to 24 hr).
2. If administering a drug incompatible with heparin, flush with 0.9% NaCl injection or sterile water for injection before and immediately after incompatible drug administered. Inject another dose of heparin lock flush solution after the final flush.
3. Observe coagulation times carefully with underlying bleeding disorders; ↑ risk for hemorrhage.
4. The presence of heparin or NSS may cause lab test interferences.
• To clear flush solution: aspirate and discard 1 mL of fluid from device before withdrawing blood sample.
• Inject 1 mL of flush solution into lock after blood samples are drawn.
• With excessively abnormal results, obtain a repeat sample from another site before initiating treatment.
5. Monitor for allergic reactions due to various biologic sources of heparin.

Client/Family Teaching

1. Review administration technique.
2. Report signs of active bleeding.
3. Report any excessive menstrual flow; may need to withhold or reduce dosage.
4. Alopecia is generally temporary.
5. Report alterations in GU function, urine color, or any injury.
6. Use an electric razor for shaving and a soft-bristle toothbrush to decrease gum irritation.
7. Arrange furniture to allow open space for unimpeded ambulation and to diminish chances of bumping into objects that may cause bruising and bleeding.
8. Use a night light to illuminate trips to the bathroom.
9. Avoid activities where excessive bumping, bruising or injury may occur.
10. Eat potassium-rich foods (e.g., baked potato, orange juice, bananas, beef, flounder, haddock, sweet potato, turkey, raw tomato).
11. Avoid eating large amounts of vitamin K foods, mostly yellow and dark green vegetables.
12. Report any increased bruising, bleeding of nose, mouth, gums, tarry stools, or GI upset.
13. Avoid alcohol, aspirin, and NSAIDs; increase anticoagulant response.

H

14. Alert all providers of therapy and wear/carry drug identification.

Outcome/Evaluate

- Clot prophylaxis/treatment
- Indwelling catheter patency

Histrelin acetate

(hiss-TREL-in)

Pregnancy Category: X

Supprelin, Synarel **(Rx)**

Classification: Gonadotropin-releasing hormone

Action/Kinetics: Histrelin contains a synthetic nonapeptide agonist of the naturally occurring GnRH. Initially the drug stimulates release of GnRH; however, chronic use desensitizes responsiveness of the pituitary gonadotropin, causing a reduction in ovarian and testicular steroidogenesis. Decreases in LH, FSH, and sex steroid levels are observed within 3 months of initiation of therapy.

Uses: To control the biochemical and clinical symptoms of central precocious puberty (either idiopathic or neurogenic) occurring before 8 years of age in girls or 9.5 years of age in boys.

Contraindications: Hypersensitivity to the product or any of its components. Lactation.

Special Concerns: Acute, serious hypersensitivity reactions may occur that require emergency medical treatment. Safety and efficacy in children less than 2 years of age have not been determined.

Side Effects: *Acute hypersensitivity reaction:* Angioedema, urticaria, ***CV collapse,*** hypotension, tachycardia, loss of consciousness, ***bronchospasm,*** dyspnea, flushing, pruritus. *CV:* Vasodilation (common), edema, palpitations, tachycardia, epistaxis, hypertension, migraine headache, pallor. *GI:* GI or abdominal pain, N&V, diarrhea, flatulence, decrease appetite, dyspepsia, GI cramps or distress, constipation, decreased appetite, thirst, gastritis. *CNS:* Headache (common), nervousness, dizziness, depression, changes in libido, mood changes, insomnia, anxiety, paresthesia, syncope, somnolence, cognitive changes, lethargy, impaired consciousness, tremor, hyperkinesia, convulsions (increased frequency), hot flashes or flushes, conduct disorder. *Endocrine:* Vaginal dryness, leukorrhea, metrorrhagia, breast pain, breast edema, decreased breast size, breast discharge, tenderness of female genitalia, anemia, goiter, hyperlipidemia, glycosuria. *Musculoskeletal:* Arthralgia, joint stiffness, muscle cramp or stiffness, myalgia, hypotonia, pain. *Respiratory:* Cough, URI, pharyngitis, respiratory congestion, asthma, breathing disorder, rhinorrhea, bronchitis, sinusitis, hyperventilation. *Dermatologic:* Commonly, redness, itching, and swelling at the injection site. Also, urticaria, sweating, keratoderma, pruritus, pain, dyschromia, alopecia, erythema. *Ophthalmologic:* Visual disturbances, abnormal pupillary function, polyopia, photophobia. *Otic:* Otalgia, hearing loss. *GU:* Vaginal bleeding (most often one episode within 1–3 weeks after starting therapy and lasting several days). Also, vaginitis, dysmenorrhea, and problems of the female genitalia including pruritus, irritation, odor, pain, infections, and hypertrophy. Dyspareunia, polyuria, dysuria, incontinence, urinary frequency, hematuria, nocturia. *Miscellaneous:* Pyrexia (common), weight gain, fatigue, viral infection, chills, various body pains, malaise, purpura.

How Supplied: *Kit:* 0.5 mg/mL, 1 mg/mL

Dosage

- **SC**

Central precocious puberty.

10 mcg/kg given as a single, daily SC injection. Doses greater than 10 mcg/kg/day have not been evaluated.

HEALTH CARE CONSIDERATIONS

Administration/Storage

1. Reevaluate if prepubertal levels of sex hormones or a prepubertal gonadotropin response to GnRH administration are not achieved within the first 3 months of therapy.
2. Rotate injection site daily.
3. Contains no preservative; store vials at 2°C–8°C (36°F–46°F) and protect from light.
4. Use vials only once; discard any unused solution.
5. Remove vial from the packaging only at the time of use. Allow vial to reach room temperature before using.

Assessment

1. Assess for histrelin-related hypersensitivity reactions.
2. Note results of physical and endocrinologic evaluation. This should include:

- Baseline height and weight
- Baseline hand and wrist X rays to determine bone age
- Sex steroid level (estradiol or testosterone)
- Adrenal steroid level (to R/O congenital hyperplasia)
- Beta-human chorionic gonadotropin level (to R/O chorionic gonadotropin-secreting tumor)
- GnRH stimulation test (to document activation of HPG [hypothalamic-pituitary-gonadal] axis)

• Pelvic ultrasound (adrenal, testicular) to R/O steroid-secreting tumor and to obtain baseline gonadal size
• CT of head (to R/O any undiagnosed intracranial tumor)

Client/Family Teaching

1. Review instructions provided with 7-day kit.
2. Drug contains no preservative; once vials entered, discard any unused solution.
3. Administer at room temperature.
4. Establish a daily administration schedule; rotate injection sites. If not administered daily, the pubertal process may be reactivated.
5. Compliance with therapy and scheduled clinical evaluations to assess progress and perform height measurements are important. Yearly bone growth determinations and serial GnRH testing document that gonadotropin responsiveness of the pituitary remains prepubertal during therapy.
6. Report any sudden swelling, dyspnea, dysphagia, rash, itching, and/or rapid heartbeat.
7. Hypogonadism may result if HPG axis reactivation fails after discontinuation of drug.
8. Drug should be discontinued when onset of puberty is desired; need F/U to assess menstrual cyclicity, reproductive function, and adult height attained.

Outcome/Evaluate: Control of biochemical/physical manifestations of puberty

COMBINATION DRUG

Hycodan Syrup and Tablets

(HY-koh-dan)
(Rx) (C-III)
Pregnancy Category: C
Classification: Antitussive

See also information on *Narcotic Analgesics* and *Cholinergic Blocking Agents*.

Content: Each tablet or 5 mL contains: *Antitussive, narcotic:* Hydrocodone bitartrate, 5 mg. *Anticholinergic:* Homatropine methylbromide, 1.5 mg.

Uses: Relief of symptoms of cough.

Special Concerns: May be habit-forming. Use with caution in children with croup, in geriatric or debilitated clients, impaired renal or hepatic function, hyperthyroidism, asthma, narrow-angle glaucoma, prostatic hypertrophy, urethral stricture, Addison's disease. Safety and effectiveness in children less than 6 years of age have not been determined.

How Supplied: See Content

Dosage

• **Tablets, Syrup**

Adults and children over 12 years: 1 tablet or 5 mL q 4–6 hr as needed, not to exceed 6 tablets or 30 mL in 24 hr. **Pediatric, 6–12 years:** ½ tablet or 2.5 mL q 4–6 hr as needed, not to exceed 3 tablets or 15 mL in 24 hr.

HEALTH CARE CONSIDERATIONS

See also *Health Care Considerations* for *Cholinergic Blocking Agents* and *Narcotic Analgesics*.

Administration/Storage

1. The single maximum dose for adults is 3 tablets or 15 mL of syrup after meals and at bedtime.
2. For children over 12 years of age, the maximum dosage is 2 tablets or 10 mL of syrup after meals and at bedtime.
3. For children 2–12 years of age, the maximum dosage is 1 tablet or 5 mL of syrup after meals and at bedtime.
4. For children less than 2 years old, the maximum dosage is ¼ tablet or 1.25 mL of syrup after meals and at bedtime.
5. Doses should be taken at least 4 hr apart.

Client/Family Teaching

1. Drug may cause drowsiness and/or dizziness; avoid tasks that require mental alertness.
2. Report if symptoms persist, change, or intensify after 3–5 days of therapy.
3. May be habit-forming if used for prolonged periods.
4. Safely store and keep out of reach of children.

Outcome/Evaluate: Relief of cough permitting uninterrupted periods of sleep

Hydralazine hydrochloride

(hy-DRAL-ah-zeen)
Pregnancy Category: C
Apo-Hydralazine ★, Apresoline, Novo-Hylazin ★, Nu-Hydral ★ **(Rx)**
Classification: Antihypertensive, direct action on vascular smooth muscle

See also *Antihypertensive Agents*.

Action/Kinetics: Exerts a direct vasodilating effect on vascular smooth muscle. Also alters cellular calcium metabolism that interferes with calcium movement within the vascular smooth muscle responsible for initiating or maintaining contraction. Preferentially dilates arterioles compared with veins; this minimizes postural hypotension and increases CO. Increases renin activity in the kidney, leading to an increase in angiotensin II, which then causes stimulation of aldosterone and thus sodium reabsorption. Because there is a reflex increase in cardiac function, hydralazine is commonly used with drugs that inhibit sympathetic activity (e.g., beta blockers, clonidine, methyldopa). Rapidly absorbed after PO use. Food increases bioavailability of the drug. **PO: Onset:** 45 min; **peak plasma level:** 1–2 hr; **duration:** 3–8 hr. **t$^1/_2$:** 3–7 hr. **IM: Onset:** 10–30 min; **peak plasma level:** 1 hr; **duration:** 2–4 hr. **IV: Onset:** 10–20 min; **maximum effect:** 10–80 min; **duration:** 2–4 hr. Metabolized in the liver and excreted through the kidney (2%–5% unchanged after PO use and 11%–14% unchanged after IV administration).

Uses: PO: In combination with other drugs for essential hypertension. **Parenteral:** Severe essential hypertension when PO use is not possible or when there is an urgent need to lower BP. Hydralazine is the drug of choice for eclampsia. *Investigational:* To reduce afterload in CHF, severe aortic insufficiency, and after valve replacement.

H

Contraindications: Coronary artery disease, angina pectoris, advanced renal disease (as in chronic renal hypertension), rheumatic heart disease (e.g., mitral valvular) and chronic glomerulonephritis.

Special Concerns: Use with caution in stroke clients, in those with pulmonary hypertension, during lactation, in clients with advanced renal disease, and in clients with tartrazine sensitivity. Safety and efficacy have not been established in children. Geriatric clients may be more sensitive to the hypotensive and hypothermic effects of hydralazine; also, a decrease in dose may be necessary in these clients due to age-related decreases in renal function.

Side Effects: *CV:* Orthostatic hypotension, hypotension, ***MI,*** angina pectoris, palpitations, paradoxical pressor reaction, tachycardia. *CNS:* Headache, dizziness, psychoses, tremors, depression, anxiety, disorientation. *GI:* N&V, diarrhea, anorexia, constipation, paralytic ileus. *Allergic:* Rash, urticaria, fever, chills, arthralgia, pruritus, eosinophilia. Rarely, hepatitis, obstructive jaundice. *Hematologic:* Decrease in hemoglobin and RBCs, purpura, agranulocytosis, leukopenia. *Other:* Peripheral neuritis (paresthesias, numbness, tingling), dyspnea, impotence, nasal congestion, edema, muscle cramps, lacrimation, flushing, conjunctivitis, difficulty in urination, lupus-like syndrome, lymphadenopathy, splenomegaly. Side effects are less severe when dosage is increased slowly. *NOTE:* Hydralazine may cause symptoms resembling SLE (e.g., arthralgia, dermatoses, fever, splenomegaly, glomerulonephritis). Residual effects may persist for several years and long-term treatment with steroids may be necessary.

OD Management of Overdose: *Symptoms:* Hypotension, tachycardia, skin flushing, headache. Also, myocardial ischemia, ***cardiac arrhythmias, MI, and severe shock.*** *Treatment:* If the CV status is stable, induce vomiting or perform gastric lavage followed by activated charcoal. Treat shock with volume expanders, without vasopressors; if a vasopressor is necessary, one should be used that is least likely to cause or aggravate tachycardia and cardiac arrhythmias. Monitor renal function.

Drug Interactions

Beta-adrenergic blocking agents / ↑ Effect of both drugs
Indomethacin / ↓ Effect of hydralazine
Methotrimeprazine / Additive hypotensive effect
Procainamide / Additive hypotensive effect
Quinidine / Additive hypotensive effect
Sympathomimetics / ↑ Risk of tachycardia and angina

How Supplied: *Injection:* 20 mg/mL; *Tablet:* 10 mg, 25 mg, 50 mg, 100 mg

Dosage

- **Tablets**

Hypertension.

Adult, initial: 10 mg q.i.d for 2–4 days; **then,** increase to 25 mg q.i.d. for rest of first week. For second and following weeks, increase to 50 mg q.i.d. **Maintenance:** individualized to lowest effective dose; do not exceed a maximum daily dose of 300 mg. **Pediatric, initial:** 0.75 mg/kg/day (25 mg/m^2/day) in two to four divided doses; dosage may be increased gradually up to 7.5 mg/kg/day (or 300 mg/day). Food increases the bioavailability of the drug.

- **IV, IM**

Hypertensive crisis.

Adults, usual: 20–40 mg, repeated as necessary. BP may fall within 5–10 min, with maximum response in 10–80 min. Usually switch to PO medication in 1–2 days. Decrease dosage in clients with renal damage. **Pediatric:** 0.1–0.2 mg/kg q 4–6 hr as needed.

Eclampsia.

5–10 mg q 20 min as an IV bolus. If no effect after 20 mg, another drug should be tried.

HEALTH CARE CONSIDERATIONS

See also *Health Care Considerations* for *Antihypertensive Agents.*

Administration/Storage

1. To enhance bioavailability, give tablets with food.

IV 2. Make parenteral injections as quickly as possible after being drawn into the syringe. Administer undiluted at a rate of 10 mg over at least 1 min.

3. A metal filter will cause a change in color.

Assessment

1. Assess VS; BP (lying, sitting, and standing).
2. Note any drug hypersensitivity.
3. List other drugs prescribed that may interact unfavorably.
4. Note any renal or CAD.
5. Record pulmonary assessment noting lung sounds, presence of rales, dyspnea, JVD, or edema.
6. Explore life-style, dietary and exercise habits; identify areas for change.

Interventions

1. During parenteral administration, take the BP q 5 min until stable, then q 15 min during crisis.
2. Monitor electrolytes and I&O; report reductions in urine output or electrolyte abnormality.
3. Take BP several times/day under standardized conditions, lying, sitting, and/or standing.
4. Clients with cardiac conditions may require closer monitoring during drug therapy.
5. Observe for development of arthralgia, dermatoses, fever, anemia, or splenomegaly; may require discontinuation of drug therapy.

Client/Family Teaching

1. Take with meals to avoid gastric irritation.
2. Headaches, palpitations, and mild postural hypotension may be experienced after the first dose; may persist for 7–10 days with continued treatment.
3. Record daily weights; report any rapid weight gain or edema.
4. Report evidence of a rheumatoid-like or influenza-like syndrome (fever, muscle, or joint aches); this requires discontinuing therapy.
5. Report tingling sensations or discomfort in the hands or feet, signs of peripheral neuropathies; may be reversed with other drugs, i.e., pyridoxine.
6. Avoid alcohol or other OTC agents that could lower BP or interact unfavorably.
7. Continue life-style modifications for BP management with diet, exercise, smoking cessation, limiting alcohol use, and reducing stress.

Outcome/Evaluate

- ↓ BP
- Improvement in S&S of CHF

Hydrochlorothiazide

(hy-droh-klor-oh-THIGH-ah-zyd)

Pregnancy Category: B

Apo-Hydro ✦, Esidrex, Ezide, Hydro-Diuril, Hydro-Par, Microzide, Novo-Hydrazide ✦, Oretic, Urozide ✦ **(Rx)**

Classification: Diuretic, thiazide type

See also *Diuretics, Thiazide.*

Action/Kinetics: Onset: 2 hr. **Peak effect:** 4–6 hr. **Duration:** 6–12 hr. **t½:** 5.6–14.8 hr.

Additional Uses: Microzide is available for once-daily, low-dose treatment for hypertension.

Special Concerns: Geriatric clients may be more sensitive to the usual adult dose.

Additional Side Effects: *CV:* Allergic myocarditis, hypotension. *Dermatologic:* Alopecia, exfoliative dermatitis, ***toxic epidermal necrolysis,*** erythema multiforme, ***Stevens-Johnson syndrome.*** *Miscellaneous:* ***Anaphylactic reactions, respiratory distress including pneumonitis and pulmonary edema.***

How Supplied: *Capsule:* 12.5 mg; *Solution:* 50 mg/5 mL; *Tablet:* 25 mg, 50 mg, 100 mg

Dosage

- **Oral Solution, Tablets**

Diuretic.

Adults, initial: 25–200 mg/day for several days until dry weight is reached; **then,** 25–100 mg/day or intermittently. Some clients may require up to 200 mg/day.

Antihypertensive.

Adults, initial: 25 mg/day as a single dose. The dose may be increased to 50 mg/day in one to two doses. Doses greater than 50 mg may cause significant reductions in serum potassium. **Pediatric, under 6 months:** 3.3 mg/kg/day in two doses; **up to 2 years of age:** 12.5–37.5 mg/day in two doses; **2–12 years of age:** 37.5–100 mg/day in two doses.

HEALTH CARE CONSIDERATIONS

See also *Health Care Considerations* for *Diuretics, Thiazide.*

Administration/Storage

1. Divide daily doses in excess of 100 mg.
2. Give b.i.d. at 6–12-hr intervals.
3. When used with other antihypertensives, the dose of hydrochlorothiazide is usually not greater than 50 mg.

Assessment: Assess for glucose intolerance; monitor electrolytes and replace potassium as needed.

Client/Family Teaching: Take once daily in the morning as directed, usually with a glass of orange juice. Report any unusual side effects.

Outcome/Evaluate

- ↓ BP
- ↑ Urine output; ↓ edema

COMBINATION DRUG

Hydrocodone bitartrate and Acetaminophen

(high-droh-KOH-dohn, ah-seat-ah-MIN-oh-fen)

Pregnancy Category: C

Anexia 5/500, Anexia 7.5/650, Anexsia 10 mg Hydrocodone bitartrate, Anexsia 660 mg Acetaminophen, Lorcet 10/650, Lorcet Plus, Lortab 10/500 10 mg Hydrocodone bitartrate, Lortab 500 mg Acetaminophen **(Rx) (C-III)**

Classification: Analgesic

See also *Narcotic Analgesics* and *Acetaminophen*.

Content: Anexia 5/500: *Narcotic analgesic:* Hydrocodone bitartrate, 5 mg, and *Nonnarcotic analgesic:* Acetaminophen, 500 mg.

Anexia 10/650 and Lorcet 10/650: *Narcotic analgesic:* Hydrocodone bitartrate, 10 mg, and *Nonnarcotic analgesic:* Acetaminophen, 650 mg. Anexia 7.5/650 and Lorcet Plus: *Narcotic analgesic:* Hydrocodone bitartrate, 7.5 mg, and *Nonnarcotic analgesic:* Acetaminophen, 650 mg. Lortab 10/500: *Narcotic analgesic:* Hydrocodone bitartrate, 10 mg, and *Nonnarcotic analgesic*: Acetaminophen, 500 mg.

Action/Kinetics: Hydrocodone produces its analgesic activity by an action on the CNS via opiate receptors. The analgesic action of acetaminophen is produced by both peripheral and central mechanisms.

Uses: Relief of moderate to moderately severe pain.

Contraindications: Hypersensitivity to acetaminophen or hydrocodone. Lactation.

Special Concerns: Use with caution, if at all, in clients with head injuries as the CSF pressure may be increased further. Use with caution in geriatric or debilitated clients; in those with impaired hepatic or renal function; in hypothyroidism, Addison's disease, prostatic hypertrophy, or urethral stricture; and in clients with pulmonary disease. Use shortly before delivery may cause respiratory depression in the newborn. Safety and efficacy have not been determined in children.

Side Effects: *CNS:* Lightheadedness, dizziness, sedation, drowsiness, mental clouding, lethargy, impaired mental and physical performance, anxiety, fear, dysphoria, psychologic dependence, mood changes. *GI:* N&V. *Respiratory:* Respiratory depression (dose-related), irregular and periodic breathing. *GU:* Ureteral spasm, spasm of vesical sphincters, urinary retention.

OD **Management of Overdose:** *Symptoms:* ***Acetaminophen overdose may result in potentially fatal hepatic necrosis.*** Also, renal tubular necrosis, hypoglycemic coma, and thrombocytopenia. Symptoms of hepatotoxic overdose include N&V, diaphoresis, and malaise. Symptoms of hydrocodone overdose include respiratory depression, somnolence progressing to stupor or ***coma,*** skeletal muscle flaccidity, cold and clammy skin, bradycardia, and hypotension. ***Severe overdose may cause apnea, circulatory collapse, cardiac arrest, and death.*** *Treatment (Acetaminophen):*

- Empty stomach promptly by lavage or induction of emesis with syrup of ipecac.
- Serum acetaminophen levels should be determined as early as possible but no sooner than 4 hr after ingestion.
- Determine liver function initially and at 24-hr intervals.
- The antidote, *N*-acetylcysteine, should be given within 16 hr of overdose for optimal results.

Treatment (Hydrocodone):

- Reestablish adequate respiratory exchange with a patent airway and assisted or controlled ventilation.
- Respiratory depression can be reversed by giving naloxone IV.
- Oxygen, IV fluids, vasopressors, and other supportive measures may be instituted as required.

Drug Interactions

Anticholinergics / ↑ Risk of paralytic ileus

CNS depressants, including other narcotic analgesics, antianxiety agents, antipsychotics, alcohol / Additive CNS depression

MAO inhibitors / ↑ Effect of either the narcotic or the antidepressant

Tricyclic antidepressants / ↑ Effect of either the narcotic or the antidepressant

How Supplied: See Content

Dosage

- **Tablets**

Analgesia.

1 tablet of Anexsia 7.5/650, Lorcet 10/650, or Lorcet Plus q 4–6 hr as needed for pain. The total 24-hr dose should not exceed 6 tablets. 1–2 tablets of Anexsia 5/500 q 4–6 hr as needed for pain. The total 24-hr dose should not exceed 8 tablets.

HEALTH CARE CONSIDERATIONS

See also *Health Care Considerations* for *Narcotic Analgesics* and *Acetaminophen*.

Assessment

1. Note onset, location, duration of symptoms, other agents prescribed, and the outcome. Determine if pain is acute or chronic; rate pain level.
2. Note history of hypothyroidism, BPH,

urethral stricture, Addison's, or pulmonary disease.
3. Monitor renal and LFTs.
4. Coadministration of an NSAID may reduce the dosage required for pain relief.

Client/Family Teaching

1. Take only as prescribed.
2. Do not perform activities that require mental alertness; causes dizziness, lethargy, and impaired physical and mental performance.
3. Report any evidence of abnormal bleeding or bruising, respiratory difficulties, N&V, urinary difficulty, or excessive sedation.
4. Avoid alcohol and any other medications without approval.
5. Store drug appropriately, away from the bedside and safely out of the reach of children.

Outcome/Evaluate: Desired pain control

COMBINATION DRUG

Hydrocodone bitartrate and Ibuprofen

(high-droh-**KOH**-dohn/eye-byou-**PROH**-fen)

Pregnancy Category: C

Vicoprofen **(Rx) (C-III)**

Classification: Narcotic analgesic and nonsteroidal anti-inflammatory drug

See also *Hydrocodone bitartrate* and *Ibuprofen*.

Content: Each tablet contains *Narcotic:* Hydrocodone bitartrate, 7.5 mg and *NSAID:* Ibuprofen, 200 mg.

Action/Kinetics: Peak plasma levels: 1.7 hr for hydrocodone and 1.8 hr for ibuprofen. **$t_{1/2}$ plasma, hydrocodone:** 4.5 hr; **ibuprofen:** 2.2 hr.

Uses: Short-term (less than 10 days) for management of acute pain.

Additional Contraindications: Use for osteoarthritis or rheumatoid arthritis. Use during labor and delivery or during lactation.

Special Concerns: Use with caution and at reduced doses in geriatric clients. Safety and efficacy have not been determined in children.

How Supplied: See Content.

Dosage

- **Tablets**

  Analgesic.

Adults: 1 tablet q 4–6 hr, as needed. Dosage should not exceed 5 tablets in a 24–hr period. Adjust dose and frequency of dosing to client needs.

HEALTH CARE CONSIDERATIONS

See also *Health Care Considerations* for *Hydrocodone bitartrate* and *Ibuprofen*.

Assessment

1. Record onset, location, and characteristics of pain; rate pain using a pain–rating scale.
2. Note any conditions that may preclude use of drug combination.

Client/Family Teaching

1. Take only as prescribed, do not exceed 5 tabs/day.
2. Drug is for short term use only, up to 10 days; may be habit forming.
3. Do not perform activities that require mental/physical alertness; may cause impairment.
4. Avoid alcohol and any other CNS depressants.
5. Report any S&S of GI bleeding, blurred vision, or other eye problems, skin rash, weight gain, or swelling of extremities.

Outcome/Evaluate: Relief of pain

Hydrocortisone (Cortisol)

(hy-droh-**KOR**-tih-zohn)

Pregnancy Category: C (topical and dental products)

Parenteral: Sterile Hydrocortisone Suspension. **Rectal:** Dermolate Anal-Itch, Cortenema ✦, Proctocort, ProctoCream.HC 2.5%, Rectocort ✦. **Retention Enema:** Cortenema, Hycort ✦, Rectocort ✦. **Roll-on Applicator:** Cortaid FastStick, Maximum Strength Cortaid Faststick, **Tablets:** Cortef, Hydrocortone. **Topical Cream:** Ala-Cort, Allercort, Alphaderm, Bactine, Cortate ✦, Cort-Dome, Cortifair, Dermacort, DermiCort, Dermolate Anti-Itch, Dermtex HC, Emo-Cort ✦, H_2Cort, Hi-Cor 1.0 and 2.5, Hydro-Tex, Hytone, Nutracort, Penecort, Prevex HC ✦, Synacort. **Topical Gel:** Extra Strength CortaGel, **Topical Liquid:** Scalpicin, T/Scalp, **Topical Lotion:** Acticort 100, Ala-Cort, Ala-Scalp, Allercort, Aquacort ✦, Cetacort, Cortate ✦, Cort-Dome, Delacort, Dermacort, Dermolate Scalp-Itch, Emo-Cort ✦, Gly-Cort, Hytone, LactiCare-HC, Lemoderm, Lexocort Forte, My Cort, Nutracort, Pentacort, Rederm, Sarna HC ✦, S-T Cort. **Topical Ointment:** Allercort, Cortoderm ✦, Cortril, Hytone, Lemoderm, Penecort. **Topical Solution:** Penecort, Emo-Cort Scalp Solution, Texacort Scalp Solution. **Topical Spray:** Cortaid, Dermolate Anti-Itch, Maximum Strength Coraid, Procort **(OTC) (Rx)**

Hydrocortisone acetate

(hy-droh-**KOR**-tih-zohn)

Pregnancy Category: C (topical and dental products)

Dental Paste: Orabase-HCA. **Intrarectal Foam:** Cortifoam. **Ophthalmic/Otic:** Cortamed ✽. **Parenteral:** Hydrocortone Acetate. **Rectal:** Cort-Dome High Potency, Cortenema, Corticaine, Cortifoam. **Suppository:** Cortiment ✽, Rectocort ✽, **Topical Cream:** CaldeCORT Light, Carmol-HC, Cortaid, Cortef Feminine Itch, Corticaine, Corticreme ✽, FoilleCort, Gynecort, Gynecort Female Cream, Hyderm ✽, Lanacort, Lanacort 10, Lanacort 5, Maximum Strength Cortaid, Pharma-Cort, Rhulicort. **Topical Lotion:** Cortaid, Rhulicort. **Topical Ointment:** Anusol HC-1, Cortef Acetate, Dermaflex HC 1% ✽, Lanacort, Lanacort 5, Nov–Hydrocort., Maximum Strength Cortaid **(OTC) (Rx)**

H

Hydrocortisone butyrate

(hy-droh-**KOR**-tih-zohn)
Pregnancy Category: C (topical products)
Topical Cream, Ointment, Solution: Locoid **(Rx)**

Hydrocortisone cypionate

(hy-droh-**KOR**-tih-zohn)
Pregnancy Category: C
Oral Suspension: Cortef **(Rx)**

Hydrocortisone probutate

(hy-droh-**KOR**-tih-zohn)
Pregnancy Category: C
Topical Cream: Pandel **(Rx)**

Hydrocortisone sodium phosphate

(hy-droh-**KOR**-tih-zohn)
Pregnancy Category: C
Parenteral: Hydrocortone Phosphate **(Rx)**

Hydrocortisone sodium succinate

(hy-droh-**KOR**-tih-zohn)
Pregnancy Category: C
Parenteral: A-hydroCort, Solu-Cortef **(Rx)**

Hydrocortisone valerate

(hy-droh-**KOR**-tih-zohn)
Pregnancy Category: C (topical products)
Topical Cream/Ointment: Westcort **(Rx)**
Classification: Corticosteroid, naturally occurring; glucocorticoid-type

See also *Corticosteroids.*
Action/Kinetics: Short-acting. **t½:** 80–118 min. Topical products are available without a prescription in strengths of 0.5% and 1%.
How Supplied: Hydrocortisone Cortisol: *Balm:* 1%; *Cream:* 0.5%, 1%, 2.5%; *Enema:* 100 mg/60 mL; *Gel/jelly:* 1%; *Liquid:* 1%; *Lotion:* 0.25%, O.5%, 1%, 2%, 2.5%; *Ointment:* 0.5%, 1%, 2.5%; *Pad:* 0.5%, 1%; *Solution:* 1%, 2.5%; *Spray:* 1%; *Tablet:* 5 mg, 10 mg, 20 mg. Hydrocortisone acetate: *Cream:* 0.5%, 1%; *Foam:* 10%; *Injection:* 50 mg/mL; *Ointment:* 0.5%, 1%; *Spray:* 0.5%; *Suppository:* 25 mg, 30 mg. Hydrocortisone butyrate: *Cream:* 0.1%; *Ointment:* 0.1%; *Solution:* 0.1%. Hydrocortisone cypionate: *Suspension:* 10 mg/5 mL. Hydrocortisone probutate: *Cream:* 0.1%. Hydrocortisone sodium phosphate: *Injection:* 50 mg/mL. Hydrocortisone sodium succinate: *Powder for injection:* 100 mg, 250 mg, 500 mg, 1 g. Hydrocortisone valerate: *Cream:* 0.2%; *Ointment:* 0.2%.

Dosage

HYDROCORTISONE
- **Tablets**

20–240 mg/day, depending on disease.
- **IM Only**

One-third to one-half the PO dose q 12 hr.
- **Rectal**

100 mg in retention enema nightly for 21 days (up to 2 months of therapy may be needed; discontinue gradually if therapy exceeds 3 weeks).
- **Topical Ointment, Cream, Gel, Lotion, Solution, Spray**

Apply sparingly to affected area and rub in lightly t.i.d.–q.i.d.

HYDROCORTISONE ACETATE
- **Intralesional, Intra-articular, Soft Tissue**

5–50 mg, depending on condition.
- **Intrarectal Foam**

1 applicatorful (90 mg) 1–2 times/day for 2–3 weeks; **then** every second day.
- **Topical**

See *Hydrocortisone.*

HYDROCORTISONE BUTYRATE
- **Topical Cream, Ointment, Solution**

Apply a thin film to the affected area b.i.d.–t.i.d.

HYDROCORTISONE PROBUTATE
- **Topical Cream**

Apply a thin film to the affected area 1–2 times/day.

HYDROCORTISONE CYPIONATE
- **Suspension**

20–240 mg/day, depending on the severity of the disease.

HYDROCORTISONE SODIUM PHOSPHATE
- **IV, IM, SC**

General uses.
Initial: 15–240 mg/day depending on use and on severity of the disease. Usually, one-half to one-third of the PO dose is given q 12 hr.

Adrenal insufficiency, acute.
Adults, initial: 100 mg IV; **then,** 100 mg q 8 hr in an IV fluid; **older children, initial:** 1–2 mg/kg by IV bolus; **then,** 150–250 mg/kg/day IV in divided doses; **infants, initial:** 1–2 mg/kg by IV bolus; **then,** 25–150 mg/kg/day in divided doses.

HYDROCORTISONE SODIUM SUCCINATE

• **IM, IV**

Initial: 100–500 mg; **then,** may be repeated at 2-, 4-, and 6-hr intervals depending on response and severity of condition.

HYDROCORTISONE VALERATE

• **Topical Cream**

See *Hydrocortisone.*

HEALTH CARE CONSIDERATIONS

See also *Health Care Considerations* for *Corticosteroids.*

Administration/Storage

1. When using topical products, wash area prior to application to increase drug penetration.
2. Do not allow topical product to come in contact with the eyes.
3. Avoid prolonged use of topical products near the genital/rectal areas and eyes, on the face, and in creases of the skin.
4. For the probutate and butyrate topical products, use an occlusive dressing only on advice of the provider if used to treat psoriasis or other deep-seated dermatoses.
5. Do not use buteprate products in the diaper area. With the butyrate products, do not use tight-fitting diapers or plastic pants.
6. No part of the intrarectal foam aerosol container should be inserted into the anus.
IV 7. Check label of parenteral hydrocortisone because IM and IV preparations are not necessarily interchangeable.
8. Give reconstituted direct IV solution at a rate of 100 mg over 30 sec. Doses larger than 500 mg should be infused over 10 min. Drug may be further diluted in 50–100 mL of dextrose or saline solutions and administered as ordered within 24 hr.

Assessment

1. Record indications for therapy, type, location, onset, and duration of symptoms.
2. List other agents used and the outcome.
3. Assess CBC, chemistry profile, liver and renal function studies.

Outcome/Evaluate

- Replacement of adrenocortical deficiency
- Restoration of skin integrity
- Relief of allergic manifestations

Hydromorphone hydrochloride

(hy-droh-**MOR**-fohn)

Pregnancy Category: C

Dilaudid, Dilaudid-HP, Dilaudid-HP-Plus ✱, Dilaudid Sterile Powder ✱, Dilaudid-XP ✱, Hydromorph Contin ✱, PMS-Hydromorphone ✱ **(C-II) (Rx)**

Classification: Narcotic analgesic, morphine type

See also *Narcotic Analgesics.*

Action/Kinetics: Hydromorphone is 7–10 times more analgesic than morphine, with a shorter duration of action. It manifests less sedation, less vomiting, and less nausea than morphine, although it induces pronounced respiratory depression. **Onset:** 15–30 min. **Peak effect:** 30–60 min. **Duration:** 4–5 hr. **t½:** 2–3 hr. Give rectally for prolonged activity.

Uses: Analgesia for moderate to severe pain (e.g., surgery, cancer, biliary colic, burns, renal colic, MI, bone trauma). Dilaudid-HP is a concentrated solution intended for those tolerant to narcotics.

Additional Contraindications: Migraine headaches. Use in children. Status asthmaticus, obstetrics, respiratory depression in absence of resuscitative equipment. Lactation.

Special Concerns: Do not confuse Dilaudid-HP with standard parenteral solutions of Dilaudid or with other narcotics as overdose and death can result. Use Dilaudid-HP with caution in clients with circulatory shock.

Additional Side Effects: Nystagmus.

How Supplied: *Injection:* 1 mg/mL, 2 mg/mL, 4 mg/mL, 10 mg/mL; *Liquid:* 1 mg/mL; *Powder for injection:* 250 mg/vial; *Suppository;* 3 mg; *Tablet:* 2 mg, 4 mg, 8 mg

Dosage

• **Tablets, Liquid**

Analgesia.

Adults: 2 mg q 4–6 hr as necessary. For severe pain, 4 or more mg q 4–6 hr.

• **Suppositories**

Analgesia.

Adults: 3 mg q 6–8 hr.

• **SC, IM, IV**

Analgesia.

Adults: 1–2 mg q 4–6 hr. For severe pain, 3–4 mg q 4–6 hr.

HEALTH CARE CONSIDERATIONS

See also *Health Care Considerations* for *Narcotic Analgesics.*

Administration/Storage

1. Refrigerate suppositories.
2. May be given as Dilaudid brand cough syrup. Be alert to an allergic response in those sensitive to yellow dye number 5.
IV 3. May be given by slow IV injection. Administer drug slowly to minimize hypotensive effects and respiratory depression. Dilute

with 5 mL of sterile water or NSS and administer at a rate of 2 mg over 5 min.

Assessment

1. Record type, location, onset, and duration of symptoms. Use a rating scale to rate pain.
2. Assess for respiratory depression; more profound with hydromorphone than with other narcotic analgesics. Encourage to turn, cough, deep breathe or use incentive spirometry every 2 hr to prevent atelectasis.
3. Drug may mask symptoms of acute pathology; assess abdomen carefully.

Client/Family Teaching

1. Use exactly as directed at the onset of pain and in the dose prescribed. Report any unusual or intolerable side effects.
2. Do not perform activities that require mental alertness or coordination.

Outcome/Evaluate: Relief of pain

H

Hydroxychloroquine sulfate

(hy-drox-ee-**KLOR**-oh-kwin)

Plaquenil Sulfate **(Rx)**

Classification: 4-Aminoquinoline, antimalarial, and antirheumatic

Action/Kinetics: Peak plasma levels: 1–3 hr. Accumulates in the liver, spleen, kidney, heart, lung, and brain. About 50% of unchanged drug excreted in the urine. Enhance excretion by acidifying the urine and decrease by alkalizing the urine.

Uses: Prophylaxis and treatment of acute attacks of malaria due to *Plasmodium vivax, P. malariae, P. ovale,* and susceptible strains of *P. falciparum*. Acute or chronic rheumatoid arthritis (not a drug of choice; discontinue after 6 months if no beneficial effects noted). Discoid and SLE. Not used as a first line of therapy.

Additional Contraindications: Long-term therapy in children, ophthalmologic changes due to 4-aminoquinolines. Pregnancy.

Special Concerns: Use with caution in alcoholism or liver disease. Use in psoriasis may precipitate an acute attack.

Additional Side Effects: The appearances of skin eruptions or of misty vision and visual halos are indications for withdrawal. Clients on long-term therapy should be examined thoroughly at regular intervals for knee and ankle reflexes and hematopoietic studies.

Drug Interactions

Digoxin / Hydroxychloroquine ↑ serum digoxin levels

Gold salts / Dermatitis and ↑ risk of severe skin reactions

Phenylbutazone / Dermatitis and ↑ risk of severe skin reactions

How Supplied: *Tablet:* 200 mg

Dosage

- **Tablets**

Acute malarial attack.

Adults, initial: 800 mg; **then,** 400 mg after 6–8 hr and 400 mg/day for next 2 days. **Children:** A total of 32 mg/kg given over a 3-day period as follows: **initial:** 12.9 mg/kg (not to exceed a single dose of 800 mg); **then,** 6.4 mg/kg (not to exceed a single dose of 400 mg) 6, 24, and 48 hr after the first dose.

Suppression of malaria.

Adults: 400 mg q 7 days. If therapy has not been initiated 14 days prior to exposure, an initial loading dose of 800 mg may be given in two divided doses 6 hr apart. **Children:** 6.4 mg/kg (not to exceed the adult dose) q 7 days. If therapy has not been initiated 14 days prior to exposure, an initial loading dose of 12.9 mg/kg may be given in two doses 6 hr apart.

Rheumatoid arthritis.

Adults: 400–600 mg/day taken with milk or meals; **maintenance** (usually after 4–12 weeks): 200–400 mg/day. Use in children is limited, but if use is warranted, a dose of 3–5 mg/kg/day, up to a maximum of 400 mg/day (given once or twice daily), may be used. (*NOTE:* Several months may be required for a beneficial effect to be seen in adults and children.)

Lupus erythematosus.

Adults, usual: 400 mg once or twice daily; **prolonged maintenance:** 200–400 mg/day.

HEALTH CARE CONSIDERATIONS

See also *General Health Care Considerations for All Anti-Infectives.*

Administration/Storage

1. Corticosteroids and salicylates may be used with hydroxychloroquine.
2. When a gradual decrease of steroid dose is indicated, reduce gradually (q 4–5 days). Reduce the dose of cortisone by no more than 5–15 mg; hydrocortisone from 5–10 mg; predisone and prednisolone from 1–2.5 mg; methylprednisolone and triamcinolone from 1–2 mg; and dexamethasone from 0.25–0.5 mg.
3. If the recommeded maintenance dose is exceeded, the incidence of retinopathy increases.

Assessment

1. Record indications for therapy, type and onset of symptoms, dates of exposure.
2. Record condition of skin; strength of ankle and knee reflexes; any joint swelling, dis-

coloration, and warmth; ROM and pain level.
3. Determine history of liver disease or alcohol abuse.
4. Monitor CBC, liver/renal function studies, and eye exams q 3 mo.

Client/Family Teaching

1. Report any skin eruptions or muscular weakness.
2. Report any visual disturbances; obtain regular eye exams; retinopathy is dose related.
3. Avoid excessive sun exposure; use sunscreen, hat, glasses, and protective clothing.
4. When given for rheumatoid arthritis:
• GI irritation may be reduced by taking with meals or a glass of milk.
• Corticosteroids and salicylates or NSAIDs may be used concomitantly; continue anti-inflammatory dose for several weeks into therapy.
• Report all side effects. Anticipate excessive side effects; may necessitate dosage reduction. After 5–10 days of reduced dosage, provider may gradually increase drug to desired level.
• Reduce dosage when desired response attained so drug will again be effective in case of flare-up.
• Benefits may not occur until 6–12 months after therapy initiated.
5. When given for lupus erythematosus, administer with evening meal.
6. Initiate suppressive antimalarial therapy 2 weeks prior to exposure; continue for 6–8 weeks after leaving endemic area. If not started prior to exposure, double the initial loading dose and take in two doses 6 hr apart.

Outcome/Evaluate

• Malarial prophylaxis
• Termination of acute malarial attack; suppression of symptoms
• ↓ Joint pain and swelling; ↑ mobility

Hydroxyurea

(hy-**DROX**-ee-you-**ree**-ah)
Pregnancy Category: D
Droxia, Hydrea (Abbreviation: HYD) **(Rx)**
Classification: Antineoplastic, antimetabolite

See also *Antineoplastic Agents.*
Action/Kinetics: Inhibits DNA synthesis but not synthesis of RNA or protein. As an antimetabolite, it interferes with the conversion of ribonucleotides to deoxyribonucleotides due to blockade of the ribonucleotide reductase system. May also inhibit incorporation of thymidine into DNA. Effectiveness in sickle cell anemia may be due to increases in hemoglobin F levels in RBCs, decrease in neutrophils, increases in the water content of RBCs, increases the deformability of sickled cells, and altered adhesion of RBCs to the endothelium. Rapidly absorbed from GI tract. **Peak serum concentration:** 1–2 hr. **t½:** 3–4 hr. Crosses the blood-brain barrier. Degraded in liver; 80% excreted through the urine with 50% unchanged; also excreted as respiratory CO_2.
Uses: Chronic, resistant, myelocytic leukemia. Carcinoma of the ovary (recurrent, inoperable, or metastatic). Melanoma. With irradiation to treat primary squamous cell carcinoma of the head and neck (but not the lip). Sickle cell anemia (Droxia). *Investigational:* Thrombocytopenia, HIV, psoriasis.
Contraindications: Leukocyte count less than 2,500/mm^3 or thrombocyte count less than 100,000/mm^3. Severe anemia.
Special Concerns: Use during pregnancy only if benefits clearly outweigh risks. Give with caution to clients with marked renal dysfunction. Geriatric clients may be more sensitive to the effects of hydroxyurea necessitating a lower dose. Dosage has not been established in children.
Laboratory Test Considerations: ↑ Serum uric acid, BUN, and creatinine.
Additional Side Effects: Erythrocyte abnormalities including megaloblastic erythropoiesis. Constipation, redness of the face, maculopapular rash.
How Supplied: *Capsule:* 200 mg, 300 mg, 400 mg, 500 mg

Dosage

• **Capsules**

Solid tumors, intermittent therapy or when used together with irradiation.
Dose individualized. Usual: 80 mg/kg as a single dose every third day. Intermittent dosage offers advantage of reduced toxicity. If effective, maintain client on drug indefinitely unless toxic effects preclude such a regimen.

Solid tumors, continuous therapy.
20–30 mg/kg/day as a single dose.

Resistant chronic myelocytic leukemia.
20–30 mg/kg/day in a single dose or two divided daily doses.

Concomitant therapy with irradiation for carinoma of the head and neck.
80 mg/kg as a single dose every third day.

Sickle cell anemia.
Initial: 15 mg once daily. Base dosage on the smaller of ideal or actual body weight. Increase dose gradually to the maximum tolerated dose or to 35 mg/kg/day.

HEALTH CARE CONSIDERATIONS

See also *Health Care Considerations* for *Antineoplastic Agents.*

Administration/Storage

1. Calculate dosage based on actual or ideal weight (whichever is less).
2. Continue therapy for at least 6 weeks before efficacy is assessed.
3. If unable to swallow a capsule, contents may be given in glass of water and drunk immediately; some material may not dissolve and may float on top of glass.
4. Start hydroxyurea at least 7 days before initiation of irradiation; continue through irradiation and indefinitely afterward as long as the client can tolerate the dose. The dosage of radiation is not usually adjusted with concomitant usage of hydroxyurea.
5. Do not store in excessive heat.

Assessment

1. Assess for exacerbation of postirradiation erythema.
2. Monitor uric acid, liver and renal function studies. With sickle cell anemia, monitor blood count q 2 weeks; adjust dosage to keep neutrophil, platelet, hemoglobin, and reticulocyte counts within acceptable ranges.
3. Initially, obtain hematologic profiles weekly. Drug may cause severe granulocyte and platelet suppression. Nadir: 7 days; recovery: 14 days.

Outcome/Evaluate

- Suppression of malignant process
- ↓ Tumor size and spread
- ↓ Occurrence of sickle cell crisis

Hydroxyzine hydrochloride

(hy-**DROX**-ih-zeen)

Apo-Hydroxyzine ✦, Atarax, Atarax 100, Multipax ✦, Novo–Hydroxyzide ✦, Nu-Hydroxyzin ✦, PMS Hydroxyzine ✦, Vistaril, Vistazine 50 **(Rx)**

Hydroxyzine pamoate

(hy-**DROX**-ih-zeen)

Vistaril **(Rx)**

Classification: Nonbenzodiazepine antianxiety agent

Action/Kinetics: Manifests anticholinergic, antiemetic, antispasmodic, local anesthetic, antihistaminic, and skeletal relaxant effects. Has mild antiarrhythmic activity and mild analgesic effects. High sedative and antiemetic effects and moderate anticholinergic activity. **Onset:** 15–30 min. **t½:** 3 hr. **Duration:** 4–6 hr. Metabolized by the liver and excreted through the urine. The pamoate salt is believed to be converted to the hydrochloride in the stomach.

Uses: PO: Symptomatic relief of anxiety and tension associated with psychoneurosis. Anxiety observed in organic disease. Prior to dental procedures, in acute emotional problems, in alcoholism, allergic conditions with strong emotional overlay (e.g., chronic urticaria and pruritus). Beneficial to the cardiac client to allay anxiety and apprehension occurring with certain types of heart disease. Pruritus caused by allergic conditions. **IM:** Acute hysteria or agitation, withdrawal symptoms (including delirium tremens) in the acute or chronic alcoholic. Pre- and postoperative and pre- and postpartum adjunct to allay anxiety, to control emesis or to allow a decrease in dosage of narcotics.

Contraindications: Pregnancy (especially early) or lactation; treatment of morning sickness during pregnancy or as sole agent for treatment of psychoses or depression. Hypersensitivity to drug. IV, SC, or intra-arterially.

Special Concerns: Possible increased anticholinergic and sedative effects in geriatric clients.

Side Effects: Low incidence at recommended dosages. Drowsiness, dryness of mouth, involuntary motor activity (rarely, tremors and convulsions), ECG abnormalities (e.g., alterations in T-waves), dizziness, urticaria, skin reactions, hypersensitivity. Worsening of porphyria. Marked discomfort, induration, and even gangrene at site of IM injection.

OD Management of Overdose: *Symptoms:* Oversedation. *Treatment:* Immediate induction of vomiting or performance of gastric lavage. General supportive care with monitoring of VS. Control hypotension with IV fluids and either norepinephrine or metaraminol (epinephrine should not be used).

Drug Interactions: Additive effects when used with other CNS depressants. See *Drug Interactions* for *Tranquilizers.*

How Supplied: Hydroxyzine hydrochloride: *Injection:* 25 mg/mL, 50 mg/mL; *Syrup:* 10 mg/5 mL; *Tablet:* 10 mg, 25 mg, 50 mg, 100 mg. Hydroxyzine pamoate: *Capsule:* 25 mg, 50 mg, 100 mg; *Suspension:* 25 mg/5 mL

Dosage

• **Capsules, Oral Suspension, Syrup, Tablets. Hydroxyzine hydrochloride and hydroxyzine pamoate**

Antianxiety.

Adults: 50–100 mg q.i.d.; **pediatric under 6 years:** 50 mg/day in divided doses; **over 6 years:** 50–100 mg/day in divided doses.

Pruritus.

Adults: 25 mg t.i.d.–q.i.d.; **children under 6 years:** 50 mg/day in divided doses; **chil-**

dren over 6 years: 50–100 mg/day in divided doses.

Preoperative or post–general anesthetic sedative.

Adults: 50–100 mg; **children:** 0.6 mg/kg.

• **IM. Hydroxyzine Hydrochloride**

Acute anxiety, including alcohol withdrawal.

Adults: 50–100 mg q.i.d.

Antiemetic/analgesia, adjunctive therapy.

Adults: 25–100 mg; **pediatric,** 1.1 mg/kg. Switch to **PO** as soon as possible.

Pruritus.

Adults: 25 mg t.i.d. or q.i.d.

Sedative, as premedication and following general anesthesia.

Adults: 50–100 mg. **Children:** 0.6 mg/kg.

HEALTH CARE CONSIDERATIONS

See also *Health Care Considerations* for *Tranquilizers/Antimanic Drugs/Hypnotics.*

Administration/Storage

1. Inject IM only. Make injection into the upper, outer quadrant of the buttocks or the midlateral muscles of the thigh. In children inject into the midlateral muscles of the thigh. In infants and small children, to minimize sciatic nerve damage, use the periphery of the upper outer quadrant of the gluteal region only when necessary (e.g., burn clients).
2. Shake suspension vigorously until it is completely resuspended.

Assessment: Record indications for therapy, type, onset, location, and duration of symptoms. Note any associated characteristics or contributing factors.

Client/Family Teaching

1. Frequent mouth rinsing, sucking hard candy, chewing sugarless gums, and increased fluid intake may relieve symptoms of dry mouth.
2. Wait and evaluate sedative effects of drug before performing tasks that require mental alertness.
3. Avoid alcohol or any other CNS depressants.
4. Drug is only for short-term management.

Outcome/Evaluate

- ↓ Anxiety and agitation
- Relief of itching/allergic S&S
- Control of N&V

Hylan G-F 20

(**HIGH**-lan)
Synvisc **(Rx)**

See *Sodium hyaluronate.*

Hyoscyamine sulfate

(high-oh-**SIGH**-ah-meen)
Pregnancy Category: C
Anaspaz, Cystospaz-M, Espasmotex, Levbid, Levsin, Levsinex, Levsin SL, Spasdel **(Rx)**
Classification: Cholinergic blocking agent

See also *Cholinergic Blocking Agents.*

Action/Kinetics: One of the belladonna alkaloids; acts by blocking the action of acetylcholine at the postganglionic nerve endings of the parasympathetic nervous system. **t½:** 3½ hr for tablets, 7 hr for extended-release capsules, and 9 hr for extended-release tablets. Majority of the drug is excreted in the urine unchanged.

Uses: To control gastric secretion, visceral spasm, and hypermotilitiy in spastic colitis, spastic bladder, cystitis, pylorospasm, and associated abdominal cramps. Adjunctive therapy to treat irritable bowel syndrome and functional GI disorders. Adjunctive therapy in neurogenic bladder and neurogenic bowel disturbances. Treat infant colic (use elixir or solution). Use with morphine or other narcotics for symptomatic relief of biliary and renal colic. In Parkinsonism to reduce rigidity and tremors and to control sialorrhea and hyperhidrosis. To treat poisoning by anticholinesterase agents. To reduce GI motility to facilitate diagnostic procedures, such as endoscopy or hypersecretion in pancreatitis. To treat selected cases of partial heart block associated with vagal activity. Used as a preoperative medication to reduce salivary, tracheobronchial, and pharyngeal secretions.

Special Concerns: Heat prostration may occur if the drug is taken in the presence of high environmental temperatures. Use with caution during lactation.

Side Effects: See *Cholinergic Blocking Agents.*

How Supplied: *Capsule, Extended Release:* 0.375 mg; *Elixir:* 0.125 mg/5 mL; *Injection:* 0.5 mg/mL; *Liquid:* 0.125 mg/mL; *Tablet:* 0.125 mg; *Tablet, Extended Release:* 0.375 mg.

Dosage

• **Extended-Release Capsules (0.375 mg) or Extended-Release Tablets (0.375 mg)**

Adults and children over 12 years of age: 0.375–0.750 mg q 12 hr, not to exceed 1.5 mg in 24 hr.

• **Tablets (0.125 mg)**

Adults and children over 12 years of age: 0.125–0.25 mg q 4 hr or as needed, not to exceed 1.5 mg in 24 hr.

• **Elixir (0.125 mg/5 mL)**

H

Adults and children over 12 years of age: 0.125 mg–0.25 mg (5–10 mL) q 4 hr, not to exceed 1.5 mg (60 mL) in 24 hr. **Children, 2 to 12 years of age:** 10 kg: 1.25 mL (0.031 mg) q 4 hr; 20 kg: 2.5 mL (0.062 mg) q 4 hr; 40 kg: 3.75 mL (0.093 mg) q 4 hr; 50 kg: 5 mL (0.125 mg) q 4 hr.

- **Drops (0.125 mg/mL)**

Adults and children over 12 years of age: 0.125–0.25 mg 5–10 mL q 4 hr, not to exceed 1.5 mg (12 mL) in 24 hr. **Children, 2 to 12 years of age:** 0.031–0.125 mg (0.251 mL) q 4 hr or as needed, not to exceed 0.75 mg (6 mL) in 24 hr. **Children, under 2 years of age:** 3.4 kg: 4 drops q 4 hr, not to exceed 24 drops in 24 hr; 5 kg: 5 drops q 4 hr, not to exceed 30 drops in 24 hr; 7 kg: 6 drops q 4 hr, not to exceed 36 drops in 24 hr; 10 kg: 8 drops q 4 hr, not to exceed 48 drops in 24 hr.

- **Injection (0.5 mg/mL)**

GI disorders.

Adults: 0.25–0.5 mg (0.5–1 mL). Some clients need only one dose while others require doses 2, 3, or 4 times a day at 4 hr intervals.

Diagnostic procedures.

Adults: 0.25–0.5 mg (0.5–1 mL) given IV 5 to 10 min prior to the procedure.

Preanesthetic medication.

Adults and children over 2 years of age: 0.005 mg/kg 30–60 min prior to induction of anesthesia. May also be given at the time the preanesthetic sedative or narcotic is given.

During surgery to reduce drug-induced bradycardia.

Adults and children over 2 years of age: Increments of 0.125 mg (0.25 mL) IV repeated as needed.

Reverse neuromuscular blockade.

Adults and children over 2 years of age: 0.2 mg (0.4 mL) for every 1 mg neostigmine or equivalent dose of physostigmine or pyridostigmine.

HEALTH CARE CONSIDERATIONS

See also *Health Care Considerations* for *Cholinergic Blocking Agents.*

Administration/Storage

1. May take hyoscyamine SL tablets sublingually, PO, or chewed. May take hyoscyamine tablets PO or sublingually.
2. Depending on the use, give the injection SC, IM, or IV.
3. Visually inspect the injectable form for particulate matter/discoloration.

Assessment

1. Record indications for therapy, type, onset, and duration of symptoms.
2. List other agents trialed and the outcome.
3. Determine any evidence of glaucoma, bladder neck or GI tract obstruction.

Client/Family Teaching

1. Take as prescribed; report any loss of symptom control so provider can adjust dose and frequency of administration.
2. Do not perform activities that require mental alertness until drug effects realized; dizziness, drowsiness, and blurred vision may occur.
3. Report diarrhea; may be symptom of intestinal obstruction, esp. with a colostomy or ileostomy.
4. Avoid excessive temperatures and activity; drug may decrease perspiration, which may cause fever, heat prostration, or stoke.
5. Stop drug and report any mental confusion, impaired gait, disorientation, or hallucinations.

Outcome/Evaluate

- ↓ GI motility
- ↓ Secretion production
- Control of pain and spasm

I

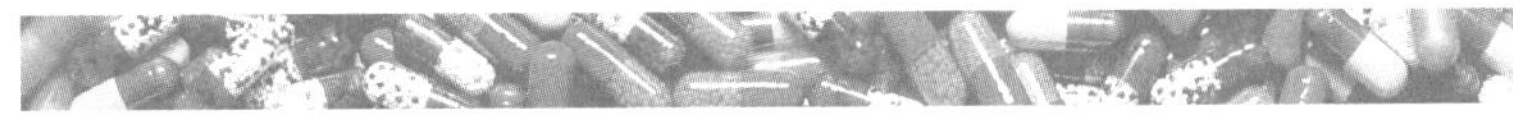

Ibuprofen

(eye-byou-**PROH**-fen)

Pregnancy Category: B (first two trimesters), D (third trimester)

Rx: Actiprofen ✤, Alti-Ibuprofen ✤, Apo-Ibuprofen ✤, Children's Advil, Children's Motrin, IBU, Ibuprohm, Motrin, Novo-Profen ✤, Nu-Ibuprofen ✤, Saleto-400, -600, and -800.

OTC: Advil Caplets and Tablets, Bayer Select Pain Relief Formula Caplets, Children's Advil Suspension, Children's Motrin Liquid Suspension, Children's Motrin Drops, Genpril Caplets and Tablets, Haltran, Ibuprin, Ibuprohm Caplets and Tablets, Junior Strength Motrin Caplets, Menadol, Midol IB, Motrin-IB Caplets and Tablets, Nuprin Caplets and Tablets, PediaCare Fever Drops, Saleto-200

Classification: Nonsteroidal anti-inflammatory drug (NSAID)

See also *Nonsteroidal Anti-Inflammatory Drugs.*

Action/Kinetics: Time to peak levels: 1–2 hr. **Onset:** 30 min for analgesia and approximately 1 week for anti-inflammatory effect. **Peak serum levels:** 1–2 hr. **t½:** 2 hr. **Duration:** 4–6 hr for analgesia and 1–2 weeks for anti-inflammatory effect. Food delays absorption rate but not total amount of drug absorbed.

Uses: Rx: Analgesic for mild to moderate pain. Primary dysmenorrhea, rheumatoid arthritis, osteoarthritis, antipyretic. *Investigational:* Resistant acne vulgaris (with tetracyclines); inflammation due to ultraviolet-B exposure (sunburn), juvenile rheumatoid arthritis. High doses to treat progressive lung deterioration in cystic fibrosis. **OTC:** Relief of fever and minor aches and pains due to colds, flu, sore throats, headaches, and toothaches.

Contraindications: Pregnancy, especially during the last trimester.

Special Concerns: Individualize dosage for children less than 12 years of age as safety and effectiveness have not been established.

Additional Side Effects: Dermatitis (maculopapular type), rash. Hypersensitivity reaction consisting of abdominal pain, fever, headache, ***meningitis,*** N&V, signs of liver damage; especially seen in clients with SLE.

Additional Drug Interactions

Furosemide / Ibuprofen ↓ diuretic effect of furosemide due to ↓ renal prostaglandin synthesis

Lithium / Ibuprofen ↑ plasma levels of lithium

Thiazide diuretics / Ibuprofen ↓ diuretic effect of furosemide due to ↓ renal prostaglandin synthesis

How Supplied: *Chew Tablet:* 50 mg, 100 mg; *Suspension:* 50 mg/1.25 mL, 100 mg/5 mL; *Tablet:* 50 mg, 100 mg, 200 mg, 300 mg, 400 mg, 600 mg, 800 mg

Dosage

• **Suspension, Chewable Tablets, Tablets**

Rheumatoid arthritis, osteoarthritis.

Either 300 mg q.i.d. or 400, 600, or 800 mg t.i.d.–q.i.d.; adjust dosage according to client response. Full therapeutic response may not be noted for 2 or more weeks.

Juvenile arthritis.

30–70 mg/kg/day in three to four divided doses (20 mg/kg/day may be adequate for mild cases).

Mild to moderate pain.

Adults: 400 mg q 4–6 hr, as needed.

Antipyretic.

Pediatric, 2–12 years of age: 5 mg/kg if baseline temperature is 102.5°F (39.1°C) or below or 10 mg/kg if baseline temperature is greater than 102.5°F (39.1°C). Maximum daily dose: 40 mg/kg.

Primary dysmenorrhea.

Adults: 400 mg q 4 hr, as needed.

• **Tablets for OTC Use**

Mild to moderate pain, antipyretic, dysmenorrhea.

200 mg q 4–6 hr; dose may be increased to 400 mg if pain or fever persist. Dose should not exceed 1,200 mg/day.

• **Suspension for OTC Use**

Pain, fever.

Children, 2–11 years: 7.5 mg/kg, up to q.i.d., to a maximum of 30 mg/kg/day.

HEALTH CARE CONSIDERATIONS

See also *Health Care Considerations* for *Nonsteroidal Anti-Inflammatory Drugs.*

Administration/Storage

1. Do not use OTC ibuprofen as an antipyretic for more than 3 days or as an analgesic for more than 10 days, unless medically cleared.
2. Do not take more than 3.2 g/day of prescription products and no more than 1.2 g/day of OTC products.

Assessment

1. Record indications for therapy, onset, location, and characteristics of symptoms.
2. Assess for evidence of lupus.
3. Obtain CBC, liver and renal function studies (X rays and eye exam) prior to initiating long-term therapy.

Client/Family Teaching

1. Take with a snack, milk, antacid, or meals to decrease GI upset. Report any N&V, diarrhea, or constipation.
2. Take the dosage prescribed for best results; report lack of response.
3. With history of CHF or compromised cardiac function, keep weight records, report edema; drug causes Na retention.
4. Report blurred vision; obtain periodic eye exams with long-term therapy.
5. Report as scheduled for follow-up evaluations: ROM, CBC, renal function, X rays, and stool for blood.

Outcome/Evaluate

- ↓ Joint pain and ↑ mobility
- ↓ Fever, ↓ Inflammation
- ↓ Uterine cramping

Idoxuridine (IDU)

(eye-dox-YOUR-ih-deen)

Pregnancy Category: C

Herplex Liquifilm, Herplex-D ✱ **(Rx)**
Classification: Antiviral agent, ophthalmic

See also *Antiviral Agents.*
Action/Kinetics: Resembles thymidine; inhibits thymidylic phosphorylase and specific DNA polymerases required for incorporation of thymidine into viral DNA. Idoxuridine, instead of thymidine, is incorporated into viral DNA, resulting in faulty DNA and the inability of the virus to infect tissue or reproduce. May also be incorporated into mammalian cells. Does not penetrate the cornea well. Rapidly inactivated by nucleotidases or deaminases.
Uses: Herpes simplex keratitis, especially for initial epithelial infections characterized by the presence of thread-like extensions. *NOTE:* Idoxuridine will control infection but will not prevent scarring, loss of vision, or vascularization. Alternative form of therapy must be instituted if no improvement is noted after 7 days or if complete reepithelialization fails to occur after 21 days of therapy.
Contraindications: Hypersensitivity; deep ulcerations involving stromal layers of cornea. Lactation. Concomitant use of corticosteroids in herpes simplex keratitis (corticosteroids may accelerate the spread of the viral infection).
Special Concerns: May be sensitizing, especially with dermal use. Safety and efficacy have not been determined in children.
Side Effects: Localized to eye. Temporary visual haze, irritation, pain, pruritus, inflammation, sensitivity to bright light, follicular conjunctivitis with preauricular adenopathy, mild edema of eyelids and cornea, allergic reactions (rare), photosensitivity, corneal clouding and stippling, small punctate defects. *NOTE:* Squamous cell carcinoma has been reported at the site of application.
OD **Management of Overdose:** *Symptoms (frequent administration):* Defects on corneal epithelium. *Treatment:* If an excess amount of drug is instilled in the eye, flush with water or normal saline.
Drug Interactions: Concurrent use of boric acid may cause irritation.
How Supplied: *Solution:* 0.1%

Dosage

- **Ophthalmic (0.1%) Solution.**

Initially: 1 gtt every hour during the day and q 2 hr during the night until definite improvement is noted (usually within 7 days). **Following improvement:** 1 gtt q 2 hr during the day and q 4 hr at night. Continue for 3–7 days after healing is complete. Alternate dosing schedule: 1 gtt q min for 5 min; repeat q 4 hr, day and night.

HEALTH CARE CONSIDERATIONS

See also *General Health Care Considerations for All Anti-Infectives.*

Administration/Storage

1. For best results, keep the infected tissues saturated with idoxuridine.
2. Store solution at 2°C–8°C (36°F–46°F); protect from light.
3. Do not mix with other meds.
4. Store ointment at 2°C–15°C (36°F–59°F).
5. Do not use drug that was improperly stored because of loss of activity and increased toxic effects.
6. Topical corticosteroids may be used with idoxuridine in the treatment of herpes simplex with corneal edema, stromal lesions, or iritis.
7. To control secondary infections, antibiotics may be used with drug.
8. Atropine may be used concomitantly with idoxuridine, if appropriate.
9. Improvement usually observed within 7–8 days; if there is continuous improvement, continue therapy for 21 days.
10. Some strains of herpes simplex may be resistant to idoxuridine; if there is no decrease in fluorescein staining after 14 days of use, another form of therapy should be used.

Client/Family Teaching

1. Review method for instillation, frequency for administration, and proper storage. Use as scheduled ATC, even during the night.
2. Report any symptoms of vision loss. Hazy vision following instillation will be of short duration.
3. *Do not* apply boric acid to the eye during idoxuridine therapy; boric acid may cause irritation.
4. Avoid using eye makeup; sharing towels and washcloths during therapy; wash hands frequently.
5. Wear dark glasses if photophobia occurs.
6. If used concurrently with corticosteroids, the idoxuridine will be continued longer than the steroid, to prevent reinfection.
7. Report for scheduled ophthalmic exams to determine drug response and to assess application site.

Outcome/Evaluate

- Control of ophthalmic infection
- Reepithelialization of eye lesions

Imipramine hydrochloride

(im-**IHP**-rah-meen)
Pregnancy Category: B
Apo-Imipramine ✱, Impril ✱, Janimine, Novo-Pramine ✱, PMS-Imipramine ✱, Tofranil **(Rx)**

Imipramine pamoate

(im-**IHP**-rah-meen)

Pregnancy Category: B

Tofranil-PM **(Rx)**

Classification: Antidepressant, tricyclic (tertiary amine)

See also *Antidepressants, Tricyclic*.

Action/Kinetics: Moderate anticholinergic and sedative effects; high orthostatic hypotensive effects. Biotransformed into its active metabolite, desmethylimipramine (desipramine). **Effective plasma level of imipramine and desmethylimipramine:** 200–350 ng/mL. **t½:** 11–25 hr. **Time to reach steady state:** 2–5 days.

Uses: Symptoms of depression. Enuresis in children. Chronic, severe neurogenic pain. Bulimia nervosa.

Laboratory Test Considerations: ↑ Metanephrine (Pisano test); ↓ Urinary 5-HIAA.

Additional Side Effects: ***High therapeutic dosage may increase frequency of seizures in epileptic clients and cause seizures in nonepileptic clients.*** Elderly and adolescent clients may have low tolerance to the drug.

How Supplied: Imipramine hydrochloride: *Tablet:* 10 mg, 25 mg, 50 mg. Imipramine pamoate: *Capsule:* 75 mg, 100 mg, 125 mg, 150 mg

Dosage

- **Tablets, Capsules**

Depression.

Hospitalized clients: 50 mg b.i.d.–t.i.d. Can be increased by 25 mg every few days up to 200 mg/day. After 2 weeks, dosage may be increased gradually to maximum of 250–300 mg/day at bedtime. **Outpatients:** 75–150 mg/day. Maximum dose for outpatients is 200 mg. Decrease when feasible to maintenance dosage: 50–150 mg/day at bedtime. **Adolescent and geriatric clients:** 30–40 mg/day up to maximum of 100 mg/day. **Pediatric:** 1.5 mg/kg/day in three divided doses; can be increased 1–1.5 mg/kg/day q 3–5 days to a maximum of 5 mg/kg/day.

Childhood enuresis.

Age 5 years and over: 25 mg/day 1 hr before bedtime. Dose can be increased to 50 mg/day up to 12 years of age and to 75 mg/day in children over 12 years of age. Dose should not exceed 2.5 mg/kg/day.

- **IM**

Antidepressant.

Adults: Up to 100 mg/day in divided doses. IM route not recommended for use in children less than 12 years of age.

HEALTH CARE CONSIDERATIONS

See also *Health Care Considerations* for *Antidepressants, Tricyclic*.

Administration/Storage

1. Total daily dose can be given once daily at bedtime.
2. Protect from direct sunlight and strong artificial light.
3. When used for the treatment of enuresis, the drug can be given in doses of 25 mg in midafternoon and 25 mg at bedtime (this regimen may increase effectiveness).
4. When used as an enuretic in children, do not exceed 2.5 mg/kg/day.

Client/Family Teaching

1. Review appropriate times and methods for administration.
2. Report any increase in frequency of seizures in epileptics and any occurrence of seizures in nonepileptics.
3. Children may experience mild N&V, unusual tiredness, nervousness, or insomnia; report if pronounced.
4. Do not perform activities that require mental alertness until drug effects realized; may cause sedation.
5. With enuresis, refer parents to regional centers with incontinence programs if bed-wetting persists.

Outcome/Evaluate

- Improvement in S&S of depression
- Prevention of bed-wetting
- Control of severe neurogenic pain
- Therapeutic serum drug levels (200–350 ng/mL)

Imiquimod

(ih-**MIH**-kwih-mod)

Pregnancy Category: B

Aldara **(Rx)**

Classification: Drug for genital and perianal warts

Action/Kinetics: May induce cytokines, including interferon-alpha and others, to modify immune response. Minimal percutaneous absorption.

Uses: External genital and perianal warts/condyloma acuminata in adults.

Contraindications: Use in urethral, intravaginal, cervical, rectal, or intra-anal human papilloma viral disease.

Special Concerns: Safety and efficacy have not been determined in clients less than 18 years of age. Use with caution during lactation.

Side Effects: *Dermatologic:* Erythema, itching, erosion, burning, excoriation/flaking, edema, pain, induration, ulceration, scabbing, vesicles, soreness. *Systemic:* Fungal infection, fatigue, fever, flu-like symptoms, headache, diarrhea, myalgia.
How Supplied: *Topical Cream:* 5%

Dosage

- **Cream**

Genital/perianal warts.
Adults: Apply 3 times/week prior to normal sleeping hours; leave on skin for 6–10 hr. Following treatment, remove by washing the area with mild soap and water. Continue treatment until there is total clearance of warts (16 weeks or less).

I

HEALTH CARE CONSIDERATIONS

Administration/Storage

1. Wash hands before and after application.
2. Apply a thin layer to the wart area and rub in until cream is not visible.
3. Avoid using excessive amounts of cream; single-use packets contain sufficient cream to cover up to 20 cm^2.
4. Due to skin reactions, rest period of several days may be necessary. Treatment may resume once reactions subside.
5. May weaken condoms or vaginal diaphragms; do not use together.
6. For external use only. Avoid contact with eyes.
7. Do not occlude treatment area with bandages or other covers/wraps. However, non-occlusive dressings (e.g., cotton gauze or underwear) can be used to manage skin reactions.
8. Do not store at temperatures greater than 30°C (86°F). Avoid freezing.

Assessment: Describe clinical presentation noting number and size of warts/condyloma, location, and condition of pretreatment area; photographs may be useful in assessing response to therapy.

Client/Family Teaching

1. Apply a thin layer of cream to completely cover each wart at bedtime, after bathing. Usually prescribed three times per week. Do not cover area with occlusive bandages or wraps.
2. Wash hands before and after treatment, avoid eye contact.
3. Drug is not cure for genital warts caused by HPV but helps clear and diminish wart area. New warts may occur during therapy.
4. Avoid sexual contact (genital, rectal, oral) while cream is on skin. Wash off before sexual activity; may also weaken condoms and diaphragms. Use extra protection and practice safe sex to avoid infecting and/or acquiring from partners.
5. May experience redness, peeling, burning, itching, and swelling in treatment area; report if severe skin reaction occurs as rest period may be needed before continuing therapy once subsided.
6. Wash application area with mild soap and water 6 to 10 hr after application.
7. Uncircumcised males treating warts under foreskin should retract foreskin and clean area daily.

Outcome/Evaluate: Clearing of genital and perianal warts/condyloma

Indapamide

(in-**DAP**-ah-myd)
Pregnancy Category: B
Apo-Indapamide ✱, Lozol, Novo-Indapamide ✱, Nu-Indapamide ✱ **(Rx)**

Indapamide Hemihydrate

(in-**DAP**-ah-myd)
Pregnancy Category: B
Gen-Indapamide ✱, Lozide ✱ **(Rx)**
Classification: Diuretic, thiazide type

See also *Diuretics, Thiazide.*
Action/Kinetics: Onset: 1–2 weeks after multiple doses. **Peak levels:** 2 hr. **Duration:** Up to 8 weeks with multiple doses. **t½:** 14 hr. Nearly 100% is absorbed from the GI tract. Excreted through the kidneys (70% with 7% unchanged) and the GI tract (23%).
Uses: Alone or in combination with other drugs for treatment of hypertension. Edema in CHF.
Special Concerns: Dosage has not been established in children. Geriatric clients may be more sensitive to the hypotensive and electrolyte effects.
How Supplied: *Tablet:* 1.25 mg, 2.5 mg

Dosage

- **Tablets**

Edema of CHF.
Adults: 2.5 mg as a single dose in the morning. If necessary, may be increased to 5 mg/day after 1 week.
Hypertension.
Adults: 1.25 mg as a single dose in the morning. If the response is not satisfactory after 4 weeks, the dose may be increased to 2.5 mg taken once daily. If the response to 2.5 mg is not satisfactory after 4 weeks, the dose may be increased to 5 mg taken once daily (however, consideration should be given to adding another antihypertensive).

HEALTH CARE CONSIDERATIONS

See also *Health Care Considerations* for *Diuretics, Thiazide* and *Antihypertensive Agents.*

Administration/Storage

1. May be combined with other antihypertensive agents if response inadequate. Initially, reduce the dose of other agents by 50%.
2. Doses greater than 5 mg/day do not increase effectiveness but may increase hypokalemia.

Assessment: Record indications for therapy, type, onset, and duration of symptoms. Note other agents trialed and the outcome.

Outcome/Evaluate

- ↓ BP
- ↑ Urinary output with ↓ edema

Indinavir sulfate

(in-**DIN**-ah-veer)

Pregnancy Category: C

Crixivan **(Rx)**

Classification: Antiviral drug, protease inhibitor

See also *Anitiviral Drugs.*

Action/Kinetics: Binds to active sites on the HIV protease enzyme resulting in inhibition of enzyme activity. Inhibition prevents cleavage of the viral polyproteins resulting in the formation of immature noninfectious viral particles. Varying degrees of cross resistance have been noted between indinavir and other HIV-protease inhibitors. Rapidly absorbed in fasting clients; **time to peak plasma levels:** Approximately 0.8 hr. Administration with a meal high in calories, fat, and protein results in a significant decrease in the amount absorbed and in the peak plasma concentration. Approximately 60% bound to plasma proteins. **t½:** 1.8 hr. Metabolized in the liver with both parent drug and metabolites excreted through the feces (over 80%) and the urine.

Uses: Treatment of HIV infection in adults when antiretroviral therapy is indicated. May be used with other anti-HIV drugs.

Contraindications: Lactation. Use with astemizole, cisapride, midazolam, rifampin, terfenadine, and triazolam. Mild to moderate liver or kidney disease.

Special Concerns: Not a cure for HIV infections; clients may continue to develop opportunistic infections and other complications of HIV disease. Not been shown to reduce the risk of transmission of HIV through sexual contact or blood contamination. No data on the effect of indinavir therapy on clinical progression of HIV infection, including survival or the incidence of opportunistic infections. Hemophiliacs treated for HIV infections with protease inhibitors may manifest spontaneous bleeding episodes. Safety and efficacy have not been determined in children.

Side Effects: *GI:* N&V, diarrhea, abdominal pain, abdominal distention, acid regurgitation, anorexia, dry mouth, aphthous stomatitis, cheilitis, cholecystitis, cholestasis, constipation, dyspepsia, eructation, flatulence, gastritis, gingivitis, glossodynia, gingival hemorrhage, increased appetite, infectious gastroenteritis, jaundice, liver cirrhosis. *CNS:* Headache, insomnia, dizziness, somnolence, agitation, anxiety, bruxism, decreased mental acuity, depression, dream abnormality, dysesthesia, excitement, fasciculation, hypesthesia, nervousness, neuralgia, neurotic disorder, paresthesia, peripheral neuropathy, sleep disorder, tremor, vertigo. *CV:* CV disorder, palpitation. *Musculoskeletal:* Back pain, arthralgia, leg pain, myalgia, muscle cramps, muscle weakness, musculoskeletal pain, shoulder pain, stiffness. *Body as a whole:* Asthenia, fatigue, flank pain, malaise, chest pain, chills, fever, flu-like illness, fungal infection, malaise, pain, syncope. *Hematologic:* Anemia, lymphadenopathy, spleen disorder. *Respiratory:* Cough, dyspnea, halitosis, pharyngeal hyperemia, pharyngitis, pneumonia, rales, rhonchi, ***respiratory failure,*** sinus disorder, sinusitis, URI. *Dermatologic:* Body odor, contact dermatitis, dermatitis, dry skin, flushing, folliculitis, herpes simplex, herpes zoster, night sweats, pruritus, seborrhea, skin disorder, skin infection, sweating, urticaria. *GU:* Nephrolithiasis, dysuria, hematuria, hydronephrosis, nocturia, PMS, proteinuria, renal colic, urinary frequency, UTI, uterine abnormality, urine sediment abnormality, urolithiasis. *Ophthalmic:* Accommodation disorder, blurred vision, eye pain, eye swelling, orbital edema. *Miscellaneous:* Asymptomatic hyperbilirubinemia, food allergy, taste disorder.

Laboratory Test Considerations: ↑ Serum transaminases (ALT, AST), total serum bilirubin, serum amylase. ↓ Hemoglobin, platelet count, neutrophils. Hyperbilirubinemia.

Drug Interactions

Astemizole / ↓ Metabolism of astemizole → possibility of cardiac arrhythmias and prolonged sedation

Cisapride / ↓ Metabolism of cisapride → possibility of cardiac arrhythmias and prolonged sedation

Clarithromycin / ↑ Plasma levels of both indinavir and clarithromycin
Didanosine / pH Dependent ↓ in absorption
Fluconazole / ↓ Plasma levels of indinavir
Isoniazid / ↑ Plasma levels of isoniazid
Ketoconazole / ↑ Plasma levels of indinavir
Midazolam / ↓ Metabolism of midazolam → possibility of cardiac arrhythmias and prolonged sedation
Oral contraceptives / ↑ Plasma levels of both estrogen and progestin components of the oral contraceptive product
Quinidine / ↑ Plasma levels of indinavir
Rifabutin / ↑ Plasma levels of rifabutin; ↓ dose by 50%
Rifampin / ↓ Plasma levels of indinavir
Stavudine / ↑ Plasma levels of stavudine
Terfenadine / ↓ Metabolism of terfenadine → possibility of cardiac arrhythmias and prolonged sedation
Triazolam / ↓ Metabolism of triazolam → possibility of cardiac arrhythmias and prolonged sedation
Trimethoprim/Sulfamethoxazole / ↑ Plasma levels of trimethoprim (no change in levels of sulfamethoxazole
Zidovudine (AZT) / ↑ Plasma levels of both indinavir and AZT

How Supplied: *Capsules*: 200 mg, 400 mg.

Dosage

- **Capsules**

  HIV infections.

Adults: 800 mg (two 400-mg capsules) q 8 hr ATC. The dosage is the same whether the drug is used alone or in combination with other retroviral agents. Reduce the dose to 600 mg q 8 hr with mild to moderate hepatic insufficiency due to cirrhosis.

HEALTH CARE CONSIDERATIONS

See also *Health Care Considerations* for *Antiviral Drugs.*

Administration/Storage

1. Capsules are sensitive to moisture. Store in the original container; keep the desiccant in the bottle. Keep in a tightly closed container protected from moisture and at a room temperature of 15°C–30°C (59°F–86°F).
2. If indinavir and didanosine are given together, give at least 1 hr apart on an empty stomach.
3. If indinavir is taken with rifabutin, reduce the dose of rifabutin to one-half the standard dose.
4. When indinavir is taken with ketoconazole, reduce the dose of indinavir to 600 mg q 8 hr.

Assessment

1. Record symptom onset, confirmation of HIV, other agents trialed with the outcome.
2. Monitor CD4 cell count, viral load, and LFTs. Anticipate reduced dosage with impaired liver function; drug is hepatically metabolized.
3. Review list of drugs currently prescribed to ensure that none interact.

Client/Family Teaching

1. Take as prescribed at 8-hr intervals ATC with water 1 hr before or 2 hr after meals for optimal absorption. May be taken with other liquids, such as skim milk, juice, coffee, or tea, or with a light meal (e.g., dry toast with jelly, juice, and coffee with skim milk and sugar; or corn flakes, skim milk, and sugar).
2. If a dose is missed by more than 2 hr, wait and take the next dose at the regularly scheduled time. If a dose is missed by less than 2 hr, take immediately.
3. Must adequately hydrate. To ensure adequate hydration, drink at least 1.5 L of liquids during a 24-hr period.
4. Report any symptoms of nephrolithiasis (e.g., flank pain with or without hematuria, including microscopic hematuria); therapy should be interrupted for 1–3 days.
5. Drug is not a cure for HIV; opportunistic infections may occur.
6. Use reliable birth control and barrier protection; drug does not decrease the risk of transmitting disease through sexual contact or blood contamination.

Outcome/Evaluate: Control of HIV infection progression

Indomethacin

(in-doh-**METH**-ah-sin)

Apo-Indomethacin ✦, Indochron E-R, Indocid ✦, Indocid Ophthalmic Suspension ✦, Indocid SR ✦, Indocin, Indocin SR, Indocollyre ✦, Indotec ✦, Novo-Methacin ✦, Nu-Indo ✦, Pro-Indo ✦, Rhodacine ✦ **(Rx)**

Indomethacin sodium trihydrate

(in-doh-**METH**-ah-sin)

Indocin I.V. **(Rx)**

Classification: Nonsteroidal anti-inflammatory drug, analgesic, antipyretic

See also *Nonsteroidal Anti-Inflammatory Drugs.*

Action/Kinetics: PO. Onset: 30 min for analgesia and up to 1 week for anti-inflammatory effect. **Peak plasma levels:** 1–2 hr (2–4 hr for sustained-release). **Peak action for gout:** 24–36 hr; swelling gradually disappears in 3–5 days. **Peak activity for antirheumatic effect:** About 4 weeks. **Duration:** 4–6 hr for analgesia and 1–2 weeks for anti-inflammatory effect. **Therapeutic plasma levels:** 10–18 mcg/mL. **t½:** Approximately 5 hr (up to 6 hr for sustained-release). **Plasma t½ following IV in infants:** 12–20 hr, depending on age and dose. Approximately 90% plasma protein bound. Metabolized in the liver and excreted in both the urine and feces.

Uses: Not a simple analgesic; use only for the conditions listed. Moderate to severe rheumatoid arthritis, osteoarthritis, and ankylosing spondylitis (drug of choice). Acute gouty arthritis and acute painful shoulder (tendinitis, bursitis). *IV:* Pharmacologic closure of persistent patent ductus arteriosus in premature infants. *Investigational:* Topically to treat cystoid macular edema (0.5% and 1% drops), sunburn, primary dysmenorrhea, prophylaxis of migraine, cluster headache, polyhydramnios.

Additional Contraindications: Pregnancy and lactation. PO indomethacin in children under 14 years of age. GI lesions or history of recurrent GI lesions. *IV use:* GI or intracranial bleeding, thrombocytopenia, renal disease, defects of coagulation, necrotizing enterocolitis. *Suppositories:* Recent rectal bleeding, history of proctitis.

Special Concerns: Restrict use in children to those unresponsive to or intolerant of other anti-inflammatory agents; efficacy has not been determined in children less than 14 years of age. Geriatric clients are at greater risk of developing CNS side effects, especially confusion. Use with caution in clients with history of epilepsy, psychiatric illness, or parkinsonism and in the elderly. Use with extreme caution in the presence of existing, controlled infections.

Additional Side Effects: Reactivation of latent infections may mask signs of infection. More marked CNS manifestations than for other drugs of this group. Aggravation of depression or other psychiatric problems, epilepsy, and parkinsonism.

Additional Drug Interactions

Captopril / Indomethacin ↓ effect of captopril, probably due to inhibition of prostaglandin synthesis

Diflunisal / ↑ Plasma levels of indomethacin; also, possible fatal GI hemorrhage

Diuretics (loop, potassium-sparing, thiazide) / Indomethacin may reduce the antihypertensive and natriuretic action of diuretics

Lisinopril / Possible ↓ effect of lisinopril

Prazosin / Indomethacin ↓ antihypertensive effects of prazosin

How Supplied: Indomethacin: *Capsule:* 25 mg, 50 mg; *Capsule, Extended Release:* 75 mg; *Suppository:* 50 mg; *Suspension:* 25 mg/5 mL Indomethacin sodium trihydrate: *Powder for injection:* 1 mg

Dosage

- **Capsules, Oral Suspension**

Moderate to severe arthritis, osteoarthritis, ankylosing spondylitis.

Adults, initial: 25 mg b.i.d.–t.i.d.; may be increased by 25–50 mg at weekly intervals, according to condition and, if tolerated, until satisfactory response is obtained. With persistent night pain or morning stiffness, a maximum of 100 mg of the total daily dose can be given at bedtime. **Maximum daily dosage:** 150–200 mg. In acute flares of chronic rheumatoid arthritis, the dose may need to be increased by 25–50 mg/day until the acute phase is under control.

Acute gouty arthritis.

Adults, initial: 50 mg t.i.d. until pain is tolerable; **then,** reduce dosage rapidly until drug is withdrawn. Pain relief usually occurs within 2–4 hr, tenderness and heat subside in 24–36 hr, and swelling disappears in 3–4 days.

Acute painful shoulder (bursitis/tendinitis).

75–150 mg/day in three to four divided doses for 1–2 weeks.

- **Sustained-Release Capsules**

Antirheumatic, anti-inflammatory.

Adults: 75 mg, of which 25 mg is released immediately, 1–2 times/day.

- **Suppositories**

Anti-inflammatory, antirheumatic, antigout.

Adults: 50 mg up to q.i.d. **Pediatric:** 1.5–2.5 mg/kg/day in three to four divided doses (up to a maximum of 4 mg/kg or 250–300 mg/day, whichever is less).

- **IV Only**

Patent ductus arteriosus.

3 IV doses, depending on age of the infant, are given at 12–24-hr intervals. **Infants less than 2 days:** first dose, 0.2 mg/kg, followed by two doses of 0.1 mg/kg each; **infants 2–7 days:** three doses of 0.2 mg/kg each; **infants more than 7 days:** first dose, 0.2 mg/kg, followed by two doses of 0.25 mg/kg each. If patent ductus arteriosus reopens, a second course of one to three doses may be given. Surgery may be required if there is no response after two courses of therapy.

HEALTH CARE CONSIDERATIONS

See also *Health Care Considerations* for *Nonsteroidal Anti-Inflammatory Drugs.*

Administration/Storage

1. Do not crush the sustained-release form; do not use for acute gouty arthritis.
2. With dysphagia, the capsule contents may be emptied into applesauce, food, or liquid to ensure that client receives the prescribed dose.
3. Suppositories (50 mg) may be used if unable to take PO medication. Store below 30°C (86°F).
4. Use the smallest effective dose, based on individual need. Adverse reactions are dose related.

Assessment

1. Note indications for therapy, type, onset, and duration of symptoms; list other agents trialed and the outcome.
2. Assess and record characteristics of involved joint(s), including goniometric measurements, ROM and rate pain.

Client/Family Teaching

1. Take with food or milk to decrease GI upset. Do not crush or break capsules; may sprinkle capsule contents on food if unable to swallow.
2. Use caution when operating potentially hazardous equipment; may cause lightheadedness and decreased alertness.
3. Withhold the drug and report if adverse side effects occur since many may be serious enough to stop therapy.
4. Record weights, especially if nausea or vomiting occur; report any abdominal pain or diarrhea.
5. Indomethacin masks infections; report any S&S of infection or fever.
6. Report for scheduled ophthalmologic exams and lab studies.
7. It will take from 2 to 4 weeks of therapy before significant improvement evident in arthritic conditions. Follow prescribed dosing regimen carefully and refrain from becoming discouraged.

Outcome/Evaluate

- ↓ Pain and inflammation; ↑ joint mobility
- Closure of patent ductus arteriosus
- Therapeutic serum drug levels (10–18 mcg/mL)

Insulin injection (crystalline zinc insulin, unmodified insulin, regular insulin)

(IN-sue-lin)

Pork: Iletin II ✦, Insulin-Toronto ✦, Regular Iletin II, Regular Purified Pork Insulin. **Beef/Pork:** Iletin ✦, Regular Iletin I. **Human:** Humulin-R ✦, Novolin ge Toronto ✦, Novolin R, Novolin R PenFill, Novolin R Prefilled, Velosulin Human BR **(OTC)**

Classification: Rapid-acting insulin

Action/Kinetics: Rarely administered as the sole agent due to its short duration of action. Injections of 100 units/mL are clear; cloudy, colored solutions should not be used. Regular insulin is the only preparation suitable for IV administration. Available only as 100 units/mL. **Onset, SC:** 30–60 min; **IV:** 10–30 min. **Peak, SC:** 2–4 hr; **IV:** 15–30 min. **Duration, SC:** 6–8 hr; **IV:** 30–60 min. *Note:* Regular beef/pork insulins are being phased out.

Uses: Suitable for treatment of diabetic coma, diabetic acidosis, or other emergency situations. Especially suitable for the client suffering from labile diabetes. During acute phase of diabetic acidosis or for the client in diabetic crisis, client is monitored by serum glucose and serum ketone levels.

How Supplied: *Injection:* 100 U/mL

Dosage

- **SC**

Diabetes.

Adults, individualized, usual, initial: 5–10 units; **pediatric:** 2–4 units. Injection is given 15–30 min before meals and at bedtime.

Diabetic ketoacidosis.

Adults: 0.1 unit/kg/hr given by continuous IV infusion.

HEALTH CARE CONSIDERATIONS

Administration/Storage

IV 1. When used IV, reduce the rate of insulin infusion when plasma glucose levels reach 250 mg/dL.
2. Due to the short half-life of regular insulin, do not give large single IV doses.

Outcome/Evaluate: Glucose and HbA1c within desired range

Insulin injection, concentrated

(IN-sue-lin)

Pregnancy Category: C

Regular (Concentrated) Iletin II U-500 **(Rx)**

Classification: Insulin, concentrated

Action/Kinetics: Concentrated insulin injection (500 U/mL). Depending on response, may be given SC or IM as a single or as two or three divided doses.

Uses: Insulin resistance requiring more than 200 units insulin/day.

Contraindications: Allergy to pork or mixed pork/beef insulin (unless client has been desensitized). IV use due to possible allergic or anaphylactoid reactions.
Special Concerns: Use with caution during lactation.
Additional Side Effects: Deep secondary hypoglycemia 18–24 hr after administration.
Drug Interactions: Do not use together with PO hypoglycemic agents.
How Supplied: *Injection:* 500 U/mL

Dosage
- **SC, IM**

Individualized, depending on severity of condition. Clients must be kept under close observation until dosage is established.

HEALTH CARE CONSIDERATIONS

Administration/Storage
1. Administer only water clear solutions (concentrated insulin may appear straw-colored).
2. Use small-caliber syringe for accuracy of measurement.
3. Deep secondary hypoglycemia may occur 18–24 hr after administration; have 10%–20% dextrose solution available.
4. Keep insulin cool or refrigerated.

Assessment
1. Observe closely for S&S of hyper- or hypoglycemia until dosage established.
2. Monitor BS frequently and HbA1c q 3 mo.

Client/Family Teaching
1. Review technique for self-administration.
2. Be alert for signs of hypoglycemia, which may indicate that responsiveness to insulin has been regained and that a reduction in dosage is warranted.

Outcome/Evaluate: Serum glucose and HbA1c to within desired range

Insulin lispro injection (rDNA origin)
(IN-sue-lin LYE-sproh)
Pregnancy Category: B
Humalog **(Rx)**
Classification: Insulin, rDNA origin

Action/Kinetics: Rapid-acting insulin derived from *Escherichia coli* that has been genetically altered by the addition of the gene for insulin lispro. Is a human insulin analog created when the amino acids at positions 28 and 29 on the insulin B-chain are reversed. Absorbed faster than regular human insulin. Compared with regular insulin, has a more rapid onset of glucose-lowering activity, an earlier peak for glucose lowering, and a shorter duration of glucose-lowering activity. However, is equipotent to human regular insulin (i.e., one unit of insulin lispro has the same glucose-lowering capacity as one unit of regular insulin). May lower the risk of nocturnal hypoglycemia in clients with type I diabetes. **Onset:** 15 min. **Peak effect:** 30–90 min. **t½:** 1 hr. **Duration:** 5 hr or less.
Uses: Diabetes mellitus.
Contraindications: Use during episodes of hypoglycemia. Hypersensitivity to insulin lispro.
Special Concerns: Since insulin lispro has a more rapid onset and shorter duration of action than regular insulin, clients with type I diabetes also require a longer acting insulin to maintain glucose control. Requirements may be decreased in impaired renal or hepatic function. Use with caution during lactation. Safety and efficacy have not been determined in children less than 12 years of age.
Side Effects: See Insulins.
Drug Interactions: See Insulins.
How Supplied: *Injection:* 100 U/mL

Dosage
- **SC**

Diabetes.

Individualized, depending on severity of the condition.

HEALTH CARE CONSIDERATIONS

Administration/Storage
1. When used as a mealtime insulin, give within 15 min before a meal as compared with human regular insulin, which is best given 30–60 min before a meal.
2. May be mixed with Humulin N, Humulin L, or Humulin U. A decrease in the rate of absorption (but not the total bioavailability) was seen when Humalog was mixed with Humulin N.
3. When Humalog is mixed with either Humulin U or Humulin N, give mixture within 15 min before a meal and immediately after mixing.
4. If Humalog is mixed with a longer acting insulin, Humalog should be drawn into the syringe first to prevent clouding of the Humalog by the longer-acting insulin.
5. Do not give mixtures IV.
6. Store in the refrigerator at 2°C–8°C (36°F–46°F). Do not freeze. If refrigeration is not possible, can be stored unrefrigerated

for up to 28 days, provided it is kept as cool as possible and away from direct heat and light.

Assessment

1. Record indications for therapy, disease onset, previous agents trialed, and the outcome.
2. Monitor CBC, HbA1c, urinalysis, and liver and renal function studies.

Client/Family Teaching

1. Review method for preparation, storage, and administration; rotate sites.
2. Drug has a more rapid onset of action and a shorter duration of action than regular insulin.
3. Take within 15 min of meals and immediately after mixing, with combined therapy.
4. Monitor FS closely until response evident. Review S&S of hypoglycemia and appropriate management.
5. Clients with type I diabetes also require a longer-acting insulin preparation for adequate glucose control.
6. Report as scheduled for follow-up labs, reinforcement of teaching, and evaluation of response to medication.

Outcome/Evaluate: BS/HbA1c within desired range

Insulin zinc suspension (Lente)

(IN-sue-lin)

Pork: Iletin II ✱, Lente Iletin II, Lente L. **Beef/Pork:** Iletin ✱, Lentin Iletin I. **Human:** Humulin L, Novolin ge Lente ✱, Novolin L **(OTC)**

Classification: Intermediate-acting insulin

Action/Kinetics: Contains 70% crystalline and 30% amorphous insulin suspension. Considered intermediate-acting. Principal advantage is the absence of a sensitizing agent such as protamine. **Onset:** 1–2.5 hr. **Peak:** 7–15 hr. **Duration:** About 22 hr. *Note:* Lente beef/pork insulins are being phased out.

Uses: Allergy to other types of insulin and in clients disposed to thrombotic phenomena in which protamine may be a factor. Not a replacement for regular insulin and is not suitable for emergency use.

How Supplied: *Injection:* 100 U/mL

Dosage

- **SC**

  Diabetes.

Adults, initial: 7–26 units 30–60 min before breakfast. Dosage is then increased by daily or weekly increments of 2–10 units until satisfactory readjustment is established. A second smaller dose may be given prior to the evening meal or at bedtime. Clients on NPH can be transferred to insulin zinc suspension on a unit-for-unit basis. Clients being transferred from regular insulin should begin zinc insulin at two-thirds to three-fourths the regular insulin dosage. If the client is being transferred from protamine zinc insulin, the dose of zinc insulin should be about 50% of that required for protamine zinc insulin.

HEALTH CARE CONSIDERATIONS

Outcome/Evaluate: Normalization of BS and HbA1c levels

Insulin zinc suspension, extended (Ultralente)

Human: Humulin-U ✱, Humulin U Ultralente, Novolin ge Ultralente ✱ **(OTC)**

Classification: Long-acting insulin

See also *Insulins.*

Action/Kinetics: Large crystals of insulin and a high content of zinc are responsible for the slow-acting properties of this preparation. **Onset:** 4–8 hr. **Peak:** 10–30 hr. **Duration:** 36 hr or longer.

Uses: Mild to moderate hyperglycemia in stabilized diabetics.

Contraindications: Use to treat diabetic coma or emergency situations

How Supplied: *Injection:* 100 U/mL

Dosage

- **SC**

  Individualized.

Usual, initial: 7–26 units as a single dose 30–60 min before breakfast. **Do not administer IV.**

HEALTH CARE CONSIDERATIONS

Outcome/Evaluate: Normalization of BS and HbA1c levels

Interferon alfa-2a recombinant (rI FN-A; IFLrA)

(in-ter-FEER-on AL-fah)

Pregnancy Category: C

Roferon-A **(Rx)**

Classification: Antineoplastic, miscellaneous agent

Action/Kinetics: Interferon alfa-2a is the product of recombinant DNA technology using strains of genetically engineered *Escherichia coli.* Activity is expressed as International Units, which are determined by comparing the antiviral activity of recombinant interferons with the activity of the international reference standard of human leukocyte interferon. Interferons bind to specific receptors on the cell surface, resulting in inhibition of virus replication in virus-infected cells, suppression of cell proliferation, increase in the phagocytic activity of macrophages, and enhancement of the toxic effects of leukocytes for target cells. **Peak serum levels:** 3.8–7.3 hr. **t½:** 3.7–8.5 hr. Metabolized by the kidney.

Uses: Hairy cell leukemia in clients older than 18 years of age. Can be used in splenectomized and nonsplenectomized clients. AIDS-related Kaposi's sarcoma in clients older than 18 years of age. Chronic myelogenous leukemia. Chronic hepatitis C. *Investigational:* The drug has been used for a large number of other conditions. Significant activity has been noted against the following neoplastic diseases: locally for superficial bladder tumors, carcinoid tumor, cutaneous T-cell lymphoma, essential thrombocythemia, low-grade non-Hodgkin's lymphoma. Limited activity has been noted in acute leukemias, cervical carcinoma, chronic lymphocytic leukemia, Hodgkin's disease, malignant gliomas, melanoma, multiple myeloma, mycosis fungoides/Sézary syndrome, nasopharyngeal carcinoma, osteosarcoma, ovarian carcinoma, renal carcinoma. Interferon alfa-2a also has significant activity against the following viral infections: chronic non-A, non-B hepatitis, condylomata acuminata, cutaneous warts, cytomegaloviruses, herpes keratoconjunctivitis; limited activity is seen against herpes simplex, HIV infection to slow progression, papillomaviruses, rhinoviruses, vaccinia virus, varicella zoster, and viral hepatitis B.

Contraindications: Lactation.

Special Concerns: Use with caution in clients with a history of unstable angina, uncontrolled CHF, COPD, diabetes mellitus prone to ketoacidosis, thrombophlebitis, pulmonary embolism, seizure disorders, severe renal and hepatic disease, compromised CNS function, and severe myelosuppression. Safety and efficacy in individuals less than 18 years of age have not been established.

Side Effects: *Flu-like symptoms:* Fever, headache, fatigue, arthralgia, myalgias, chills, weight loss, dizziness. *CV:* Hypotension, ***arrhythmias,*** syncope, hypertension, edema, palpitations, transient ischemic attacks, pulmonary edema, CHF, cardiac murmur, ***MI, stroke, cardiomyopathy,*** hot flashes, Raynaud's phenomenon, thrombophlebitis. *Respiratory:* Coughing, dyspnea, dryness or inflammation of oropharynx, chest pain or congestion, ***bronchospasm,*** pneumonia, tachypnea, rhinitis, rhinorrhea, sinusitis. *CNS:* Depression, confusion, dizziness, headache, paresthesia, anxiety, ataxia, aphasia, aphonia, dysarthria, amnesia, weakness, nervousness, emotional lability, impotence, numbness, lethargy, sleep disturbances, visual disturbances, vertigo, decreased mental status, memory loss, disturbances of libido, involuntary movements, ***suicidal ideation, seizures,*** forgetfulness, neuropathy, tremor. *GI:* Anorexia, N&V, diarrhea, emesis, abdominal pain, hypermotility, abdominal fullness, abdominal pain, flatulence, constipation, gastric distress. *Hematologic:* Thrombocytopenia, neutropenia, leukopenia, decreased hemoglobin, severe anemia, severe cytopenias, coagulopathy, Coombs' positive hemolytic anemia, aplastic anemia. *Musculoskeletal:* Joint or bone pain, arthritis, polyarthritis, poor coordination, muscle contractions, gait disturbances. *Dermatologic:* Rash, pruritus, dry skin, ecchymosis, petechiae, skin flushing, alopecia, urticaria, diaphoresis, cyanosis, bruising. *Miscellaneous:* Generalized pain, back pain, inflammation at injection site, epistaxis, bleeding gums, weight loss, alteration of taste, altered hearing, edema, night sweats, earache, eye irritation, hypothyroidism, hypertriglyceridemia.

Laboratory Test Considerations: ↑ AST, ALT, LDH, BUN, serum creatinine, alkaline phosphatase, bilirubin, uric acid, serum glucose, serum phosphorus. ↓ H&H. Hypocalcemia, proteinuria.

Drug Interactions

Interleukin-2 / ↑ Risk of renal failure
Theophylline / ↓ Clearance of theophylline

How Supplied: *Injection:* 3 million IU/0.5 mL, 3 million IU/mL, 6 million IU/0.5 mL, 6 million IU/mL, 9 million IU/0.5 mL, 9 million IU/0.9 mL, 36 million IU/mL

Dosage

- **IM, SC**

Hairy cell leukemia.

Induction: 3 million IU/day for 16–24 weeks; **maintenance,** 3 million IU 3 times/week. Doses higher than 3 million IU are not recommended.

AIDS-related Kaposi's sarcoma.

Induction: 36 million IU/day for 10–12 weeks; or, 3 million IU/day on days 1–3; 9 million IU/day on days 4–6; and 18 million IU/day on days 7–9 followed by 36 million IU/day for the remainder of the 10 to 12-week induction period. **Maintenance:** 36 million IU 3 times/week. If severe side effects occur, the dose can be withheld or reduced by one-half.

Chronic myelogenous leukemia.

Induction: 9 million IU/day. The dose can be graded during the first week of therapy to improve short-term tolerance by giving 3 million IU/day for 3 days to 6 million IU/day for 3 days and then to the target dose of 9 million IU/day. **Maintenance:** Optimal dose and duration of therapy have not been determined. Continue the regimen until the disease progresses.

Chronic hepatitis C.

3 million IU, SC or IM, 3 times/week for 12 months.

HEALTH CARE CONSIDERATIONS

Administration/Storage

1. Discontinue treatment if leukemia does not respond within 6 mo.
2. If severe reactions occur, reduce dose of drug by one-half or withhold individual doses. Assess effect on bone marrow of previous radiation or chemotherapy.
3. Although optimal treatment duration has not been established, clients have been treated for up to 20 consecutive mo. Nadir: leukocytes, 20–40 days; platelets, 15–20 days.
4. Consider SC route with a platelet count less than 50,000/mm^3.
5. Although not approved by the FDA, interferon alfa-2a has been given by continuous or intermittent IV infusion as well as ophthalmically and intravaginally.
6. The reconstituted solution is stable for 30 days when stored at 2°C–8°C (36°F–46°F) and for 24 hr when stored at room temperature. The undiluted drug is not stable in syringes due to adhesion to syringe surfaces.

Client/Family Teaching

1. Review appropriate method for administration, care and safe storage of drug and equipment.
2. Most common side effects are flu-like symptoms, such as fever, fatigue, headache, chills, nausea, and loss of appetite; may be minimized by taking at bedtime.
3. Flu-like symptoms usually diminish in severity as treatment continues. Acetaminophen may be used for fever and headache.
4. Drink plenty of fluids (2–3 L/day).
5. Hypotension may occur up to 2 days following drug therapy; sit before standing and rise slowly.
6. Do not change brands of interferon without approval; changes in dosage may occur with different brands.
7. Report for CBC, electrolytes, and liver function studies as scheduled.
8. Report any evidence of neurologic or psychologic disturbances.
9. Hair loss may occur.
10. Practice safe sex and birth control.
11. Avoid alcohol and any other unprescribed CNS depressants.

Outcome/Evaluate

- ↓ Tumor size and spread
- Inhibition of viral replication
- ↓ Lesions with Kaposi's sarcoma

Interferon alfa-2b recombinant (rI FN-α2; α-2-interferon)

(in-ter-**FEER**-on **AL**-fah)

Pregnancy Category: C

Intron A **(Rx)**

Classification: Antineoplastic, miscellaneous agent

Action/Kinetics: A product of recombinant DNA technology using strains of genetically engineered *Escherichia coli*. The activity is expressed as IU, which are determined by comparing the antiviral activity of the recombinant interferon with the activity of the international reference standard of human leukocyte interferon. Interferons bind to specific receptors on the cell surface, resulting in inhibition of virus replication in virus-infected cells, suppression of cell proliferation, increase in the phagocytic activity of macrophages, and enhancement of the toxic effects of leukocytes for target cells. **Peak serum levels after IM, SC:** 18–116 IU/mL after 3–12 hr. **t½, IM, SC:** 2–3 hr. **Peak serum levels after IV infusion:** 135–270 IU/mL at the end of the infusion. **t½, IV:** 2 hr. The main site of metabolism may be the kidney.

Uses: Hairy cell leukemia in clients older than 18 years of age (in both splenectomized and nonsplenectomized clients). Intralesional use for genital or venereal warts (*Condylomata acuminata.*) AIDS-related Kaposi's sarcoma in clients over 18 years of age. Chronic hepatitis C in clients at least 18 years of age with compensated liver disease and a history of blood or blood product exposure or who are HCV antibody positive. Chronic hepatitis B in clients over 18 years of age with compensated liver disease and HBV replication (clients must be serum HBsAg positive for at least 6 months and have HBV replication with elevated serum ALT). Adjunct therapy for malignant melanoma in those who are 18 years of age or older who are free of the disease but at a high risk for recurrence within 56 days of surgery. With an anthracycline drug for the initial treatment of clinically aggressive non-Hodgkin's lymphoma.

Investigational: The drug has been used for a large number of conditions. Significant activity has been noted against the following neoplastic diseases: locally for superficial bladder tumors, carcinoid tumor, chronic myelogenous leukemia, cutaneous T-cell lymphoma, essential thrombocythemia, low-grade non-Hodgkin's lymphoma, and chronic granulocytic leukemia. Limited activity has been noted in acute leukemias, cervical carcinoma, chronic lymphocytic leukemia, Hodgkin's disease, malignant gliomas, melanoma, multiple myeloma, nasopharyngeal carcinoma, osteosarcoma, ovarian carcinoma, renal carcinoma, and chronic granulomatous disease. Interferon alfa-2b has also been used to treat the following viral infections: Significant activity has been seen against cutaneous warts, CMVs, herpes keratoconjunctivitis, and herpes simplex. Limited activity has been noted against papillomaviruses, rhinoviruses, vaccinia virus, varicella zoster, and HIV (used with foscarnet/AZT). It has also been used to treat multiple sclerosis.

Contraindications: Lactation. Use to treat rapidly progressive visceral disease in AIDS-related Kaposi's sarcoma. Use in clients with decompensated liver disease, autoimmune hepatitis, history of autoimmune disease, or immunosuppressed transplant clients.

Special Concerns: Use with caution in clients with a history of unstable angina, uncontrolled CHF, COPD, diabetes mellitus prone to ketoacidosis, thrombophlebitis, pulmonary embolism, seizure disorders, severe renal and hepatic disease, compromised CNS function, and severe myelosuppression. Safety and efficacy in individuals less than 18 years of age have not been established.

Side Effects: *Flu-like symptoms:* Fever, headache, fatigue, myalgia, chills. *CV:* Hypotension, ***arrhythmias,*** tachycardia, syncope, hypertension, coagulation disorders, chest pain, palpitations, flushing, atrial fibrillation, bradycardia, ***cardiac failure, cardiomyopathy,*** extrasystoles, postural hypotension. *CNS:* Depression, confusion, somnolence, migraine, dizziness, ataxia, insomnia, irritability, paresthesia, anxiety, nervousness, emotional lability, amnesia, impaired concentration, weakness, tremor, syncope, abnormal coordination, hypoesthesia, hypesthesia, abnormal coordination, aggravated depression, aggressive reaction, hypertonia, hypokinesia, impaired consciousness, neuropathy, agitation, apathy, aphasia, dysphonia, extrapyramidal disorder, hot flashes, hyperesthesia, hyperkinesia, neurosis, paresis, paroniria, parosmia, personality disorder, ***seizures, coma,*** polyneuropathy, ***suicide attempt.*** *GI:* N&V, diarrhea, stomatitis, weight loss, anorexia, flatulence, thirst, dehydration, constipation, eructation, abdominal pain, loose stools, abdominal distention, dysphagia, esophagitis, gastric ulcer, ***GI hemorrhage,*** GI mucosal discoloration, gum hyperplasia, gingival bleeding, gingivitis, increased saliva, increased appetite, melena, oral leukoplakia, rectal bleeding after stool, ***rectal hemorrhage,*** ulcerative stomatitis, ascites, gallstones, gastroenteritis, halitosis. *Hematologic:* Thrombocytopenia, granulocytopenia, anemia, ***hemolytic anemia,*** leukopenia. *Musculoskeletal:* Arthralgia, leg cramps, asthenia, arthrosis, arthritis, muscle pain or weakness, back pain, bone pain, rigors, CTS. *Respiratory:* Pharyngitis, coughing, dyspnea, sinusitis, rhinitis, epistaxis, nasal congestion, dry mouth, ***bronchospasm,*** pleural pain, pneumonia, rhinorrhea, sneezing, wheezing, bronchitis, cyanosis, lung fibrosis. *EENT:* Alteration or loss of taste, tinnitus, hearing disorders, conjunctivitis, photophobia, vision disorders, eye pain, diplopia, dry eyes, earache, lacrimal gland disorder, periorbital edema, vertigo, speech disorder. *Dermatologic:* Rash, pruritus, alopecia, urticaria, dry skin, dermatitis, purpura, photosensitivity, acne, nail disorder, facial edema, moniliasis, reaction at injection site, abnormal hair texture, cold/clammy skin, cyanosis of the hand, epidermal necrolysis, dermatitis lichenoides, furunculosis, increased hair growth, erythema, melanosis, nonherpetic cold sores, peripheral ischemia, skin depigmentation or discoloration, vitiligo, folliculitis, lipoma, psoriasis. *GU:* Amenorrhea, hematuria, impotence, leukorrhea, menorrhagia, urinary frequency, nocturia, polyuria, uterine bleeding, increased BUN, incontinence, pelvic pain. *Endocrine:* Gynecomastia, thyroid disorder, aggravation of diabetes mellitus, virilism. *Hepatic:* Jaundice, upper right quadrant pain, ***hepatic encephalopathy, hepatic failure.*** *Other:* Pain, increased sweating, malaise, decreased libido, herpes simplex, lymphadenopathy, chest pain, abscess, cachexia, hypercalcemia, peripheral edema, stye, substernal chest pain, weakness, sepsis, dehydration, fungal infection, herpes zoster, viral infection, trichomoniasis.

Laboratory Test Considerations: ↑ AST, ALT, LDH, BUN, serum creatinine, alkaline phosphatase. ↓ H&H. Abnormal hepatic function tests, bilirubinemia.

Drug Interactions

Aminophylline / ↓ Clearance of aminophylline due to ↓ breakdown by the liver

Zidovudine (AZT) / ↑ Risk of neutropenia

How Supplied: *Solution for Injection:* 3 million IU/vial, 5 million IU/vial, 10 million IU/vial, 18 million IU/vial, 25 million IU/vial; *Powder for injection:* 3 million IU/vial, 5 million IU/vial, 10 million IU/vial, 18 million IU/vial, 25 million IU/vial.

Dosage

- **IM, SC**

Hairy cell leukemia.

2 million IU/m² 3 times/week. Higher doses are not recommended. May require 6 or more months of therapy for improvement. Do not use the 50-million-IU strength of the powder for injection for treating hairy cell leukemia.

AIDS-related Kaposi's sarcoma

30 million IU/m² 3 times/week SC or IM using only the 50-million-IU vial. Using this dose, clients should tolerate an average dose of 110 million IU/week at the end of 12 weeks of therapy and 75 million IU/week at the end of 24 weeks of therapy.

Chronic hepatitis C.

3 million IU 3 times/week for 16 weeks. At 16 weeks, extend treatment to 18 to 24 months at 3 million IU 3 times/week to improve the sustained response of normalization of ALT. Discontinue therapy if there is no response after 16 weeks.

Chronic hepatitis B.

30–35 million IU/week SC or IM, given as either 5 million IU/day or 10 million IU 3 times/week for 16 weeks. If serious side effects occur, the dose may be decreased by 50%.

- **IV**

Malignant melanoma.

20 million IU/m² IV on 5 consecutive days/week for 4 weeks. **Maintenance:** 10 million IU/m² SC 3 times/week for 48 weeks.

- **Intralesional**

Condylomata acuminata (genital or venereal warts).

1 million IU/lesion 3 times/week for 3 weeks. For this purpose, use only the vial containing 10 million units and reconstitute using no more than 1 mL diluent. To reduce side effects, give in the evening with acetaminophen. Maximum response usually occurs within 4–8 weeks. If results are unsatisfactory after 12–16 weeks, a second course may be started.

HEALTH CARE CONSIDERATIONS

See also *Health Care Considerations* for *Interferon alfa-2a recombinant* and *Interferon alfa-n3.*

Administration/Storage

1. Prior to administration, the drug must be reconstituted with bacteriostatic water for injection, which is provided. Consult the chart provided by the manufacturer to prepare the powder for injection based on the use. The client may self-administer the dose at bedime.
2. If severe side effects occur, the dose can be reduced as much as 50% or therapy can be discontinued until side effects subside. For example, if the granulocyte count is less than 750/mm³ and the platelet count is less than 50,000/mm³, reduce the dose by 50%; if the granulocyte count is less than 500/mm³ and the platelet count is less than 30,000/mm³, interrupt drug therapy until counts return to normal or baseline levels. Nadir: 3–5 days.
3. Discontinue treatment for leukemia if no response within 6 mo.
4. When used for venereal or genital warts, maximum response usually occurs 4–8 weeks after therapy is initiated. If results not satisfactory after 12–16 weeks, a second course of therapy may be undertaken.
5. Although the optimal duration of treatment has not been established, clients have been treated for up to 20 consecutive months.
6. If the platelet count is less than 50,000/mm³, give SC rather than IM.
7. Use a tuberculin or similar syringe with a 25- to 30-gauge needle for intralesion administration. Do not give beneath the lesion too deeply or inject too superficially. As many as five lesions can be treated at one time.
8. Store powder from 2°C–8°C (36°F–46°F). The reconstituted solution is stable for 30 days when stored from 2°C–8°C (36°F–46°F). The solution for injection is stable at 35°C (95°F) for up to 7 days and at 30°C (86°F) for up to 14 days. The undiluted drug is not stable in syringes due to adhesion to syringe surfaces.
9. IV Although not approved by the FDA, interferon alfa-2a has been given by continuous or intermittent IV infusion as well as ophthalmically and intravaginally.
10. For infusion solutions, after reconstitution, withdraw the appropriate dose and inject into a 100-mL bag of 0.9% NaCl injection. The final concentration should be 10 million IU/10 mL or more. Infuse over a 20-min period. Prepare solution immediately prior to use.

Client/Family Teaching

1. Flu-like symptoms may be minimized by administering the drug at bedtime. Use acetaminophen for fever and headache.

2. Consume 2–3 L/day of fluids.
3. Report for labs and bone marrow hairy cell determinations.

Outcome/Evaluate

- Improved hematologic response with disease regression
- ↓ Size and number of genital/venereal warts

Interferon alfacon-1

(in-ter-**FEER**-on **AL**-fah-kon)
Pregnancy Category: C
Infergen **(Rx)**
Classification: Drug for chronic hepatitis

See also *Interferon alfa-2a* and *Interferon-alfa 2b.*

Action/Kinetics: Prepared by recombinant technology. Has antiviral, antiproliferative, and immunomodulatory effects. Plasma levels are too small to measure.

Uses: Treatment of chronic hepatitis C infections in those over 18 years of age with compensated liver disease. *Investigational:* With G-CSF therapy to treat hairy-cell leukemia.

Contraindications: Hypersensitivity to alpha interferons or to products derived from *E. coli.* Use in autoimmune hepatitis or in decompensated hepatic disease.

Special Concerns: Use with caution during lactation and in preexisting cardiac disease, in depression, in those with abnormally low peripheral blood cell counts, in those receiving myelosuppressive agents, and in autoimmune disorder. Safety and efficacy have not been determined in children less than 18 years of age.

Side Effects: *Flu-like symptoms:* Headache, fatigue, fever, myalgia, rigors, arthralgia, increased sweating. *Body as a whole:* Body pain, hot flushes, non-cardiac chest pain, malaise, asthenia, peripheral edema, access pain, allergic reactions, weight loss. *Hypersensitivity:* Urticaria, angioedema, bronchoconstriction, ***anaphylaxis.*** *CNS:* Insomnia, dizziness, paresthesia, amnesia, hypoesthesia, hypertonia, nervousness, depression, anxiety, emotional lability, abnormal thinking, agitation, decreased libido. *GI:* Abdominal pain, N&V, diarrhea, anorexia, dyspepsia, constipation, flatulence, toothache, hemorrhoids, decreased saliva, tender liver. *CV:* Hypertension, palpitation. *Hematologic:* Granulocytopenia, thrombocytopenia, leukopenia, ecchymosis, lymphadenopathy, lymphocytosis. *Respiratory:* Pharyngitis, URI, cough, sinusitis, rhinitis, respiratory tract congestion, upper respiratory tract congestion, epistaxis, dyspnea, bronchitis. *Dermatologic:* Alopecia, pruritus, rash, erythema, dry skin. *Musculoskeletal:* Back, limb, neck, or skeletal pain. *GU:* Dysmenorrhea, vaginitis, menstrual disorder. *Ophthalmic:* Conjunctivitis, eye pain. *Otic:* Tinnitus, earache.

Laboratory Test Considerations: ↑ TSH, triglycerides. ↓ Hemoglobin, hematocrit. Abnormal thyroid tests.

How Supplied: *Injection:* 30 mcg/mL

Dosage

- **SC Injection**

Chronic hepatitis C infection.

Adults over 18 years of age: 9 mcg SC as a single injection three times a week for 24 weeks. At least 48 hr should elapse between doses. Those who tolerate therapy but did not respond or relapsed following discontinuation may be subsequently treated with 15 mcg three times a week for 6 months.

HEALTH CARE CONSIDERATIONS

See also *Health Care Considerations* for *Interferon alfa-2a* and *Interferon alfa-*2b.

Administration/Storage

1. Do not give 15 mcg three times a week if client has not received or has not tolerated an initial course of therapy.
2. Reduce dose to 7.5 mcg following an intolerable adverse reaction. If adverse effects continue at reduced dosage, discontinue therapy or reduce dose further.
3. Store refrigerated but do not freeze. Avoid vigorous shaking.

Assessment

1. Note any cardiac disease, hypertension, or severe psychiatric disorders as these preclude drug therapy.
2. Monitor CBC, TSH, HCV RNA, liver and renal function studies.

Client/Family Teaching

1. Review dose and method of administration (SC); usually administered 3 times per week with 48 hr between doses.
2. May experience flu-like symptoms, including headache, fatigue, fever, muscle/joint pain, rigors, and increased sweating.
3. Stop drug and report any S&S of depression, suicide thoughts/attempt.
4. Do not change brands of interferon without provider approval.

Outcome/Evaluate: Improvement in LFTs

Interferon alfa-n1 lymphoblastoid

(in-ter-**FEER**-on **AL**-fah)

Pregnancy Category: C

Wellferon **(Rx)**

Classification: Interferon for hepatitis C

Action/Kinetics: A mixture of alpha interferons isolated from a human cell line. Natural alpha interferons are derived from leukocytes. They bind to a high-affinity type I receptor and produce immunomodulatory, antiviral, and antiproliferative effects. After binding to the cell membrane, interferon initiates a complex sequence of intracellular events that cause induction of certain enzymes, inhibition of virus replication, suppression of cell proliferation, enhancement of macrophage phagocytic activity, and enhancement of lymphocyte cytotoxicity. The mechanism in the treatment of chronic hepatitis C is not known. **Time to peak levels:** 6–9 hr. **t½, elimination:** 7–10 hr. Clearance is mainly through the kidney and cellular catabolism.

Uses: Treatment of chronic hepatitis C in clients 18 years and older without decompensated liver disease.

Contraindications: Hypersensitivity to alpha interferons, history of anaphylaxis to bovine or ovine immunoglobulins, egg protein, polymyxin B, or neomycin sulfate. Use in clients with decompensated liver disease or autoimmune hepatitis because of the potential for worsening of disease symptoms. Lactation.

Special Concerns: Use with caution in the elderly; in preexisting cardiac disease; clinically significant, preexisting depressive disorders; severe, preexisting autoimmune, renal, or hepatic disease; seizure disorders or compromised CNS function; leukopenia or thrombocytopenia or in those receiving myelosuppressive drugs; pulmonary dysfunction, including unstable asthma or other conditions. Safety and efficacy have not been determined in children.

Side Effects: *Flu-like symptoms:* Asthenia, headache, fever, myalgia, chills, nausea. *GI:* Nausea, diarrhea, abdominal pain, anorexia, vomiting, weight loss, cholecystitis, abnormal liver function, liver tenderness, hepatotoxicity, peritonitis, ruptured spleen. *CNS:* Nervousness, agitation, hostility, emotional lability, insomnia, somnolence, sleep disorder, depression, dizziness (including vertigo), confusion, abnormal thinking, amnesia, paresthesia, convulsions, hallucinations, migraine, suicidal ideation/attempts, decrease in mental status, dizziness, impaired memory, manic behavior, psychotic reactions. *Hematologic:* Thrombocytopenia, decreased WBC count and absolute neutrophil count, leukopenia, myelosuppression, leukocytosis. *CV:* Arrhythmia, angina, hypotension, hypertension, myocardial ischemia, atrial fibrillation. *Hypersensitivity:* Urticaria, angioedema, ***bronchoconstriction, anaphylaxis.*** *Respiratory:* Cough, bronchitis, dyspnea, pneumonia, rhinitis, pharyngitis; respiratory, lung, and pleural disorders. *Musculoskeletal:* Myalgia, arthralgia. *Dermatologic:* Alopecia, rash, pruritus, dry skin, urticaria, sweating, herpes simplex, photosensitivity, psoriasis, worsening of cellulitis and dermatitis. *GU:* Abnormal ejaculation, UTI, decreased libido, menstrual irregularities, renal hemorrhage. *Endocrine:* Thyroid carcinoma, altered hormone levels, hyperglycemia, hypothyroidism, hyperthyroidism, development or exacerbation of preexisting diabetes mellitus. *Injection site reaction:* Pain, edema, hemorrhage, inflammation of injection site. *Autoimmunity disease:* Vasculitis, Raynaud''s disease, rheumatoid arthritis, lupus erythematosus, rhabdomyolysis. *Ophthalmic:* Amblyopia, retinal vein thrombosis, retinal artery or vein obstruction. *Miscellaneous:* Pain, back pain, cyst, peripheral edema, accidental injury, cotton-wool spots.

Laboratory Test Considerations: ↑ Creatinine. ↓ Hemoglobin, hematocrit. Thrombocytopenia, neutropenia. Abnormal TSH and T4. Hyperglycemia.

OD **Management of Overdose:** *Symptoms:* Profound lethargy, prostration, coma, neurotoxicity, EEG abnormalities, seizures. Transient abnormalities in serum LFTs, hyperkalemia, elevations of serum BUN and creatinine, proteinuria, nephrotic syndromes, renal insufficiency, renal failure. *Treatment:* Symptomatic, supportive treatment.

Drug Interactions: Use with caution when giving interferon alfa-n1 with other drugs metabolized by the cytochrome P450 enzyme system (e.g., vinblastine, zidovudine, theophylline).

How Supplied: *Solution:* 3 MU/mL

Dosage

- **IM, SC**

Chronic hepatitis C virus.

Adults: 3 MU SC or IM 3 times a week for 48 weeks.

HEALTH CARE CONSIDERATIONS

Administration/Storage

1. Clients who do not show a reduction in serum ALT or HCV load within the first 16 weeks are not likely to benefit from additional treatment.

2. Reduce dosage by 50% in those who do not tolerate therapy; discontinue therapy in those who continue not to tolerate therapy after dosage reduction.
3. Give proper instructions if home administration is desired.
4. After administration, it is essential to dispose of syringes and needles properly.
5. Store in the refrigerator at 2–8°C (36–46°F). Protect from light. Do not freeze or shake vial.

Assessment

1. Note cause of hepatitis C, other agents trialed and any evidence of severe depression.
2. Before beginning therapy, exclude other causes of hepatitis, including hepatitis B; ensure titer negative.
3. Determine any sensitivity to bovine/ovine immunoglobulins, egg protein, polymyxin B, or neomycin sulfate.
4. Obtain baseline labs and set up a schedule for regular blood draws to evaluate drug effects.

Client/Family Teaching

1. Review method for self injection; frequency of administration, dosage and proper storage and disposal of meds and equipment.
2. Drug is generally used for 12 mo and given three times per week.
3. Report if unable to tolerate side effects as provider may decrease dose by as much as 50 % until S&S resolve.
4. If no reduction in serum ALT or HCV viral load within first 16 weeks of therapy, then unlikely to benefit from continued treatment.
5. Ensure adequate hydration especially during initial treatment stages.
6. May use antiinflammatory analgesics to reduce drug induced discomfort.
7. Practice safe sex as drug does not decrease the risk of disease transmission through blood or sexual contact.
8. With hepatitis C, avoid Tylenol, or Tylenol containing products, alcohol, unprotected sex and do not share toothbrush, clippers, or razors.
9. Identify support groups for counselling and assistance.

Outcome/Evaluate: Treatment of hepatitis C with reduction of viral load and prevention of cirrhosis/hepatic carcinoma R/T hepatitis C

Interferon alfa-n3

(in-ter-**FEER**-on **AL**-fah)

Pregnancy Category: C

Alferon N **(Rx)**

Classification: Antineoplastic

Action/Kinetics: Made from pooled human leukocytes induced by incomplete infection with Sendai (avian) virus. Is a sterile, aqueous formulation of purified, natural, human interferon alpha proteins. Binds to receptors on cell surfaces leading to a sequence of events including inhibition of virus replication and suppression of cell proliferation. Also, causes immunomodulation characterized by enhanced phagocytosis by macrophages, augmentation of the cytotoxicity of lymphocytes, and enhancement of human leukocyte antigen expression. Intralesional use of interferon alfa-n3 does not result in detectable plasma levels of the drug.

Uses: Intralesional treatment of refractory or recurring external condylomata acuminata (genital or venereal warts) in clients 18 years of age or older. *Investigational:* Alpha interferons are being tested for use in a large number of neoplastic diseases and viral infections.

Contraindications: Hypersensitivity to human interferon alpha; clients who are allergic to mouse immunoglobulin (IgG), egg protein, or neomycin (the production process involves a nutrient medium containing neomycin although it has not been detected in the final product). Lactation.

Special Concerns: Due to fever and flu-like symptoms with use of interferon alfa-n3, use with caution in clients with debilitating diseases, including unstable angina, uncontrolled CHF, COPD, diabetes mellitus with ketoacidosis, thrombophlebitis, pulmonary embolism, hemophilia, severe myelosuppression, or seizure disorders. Safety and effectiveness have not been determined in children less than 18 years of age.

Side Effects: *Flu-like symptoms:* Commonly, fever, headache, myalgias which decrease with repeated doses. Also, chills, fatigue, malaise. *CNS:* Dizziness, lightheadedness, insomnia, depression, nervousness, decreased ability to concentrate. *GI:* N&V, heartburn, diarrhea, tongue hyperesthesia, thirst, altered taste, increased salivation. *Musculoskeletal/Skin:* Arthralgia, back pain, hot sensation at bottom of feet, tingling of legs/feet, muscle cramps. *Respiratory:* Nose or sinus drainage, nose bleed, throat tightness, pharyngitis. *Miscellaneous:* Pruritus, swollen lymph nodes, heat intolerance, visual disturbances, sensitivity to allergens, papular rash on neck, hot flashes, herpes labialis, dysuria, photosensitivity, decreased WBC count.

NOTE: When used for treatment of cancer, the incidence of many of the preceding side effects was increased. Additional side effects were noted including: *GI:* Constipation, anorexia, stomatitis, dry mouth, mucositis, sore mouth. *Laboratory Test Values:* Abnormal hemoglobin, WBC count, alkaline phosphatase, total bilirubin, platelet count, AST, and GGT. *Miscellaneous:* Insomnia, blurred vision, ocular rotation pain, sore injection site, chest pains, low BP.

How Supplied: *Injection:* 5 million IU/mL

Dosage

- **Intralesional Injection**

Condylomata acuminata.

0.05 mL (250,000 IU)/wart twice a week for up to 8 weeks. The maximum recommended dose per treatment session is 0.5 mL (2.5 million IU). The safety and effectiveness of a second course of treatment have not been determined.

HEALTH CARE CONSIDERATIONS

See also *Health Care Considerations* for *Interferon alfa-2a* and *Interferon alfa-2b Recombinant.*

Administration/Storage

1. Inject drug into the base of the wart using a 30-gauge needle.
2. For large warts, inject at several points around the periphery of the wart using a total dose of 0.05 mL/wart.
3. Store drug at 2°C–8°C (36°F–46°F). Do not freeze or shake.

Assessment

1. Note any allergic reactions to egg protein or neomycin; may have increased sensitivity to drug.
2. Determine any preexisting debilitating diseases; note functional level.
3. For condylomata therapy, measure and document size and number of lesions.

Client/Family Teaching

1. Intralesional treatment should be continued for 8 weeks.
2. Genital warts may disappear both during and after treatment has been completed. When this occurs, unless new warts appear or warts become enlarged, there should be a 3-month waiting period after the first 8-week course of therapy.
3. Do not change brands of interferon without approval; manufacturing process, strength, and type of interferon may vary.
4. Fertile women should practice contraception.
5. Report early signs of hypersensitivity reactions (e.g., hives, chest tightness, generalized urticaria, hypotension, wheezing, anaphylaxis).

Outcome/Evaluate

- ↓ Pain, number of genital warts
- Suppression of malignant cell proliferation

Interferon beta-1a

Interferon beta-1b (r1FN-B)

(in-ter-**FEER**-on **BAY**-tah)

Pregnancy Category: C

Avonex (Interferon beta-1a), Betaseron (Interferon beta-1b) **(Rx)**

Classification: Drug for multiple sclerosis (MS)

Action/Kinetics: Interferon beta-1a is produced by mammalian cells into which the human interferon beta gene has been introduced. Interferon beta-1b is made by bacterial fermentation of a strain of *Escherichia coli* that is a genetically engineered plasmid containing the gene for human interferon $beta_{ser17}$. Interferon betas have antiviral, antiproliferative, and immunoregulatory effects. Mechanism for the beneficial effect in MS is unknown, although the effects are mediated through combination with specific cell receptors located on the cell membrane. The receptor-drug complex induces the expression of a number of interferon-induced gene products that are thought to be the mediators of the biologic effects of interferon beta-1a and beta-1b. **t½, interferon beta-1a:** 10 hr. Kinetic information is not available for interferon beta-1b since serum levels are low or not detectable following SC administration to MS clients. **Peak serum levels of beta-1b:** Within 1–8 hr with a mean serum concentration of 40 IU/mL. Mean terminal half-lives ranged from 8 min to 4.3 hr.

Uses: Interferon beta-1a: Treatment of relapsing forms of MS to slow the appearance of physical disability and decrease the frequency of clinical exacerbations. **Interferon beta-1b:** Treatment of ambulatory clients with relapsing-remitting MS to reduce the frequency of clinical exacerbations. Remitting-relapsing MS is manifested by recurrent attacks of neurologic dysfunction followed by complete or incomplete recovery. *Investigational:* Treatment of AIDS, AIDS-related Kaposi's sarcoma, metastatic renal cell carcinoma, herpes of the lips or genitals, malignant melanoma, cutaneous T-cell lymphoma, and acute non-A/non-B hepatitis.

Contraindications: Hypersensitivity to natural or recombinant interferon beta or human albumin. Lactation.

Special Concerns: The safety and efficacy for use in chronic progressive MS and in children less than 18 years of age have not been studied. Depression and attempted suicide and suicide have occurred. Potential to be an abortifacient. Use with caution in those with preexisting seizure disorder.

Side Effects: Side effects common to interferon beta-1a and beta-1b. *Body as a whole:* Headache, fever, flu-like symptoms, pain, asthenia, chills, reaction at injection site (including necrosis/inflammation), malaise. *GI:* Abdominal pain, diarrhea, dry mouth, ***GI hemorrhage,*** gingivitis, hepatomegaly, intestinal obstruction, periodontal abscess, proctitis. *CV:* Arrhythmia, hypotension, postural hypotension. *CNS:* Dizziness, speech disorder, convulsion, suicide attempt, abnormal gait, depersonalization, facial paralysis, hyperesthesia, neurosis, psychosis. *Respiratory:* Sinusitis, dyspnea, hemoptysis, hyperventilation. *Musculoskeletal:* Myalgia, arthritis. *Dermatologic:* Contact dermatitis, furunculosis, seborrhea, skin ulcer. *GU:* Epididymitis, gynecomastia, hematuria, kidney calculus, nocturia, vaginal hemorrhage, ovarian cyst. *Miscellaneous:* Abscess, ascites, cellulitis, hernia, hypothyroidism, ***sepsis,*** hiccoughs, thirst, leukorrhea.

Interferon beta-1a. *Body as a whole:* Infection. *GI:* Nausea, dyspepsia, anorexia, blood in stool, colitis, constipation, diverticulitis, gall bladder disorder, gastritis, gum hemorrhage, hepatoma, increased appetite, ***intestinal perforation,*** periodontitis, tongue disorder. *CV:* Syncope, vasodilation, arteritis, ***heart arrest, hemorrhage, pulmonary embolus,*** palpitation, pericarditis, peripheral ischemia, peripheral vascular disorder, spider angioma, telangiectasia. *CNS:* Sleep difficulty, muscle spasm, ataxia, amnesia, Bell's palsy, clumsiness, drug dependence, increased libido. *Respiratory:* URTI, emphysema, laryngitis, pharyngeal edema, pneumonia. *Musculoskeletal:* Arthralgia, bone pain, myasthenia, osteonecrosis, synovitis. *Dermatologic:* Urticaria, alopecia, nevus, herpes zoster, herpes simplex, basal cell carcinoma, blisters, cold clammy skin, erythema, genital pruritus, skin discoloration. *GU:* Vaginitis, breast fibroadenosis, breast mass, dysuria, fibrocystic change of the breast, fibroids, kidney pain, menopause, pelvic inflammatory disease, penis disorder, Peyronie's disease, polyuria, postmenopausal hemorrhage, prostatic disorder, pyelonephritis, testis disorder, urethral pain, urinary urgency, urinary retention, urinary incontinence. *Hematologic:* Anemia, ecchymosis at injection site, eosinophils greater than 10%, hematocrit less than 37%, increased coagulation time, ecchymosis, lymphadenopathy, petechia. *Metabolic:* Dehydration, hypoglycemia, hypomagnesemia, hypokalemia. *Ophthalmic:* Abnormal vision, conjunctivitis, eye pain, vitreous floaters. *Miscellaneous:* Otitis media, decreased hearing, facial edema, fibrosis at injection site, hypersensitivity at injection site, lipoma, neoplasm, photosensitivity, toothache, sinus headache, chest pain.

Interferon beta-1b. *Body as a whole:* Generalized edema, hypothermia, ***anaphylaxis, shock,*** adenoma, sarcoma. *GI:* Constipation, vomiting, GI disorder, aphthous stomatitis, cardiospasm, cheilitis, cholecystitis, cholelithiasis, duodenal ulcer, enteritis, esophagitis, fecal impaction or incontinence, flatulence, gastritis, glossitis, hematemesis, hepatic neoplasia, hepatitis, ileus, increased salivation, melena, nausea, oral leukoplakia, oral moniliasis, ***pancreatitis, rectal hemorrhage,*** salivary gland enlargement, stomach ulcer, peritonitis, tenesmus. *CV:* Migraine, palpitation, hypertension, tachycardia, peripheral vascular disorder, ***hemorrhage,*** angina pectoris, atrial fibrillation, cardiomegaly, ***cardiac arrest, cerebral hemorrhage, heart failure, MI, pulmonary embolus, ventricular fibrillation*** cerebral ischemia, endocarditis, pericardial effusion, spider angioma, subarachnoid hemorrhage, syncope, thrombophlebitis, thrombosis, varicose veins, vasospasm, venous pressure increase, ventricular extrasystoles. *CNS:* Mental symptoms, hypertonia, somnolence, hyperkinesia, acute/chronic brain syndrome, agitation, apathy, aphasia, ataxia, brain edema, ***coma,*** delirium, delusions, dementia, dystonia, encephalopathy, euphoria, hallucinations, hemiplegia, hypalgesia, incoordination, intracranial hypertension, decreased libido, manic reaction, meningitis, neuralgia, neuropathy, paralysis, paranoid reaction, decreased reflexes, stupor, subdural hematoma, torticollis, tremor. *Respiratory:* Laryngitis, apnea, asthma, atelectasis, lung carcinoma, hypoventilation, interstitial pneumonia, lung edema, pleural effusion, pneumothorax. *Musculoskeletal:* Myasthenia, arthrosis, bursitis, leg cramps, muscle atrophy, myopathy, myositis, ptosis, tenosynovitis. *Dermatologic:* Sweating, alopecia, erythema nodosum, exfoliative dermatitis, hirsutism, leukoderma, lichenoid dermatitis, maculopapular rash, photosensitivity, psoriasis, benign skin neoplasm, skin carcinoma, skin hypertrophy, skin necrosis, urticaria, vesiculobullous rash. *GU:* Dysmenorrhea, menstrual disorder, metrorrhagia, cystitis, breast pain, menorrhagia, urinary urgency, fibrocystic breast, breast neoplasm, urinary retention, anuria, balanitis, breast engorgement, cervicitis, impotence, kidney failure, tubular disorder, nephritis, oliguria, polyuria, salpingitis, urethritis, urinary incontinence, enlarged uterine fibroids, uterine neoplasm. *Hematologic:* Lymphocytes less than 1500/mm^3, active neutrophil count less than 1500/mm^3, WBCs less than 3000/mm^3, lymphadenopathy, chronic lymphocytic leukemia, petechia, hemoglobin less than 9.4 g/dL, platelets less than 75,000/mm^3, splenomegaly. *Metabolic:* Weight gain, weight loss, goiter, glucose less than 55 mg/dL or greater than 160 mg/dL, AST or ALT greater than 5 times baseline, total bilirubin greater than 2.5 times baseline, urine protein greater than 1+, alkaline phosphatase greater than 5 times baseline, BUN greater than 40 mg/dL, calcium greater than 11.5 mg/dL, cyanosis, edema, glycosuria, hypoglycemic reaction, hypoxia, ketosis. *Ophthalmic:* Conjunctivitis, abnormal vision, diplopia, nystagmus, oculogyric crisis, papilledema, blepharitis, blindness, dry eyes, iritis, keratoconjunctivitis, mydriasis, photophobia, retinitis, visual field defect. *Miscellaneous:* Pelvic pain, hydrocephalus, alcohol intolerance, otitis externa, otitis media, parosmia, taste loss, taste perversion.

Laboratory Test Considerations: ↑ ALT, total bilirubin, AST, BUN, urine protein. Hypoglycemia or hyperglycemia. Ketosis.

How Supplied: *Kit:* 33 mcg; *Powder for injection:* 0.3 mg

Dosage

- **Interferon beta-1a: IM**

  Relapsing forms of MS.

30 mcg IM once a week.

- **Inteferon beta-1b: SC**

  Relapsing-remitting MS clients.

0.25 mg (8 mIU) every other day.

HEALTH CARE CONSIDERATIONS

Administration/Storage

1. Effectiveness beyond 2 years of use is not known.
2. To reconstitute and use interferon beta-1a, use the following process:
- Reconstitute with 1.1 mL of diluent and swirl gently to dissolve.
- Vials must be stored in a refrigerator at 2°C–8°C (36°F–46°F).
- Following reconstitution, use within 6 hr and store at the same temperatures as the unreconstituted drug.

3. To reconstitute and use interferon beta-1b, use the following process:
- Using a sterile syringe and needle, inject 1.2 mL of diluent provided (0.54% NaCl) into the vial. Swirl gently to dissolve the drug completely. (Do not shake.)
- Visually inspect reconstituted product; discard if it contains particulate matter or is discolored.
- Withdraw 1 mL of the reconstituted solution from the vial into a sterile syringe fitted with a 27-gauge needle and inject SC. Injection sites include the arms, abdomen, hips, and thighs.
- Since the reconstituted product contains no preservative, discard any unused portions after one use.
- Before and after reconstitution with diluent, store the drug at 2°C–8°C (36°F–46°F). Use the product within 3 hr of reconstitution.

Assessment

1. Record age of diagnosis, frequency of exacerbations, other therapies prescribed and the outcome.
2. Note any hypersensitivity to human albumin or interferon beta.
3. Determine if pregnant; drug has abortifacient properties.
4. Monitor hematologic profile and hepatic enzyme levels q 3 mo.

Client/Family Teaching

1. Review guidelines for drug reconstitution, proper dose, administration, and care and disposal of equipment.
2. Do not change dose or administration schedule without approval.
3. Flu-like symptoms are common; acetaminophen may help.
4. Report any mental changes, depression, or suicide thoughts.
5. Practice reliable birth control; drug may harm fetus.
6. May cause photosensitivity reactions; wear protective clothing, sunscreen, sun glasses, and a hat.
7. Avoid alcohol in any form.
8. With diabetes, monitor FS and report any overt changes.
9. Identify support groups that may assist to cope with chronic diseases.

Outcome/Evaluate: ↓ Frequency and severity of MS exacerbations

Interferon gamma-1b

(in-ter-**FEER**-on **GAM**-uh)

Pregnancy Category: C

Actimmune **(Rx)**

Classification: Interferon

Action/Kinetics: Consists of a single-chain polypeptide of 140 amino acids. Produced by fermentation of a genetically engineered *Escherichia coli* bacterium containing the DNA that encodes for the human protein. Manifests potent phagocyte-activating effects including generation of toxic oxygen metabolites within phagocytes. Such metabolites result in the death of microorganisms such as *Staphylococcus aureus, Toxoplasma gondii, Leishmania donovani, Listeria monocytogenes,* and *Mycobacterium avium intracellulare.* Since interferon gamma regulates activity of immune cells, it is characterized as a lymphokine of the interleukin type. Interferon gamma interacts functionally with other interleukin molecules (e.g., interleukin-2) and all interleukins form part of a complex, lymphokine regulatory network. As an example, interferon gamma and interleukin-4 may interact reciprocally to regulate murine IgE levels; interferon gamma can suppress IgE levels and inhibit the production of collagen at the transcription level in humans. Slowly absorbed after SC injection. **t½, elimination: SC,** 5.9 hr. **Peak plasma levels:** 7 hr after SC.

Uses: Decrease the frequency and severity of serious infections associated with chronic granulomatous disease.

Contraindications: Hypersensitivity to interferon gamma or *E. coli*-derived products. Lactation.

Special Concerns: Safety and effectiveness have not been determined in children less than 1 year of age. Use with caution in clients with preexisting cardiac disease, including symptoms of ischemia, arrhythmia, or CHF, and in clients with myelosuppression, seizure disorders, or compromised CNS function.

Side Effects: The following side effects were noted in clients with chronic granulomatous disease receiving the drug SC. *GI:* Diarrhea, vomiting, nausea, abdominal pain, anorexia. *CNS:* Fever (over 50%), headache, fatigue, depression. *Miscellaneous:* Rash, chills, erythema or tenderness at injection site, pain at injection site, weight loss, myalgia, arthralgia, back pain.

When used in clients other than those with chronic granulomatous disease, in addition to the preceding, the following side effects were reported. *GI:* ***GI bleeding,*** pancreatitis, hepatic insufficiency. *CV:* Hypotension, heart block, ***heart failure,*** syncope, ***tachyarrhythmia, MI.*** *CNS:* Confusion, disorientation, symptoms of parkinsonism, gait disturbance, ***seizures,*** hallucinations, transient ischemic attacks. *Hematologic:* ***Deep venous thrombosis, pulmonary embolism.*** *Respiratory:* ***Bronchospasm,*** tachypnea, interstitial pneumonitis. *Metabolic:* Hyperglycemia, hyponatremia. *Miscellaneous:* Reversible renal insufficiency, worsening of dermatomyositis.

How Supplied: *Injection:* 3 million U/0.5 mL

Dosage

- **SC**

Chronic granulomatous disease.

50 mcg/m² (1.5 million units/m²) for clients whose body surface is greater than 0.5 m². If the body surface is less than 0.5 m², the dose of interferon gamma should be 1.5 mcg/kg/dose. The drug is given 3 times/ week (e.g., Monday, Wednesday, Friday).

HEALTH CARE CONSIDERATIONS

Administration/Storage

1. Preferred injection sites are the right and left deltoid and anterior thigh.
2. Does not contain a preservative. Use the vial only for a single dose and discard any unused portion.
3. Safety and effectiveness have not been determined for doses greater or less than 50 mcg/m².
4. If severe side effects occur, dose can be reduced by 50% or therapy can be discontinued until these subside.
5. May be administered using either sterilized glass or plastic disposable syringes.
6. Do not shake the vial; avoid vigorous agitation.
7. Vials must be stored at 2°C–8°C (36°F–46°F) to assure optimal retention of activity. Do not freeze vial.
8. Discard vials stored at room temperature for more than 12 hr.
9. Do not store undiluted drug in syringes due to syringe adhesion.
10. IV Although not approved by the FDA, the drug has been given by continuous (10 days to 8 weeks) or intermittent (at 1, 6, or 24 hr) IV infusion as well as by IM injection.

Assessment

1. Determine age with onset of chronic granulomatous disease and what if any treatments in the past were used to reduce frequency and severity of infections.
2. Note history of CAD or CNS disorders; assess for symptoms.
3. Monitor urinalysis, CBC, liver and renal function studies q 3 mo.

Client/Family Teaching

1. Review appropriate method for administration, reconstitution, storage, and disposal of drug/equipment.

2. Keep drug in the refrigerator; do *not* shake container.
3. Take at bedtime with acetaminophen to minimize flu-like symptoms (fever and headaches).
4. Consume 2–3 L/day of fluids.
5. Avoid alcohol and any other CNS depressants.
6. Close medical supervision is imperative with this disease and genetically engineered drug therapy as dosage may require frequent adjustments. Report all concerns and any adverse effects.

Outcome/Evaluate: Suppression of infective organisms associated with chronic granulomatous disease

I

Ipecac syrup

(IP-eh-kak)
Pregnancy Category: C
PMS Ipecac Syrup ✱ **(OTC)**
Classification: Emetic

Action/Kinetics: Acts both locally on the gastric mucosa as an irritant and centrally to stimulate the CTZ. The central effect is caused by emetine and cephaeline, which are two alkaloids in the product. **Onset:** 20 min. **Duration:** 20–25 min. In contrast to apomorphine, a second dose may be given if necessary. **Ipecac syrup must not be confused with ipecac fluid extract, which is 14 times as potent.** Syrup of ipecac can be purchased without a prescription.
Uses: To empty the stomach promptly and completely after oral poisoning or drug overdose.
Contraindications: With corrosives or petroleum distillates, in individuals who are unconscious or semicomatose, severely inebriated, or in shock. Infants under 6 months of age.
Special Concerns: Use with caution during lactation. If used in children less than 12 months of age, there is an increased risk of aspiration of vomitus. Abuse may occur in anorexic or bulemic clients and its use in these groups has been associated with severe cardiomyopathies and death.
Side Effects: Diarrhea, drowsiness, coughing, or choking with emesis, mild CNS depression, GU upset (may last several hours) after emesis. Can be cardiotoxic if not vomited and allowed to be absorbed. Cardiotoxic effects include heart conduction disturbances, atrial fibrillation, or fatal myocarditis.
OD Management of Overdose: *Symptoms:* If absorbed into the general circulation, symptoms may include cardiac conduction disturbances, bradycardia, atrial fibrillation, hypotension, or ***fatal myocarditis.*** *Treatment:* Activated charcoal to absorb ipecac syrup. Gastric lavage. Support the CV system with symptomatic treatment.
Drug Interactions: Activated charcoal adsorbs ipecac syrup, thus decreasing its effect.
How Supplied: *Syrup*

Dosage

- **Syrup**

  Emetic.

Adults and children over 12 years: 15–30 mL followed by 240 mL of water; **infants up to 1 year:** 5–10 mL followed by one-half to one glass of water; **pediatric, 1–12 years:** 15 mL followed by one to two glasses of water.

HEALTH CARE CONSIDERATIONS

Administration/Storage
1. Check label of medication closely so that the syrup and the fluid extract are not confused.
2. Dosage may be repeated in children over 1 year of age and adults once if vomiting does not occur within 30 min. Consider gastric lavage if vomiting does not occur within 15 min of second dose.
3. Administer ipecac syrup with 200–300 mL of water.
4. There is controversy as to whether ipecac should be given to children less than 1 year old. It appears to be both safe and effective.

Assessment
1. Estimate amount and time of ingestion and compare with plasma level of agent ingested.
2. Do not use if intoxicant is a convulsant (i.e., TCAs); may trigger seizures abruptly.
3. Do not use for petroleum-based or caustic substances such as kerosene, lye, Drano, or gasoline.
4. Assess respiratory status and level of consciousness; do not use if there is no gag reflex or if semicomatose.

Client/Family Teaching
1. For use in the event of accidental poisoning.
2. Before administering ipecac syrup, contact regional poison control center or local hospital.
3. Store in a locked closet, out of the reach of children. Check expiration date periodically and always before use.
4. Review abuse potential, such as to induce vomiting after meals for weight reduction and its potential cardiac toxic effects. (Some states have banned OTC sales.)

Outcome/Evaluate: Inducement of vomiting following drug overdose or poisoning

Ipratropium bromide

(eye-prah-**TROH**-pee-um)

Pregnancy Category: B

Alti-Ipratropium Bromide ✱, Apo-Ipravent ✱, Atrovent, Novo-Ipramide ✱, PMS-Ipratropium ✱ **(Rx)**

Classification: Anticholinergic, quaternary ammonium compound

See also *Cholinergic Blocking Agents.*

Action/Kinetics: Chemically related to atropine. Antagonizes the action of acetylcholine. Prevents the increase in intracellular levels of cyclic guanosine monophosphate, which is caused by the interaction of acetylcholine with muscarinic receptors in bronchial smooth muscle; this leads to bronchodilation which is primarily a local, site-specific effect. Not easily absorbed into the systemic circulation; excreted through the feces. **t½, elimination:** 2 hr after inhalation.

Uses: Aerosol or solution: Bronchodilation in COPD, including chronic bronchitis and emphysema. **Nasal spray:** Symptomatic relief (using 0.03%) of rhinorrhea associated with allergic and nonallergic perennial rhinitis in clients over 6 years of age. Symptomatic relief (using 0.03%) of rhinorrhea associated with the common cold in those over 12 years of age. *NOTE:* The use of ipratropium with sympathomimetic bronchodilators, methylxanthines, steroids, or cromolyn sodium (all of which are used in treating COPD) are without side effects.

Contraindications: Hypersensitivity to atropine, ipratropium, or derivatives. Hypersensitivity to soya lecithin or related food products, including soy bean or peanut (inhalation aerosol).

Special Concerns: Use with caution in clients with narrow-angle glaucoma, prostatic hypertrophy, or bladder neck obstruction and during lactation. Safety and efficacy have not been determined in children. Use of ipratropium as a single agent for the relief of bronchospasm in acute COPD has not been studied adequately.

Side Effects: *Inhalation aerosol. CNS:* Cough, nervousness, dizziness, headache, fatigue, insomnia, drowsiness, difficulty in coordination, tremor. *GI:* Dryness of oropharynx, GI distress, dry mouth, nausea, constipation. *CV:* Palpitations, tachycardia, flushing. *Dermatologic:* Itching, hives, alopecia. *Miscellaneous:* Irritation from aerosol, worsening of symptoms, rash, hoarseness, blurred vision, difficulty in accommodation, drying of secretions, urinary difficulty, paresthesias, mucosal ulcers.

Inhalation solution. CNS: Dizziness, insomnia, nervousness, tremor, headache. *GI:* Dry mouth, nausea, constipation. *CV:* Hypertension, aggravation of hypertension, tachycardia, palpitations. *Respiratory:* Worsening of COPD symptoms, coughing, dyspnea, bronchitis, bronchospasm, increased sputum, URI, pharyngitis, rhinitis, sinusitis. *Miscellaneous:* Urinary retention, UTIs, urticaria, pain, flulike symptoms, back or chest pain, arthritis.

Nasal spray. CNS: Headache, dizziness. *GI:* Nausea, dry mouth, taste perversion. *CV:* Palpitation, tachycardia. *Respiratory:* URI, epistaxis, pharyngitis, nasal dryness, miscellaneous nasal symptoms, nasal irritation, blood-tinged mucus, dry throat, cough, nasal congestion, nasal burning, coughing. *Ophthalmic:* Ocular irritation, blurred vision, conjunctivitis. *Miscellaneous:* Hoarseness, thirst, tinnitis, urinary retention.

All products. Allergic: Skin rash; angioedema of the tongue, throat, lips, and face; urticaria, laryngospasm, ***anaphylaxis.*** *Anticholinergic reactions:* Precipitation or worsening of narrow angle glaucoma, prostatic disorders, tachycardia, urinary retention, constipation, and bowel obstruction.

How Supplied: *Aerosol:* 0.018 mg/inh; *Nasal Spray:* 0.03%; *Solution for Inhalation:* 0.02%

Dosage

- **Respiratory Aerosol**

  Treat bronchospasms.

Adults: 2 inhalations (36 mcg) q.i.d. Additional inhalations may be required but should not exceed 12 inhalations/day.

- **Solution for Inhalation**

  Treat bronchospasms.

Adults: 500 mcg (1-unit-dose vial) administered t.i.d.–q.i.d. by oral nebulization with doses 6–8 hr apart.

- **Nasal Spray, 0.03%**

  Perennial rhinitis.

2 sprays (42 mcg) per nostril b.i.d.–t.i.d. for a total daily dose of 168–252 mcg/day.

- **Nasal Spray, 0.06%**

  Rhinitis due to the common cold.

2 sprays (84 mcg) per nostril t.i.d.–q.i.d. for a total daily dose of 504–672 mcg/day. The safety and efficacy for use for the common cold for more than 4 days have not been determined.

HEALTH CARE CONSIDERATIONS

See also *Health Care Considerations* for *Cholinergic Blocking Agents.*

Administration/Storage

1. If also taking albuterol, ipratropium may be

mixed in the nebulizer with albuterol if used within 1 hr.
2. Store the aerosol below 30°C (86°F); avoid excessive humidity.
3. Store the solution between 15°C and 30°C (59°F and 86°F); protect from light. Store unused vials in the foil pouch.
4. Store the nasal spray tightly closed between 15°C and 30°C (59°F and 86°F). Avoid freezing.

Assessment

1. Record type, onset, characteristics of symptoms, any other agents used and the results.
2. Perform full pulmonary assessment; review PFTs and X-rays.
3. Note any prostate enlargement or difficulty urinating.

Client/Family Teaching

1. Take only as directed; shake well before using. Review administration technique and rinse mouth after use.
2. If using more than one inhalation per dose, wait 3 min before administering the second inhalation.
3. Drug is not for use in terminating an acute attack; effects take up to 15 min. Have another prescribed agent readily available in this event.
4. Avoid contact with the eyes. A spacer may be useful with the inhaler and a mouthpiece with the nebulizer to help prevent solution (mist) contact with the eyes.
5. May experience a bitter taste and dry mouth; use frequent mouth rinses and hard candy to relieve.
6. Transient dizziness, insomnia, blurred vision, or excessive weakness may occur.
7. Stop smoking now to preserve current level of lung function and to prevent further damage; utilize smoking cessation program.

Outcome/Evaluate

- Improved airway exchange and breathing patterns
- ↓ Wheezing, dyspnea
- Relief of rhinorrhea

Ipratropium bromide and Albuterol sulfate

(eye-prah-**TROH**-pee-um/ al-**BYOU**-ter-ohl)

Pregnancy Category: C
Combivent **(Rx)**
Classification: Drug for chronic obstructive pulmonary disease

See also *Ipratropium bromide* and *Albuterol sulfate.*

Content: Each actuation of metered dose inhaler delivers: *Cholinergic blocking drug:* Ipratropium bromide, 18 mcg; and *Sympathomimetic:* Albuterol sulfate, 103 mcg.
Uses: Treatment of COPD in those who are on regular aerosol bronchodilator therapy and who require a second bronchodilator.
Contraindications: History of hypersensitivity to soya lecithin or related food products, such as soybean and peanuts. Lactation.
Special Concerns: Use with caution in CV disorders, especially coronary insufficiency, cardiac arrhythmias, and hypertension. Use with caution in narrow-angle glaucoma, prostatic hypertrophy, bladder-neck obstruction, convulsive disorders, hyperthyroidism, diabetes mellitus, in those unusually responsive to sympathomimetic amines, and renal or hepatic disease. Safety and efficacy have not been determined in children.
Side Effects: *Respiratory:* ***Paradoxical bronchospasm,*** bronchitis, dyspnea, coughing, respiratory disorders, pneumonia, URTI, pharyngitis, sinusitis, rhinitis. *CV:* ECG changes including flattening of T wave, prolongation of QTc interval, and ST segment depression. Also, arrhythmias, palpitation, tachycardia, angina, hypertension. *Hypersensitivity, immediate:* Urticaria, ***angioedema, bronchospasm, anaphylaxis, oropharyngeal edema.*** *Body as a whole:* Headache, pain, flu, chest pain, edema, fatigue. *GI:* N&V, dry mouth, diarrhea, dyspepsia. *CNS:* Dizziness, nervousness, paresthesia, tremor, dysphonia, insomnia. *Miscellaneous:* Arthralgia, increased sputum, taste perversion, UTI, dysuria.
Drug Interactions: See individual drugs.
How Supplied: See Content

Dosage

- **Inhalation**

COPD.

2 inhalations q 6 hr not to exceed 12 inhalations/24-hr.

HEALTH CARE CONSIDERATIONS

See also *Health Care Considerations* for *Ipratropium bromide* and *Albuterol sulfate.*

Administration/Storage

1. Canister provides sufficient medication for 200 inhalations.
2. Discard canister after labeled number of inhalations have been used.
3. Store between 15°C–30°C (59°F–86°F).

Assessment

1. Assess for any soybean or peanut allergy.
2. Note indications for therapy, characteristics and frequency of symptoms, other agents trialed, and outcome.

3. Assess breath sounds and PFTs.

Client/Family Teaching

1. Use as directed; do not increase dose or frequency of administration unless specifically directed.
2. Avoid excessive humidity. For best results, have canister at room temperature before use.
3. Shake canister well before using.
4. Test spray 3 times before first use and again if the canister has not been used for 24 hr.
5. Report any loss of effectiveness.
6. Avoid eye contact; report any visual disturbances or eye irritation.
7. Drug is not for use in terminating an acute attack; effects take up to 15 min. Have another prescribed agent readily available in this event.
8. Stop smoking now to preserve current level of lung function and to prevent further damage; utilize smoking cessation program.

Outcome/Evaluate: Improved airway exchange

Irbesartan

(ihr-beh-**SAR**-tan)

Pregnancy Category: C (first trimester), D (second and third trimesters)

Avapro **(Rx)**

Classification: Antihypertensive, angiotensin II receptor antagonist

---

See also *Antihypertensive Drugs.*

Action/Kinetics: By binding to AT_1 angiotensin II receptor, blocks vasoconstrictor and aldosterone-secreting effects of angiotensin II. Rapid absorption after PO use. **Peak plasma levels:** 1.5–2 hr. Food does not affect bioavailability. **t½, terminal elimination:** 11–15 hr. Over 90% bound to plasma proteins. Metabolized in liver and both unchanged drug and metabolites excreted through urine and feces.

Uses: Treat hypertension alone or in combination with other antihypertensives. *Investigational:* Heart failure, reduce rate of progression of renal disease and adverse clinical sequelae in hypertensives with diabetic nephropathy.

Special Concerns: Safety and efficacy have not been determined in children.

Side Effects: *GI:* Diarrhea, dyspepsia, heartburn, abdominal pain, N&V, constipation, oral lesion, gastroenteritis, flatulence, abdominal distention. *CV:* Tachycardia, syncope, orthostatic hypotension, hypotension (especially in volume- or salt-depletion), flushing, hypertension, cardiac murmur, ***MI, cardio-respiratory arrest, heart failure, hypertensive crisis, CVA,*** angina pectoris, arrhythmias, conduction disorder, transient ischemic attack. *CNS:* Sleep disturbance, anxiety, nervousness, dizziness, numbness, somnolence, emotional disturbance, depression, paresthesia, tremor. *Musculoskeletal:* Extremity swelling, muscle cramp, arthritis, muscle ache, musculoskeletal pain, musculoskeletal chest pain, joint stiffness, bursitis, muscle weakness. *Respiratory:* Epistaxis, tracheobronchitis, congestion, pulmonary congestion, dyspnea, wheezing, upper respiratory infection, rhinitis, pharyngitis, sinus abnormality. *GU:* Abnormal urination, prostate disorder, UTI, sexual dysfunction, libido change. *Dermatologic:* Pruritus, dermatitis, ecchymosis, facial erythema, urticaria. *Ophthalmic:* Vision disturbance, conjunctivitis, eyelid abnormality. *Otic:* Hearing abnormality, ear infection, ear pain, ear abnormality. *Miscellaneous:* Gout, fever, fatigue, chills, facial edema, upper extremity edema, headache, influenza, rash, chest pain.

Laboratory Test Considerations: ↑ BUN (minor), serum creatinine.

How Supplied: *Tablet:* 75 mg, 150 mg, 300 mg

Dosage

- **Tablets**

Hypertension.

150 mg once daily, up to 300 mg once daily. Lower initial dose of 75 mg is recommended for clients with depleted intravascular volume or salt. If BP is not controlled by irbesartan alone, hydrochlorothiazide may have an additive effect. Clients not adequately treated by 300 mg irbesartan are unlikely to get benefit from higher dose or b.i.d. dosing.

HEALTH CARE CONSIDERATIONS

See also *Health Care Considerations* for *Antihypertensive Drugs.*

Administration/Storage

1. Adjustment of dose is not required in geriatric clients or in hepatic or renal impairment.
2. May be given with other antihypertensive drugs.

Assessment

1. Record indications for therapy, onset, duration, characteristics of symptoms, and other agents trialed.
2. Observe infants exposed to an angiotensin II inhibitor in utero for hypotension, oliguria, and ↑ K.

Client/Family Teaching
1. Take only as directed. May take with or without food.
2. Continue low-fat, low-cholesterol diet, regular exercise, tobacco cessation, salt restriction and life-style changes necessary to maintain lowered BP.
3. Practice reliable contraception. Stop drug and report if pregnancy suspected.
Outcome/Evaluate: ↓ BP

Iron dextran parenteral

Pregnancy Category: C
InFeD, DexFerrum **(Rx)**
Classification: Iron product

I

Action/Kinetics: A complex of ferric hydroxide and dextran. Is removed from the plasma by the reticuloendothelial system which splits the complex into iron and dextran. The iron is bound to protein to form hemosiderin or ferritin, which replenishes hemoglobin and depleted iron stores. After IM, most absorbed within 72 hr and the rest over 3–4 weeks. Negligible amounts of iron in iron dextran are lost via the urine and feces.
Uses: Treatment of documented iron deficiency where oral use is unsatisfactory or impossible. *Investigational:* Iron supplementation in clients receiving epoetin therapy.
Contraindications: All anemias not associated with iron deficiency. Acute phase of infectious kidney disease. Use in infants less than 4 months of age.
Special Concerns: Use with extreme caution in seriously impaired liver function. Use with caution during lactation and in clients with a history of significant allergies/asthma. Rheumatoid arthritis clients may have an acute exacerbation of joint pain and swelling after iron dextran. Side effects may exacerbate CV complications in clients with preexisting CV disease. Unwarranted therapy will cause excess storage of iron with the possibility of exogenous hemosiderosis.

Large IV or IM doses may cause arthralgia, backache, chills, dizziness, moderate to high fever, headache, malaise, myalgia, N&V (onset is 24–48 hr; symptoms usually subside within 3–4 days after IV and within 3–7 days after IM).
Side Effects: *Delayed reactions:* Arthralgia, backache, chills, dizziness, fever, headache, malaise, myalgia, N&V. *Hypersensitivity:* ***Anaphylaxis.*** *GI:* Abdominal pain, N&V, diarrhea. *CNS:* Convulsions, syncope, headache, weakness, unresponsiveness, paresthesia, febrile episodes, chills, dizziness, disorientation, numbness, unconsciousness. *CV:* Chest pain, chest tightness, shock, ***cardiac arrest,*** hypotension, hypertension, tachycardia, bradycardia, flushing, arrhythmias. Also, flushing and hypotension from too rapid IV injection. *Respiratory:* Dyspnea, bronchospasm, wheezing, ***respiratory arrest.*** *Musculoskeletal:* Arthralgia, arthritis (including reactivation), myalgia, backache, sterile abscess, atrophy/fibrosis (at IM injection site), soreness or pain at or near IM injection site, cellulitis, swelling, inflammation, local phlebitis at or near IV injection site. *Hematologic:* Leukocytosis, lymphadenopathy. *Dermatologic:* Urticaria, pruritus, purpura, rash, cyanosis. *Miscellaneous:* Hematuria, febrile episodes, sweating, shivering, chills, malaise, altered taste.
Drug Interactions: If taken with chloramphenicol, may see ↑ serum iron levels R/T ↓ iron clearance and erythropoiesis due to direct bone marrow toxicity.
How Supplied: *Injection:* 50 mg iron/mL (as dextran)

Dosage

Dosage is based on results of hematology data. The table in the package insert must be used to estimate the total iron required to restore hemoglobin to normal or near normal levels plus an additional allowance to replenish iron stores. The information in the table is to be used only in clients with iron deficiency anemia; they are not to be used to determine dosage in those needing iron replacement for blood loss.

IV injection. Prior to the first therapeutic dose, give an IV test dose of 0.5 mL slowly (over 30 seconds for InFeD or 5 minutes or more for DexFerrum). To ensure the client does not experience an anaphylactic reaction, allow 1 hr or more to elapse before the remainder of the initial therapeutic dose is given. Individual doses of 2 mL or less may be given daily until the calculated total amount of iron required has been administered. Give undiluted and slowly 50 mg or less/min (1 mL or less/min).

IM injection. As with IV administration, give a 0.5 mL test dose as described above. If no side effects occur, give injections as follows until the calculated total amount of iron has been administered. Do not exceed a daily dose of 25 mg iron (i.e., 0.5 mL) for infants less than 5 kg, 50 mg iron (i.e., 1 mL) for children less than 10 kg, and 100 mg iron (i.e., 2 mL) for all others.

HEALTH CARE CONSIDERATIONS

Administration/Storage

1. For IM, inject into the upper outer quadrant of the buttock; never inject into the arm or other exposed areas. Inject deeply with a 2 or 3 inch 19 or 20 gauge needle.
2. If the client is standing, have them bear weight on the leg opposite the injection site. If in bed, have them lie in a lateral position with injection site uppermost.
3. To avoid leakage or injection into SC tissue, use a Z-track technique.

IV 4. Do not mix iron dextran with other drugs or add to parenteral nutrition solutions for IV infusion.

Assessment

1. Record indications for therapy (ensure iron deficieny anemia), onset, reason oral replacement not used and previous therapies trialed.
2. Assess for any CAD, significant allergies or asthma.
3. Those with rheumatoid arthritis may experience acute exacerbation of joint swelling /pain after receiving dose.
4. Ensure that test dose performed as directed.
5. Serum iron levels not useful until 3 weeks, ferritin peaks in 7-9 days and reliable at 3 weeks.
6. May alter bone scans and discolor blood brown in samples drawn 4 hr after treatment.
7. May falsely elevate bilirubin and decrease calcium. Keep this in mind when monitoring lab values.

Outcome/Evaluate: Desired iron replacement with iron deficiency anemia. Improved lab values.

Isoetharine hydrochloride

(eye-so-ETH-ah-reen)

Pregnancy Category: C

(Rx)

Classification: Adrenergic agent, bronchodilator

See also *Sympathomimetic Drugs.*

Action/Kinetics: Has a greater stimulating activity on beta-2 receptors of the bronchi than on beta-1 receptors of the heart. Causes relief of bronchospasms. **Inhalation: Onset,** 1–6 min; **peak effect:** 15–60 min; **duration:** 1–3 hr. Partially metabolized; excreted in urine.

Uses: Bronchial asthma, bronchospasms due to chronic bronchitis or emphysema, bronchiectasis, pulmonary obstructive disease.

Special Concerns: Dosage has not been established in children less than 12 years of age.

How Supplied: Isoetharine hydrochloride: *Solution:* 1%

Dosage

- **Inhalation Solution**

  Hand nebulizer.

Adults: 3–7 inhalations (use undiluted) of the 0.5% or 1% solution.

Oxygen aerosolization or IPPB.

Adults: Dose depends on strength of solution used (range: 0.062%–1%) and whether the solution is used undiluted or diluted according to the following: **1%:** 0.25–1 mL by IPPB or 0.25–0.5 mL by oxygen aerosolization diluted 1:3 with saline or other diluent. **0.2–0.5%:** 2 mL used undiluted; **0.2%:** 1.25–2.5 mL used undiluted; **0.167 or 0.17%:** 3 mL used undiluted; **0.125%:** 2–4 mL used undiluted; **0.1%:** 2.5-5 mL used undiluted; **0.08%:** 3 mL used undiluted; **0.062%:** 4 mL used undiluted.

HEALTH CARE CONSIDERATIONS

See *Special Health Care Considerations for Adrenergic Bronchodilators* under *Sympathomimetic Drugs.*

Administration/Storage

1. One or 2 inhalations are usually sufficient; wait 1 min after initial dose to determine if another dose needed.
2. Usually does not need to be repeated more than q 4 hr.
3. Do not use if solution contains a precipitate or is brown.

Assessment: Record indications for therapy, pulmonary assessments, X-rays and review PFTs; note any allergy to sulfites.

Client/Family Teaching

1. Review proper technique for administration.
2. Stop smoking; enroll in smoking cessation program.

Outcome/Evaluate: Improved airway exchange; ↓ airway resistance

Isoniazid (INH, Isonicotinic acid hydrazide)

(eye-so-NYE-ah-zid)

Pregnancy Category: C

Dom-Isoniazide ✦, Isotamine ✦, Laniazid, Laniazid C.T., Nydrazid Injection, PMS-Isoniazid ✦ **(Rx)**
Classification: Primary antitubercular agent

Action/Kinetics: The most effective tuberculostatic agent. Probably interferes with lipid and nucleic acid metabolism of growing bacteria, resulting in alteration of the bacterial wall. Is tuberculostatic. Readily absorbed after PO and parenteral (IM) administration and widely distributed in body tissues, including cerebrospinal, pleural, and ascitic fluids. **Peak plasma concentration: PO,** 1–2 hr. **t½, fast acetylators:** 0.5–6 hr; **t½, slow acetylators:** 2–5 hr. Liver and kidney impairment increase these values. Metabolized in liver and excreted primarily in urine.

The metabolism of isoniazid is genetically determined. Clients fall into two groups, depending on the rapidity with which they metabolize isoniazid. As a rule, 50% of whites and blacks inactivate the drug slowly, whereas the majority of American Indians, Eskimos, Japanese, and Chinese are rapid acetylators (inactivators).

1. **Slow acetylators:** These clients show earlier, favorable response but have more toxic reactions (e.g., neuropathies because of higher blood levels of drug).
2. **Rapid acetylators:** These clients have possible poor clinical response due to rapid inactivation, which is 5–6 times faster than slow acetylators. This group requires an increased daily dose of the drug. They are more likely to develop hepatitis.

Uses: Tuberculosis caused by human, bovine, and BCG strains of *Mycobacterium tuberculosis*. Not to be used as the sole tuberculostatic agent. Prophylaxis of tuberculosis. *Investigational:* To improve severe tremor in clients with multiple sclerosis.

Contraindications: Severe hypersensitivity to isoniazid or in clients with previous isoniazid-associated hepatic injury or side effects.

Special Concerns: Severe and sometimes fatal hepatitis may occur even after several months of therapy; incidence is age-related and current alcohol use increases the risk. Increased risk of fatal hepatitis in minority women, especially blacks and Hispanics; also increased risk postpartum. Extreme caution should be exercised in clients with convulsive disorders, in whom the drug should be administered only when the client is adequately controlled by anticonvulsant medication. Also, use with caution for the treatment of renal tuberculosis and, in the lowest dose possible, in clients with impaired renal function and in alcoholics.

Side Effects: *Neurologic:* Peripheral neuropathy characterized by symmetrical numbness and tingling of extremities (dose-related). Rarely, toxic encephalopathy, optic neuritis, optic atrophy, ***seizures,*** impaired memory, toxic psychosis. *GI:* N&V, epigastric distress, xerostomia. *Hypersensitivity:* Fever, skin rashes and eruptions, vasculitis, lymphadenopathy. *Hepatic:* Liver dysfunction, jaundice, bilirubinemia, bilirubinuria, ***serious and sometimes fatal hepatitis (especially in clients over 50 years of age).*** Increases in serum AST and ALT. *Hematologic:* ***Agranulocytosis,*** eosinophilia, thrombocytopenia, ***hemolytic, sideroblastic, or aplastic anemia.*** *Metabolic/Endocrine:* Metabolic acidosis, pyridoxine deficiency, pellagra, hyperglycemia, gynecomastia. *Miscellaneous:* Tinnitus, urinary retention, rheumatic syndrome, lupus-like syndrome, arthralgia.

NOTE: Pyridoxine, 10–50 mg/day, may be given concomitantly with isoniazid to decrease CNS side effects. Ophthalmologic and liver function tests are recommended periodically.

Laboratory Test Considerations: Altered liver function tests. False + or ↑ potassium, AST, ALT, urine glucose (Benedict's test, Clinitest).

OD **Management of Overdose:** *Symptoms:* N&V, dizziness, blurred vision, slurred speech, visual hallucinations within 30–180 min. Severe overdosage may cause respiratory distress, ***CNS depression (coma can occur), severe seizures,*** metabolic acidosis, acetonuria, hyperglycemia. *Treatment:* Maintain respiration and undertake gastric lavage (within first 2–3 hr providing seizures are not present). To control seizures, give diazepam or a short-acting IV barbiturate followed by pyridoxine (1 mg IV/1 mg isoniazid ingested). Sodium bicarbonate, IV, to correct metabolic acidosis. Forced osmotic diuresis; monitor fluid I&O. For severe cases, consider hemodialysis or peritoneal dialysis.

Drug Interactions
Aluminum salts / ↓ Effect of isoniazid due to ↓ absorption from GI tract
Aminosalicylate sodium / ↑ Effect of isoniazid by ↑ blood levels
Anticoagulants, oral / ↓ Anticoagulant effect
Atropine / ↑ Side effects of isoniazid
Benzodiazepines / ↑ Effect of benzodiazepines that undergo oxidative metabolism (e.g., diazepam, triazolam)
Carbamazepine / ↑ Risk of both carbamazepine and isoniazid toxicity
Cycloserine / ↑ Risk of cycloserine CNS side effects

Disulfiram / ↑ Risk of acute behavioral and coordination changes
Enflurane / Isoniazid may produce high levels of hydrazine, which increases defluorination of enflurane
Ethanol / ↑ Chance of isoniazid-induced hepatitis
Halothane / ↑ Risk of hepatotoxicity and hepatic encephalopathy
Hydantoins (phenytoin) / ↑ Effect of hydantoins due to ↓ breakdown in liver
Ketoconazole / ↓ Serum levels of ketoconazole → ↓ effect
Meperidine / ↑ Risk of hypotension or CNS depression
Rifampin / Additive liver toxicity
How Supplied: *Syrup:* 50 mg/5 mL; *Tablet:* 100 mg, 300 mg; *Injection:* 100 mg/mL

Dosage

- **Syrup, Tablets**

Active tuberculosis.

Adults: 5 mg/kg/day (up to 300 mg/day) as a single dose; **children and infants:** 10–20 mg/kg/day (up to 300 mg total) in a single dose.

Prophylaxis.

Adults: 300 mg/day in a single dose; **children and infants:** 10 mg/kg/day (up to 300 mg total) in a single dose.

- **IM**

Active tuberculosis.

Adults: 5 mg/kg (up to 300 mg) once daily. **Pediatric:** 10–20 mg/kg (up to 300 mg) once daily.

Prophylaxis.

Adults/adolescents: 300 mg/day. **Pediatric:** 10 mg/kg/day.

NOTE: Pyridoxine, 6–50 mg/day, is recommended in the malnourished and those prone to neuropathy (e.g., alcoholics, diabetics).

HEALTH CARE CONSIDERATIONS

See also *General Health Care Considerations for All Anti-Infectives.*

Administration/Storage

1. Store in dark, tightly closed containers.
2. Solutions for IM injection may crystallize at low temperature; warm to room temperature if precipitation is evident.
3. Anticipate a slight local irritation at the site of injection. Rotate and document injection sites.
4. Administer with pyridoxine, 10–50 mg/day, in malnourished, alcoholic, or diabetic clients to prevent symptoms of peripheral neuropathy.

Assessment

1. Record indications for therapy, type and onset of symptoms. List other therapies used and the outcome.
2. Obtain baseline labs, CXR, and AFB sputums; note date of PPD conversion. Monitor renal and LFTs; reduce dose with dysfunction.
3. Perform pulmonary assessment; describe cough/sputum characteristics.

Client/Family Teaching

1. Take on an empty stomach 1 hr before or 2 hr after meals.
2. Consume 2–3 L/day of fluids to ensure adequate hydration.
3. Pyridoxine is given to prevent neurotoxic drug effects (peripheral neuritis).
4. Avoid alcohol to prevent hepatic toxicity.
5. Withhold drug and report fatigue, weakness, malaise, and anorexia (S&S of hepatitis).
6. Report any visual disturbances; may precede optic neuritis.
7. With diabetes, monitor FS closely.
8. Take drugs as ordered; report for periodic lab and eye exams.

Outcome/Evaluate

- Negative sputum cultures for AFB
- ↓ Neurotoxic drug effects
- Symptomatic improvement (↓ fever, ↓ secretions, ↑ appetite)

Isophane insulin suspension (NPH)

(EYE-so-fayn IN-sue-lin)

Pork: Iletin II NPH ✱, NPH-N, NPH Iletin II. **Beef/Pork:** Iletin NPH ✱, NPH Iletin I. **Human:** Humulin N, Novolin ge NPH ✱, Novolin N, Novolin N PenFill, Novolin N Prefilled **(OTC)**

Classification: Intermediate-acting insulin

Action/Kinetics: Contains zinc insulin crystals modified by protamine, appearing as a cloudy or milky suspension. Not recommended for emergency use. Not suitable for IV administration or in the presence of ketosis. **Onset:** 1–1.5 hr. **Peak:** 4–12 hr. **Duration:** Up to 24 hr. *NOTE:* NPH beef/pork insulins are being phased out.
How Supplied: *Injection:* 100 U/mL

Dosage

- **SC**

Diabetes.

Adult, individualized, usual, initial: 7–26 units as a single dose 30–60 min before breakfast. A second smaller dose may be given, if needed, prior to the evening meal or at bedtime. If necessary, the daily dose may be increased in increments of 2–10 units at daily or weekly intervals until desired control is achieved.

Clients on insulin zinc may be transferred directly to isophane insulin on a unit-for-unit basis. If client is being transferred from regular insulin, the initial dose of isophane should be from two-thirds to three-fourths the dose of regular insulin.

HEALTH CARE CONSIDERATIONS

Outcome/Evaluate

- Normalization of BS and HbA1c
- Control of diabetes; ↓ organ damage

COMBINATION DRUG

Isophane insulin suspension and insulin injection

(EYE-so-fayn IN-sue-lin)

Human: Humulin 10/90 🍁, Humulin ge 10/90 🍁, Humulin 20/80 🍁, Humulin ge 20/80 🍁, Humulin 30/70 🍁, Humulin ge 30/70 🍁, Humulin 40/60 🍁, Humulin ge 40/60 🍁, Humulin 50/50, Humulin ge 50/50 🍁, Humulin 70/30, Novolin 70/30, Novolin 70/30 PenFill, Novolin 70/30 Prefilled **(OTC)**

Classification: Mixture of insulins to achieve variable duration of action

---

Content: Contains from 10% to 50% insulin injection and from 50% to 70% isophane insulin. Except for Humulin 50/50 and Novolin ge 50/50, the larger number in the product refers to the percentage of isophane insulin suspension.

Action/Kinetics: This combination allows for a rapid onset (30–60 min) due to insulin injection and a long duration (24 hr) due to isophane insulin. **Peak effect:** 4–8 hr.

How Supplied: See Content

Dosage

- **SC**

Diabetes.

Adults: Individualized and given once daily 15–30 min before breakfast, or as directed. **Children:** Individualized according to client size.

HEALTH CARE CONSIDERATIONS

Outcome/Evaluate: Normalization of BS and HbA1c

Isoproterenol hydrochloride

(eye-so-proh-TER-ih-nohl)

Pregnancy Category: C

Dispos-a-Med Isoproterenol HCl, Isuprel, Isuprel Mistometer, Norisodrine Aerotrol **(Rx)**

Isoproterenol sulfate

(eye-so-proh-TER-ih-nohl)

Pregnancy Category: C

Medihaler-Iso **(Rx)**

Classification: Sympathomimetic, direct-acting

See also *Sympathomimetic Drugs*.

Action/Kinetics: Produces pronounced stimulation of both beta-1 and beta-2 receptors of the heart, bronchi, skeletal muscle vasculature, and the GI tract. Has both positive inotropic and chronotropic activity; systolic BP may increase while diastolic BP may decrease. Thus, mean arterial BP may not change or may be decreased. Causes less hyperglycemia than epinephrine, but produces bronchodilation and the same degree of CNS excitation. **Inhalation: Onset,** 2–5 min; **peak effect:** 3–5 min; **duration:** 30–120 min. **IV: Onset,** immediate; **duration:** less than 1 hr. **Sublingual: Onset,** 15–30 min; **duration:** 1–2 hr. Partially metabolized; excreted in urine.

Uses: Bronchodilator in asthma, chronic pulmonary emphysema, bronchiectasis, bronchitis, and other conditions involving bronchospasms (e.g., during surgery). Treat bronchospasms during anesthesia. Cardiac arrest, heart block, syncope due to complete heart block, Adams-Stokes syndrome. Certain cardiac arrhythmias including ventricular tachycardia, ventricular arrhythmias; syncope due to carotid sinus hypersensitivity. Hypoperfusion shock syndrome. Hypovolemic and septic shock as an adjunct to fluid and electrolyte replacement. Use in cardiac arrest until electric shock or pacemaker therapy is available.

Contraindications: Tachyarrhythmias, tachycardia, or heart block caused by digitalis intoxication, ventricular arrhythmias that require inotropic therapy, and angina pectoris.

Special Concerns: Use with caution during lactation and in the presence of tuberculosis. Safety and effectiveness have not been determined in children less than 12 years of age.

Additional Side Effects: *CV:* ***Cardiac arrest,*** Adams-Stokes attack, hypotension, precordial pain or distress. *CNS:* Hyperactivity, hyperkinesia. *Respiratory:* Wheezing, bronchitis, increase in sputum, ***bronchial edema and inflammation, pulmonary edema, paradoxical airway resistance.*** Excessive inhalation causes refractory bronchial obstruction. *Miscellaneous:* Flushing, sweating, swelling of the parotid gland. Sublingual administration may cause buccal ulceration. Side effects of drug are less severe after inhalation.

Drug Interactions
Bretylium / Possibility of arrhythmias
Guanethidine / ↑ Pressor response of isoproterenol
Halogenated hydrocarbon anesthetics / Sensitization of the heart to catecholamines which may cause serious arrhythmias
Oxytocic drugs / Possibility of severe, persistent hypertension
Tricyclic antidepressants / Potentiation of pressor effect

How Supplied: Isoproterenol Hydrochloride: *Metered dose inhaler:* 0.131 mg/inh; *Injection:* 0.02 mg/mL, 0.2 mg/mL; *Solution:* 0.25%, 0.5%, 1% Isoproterenol Sulfate: *Metered dose inhaler:* 0.08 mg/inh

Dosage

ISOPROTERENOL HYDROCHLORIDE

• **IV Infusion**

Shock.

5 mcg/min (1.25 mL/min of solution prepared by diluting 10 mL of 1:5,000 solution in 500 mL of D5W or 5 mL of 1:5,000 solution in 250 mL of D5W).

Cardiac standstill and cardiac arrhythmias.

Adults: 5 mcg/min (1.25 mL of either 1.25 mL/min of solution prepared by diluting 10 mL of 1:5,000 solution in 500 mL of D5W or 5 mL of 1:5,000 solution in 250 mL of D5W).

• **IV**

Cardiac standstill and cardiac arrhythmias.

1–3 mL (0.02–0.06 mg) of solution prepared by diluting 1 mL of 1:5,000 solution to 10 mL with NaCl or 5% dextrose solution. Dosage range: 0.01–0.2 mg.

Bronchospasm during anesthesia.

Adults: Dilute 1 mL of the 1:5,000 solution to 10 mL with NaCl injection or D5 solution and given an initial dose of 0.01–0.02 mg IV; repeat when necessary.

• **IM, SC**

Cardiac standstill and cardiac arrhythmias.

Adults: 1 mL (0.2 mg) of 1:5,000 solution (range: 0.02–1 mg).

Intracardiac (in extreme emergencies): 0.1 mL (0.02 mg) of 1:5,000 solution.

• **Hand Bulb Nebulizer**

Acute bronchial asthma.

Adults and children: 5–15 deep inhalations of the 1:200 solution. In adults 3–7 inhalations of the 1:100 solution may be useful. If there is no relief after 5–10 min, the doses may be repeated one more time. Repeat treatment up to 5 times/day may be necessary if there are repeat attacks.

Bronchospasm in chronic obstructive lung disease.

Adults and children: 5–15 deep inhalations of the 1:200 solution (in clients with severe attacks, 3–7 inhalations of the 1:100 solution may be useful). An interval of 3–4 hr should elapse between uses.

• **Metered-Dose Inhalation**

Acute bronchial asthma.

Adults, usual: 1–2 inhalations beginning with 1 inhalation, and if no relief occurs within 2–5 min, a second inhalation may be used. **Maintenance:** 1–2 inhalations 4–6 times/day. No more than 2 inhalations at any one time or more than 6 inhalations in 1 hr should be taken.

Bronchospasm in COPD.

Adults and children: 1–2 inhalations repeated at no less than 3–4 hr intervals (i.e., 4–6 times/day).

• **Nebulization by Compressed Air or Oxygen**

Bronchospasms in COPD.

Adults and children: 0.5 mL of the 1:200 solution is diluted to 2–2.5 mL (for a concentration of 1:800–1:1,000). The solution is delivered over 15–20 min and may be repeated up to 5 times/day.

• **IPPB**

Bronchospasms in COPD.

Adults and children: 0.5 mL of a 1:200 solution diluted to 2–2.5 mL with water or isotonic saline. The solution is delivered over 10–20 min and may be repeated up to 5 times/day.

ISOPROTERENOL SULFATE

Dispensed from metered aerosol inhaler for bronchospasms. See preceding dosage for *Hydrochloride*.

HEALTH CARE CONSIDERATIONS

See also *Special Health Care Considerations for Adrenergic Bronchodilators* under *Sympathomimetic Drugs*.

Administration/Storage

1. Administration to children, except where noted, is the same as that for adults, because a child's smaller ventilatory exchange capacity will permit a proportionally smaller aerosol intake. For acute bronchospasms in children, use 1:200 solution.
2. In children, no more than 0.25 mL of the 1:200 solution should be used for each 10–15 min of programmed treatment.

3. Elderly clients usually receive a lower dose.
4. Do not crush or chew sublingual tablets; place under the tongue and allow to disintegrate. Do not swallow saliva until absorption has taken place.
IV 5. Do not use the injection if it is pinkish to brownish in color. Protect from light and store at 15°C–30°C (59°F–86°F).

Assessment

1. Record indications for therapy, causative factors, type and onset of symptoms.
2. Perform pulmonary assessment; note PFTs and CXRs. Report respiratory problems that worsen after administration; refractory reactions may necessitate drug withdrawal.
3. Identify arrhythmias (especially ventricular) and angina; may preclude drug therapy.

Client/Family Teaching

1. Review method for inhaler use; a spacer enhances dispersion.
2. Rinse mouth and equipment with water; removes drug residue and minimizes dryness after inhalation.
3. Maintain fluid intake of 2–3 L/day; liquefies secretions.
4. Sputum and saliva may appear pink after inhalation therapy; do not become alarmed.
5. When also taking inhalant glucocorticoids, take isoproterenol first and wait 15 min before using the second inhaler.
6. Do not use more often than prescribed; over use can cause severe cardiac and respiratory problems.
7. Identify parotid gland; withhold drug and report if enlarged.
8. Stop smoking now to preserve current level of lung function; enroll in smoking cessation program.

Outcome/Evaluate

- Improved airway exchange
- ↓ Bronchoconstriction/bronchospasms
- Stable cardiac rhythm

Isosorbide dinitrate chewable tablets

(eye-so-**SOR**-byd)
Pregnancy Category: C
Sorbitrate **(Rx)**

Isosorbide dinitrate extended-release capsules

(eye-so-**SOR**-byd)
Pregnancy Category: C
Dilatrate-SR, Isordil Tembids **(Rx)**

Isosorbide dinitrate extended-release tablets

(eye-so-**SOR**-byd)
Pregnancy Category: C
Cedocard-SR ✱, Coradur ✱, Isordil Tembids **(Rx)**

Isosorbide dinitrate sublingual tablets

(eye-so-**SOR**-byd)
Pregnancy Category: C
Apo-ISDN ✱, Isordil, Sorbitrate **(Rx)**

Isosorbide dinitrate tablets

(eye-so-**SOR**-byd)
Pregnancy Category: C
Apo-ISDN ✱, Isordil Titradose, Sorbitrate **(Rx)**
Classification: Coronary vasodilator, antianginal drug

See also *Antianginal Drugs, Nitrates/Nitrites.*

Action/Kinetics: Sublingual, chewable. Onset: 2–5 min; **duration:** 1–3 hr. **Oral Capsules/Tablets. Onset:** 20–40 min; **duration:** 4–6 hr. **Extended-release. Onset:** up to 4 hr; **duration:** 6–8 hr.

Additional Uses: Diffuse esophageal spasm. Oral tablets are only for prophylaxis while sublingual and chewable forms may be used to terminate acute attacks of angina.

Special Concerns: Use with caution during lactation. Safety and efficacy have not been established in children.

Additional Side Effects: Vascular headaches occur especially frequently.

Additional Drug Interactions

Acetylcholine / Isosorbide antagonizes the effect of acetylcholine
Norepinephrine / Isosorbide antagonizes the effect of norepinephrine

How Supplied: *Chew Tablet:* 5 mg, 10 mg; *Capsule, Extended Release:* 40 mg; *Tablet, Extended Release:* 40 mg; *Sublingual tablet:* 2.5 mg, 5 mg, 10 mg; *Tablet:* 5 mg, 10 mg, 20 mg, 30 mg, 40 mg

Dosage

- **Tablets**
  Antianginal.

Initial: 5–20 mg q 6 hr; **maintenance:** 10–40 mg q 6 hr (usual: 20–40 mg q.i.d.

- **Chewable Tablets**
  Antianginal, acute attack.

Initial: 5 mg q 2–3 hr. The dose can be titrated upward until angina is relieved or side effects occur.

Prophylaxis.

5–10 mg q 2–3 hr.

- **Extended-Release Capsules**
  Antianginal.

Initial: 40 mg; **maintenance:** 40–80 mg q 8–12 hr.

- **Extended-Release Tablets**
  Antianginal.

Initial: 40 mg; **maintenance:** 40–80 mg q 8–12 hr.

- **Sublingual**

Acute attack.

2.5–5 mg q 2–3 hr as required. The dose can be titrated upward until angina is relieved or side effects occur.

Prophylaxis.

5–10 mg q 2–3 hr.

HEALTH CARE CONSIDERATIONS

See also *Health Care Considerations* for *Antianginal Drugs, Nitrates/Nitrites.*

Client/Family Teaching

1. Administer with meals to eliminate or reduce headaches; otherwise, take on an empty stomach to facilitate absorption.
2. Tolerance may develop. Short-acting products can be given b.i.d.–t.i.d. with the last dose no later than 7:00 p.m. while the extended-release products can be given once or twice daily at 8:00 a.m. and 2:00 p.m.
3. None of the products should be crushed or chewed, unless ordered.
4. Review method for administration; do not chew SL tablets.
5. Hold chewable tablets in the mouth for 1–2 min; allows absorption through buccal membranes.
6. Avoid alcohol or alcohol-containing products.
7. Acetaminophen may assist to relieve drug-induced headaches.

Outcome/Evaluate

- ↓ Frequency and severity of anginal attacks
- ↑ Exercise tolerance
- Resolution of esophageal spasm

Isosorbide mononitrate, oral

(eye-so-**SOR**-byd)

Pregnancy Category: C

Imdur, ISMO, Monoket **(Rx)**

Classification: Coronary vasodilator, antianginal drug

See also *Antianginal Drugs, Nitrates/Nitrites* and *Isosorbide dinitrate.*

Action/Kinetics: Isosorbide mononitrate is the major metabolite of isosorbide dinitrate. The mononitrate is not subject to first-pass metabolism. Bioavailability is nearly 100%. **Onset:** 30–60 min. **t½:** About 5 hr.

Uses: Prophylaxis of angina pectoris.

Contraindications: To abort acute anginal attacks. Use in acute MI or CHF.

Special Concerns: Use with caution during lactation and in clients who may be volume depleted or who are already hypotensive. Safety and effectiveness have not been determined in children. The benefits have not been established in acute MI or CHF.

Side Effects: *CV:* Hypotension (may be accompanied by paradoxical bradycardia and increased angina pectoris). *CNS:* Headache, lightheadedness, dizziness. *GI:* N&V. *Miscellaneous:* Possibility of methemoglobinemia.

OD **Management of Overdose:** *Symptoms:* Increased intracranial pressure manifested by throbbing headache, confusion, moderate fever. Also, vertigo, palpitations, visual disturbances, N&V, syncope, air hunger, dyspnea (followed by reduced ventilatory effort), diaphoresis, skin either flushed or cold and clammy, heart block, bradycardia, paralysis, ***coma, seizures, death.*** *Treatment:* Direct therapy toward an increase in central fluid volume. Do *not* use vasoconstrictors.

Drug Interactions

Calcium channel blockers / Severe orthostatic hypotension

Ethanol / Additive vasodilation

Organic nitrates / Severe orthostatic hypotension

How Supplied: *Tablet:* 10 mg, 20 mg; *Tablet, Extended Release:* 30 mg, 60 mg, 120 mg

Dosage

IMDUR TABLETS

Prophylaxis of angina.

Initial: 30 mg (given as one-half of the 60-mg tablet) or 60 mg once daily; **then,** dosage may be increased to 120 mg given as 2–60-mg tablets once daily. Rarely, 240 mg daily may be needed.

ISMO, MONOKET TABLETS

Prevention and treatment of angina.

Adults: 20 mg b.i.d. with the doses 7 hr apart (it is preferable that first dose be given on awakening). An initial dose of 5 mg may be best for clients of small stature; increase the dose to at least 10 mg by the second or third day of therapy.

HEALTH CARE CONSIDERATIONS

See also *Health Care Considerations* for *Antianginal Drugs, Nitrates/Nitrites* and *Isosorbide dinitrate.*

Administration/Storage: The treatment regimen minimizes the development of refractory tolerance.

Client/Family Teaching

1. Consume 1–2 L/day of fluids to ensure adequate hydration.

2. Take the extended-release tablet in the morning upon arising. Do not crush or chew; take with a half glass of water.
3. May cause marked hypotension.
4. Report if angina persists/recurs.

Outcome/Evaluate: Angina prophylaxis

Isotretinoin

(eye-so-**TRET**-ih-noyn)

Pregnancy Category: X

Accutane, Accutane Roche ✱, Isotrex ✱ **(Rx)**

Classification: Vitamin A metabolite (antiacne, keratinization stabilizer)

Action/Kinetics: Reduces sebaceous gland size, decreases sebum secretion, and inhibits abnormal keratinization. Approximately 25% of the PO dosage form is bioavailable. **Peak plasma levels:** 3 hr. **Steady-state blood levels following 80 mg/day:** 160 ng/mL. Nearly 100% bound to plasma protein. **t½:** 10–20 hr. Metabolized in the liver to 4-oxo-isotretinoin, which is also active. Approximately equal amounts are excreted through the urine and in the feces.

Uses: Severe recalcitrant cystic acne unresponsive to other therapy. *Investigational:* Cutaneous disorders of keratinization, cutaneous T-cell lymphoma (mycosis fungoides), leukoplakia, prevention of secondary primary tumors in those treated for squamous-cell carcinoma of the head and neck.

Contraindications: Due to the possibility of fetal abnormalities or spontaneous abortion, women who are pregnant or intend to become pregnant should not use the drug. Certain conditions for use should be met in women with childbearing potential (see package insert). Use during lactation and in children.

Special Concerns: Intolerance to contact lenses may develop.

Side Effects: *Skin:* Cheilitis, skin fragility, pruritus, dry skin, desquamation of facial skin, drying of mucous membranes, brittle nails, photosensitivity, rash, hypo- or hyperpigmentation, urticaria, erythema nodosum, hirsutism, excess granulation of tissues as a result of healing, petechiae, peeling of palms and soles, skin infections, paronychia, thinning of hair, nail dystrophy, pyogenic granuloma, bruising. *CNS:* Headache, fatigue, pseudotumor cerebri (i.e., headaches, papilledema, disturbances in vision), depression. *Ocular:* Conjunctivitis, optic neuritis, corneal opacities, dry eyes, decrease in acuity of night vision, photophobia, eyelid inflammation, cataracts, visual disturbances. *GI:* Dry mouth, N&V, abdominal pain, nonspecific GI symptoms, inflammatory bowel disease (including regional enteritis), anorexia, weight loss, inflammation and bleeding of gums. *Neuromuscular:* Arthralgia, muscle pain, bone and joint pain and stiffness, skeletal hyperostosis. *CV:* Flushing, palpitation, tachycardia. *GU:* White cells in urine, proteinuria, nonspecific urogenital findings, microscopic or gross hematuria, abnormal menses. *Other:* Epistaxis, dry nose and mouth, respiratory infections, disseminated herpes simplex, edema, transient chest pain, development of diabetes, hepatitis, hepatotoxicity, vasculitis, anemia, lymphadenopathy, flushing, palpitations.

Laboratory Test Considerations: ↑ Plasma triglycerides, sedimentation rate, platelet counts, alkaline phosphatase, AST, ALT, GGTP, LDH, fasting blood glucose, uric acid in blood, cholesterol, CPK levels in clients who exercise vigorously. ↓ HDL, RBC parameters, WBC counts.

OD Management of Overdose: *Symptoms:* Abdominal pain, ataxia, cheilosis, dizziness, facial flushing, headache, vomiting. Symptoms are transient. *Treatment:* Symptoms are quickly resolved with drug cessation or decrease in dose.

Drug Interactions

Alcohol / Potentiation of ↑ in serum triglycerides
Benzoyl peroxide / ↑ Drying effects of isotretinoin
Carbamazepine / ↓ Carbamazepine plasma levels
Minocycline / ↑ Risk of development of pseudotumor cerebri or papilledema
Tetracycline / ↑ Risk of development of pseudotumor cerebri or papilledema
Tretinoin / ↑ Drying effects of isotretinoin
Vitamin A / ↑ Risk of toxicity

How Supplied: *Capsule:* 10 mg, 20 mg, 40 mg

Dosage

• **Capsules**

Recalcitrant cystic acne.

Adults, individualized, initial: 0.5–1 mg/kg/day (range: 0.5–2 mg/kg/day) divided in two doses for 15–20 weeks. Adjust dose based on toxicity and clinical response; if cyst count decreases by 70% or more, drug may be discontinued. If necessary, a second course of therapy may be instituted after a rest period of 2 months. Doses of 0.05–0.5 mg/kg/day are effective but result in higher frequency of relapses.

Keratinization disorders.

Doses up to 4 mg/kg/day have been used.

Prevent second tumors in squamous-cell carcinoma of the head and neck.

50–100 mg/m^2.

HEALTH CARE CONSIDERATIONS

Administration/Storage

1. Do not crush capsules.
2. To enhance absorption, administer with meals.
3. Before using drug, have client complete consent form included with the package insert.
4. A rest period of 2 months is recommended if a second course of therapy is needed.

Assessment

1. Record clinical presentation; photos may help.
2. Perform a pregnancy test on all sexually active women of childbearing age.
3. Determine other agents used and the outcome.
4. Monitor serum glucose levels, chemistry, CBC, urinalysis, and LFTs, especially lipoprotein, cholesterol, and triglycerides.

Client/Family Teaching

1. Do not crush capsules. To enhance absorption, administer with meals.
2. Avoid donating blood for 30 days after discontinuing drug therapy.
3. Drug is teratogenic; perform monthly pregnancy test. Females of childbearing age should practice reliable birth control 1 mo before, during, and 1 mo following therapy; severe fetal damage may occur.
4. A 30-day prescription will be dispensed to ensure compliance.
5. Report if persistent headache, N&V, or visual disturbances occur. Lubricants may help diminish symptoms of dry, chapped skin and lips.
6. Contact lens wearers may develop sensitivity to contacts during and after therapy. Excessively dry eyes may require an eye lubricant.
7. Condition may become worse before healing starts.
8. Avoid OTC meds, especially vitamin A, without consent.
9. Eliminate or markedly reduce consumption of alcohol; may increase triglyceride levels.
10. Avoid prolonged sunlight exposure; may cause photosensitivity. Wear protective clothing, sunscreen, and sunglasses when exposed.

Outcome/Evaluate: ↓ Number/severity of cystic acne lesions

Isradipine

(iss-**RAD**-ih-peen)

Pregnancy Category: C

DynaCirc, DynaCirc CR **(Rx)**

Classification: Calcium channel blocking agent

See also *Calcium Channel Blocking Agents*.

Action/Kinetics: Binds to calcium channels resulting in the inhibition of calcium influx into cardiac and smooth muscle and subsequent arteriolar vasodilation. Reduced systemic resistance leads to a decrease in BP with a small increase in resting HR. In clients with normal ventricular function, the drug reduces afterload leading to some increase in CO. Well absorbed from the GI tract, although it undergoes significant first-pass metabolism. **Peak plasma levels:** 1 ng/mL after 1.5 hr. **Onset:** 2–3 hr. Food increases the time to peak effect by about 1 hr, although the total bioavailability does not change. **t½, initial:** 1.5–2 hr; **terminal,** 8 hr. Completely metabolized in the liver with 60%–65% excreted through the kidneys and 25%–30% through the feces. Maximum effect may not be observed for 2–4 wks.

Uses: Alone or with thiazide diuretics in the management of essential hypertension. *Investigational:* Chronic stable angina.

Contraindications: Lactation.

Special Concerns: Safety and effectiveness have not been determined in children. Use with caution in clients with CHF, especially those taking a beta-adrenergic blocking agent. Bioavailability increases in those over 65 years of age, in impaired hepatic function, and in mild renal impairment.

Side Effects: *CV:* Palpitations, edema, flushing, tachycardia, SOB, hypotension, transient ischemic attack, ***stroke,*** atrial fibrillation, ***ventricular fibrillation, MI,*** CHF, angina. *CNS:* Headache, dizziness, fatigue, drowsiness, insomnia, lethargy, nervousness, depression, syncope, amnesia, psychosis, hallucinations, weakness, jitteriness, paresthesia. *GI:* Nausea, abdominal discomfort, diarrhea, vomiting, constipation, dry mouth. *Respiratory:* Dyspnea, cough. *Dermatologic:* Pruritus, urticaria. *Miscellaneous:* Chest pain, rash, pollakiuria, cramps of the legs and feet, nocturia, polyuria, hyperhidrosis, visual disturbances, numbness, throat discomfort, leukopenia, sexual difficulties.

Laboratory Test Considerations: ↑ LFTs.

Drug Interactions: Severe hypotension has been observed during fentanyl anesthesia with concomitant use of a beta-blocker and a calcium channel blocking agent.

How Supplied: *Capsule:* 2.5 mg, 5 mg; *Tablet, Extended Release:* 5 mg, 10 mg

Dosage

- **Capsules**

Hypertension.

Adults, initial: 2.5 mg b.i.d. alone or in combination with a thiazide diuretic. If BP is not decreased satisfactorily after 2–4 weeks, the dose may be increased in increments of 5 mg/day at 2 *to* 4-week intervals up to a maximum of 20 mg/day. Adverse effects increase at doses above 10 mg/day.

- **Tablets, Controlled-Release**

Hypertension.

Adults: 5–10 mg once daily.

HEALTH CARE CONSIDERATIONS

See *Health Care Considerations* for *Calcium Channel Blocking Agents.*

Administration/Storage: Store in a tight container protected from light.

Client/Family Teaching

1. Use caution, may cause dizziness and confusion; assess drug effects.
2. Report for scheduled lab tests: liver and renal function studies every 3–6 months.

Outcome/Evaluate: ↓ BP; control of hypertension

Itraconazole

(ih-trah-KON-ah-zohl)

Pregnancy Category: C

Sporanox **(Rx)**

Classification: Antifungal

Action/Kinetics: Believed to inhibit cytochrome P-450-dependent synthesis of ergosterol, a necessary component of fungal cell membranes. Absorption appears to increase when taken with a cola beverage. Concentrates in fatty tissues, omentum, liver, kidney, and skin. **t½, at steady-state:** 64 hr. Extensively metabolized by the liver; the major metabolite is hydroxyitraconazole, which also has antifungal activity. The drug and major metabolite are extensively bound (over 99%) to plasma proteins. Metabolites are excreted in both the urine and feces.

Uses: Treatment of blastomycosis (pulmonary and extrapulmonary) and histoplasmosis (including chronic cavitary pulmonary disease and disseminated, nonmeningeal histoplasmosis) in both immunocompromised and nonimmunocompromised clients. To treat aspergillus infections (pulmonary and extrapulmonary) in clients intolerant or refractory to amphotericin B. Onychomycosis due to tinea unguium of the toenail with or without fingernail involvement. The drug is effective against *Blastomyces dermatitidis, Histoplasma capsulatum* and *H. duboisii, Aspergillus flavus* and *A. fumigatis,* and *Cryptococcus neoformans.* Oropharyngeal and esophageal candidiasis. In vitro activity has also been found for a number of other organisms, including *Sporothirx scheneckii, Trochophyton* species, *Candida albicans,* and *Candida species. Investigational:* (1) Superficial mycoses including dermatophytoses (tinea capitis, tinea corporis, tinea cruris, tinea pedis, and tinea manuum), pityriasis versicolor, candidiasis (vaginal, oral, chronic mucocutaneous), and sebopsoriasis. (2) Systemic mycoses including dimorphic infections (paracoccidioidomycosis, coccidioidomycosis), cryptococcal infections (meningitis, disseminated), and candidiasis. (3) Miscellaneous mycoses including fungal keratitis, alternariosis, leishmaniasis (cutaneous), subcutaneous mycoses (chromomycosis, sporotrichosis), and zygomycosis.

Contraindications: Concomitant use of astemizole, cisapride, triazolam, oral midazolam, or terfenadine. Hypersensitivity to the drug or its excipients. Lactation. Use for the treatment of onychomycosis in pregnant women or in women wishing to become pregnant.

Special Concerns: Safety and efficacy have not been determined in children although pediatric clients have been treated for systemic fungal infections.

Side Effects: *GI:* N&V, diarrhea, abdominal pain, anorexia, general GI disorders, flatulence, constipation, gastritis. *CNS:* Headache, dizziness, vertigo, insomnia, decreased libido, somnolence, depression. *CV:* Hypertension, orthostatic hypotension, vasculitis. *Dermatologic:* Rash (occurs more frequently in immunocompromised clients also taking immunosuppressant drugs), pruritus. *Allergic:* Rash, pruritus, urticaria, angioedema, and rarely, ***anaphylaxis and Stevens-Johnson syndrome.*** *Miscellaneous:* Edema, fatigue, fever, malaise, abnormal hepatic function, hypokalemia, albuminuria, tinnitus, impotence, adrenal insufficiency, gynecomastia, breast pain in males, menstrual disorder, hepatitis (rare), neuropathy (rare).

Laboratory Test Considerations: ↑ Liver enzymes

OD **Management of Overdose:** *Symptoms:* Extension of side effects. *Treatment:* Use supportive measures, including gastric lavage and sodium bicarbonate. Dialysis will not remove itraconazole.

Drug Interactions

Astemizole / ↑ Astemizole levels → serious CV toxicity including ventricular tachycardia, torsades de pointes, and death.

Calcium blockers (especially amlodipine and nifedipine) / Development of edema
Cisapride / Cisapride levels serious CV toxicity including ventricular tachycardia, torsades de pointes, and death.
Cyclosporine and HMG-CoA reductase inhibitors / Possible development of rhabdomyolysis. ↑ Cyclosporine levels (dose of cyclosporine should be ↓ by 50% if itraconazole doses are much greater than 100 mg/day)
Digoxin / ↑ Digoxin levels
H_2 Antagonists / ↓ Plasma levels of itraconazole
Midazolam, oral / ↑ Levels of oral midazolam → potentiation of sedative and hypnotic effects
Isoniazid / ↓ Plasma levels of itraconazole
Phenytoin / ↓ Plasma levels of itraconazole; also, metabolism of phenytoin may be altered
Quinidine / Tinnitus and decreased hearing
Rifampin / ↓ Plasma levels of itraconazole
Sulfonylureas / ↑ Risk of hypoglycemia
Tacrolimus / ↑ Levels of tacrolimus
Terfenadine / ↑ Terfenadine levels → serious CV toxicity including ventricular tachycardia, torsades de pointes, and death
Triazolam / Levels of triazolam potentiation of sedative and hypnotic effects
Warfarin / ↑ Anticoagulant effect of warfarin

How Supplied: *Capsule:* 100 mg; *Oral Solution:* 10 mg/mL

Dosage

• **Capsules**

Blastomycosis or histoplasmosis.

Adults: 200 mg once daily. If there is no improvement or the disease is progressive, the dose may be increased in 100-mg increments to a maximum of 400 mg/day. **Children, 3–16 years of age:** 100 mg/day (for systemic fungal infections).

Aspergillosis.

200–400 mg daily.

Life-threatening infections.

Adults: A loading dose of 200 mg t.i.d. for the first 3 days should be given.

Onychomycosis.

200 mg once a day for 12 consecutive weeks. Alternatively, for fingernail fungus, 200 mg b.i.d. for 1 week, followed by a 3-week rest and then a second 1-week course of 200 mg b.i.d.

Unlabeled uses.

Adults: 50–400 mg/day for 1 day to more than 6 months, depending on the condition and the response.

• **Oral Solution**

Oropharyngeal candidiasis.

200 mg/day for 1–2 weeks.

Esophageal candidiasis.

100 mg/day for a minimum of 3 weeks.

HEALTH CARE CONSIDERATIONS

Administration/Storage

1. Take with food to ensure maximal absorption.
2. Give daily doses greater than 200 mg in two divided doses.
3. Continue treatment for a minimum of 3 mo until symptoms and lab tests indicate the active fungal infection has subsided. Recurrence of active infection may occur with inadequate treatment period.

Assessment

1. Record indications for therapy, onset, duration of symptoms, and other agents prescribed, noting compliance and outcome. Drug is extremely expensive and should not be used as first-line therapy with typical fungal infections.
2. List drugs currently prescribed to prevent any unfavorable effects.
3. Monitor CBC, electrolytes, fungal cultures/scrapings, renal and LFTs.
4. Drug is not intended for pregnant or nursing mothers.
5. The response rate of histoplasmosis in HIV-infected clients is similar to non-HIV-infected clients, although the clinical course in HIV-infected clients is more severe and usually requires maintenance therapy to prevent relapse.
6. Absorption may be decreased in HIV-infected clients with hypochlorhydria.

Client/Family Teaching

1. Take with food to enhance absorption and only as directed (usually for 3 months). Noncompliance or inadequate treatment period may lead to recurrence of active infection.
2. Report S&S suggesting liver dysfunction; i.e., anorexia, unusual fatigue, N&V, diarrhea, yellow skin/eyes, or dark urine.
3. Report symptoms that may indicate reactivation of histoplasmosis, such as weight loss, chest pain, SOB, fever, rales, and pain.
4. S&S of blastomycosis include SOB, rales, hemoptysis, chest pain, fever, cough, skin lesions, rashes, and weight loss; requires immediate attention.

Outcome/Evaluate: Eradication of infecting organisms; symptom relief

I

Ivermectin

(eye-ver-**MEK**-tin)
Pregnancy Category: C
Stromectol **(Rx)**
Classification: Anthelmintic

Action/Kinetics: Binds selectively to glutamate-gated chloride channels that occur in invertebrate nerve and muscle cells. This leads to increase in permeability of cell membrane to chloride ions and hyperpolarization of nerve or muscle cell, resulting in paralysis and death of parasite. **Peak plasma levels:** About 4 hr. **t½:** About 19 hr. Metabolized in liver and excreted through feces.

Uses: Intestinal strongyloidiasis due to *Strongyloides stercoralis*. Onchocerciasis due to *Onchocerca volvulus*.

Special Concerns: Use during lactation only if benefits outweigh risks. Those with hyperreactive onchodermatitis (sowdah) may be more likely to have severe side effects. Control of extraintestinal strongyloidiasis is difficult in immunocompromised clients.

Side Effects: When used to treat strongyloidiasis. *GI:* Diarrhea, nausea, anorexia, constipation, vomiting, abdominal pain. *CNS:* Dizziness, somnolence, tremor, vertigo. *Dermatologic:* Pruritus, rash, urticaria. *Miscellaneous:* Asthenia, fatigue.

When used to treat onchocerciasis. *Mazzotti reaction:* Pruritus, edema, papular and pustular or frank urticarial rash, fever, inguinal lymph node enlargement and tenderness, axillary lymph node enlargement and tenderness, arthralgia, synovitis, cervical lymph node enlargement and tenderness. *Ophthalmic:* Limbitis, punctate opacity, abnormal sensation in the eyes, anterior uveitis, chorioretinitis, choroiditis, conjunctivitis, eyelid edema, keratitis. *Miscellaneous:* Tachycardia, peripheral edema, facial edema, orthostatic hypotension, headache, myalgia, worsening of bronchial asthma.

Laboratory Test Considerations: ↑ ALT, AST, hemoglobin. ↓ Leukocyte count. Eosinophilia.

OD **Management of Overdose:** *Symptoms:* Asthenia, diarrhea, dizziness, edema, headache, nausea, rash, vomiting, abdominal pain, ataxia, dyspnea, paresthesia, seizure, urticaria. *Treatment:* Supportive therapy, including parenteral fluids and electrolytes, respiratory support, and pressor agents (if significant hypotension). Induce emesis or gastric lavage as soon as possible, followed by laxatives and other anti-poison measures.

How Supplied: *Tablet:* 6 mg

Dosage

• **Tablets**

Strongyloidiasis.

Single oral dose to provide about 200 mcg/kg: **15–24 kg:** 0.5 tablet; **25–35 kg:** 1 tablet; **36–50 kg:** 1.5 tablets; **51–65 kg:** 2 tablets; **66–79 kg:** 2.5 tablets.

Onchocerciasis.

Single oral dose to provide about 150 mcg/kg: **15–25 kg:** 0.5 tablet; **26–44 kg:** 1 tablet; **45–64 kg:** 1.5 tablets; **65–84 kg:** 2 tablets.

HEALTH CARE CONSIDERATIONS

Administration/Storage

1. For either use, take with water.
2. For strongyloidiasis, perform follow-up stool examinations to verify eradication of infection.
3. For onchocerciasis, may retreat at intervals as short as 3 mo.

Assessment: Determine dates of exposure, onset, duration, and characteristics of symptoms, and lab confirmation of parasitic nematode.

Client/Family Teaching

1. Take as directed with a full glass of water.
2. Report if abdominal pain, chest discomfort, severe rash, joint inflammation, or vision alterations occur.
3. Must bring consecutive F/U stool specimens to lab to verify eradication of strongyloides parasite. With onchocerciasis, the adult parasite is not killed, thus retreatment is usually required.

Outcome/Evaluate: Control/eradication of extraintestinal strongyloidiasis/onchocerciasis

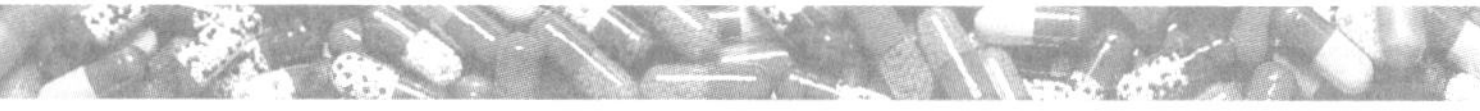

Kanamycin sulfate

(kan-ah-**MY**-sin)
Pregnancy Category: D
Kantrex, Klebcil **(Rx)**
Classification: Aminoglycoside antibiotic and antitubercular agent (tertiary)

See also *Anti-Infectives* and *Aminoglycosides*.

Action/Kinetics: Activity resembles that of neomycin and streptomycin. **Peak therapeutic serum levels: IM,** 15–40 mcg/mL.

t½: 2–3 hr. Toxic serum levels: >35 mcg/mL (peak) and >10 mcg/mL (trough).
Uses: Parenteral: Initial therapy for infections due to *Escherichia coli, Proteus, Enterobacter aerogenes, Klebsiella pneumoniae, Serratia marcescens,* and *Acinetobacter.* May be combined with a penicillin or cephalosporin before knowing results of susceptibility tests. *Investigational:* As part of a multiple-drug regimen for *Mycobacterium avium* complex in AIDS clients.

PO: Adjunct to mechanical cleansing of large bowel for suppression of intestinal bacteria; hepatic coma.
Special Concerns: Use with caution in premature infants and neonates.
Additional Side Effects: Sprue-like syndrome with steatorrhea, malabsorption, and electrolyte imbalance.
Additional Drug Interactions: *Procainamide* / ↑ muscle relaxation.
How Supplied: *Capsule:* 500 mg; *Injection:* 1 g/3 mL, 75 mg/2 mL, 500 mg/2 mL

Dosage

- **Capsules**

Intestinal bacteria suppression.

1 g every hour for 4 hr; **then,** 1 g q 6 hr for 36–72 hr.

Hepatic coma.

8–12 g/day in divided doses.

- **IM, IV**

Adults and children: 15 mg/kg/day in two to three equal doses. Maximum daily dose should not exceed 1.5 g regardless of route of administration.

For calculating dosage interval (in hr) in clients with impaired renal function, multiply serum creatinine (mg/100 mL) by 9.

- **IM**

Tuberculosis.

Adults: 15 mg/kg/day. Not recommended for use in children.

- **Intraperitoneal**

500 mg diluted in 20 mL sterile distilled water.

- **Inhalation**

250 mg in saline—nebulize b.i.d.–q.i.d.

Irrigation of abscess cavities, pleural space, ventricular cavities.

0.25% solution.

HEALTH CARE CONSIDERATIONS

See also *General Health Care Considerations for All Anti-Infectives* and *Aminoglycosides.*

Assessment: Record indications for therapy, onset, duration, and characteristics of symptoms; reduce dose with renal dysfunction.

Outcome/Evaluate

- Negative culture reports
- Desired bowel cleansing

Ketoconazole

(kee-toe-**KON**-ah-zohl)

Pregnancy Category: C
Nizoral **(Rx)**, Nizoral AD **(OTC)**
Classification: Broad-spectrum antifungal

See also *Anti-Infectives.*
Action/Kinetics: Inhibits synthesis of sterols (e.g., ergosterol), damaging the cell membrane and resulting in loss of essential intracellular material. Also inhibits biosynthesis of triglycerides and phospholipids and inhibits oxidative and peroxidative enzyme activity. When used to treat *Candida albicans,* it inhibits transformation of blastospores into the invasive mycelial form. Use in Cushing's syndrome is due to its ability to inhibit adrenal steroidogenesis. **Peak plasma levels:** 3.5 mcg/mL after 1–2 hr after a 200-mg dose. **t½ [biphasic]:** first, 2 hr; second, 8 hr. Requires acidity for dissolution. Metabolized in liver to inactive metabolites and most excreted through feces.
Uses: PO: Candidiasis, chronic mucocutaneous candidiasis, candiduria, histoplasmosis, chromomycosis, oral thrush, blastomycosis, coccidioidomycosis, paracoccidioidomycosis. Recalcitrant cutaneous dermatophyte infections not responding to other therapy. **Cream:** Tinea pedis. Tinea corporis and tinea cruris due to *Trichophyton rubrum, T. mentagrophytes,* and *Epidermophyton floccosum.* Tinea versicolor caused by *Microsporum furfur;* cutaneous candidiasis caused by *Candida* species; seborrheic dermatitis. **Shampoo:** To reduce scaling due to dandruff and tinea versicolor. *Investigational:* Onychomycosis due to *Candida* and *Trichophyton.* High doses to treat CNS fungal infections. Advanced prostate cancer, Cushing's syndrome.
Contraindications: Hypersensitivity, fungal meningitis. Topical product not for ophthalmic use. Use during lactation.
Special Concerns: Use tablets with caution in children less than 2 years of age. The safety and effectiveness of the shampoo and cream have not been determined in children. Use with caution during lactation.
Side Effects: *GI:* N&V, abdominal pain, diarrhea. *CNS:* Headache, dizziness, somnolence, fever, chills, suicidal tendencies, depres-

K

sion (rare). *Hematologic:* Thrombocytopenia, leukopenia, ***hemolytic anemia.*** *Miscellaneous:* Hepatotoxicity, photophobia, pruritus, gynecomastia, impotence, bulging fontanelles, urticaria, decreased serum testosterone levels, anaphylaxis (rare). *Topical cream:* Stinging, irritation, pruritus. *Shampoo:* Increased hair loss, irritation, abnormal hair texture, itching, oiliness or dryness of the scalp and hair, scalp pustules.

Laboratory Test Considerations: Transient ↑ serum liver enzymes. ↓ Serum testosterone.

Drug Interactions

Antacids / ↓ Absorption of ketoconazole due to ↑ pH induced by these drugs
Anticholinergics / ↓ Absorption of ketoconazole due to ↑ pH induced by these drugs
Anticoagulants / ↑ Effect of anticoagulants
Astemizole / ↑ Plasma levels of astemizole → serious CV effects
Cisapride / ↑ Risk of serious cardiac arrhythmias
Corticosteroids / ↑ Risk of corticosteroid toxicity due to ↑ bioavailability
Cyclosporine / ↑ Levels of cyclosporine (may be used therapeutically to decrease the dose of cyclosporine)
Histamine H_2 antagonists / ↓ Absorption of ketoconazole due to ↑ pH induced by these drugs
Isoniazid / ↓ Bioavailability of ketoconazole
Rifampin / ↓ Serum levels of both drugs
Terfenadine / ↑ Plasma levels of terfenadine → serious CV effects
Theophyllines / ↓ Serum levels of theophylline

How Supplied: *Cream:* 2%; *Shampoo:* 2%; *Tablet:* 200 mg

Dosage

• **Tablets**

Fungal infections.

Adults: 200 mg once daily; in serious infections or if response is not sufficient, increase to 400 mg once daily. **Pediatric, over 2 years:** 3.3–6.6 mg/kg once daily. Dosage has not been established for children less than 2 years of age.

CNS fungal infections.

Adults: 800–1,200 mg/day.

Advanced prostate cancer.

400 mg q 8 hr.

Cushing's syndrome.

800–1,200 mg/day.

• **Topical Cream (2%)**

Tinea corporis, tinea cruris, tinea versicolor, tinea pedis, cutaneous candidiasis.

Cover the affected and immediate surrounding areas once daily (twice daily for more resistant cases). Duration of treatment is usually 2 weeks.

Seborrheic dermatitis.

Apply to affected area b.i.d. for 4 weeks or until symptoms clear.

• **Shampoo (1%, 2%)**

Use twice a week for 4 weeks with at least 3 days between each shampooing. **Then,** use as required to maintain control.

HEALTH CARE CONSIDERATIONS

See also *General Health Care Considerations for All Anti-Infectives.*

Administration/Storage

1. Give a minimum of 2 hr before administration of drugs that increase gastric pH (such as antacids, anticholinergics, or H_2 blockers; avoid cisapride). Delay any antacid administration by 2 hr.
2. The minimum treatment for candidiasis (using tablets) is 1–2 weeks; for other systemic mycoses 6 mo. The minimum treatment for recalcitrant dermatophyte infections is 4 weeks in cases involving glabrous skin; palmar and plantar infections may respond more slowly.

Client/Family Teaching

1. Take tablets with food to decrease GI upset. Take 2 hr before drugs that alter gastric pH.
2. Apply shampoo to wet hair in sufficient quantities to cover the entire scalp for 1 min. Rinse with warm water; repeat, leaving shampoo on the scalp for 3 min. After the second washing, rinse thoroughly and dry hair with towel or warm air flow.
3. Report persistent fever, pain, or diarrhea.
4. With lack of stomach acid, dissolve each tablet in 4 mL aqueous solution of 0.2 N HCl; use a straw to avoid contact with teeth. Follow by drinking a glass of tap water.
5. Use caution when driving or performing hazardous tasks; may cause headaches, dizziness, and drowsiness.
6. Avoid alcohol or alcohol-containing products.
7. Wear sunglasses, sunscreen, and protective clothing, avoid sun exposure to prevent photosensitivity reactions.

Outcome/Evaluate

- Eradication of fungal infections
- Clearing of skin lesions
- Control of dandruff with ↓ scaling

Ketoprofen

(kee-toe-**PROH**-fen)

Pregnancy Category: B

Rx: Apo-Keto ✱, Apo-Keto-E ✱, Apo-Keto-SR ✱, Novo-Keto ✱, Novo-Keto-EC ✱, Nu-

Ketoprofen ✱, Nu-Ketoprofen-E ✱, Orafen ✱, Orudis, Orudis-E ✱, Orudis-SR ✱, Oruvail, PMS-Ketoprofen ✱, PMS-Ketoprofen-E ✱, Rhodis ✱, Rhodis-EC ✱, Rhodis SR ✱, Rhovail ✱, **OTC:** Actron, Orudis KT.
Classification: Nonsteroidal anti-inflammatory drug

See also *Nonsteroidal Anti-Inflammatory Drugs.*
Action/Kinetics: Possesses anti-inflammatory, antipyretic, and analgesic properties. Known to inhibit both prostaglandin and leukotriene synthesis, to have antibradykinin activity, and to stabilize lysosomal membranes. **Onset:** 15–30 min. **Peak plasma levels:** 0.5–2 hr. **Duration:** 4–6 hr. **t½:** 2–4 hr. **t½, geriatrics:** Approximately 5 hr. Is 99% bound to plasma proteins. Food does not alter the bioavailability; however, the rate of absorption is reduced.
Uses: Rx: Acute or chronic rheumatoid arthritis and osteoarthritis (both capsules and sustained-release capsules). Primary dysmenorrhea. Analgesic for mild to moderate pain.
OTC: Temporary relief of aches and pains associated with the common cold, toothache, headache, muscle aches, backache, menstrual cramps, reduction of fever, and minor pain of arthritis.
Investigational: Juvenile rheumatoid arthritis, sunburn, prophylaxis of migraine, migraine due to menses.
Contraindications: Use during late pregnancy, in children, and during lactation. Use of the extended-release product for acute pain in any client or for initial therapy in clients who are small, elderly, or who have renal or hepatic impairment.
Special Concerns: Safety and effectiveness have not been established in children. Geriatric clients may manifest increased and prolonged serum levels due to decreased protein binding and clearance. Use with caution in clients with a history of GI tract disorders, in fluid retention, hypertension, and heart failure.
Additional Side Effects: *GI:* Peptic ulcer, ***GI bleeding,*** dyspepsia, nausea, diarrhea, constipation, abdominal pain, flatulence, anorexia, vomiting, stomatitis. *CNS:* Headache. *CV:* Peripheral edema, fluid retention.
Additional Drug Interactions
Acetylsalicylic acid / ↑ Plasma ketoprofen levels due to ↓ plasma protein binding
Hydrochlorothiazide / ↓ Chloride and potassium excretion
Methotrexate / Concomitant use → toxic plasma levels of methotrexate
Probenecid / ↓ Plasma clearance of ketoprofen and ↓ plasma protein binding
Warfarin / Additive effect to cause bleeding
How Supplied: *Capsule:* 25 mg, 50 mg, 75 mg; *Capsule, Extended Release:* 100 mg, 150 mg, 200 mg; *Tablet:* 12.5 mg

Dosage
- **Rx: Extended Release Capsules, Capsules**

Rheumatoid arthritis, osteoarthritis.
Adults, initial: 75 mg t.i.d. or 50 mg q.i.d.; **maintenance:** 150–300 mg in three to four divided doses daily. Doses above 300 mg/day are not recommended. Alternatively, 200 mg once daily using the sustained-release formulation (Oruvail). Decrease dose by one-half to one-third in clients with impaired renal function or in geriatric clients.
Mild to moderate pain, dysmenorrhea.
Adults: 25–50 mg q 6–8 hr as required, not to exceed 300 mg/day. Reduce dose in smaller or geriatric clients and in those with liver or renal dysfunction. Doses greater than 75 mg do not provide any added therapeutic effect.
- **OTC: Tablets**

Adults, over 16 years of age: 12.5 mg with a full glass of liquid every 4 to 6 hr. If pain or fever persists after 1 hr follow with an additional 12.5 mg. Experience may determine that an initial dose of 25 mg gives a better effect. Do not exceed a dose of 25 mg in a 4- to 6-hr period or 75 mg in a 24-hr period.

HEALTH CARE CONSIDERATIONS

See also *Health Care Considerations* for *Nonsteroidal Anti-Inflammatory Drugs.*
Assessment
1. Record indications for therapy, type, onset, location, intensity, and symptom characteristics.
2. Note history of GI disorders, cardiac failure, hypertension, or edema.
3. Determine if pregnant. Not for children under age 12.
4. Monitor hematologic profiles, renal and LFTs. In high doses, may prolong bleeding times by decreasing platelet aggregation. Reduce dose in the elderly and those with impaired renal function.
Client/Family Teaching
1. GI side effects may be minimized by taking with antacids, milk, or food.
2. Avoid alcohol.
3. Do not take any aspirin products unless specifically prescribed.

4. Report any new symptoms such as rash, headaches, black stools, disturbances in vision, petechiae, unexplained bruising, bleeding from the gums, or nose bleeds.
5. Report any S&S of liver dysfunction such as fatigue, upper right quadrant pain, clay-colored stools, or yellowing of the skin and sclera.

Outcome/Evaluate
- ↓ Joint pain, inflammation; ↑ mobility
- ↓ Uterine cramping

Ketorolac tromethamine

(kee-toh-**ROH**-lack)
Pregnancy Category: C
Acular, Acular PF, Toradol, Toradol IM **(Rx)**
Classification: Nonsteroidal anti-inflammatory drug

See also *Nonsteroidal Anti-Inflammatory Drugs*.

Action/Kinetics: Possesses anti-inflammatory, analgesic, and antipyretic effects. Completely absorbed following IM use. **Onset:** Within 30 min. **Maximum effect:** 1–2 hr after IV or IM dosing. **Duration:** 4–6 hr. **Peak plasma levels:** 2.2–3.0 mcg/mL 50 min after a dose of 30 mg. **t½, terminal:** 3.8–6.3 hr in young adults and 4.7–8.6 hr in geriatric clients. Over 99% is bound to plasma proteins. Metabolized in the liver with over 90% excreted in the urine and the remainder excreted in the feces.

Uses: PO: Short-term (up to 5 days) management of severe, acute pain that requires analgesia at the opiate level. Always initiate therapy with IV or IM followed by PO only as continuation treatment, if necessary. **IM/IV:** Ketorolac has been used with morphine and meperidine and shows an opioid-sharing effect. The combination can be used for break through pain. **Ophthalmic:** Relieve itching caused by seasonal allergic conjunctivitis. Reduce ocular pain and photophobia following incisional refractive surgery (Acular PF).

Contraindications: Hypersensitivity to the drug, incomplete or partial syndrome of nasal polyps, angioedema, and bronchospasm due to aspirin or other NSAIDs. Use in clients with advanced renal impairment or in those at risk for renal failure due to volume depletion. Use in suspected or confirmed cardiovascular bleeding, hemorrhagic diathesis, or incomplete hemostasis and in those with a high risk of bleeding. Use as an obstetric preoperative medication or for obstetric analgesia. Routine use with other NSAIDs. Intrathecal or epidural administration. Use in labor and delivery. Use of the ophthalmic solution in clients wearing soft contact lenses.

Special Concerns: Use with caution in impaired hepatic or renal function, during lactation, in geriatric clients, and in clients on high-dose salicylate regimens. The age, dosage, and duration of therapy should receive special consideration when using this drug. Safety and effectiveness have not been determined in children.

Additional Side Effects: *CV:* Vasodilation, pallor. *GI:* GI pain, peptic ulcers, nausea, dyspepsia, flatulence, GI fullness, stomatitis, excessive thirst, GI bleeding (higher risk in geriatric clients), ***perforation***. *CNS:* Headache, nervousness, abnormal thinking, depression, euphoria. *Hypersensitivity:* ***Bronchospasm, anaphylaxis.*** *Miscellaneous:* Purpura, asthma, abnormal vision, abnormal liver function.

Ophthalmic solution: Transient stinging and burning following instillation, ocular irritation, allergic reactions, superficial ocular infections, superficial keratitis.

Drug Interactions: Ketorolac may ↑ plasma levels of salicylates due to ↓ plasma protein binding.

How Supplied: *Injection:* 15 mg/mL, 30 mg/mL; *Ophthalmic solution:* 0.5%; *Tablet:* 10 mg

Dosage

- **IM**

Analgesic, single dose.

Adults: less than 65 years of age: One 60-mg dose. **Adults, over 65 years of age, in renal impairment, or weight less than 50 kg:** One 30-mg dose.

Analgesic, multiple dose.

Adults, less than 65 years of age: 30 mg q 6 hr, not to exceed 120 mg daily. **Adults, over 65 years of age, in renal impairment, or weight less than 50 kg:** 15 mg q 6 hr, not to exceed 60 mg daily.

- **IV**

Analgesic, single dose.

Adults, less than 65 years of age: One 30-mg dose. **Adults, over 65 years of age, in renal impairment, or weight less than 50 kg:** One 15-mg dose.

- **Tablets**

Transition from IV/IM to PO.

Adults less than 65 years of age: 20 mg as a first PO dose for clients who received 60 mg IM single dose, 30 mg IV single dose, or 30 mg multiple dose IV/IM; **then,** 10 mg q 4–6 hr, not to exceed 40 mg in a 24-hr period. **Adults, over 65 years of age, in renal impairment, or weight less than 50 kg:** 10 mg as a first PO dose for those who received a 30-mg IM single dose, a 15-mg IV single dose, or a 15-mg multiple dose IV/IM; **then,** 10 mg q 4–6 hr, not to exceed 40 mg in a 24-hr period.

- **Ophthalmic Solution**

Seasonal allergic conjunctivitis.

1 gtt (0.25 mg) q.i.d. Efficacy has not been determined beyond 1 week of use.

Following cataract extraction.

1 gtt to the affected eye(s) q.i.d. beginning 24 hr after surgery and continuing for 2 weeks postoperatively.

Ocular pain and photophobia after incisional refractive surgery.

1 gtt (0.25 mg) q.i.d. for up to 3 days after surgery.

HEALTH CARE CONSIDERATIONS

See also *Health Care Considerations* for *Nonsteroidal Anti-Inflammatory Drugs.*

Administration/Storage

1. Use as part of a regular analgesic schedule rather than on an as needed basis.
2. If given on p.r.n. basis, base the size of a repeat dose on the duration of pain relief from the previous dose. If the pain returns within 3–5 hr, the next dose can be increased by up to 50% (as long as the total daily dose is not exceeded). If the pain does not return for 8–12 hr, the next dose can be decreased by as much as 50% or the dosing interval could be increased to q 8–12 hr.
3. Shortening the dosing intervals recommended will lead to an increased frequency and duration of side effects.
4. Correct hypovolemia prior to administering.
5. IV Do not mix IV/IM ketorolac in a small volume (i.e., a syringe) with morphine sulfate, meperidine HCl, promethazine HCl, or hydroxyzine HCl; will precipitate from solution.
6. When used IM/IV, the IV bolus must be given over no less than 15 sec. Give IM slowly and deeply into the muscle.
7. Protect the injection from light.

Assessment

1. Record indications for therapy, type, location, intensity, duration, and onset of symptoms.
2. Note any previous experience with NSAIDs and the results.
3. Determine any liver or renal dysfunction; assess hydration.

Client/Family Teaching

1. Take only as directed; do not exceed prescribed dosage. Report if symptoms unrelieved.
2. Drug may cause drowsiness and dizziness.
3. Avoid alcohol and all OTC agents without approval.
4. With eye drops, do not wear soft contact lens; report ocular reactions that do not subside with therapy.

Outcome/Evaluate

- Effective pain control
- ↓ Ocular allergic manifestations
- ↓ Ocular pain/photophobia

Ketotifen fumarate

(kee-**TOHT**-ih-fen)

Pregnancy Category: C

Zaditor **(Rx)**

Classification: Ophthalmic decongestant

Action/Kinetics: Selective, non-competitive histamine H_1 receptor antagonist and mast cell stabilizer. Inhibits release of mediators from cells involved in hypersensitivity reactions. Decreased chemotaxis and activation of eosinophils. Rapid acting; effect seen within minutes of administration.

Uses: Temporary prophylaxis of itching of the eye due to allergic conjunctivitis.

Contraindications: Use orally or by injection. Use to treat contact lens-related irritation.

Special Concerns: Use with caution during lactation. Safety and efficacy have not been determined in children less than 3 years of age.

Side Effects: *Ophthalmic:* Burning, stinging, conjunctivitis, conjunctival injection, discharge, dry eyes, eye pain, eyelid disorder, itching, keratitis, lacrimation disorder, mydriasis, photophobia. *Miscellaneous:* Headache, rhinitis, allergic reactions, rash, flu syndrome, pharyngitis.

How Supplied: *Solution:* 0.025%

Dosage

- **Solution, Ophthalmic**

Allergic conjunctivitis.

1 gtt in the affected eye(s) q 8–12 hr.

HEALTH CARE CONSIDERATIONS

Assessment

1. Record indications for therapy, onset, and characteristics of symptoms.
2. Assist to identify triggers; practice avoidance.

Client/Family Teaching

1. To prevent contaminating the dropper tip and solution, do not touch the eyelids or surrounding areas with the dropper tip.
2. For topical use only. Keep bottle tightly closed when not in use.

3. Not for use with contact lens related irritation; do not wear contact lenses if eyes are red.
4. Benzalkonium chloride, the preservative in the product, may be absorbed by soft contact lenses. For those who wear soft contact lenses and whose eyes are not red, wait 10 min or longer after instilling ketotifen before inserting contact lenses.
5. May experience burning, stinging and inflammation with instillation; notify provider if persistent.

Outcome/Evaluate: Relief of S&S allergic conjunctivitis

L

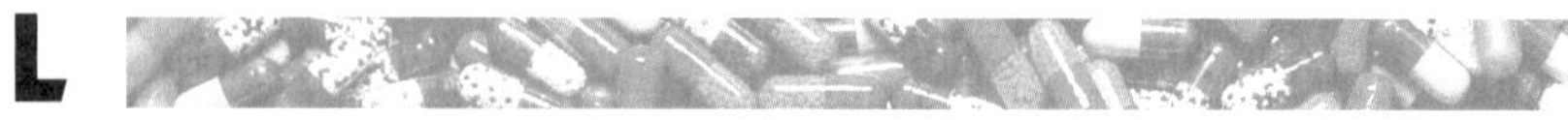

Labetalol hydrochloride

(lah-**BET**-ah-lohl)

Pregnancy Category: C

Normodyne, Trandate **(Rx)**

Classification: Alpha- and beta-adrenergic blocking agent

See also *Beta-Adrenergic Blocking Agents* and *Antihypertensive Agents*.

Action/Kinetics: Decreases BP by blocking both alpha- and beta-adrenergic receptors. Standing BP is lowered more than supine. Significant reflex tachycardia and bradycardia do not occur although AV conduction may be prolonged. **Onset: PO,** 2–4 hr; **IV,** 5 min. **Peak plasma levels, PO:** 1–2 hr. **Peak effects, PO:** 2–4 hr. **Duration: PO,** 8–12 hr. **t½: PO,** 6–8 hr; **IV,** 5.5 hr. Significant first-pass effect; metabolized in liver. Food increases bioavailability of the drug.

Uses: PO: Alone or in combination with other drugs for hypertension. **IV:** Hypertensive emergencies. *Investigational:* Pheochromocytoma, clonidine withdrawal hypertension.

Contraindications: Cardiogenic shock, cardiac failure, bronchial asthma, bradycardia, greater than first-degree heart block.

Special Concerns: Use with caution during lactation, in impaired renal and hepatic function, in chronic bronchitis and emphysema, and in diabetes (may prevent premonitory signs of acute hypoglycemia). Safety and efficacy in children have not been established.

Side Effects: See also *Beta-Adrenergic Blocking Agents*. **After PO Use.** *GI:* Diarrhea, cholestasis with or without jaundice. *CNS:* Fatigue, drowsiness, paresthesias, headache, syncope (rare). *GU:* Impotence, priapism, ejaculation failure, difficulty in micturition, Peyronie's disease, acute urinary bladder retention. *Respiratory:* Dyspnea, bronchospasm. *Musculoskeletal:* Muscle cramps, asthenia, toxic myopathy. *Dermatologic:* Generalized maculopapular, lichenoid, or urticarial rashes; bullous lichen planus, psoriasis, facial erythema, reversible alopecia. *Ophthalmic:* Abnormal vision, dry eyes. *Miscellaneous:* SLE, positive antinuclear factor, antimitochondrial antibiodies, fever, edema, nasal stuffiness.

After parenteral use. *CV:* Ventricular arrhythmias. *CNS:* Numbness, somnolence, yawning. *Miscellaneous:* Pruritus, flushing, wheezing.

After PO or parenteral use. *GI:* N&V, dyspepsia, taste distortion. *CNS:* Dizziness, tingling of skin or scalp, vertigo. *Miscellaneous:* Postural hypotension, increased sweating.

Laboratory Test Considerations: False + increase in urinary catecholamines. Transient ↑ serum transaminases, BUN, serum creatinine.

OD Management of Overdose: *Symptoms:* Excessive hypotension and bradycardia. *Treatment:* Induce vomiting or perform gastric lavage. Place clients in a supine position with legs elevated. If required, the following treatment can be used:

- Epinephrine or a beta-2 agonist (aerosol) to treat bronchospasm.
- Atropine or epinephrine to treat bradycardia.
- Digitalis glycoside and a diuretic for cardiac failure; dopamine or dobutamine may also be used.
- Diazepam to treat seizures.
- Norepinephrine (or another vasopressor) to treat hypotension.
- Administration of glucagon (5–10 mg rapidly over 30 sec), followed by continuous infusion of 5 mg/hr, may be effective in treating severe hypotension and bradycardia.

Drug Interactions

Beta-adrenergic bronchodilators / Labetalol ↓ bronchodilator effect of these drugs
Cimetidine / ↑ Bioavailability of PO labetalol
Glutethimide / ↓ Effects of labetalol due to ↑ breakdown by liver
Halothane / ↑ Risk of severe myocardial depression → hypotension
Nitroglycerin / Additive hypotension
Tricyclic antidepressants / ↑ Risk of tremors

How Supplied: *Injection:* 5 mg/mL; *Tablet:* 100 mg, 200 mg, 300 mg

Dosage

- **Tablets**

  Hypertension.

Individualize. Initial: 100 mg b.i.d. alone or with a diuretic; **maintenance:** 200–400 mg b.i.d. up to 1,200–2,400 mg/day for severe cases.

- **IV**

  Hypertension.

Individualize. Initial: 20 mg slowly over 2 min; **then,** 40–80 mg q 10 min until desired effect occurs or a total of 300 mg has been given.

- **IV Infusion**

  Hypertension.

Initial: 2 mg/min; **then,** adjust rate according to response. **Usual dose range:** 50–300 mg.

Transfer from IV to PO therapy.

Initial: 200 mg; **then,** 200–400 mg 6–12 hr later, depending on response. Thereafter, dosage based on response.

HEALTH CARE CONSIDERATIONS

See also *Health Care Considerations* for *Beta-Adrenergic Blocking Agents,* and *Antihypertensive Agents.*

Administration/Storage

1. When transferring to PO labetalol from other antihypertensive therapy, slowly reduce dosage of current therapy.
2. Full antihypertensive effect is usually seen within the first 1–3 hr after the initial dose or dose increment.
3. IV To transfer from IV to PO therapy in hospitalized clients, begin when supine BP begins to increase.
4. Not compatible with 5% sodium bicarbonate injection.
5. May give IV undiluted (20 mg over 2 min) or reconstituted with dextrose or saline solutions (infuse at a rate of 2 mg/min). When given by IV infusion, use a device that allows precise control of flow rate.

Assessment

1. Assess effect of labetalol tablets on standing BP before hospital discharge. Obtain standing BP at different times during the day to assess full effects.
2. To reduce chance of orthostatic hypotension, keep clients supine for 3 hr after receiving parenteral labetalol.

Client/Family Teaching

1. Use caution; may precipitate orthostatic hypotension and cause dizziness.
2. May cause increased sensitivity to cold; dress appropriately.

Outcome/Evaluate: ↓ BP

Lactulose

(LAK-tyou-lohs)

Pregnancy Category: B

Acilac ✦, Cephulac, Cholac, Chronulac, Constilac, Constulose, Duphalac, Gen-Lac ✦, Enulose, Evalose, Heptalac, Lactulax ✦, Laxilose ✦, PMS Lactulose ✦ **(Rx)**

Classification: Ammonia detoxicant, laxative

Action/Kinetics: A disaccharide containing both lactose and galactose; causes a decrease in the blood concentration of ammonia in clients suffering from portal-systemic encephalopathy. Due to bacteria-induced degradation of lactulose in the colon, resulting in an acid medium. Ammonia will then migrate from the blood to the colon to form ammonium ion, which is trapped and cannot be absorbed. A laxative action due to increased osmotic pressure from lactic, formic, and acetic acids then expels the trapped ammonium. The decrease in blood ammonia concentration improves the mental state, EEG tracing, and diet protein tolerance of clients. The increased osmotic pressure also results in a laxative effect, which may take up to 24 hr. Partly absorbed from the GI tract. **Onset:** 24–48 hr.

Uses: Prevention and treatment of portal-systemic encephalopathy, including hepatic and prehepatic coma (Cephylac, Cholac, Enulose, Evalose, Heptalac are used). Chronic constipation (Chronulac, Constilac, Duphalac are used).

Contraindications: Clients on galactose-restricted diets.

Special Concerns: Safe use during lactation and in children has not been established. Infants who have been given lactulose have developed hyponatremia and dehydration. Use with caution in presence of diabetes mellitus.

Side Effects: *GI:* N&V, diarrhea, cramps, flatulence, gaseous distention, belching.

Drug Interactions

Antacids / May inhibit the drop in pH of the colon required for lactulose activity
Neomycin / May cause ↓ degradation of lactulose due to neomycin-induced ↑ in elimination of certain bacteria in the colon

How Supplied: *Oral Solution:* 10g/15 mL ; *Syrup:* 10 g/15 mL

Dosage

- **Syrup, Oral Solution**

  Encephalopathy.

Adults, initial: 30–45 mL (20–30 g) t.i.d.–q.i.d.; adjust q 2–3 days to obtain two or three soft stools daily. Long-term therapy may be required in portal-systemic encephalopathy; **infants:** 2.5–10 mL/day (1.6–6.6 g/day) in divided doses; **older children and adolescents:** 40–90 mL/day (26.6–60 g/day) in divided doses.

During acute episodes of constipation.
30–45 mL (20–30 g) q 1–2 hr to induce rapid initial laxation.

Chronic constipation.
Adults and children: 15–30 mL/day (10–20 g/day) as a single dose after breakfast (up to 60 mL/day may be required).

HEALTH CARE CONSIDERATIONS

Administration/Storage

1. To minimize sweet taste, dilute with water/juice or add to desserts.
2. When given by gastric tube, dilute well to prevent vomiting and possibility of aspiration pneumonia.
3. Use a rectal balloon catheter to assist with enema retention.
4. Do not take with other laxatives.
5. Store below 30°C (86°F). Avoid freezing.

Assessment: Record mental status; monitor serum ammonia and potassium levels during therapy for encephalopathy. May also cause further potassium loss that will intensify disease symptoms.

Client/Family Teaching

1. Report any GI distress; may subside or dose may need to be reduced.
2. Medication contains carbohydrate; report flushed, dry skin, complaints of dry mouth and intense thirst, a fruity odor to the breath, abdominal pain, and low BP (S&S of hyperglycemia; more likely to occur with diabetes).
3. Keep skin clean and dry; reposition frequently because skin breakdown may occur rapidly.

Outcome/Evaluate

- Improved level of consciousness
- ↓ Serum ammonia levels
- Relief of constipation

Lamivudine (3TC)

(lah-**MIH**-vyou-deen)

Pregnancy Category: C

3TC ✦, Epivir **(Rx)**

Classification: Antiviral drug

See also *Antiviral Drugs.*

Action/Kinetics: Synthetic nucleoside analog effective against HIV. Converted to active 5'-triphosphate (L-TP) metabolite which inhibits HIV reverse transcription via viral DNA chain termination. L-TP also inhibits the RNA- and DNA-dependent DNA polymerase activities of reverse transcriptase. Rapidly absorbed after PO administration. Most eliminated unchanged through the urine.

Uses: In combination with AZT for the treatment of HIV infection, based on clinical or immunologic evidence of progression of the disease. There are no data on the effect of lamivudine and AZT on clinical progression of HIV infection, such as the incidence of opportunistic infections or survival.

Contraindications: Lactation.

Special Concerns: Clients taking lamivudine and AZT may continue to develop opportunistic infections and other complications of HIV infection. Use with caution and at a reduced dose in those with impaired renal function. Data on the use of lamivudine and AZT in pediatric clients are lacking; however, use the combination with extreme caution in children with pancreatitis.

Side Effects: Side effects are for the combination of lamivudine plus AZT. *GI:* N&V, diarrhea, anorexia, or decreased appetite, abdominal pain, abdominal cramps, dyspepsia. *CNS:* Neuropathy, insomnia or other sleep disorders, dizziness, depressive disorders, paresthesias, peripheral neuropathies. *Respiratory:* Nasal signs and symptoms, cough. *Musculoskeletal:* Musculoskeletal pain, myalgia, arthralgia. *Body as a whole:* Headache, malaise, fatigue, fever or chills, skin rashes. *NOTE:* Pediatric clients have an increased risk to develop ***pancreatitis.***

Drug Interactions: Use of lamivudine with trimethoprim-sulfamethoxazole resulted in a significant increase in lamivudine levels.

How Supplied: *Tablet:* 150 mg; *Solution:* 10 mg/mL

Dosage

- **Oral Solution, Tablets**

HIV infection.

Adults and adolescents, aged 12–16 years: 150 mg b.i.d. in combination with AZT. For adults with low body weight (less than 50 kg), the recommended dose is 2 mg/kg b.i.d. in combination with AZT. **Children, 3 months to 12 years of age:** 4 mg/kg b.i.d. (up to a maximum of 150 mg b.i.d.) in combination with AZT. In clients over 16 years of age, adjust the dose as follows in impaired renal function: C_{CR} less than 50 mL/min: 150 mg b.i.d.; C_{CR} 30–49 mL/min: 150 mg once daily; C_{CR} 15–29 mL/min: 150 mg for the first dose followed by 100 mg once daily; C_{CR} 5–14 mL/min: 150 mg for the first dose followed by 50 mg once daily; C_{CR} less than 5 mL/min: 50 mg for the first dose followed by 25 mg once daily.

HEALTH CARE CONSIDERATIONS

See also *Health Care Considerations* for *Antiviral Drugs.*

Administration/Storage

1. Consult AZT prescribing information before using with lamivudine.
2. Store PO solution at 2°C–25°C (36°F–77°F).

Assessment

1. Note disease confirmation, other agents trialed, and the outcome.
2. Monitor children for clinical symptoms of pancreatitis.
3. Monitor liver, renal, and hematologic parameters, including CD_4 and viral load. Adjust dose with impaired renal function.

Client/Family Teaching

1. Take exactly as prescribed with AZT twice a day.
2. May be taken without regard to food.
3. Drug is not a cure; may continue to experience illnesses and opportunistic infections associated with HIV.
4. Use barrier protection with sexual partners to prevent HIV transmission.
5. With children, report symptoms of pancreatitis (i.e., abdominal pain, N&V, fever, loss of appetite, yellow skin discoloration).

Outcome/Evaluate: Control of HIV disease progression with AZT

COMBINATION DRUG

Lamivudine/Zidovudine

[(lah-**MIH**-vyou-deen, zye-**DOH**-vyou-deen)]

Pregnancy Category: C

Combivir **(Rx)**

Classification: Antiviral drug combination

See also *Lamivudine, Zidovudine,* and *Antiviral Drugs.*

Content: Each Combivir tablet contains: *Antiviral:* Lamivudine, 150 mg and *Antiviral:* Zidovudine, 300 mg.

Action/Kinetics: Both drugs are reverse transcriptase inhibitors with activity against HIV. Combination results in synergistic antiretroviral effect. Each drug is rapidly absorbed.

Uses: Treatment of HIV infection.

Contraindications: Use in clients requiring dosage reduction, children less than 12 years of age, C_{CR} less than 50 mL/min, body weight less than 50 kg, and in those experiencing dose-limiting side effects.

Side Effects: See individual drugs.

How Supplied: See Content

Dosage

- **Tablets**

  HIV infection.

Adults and children over 12 years of age: One combination tablet—150 mg lamivudine/300 mg zidovudine—b.i.d.

HEALTH CARE CONSIDERATIONS

See also *Health Care Considerations* for *Lamivudine, Zidovudine,* and *Antiviral Drugs.*

Administration/Storage: May be taken without regard to food.

Assessment

1. Record disease onset, clinical characteristics, other agents trialed, and outcome.
2. Weigh client; not for use in those with low body weight or C_{CR} less than 50 mL/min.
3. Monitor CBC, renal and LFTs; report dysfunction.
4. Assess for hepatomegaly and lactic acidosis (pH < 7.35 or serum lactate > 5-6 mEq/L).

Client/Family Teaching

1. Take as directed, with or without food, twice daily.
2. Report any severe fatigue, SOB, dizziness, or muscle pain; drug may cause neutropenia and anemia.
3. Drug is not a cure, may continue to experience opportunistic infections.
4. Practice safe sex; drug does not prevent disease transmission.

Outcome/Evaluate: Control of HIV; ↓ viral load

Lamotrigine

(lah-**MAH**-trih-jeen)

Pregnancy Category: C

Lamictal **(Rx)**

Classification: Anticonvulsant

See also *Anticonvulsants.*

Action/Kinetics: Mechanism of anticonvulsant action not known. May act to inhibit voltage-sensitive sodium channels. This effect stabilizes neuronal membranes and modulates presynaptic transmitter release of excitatory amino acids such as glutamate and aspartate. Rapidly and completely absorbed after PO use. **Peak plasma levels:** 1.4–4.8 hr. **t½, after repeated doses: About 33 hr.** Metabolized by the liver with metabolites and unchanged drug excreted mainly through the urine (94%). Lamotrigine induces its own metabolism. Eliminated more rapidly in clients who have been taking antiepileptic drugs that induce liver enzymes.

L

However, valproic acid decreases the clearance of lamotrigine.

Uses: Adjunct in the treatment of partial seizures in adults with epilepsy. For add-on treatment of generalized seizures in adults and children with Lennox-Gastaut syndrome. *Investigational:* Adults with generalized clonic-tonic, absence, atypical absence, and myoclonic seizures.

Contraindications: Use during lactation and in children less than 16 years of age.

Special Concerns: Use with caution in clients with diseases or conditions that could affect metabolism or elimination of the drug, such as in impaired renal, hepatic, or cardiac function.

Side Effects: Side effects listed are those with an incidence of 0.1% or greater. *CNS:* Dizziness, ataxia, somnolence, headache, incoordination, insomnia, tremor, depression, anxiety, irritability, decreased memory, speech disorder, confusion, disturbed concentration, sleep disorder, emotional lability, vertigo, mind racing, amnesia, nervousness, abnormal thinking, abnormal dreams, agitation, akathisia, aphasia, CNS depression, depersonalization, dyskinesia, dysphoria, euphoria, faintness, hallucinations, hostility, hyperkinesia, hypesthesia, myoclonus, panic attack, paranoid reaction, personality disorder, psychosis, stupor. *GI:* N&V, diarrhea, dyspepsia, constipation, tooth disorder, anorexia, dry mouth, abdominal pain, dysphagia, flatulence, gingivitis, gum hyperplasia, increased appetite, increased salivation, abnormal liver function tests, mouth ulceration, stomatitis, thirst. *CV:* Hot flashes, palpitations, flushing, migraine, syncope, tachycardia, vasodilation. *Musculoskeletal:* Arthralgia, joint disorder, myasthenia, dysarthria, muscle spasm, twitching. *Hematologic:* Anemia, ecchymosis, leukocytosis, leukopenia, lymphadenopathy, petechiae. *Respiratory:* Rhinitis, pharyngitis, increased cough, dyspnea, epistaxis, hyperventilation. *Dermatologic:* ***Stevens-Johnson syndrome, toxic epidermal necrolysis,*** pruritus, alopecia, acne, dry skin, eczema, erythema, hirsutism, maculopapular rash, sweating, urticaria. *Ophthalmologic:* Diplopia, blurred vision, nystagmus, abnormal vision, abnormal accommodation, conjunctivitis, oscillopsia, photophobia. *GU:* Dysmenorrhea, vaginitis, amenorrhea, female lactation, hematuria, polyuria, urinary frequency or incontinence, UTI, vaginal moniliasis. *Body as a whole:* ***Possibility of sudden unexplained death in epilepsy,*** flu syndrome, fever, infection, neck pain, malaise, ***seizure exacerbation,*** chills, halitosis, facial edema, weight gain or loss, peripheral edema, hyperglycemia. *Miscellaneous:* Ear pain, tinnitus, taste perversion.

OD **Management of Overdose:** *Symptoms:* Possibility of dizziness, headache, somnolence, coma. *Treatment:* Hospitalization with general supportive care. If indicated, induce emesis or perform gastric lavage. Protect the airway.

Drug Interactions

Acetaminophen / ↓ Serum lamotrigine levels

Carbamazepine / Lamotrigine concentration is ↓ by about 40%

Phenobarbital / Lamotrigine concentration is ↓ by about 40%

Phenytoin / Lamotrigine concentration is ↓ by 45%–54%

Primidone / Lamotrigine concentration is ↓ by about 40%

Valproic acid / Lamotrigine concentration is ↑ twofold while valproic acid concentration is ↓ by 25%

How Supplied: *Chewable Tablet:* 5 mg, 25 mg; *Tablet:* 25 mg, 100 mg, 150 mg, 200 mg

Dosage

- **Tablets**

Treatment of partial seizures.

Adults and children over 16 years of age who are taking enzyme-inducing antiepileptic drugs, but not valproate: 50 mg once a day for weeks 1 and 2, followed by 100 mg/day in two divided doses for weeks 3 and 4. **Maintenance dose:** 300–500 mg/day given in two divided doses. The dose should be increased by 100 mg/day every week until maintenance levels are reached. **Adults and children over 16 years of age who are taking enzyme-inducing antiepileptic drugs plus valproic acid:** 25 mg every other day for weeks 1 and 2, followed by 25 mg once daily for weeks 3 and 4. **Maintenance dose:** 100–150 mg/day in two divided doses. The dose should be increased by 25–50 mg/day every 1–2 weeks.

HEALTH CARE CONSIDERATIONS

See also *Health Care Considerations* for *Anticonvulsants.*

Administration/Storage

1. Base dose on the therapeutic response since a therapeutic plasma level has not been determined.
2. If a change in seizure control or worsening of side effects is noted in clients receiving lamotrigine in combination with other antiepileptic drugs, reevaluate all drugs in the regimen.
3. Discontinuing an enzyme-inducing antiepileptic drug should prolong the half-life of lamotrigine, whereas discontinuing valproic acid should shorten the half-life of lamotrigine.

4. If it is decided to discontinue lamotrigine therapy, a stepwise reduction of dose over 2 weeks (about 50% per week) is recommended unless safety concerns mandate a more rapid withdrawal.

Assessment

1. Record type, onset, and duration of symptoms, previous agents used, and the outcome.
2. If also prescribed other anticonvulsant agents (i.e., valproate, carbamazepine), monitor closely for adverse effects.
3. Monitor CBC, renal and LFTs; reduce dose with dysfunction.

Client/Family Teaching

1. Do not stop abruptly; may cause increased seizure frequency. Drug should be gradually decreased over at least 2 weeks unless safety concerns require rapid withdrawal.
2. Do not perform activities that require mental alertness and/or coordination until drug effects realized; may cause dizziness, ataxia, somnolence, headache, and blurred vision.
3. Report loss of seizure control or if a rash occurs.
4. Photosensitization may occur; wear protective clothing, sunscreen, and sunglasses until tolerance determined.

Outcome/Evaluate: Control of seizures

Lansoprazole

(lan-**SAHP**-rah-zohl)
Pregnancy Category: B
Prevacid **(Rx)**
Classification: GI drug, proton pump inhibitor

Action/Kinetics: Suppresses gastric acid secretion by inhibition of the (H^+, K^+)-ATPase system located at the secretory surface of the parietal cells in the stomach. Drug is a gastric acid (proton) pump inhibitor in that it blocks the final step of acid production. Both basal and stimulated gastric acid secretion are inhibited, regardless of the stimulus. May have antimicrobial activity against *Helicobacter pylori*. Absorption begins only after lansoprazole granules leave the stomach, but absorption is rapid. **Peak plasma levels:** 1.7 hr. **Mean plasma t½:** 1.5 hr. Over 97% bound to plasma proteins. Food does not appear to affect the rate of absorption, if given before meals. Metabolized in the liver with metabolites excreted through both the urine (33%) and feces (66%).

Uses: Short-term treatment (up to 4 weeks) for healing and symptomatic relief of active duodenal ulcer. Maintain healing of duodenal ulcer. With clarithromycin and/or amoxicillin to eradicate *Helicobacter pylori* infection in active or recurrent duodenal ulcers. Short-term treatment (up to 8 weeks) for healing and symptomatic relief of benign gastric ulcer. Short-term treatment (up to 8 weeks) for healing and symptomatic relief of all grades of erosive esophagitis. Maintain healing of erosive esophagitis. Long-term treatment of pathologic hypersecretory conditions, including Zollinger-Ellison syndrome. Short-term treatment of symptomatic GERD.

Contraindications: Lactation.

Special Concerns: Reduce dosage in impaired hepatic function. Symptomatic relief does not preclude the presence of gastric malignancy. Safety and efficacy have not been determined in children less than 18 years of age.

Side Effects: *GI:* Diarrhea, abdominal pain, nausea, melena, anorexia, bezoar, cardiospasm, cholelithiasis, constipation, dry mouth, thirst, dyspepsia, dysphagia, eructation, esophageal stenosis, esophageal ulcer, esophagitis, fecal discoloration, flatulence, gastric nodules, fundic gland polyps, gastroenteritis, ***GI hemorrhage, rectal hemorrhage,*** hematemesis, increased appetite, increased salivation, stomatitis, tenesmus, vomiting, ulcerative colitis. *CV:* Angina, hypertension or hypotension, ***CVA, MI, shock,*** palpitations, vasodilation. *CNS:* Headache, agitation, amnesia, anxiety, apathy, confusion, depression, syncope, dizziness, hallucinations, hemiplegia, aggravated hostility, decreased libido, nervousness, paresthesia, abnormal thinking. *GU:* Abnormal menses, breast enlargement, gynecomastia, breast tenderness, hematuria, albuminuria, glycosuria, impotence, kidney calculus. *Respiratory:* Asthma, bronchitis, increased cough, dyspnea, epistaxis, hemoptysis, hiccoughs, pneumonia, upper respiratory inflammation or infection. *Endocrine:* Diabetes mellitus, goiter, hypoglycemia or hyperglycemia. *Hematologic:* Anemia, eosinophilia, hemolysis. *Musculoskeletal:* Arthritis, arthralgia, musculoskeletal pain, myalgia. *Dermatologic:* Acne, alopecia, pruritus, rash, urticaria. *Ophthalmologic:* Amblyopia, eye pain, visual field defect. *Otic:* Deafness, otitis media, tinnitus. *Miscellaneous:* Gout, weight loss or gain, taste perversion, asthenia, candidiasis, chest pain, edema, fever, flu syndrome, halitosis, infection, malaise.

Laboratory Test Considerations: Abnormal LFTs. ↑ AST, ALT, creatinine, alkaline phosphatase, globulins, GGTP, glucocorticoids, LDH, gastrin. ↑ or ↓ or abnormal WBC and platelets. Abnormal AG ratio,

L

RBC. Bilirubinemia, hyperlipemia. ↑ or ↓ Electrolytes or cholesterol.

Drug Interactions

Ampicillin / ↓ Effect of ampicillin due to ↓ absorption

Digoxin / ↓ Effect of digoxin due to ↓ absorption

Iron salts / ↓ Effect of iron salts due to ↓ absorption

Ketoconazole / ↓ Effect of ketoconazole due to ↓ absorption

Sucralfate / Delayed absorption of lansoprazole

How Supplied: *Enteric-coated capsule:* 15 mg, 30 mg

Dosage

- **Capsules, Delayed Release**

Treatment of duodenal ulcer.

Adults: 15 mg once daily before breakfast for 4 weeks.

Maintenance of healed duodenal ulcer.

Adults: 15 mg once daily.

Duodenal ulcers associated with H. pylori.

Triple therapy: Lansoprazole, 30 mg, plus clarithromycin, 500 mg, and amoxicilin, 1 g, b.i.d. for 10 to 14 days. **Double therapy:** Lansoprazole, 30 mg, plus amoxicillin, 1 g, t.i.d. for 14 days in those intolerant or resistant to clarithromycin.

Treatment of gastric ulcer.

30 mg once daily for up to 8 weeks.

Treatment of erosive esophagitis.

30 mg before eating for up to 8 weeks. If the client does not heal in 8 weeks, an additional 8 weeks of therapy may be given. If there is a recurrence, an additional 8-week course may be considered.

Maintenance of healed erosive esophagitis.

15 mg once daily for up to 12 months.

Pathologic hypersecretory conditions.

Initial: 60 mg once daily. Adjust the dose to client need. Dosage may be continued as long as necessary. Doses up to 90 or 120 mg (in divided doses) daily have been given.

Treatment of GERD.

15 mg once daily.

HEALTH CARE CONSIDERATIONS

Administration/Storage

1. There is no significant effect on the amount or rate of absorption if lansoprazole is given before meals.
2. For those unable to swallow capsules, open the delayed-release capsule and sprinkle the contents on a tablespoon of applesauce. Do not chew or crush the granules.
3. To give with a NG tube in place, open the capsule and mix intact granules with 40 mL of apple juice. Instill through the NG tube into the stomach, flushing with additional apple juice to clear the tube.
4. Adjust dosage in severe liver disease.
5. Store in a tight container protected from moisture. Store between 15°C and 30°C (59°F and 86°F).

Assessment

1. Record indications for therapy, onset, duration of symptoms, and any other agents trialed.
2. Note findings of upper GI, barium swallow, or endoscopy.
3. Monitor CBC, electrolytes, triglycerides, renal and LFTs; reduce dose with severe liver disease.

Client/Family Teaching

1. Take exactly as prescribed; do not exceed dose or share meds.
2. Follow prescribed diet and activities to control S&S of GERD.
3. Keep scheduled appointments. Drug is generally for short-term therapy and discontinued once condition is healed. Long-term effects are not known; users should be assessed for gastric malignancy.

Outcome/Evaluate

- Suppression of acid secretion
- Healing of ulcer/erosive esophagitis
- ↓ Pain; relief of heartburn

Latanoprost

(lah-**TAH**-noh-prost)

Pregnancy Category: C

Xalatan **(Rx)**

Classification: Prostaglandin agonist

Action/Kinetics: A prostaglandin $F_2\alpha$ analog that decreases intraocular pressure by increasing the outflow of aqueous humor. Absorbed through the cornea where it is hydrolyzed by esterases to the active acid. **Peak levels in aqueous humor:** 2 hr. **Onset:** 3–4 hr. **Maximum effect:** 8–12 hr. The active acid is metabolized in the liver and excreted in the urine. **t½, elimination:** 17 min.

Uses: To reduce intraocular pressure in open-angle glaucoma and ocular hypertension in clients who are intolerant of other drugs to reduce intraocular pressure or who have been unresponsive to other drug therapy.

Contraindications: Use while wearing contact lenses.

Special Concerns: May gradually change eye color by increasing the amount of brown pigment in the iris; the resultant color changes may be permanent. Use with caution during lactation. The drug product contains benzalkonium chloride, which may

be absorbed by contact lenses. Safety and efficacy have not been determined in children.
Side Effects: *Ophthalmic:* Blurred vision, burning, stinging, conjunctival hyperemia, foreign body sensation, itching, increased pigmentation of the iris, punctate epithelial keratopathy, dry eye, excessive tearing, eye pain, lid crusting, lid edema, lid erythema, lid discomfort or pain, photophobia, conjunctivitis, diplopia, discharge from the eye, retinal artery embolus, retinal detachment, vitreous hemorrhage from diabetic retinopathy (rare). *Systemic:* URTI (e.g., cold, flu), pain in muscles/joints/back, chest pain/angina pectoris, rash, allergic skin reactions.
Drug Interactions: A precipitate may form if latanoprost is used with eye drops containing thimerosal.
How Supplied: *Ophthalmic solution:* 0.005%

Dosage

- **Solution, 0.005%**

  Elevated intraocular pressure.

1 gtt (1.5 mcg) in the affected eye(s) once daily in the evening. More frequent use may decrease the intraocular pressure lowering effect.

HEALTH CARE CONSIDERATIONS

Administration/Storage

1. At least 5 min should elapse between administration of latanoprost and other topical ophthalmic drugs; esp. drops containing thimerosal.
2. Prior to administration, remove contact lenses. Reinsert 15 min following administration.
3. Protect from light. Refrigerate unopened bottles. Once opened, may store container at room temperature (up to 25°C; 77°F) for 6 weeks.

Client/Family Teaching

1. Wash hands before and after use. Avoid touching any part of the eye with the container tip to prevent contamination and eye infections. Contaminated solutions may cause eye damage and loss of vision.
2. Use once daily, in the evening.
3. Remove contact lenses and do not reinsert for at least 15 min after administration.
4. Report any lid or eye reactions, especially conjunctivitis.
5. Iris color changes may occur due to an increase of brown pigment in the iris; this may be permanent.

Outcome/Evaluate: ↓ Intraocular pressure

Leflunomide

(leh-**FLOON**-oh-myd)
Pregnancy Category: X
Arava **(Rx)**
Classification: Anti-arthritic drug

Action/Kinetics: Inhibits dihydroorotate dehydrogenase, an enzyme involved in de novo pyrimidine synthesis; has antiproliferative activity and an anti-inflammatory effect. After PO, is metabolized to an active metabolite (M1). **Peak levels, M1:** 6–12 hr. **t½, M1:** About 2 weeks. M1 is extensively bound to albumin. M1 is further metabolized and excreted through the kidney (more significant over the first 96 hr) and bile.
Uses: Treatment of active rheumatoid arthritis in adults, including to retard structural damage.
Contraindications: Use in pregnancy, lactation, in children less than 18 years of age, in hepatic insufficiency, or positive hepatitis B or C. Also, use in those with severe immunodeficiency, bone marrow dysplasia, severe uncontrolled infections, or vaccination with live vaccines.
Special Concerns: Use with caution in those with renal insufficiency.
Side Effects: *GI:* Diarrhea, N&V, dyspepsia, abnormal liver enzymes, GI/abdominal pain, anorexia, dry mouth, gastroenteritis, mouth ulcer, cholelithiasis, colitis, constipation, esophagitis, flatulence, gastritis, gingivitis, melena, oral moniliasis, pharyngitis, enlarged salivary gland, stomatitis or aphthous stomatitis, tooth disorder. *CNS:* Headache, dizziness, paresthesia, anxiety, depression, insomnia, neuralgia, neuritis, sleep disorder, sweat, vertigo. *CV:* Hypertension (as pre-existing condition was over represented in drug treatment groups), chest pain, angina pectoris, migraine, palpitation, tachycardia, vasculitis, vasodilation, varicose vein. *Dermatologic:* Alopecia, rash, pruritus, eczema, dry skin, acne, contact dermatitis, fungal dermatitis, hair discoloration, hematoma, herpes simplex, herpes zoster, nail disorder, skin nodule, subcutaneous nodule, maculopapular rash, skin disorder, skin discoloration, skin ulcer. *Musculoskeletal:* Joint disorder, tenosynovitis, synovitis, arthralgia, leg cramps, arthrosis, bursitis, muscle cramps, myalgia, bone necrosis, bone pain, tendon rupture. *Respiratory:* Respiratory infection, bronchitis, increased cough, pharyngitis, pneumonia, rhinitis, sinusitis, asthma, dyspnea, epistaxis, lung disorder. *GU:* Albuminu-

L

ria, cystitis, dysuria, hematuria, menstrual disorder, vaginal moniliasis, prostate disorder, urinary frequency, UTI. *Hematologic:* Anemia, including iron deficiency anemia; ecchymosis. *Metabolic:* Weight loss, hypokalemia, peripheral edema, hyperglycemia, hyperlipidemia. *Ophthalmic:* Blurred vision, cataract, conjunctivitis, eye disorder. *Miscellaneous:* Diabetes mellitus, hyperthyroidism, taste perversion, back pain, injury accident, infection, asthenia, allergic reaction, flu syndrome, pain, abscess, cyst, fever, hernia, malaise, neck pain, pelvic pain.

Laboratory Test Considerations: ↑ ALT, AST, creatine phosphokinase. Uricosuric effect, hypophosphatemia.

OD **Management of Overdose:** *Symptoms:* See Side Effects. *Treatment:* Give cholestyramine or charcoal. Dose of cholestyramine is 8 g t.i.d. PO for 24 hr. Dose of charcoal is 50 g made into a suspension for PO or NGT given q 6 hr for 24 hr.

Drug Interactions

Charcoal / Rapid and significant ↓ in active M1 metabolite of leflunomide
Cholestyramine / Rapid and significant ↓ in active M1 metabolite of leflunomide
Hepatotoxic drugs / ↑ Side effects
Rifampin / ↑ M1 peak levels

How Supplied: *Tablets:* 10 mg, 20 mg, 100 mg

Dosage

- **Tablets**

Rheumatoid arthritis.

Loading dose: 100 mg/day PO for 3 days. **Maintenance:** 20 mg/day; if this dose is not well tolerated, decrease to 10 mg/day. Doses greater than 20 mg/day are not recommended due to increased risk of side effects.

HEALTH CARE CONSIDERATIONS

Administration/Storage

1. Aspirin, NSAIDs, or low dose corticosteroids may be continued during leflunomide therapy.
2. To achieve nondetectable plasma levels (less than 0.02 mcg/mL) after stopping treatment, give cholestyramine, 8 g t.i.d. for 11 days (do not need to be consecutive unless there is a need to lower plasma levels rapidly). Verify plasma levels by 2 separate tests at least 14 days apart. Without the drug elimination procedure, it may taken 2 years or less to reach plasma M1 levels of 0.02 mcg/mL due to variations in drug clearance.

Assessment

1. Assess for liver dysfunction and hepatitis B or C.
2. Obtain negative pregnancy test.
3. Monitor SGPT (ALT) and AST monthly and adjust dosage with elevations. If elevations persist 2-3x ULN and continued therapy is desired, may consider liver biopsy.
4. Drug metabolite M1 has an extremely long half-life (up to 2 years). Cholestyramine may accelerate drug elimination. Women of childbearing age desiring pregnancy should undergo the drug elimination procedure that has been established to prevent fetal death or damage.

Client/Family Teaching

1. Therapy consists of a three day loading dose and then a daily maintenance dose.
2. Drug will cause fetal damage. Practice reliable birth control. If pregnancy desired or suspected in females or males wish to father a child, report immediately so drug elimination procedure can be initiated.
3. Avoid live vaccines.
4. May experience diarrhea, nausea, GI upset, URI, headache and rash; report if persistent or intolerable.
5. Report as scheduled for monthly liver function studies.

Outcome/Evaluate

- ↓ Bone erosion and joint narrowing
- Slowing of RA disease progression

Letrozole

(LET-roh-zohl)

Pregnancy Category: D

Femara **(Rx)**

Classification: Antineoplastic, hormone

See also *Antineoplastic Agents.*

Action/Kinetics: A nonsteroidal competitive inhibitor of aromatase, resulting in inhibition of conversion of androgens to estrogens. It acts by competitively binding to heme of cytochrome P450 subunit of aromatase, leading to decreased biosynthesis of estrogen in all tissues. Does not cause increase in serum FSH and does not affect synthesis of adrenocorticosteroids, aldosterone, or thyroid hormones. **t½, elimination:** About 2 days. Steady state plasma levels after daily doses of 2.5 mg reached in 2 to 6 weeks. Inactive metabolites are excreted in urine.

Uses: Advanced breast cancer in postmenopausal women with disease progression following antiestrogen therapy.

Special Concerns: Use with caution during lactation and in those with severely impaired hepatic function. Safety and efficacy have not been determined in children.

Side Effects: *CNS:* Headache, somnolence, dizziness, vertigo, depression, anxiety. *GI:* N&V, constipation, diarrhea, abdominal

pain, anorexia, dyspepsia. *Body as a whole:* Fatigue, viral infections, peripheral edema, asthenia, decreased weight. *Dermatologic:* Hot flashes, rash, pruritus, alopecia, increased sweating. *Respiratory:* Dyspnea, coughing, pleural effusion. *Miscellaneous:* Chest pain, hypertension, arthralgia, fracture.
Laboratory Test Considerations: ↑ AST, ALT, GGT. ↓ Lymphocyte counts. Hypercholesterolemia, hypercalcemia.
How Supplied: *Tablet:* 2.5 mg

Dosage

- **Tablets**

Advanced breast cancer.
Adults and elderly: 2.5 mg once/day. Continue until tumor progression is evident. Dosage adjustment is not needed in renal impairment if C_{CR} is greater than or equal to 10 mL/min.

HEALTH CARE CONSIDERATIONS

See also *Health Care Considerations* for *Antineoplastic Agents.*

Assessment
1. Note disease onset, clinical findings, previous antiestrogen therapy, and response.
2. Monitor renal and LFTs.

Client/Family Teaching
1. Take as directed; may take without regard to meals.
2. Report any severe rash, diarrhea, pain, dyspnea, or chest pain.

Outcome/Evaluate: ↓ Tumor mass; ↓ malignant cell proliferation

Leucovorin calcium (Citrovorum factor, Folinic acid)

(loo-koh-**VOR**-in)
Pregnancy Category: C
Lederle Leucovorin Calcium ✱, Wellcovorin
(Rx)
Classification: Folic acid derivative

Action/Kinetics: Derivative of folic acid; is a mixture of the diasterioisomers of the 5-formyl derivative of tetrahydrofolic acid. Does not require reduction by dihydrofolate reductase to be active in intracellular metabolism; thus, it is not affected by dihydrofolate inhibitors. Rapidly absorbed following PO administration. Quickly metabolized to 1,5-methyltetrahydrofolate, which is then metabolized by other pathways back to 5,10-methylene-tetrahydrofolate and then converted to 5-methyltetrahydrofolate using the cofactors $FADH_2$ and NADPH. Leucovorin can counteract the therapeutic and toxic effects of methotrexate (acts by inhibiting dihydrofolate reductase) but can enhance the effects of 5-fluorouracil (5-FU). Is rapidly absorbed. **Peak serum levels, PO:** Approximately 2.3 hr; **after IM:** 52 min; **after IV:** 10 min. **Onset, PO:** 20–30 min; **IM:** 10–20 min; **IV: < 5 min. Terminal t½: 5.7 hr (PO), 6.2 hr (IM and IV). Duration:** 3–6 hr. Excreted by the kidney.
Uses: PO and Parenteral: Prophylaxis and treatment of toxicity due to methotrexate and folic acid antagonists (e.g., pyrimethamine and trimethoprim). Leucovorin rescue following high doses of methotrexate for osteosarcoma. **Parenteral:** Megaloblastic anemias due to nutritional deficiency, sprue, pregnancy, and infancy when oral folic acid is not appropriate. Adjunct with 5-FU to prolong survival in the palliative treatment of metastatic colorectal carcinoma. *Note:* It is recommended for megaloblastic anemia caused by pregnancy even though the drug is pregnancy category C.
Contraindications: Pernicious anemia or megaloblastic anemia due to vitamin B_{12} deficiency.
Special Concerns: Use with caution during lactation. May increase the frequency of seizures in susceptible children. When leucovorin is used with 5-FU for advanced colorectal cancer, the dosage of 5-FU must be lower than usual as leucovorin enhances the toxicity of 5-FU. The benzyl alcohol in the parenteral form may cause a fatal gasping syndrome in premature infants.
Side Effects: Leucovorin alone. Allergic reactions, including urticaria and ***anaphylaxis.***

Leucovorin and 5-FU. *GI:* N&V, diarrhea, stomatitis, constipation, anorexia. *Hematologic:* Leukopenia, thrombocytopenia. *CNS:* Fatigue, lethargy, malaise. *Miscellaneous:* Infection, alopecia, dermatitis.

Drug Interactions
5-FU / ↑ Toxicity of 5-FU
Aminosalicylate sodium / ↓ Serum folate levels → folic acid deficiency
Methotrexate / High doses of leucovorin ↓ effect of intrathecally administered methotrexate
Phenobarbital / ↓ Effect of phenobarbital → ↑ frequency of seizures, especially in children
Phenytoin / ↓ Effect of phenytoin due to ↑ rate of breakdown by liver; also, phenytoin may ↓ plasma folate levels

Primidone / ↓ Effect of primidone → ↑ frequency of seizures, especially in children
Sulfasalazine / ↓ Serum folate levels → folic acid deficiency

How Supplied: *Injection:* 10 mg/mL; *Powder for injection:* 50 mg, 100 mg, 200 mg, 350 mg; *Tablet:* 5 mg, 10 mg, 15 mg, 25 mg

Dosage

- **IM, IV, Tablets**

Advanced colorectal cancer.

Either leucovorin, 200 mg/m² by slow IV over a minimum of 3 min followed by 5-FU, 370 mg/m² IV **or** leucovorin 20 mg/m² IV followed by 5-FU, 425 mg/m² IV. Treatment is repeated daily for 5 days with the 5-day treatment course repeated at 28-day intervals for two courses and then repeated at 4- to 5-week intervals as long as the client has recovered from the toxic effects.

Leucovorin rescue after high-dose methotrexate therapy.

The dose of leucovorin is based on a methotrexate dose of 12–15 mg/m² given by IV infusion over 4 hr. The dose of leucovorin is 15 mg (10 mg/m²) PO, IM, or IV q 6 hr for 10 doses starting 24 hr after the start of the methotrexate infusion. Give leucovorin parenterally if there is nausea, vomiting, or GI toxicity. If serum methotrexate levels are greater than 0.2 µM at 72 hr and greater than 0.05 µM at 96 hr after administration, leucovorin should be continued at a dose of 15 mg PO, IM, or IV q 6 hr until methotrexate levels are less than 0.05 µM. If serum methotrexate levels are equal to or greater than 50 µM at 24 hr or equal to or greater than 5 µM at 48 hr after administration or if there is a 100% or greater increase in serum creatinine levels at 24 hr after methotrexate administration, the dose of leucovorin should be 150 mg IV q 3 hr until methotrexate levels are less than 1 µM; **then,** give leucovorin, 15 mg IV q 3 hr until methotrexate levels are less than 0.05 µM. If significant clinical toxicity is seen following methotrexate, leucovorin rescue should total 14 doses over 84 hr in subsequent courses of methotrexate therapy.

Impaired methotrexate elimination or accidental overdose.

Start leucovorin rescue as soon as the overdose is discovered and within 24 hr of methotrexate administration when excretion is impaired. Give leucovorin, 10 mg/m² PO, IM, or IV q 6 hr until serum methotrexate levels are less than 10^{-8} M. If the 24-hr serum creatinine has increased 50% over baseline or if the 24- or 48-hr methotrexate level is more than 5×10^{-6} M or greater than 9×10^{-7} M, respectively, the dose of leucovorin should be increased to 100 mg/m² IV q 3 hr until the methotrexate level is less than 10^{-8} M. Urinary alkalinization with sodium bicarbonate solution (to maintain urine pH at 7 or greater) and hydration with 3 L/day should be undertaken at the same time.

Overdosage of folic acid antagonists.

5–15 mg/day.

Megaloblastic anemia due to folic acid deficiency.

Adults and children: Up to 1 mg/day.

HEALTH CARE CONSIDERATIONS

Administration/Storage

1. The oral solution is stable for 14 days if refrigerated or for 7 days if stored at room temperature.

Assessment

1. Record indications for therapy: replacement or rescue. If for rescue therapy, administer promptly (first dose within 1 hr) following a high dose of folic acid antagonists; follow dosage exactly to be effective.
2. Note history of B_{12} deficiency that has resulted in pernicious or megaloblastic anemia. Leucovorin may obscure the diagnosis of pernicious anemia if previously undiagnosed.
3. Determine any history of seizure disorders; assess for recurrence.
4. Monitor renal, B_{12}, folic acid, and hematologic values. Creatinine increases of 50% over pretreatment levels indicate severe renal toxicity.
5. Urine pH should be greater than 7.0; monitor q 6 hr during therapy. Urine alkalinization with $NaHCO_3$ or acetazolamide may be necessary to prevent nephrotoxic effects.

Client/Family Teaching

1. Report immediately any skin rash, itching, malaise, or difficulty breathing.
2. Parenteral therapy generally is used following chemotherapy; N&V may prevent oral absorption.
3. When high-dose therapy is used, be alert for mental confusion and impaired judgment. Safety measures and supervision help to ensure safety and protection.
4. Consume 3 L/day of fluids with rescue therapy.

Outcome/Evaluate

- Symptomatic improvement (↓ fatigue, ↑ weight, improved orientation)
- ↑ Normoblasts (with megaloblastic anemias)
- Prevention/reversal of GI, renal, and bone marrow toxicity in methotrexate therapy or during overdosage of folic acid antagonists

Leuprolide acetate

(loo-**PROH**-lyd)

Pregnancy Category: X

Lupron, Lupron/Lupron Depot ✹, Lupron/Lupron Depot 7.5 mg/22.5 mg ✹, Lupron Depot 3.75 mg ✹, Lupron Depot, Lupron Depot—3 Month, Lupron Depot—4 Month, Lupron Depot-Ped, Lupron for Pediatric Use **(Rx)**

Classification: Antineoplastic agent, hormonal

See also *Antineoplastic Agents.*

Action/Kinetics: Related to the naturally occurring GnRH. By desensitizing GnRH receptors, gonadotropin secretion is inhibited. Initially, however, LH and FSH levels increase, leading to increases of sex hormones. However, decreases in these hormones will be observed within 2–4 weeks. **Peak plasma levels:** 4 hr for various doses. **t½:** 3 hr.

Uses: Palliative treatment in advanced prostatic cancer when orchiectomy or estrogen treatment are not appropriate. Endometriosis (use depot form). Central precocious puberty (use depot-PED form). In combination with iron supplements for the presurgical treatment of anemia caused by uterine fibroid tumors (use depot form). *Investigational:* With flutamide for metastatic prostatic cancer.

Contraindications: Pregnancy, in women who may become pregnant while receiving the drug, and during lactation. Sensitivity to benzyl alcohol (found in leuprolide injection). Undiagnosed abnormal vaginal bleeding. Hypersensitivity to GnRH or GnRH agonist analogs. The 30-mg depot in women.

Special Concerns: Safety and efficacy have not been determined in children (except depot-PED). May cause increased bone pain and difficulty in urination during the first few weeks of therapy for prostatic cancer.

Side Effects: Injection and Depot. *GI:* N&V, anorexia, diarrhea, constipation, taste disorders/perversion, gingivitis, dysphagia, hepatic dysfunction. *CNS:* Pain, depression, emotional lability, insomnia, headache, dizziness, nervousness, paresthesias, anxiety, memory disorder, syncope, personality disorder, somnolence, spinal fracture/paralysis. *CV:* Peripheral edema, angina, ***cardiac arrhythmias, TIA/stroke,*** hypotension, vasodilation. *GU:* Hematuria, urinary frequency or urgency, dysuria, testicular pain, incontinence, cervix disorder, penile swelling, prostate pain. *Respiratory:* Dyspnea, hemoptysis, pneumonia, epistaxis, pulmonary infiltrates. *Endocrine:* Gynecomastia, breast tenderness, impotency, hot flashes, sweating, decreased testicular size, increased or decreased libido. *Musculoskeletal:* Myalgia, bone pain, pelvic fibrosis, ankylosing spondylosis. *Dermatologic:* Dermatitis, skin reactions, acne, seborrhea, hair growth, ecchymosis, hair loss, skin striae, erythema multiforme and other rashes, androgen-like effects. *Ophthalmic:* Ophthalmic disorder, abnormal vision. *Other:* Asthenia, diabetes, fever, chills, tinnitus, infection, body odor, hard nodule in throat, accelerated sexual maturation, hearing disorder, peripheral neuropathy.

Injection. *CV:* ***MI, pulmonary emboli.*** *GI:* ***GI bleeding,*** rectal polyps, peptic ulcer. *CNS:* Lethargy, mood swings, numbness, blackouts, fatigue. *Respiratory:* Cough, ***pulmonary fibrosis,*** pleural rub. *Dermatologic:* Carcinoma of the skin/ear, itching, dry skin, pigmentation, skin lesions. *GU:* Bladder spasms, urinary obstruction. *Miscellaneous:* Enlarged thyroid, inflammation, temporal bone swelling, blurred vision.

Depot. *CV:* Tachycardia, bradycardia, ***heart failure,*** varicose vein, palpitations. *GI:* Dysphagia, gingivitis. *CNS:* Delusions, confusion, hypesthesia. *GI:* Duodenal ulcer, dry mouth, thirst, appetite changes. *Respiratory:* Rhinitis, pharyngitis, pleural effusion. *Endocrine:* Lactation, menstrual disorder. *GU:* Penis disorder, testis disorder. *Ophthalmic:* Conjunctivitis, amblyopia, dry eyes. *Miscellaneous:* Nail disorder, flu syndrome, enlarged abdomen, lymphedema, dehydration, lymphadenopathy.

Laboratory Test Considerations: Injection and Depot. ↑ Calcium. ↓ WBC. Hypoproteinemia. **Injection:** ↑ BUN, creatinine. **Depot:** ↑ LDH, alkaline phosphatase, AST, uric acid, cholesterol, LDL, triglycerides, PT, PTT, glucose, WBC. ↓ Platelets, potassium. Hyperphosphatemia, abnormal LFTs. Misleading results from tests of pituitary gonadotropic and gonadal function up to 4–8 weeks after discontinuing depot therapy.

How Supplied: *Injection:* 5 mg/mL; *Kit:* 5 mg/mL, 7.5 mg, 11.25 mg, 15 mg, 22.5 mg; *Powder for injection:* 3.75 mg, 7.5 mg. 11.5 mg, 15 mg, 30 mg

Dosage

- **Depot, Injection**

Advanced prostatic cancer.

Injection: 1 mg/day SC using the syringes provided. Depot (IM): 7.5 mg monthly, 22.5 mg q 3 months, or 30 mg q 4 months.

Central precocious puberty.

Injection: **Initial:** 50 mcg/kg/day SC as a single dose. Dose may increased by 10 mcg/kg/day, which is the maintenance dose. Depot-Ped: **Initial:** 0.3 mg/kg/4 weeks (minimum 7.5 mg) as a single IM dose.

Endometriosis, uterine fibroids.

3.75 mg IM once a month for at least 6 months for endometriosis and 3 months or less for uterine fibroids. If further treatment is contemplated, assess bone density prior to beginning therapy.

HEALTH CARE CONSIDERATIONS

See also *Health Care Considerations* for *Antineoplastic Agents.*

Administration/Storage

1. Follow manufacturer's guidelines carefully to prepare the depot form. Reconstitute only with the diluent provided; after reconstitution, the preparation is stable for 24 hr. There is no preservative so discard if not used immediately.
2. When injecting depot form, do not use needles smaller than 22 gauge.
3. Give the injection using only the syringes provided.
4. Injection: Store below room temperature at 25°C (77°F) or less. Avoid freezing and protect from light. Store vial in carton until use.
5. Depot may be stored at room temperature.

Assessment: Record indications for therapy, onset of symptoms, other agents trialed, and the outcome.

Client/Family Teaching

1. Hot flashes may occur with drug therapy.
2. Record weight; report gains of more than 2 lb/day.
3. Immediately report any weakness, numbness, respiratory difficulty, or impaired urination.
4. Altered sexual effects (impotence, decreased testes size) may occur; identify appropriate resources for counseling and support.
5. Increased bone pain may be evident at the start of therapy; analgesics may be used for pain control.

Outcome/Evaluate

- ↓ Tumor size and spread
- Improved symptoms with endometriosis

Levamisole hydrochloride

(lee-**VAM**-ih-sohl)

Pregnancy Category: C

Ergamisol, Novo-Levamisole ✱ **(Rx)**

Classification: Antineoplastic, adjunct

Action/Kinetics: Used in combination with fluorouracil; considered to be an immunomodulator. It restores depressed immune function. As such, it stimulates formation of antibodies, stimulates T-cell activation and proliferation, potentiates monocyte and macrophage function (including phagocytosis and chemotaxis), and increases mobility adherence and chemotaxis of neutrophils. Rapidly absorbed from the GI tract. **Peak plasma levels:** 0.13 mcg/mL after 1.5–2 hr. **t½:** 3–4 hr. Metabolized by the liver and excreted mainly in the urine.

Uses: In combination with fluorouracil to treat clients with Dukes' stage C colon cancer following surgical resection.

Contraindications: Lactation.

Special Concerns: Safety and effectiveness have not been demonstrated in children. Agranulocytosis, caused by levamisole, may be accompanied by a flu-like syndrome, or it may be asymptomatic. Thus, hematologic monitoring is required.

Side Effects: *GI:* Commonly nausea and diarrhea; vomiting, stomatitis, anorexia, abdominal pain, constipation, flatulence, dyspepsia. *Hematologic:* Leukopenia, thrombocytopenia, anemia, granulocytopenia. *Dermatologic:* Commonly: dermatitis and pruritus; alopecia, skin discoloration. *CNS:* Dizziness, headache, inability to concentrate, weakness, memory loss, paresthesia, ataxia, somnolence, depression, insomnia, confusion, nervousness, anxiety, forgetfulness. *Musculoskeletal:* Arthralgia, myalgia. *Ophthalmologic:* Abnormal tearing, conjunctivitis, blurred vision. *Miscellaneous:* Fatigue, fever, rigors, chest pain, edema, taste perversion, altered sense of smell, infection, hyperbilirubinemia, epistaxis.

Drug Interactions

Ethanol / Disulfiram-like reaction when used with levamisole

Phenytoin / ↑ Phenytoin plasma levels

How Supplied: *Tablet:* 50 mg

Dosage

- **Tablets**

Adults, initial: Levamisole, 50 mg q 8 hr for 3 days (starting 7–30 days after surgery) given together with fluorouracil, 450 mg/m²/day by IV push for 5 days (starting 21–34 days after surgery). **Maintenance:** Levamisole, 50 mg q 8 hr for 3 days q 2 weeks for 1 year; fluorouracil, 450 mg/m²/day by IV push once a week beginning 28 days after the beginning of the 5-day course and continuing for 1 year.

HEALTH CARE CONSIDERATIONS

Administration/Storage

1. Start levamisole no earlier than 7 and no later than 30 days after surgery; initiate fluorouracil therapy no earlier than 21 days and no later than 35 days after surgery. Before flu-

orouracil therapy is started, have client out of the hospital, ambulatory, eating normally, have well-healed wounds, and recovered from any postoperative complications.
2. If levamisole therapy has been started 7–20 days after surgery, start fluorouracil therapy at the same time as the second course of levamisole (i.e., 21–34 days after surgery).

Assessment

1. Record indications for therapy, symptom onset, and any previous treatments.
2. Give concomitantly with IV fluorouracil.
3. Monitor CBC, electrolytes, and LFTs.

• Consider granulocyte colony-stimulating factors.
• If WBC is between 2,500 and 3,500/mm^3, hold fluorouracil until WBC is 3,500/mm^3.
• If WBC is less than 2,500/mm^3, hold until 3,500/mm^3 and then reinstitute fluorouracil at a dose reduced by 20%.
• If the WBC is less than 2,500/mm^3 for more than 10 days even though fluorouracil has not been given, and despite Neupogen, the administration of levamisole should be discontinued.
• Administration of both levamisole and fluorouracil should be deferred until the platelet count is restored.

Client/Family Teaching

1. Report immediately any malaise, confusion, fever, or chills (flu-like symptoms).
2. Avoid alcohol; may cause a disulfiram-like effect.
3. Female clients of childbearing age should practice safe contraception.
4. Report any stomatitis or diarrhea after fluorouracil administration; drug should be discontinued before the full five doses are given.
5. Need weekly lab studies for CBC prior to therapy and electrolyte and LFTs every 3 months for 1 year.

Outcome/Evaluate

• Control of tumor size and spread
• Restoration of immune function; inhibition of malignant cell proliferation

Levetiracetam

(lehv-ah-ter-ASS-ah-tam)
Pregnancy Category: C
Keppra **(Rx)**
Classification: Anticonvulsant

Action/Kinetics: Precise mechanism unknown. May act in synaptic plasma membranes in the CNS to inhibit burst firing without affecting normal neuronal excitability. Thus, it may selectively prevent hypersynchronization of epileptiform burst firing and propagation of seizure activity. Rapidly absorbed. **Peak plasma levels:** 1 hr during fasting. Metabolized in the liver. **t½:** 7 hr. Excreted through the urine as metabolites and unchanged drug.

Uses: Adjunctive treatment of partial onset seizures in adults with epilepsy.

Special Concerns: Reduce dosage in clients with impaired renal function. Clearance is increased in children. Half-life is prolonged in the elderly. Use with caution during lactation. Safety and efficacy have not been determined in children less than 16 years of age.

Side Effects: *CNS:* Somnolence, dizziness, depression, nervousness, ataxia, vertigo, amnesia, anxiety, hostility, paresthesia, emotional lability, psychotic symptoms, withdrawal seizures. *Respiratory:* Pharyngitis, rhinitis, sinusitis, increased cough. *GI:* Abdominal pain, constipation, diarrhea, dyspepsia, gastroenteritis, gingivitis, N&V. *Miscellaneous:* Asthenia, headache, infection, pain, anorexia, diplopia, coordination difficulties.

Laboratory Test Considerations: Infrequent abnormalities in hematologic parameters and LFTs.

OD **Management of Overdose:** *Symptom:* Drowsiness. *Treatment:* Emesis or gastric lavage; maintain airway. General supportive care. Monitor VS. Hemodialysis may be beneficial.

How Supplied: *Tablets:* 250 mg, 500 mg, 750 mg

Dosage

• **Tablets**

Partial onset seizures in adults.

Initial: 500 mg b.i.d. Can increase dose by 1,000 mg/day q 2 weeks up to a maximum daily dose of 3,000 mg. For impaired renal function, use the following doses: **C_{CR}, 50–80 mL/min:** 500–1,000 mg q 12 hr; **C_{CR}, 30–50 mL/min:** 250–750 mg q 12 hr; **C_{CR}, less than 30 mL/min:** 250–500 mg q 12 hr.

HEALTH CARE CONSIDERATIONS

Assessment

1. Record history and characteristics of seizures.
2. Monitor CBC, renal and LFTs; with impaired renal function, drug dose based on creatinine clearance.

Client/Family Teaching

1. Take exactly as directed.
2. May cause dizziness and sleepiness. Do not

L

engage in activities that require mental alertness until drug effects realized.
3. Use reliable birth control. Notify provider if pregnant or planning to become pregnant.
4. Report any unusual side effects or loss of seizure control.
Outcome/Evaluate: Control of seizures

Levobetaxolol

(lee-voh-beh-TAX-oh-lohl)
Pregnancy Category: C
Betaxon **(Rx)**
Classification: Beta-adrenergic blocking agent, Ophthalmic

See also *Beta-Adrenergic Blocking Agents*
Action/Kinetics: Levobetaxolol is a cardioselective, $beta_1$-adrenergic receptor blocking agent. Levobetaxolol is the more active enatiomer of betaxolol. Intraocular pressure is decreased by reducing the production of aqueous humor. **t½:** 20 hours
Uses: Lowers IOP in patients with chronic open-angle glaucoma or ocular hypertension.
Contraindications: Hypersensitivity to levobetaxolol or any component; sinus bradycardia; greater than first degree heart block (without a functional pacemaker); cardiogenic shock; decompensated heart failure.
Special Concerns: Observe for bronchospasm, bradycardia, or heart failure since topically applied beta-blockers can sometimes be absorbed systemically. Caution should be used in patients with a history of heart failure, heart block (without functional pacemaker), or pulmonary dysfunction. Also, use with caution in labile diabetic patients as beta-blockers may mask signs of hypoglycemia and hyperthyroidism. May increase muscle weakness in myasthenia.
Side Effects: *Ophthalmic:*Transient eye discomfort (>10%), blurred vision (<10%). *CV:* Watch for bradycardia, heart block, hypertension, hypotension, tachycardia (<2%).
OD Management of Overdose: Overdose is not documented in humans. See special concerns for probable events. Treatment should be symptomatic and supportive.
Drug Interactions: Increased toxicity (hypotension): systemic beta-blockers, catecholamine-depleting agents (reserpine), adrenergic psychotropic agents.
How Supplied: *Ophthalmic solution:* 0.5%; 5mL, 10mL, 15mL.

Dosage

- **Ophthalmic solution**

Chronic open-angle glaucoma; ocular hypertension

Adults: Instill 1 drop in affected eye(s) twice daily.

HEALTH CARE CONSIDERATIONS

Administration/Storage
1. Store upright 4°C to 25°C (39°F to 77°F).
2. Protect from light.
3. Apply gentle pressure to the inside corner of the eye during and immediately after instillation to avoid systemic absorption.

Assessment: Monitor and record IOP.

Client/Family Teaching
1. Apply gentle pressure to inside corner of the eye during and immediately following placing medication in the eye to avoid systemic absorption.
2. Do not use with contact lens in the eye.
3. Stop the medicine if breathing problems occur and contact healthcare provider.
4. May sting eyes; do not touch dropper tip to eye; vision may be blurred briefly.
5. Shake well before use.

Outcome/Evaluate: Monitor IOP: IOP should be within acceptable range.

Levobunolol hydrochloride

(lee-voh-BYOU-no-lohl)
Pregnancy Category: C
AKBeta, Betagan ✱, Betagan Liquifilm, Novo-Levobunolol ✱, Ophtho-Bunolol ✱ **(Rx)**
Classification: Beta-adrenergic blocking agent

See also *Beta-Adrenergic Blocking Agents.*
Action/Kinetics: Both beta-1- and beta-2-adrenergic receptor agonist. May act by decreasing the formation of aqueous humor. **Onset:** <60 min. **Peak effect:** 2–6 hr. **Duration:** 24 hr.
Uses: To decrease IOP in chronic open-angle glaucoma or ocular hypertension.
Special Concerns: Safety and effectiveness have not been determined in children. Significant absorption in geriatric clients may result in myocardial depression. Also, use with caution in angle-closure glaucoma (use with a miotic), in clients with muscle weaknesses, and in those with decreased pulmonary function.
Additional Side Effects: *Ophthalmic:* Stinging and burning (transient), decreased corneal sensitivity, blepharoconjunctivitis. *Dermatologic:* Urticaria, pruritus.
How Supplied: *Ophthalmic Solution:* 0.25%, 0.5%

Dosage

- **Ophthalmic Solution (0.25%, 0.5%)**

Adults, usual: 1 gtt of 0.25% or 0.5% solution in affected eye(s) 1–2 times/day (depending on variations in diurnal intraocular pressure).

HEALTH CARE CONSIDERATIONS

See also *Health Care Considerations* for *Beta-Adrenergic Blocking Agents*.

Administration/Storage

1. If IOP is not decreased sufficiently, pilocarpine, epinephrine, or systemic carbonic anhydrase inhibitors may be used.
2. Due to diurnal intraocular pressure variations, a satisfactory response to twice daily therapy is best determined by measuring intraocular pressure at different times during the day.

Client/Family Teaching

1. Used to lower pressures in the eye and to prevent vision loss.
2. Apply gentle pressure to the inside corner of the eye for approximately 60 sec following instillation.
3. Wait at least 5 min before instilling other eye drops.
4. Do not close the eyes tightly or blink more frequently than usual after instillation of the drug.
5. Return for evaluation of IOP and drug's effectiveness.

Outcome/Evaluate: ↓ IOP

Levocabastine hydrochloride

(lee-voh-kah-**BASS**-teen)

Pregnancy Category: C

Livostin Eye Drops ✦, Livostin Nasal Spray **(Rx)**

Classification: Ophthalmic antihistamine

Action/Kinetics: A histamine H_1 receptor antagonist. **Duration:** 2 hr. A small amount of the drug is absorbed into the systemic circulation.

Uses: Temporary relief of seasonal allergic conjunctivitis.

Contraindications: Use while soft contact lenses are being worn.

Special Concerns: The drug is only for ophthalmic use. Safety and efficacy have not been determined in children less than 12 years of age.

Side Effects: *Ophthalmologic:* Transient stinging and burning, visual disturbances, eye pain, eye dryness, red eyes, lacrimation, discharge from eyes, eyelid edema. *CNS:* Headache, fatigue, somnolence. *Miscellaneous:* Pharyngitis, cough, nausea, rash, erythema, dyspnea.

How Supplied: *Ophthalmic Suspension:* 0.05%

Dosage

- **Ophthalmic Suspension**

Allergic conjunctivitis.

1 gtt instilled in affected eye(s) q.i.d. for up to 2 weeks.

HEALTH CARE CONSIDERATIONS

Administration/Storage: Keep the bottle tightly closed. Store at room temperature (15°C–30°C or 59°F–86°F) and do not freeze.

Assessment

1. Note other agents prescribed and the outcome.
2. Assess for evidence of infection or abnormal drainage from the eye.
3. Determine any changes in or loss of vision.

Client/Family Teaching

1. Thoroughly mix/shake suspension before using. Do not use if it is discolored.
2. Soft contact lens *cannot* be worn during this therapy.
3. Do not permit dropper tip to touch the eyelids or surrounding areas; this prevents contamination to the dropper tip and suspension.
4. Some burning and stinging may be evident but should subside.
5. Report if symptoms do not improve or if they become worse after 2–4 days of therapy.

Outcome/Evaluate: Relief of ocular itching with allergic conjunctivitis

Levodopa

(lee-voh-**DOH**-pah)

Dopar, Larodopa, L-Dopa **(Rx)**

Classification: Antiparkinson agent

Action/Kinetics: Depletion of dopamine in the striatum of the brain is thought to cause the symptoms of Parkinson's disease. Levodopa, a dopamine precursor, is able to cross the blood-brain barrier to enter the CNS. It is decarboxylated to dopamine in the basal ganglia, thus replenishing depleted dopamine stores. **Peak plasma levels:** 0.5–2 hr (may be delayed if ingested with food). **t½, plasma:** 1–3 hr. **Onset:** 2–3 weeks, although some clients may require up to 6 months. Extensively metabolized both in the GI tract and the liver; metabolites are excreted in the urine.

Uses: Idiopathic, arteriosclerotic, or postencephalitic parkinsonism due to carbon monoxide or manganese intoxication and in the elderly associated with cerebral arteriosclerosis. Levodopa only provides symptomatic relief and does not alter the course of the disease. When effective, it relieves rigidity, bradykinesia, tremors, dysphagia, seborrhea,

L

sialorrhea, and postural instability. Used in combination with carbidopa. *Investigational:* Pain from herpes zoster; restless legs syndrome.

Contraindications: Concomitant use with MAO inhibitors, except MAO-B inhibitors (e.g., selegiline). History of melanoma or in clients with undiagnosed skin lesions. Lactation. Hypersensitivity to drug, narrow-angle glaucoma, blood dyscrasias, hypertension, coronary sclerosis.

Special Concerns: Use with extreme caution in clients with history of MIs, convulsions, arrhythmias, bronchial asthma, emphysema, active peptic ulcer, psychosis or neurosis, wide-angle glaucoma, and renal, hepatic, or endocrine diseases. Use during pregnancy only if benefits clearly outweigh risks. Safety has not been established in children less than 12 years of age. Geriatric clients may require a lower dose as they have a reduced tolerance for the drug and its side effects (including cardiac effects). Clients may experience an "on-off" phenomenon in which they experience an improved clinical status followed by loss of therapeutic effect.

L

Side Effects: The side effects of levodopa are numerous and usually dose related. Some may abate with usage. *CNS:* Choreiform and/or dystonic movements, paranoid ideation, psychotic episodes, ***depression (with possibility of suicidal tendencies),*** dementia, ***seizures (rare),*** dizziness, headache, faintness, confusion, insomnia, nightmares, hallucinations, delusions, agitation, anxiety, malaise, fatigue, euphoria. *GI:* N&V, anorexia, abdominal pain, dry mouth, sialorrhea, dysphagia, dysgeusia, hiccups, diarrhea, constipation, burning sensation of tongue, bitter taste, flatulence, weight gain or loss, GI bleeding (rare), duodenal ulcer (rare). *CV:* Cardiac irregularities, palpitations, orthostatic hypotension, hypertension, phlebitis, hot flashes. *Ophthalmologic:* Diplopia, dilated pupils, blurred vision, development of Horner's syndrome, oculogyric crisis. *Hematologic:* ***Hemolytic anemia, agranulocytosis,*** leukopenia. *Musculoskeletal:* Muscle twitching (early sign of overdose), tonic contraction of the muscles of mastication, increased hand tremor, ataxia. *Miscellaneous:* Blepharospasm (early sign of overdose), urinary retention, urinary incontinence, increased sweating, unusual breathing patterns, weakness, numbness, bruxism, alopecia, priapism, hoarseness, edema, dark sweat and/or urine, flushing, skin rash, sense of stimulation. Levodopa interacts with many other drugs (see what follows) and must be administered cautiously.

Laboratory Test Considerations: ↑ BUN, AST, LDH, ALT, bilirubin, alkaline phosphatase, protein-bound iodine, uric acid (with colorimetric test). ↓ H&H, WBCs. False + Coombs' test. Interference with tests for urinary glucose and ketones.

OD **Management of Overdose:** *Symptoms:* Muscle twitching, blepharospasm. Also see *Side Effects. Treatment:* Immediate gastric lavage for acute overdose. Maintain airway and give IV fluids carefully. General supportive measures.

Drug Interactions

Antacids / ↑ Effect of levodopa due to ↑ absorption from GI tract
Anticholinergic drugs / Possible ↓ effect of levodopa due to ↑ breakdown of levodopa in stomach (due to delayed gastric emptying time)
Antidepressants, tricyclic / ↓ Effect of levodopa due to ↓ absorption from GI tract; also, ↑ risk of hypertension
Benzodiazepines / ↓ Effect of levodopa
Clonidine / ↓ Effect of levodopa
Digoxin / ↓ Effect of digoxin
Furazolidone / ↑ Effect of levodopa due to ↓ breakdown by liver
Guanethidine / ↑ Hypotensive effect of guanethidine
Hypoglycemic drugs / Levodopa upsets diabetic control with hypoglycemic agents
MAO inhibitors / Concomitant administration may result in hypertension, lightheadedness, and flushing due to ↓ breakdown of dopamine and norepinephrine formed from levodopa
Methionine / ↓ Effect of levodopa
Methyldopa / Additive effects including hypotension
Metoclopramide / ↑ Bioavailability of levodopa; ↓ effect of metoclopramide
Papaverine / ↓ Effect of levodopa
Phenothiazines / ↓ Effect of levodopa due to ↓ uptake of dopamine into neurons
Phenytoin / Antagonizes the effect of levodopa
Propranolol / May antagonize the hypotensive and positive inotropic effect of levodopa
Pyridoxine / Reverses levodopa-induced improvement in Parkinson's disease
Thioxanthines / ↓ Effect of levodopa in Parkinson clients
Tricyclic antidepressants / ↓ Absorption of levodopa → ↓ effect

How Supplied: *Capsule:* 250 mg; *Tablet:* 100 mg, 250 mg, 500 mg

Dosage

- **Capsules, Tablets**

  Parkinsonism.

Adults, initial: 250 mg b.i.d.–q.i.d. taken with food; **then,** increase total daily dose by 100–750 mg/3–7 days until optimum dosage reached (should not exceed 8 g/day). Up to 6 months may be required to achieve a significant therapeutic effect.

HEALTH CARE CONSIDERATIONS

See also *Health Care Considerations* for *Cholinergic Blocking Agents*.

Administration/Storage

1. If unable to swallow tablets or capsules, crush tablets or empty the capsule into a small amount of fruit juice at the time of administration.
2. Often administered together with an anticholinergic agent.

Assessment

1. Review medical history for any contraindications to therapy. Stop drug 24 hr before surgery and note when drug is to be restarted.
2. Assess and record baseline rigidity, tremors, motor function, and involuntary movements. Note mental status.
3. Note adverse side effects that may require ↓ drug dose or "drug holiday".
4. Monitor ECG, CBC, liver/renal function studies, and protein bound iodine tests.

Client/Family Teaching

1. Take with food to decrease GI upset.
2. Report headaches; may indicate drug-induced glaucoma. Twitching or eye spasms may indicate toxicity.
3. Dosage should not exceed 8 g/day; do not stop abruptly.
4. Avoid taking multivitamin preparations containing 10–25 mg of B_6; reverses the antiparkinson effect.
5. Significant results may take up to 6 months to be realized.
6. May cause dizziness or drowsiness. Do not perform tasks that require mental alertness until drug effects realized.
7. Sweat and urine may appear dark; this is not harmful.
8. Sustained erection may occur; report immediately.
9. Report any evidence of depression or psychosis or other unusual mental or behavioral changes.
10. Report for all scheduled visits so that drug effectiveness can be evaluated and dosage adjusted as needed.
11. Identify appropriate support services.

Outcome/Evaluate: Improvement in motor function, reflexes, gait, strength of grip, and amount of tremor

Levofloxacin

(lee-voh-**FLOX**-ah-sin)
Pregnancy Category: C
Levaquin **(Rx)**
Classification: Fluoroquinolone antibiotic

See also *Fluoroquinolones*.

Uses: Acute maxillary sinusitis due to *Streptococcus pneumoniae, Haemophilus influenzae,* or *Moraxella catarrhalis*. Acute bacterial exacerbation of chronic bronchitis due to *Staphylococcus aureus, S. pneumoniae, H. influenzae, Haemophilus parainfluenzae,* or *M. catarrhalis*. Community acquired pneumonia due to *S. aureus, S. pneumoniae, H. influenzae, H. parainfluenzae, Klebsiella pneumoniae, M. catarrhalis, Chlamydia pneumoniae, Legionella pneumophila,* or *Mycoplasma pneumoniae*. Uncomplicated mild to moderate infections of the skin and skin structures, including abscesses, cellulitis, furuncies, impetigo, pyoderma, and wound infections due to *S. aureus* or *Streptococcus pyogenes*. Mild to moderate complicated UTIs due to *Enterococcus faecalis, Enterobacter cloacae, Escherichia coli, Klebsiella pneumoniae, Proteus mirabilis,* or *Pseudomonas aeruginosa*. Acute mild to moderate pyelonephritis due to *E. coli*.

Contraindications: Lactation.

Special Concerns: The dose must be reduced with impaired renal function. (See *Administration/Storage*.) Safety and efficacy have not been determined in those less than 18 years of age.

How Supplied: *Injection:* 500 mg; *Injection (premix):* 250 mg, 500 mg; *Tablets:* 250 mg, 500 mg.

Dosage

- **Injection, Tablets**

Acute maxillary sinusitis.
500 mg once daily for 10–14 days.

Acute bacterial exacerbation of chronic bronchitis.
500 mg once daily for 7 days.

Community acquired pneumonia.
500 mg once daily for 7–14 days.

Uncomplicated skin and skin structure infections.
500 mg once daily for 7–10 days.

Complicated UTIs.
250 mg once daily for 10 days.

Acute pyelonephritis.
250 mg once daily for 10 days.

L

HEALTH CARE CONSIDERATIONS

See also *Health Care Considerations* for *Fluoroquinolones*.

Administration/Storage

1. Reduce dose with impaired renal function when used for acute maxillary sinusitis, acute bacterial exacerbation of chronic bronchitis, community acquired pneumonia, and uncomplicated skin and skin structure infections. If C_{CR} is between 20 and 49 mL/min, the initial dose is 500 mg and subsequent doses are 250 mg q 24 hr. If C_{CR} is between 10 and 19 mL/min, the initial dose is 500 mg and subsequent doses are 250 mg q 48 hr. If the client is on hemodialysis or chronic ambulatory peritoneal dialysis, the initial dose is 500 mg and subsequent doses are 250 mg q 48 hr.
2. Oral doses are given at least 2 hr before or 2 hr after antacids containing magnesium or aluminum, as well as sucralfate, iron products, and multivitamin preparations containing zinc.
3. Store tablets in a tight container at 15°C–30°C (59°F–85°F).
4. **IV** The injectable form may be mixed with 0.9% NaCl injection, D5W, D5/0.9% NaCl, D5/RL, Plasma-Lyte 56/5% dextrose injection, D5/0.45% NaCl, 0.15% KCl injection, or M/6 sodium lactate injection.
5. Diluted solutions for IV use are stable for 72 hr up to a concentration of 5 mg/mL when stored in IV containers at 25°C or less (77°F or less). Such solutions are stable for 14 days when stored under refrigeration at 5°C (41°F). Diluted solutions that are frozen in glass bottles or plastic IV containers are stable for 6 months when stored at –20°C (–4°F).
6. Thaw frozen solutions at room temperature or in a refrigerator. Do not thaw in a microwave or by bath immersion. After initial thawing, do not refreeze.

Client/Family Teaching

1. Take only as directed; complete entire prescription.
2. Avoid multivitamins with zinc, iron products, sucralfate, and Mg- or aluminum-containing antacids 2 hr before and after dose.
3. Practice reliable birth control.
4. Use caution until drug effects realized; may experience dizziness, drowsiness or visual changes.
5. Report if symptoms do not improve or worsen after 72 hr of therapy.

Outcome/Evaluate

- Symptomatic improvement
- Resolution of infective organism

L

Levonorgestrel Implants

(lee-voh-nor-JES-trel)
Pregnancy Category: X
Norgestrel II, Norplant System **(Rx)**
Classification: Progestin, contraceptive system

See also *Progesterone and Progestins*.

Action/Kinetics: Levonorgestrel implants are marketed either in a set of six flexible Silastic capsules each containing 36 mg of levonorgestrel (Norplant) or two rods containing 150 mg of levonorgestrel (Norgestrel II); the provider receives an insertion kit to assist with implantation. Small amounts of the drug slowly diffuse through the wall of each capsule resulting in blood levels of levonorgestrel that are lower than those seen when levonorgestrel or norgestrel is taken as oral contraceptive. The dose released is initially 85 mcg/day, followed by a decrease to approximately 50 mcg/day after 9 months, to 35 mcg/day after 18 months, and then leveling off to 30 mcg/day thereafter. Blood levels of levonorgestrel vary over a wide range and cannot be used as the sole measure of the risk of pregnancy. If used properly, the risk of pregnancy is less than 1 for every 100 users. Does not have any estrogenic effects. The implant system lasts up to 5 years and the contraceptive effect is rapidly reversed if the system is removed from the body.

Uses: Prevention of pregnancy (system lasts for up to 5 years). A new system may be inserted after 5 years if continuing contraception is desired.

Contraindications: Active thrombophlebitis, thromboembolic disorders, undiagnosed abnormal genital bleeding, acute liver disease, benign or malignant liver tumors, known or suspected breast carcinoma, confirmed or suspected pregnancy.

Special Concerns: Menstrual bleeding irregularities are commonly observed. Monitor carefully women who have a family history of breast cancer or who have breast nodules. Monitor closely women being treated for hyperlipidemias because an increase in LDL levels may occur. Use with caution in individuals in whom fluid retention might be dangerous and in those with a history of depression. Do not insert until 6 weeks after parturition in women who are breast-feeding.

Side Effects: *Menstrual irregularities:* Prolonged menses, spotting, irregular onset of menses, frequent menses, amenorrhea, scanty bleeding, cervicitis, vaginitis. *At implant site:* Pain or itching, infection, bruising following insertion or removal, hyperpigmentation (reversible upon removal). *GI:* Abdominal discomfort, nausea, change of appetite, weight gain. *CNS:* Headache, nervousness, dizziness. *Dermatologic:* Dermatitis, acne, hirsutism, scalp hair loss, excess hair growth. *Miscellaneous:* Breast discharge, breast pain, leukorrhea, musculoskeletal pain, fluid retention, possibility of ectopic pregnancy in long-term users, delayed follicular atresia.

Laboratory Test Considerations: ↓ Sex hormone binding globulin levels, T_4 levels (slight). ↑ Uptake of T_3.

OD **Management of Overdose:** *Symptoms:* Overdosage can result if more than six capsules are inserted. Symptoms include fluid retention and uterine bleeding irregularities. *Treatment:* All capsules should be removed.

Drug Interactions

Carbamazepine / ↓ Effectiveness → ↑ risk of pregnancy

Phenytoin / ↓ Effectiveness → ↑ risk of pregnancy

How Supplied: *Kit:* 36 mg/implant, 150 mg/implant

Dosage

- **Silastic Capsules, Rods**

Six Silastic capsules (36 mg levonorgestrel each) or two rods (150 mg levonorgestrel each) implanted subdermally in the midportion of the upper arm (8–10 cm above the elbow crease). Capsules are distributed in a fan-like pattern 15° apart (total of 75°).

HEALTH CARE CONSIDERATIONS

See also *Health Care Considerations* for *Progesterone and Progestins.*

Administration/Storage

1. To ensure effectiveness and to be sure not pregnant at the time of capsule implantation, implant during the first 7 days of the cycle or immediately after an abortion.
2. The system should be inserted only by individuals instructed on the proper procedure for insertion. If capsules are placed too deeply, they may be more difficult to remove.
3. If all capsules cannot be removed at the first attempt, allow the site to heal before another attempt is made.
4. Expulsion is not common but may occur if capsules are placed too shallow/too close to the incision or if infection occurs.
5. If infection occurs, treat and cure before replacing capsules.
6. After 5 years, remove capsules; if additional contraception desired, a new system can be inserted.

Assessment

1. A complete medical history, physical and gynecologic exam should be performed prior to implantation or reimplantation and annually during use.
2. Ensure not pregnant at the time of implantation.
3. Determine if breast-feeding; do not insert until 6 weeks after delivery.
4. Note any history of thromboembolic disorders or depression.
5. Assess liver function and for evidence of hyperlipidemia.
6. Assess for family history of breast cancer. Record presence of breast nodules and carefully monitor.
7. Obtain weight; effectiveness of levonorgestrel may be slightly decreased with weights exceeding 70.5 kg.

Client/Family Teaching

1. Review procedure for wound care postinsertion and report symptoms of infection/rejection. A small scar may be evident at the insertion site.
2. Expect some irregularity with the menstrual cycle such as longer periods, missed periods, and spotting in between during the first year of implantation.
3. Report for regularly scheduled F/U visits so that therapy can be carefully evaluated.
4. The system may be removed at any time if necessary; pregnancy can occur after the next menstrual cycle.
5. Additional protection must be used to prevent STDs.

Outcome/Evaluate: Effective contraception

L

Levothyroxine sodium (T_4)

(lee-voh-thigh-**ROX**-een)

Pregnancy Category: A

Eltroxin, Euthyrox, Levo-T, Levothroid, Levoxyl, PMS-Levothyroxine ✦, Synthroid, L-Thyroxine Sodium **(Rx)**

Classification: Thyroid preparation

See also *Thyroid Drugs.*

Action/Kinetics: Levothyroxine is the synthetic sodium salt of the levoisomer of T_4 (tetraiodothyronine). Levothyroxine, 0.05–0.6 mg equals approximately 60 mg (1 grain) of thyroid. Absorption from the GI tract is incomplete and variable, especially when taken with food. Has a slower onset but a longer duration than sodium liothyronine. More active on a weight basis than thyroid. Is usually the drug of choice. Effect is predictable as thyroid content is standard. **Time to peak therapeutic effect:** 3–4 weeks. **t½:** 6–7 days in a euthyroid person, 9–10 days in a hypothyroid

client, and 3–4 days in a hyperthyroid client. Is 99% protein bound. **Duration:** 1–3 weeks after withdrawal of chronic therapy. *NOTE:* All levothyroxine products are not bioequivalent; thus, changing brands is not recommended.
Drug Interactions: Concurrent use of aluminum hydroxide and levothyroxine may result in adsorption of levothyroxine to the aluminum and increased fecal elimination of levothyroxine.
How Supplied: *Powder for injection:* 0.2 mg, 0.5 mg; *Tablet:* 0.025 mg, 0.05 mg, 0.075 mg, 0.088 mg, 0.1 mg, 0.112 mg, 0.125 mg, 0.137 mg, 0.15 mg, 0.175 mg, 0.2 mg, 0.3 mg, 0.5 mg

Dosage

- **Tablets**

Mild hypothyroidism.

Adults, initial: 50 mcg once daily; **then,** increase by 25–50 mcg q 2–3 weeks until desired clinical response is attained; **maintenance, usual:** 75–125 mcg/day (although doses up to 200 mcg/day may be required in some clients).

Severe hypothyroidism.

Adults, initial: 12.5–25 mcg once daily; **then,** increase dose, as necessary, in increments of 25 mcg at 2- to 3-week intervals.

Congenital hypothyroidism.

Pediatric, 12 years and older: 2–3 mcg/kg once daily until the adult daily dose (usually 150 mcg) is reached. **6–12 years of age:** 4–5 mcg/kg/day or 100–150 mcg once daily. **1–5 years of age:** 5–6 mcg/kg/day or 75–100 mcg once daily. **6–12 months of age:** 6–8 mcg/kg/day or 50–75 mcg once daily. **Less than 6 months of age:** 8–10 mcg/kg/day or 25–50 mcg once daily.

- **IM, IV**

Myxedematous coma.

Adults, initial: 400 mcg by rapid IV injection, even in geriatric clients; **then,** 100–200 mcg/day, IV. **Maintenance:** 100–200 mcg/day, IV. Smaller daily doses should be given until client can tolerate PO medication.

Hypothyroidism.

Adults: 50–100 mcg once daily; **pediatric, IV, IM:** A dose of 75% of the usual PO pediatric dose should be given.

HEALTH CARE CONSIDERATIONS

See also *Health Care Considerations* for *Thyroid Drugs.*

Administration/Storage

1. In infants and children who cannot swallow tablets, the correct dosage tablet may be crushed and suspended in a small amount of formula or water and given by dropper or spoon. The crushed tablet may also be sprinkled over cooked cereal or applesauce.
2. Transfer from liothyronine to levothyroxine: administer replacement drug for several days before discontinuing liothyronine. Transfer from levothyroxine to liothyronine: discontinue levothyroxine before starting low daily dose of liothyronine.
3. IV Prepare solution for injection immediately before administration. Reconstitute by adding 5 mL of 0.9% NaCl injection or bacteriostatic NaCl injection and shake vial to ensure complete mixing.
4. Discard any unused portion of the IV medication.
5. Do not mix with other IV infusion solutions.

Assessment

1. Elderly clients are likely to have undetected cardiac problems. Obtain ECG prior to initiating therapy.
2. Monitor thyroid profile.
3. If pregnant, must continue taking thyroid preparations throughout the pregnancy.
4. Note height, weight, and psychomotor development in child.
5. List drugs currently consumed to ensure none interact unfavorably.

Client/Family Teaching

1. Do not switch brands; bioavailability may change.
2. Do not take with food unless specifically instructed; may interfere with absorption.
3. Report any persistent headaches, increased HR (hold if resting HR is greater than 100), chest pain, diarrhea, irritability, excitability, more than 5 lb/week weight loss, and excessive sweating.
4. Avoid iodine-rich foods.
5. Drug is not a cure for hypothyroidism; must be taken for lifetime to control symptoms.

Outcome/Evaluate

- Promotion of normal metabolism
- ↑ Levels of T_3 and T_4, ↓ TSH

COMBINATION DRUG

Librax

(LIB-rax)

Pregnancy Category: Do not use during pregnancy, especially first trimester.
(Rx)
Classification: Antianxiety agent

See also *Tranquilizers, Antimanic Drugs, and Hypnotics* and *Cholinergic Blocking Agents.*
Content: *Antianxiety agent:* Chlordiazepoxide, 5 mg. *Anticholinergic agent:* Clidinium bromide, 2.5 mg. See also information on individual components.

Uses: Possibly effective as an adjunct in the treatment of irritable colon, spastic colon, mucous colitis, and acute enterocolitis.
Contraindications: Pregnancy, glaucoma, prostatic hypertrophy.
How Supplied: See Content

Dosage

- **Capsules**

Individualized. Adults, usual: 1–2 capsules t.i.d.–q.i.d. before meals and at bedtime.

HEALTH CARE CONSIDERATIONS

See *Health Care Considerations* for *Tranquilizers, Antimanic Drugs, and Hypnotics* and *Cholinergic Blocking Agents*.

Outcome/Evaluate

- Restoration of normal bowel motility and relief of pain
- Symptomatic improvement

Lidocaine hydrochloride

(LYE-doh-kayn)
Pregnancy Category: B
IM: LidoPen Auto-Injector, **(Rx)**. **Direct IV or IV Admixtures:** Lidocaine HCl for Cardiac Arrhythmias, Xylocaine HCl IV for Cardiac Arrhythmias, Xylocard ✦ **(Rx)**. **IV Infusion:** Lidocaine HCl in 5% Dextrose **(Rx)**
Classification: Antiarrhythmic, class IB

See also *Antiarrhythmic Agents*.
Action/Kinetics: Shortens the refractory period and suppresses the automaticity of ectopic foci without affecting conduction of impulses through cardiac tissue. Increases the electrical stimulation threshold of the ventricle during diastole. It does not affect BP, CO, or myocardial contractility. **IV: Onset,** 45–90 sec; **duration:** 10–20 min. **IM, Onset,** 5–15 min; **duration,** 60–90 min. **t½:** 1–2 hr. **Therapeutic serum levels:** 1.5–6 mcg/mL. **Time to steady-state plasma levels:** 3–4 hr (8–10 hr in clients with AMI). **Protein-binding:** 40%–80%. Ninety percent is rapidly metabolized in the liver to active metabolites. Since lidocaine has little effect on conduction at normal antiarrhythmic doses, use in acute situations (instead of procainamide) in instances in which heart block might occur.
Uses: IV: Treatment of acute ventricular arrhythmias such as those following MIs or occurring during surgery. The drug is ineffective against atrial arrhythmias. **IM:** Certain emergency situations (e.g., ECG equipment not available; mobile coronary care unit, under advice of a physician).

Investigational: IV in children who develop ventricular couplets or frequent premature ventricular beats.
Contraindications: Hypersensitivity to amide-type local anesthetics, Stokes-Adams syndrome, Wolff-Parkinson-White syndrome, severe SA, AV, or intraventricular block (when no pacemaker is present). Use of the IM autoinjector for children.
Special Concerns: Use with caution during labor and delivery, during lactation, and in the presence of liver or severe kidney disease, CHF, marked hypoxia, digitalis toxicity with AV block, severe respiratory depression, or shock. In geriatric clients, the rate and dose for IV infusion should be decreased by one-half and slowly adjusted. Safety and efficacy have not been determined in children.
Side Effects: *Body as a whole:* Malignant hyperthermia characterized by tachycardia, tachypnea, labile BP, metabolic acidosis, temperature elevation. *CV:* ***Precipitation or aggravation of arrhythmias (following IV use),*** hypotension, ***bradycardia (with possible cardiac arrest), CV collapse.*** *CNS:* Dizziness, apprehension, euphoria, lightheadedness, nervousness, drowsiness, confusion, changes in mood, hallucinations, twitching, "doom anxiety," ***convulsions,*** unconsciousness. *Respiratory:* Difficulties in breathing or swallowing, ***respiratory depression or arrest.*** *Allergic:* Rash, cutaneous lesions, urticaria, edema, ***anaphylaxis.*** *Other:* Tinnitus, blurred or double vision, vomiting, numbness, sensation of heat or cold, twitching, tremors, soreness at IM injection site, fever, ***venous thrombosis or phlebitis (extending from site of injection),*** extravasation. During anesthesia, CV depression may be the first sign of lidocaine toxicity. During other usage, convulsions are the first sign of lidocaine toxicity.
OD **Management of Overdose:** *Symptoms:* Dependent on plasma levels. If plasma levels range from 4 to 6 mcg/mL, mild CNS effects are observed. Levels of 6 to 8 mcg/mL may result in significant CNS and CV depression while levels greater than 8 mcg/mL cause hypotension, decreased CO, respiratory depression, obtundation, ***seizures, and coma.*** *Treatment:* Discontinue the drug and begin emergency resuscitative procedures. Seizures can be treated with diazepam, thiopental, or thiamylal. Succinylcholine, IV, may be used if the client is anesthetized. IV fluids, vasopressors, and CPR are used to correct circulatory depression.
Drug Interactions
Aminoglycosides / ↑ Neuromuscular blockade

L

Beta-adrenergic blockers / ↑ Lidocaine levels with possible toxicity
Cimetidine / ↓ Clearance of lidocaine → possible toxicity
Phenytoin / IV phenytoin → excessive cardiac depression
Procainamide / Additive cardiodepressant effects
Succinylcholine / ↑ Action of succinylcholine by ↓ plasma protein binding
Tocainide / ↑ Risk of side effects
Tubocurarine / ↑ Neuromuscular blockade
How Supplied: *Dextrose/Lidocaine Hydrochloride—Injection:* 5%-0.2%, 5%-0.4%, 5%-0.8%, 7.5%-5%; *Lidocaine Hydrochloride—Injection:* 0.5%, 1%, 1.5%, 2%, 10%, 20%; *Kit:* 2%

Dosage

- **IV Bolus**

Antiarrhythmic.

Adults: 50–100 mg at rate of 25–50 mg/min. Bolus is used to establish rapid therapeutic plasma levels. Repeat if necessary after 5-min interval. Onset of action is 10 sec. **Maximum dose/hr:** 200–300 mg.

- **Infusion**

Antiarrhythmic.

20–50 mcg/kg at a rate of 1–4 mg/min. No more than 200–300 mg/hr should be given. **Pediatric, loading dose:** 1 mg/kg IV or intratracheally q 5–10 min until desired effect reached (maximum total dose: 5 mg/kg).

- **IV Continuous Infusion**

Maintain therapeutic plasma levels following loading doses.

Adults: Give at a rate of 1–4 mg/min (20–50 mcg/kg/min). Reduce the dose in clients with heart failure, with liver disease, or who are taking drugs that interact with lidocaine. **Pediatric:** 20–50 mcg/kg/min (usual is 30 mcg/kg/min).

- **IM**

Antiarrhythmic.

Adults: 4.5 mg/kg (approximately 300 mg for a 70-kg adult). Switch to IV lidocaine or oral antiarrhythmics as soon as possible although an additional IM dose may be given after 60–90 min.

HEALTH CARE CONSIDERATIONS

See also *Health Care Considerations* for *Antiarrhythmic Agents.*

Administration/Storage

IV 1. Do not add lidocaine to blood transfusion assembly.
2. Do not use lidocaine solutions that contain epinephrine to treat arrhythmias. Make certain that vial states, "For Cardiac Arrhythmias." Check prefilled syringes closely to ensure appropriate dose has been obtained. (Lidocaine prefilled syringes come in both milligrams and grams.)
3. Use D5W to prepare solution; this is stable for 24 hr. Administer with an electronic infusion device.
4. Reduce IV bolus dosage in clients over 70 years old, with CHF or liver disease, and if taking cimetidine or propranolol (i.e., where metabolism of lidocaine is reduced).

Assessment

1. Note any hypersensitivity to amide-type local anesthetics.
2. Elderly clients who have hepatic or renal disease or who weigh less than 45.5 kg will need to be watched especially closely for adverse side effects; adjust dosage as directed.
3. Record CNS status; report sudden changes in mental status, dizziness, visual disturbances, twitching, and tremors. These symptoms may precede convulsions. Note pulmonary findings; assess for respiratory depression, characterized by slow, shallow respirations. Monitor liver and renal function studies, electrolytes, and ECG; assess for hypotension and cardiac collapse.
4. View monitor strips for myocardial depression, variations of rhythm, or aggravation of arrhythmia.

Outcome/Evaluate

- Control of ventricular arrhythmias
- Therapeutic serum drug levels (1.5–6 mcg/mL)

Lincomycin hydrochloride

(link-oh-**MY**-sin)
Pregnancy Category: B
Lincocin, Lincorex **(Rx)**
Classification: Anti-infective

See also *Anti-Infectives.*
Action/Kinetics: Isolated from *Streptomyces lincolnensis.* Suppresses protein synthesis by microorganisms by binding to ribosomes (50S subunit), which is essential for transmittal of genetic information. Both bacteriostatic and bactericidal. Rapidly absorbed from the GI tract and is widely distributed. **Peak serum levels: PO,** 1.8–5.3 mcg/mL after 500 mg; **IM,** 9.3–18.5 mcg/mL after 600 mg; **IV,** 15.9–20.9 mcg/mL after 600 mg. **t½:** 4.4–6.4 hr. Metabolized by the liver; about 60% excreted through the urine and 40% in the feces. Do not use for trivial infections.
Uses: Not a first-choice drug but useful for clients allergic to penicillin. Spectrum resembles that of the erythromycins. Used for serious respiratory tract, skin, and soft tissue infections due to staphylococci, streptococci, or pneu-

mococci and some gram-negative organisms. Septicemia. In conjunction with diphtheria antitoxin in the treatment of diphtheria.
Contraindications: Hypersensitivity to drugs. Use in pre-existing liver disease, in infants up to 1 month of age, or in treating viral and minor bacterial infections.
Special Concerns: Safe use during pregnancy has not been established. Use with caution in clients with GI disease, liver or renal disease, or a history of allergy or asthma.
Side Effects: *GI:* N&V, diarrhea (may be severe), abdominal pain, tenesmus, flatulence, bloating, anorexia, weight loss, esophagitis, pruritus ani. Nonspecific colitis, pseudomembranous colitis (may be severe). *Allergic:* Morbilliform rash (most common). Also, maculopapular rash, urticaria, pruritus, fever, hypotension. Rarely, polyarteritis, ***anaphylaxis,*** erythema multiforme. *Hematologic:* Leukopenia, neutropenia, eosinophilia, thrombocytopenia, ***agranulocytosis.*** *Miscellaneous:* Superinfection.

Following IV use: Thrombophlebitis, erythema, pain, swelling. IV lincomycin may cause hypotension, syncope, and ***cardiac arrest*** (rare). *Following IM use:* Pain, induration, sterile abscesses. *Following topical use:* Erythema, irritation, dryness, peeling, itching, burning, oiliness. Also, sore throat, fatigue, urinary frequency, headache.

NOTE: The injection contains benzyl alcohol, which has been associated with a fatal gasping syndrome in infants.
Laboratory Test Considerations: ↓ Levels of AST, ALT, NPN, alkaline phosphatase, bilirubin, BSP retention, and ↓ platelet count.
Drug Interactions
Antiperistaltic antidiarrheals (opiates, Lomotil) / ↑ Diarrhea due to ↓ removal of toxins from colon
Erythromycin / Cross-interference → ↓ effect of both drugs
Kaolin (e.g., Kaopectate) / ↓ Effect due to ↓ absorption from GI tract
Neuromuscular blocking agents / ↑ Effect of blocking agents; possible severe respiratory depression
How Supplied: *Capsule:* 500 mg; *Injection:* 300 mg/mL

Dosage
- **Capsules**

Infections.
Adults: 500 mg t.i.d. for serious infections. **Adults:** 500 mg or more q 6 hr for more severe infections. Continue treatment for at least 10 days with β–hemolytic streptococcal infections. **Children over 1 month of age:** 30–60 mg/kg/day in three to four divided doses, depending on severity of infection.
- **IM**

Infections.
Adults: 600 mg q 24 hr for serious infections and every 12 hr or more for more severe infections. **Children over 1 month of age:** 10 mg/kg q 12–24 hr, depending on severity of infection.
- **IV**

Infections.
Adults: 0.6–1.0 g q 8–12 hr up to 8 g/day, depending on severity of infection. **Children over 1 month of age:** 10–20 mg/kg/day, depending on severity of infection.

NOTE: In impaired renal function, reduce dosage by 70%–75%.
- **Subconjunctival Injection**

0.75 mg/0.25 mL.

HEALTH CARE CONSIDERATIONS

See also *General Health Care Considerations for All Anti-Infectives.*

Administration/Storage
1. Prepare drug for administration as directed on package insert.
2. Administer slowly IM to minimize pain.
3. IV For IV use, carefully follow concentration and recommended rate for administration to prevent severe cardiopulmonary reactions.
4. Injection contains benzyl alcohol.

Assessment
1. Manage colitis by providing fluids, electrolytes, protein supplements, systemic corticosteroids, and vancomycin (may occur 2–9 days to several weeks after therapy).
2. Assess for transient flushing, sensations of warmth and cardiac disturbances, with IV infusions.
3. Monitor VS, CBC, and LFTs. Note any liver dysfunction/disease.

Client/Family Teaching
1. Take on an empty stomach between meals and not with a sugar substitute, to ensure optimum absorption. Report GI disturbances, including abdominal pain, diarrhea, anorexia, N&V, bloody or tarry stools, and excessive flatulence.
2. Do not use antiperistaltic agents if diarrhea occurs; may prolong or aggravate condition.
3. Avoid acne or topical mercury preparations containing a peeling agent in area affected by medication; severe irritation can occur.
4. Do not take kaolin concomitantly; will reduce absorption of lincomycin. If kaolin is required, administer 3 hr before.

Outcome/Evaluate

- Negative culture reports
- Resolution of infection

Linezolid

(lih-**NAY**-zoh-lid)

Pregnancy Category: C

Zyvox **(Rx)**

Classification: Antibiotic, Oxazolidinone

Action/Kinetics: Inhibits bacterial protein synthesis by binding to bacterial 23_s ribosomal RNA of the 50_s subunit. This action prevents the formation of a functional 70_sinitiation complex that is essential for the bacterial translation process. Linezolid is bacteriostatic against enterococci, staphylococci; bactericidal against most strains of streptococci. **t½:** 4-5 hours. **Peak:** 1-2 hours. Hepatic metabolism; does not involve cytochrome P-450 isoenzymes. 65% nonrenal elimination for linezolid; 30% renally as linezolid.

Uses: Treatment of vancomycin-resistant *Enterococcus faecium* (VRE) infections, nosocomial pneumonia caused by *Staphylococcus aureus* including MRSA or *Streptococcus pneumoniae* (penicillin-susceptible strains only), complicated and uncomplicated skin structure infections, and community-acquired pneumonia caused by susceptible gram-positive organisms.

Contraindications: Allergy to linezolid or any other component.

Special Concerns: Linezolid has mild monoamine oxidase inhibitor properties and has the potential to have the same interactions as other MAOIs: use cautiously in uncontrolled hypertension, pheochromocytoma, carcinoid syndrome, or untreated hyperthyroidism; thrombocytopenia has been reported and may be dependent on duration of therapy (generally >2 weeks of treatment); avoid use with serotonergic agents such as TCAs, venlafaxine, trazodone, sibutramine, meperidine, dextromethorphan, and SSRIs; consider alternatives before initiating outpatient treatment (unnecessary use may lead to the development of organism resistance to linezolid).

Side Effects: Rash, nausea, diarrhea, thrombocytopenia.

Laboratory Test Considerations: The following lab values may be abnormal: Hemoglobin, platelet count, WBCs, neutrophils, AST, ALT, LOH, alkaline phosphates, lipase, amaylase, total bilirubin, BUN, creatinine.

OD **Management of Overdose:** *Symptoms: Treatment:* Supportive care; hemodialysis may improve elimination (30% of a dose is removed during a 3-hour hemodialysis treatment).

Drug Interactions: Linezolid is a reversible, nonselective inhibitor of monoamine oxidase (MAO). Sertonergic agents (i.e.SSRIs, TCAs, venlafaxine, trazodone, sibutramine, meperidine, dextromethorphan) may cause serotonin syndrome (hyperpyrexia, cognitive dysfunction) when used together. Adrenergic agents (i.e. phenylpropanolamine, pseudoephedrine, sympathomimetic agents, vasopressor or dopaminergic agents) may cause hypertension.

How Supplied: *Tablet:* 400 mg, 600 mg; *Oral Suspension:* 20 mg/mL (150 mL) (orange-flavored); *I.V. Infusion:* 200mg (100 mL); 400 mg (200 mL); 600 mg (300 mL).

Dosage

Adult: Oral, I.V.: Vancomycin-resistant *Enterococcus faecium* (VRE): 600 mg every 12 hours for 14-28 days. Nosocomial pneumonia, complicated skin and skin structure infections, community-acquired pneumonia including concurrent bacteremia: 600 mg every 12 hours for 10-14 days.

Oral: Uncomplicated skin and skin structure infections: 400 mg every 12 hours for 10-14 days.

HEALTH CARE CONSIDERATIONS

Administration/Storage

1. Suspension contains 20 mg phenylalanine per teaspoonful.
2. Mix suspension gently; store at room temperature.
3. **IV** Administer I.V. solution over 30-120 minutes.
4. Do not mix or infuse with other medications.
5. The yellow color of the solution may become darker over time without affecting potency.

Assessment

1. Record onset, type, severity and duration of symptoms.
2. Ask about drug allergies.

Client/Family Teaching

1. Take all of the medication; do not skip doses.
2. Take with or without food; take with food if medicine causes stomach upset.
3. Tell your healthcare provider if you have hypertension or are taking any cold remedy or decongestant.
4. Limit tyramine-containing foods
5. Store at room temperature; suspension should be mixed gently before administration.

L

Outcome/Evaluate: Resolution of infection.

Liothyronine sodium (T_3)

(lye-oh-THIGH-roh-neen)

Pregnancy Category: A

Cytomel, Sodium-L-Triiodothyronine, Triostat **(Rx)**

Classification: Thyroid preparation

See also *Thyroid Drugs.*

Action/Kinetics: Synthetic sodium salt of levoisomer of T_3. Has more predictable effects due to standard hormone content. From 15 to 37.5 mcg is equivalent to about 60 mg of desiccated thyroid. May be preferred when a rapid effect or rapidly reversible effect is required. Has a rapid onset, which may result in difficulty in controlling the dosage as well as the possibility of cardiac side effects and changes in metabolic demands. However, its short duration allows quick adjustment of dosage and helps control overdosage. **t½:** 24 hr for euthyroid clients, approximately 34 hr in hypothyroid clients, and approximately 14 hr in hyperthyroid clients. **Duration:** Up to 72 hr. Is 99% protein bound.

Additional Contraindications: Use in children with cretinism because there is some question about whether the hormone crosses the blood-brain barrier.

How Supplied: *Injection:* 10 mcg/mL; *Tablet:* 5 mcg, 25 mcg, 50 mcg

Dosage

- **Tablets**

Mild hypothyroidism.

Adults, individualized, initial: 25 mcg/day. Increase by 12.5–25 mcg q 1–2 weeks until satisfactory response has been obtained. **Usual maintenance:** 25–75 mcg/day (100 mcg may be required in some clients). Use lower initial dosage (5 mcg/day) for the elderly, children, and clients with CV disease. Increase only by 5-mcg increments.

Myxedema.

Adults, initial: 5 mcg/day increased by 5–10 mcg/day q 1–2 weeks until 25 mcg/day is reached; **then,** increase q 1–2 weeks by 12.5–50 mcg. **Usual maintenance:** 50–100 mcg/day.

Simple (nontoxic) goiter.

Adults, initial: 5 mcg/day; **then,** increase q 1–2 weeks by 5–10 mcg until 25 mcg/day is reached; **then,** dose can be increased by 12.5–25 mcg/week until the maintenance dose of 50–100 mcg/day is reached (usual is 75 mcg/day).

T_3 suppression test.

75–100 mcg/day for 7 days followed by a repeat of the I^{131} thyroid uptake test (a 50% or greater suppression of uptake indicates a normal thyroid-pituitary axis).

Congenital hypothyroidism.

Adults and children, initial: 5 mcg/day; **then,** increase by 5 mcg/day q 3–4 days until the desired effect is achieved. Approximately 20 mcg/day may be sufficient for infants a few months of age while children 1 year of age may require 50 mcg/day. Children above 3 years may require the full adult dose.

- **IV Only**

Myxedema coma, precoma.

Adults, initial: 25–50 mcg. Base subsequent doses on continuous monitoring of client's clinical status and response. Doses should be given at least 4 hr, and no more than 12 hr, apart. Total daily doses of 65 mcg in initial days of therapy are associated with a lower incidence of mortality. In cases of known CV disease, give an initial dose of 10–20 mcg.

HEALTH CARE CONSIDERATIONS

See also *Health Care Considerations* for *Thyroid Drugs.*

Administration/Storage

1. *Transfer from other thyroid preparations to liothyronine:* Discontinue old preparation before starting on low daily dose of liothyronine. *Transfer from liothyronine to another thyroid preparation:* Start therapy with replacement drug several days prior to complete withdrawal of sodium liothyronine.
2. If symptoms of hyperthyroidism noted, the drug can be withdrawn for 2–3 days and can be reinstituted at a lower dose.
3. IV A Cytomel injection kit is available for the emergency treatment of myxedema coma.

Outcome/Evaluate: Thyroid hormone replacement

Liotrix

(LYE-oh-trix)

Pregnancy Category: A

Thyrolar **(Rx)**

Classification: Thyroid preparation

See also *Thyroid Drugs.*

Action/Kinetics: Mixture of synthetic levothyroxine sodium (T_4) and liothyronine (T_3) in a 4:1 ratio by weight and in a 1:1 ratio by biologic activity.

How Supplied: *Tablet:* 15 mg, 30 mg, 60 mg, 120 mg, 180 mg

Dosage

- **Tablets**

Hypothyroidism.

Adults and children, initial: 50 mcg levothyroxine and 12.5 mcg liothyronine (Thyrolar); **then,** at monthly intervals, increments of like amounts can be made until the desired effect is achieved. **Usual maintenance:** 50–100 mcg of levothyroxine and 12.5–25 mcg liothyronine daily.

Congenital hypothyroidism.

Children, 0–6 months: 8–10 mcg T_4/kg/day (25–50 mcg/day); **6–12 months:** 6–8 mcg T_4/kg/day (50–75 mcg/day); **1–5 years:** 5–6 mcg T_4/kg/day (75–100 mcg/day); **6–12 years:** 4–5 mcg T_4/kg/day (100–150 mcg/day); **over 12 years:** 2–3 mcg T_4/kg/day (over 150 mcg/day).

HEALTH CARE CONSIDERATIONS

See also *Health Care Considerations* for *Thyroid Drugs*.

Administration/Storage

1. The initial dose for geriatric clients is ½ the usual adult dose; this can be doubled q 6–8 weeks until desired effect is attained.
2. In children, make dosing increments q 2 weeks until desired response attained.
3. Always do thyroid function tests before initiating dosage changes.
4. Administer as a single dose before breakfast.
5. Protect tablets from light, heat, and moisture.
6. Due to differences in the amounts of hormones between Euthroid and Thyrolar, do not switch brands once started on a particular brand.

Outcome/Evaluate: Thyroid hormone replacement

Lisinopril

(lie-**SIN**-oh-prill)

Pregnancy Category: C

Apo-Lisinopril ✦, Prinivil, Zestril **(Rx)**

Classification: Antihypertensive, ACE inhibitor

See also *Angiotensin-Converting Enzyme Inhibitors*.

Action/Kinetics: Both supine and standing BPs are reduced, although the drug is less effective in blacks than in Caucasians. Although food does not alter the bioavailability of lisinopril, only 25% of a PO dose is absorbed. **Onset:** 1 hr. **Peak serum levels:** 7 hr. **Duration:** 24 hr. **t½:** 12 hr. 100% of the drug is excreted unchanged in the urine.

Uses: Alone or in combination with a diuretic (usually a thiazide) to treat hypertension. In combination with digitalis and a diuretic for treating CHF not responding to other therapy. Use within 24 hr of acute MI to improve survival in hemodynamically stable clients (clients should receive the standard treatment, including thrombolytics, aspirin, and beta blockers).

Special Concerns: Use with caution during lactation. Safety and efficacy have not been established in children. Geriatric clients may manifest higher blood levels. Reduce the dosage in clients with impaired renal function.

Side Effects: *CV:* Hypotension, orthostatic hypotension, angina, tachycardia, palpitations, rhythm disturbances, ***stroke,*** chest pain, orthostatic effects, peripheral edema, ***MI, CVA,*** worsening of heart failure, chest sound abnormalities, PVCs, TIAs, decreased blood pressure, atrial fibrillation. *CNS:* Dizziness, headache, fatigue, vertigo, insomnia, depression, sleepiness, paresthesias, malaise, nervousness, confusion, ataxia, impaired memory, tremor, irritability, hypersomnia, peripheral neuropathy, spasm. *GI:* Diarrhea, N&V, dyspepsia, anorexia, constipation, dysgeusia, dry mouth, abdominal pain, flatulence, dry mouth, gastritis, heartburn, GI cramps, weight loss/gain, taste alterations, increased salivation. *Respiratory:* Cough, dyspnea, bronchitis, upper respiratory symptoms, nasal congestion, sinusitis, pharyngeal pain, ***bronchospasm, asthma,*** pulmonary edema, ***pulmonary embolism, pulmonary infarction,*** paroxysmal nocturnal dyspnea, chest discomfort, common cold, nasal congestion, pulmonary infiltrates, pleural effusion, wheezing, painful respiration, epistaxis, laryngitis, pharyngitis, rhinitis, rhinorrhea, orthopnea. *Musculoskeletal:* Asthenia, muscle cramps, neck/hip/leg/knee/arm/joint/shoulder/back/pelvic/flank pain, myalgia, arthralgia, arthritis, lumbago. *Hepatic:* Hepatitis, hepatocellular/cholestatic jaundice, pancreatitis, hepatomegaly. *Dermatologic:* Rash, pruritus, flushing, increased sweating, urticaria, alopecia, erythema multiforme, photophobia. *GU:* Impotence, oliguria, progressive azotemia, acute renal failure, UTI, anuria, uremia, renal dysfunction, pyelonephritis, dysuria. *Ophthalmic:* Blurred vision, visual loss, diplopia. *Miscellaneous:* ***Angioedema (may be fatal if laryngeal edema occurs),*** hyperkalemia, neutropenia, anemia, ***bone marrow depression,*** decreased libido, fever, syncope, vasculitis of the legs, gout, eosinophilia, fluid overload, dehydration, diabetes mellitus, chills, virus infection, edema, ***anaphylactoid reaction,*** malignant lung neoplasms, hemoptysis, breast pain.

Laboratory Test Considerations: ↑ Serum potassium, BUN, serum creatinine. ↓ H&H.

OD Management of Overdose: *Symptoms:* Hypotension. *Treatment:* Supportive. To correct hypotension, IV normal saline is treatment of choice. Lisinopril may be removed by hemodialysis.

Drug Interactions

Diuretics / Excess ↓ BP

Indomethacin / Possible ↓ effect of lisinopril

Potassium-sparing diuretics / Significant ↑ serum potassium

How Supplied: *Tablet:* 2.5 mg, 5 mg, 10 mg, 20 mg, 40 mg

Dosage

• **Tablets**

Essential hypertension, used alone.

10 mg once daily. Adjust dosage depending on response (range: 20–40 mg/day given as a single dose). Doses greater than 80 mg/day do not give a greater effect.

Essential hypertension in combination with a diuretic.

Initial: 5 mg. The BP-lowering effects of the combination are additive. Reduce dosage in renal impairment.

CHF.

Initial: 5 mg once daily (2.5 mg/day in clients with hyponatremia) in combination with diuretics and digitalis. **Dosage range:** 5–20 mg/day as a single dose.

Acute MI.

First dose: 5 mg; **then,** 5 mg after 24 hr, 10 mg after 48 hr, and then 10 mg daily. Continue dosing for 6 weeks. In clients with a systolic pressure less than 120 mm Hg when treatment is started or within 3 days after the infarct should be given 2.5 mg. If hypotension occurs (systolic BP less than 100 mm Hg), the dose may be temporarily reduced to 2.5 mg. If prolonged hypotension occurs, withdraw the drug.

HEALTH CARE CONSIDERATIONS

See also *Health Care Considerations* for *Angiotensin-Converting Enzyme Inhibitors* and *Antihypertensive Agents.*

Administration/Storage

1. When considering use of lisinopril in a client taking diuretics, discontinue the diuretic, if possible, 2–3 days before beginning lisinopril therapy. If the diuretic cannot be discontinued, the initial dose of lisinopril should be 5 mg; observe closely for at least 2 hr.
2. Maximum antihypertensive effects may not be observed for 2–4 weeks in some.
3. When starting treatment for CHF, give under medical supervision, especially if SBP less than 100 mm Hg.
4. With clients whose BP is controlled with lisinopril, 20 mg plus hydrochlorothiazide 25 mg, given separately should trial Prinzide 12.5 mg or Zestoretic 20–12.5 mg before Prinzide 25 mg or Zestoretic 20–25 mg is used.
5. The maximum recommended daily dose of lisinopril is 80 mg in a single daily dose. Clients usually do not require hydrochlorothiazide in doses exceeding 50 mg/day, especially if combined with other antihypertensives.
6. Use of potassium supplements, potassium-sparing diuretics, or potassium salt substitutes with Prinzide or Zestoretic may lead to increases in serum potassium.
7. Prinzide or Zestoretic is recommended for those with a C_{CR} greater than 30 mL/min.
8. Anticipate reduced dosage with renal insufficiency—initial dose of 10 mg/day if C_{CR} is greater than 30 mL/min, 5 mg/day if C_{CR} is between 10 and 30 mL/min, and 2.5 mg/day in dialysis clients (i.e., C_{CR} less than 10 mL/min).

Assessment

1. Record indications for therapy, agents trialed and the outcome,
2. Perform physical exam noting cardio-pulmonary status, review history for any existing conditions, and assess labs for any organ dysfunction.
3. Obtain ECG, CXR, and baseline labs. Reduce dose with renal dysfunction.

Client/Family Teaching

1. Avoid symptoms of orthostatic hypotension (i.e., rise slowly from sitting or lying position and wait until symptoms subside).
2. Avoid all potassium supplements as well as foods high in potassium.
3. Review drug side effects; report for BP check, ECG, and lab studies.
4. Report any new or unusual side effects or any aggravation of existing conditions.

Outcome/Evaluate

• ↓ BP
• Improved survival with acute MI

COMBINATION DRUG

Lisinopril and Hydrochlorothiazide

(lie-**SIN**-oh-pril, hy-droh-kloh-roh-**THIGH**-ah-zyd)

Pregnancy Category: C

Prinzide, Zestoretic **(Rx)**
Classification: Antihypertensive

See also *Lisinopril* and *Hydrochlorothiazide*.
Content: Lisinopril is an ACE inhibitor and hydrochlorothiazide is a diuretic. Prinzide 12.5 and Zestoretic 20–12.5: Lisinopril, 20 mg, and hydrochlorothiazide, 12.5 mg. Prinzide 25 and Zestoretic 20–25: Lisinopril, 20 mg, and hydrochlorothiazide, 25 mg.
Uses: Hypertension in clients in whom combination therapy is appropriate. Not for initial therapy.
How Supplied: See Content

Dosage
- **Tablets**

  Hypertension.

Individualized. Usual: 1 or 2 tablets once daily of Prinzide 12.5, Prinzide 25, Zestoretic 20–12.5, or Zestoretic 20–25.

HEALTH CARE CONSIDERATIONS

L

See also *Health Care Considerations* for *Antihypertensive Agents, Lisinopril,* and *Hydrochlorothiazide*.
Administration/Storage
1. With clients whose BP is controlled with lisinopril 20 mg plus hydrochlorothiazide 25 mg, given separately, trial Prinzide 12.5 or Zestoretic 20–12.5 before Prinzide 25 or Zestoretic 20–25 mg is used.
2. Maximum recommended daily dose of lisinopril is 80 mg in a single daily dose. Clients usually do not require hydrochlorothiazide in doses exceeding 50 mg/day, especially if combined with other antihypertensives.
3. Use of potassium supplements, potassium-sparing diuretics, or potassium salt substitutes with Prinzide or Zestoretic may lead to increases in serum potassium.
4. Prinzide or Zestoretic is recommended for those with a C_{CR} greater than 30 mL/min.

Client/Family Teaching
1. Take BP and maintain written record for review.
2. Avoid symptoms of orthostatic hypotension (i.e., rise slowly from sitting or lying position and wait until symptoms subside).
3. Avoid all potassium supplements as well as foods high in potassium.
4. Report for BP check, ECG, and labs.
5. Report any new or unusual side effects or any aggravation of existing conditions.

Outcome/Evaluate: Control of hypertension

Lithium carbonate
(LITH-ee-um)
Pregnancy Category: D
Carbolith ✤, Duralith ✤, Eskalith, Eskalith CR, Lithane ✤, Lithobid, Lithonate, Lithotabs, PMS-Lithium Carbonate ✤ **(Rx)**

Lithium citrate
(LITH-ee-um)
Pregnancy Category: D
PMS-Lithium Citrate ✤
Classification: Antipsychotic agent, miscellaneous

Action/Kinetics: Mechanism for the antimanic effect of lithium is unknown. Various hypotheses include: (a) a decrease in catecholamine neurotransmitter levels caused by lithium's effect on Na^+–K^+ ATPase to improve transneuronal membrane transport of sodium ion; (b) a decrease in cyclic AMP levels caused by lithium which decreases sensitivity of hormonal-sensitive adenyl cyclase receptors; or (c) interference by lithium with lipid inositol metabolism ultimately leading to insensitivity of cells in the CNS to stimulation by inositol.

Affects the distribution of calcium, magnesium, and sodium ions and affects glucose metabolism. **Peak serum levels** (regular release): 1–4 hr; (slow-release): 4–6 hr. **Onset:** 5–14 days. **Therapeutic serum levels:** 0.4–1.0 mEq/L (must be carefully monitored because toxic effects may occur at these levels and significant toxic reactions occur at serum lithium levels of 2 mEq/L). **t½ (plasma):** 24 hr (longer in presence of renal impairment and in the elderly). Lithium and sodium are excreted by the same mechanism in the proximal tubule. Thus, to reduce the danger of lithium intoxication, sodium intake must remain at normal levels.
Uses: Control of mania in manic-depressive clients. *Investigational:* To reverse neutropenia induced by cancer chemotherapy, in children with chronic neutropenia, and in AIDs clients receiving AZT. Prophylaxis of cluster headaches. Also for premenstrual tension, alcoholism accompanied by depression, tardive dyskinesia, bulimia, hyperthyroidism, excess ADH secretion, postpartum affective psychosis, corticosteroid-induced psychosis. Lithium succinate, in a topical form, has been used for the treatment of genital herpes and seborrheic dermatitis.
Contraindications: Cardiovascular or renal disease. Brain damage. Dehydration, sodium depletion, clients receiving diuretics. Lactation.
Special Concerns: Safety and efficacy have not been established for children less than 12 years of age. Use with caution in geriatric clients because lithium is more toxic to the CNS in these clients; also, geriatric clients are more likely to develop lithium-induced

goiter and clinical hypothyroidism and are more likely to manifest excessive thirst and larger volumes of urine.

Side Effects: *Due to initial therapy:* Fine hand tremor, polyuria, thirst, transient and mild nausea, general discomfort. The following side effects are dependent on the serum level of lithium. *CV:* Arrhythmia, hypotension, ***peripheral circulatory collapse,*** bradycardia, sinus node dysfunction with severe bradycardia causing syncope; reversible flattening, isoelectricity, or inversion of T waves. *CNS:* Blackout spells, epileptiform seizures, slurred speech, dizziness, vertigo, somnolence, psychomotor retardation, restlessness, sleepiness, confusion, stupor, coma, acute dystonia, startled response, hypertonicity, slowed intellectual functioning, hallucinations, poor memory, tics, cog wheel rigidity, tongue movements. Pseudotumor cerebri leading to increased intracranial pressure and papilledema; if undetected may cause enlargement of the blind spot, constriction of visual fields, and eventual blindness. Diffuse slowing of EEG; widening of frequency spectrum of EEG; disorganization of background rhythm of EEG. *GI:* Anorexia, N&V, diarrhea, dry mouth, gastritis, salivary gland swelling, abdominal pain, excessive salivation, flatulence, indigestion, incontinence of urine or feces, dysgeusia/taste distortion, salty taste, swollen lips, denal caries. *Dermatologic:* Drying and thinning of hair, anesthesia of skin, chronic folliculitis, xerosis cutis, alopecia, exacerbation of psoriasis, acne, angioedema. *Neuromuscular:* Tremor, muscle hyperirritability (fasciculations, twitching, clonic movements), ataxia, choreo-athetotic movements, hyperactive DTRs, polyarthralgia. *GU:* Albuminuria, oliguria, polyuria, glycosuria, decreased C_{CR}, symptoms of nephrogenic diabetes, impotence/sexual dysfunction. *Thyroid:* Euthyroid goiter or hypothyroidism, including myxedema, accompanied by lower T_3 and T_4. *Miscellaneous:* Fatigue, lethargy, dehydration, weight loss, transient scotomata, tightness in chest, hypercalcemia, hyperparathyroidism, thirst, swollen painful joints, fever.

The following symptoms are unrelated to lithium dosage. Transient EEG and ECG changes, leukocytosis, headache, diffuse nontoxic goiter with or without hypothyroidism, transient hyperglycemia, generalized pruritus with or without rash, cutaneous ulcers, albuminuria, worsening of organic brain syndrome, excessive weight gain, edematous swelling of ankles or wrists, thirst or polyuria (may resemble diabetes mellitus), metallic taste, symptoms similar to Raynaud's phenomenon.

Laboratory Test Considerations: False + urinary glucose test (Benedict's), ↑ serum glucose, creatinine kinase. False – or ↓ serum PBI, uric acid; ↑ TSH, I^{131} uptake; ↓ T_3, T4

OD Management of Overdose: *Symptoms:* Symptoms dependent on serum lithium levels. Levels less than 2 mEq/L: N&V, diarrhea, muscle weakness, drowsiness, loss of coordination.

Levels of 2–3 mEq/L: Agitation, ataxia, blackouts, blurred vision, choreoathetoid movements, confusion, dysarthria, fasciculations, giddiness, hyperreflexia, hypertonia, agitation or manic-like behavior, myoclonic twitching or movement of entire limbs, slurred speech, tinnitus, urinary or fecal incontinence, vertigo.

Levels over 3 mEq/L: Complex clinical picture involving multiple organs and organ systems. ***Arrhythmias, coma,*** hypotension, ***peripheral vascular collapse, seizures (focal and generalized),*** spasticity, stupor, twitching of muscle groups.

Treatment: Early symptoms are treated by decreasing the dose or stopping treatment for 24–48 hr:

- Use gastric lavage.
- Restore fluid and electrolyte balance (can use saline) and maintain kidney function.
- Increase lithium excretion by giving aminophylline, mannitol, or urea.
- Prevent infection. Maintain adequate respiration.
- Monitor thyroid function.
- Institute hemodialysis.

Drug Interactions

Acetazolamide / ↓ Lithium effect by ↑ renal excretion
Bumetanide / ↑ Lithium toxicity due to ↓ renal clearance
Carbamazepine / ↑ Risk of lithium toxicity
Diazepam / ↑ Risk of hypothermia
Ethacrynic acid / ↑ Lithium toxicity due to ↓ renal clearance
Fluoxetine / ↑ Serum levels of lithium
Furosemide / ↑ Lithium toxicity due to ↓ renal clearance
Haloperidol / ↑ Risk of neurologic toxicity
Iodide salts / Additive effect to cause hypothyroidism
Mannitol / ↓ Lithium effect by ↑ renal excretion
Mazindol / ↑ Chance of lithium toxicity due to ↑ serum levels
Methyldopa / ↑ Chance of neurotoxic effects with or without ↑ lithium serum levels

Neuromuscular blocking agents / Lithium ↑ effect of these agents → severe respiratory depression and apnea
NSAIDs / ↓ Renal clearance of lithium, possibly due to inhibition of renal prostaglandin synthesis
Phenothiazines / ↓ Levels of phenothiazines or ↑ lithium levels
Phenytoin / ↑ Chance of lithium toxicity
Probenecid / ↑ Chance of lithium toxicity due to ↑ serum levels
Sodium chloride / Excretion of lithium is proportional to amount of sodium chloride ingested; if client is on salt-free diet, may develop lithium toxicity since less lithium excreted
Sympathomimetics / ↓ Pressor effect of sympathomimetics
Theophyllines, including Aminophylline / ↓ Effect of lithium due to ↑ renal excretion
Thiazide diuretics, triamterene / ↑ Chance of lithium toxicity due to ↓ renal clearance
Tricyclic antidepressants / ↑ Effect of tricyclic antidepressants
Urea / ↓ Lithium effect by ↑ renal excretion
Urinary alkalinizers / ↓ Lithium effect by ↑ renal excretion
Verapamil / ↓ Lithium levels and toxicity

How Supplied: Lithium carbonate: *Capsule:* 150 mg, 300 mg, 600 mg; *Tablet:* 300 mg; *Tablet, Extended Release:* 300 mg, 450 mg; Lithium citrate: *Syrup:* 300 mg/5 mL

Dosage

• **Capsules, Tablets, Extended-Release Tablets, Syrup**

Acute mania.

Adults: Individualized and according to lithium serum level (not to exceed 1.4 mEq/L) and clinical response. **Usual initial:** 300–600 mg t.i.d. or 600–900 mg b.i.d. of slow-release form; **elderly and debilitated clients:** 0.6–1.2 g/day in three doses. **Maintenance:** 300 mg t.i.d.–q.i.d.

Administration of drug is discontinued when lithium serum level exceeds 1.2 mEq/L and resumed 24 hr after it has fallen below that level.

To reverse neutropenia.

300–1,000 mg/day (to achieve serum levels of 0.5–1.0 mEq/L) for 7–10 days.

Prophylaxis of cluster headaches.

600–900 mg/day.

HEALTH CARE CONSIDERATIONS

Administration/Storage

1. To prevent toxic serum levels, determine blood levels 1–2 times/week during initiation of therapy, and monthly thereafter, on blood samples taken 8–12 hr after dosage.
2. Full beneficial drug effects may not be noted for 6–10 days.

Assessment

1. Conduct a drug history; determine if taking other medications likely to interact.
2. With arthritic conditions, document anti-inflammatory agent use.
3. Monitor thyroid function studies; assess for decreased function.
4. Record mental status; monitor CV function, chemistry, urinalysis, weight, and ECG.

Client/Family Teaching

1. Take with food or immediately after meals. Avoid any caffeinated beverages/foods because these may aggravate mania.
2. Report any persistent diarrhea; may need supplemental fluids or salt.
3. Maintain a constant level of salt intake to avoid fluctuations in lithium activity. Weight gain and edema may be related to sodium retention; report if excessive.
4. Drink 10–12 glasses of water each day; avoid dehydration (e.g., vigorous exercise, sunbathing, sauna) to prevent increased concentrations of lithium in urine.
5. Review goals of therapy, drug interactions and side effects. Report diarrhea, vomiting with drowsiness, muscular weakness, or lack of coordination.
6. Do not engage in physical activities that require alertness or physical coordination until drug effects are realized; may cause drowsiness.
7. Will take several weeks to realize a behavioral benefit from therapy.
8. Do not change brands of drug. Avoid all OTCs unless prescribed.
9. Lithium works well in the manic phase; use with antidepressant may be necessary during depressive phases.
10. Transient acneiform eruptions, folliculitis, and altered sexual function in men may occur.
11. Carry name and telephone number of persons to contact if needed or if family members note behavioral changes or physical changes contrary to expectations. Carry ID, noting diagnosis and prescribed meds.

Outcome/Evaluate

- Stabilization of mood swings
- ↓ Symptoms of mania (↓ hyperactivity, ↓ sleeplessness, and improved judgment)
- Therapeutic serum drug levels (0.4–1.0 mEq/L)

Lodoxamide tromethamine

(loh-**DOX**-ah-myd)

Pregnancy Category: B

Alomide **(Rx)**

Classification: Antiallergenic ophthalmic

Action/Kinetics: Mast cell stabilizer that prevents the release of mast cell inflammatory mediators, including slow-reacting substances of anaphylaxis (peptidoleukotrienes), and inhibits eosinophil chemotaxis. Beneficial effect may be due to prevention of calcium influx into mast cells upon stimulation by antigens. **Elimination t½:** 8.5 hr. Excreted mainly through the urine.
Uses: To treat ocular disorders such as vernal keratoconjunctivitis, vernal conjunctivitis, and vernal keratitis.
Contraindications: Use in clients wearing soft contact lenses.
Special Concerns: Use with caution during lactation. The drug is for ophthalmic use only and should not be injected. Safety and efficacy have not been determined for use in children less than 2 years of age.
Side Effects: *Ophthalmologic:* Transient burning, stinging, or discomfort upon instillation. Ocular itching or pruritus, blurred vision, dry eye, tearing, discharge from eyes, hyperemia, crystalline deposits in eye, foreign body sensation, corneal erosion or ulcer, scales on lid or lash, eye pain, ocular edema or swelling, ocular warming sensation, ocular fatigue, chemosis, corneal abrasion, anterior chamber cells, keratopathy, keratitis, blepharitis, allergy, sticky sensation, epitheliopathy. *CNS:* Headache, dizziness, somnolence. *GI:* Nausea, stomach discomfort. *Miscellaneous:* Heat sensation, sneezing, dry nose, rash.
How Supplied: *Solution:* 0.1%

Dosage

- **Ophthalmic Solution**

Ocular disorders.

Adults and children over 2 years of age: 1–2 gtt in each affected eye q.i.d. for up to 3 months.

HEALTH CARE CONSIDERATIONS

Assessment: Determine onset and symptoms; list other agents trialed.

Client/Family Teaching

1. Review appropriate method and frequency for administration. Some stinging and burning may be evident on instillation; report if symptoms persist after instillation.
2. Soft contact lenses *cannot* be worn during therapy.

Outcome/Evaluate: ↓ Ocular inflammation

Lomefloxacin hydrochloride

(loh-meh-FLOX-ah-sin)
Pregnancy Category: C
Maxaquin **(Rx)**
Classification: Antibacterial, fluoroquinolone derivative

See also *Fluoroquinolones.*
Action/Kinetics: Mean peak plasma levels: 4.2 mcg/mL after a 400-mg dose. The rate and extent of absorption are decreased if taken with food. **t½:** 8 hr. Metabolized in the liver with 65% excreted unchanged through the urine and 10% excreted unchanged in the feces.
Uses: Acute bacterial exacerbation of chronic bronchitis caused by *Haemophilus influenzae* or *Morazella catarrhalis.* Uncomplicated UTIs due to *Escherichia coli, Klebsiella pneumoniae, Proteus mirabilis,* or *Staphylococcus saprophyticus.* Complicated UTIs due to *E. coli, K. pneumoniae, P. mirabilis, Pseudomonas aeruginosa, Citrobacter diversus,* or *Enterobacter cloacae.* Preoperatively to decrease the incidence of UTIs 3–5 days after surgery in clients undergoing transurethral procedures. Uncomplicated gonococcal infections. Prevent infection in preoperative transrectal prostate biopsy.
Contraindications: Use in minor urologic procedures for which prophylaxis is not indicated (e.g., simple cystoscopy, retrograde pyelography). Use for the empiric treatment of acute bacterial exacerbation of chronic bronchitis due to *Streptococcus pneumoniae.* Lactation.
Special Concerns: Plasma clearance is reduced in the elderly. Safety and efficacy have not been determined in children less than 18 years of age. Serious hypersensitivity reactions that are occasionally fatal have occurred, even with the first dose. No dosage adjustment is needed for elderly clients with normal renal function. Not efficiently removed from the body by hemodialysis or peritoneal dialysis.
Laboratory Test Considerations: ↑ ALT, AST, alkaline phosphatase, bilirubin, BUN, gamma-glutamyltransferase. ↑ or ↓ Potassium. Abnormalities of urine specific gravity or serum electrolytes.
Additional Side Effects: *CNS:* Confusion, tremor, vertigo, nervousness, anxiety, hyperkinesia, anorexia, agitation, increased appetite, depersonalization, paranoia, ***coma.*** *GI:* GI inflammation or bleeding, dysphagia, tongue discoloration, bad taste in mouth. *GU:* Dysuria, hematuria, micturition disorder, anuria, strangury, leukorrhea, intermenstrual bleeding perineal pain, vaginal moniliasis, orchitis, epididymitis, proteinuria, albuminuria. *Hypersensitivity Reactions:* Urticaria, itching, pharyngeal or facial edema, ***CV collapse,*** tin-

gling, loss of consciousness, dyspnea. *CV:* Hypotension, tachycardia, bradycardia, extrasystoles, cyanosis, ***arrhythmia, cardiac failure,*** angina pectoris, ***MI, pulmonary embolism, cardiomyopathy,*** phlebitis, cerebrovascular disorder. *Respiratory:* Dyspnea, respiratory infection, epistaxis, ***bronchospasm,*** cough, increased sputum, respiratory disorder, stridor. *Hematologic:* Eosinophilia, leukopenia, increase or decrease in platelets, increase in ESR, lymphocytopenia, decreased hemoglobin, anemia, bleeding, increased PT, increase in monocytes. *Dermatologic:* Urticaria, eczema, skin exfoliation, skin disorder. *Ophthalmologic:* Conjunctivitis, eye pain. *Otic:* Earache, tinnitus. *Musculoskeletal:* Back or chest pain, asthenia, leg cramps, arthralgia, myalgia. *Miscellaneous:* Increase or decrease in blood glucose, flushing, increased sweating, facial edema, influenza-like symptoms, decreased heat tolerance, purpura, lymphadenopathy, increased fibrinolysis, thirst, gout, hypoglycemia, phototoxicity.

How Supplied: *Tablet:* 400 mg

L

Dosage

- **Tablets**

Acute bacterial exacerbation of chronic bronchitis. Cystitis.

Adults: 400 mg once daily for 10 days.

Complicated UTIs.

Adults: 400 mg once daily for 14 days.

Uncomplicated UTIs.

400 mg once daily for 3 days.

Prophylaxis of infection before surgery for transurethral procedures.

Single 400-mg dose 2–6 hr before surgery.

Uncomplicated gonococcal infections.

400 mg as a single dose (as an alternative to ciprofloxacin or ofloxacin).

HEALTH CARE CONSIDERATIONS

See also *General Health Care Considerations for All Anti-Infectives* and *Fluoroquinolones.*

Administration/Storage

1. May take without regard for meals.
2. Dosage modification is required for clients with C_{CR} less than 40 mL/min/1.73 m^2 and more than 10 mL/min/1.73 m^2. Following an initial loading dose of 40 mg, give daily maintenance doses of 200 mg for the duration of treatment. Assess lomefloxacin levels to determine any need to alter dosing interval. Follow this same regimen for clients on hemodialysis.

Assessment

1. Record indications for therapy, type and onset of symptoms.
2. Obtain cultures and renal function studies; modify dosage with renal dysfunction.

Outcome/Evaluate

- UTI prophylaxis
- Symptomatic relief
- Improved breathing patterns

Lomustine

(loh-**MUS**-teen)

Pregnancy Category: D

CeeNu (Abbreviation: CCNU) **(Rx)**

Classification: Antineoplastic, alkylating agent

See also *Antineoplastic Agents* and *Alkylating Agents.*

Action/Kinetics: Alkylating agent that inhibits DNA and RNA synthesis through DNA alkylation. It also affects other cellular processes, includling RNA, protein synthesis and the processing of ribosomal and nucleoplasmic messenger RNA; DNA base component structure; the rate of DNA synthesis and DNA polymerase activity. Is cell cycle nonspecific. Rapidly absorbed from the GI tract; crosses the blood-brain barrier resulting in concentrations higher than in plasma. **Peak plasma level:** 1–6 hr; **t½:** biphasic; **initial,** 6 hr; **postdistribution:** 1–2 days. From 15% to 20% of drug remains in body after 5 days. Fifty percent of drug excreted within 12 hr through the kidney, 75% within 4 days. Small amounts are excreted through the lungs and feces. Metabolites present in milk.

Uses: Used alone or in combination to treat primary and metastatic brain tumors. Secondary therapy in Hodgkin's disease (in combination with other antineoplastics).

Contraindications: Lactation.

Laboratory Test Considerations: ↑ LFTs (reversible).

Additional Side Effects: High incidence of N&V 3–6 hr after administration and lasting for 24 hr. Renal and pulmonary toxicity. Dysarthria. ***Delayed bone marrow suppression*** may occur due to cumulative bone marrow toxicity. ***Thrombocytopenia and leukopenia may lead to bleeding and overwhelming infections.*** Secondary malignancies.

How Supplied: *Capsule:* 10 mg, 40 mg, 100 mg

Dosage

- **Capsules**

Adults and children, initial: 130 mg/m^2 as a single dose q 6 weeks. If bone marrow function is reduced, decrease dose to 100 mg/m^2 q 6 weeks. Subsequent dosage based on blood counts of clients (platelet count above 100,000/mm^3 and leukocyte count above 4,000/mm^3). Undertake weekly blood tests and do not repeat therapy before 6 weeks.

HEALTH CARE CONSIDERATIONS

See also *Health Care Considerations* for *Antineoplastic Agents.*

Administration/Storage

1. Store below 40°C (104°F).
2. Given alone or in combination with other drugs, surgery, or XRT.
3. Causes platelet and leukocyte suppression. Nadir: 3–7 weeks.

Client/Family Teaching

1. Medication comes in capsules of three strengths and a combination of capsules will make up the correct dose; take all at one time.
2. May have N&V up to 36 hr after treatment; may be followed by 2–3 days of anorexia. Take antiemetics as prescribed. GI distress may be reduced by taking antiemetics before drug administration or by taking the drug after fasting.
3. Report feelings of depression caused by prolonged N&V so that various antiemetics can be tried and to ensure that psychological support is available as needed.
4. Report abnormal bruising or bleeding, sore throat or flu symptoms.
5. Avoid all OTC agents.
6. Intervals of 6 weeks are necessary between doses for optimum effect with minimal toxicity; hematologic profiles should be assessed weekly.

Outcome/Evaluate: Control/remission of metastatic processes

Loperamide hydrochloride

(loh-**PER**-ah-myd)

Pregnancy Category: B

Apo-Loperamide ✱, Diarr-Eze ✱, Imodium, Imodium A-D Caplets, Kaopectate II Caplets, Loperacap ✱, Maalox Anti-Diarrheal Caplets, Novo-Loperamide ✱, Pepto Diarrhea Control, PMS-Loperamide Hydrochloride ✱ (Imodium is Rx, all others are OTC)

Classification: Antidiarrheal agent, systemic

Action/Kinetics: Slows intestinal motility by acting on the nerve endings and/or intramural ganglia embedded in the intestinal wall. The prolonged retention of the feces in the intestine results in reducing the volume of the stools, increasing viscosity, and decreasing fluid and electrolyte loss. Reportedly more effective than diphenoxylate. **Time to peak effect, capsules:** 5 hr; **PO solution:** 2.5 hr. **t½:** 9.1–14.4 hr. Twenty-five percent excreted unchanged in the feces.

Uses: Rx: Symptomatic relief of acute nonspecific diarrhea and of chronic diarrhea associated with inflammatory bowel disease. Decrease the volume of discharge from ileostomies.

OTC: Control symptoms of diarrhea, including traveler's diarrhea. *Investigational:* With trimethoprim-sulfamethoxazole to treat traveler's diarrhea.

Contraindications: In clients in whom constipation should be avoided. OTC if body temperature is over 101°F (38°C) and in presence of bloody diarrhea. Use in acute diarrhea associated with organisms that penetrate the intestinal mucosa, such as *E. coli, Salmonella,* and Shigella.

Special Concerns: Safe use in children under 2 years of age and during lactation has not been established. Fluid and electrolyte depletion may occur in clients with diarrhea. Children less than 3 years of age are more sensitive to the narcotic effects of loperamide.

Side Effects: *GI:* Abdominal pain, distention, or discomfort. Constipation, dry mouth, N&V, epigastric distress. Toxic megacolon in clients with acute colitis. *CNS:* Drowsiness, dizziness, fatigue. *Other:* Allergic skin rashes.

OD Management of Overdose: *Symptoms:* Constipation, CNS depression, GI irritation. *Treatment:* Give activated charcoal (it will reduce absorption up to ninefold). If vomiting has not occurred, perform gastric lavage followed by activated charcoal, 100 g, through a gastric tube. Give naloxone for respiratory depression.

How Supplied: *Capsule:* 2 mg; *Liquid:* 1 mg/5 mL; *Tablet:* 2 mg

Dosage

- **Rx Capsules, Liquid**

Acute diarrhea.

Adults, initial: 4 mg, followed by 2 mg after each unformed stool, up to maximum of 16 mg/day. **Pediatric:** *Day 1 doses:* **8–12 years:** 2 mg t.i.d.; **6–8 years:** 2 mg b.i.d.; **2–5 years:** 1 mg t.i.d. using only the liquid. *After day 1:* 1 mg/10 kg after a loose stool (total daily dosage should not exceed day 1 recommended doses).

Chronic diarrhea.

Adults: 4–8 mg/day as a single or divided dose. Dosage not established for chronic diarrhea in children.

- **OTC Oral Solution, Tablets**

Acute diarrhea.

Adults: 4 mg after the first loose bowel movement followed by 2 mg after each subsequent bowel movement to a maximum of 8 mg/day for no more than 2 days. **Pediatric,**

L

9–11 years: 2 mg after the first loose bowel movement followed by 1 mg after each subsequent loose bowel movement, not to exceed 6 mg/day for no more than 2 days. **Pediatric, 6–8 years:** 1 mg after the first bowel movement followed by 1 mg after each subsequent loose bowel movement, not to exceed 4 mg/day for no more than 2 days.

HEALTH CARE CONSIDERATIONS

Assessment

1. Note any allergy to piperidine derivatives.
2. Record indications for therapy, onset, frequency, and duration of symptoms. Identify any contributing causative factors.
3. Discontinue drug promptly and report if abdominal distention develops in clients with acute ulcerative colitis.

Client/Family Teaching

1. May cause a dry mouth; try ice, sugarless gum, and candy to alleviate.
2. Use caution while driving or performing tasks requiring alertness; may cause dizziness/drowsiness.
3. OTC products are not intended for use in children less than 6 years of age unless physician prescribed.
4. Record the number, frequency, and consistency of stools per day and the amount of medication consumed. Report if diarrhea lasts up to 5 days without relief.
5. In *acute diarrhea,* discontinue after 48 hr and report if ineffective.
6. If no improvement within 10 days after using up to 16 mg/day for *chronic diarrhea,* symptoms are not likely to improve with further use. Seek medical intervention.
7. Report if fever, nausea, abdominal pain, or abdominal distention occurs; may require dosage adjustment.
8. Dietary treatment of diarrhea is preferred, if possible, in children (avoid apple juices, high-fat and highly spiced foods).

Outcome/Evaluate: ↓ Diarrhea

Loracarbef

(lor-ah-KAR-bef)
Pregnancy Category: B
Lorabid **(Rx)**
Classification: Beta-lactam antibiotic

See also *Anti-Infectives.*

Action/Kinetics: Related chemically to cephalosporins. Acts by inhibiting cell wall synthesis. Stable in the presence of certain bacterial beta-lactamases. **Average peak plasma levels:** 8 mcg/mL following a single 200-mg dose in a fasting subject after 90 min and 14 mcg/mL following a single 400-mg dose in a fasting subject after 90 min. Following doses of 7.5 mg/kg and 15 mg/kg of the oral suspension to children, average peak plasma levels were 13 and 19 mcg/mL, respectively, within 40–60 min. **Elimination t½:** 1 hr (increased to 5.6 hr in clients with a C_{CR} from 10 to 50 mL/min/1.73 m^2 and to 32 hr in clients with a C_{CR} of less than 10 mL/min/1.73 m^2). Over 90% excreted unchanged in the urine.

Uses: Secondary bacterial infections of acute bronchitis and acute bacterial exacerbations of chronic bronchitiscaused by *Streptococcus pneumoniae, Haemophilus influenzae,* or *Morazella catarrhalis* (including beta-lactamase-producing strains of both organisms). Pneumonia caused by *S. pneumoniae* or *H. influenzae* (only non-beta-lactamase-producing strains). Otitis media caused by *S. pneumoniae, Streptococcus pyogenes, H. influenzae,* or *M. catarrhalis* (including beta-lactamase-producing strains of both organisms). Acute maxillary sinusitis caused by *S. pneumoniae, H. influenzae* (only non-beta-lactamase-producing strains), or *M. catarrhalis* (including beta-lactamase-producing strains). Pharyngitis and tonsillitis caused by *S. pyogenes.* Uncomplicated skin and skin structure infections caused by *Staphylococcus aureus* (including penicillinase-producing strains) or *S. pyogenes.* Uncomplicated UTIs caused by *Escherichia coli* or *Staphylococcus saprophyticus.* Uncomplicated pyelonephritis caused by *E. coli.*

Contraindications: Hypersensitivity to loracarbef or cephalosporin-class antibiotics.

Special Concerns: Use during labor and delivery only if clearly needed. Pseudomembranous colitis is possible with most antibacterial agents. Use with caution and at reduced dosage in clients with impaired renal function, in those with a history of colitis, in clients receiving concurrent treatment with potent diuretics, during lactation, and in clients with known penicillin allergies. Safety and efficacy in children less than 6 months of age have not been determined.

Side Effects: The incidence of certain side effects is different in the pediatric population compared with the adult population. *GI:* Diarrhea, N&V, abdominal pain, anorexia, pseudomembranous colitis. *Hypersensitivity:* Skin rashes, urticaria, pruritus, erythema multiforme. *CNS:* Headache, somnolence, nervousness, insomnia, dizziness. *Hematologic:* Transient thrombocytopenia, leukopenia, eosinophilia. *Miscellaneous:* Vasodilation, vaginitis, vaginal moniliasis, rhinitis.

OD **Management of Overdose:** *Symptoms:* N&V, epigastric distress, diarrhea. *Treatment:* Hemodialysis may be effective in increasing the elimination of loracarbef from plasma from clients with chronic renal failure.

Drug Interactions

Diuretics, potent / ↑ Risk of renal dysfunction

Probenecid / ↓ Renal excretion resulting in ↑ plasma levels of loracarbef

How Supplied: *Capsule:* 200 mg, 400 mg; *Powder for reconstitution:* 100 mg/5 mL, 200 mg/5 mL

Dosage

- **Capsules, Oral Suspension**

Secondary bacterial infection of acute bronchitis.

Adults 13 years of age and older: 200–400 mg q 12 hr for 7 days.

Acute bacterial exacerbation of chronic bronchitis.

Adults 13 years of age and older: 400 mg q 12 hr for 7 days.

Pneumonia.

Adults 13 years of age and older: 400 q 12 hr for 14 days.

Pharyngitis, tonsillitis.

Adults 13 years of age and older: 200 mg q 12 hr for 10 days (longer for *S. pyogenes* infections). **Infants and children, 6 months–12 years:** 15 mg/kg/day in divided doses q 12 hr for 10 days (longer for *S. pyogenes* infections).

Sinusitis.

Adults 13 years of age and older: 400 mg q 12 hr for 10 days.

Acute otitis media, Acute maxillary sinusitis.

Infants and children, 6 months–12 years: 30 mg/kg/day in divided doses q 12 hr for 10 days. Use the suspension as it is more rapidly absorbed than the capsules, resulting in higher peak plasma levels when given at the same dose.

Skin and skin structure infections (impetigo).

Adults: 200 mg q 12 hr for 7 days. **Infants and children, 6 months–12 years:** 15 mg/kg/day in divided doses q 12 hr for 7 days.

Uncomplicated cystitis.

Adults 13 years of age and older: 200 mg q 24 hr for 7 days.

Uncomplicated pyelonephritis.

Adults 13 years of age and older: 400 mg q 12 hr for 14 days.

HEALTH CARE CONSIDERATIONS

See also *General Health Care Considerations for All Anti-Infectives.*

Administration/Storage

1. The manufacturer provides a chart to assist with establishing the dosage regimen for pediatric clients.
2. Clients with C_{CR} levels of 10–49 mL/min may be given one-half the recommended dose at the usual dosage interval. Clients with C_{CR} less than 10 mL/min may be treated with the recommended dose given every 3–5 days. Clients on hemodialysis should receive another dose following dialysis.
3. Reconstitute the oral suspension by adding 30 mL water to the 50-mL bottle or 60 mL water to the 100-mL bottle. After mixing, the suspension may be kept at room temperature for 14 days without significant loss of potency. Keep tightly closed and discard any unused portion after 14 days.

Assessment

1. Record indications for therapy and any sensitivity to cephalosporins and penicillin derivatives.
2. List drugs currently prescribed to ensure none interact unfavorably.
3. Obtain baseline cultures and renal function studies. Adjust dosage with dysfunction.

Client/Family Teaching

1. Take at least 1 hr before or at least 2 hr after meals. Complete entire prescription.
2. Report persistent diarrhea, which may be secondary to pseudomembranous colitis and requires medical intervention.
3. Lack of response or worsening of symptoms as well as any unusual side effects should be reported.

Outcome/Evaluate

- Negative C&S reports
- Relief of ear/throat pain
- Improved breathing patterns
- Evidence of wound healing

Loratidine

(loh-**RAH**-tih-deen)

Pregnancy Category: B

Claritin, Claritin Reditabs **(Rx)**

Classification: Antihistamine

See also *Antihistamines.*

Action/Kinetics: Metabolized in the liver to active metabolite descarboethoxyloratidine. Low to no sedative and anticholinergic effects. Does not alter cardiac repolarization and has not been linked to development of

L

torsades de pointes as seen with astemizole and terfenadine. **Onset:** 1–3 hr. **Maximum effect:** 8–12 hr. Food delays absorption. **t½, loratidine:** 8.4 hr; **t½, descarboethoxyloratidine:** 28 hr. **Duration:** 24 hr. Excreted through both the urine and feces.
Uses: Relief of nasal and nonnasal symptoms of seasonal allergic rhinitis, including runny nose, itchy and watery eyes, itchy palate, and sneezing. Treatment of chronic idiopathic urticaria in clients 6 years of age and older.
Special Concerns: Use with caution, if at all, during lactation. Give a lower initial dose in liver impairment. Safety and efficacy have not been determined in children less than 2 years of age.
Side Effects: Most commonly, headache, somnolence, fatigue, and dry mouth. *GI:* Altered salivation, gastritis, dyspepsia, stomatitis, tooth ache, thirst, altered taste, flatulence. *CNS:* Hypoesthesia, hyperkinesia, migraine, anxiety, depression, agitation, paroniria, amnesia, impaired concentration. *Ophthalmologic:* Altered lacrimation, conjunctivitis, blurred vision, eye pain, blepharospasm. *Respiratory:* Upper respiratory infection, epistaxis, pharyngitis, dyspnea, coughing, rhinitis, sinusitis, sneezing, bronchitis, ***bronchospasm,*** hemoptysis, laryngitis. *Body as a whole:* Asthenia, increased sweating, flushing, malaise, rigors, fever, dry skin, aggravated allergy, pruritus, purpura. *Musculoskeletal:* Back/chest pain, leg cramps, arthralgia, myalgia. *GU:* Breast pain, menorrhagia, dysmenorrhea, vaginitis. *Miscellaneous:* Earache, dysphonia, dry hair, urinary discoloration.
How Supplied: *Syrup:* 5 mg/5 mL; *Tablet:* 10 mg

Dosage

- **Syrup, Tablets**

Allergic rhinitis, chronic idiopathic urticaria.

Adults and children over 12 years of age: 10 mg once daily on an empty stomach. **Children, 6 to 11 years of age:** 10 mg (10 mL) once daily. *In clients with impaired liver function (GFR less than 30 mL/min):* 10 mg every other day.

HEALTH CARE CONSIDERATIONS

See also *Health Care Considerations* for *Antihistamines*.

Administration/Storage

1. Use the syrup or rapid-distintegrating tablets for children 6 to 11 years of age.
2. Use caution. The concentration of the syrup is 10 mg/10 mL.

Assessment

1. Record indications for therapy, type, onset, and duration of symptoms. List other agents trialed and the outcome.
2. Monitor LFTs; reduce dose with dysfunction. Assess the elderly and clients with hepatic and renal impairment for increasing somnolence.
3. Record pulmonary findings; assess throat, nodes, and turbinates.
4. Perform a drug profile. Cautiously coadminister with drugs that inhibit hepatic metabolism (i.e., macrolide antibiotics, cimetidine, ranitidine, ketoconazole, or theophylline).

Client/Family Teaching

1. Take on an empty stomach; food may delay absorption.
2. If using rapid-disintegrating tablets, place under the tongue. Disintegration occurs within seconds, after which the tablet contents may be swallowed with or without water.
3. Use rapid-disintegrating tablets within 6 months of opening the foil pouch and immediately after opening the individual tablet blister.
4. Do not perform activities that require mental alertness until drug effects realized; should not cause drowsiness.
5. Identify triggers, i.e., foods, detergents, or materials that may have induced urticarial response.

Outcome/Evaluate

- Relief of nasal congestion and seasonal allergic manifestations
- Control of skin eruption R/T antigenic offender

COMBINATION DRUG

Loratidine and Pseudoephedrine sulfate

(loh-**RAH**-tih-deen, **soo**-doh-eh-**FED**-rin)
Pregnancy Category: B
Chlor-Tripolon N.D. ✤, Claritin-D, Claritin-D 24 Hour Extended Release Tablets, Claritin-D 24 hour, Claritin Extra ✤ **(Rx)**
Classification: Antihistamine/decongestant

See also *Loratidine* and *Pseudoephedrine sulfate.*
Content: Each tablet of Claritin-D contains: *Antihistamine:* Loratidine, 5 mg. *Decongestant:* Pseudoephedrine sulfate, 120 mg. The product is formulated such that loratidine is released immediately and pseudoephedrine is released both immediately and over time.

Each tablet of Claritin-D 24 Hour Extended Release contains: *Antihistamine:* Loratidine, 10 mg. *Decongestant:* Pseudoephedrine sulfate, 240 mg. Tablet Extended Relaease 10 mg-240 mg.

Uses: To relieve symptoms of seasonal allergic rhinitis, including those with asthma.
Contraindications: Clients with narrow-angle glaucoma or urinary retention and in those receiving MAO inhibitors and within 14 days of such treatment. In clients with severe hypertension, severe CAD, hepatic insufficiency, and hypersensitivity to the components. In those who have difficulty swallowing due to possibility of upper GI tract obstruction.
Special Concerns: Use with caution in clients with hypertension, diabetes mellitus, ischemic heart disease, increased intraocular pressure, hyperthyroidism, renal impairment, or prostatic hypertrophy. The safety and efficacy in clients over 60 years of age and below 12 years of age have not been determined. Use with caution during lactation.
Side Effects: See individual components. The most common side effects for this product are: *CNS:* Headache, insomnia, somnolence, nervousness, dizziness, fatigue. *GI:* Dry mouth, dyspepsia, nausea. *Miscellaneous:* Pharyngitis, anorexia, thirst.
How Supplied: See Content

Dosage

- **Tablets**

  Allergic rhinitis.

Adults and children over 12 years of age: 1 tablet q 12 hr given on an empty stomach. Clients with a GFR less than 30 mL/min should receive 1 tablet daily.

- **Extended Release Tablets**

  Allergic rhinitis.

Adults: One 24 Hour Extended Release Tablet daily.

HEALTH CARE CONSIDERATIONS

See also *Health Care Considerations* for *Antihistamines* and individual agents.
Administration/Storage: Store away from heat, moisture, and direct light.
Assessment
1. List indications for therapy.
2. Note any history of hypertension, CAD, and renal and hepatic dysfunction.
3. Drug is contraindicated with glaucoma, MAO therapy (or within 14 days of stopping), urinary retention, and seizures.
4. Monitor blood pressure throughout long-term therapy.

Client/Family Teaching
1. May take with food or milk to decrease GI upset.
2. Take in the morning upon first arising to prevent bedtime insomnia.
3. Drug may cause nervousness and dizziness; do not perform activities that require mental and physical alertness until drug effects realized.
4. Avoid alcohol, CNS depressants, and any OTC agents for sleep or pain.

Outcome/Evaluate: Relief of nasal and sinus allergy S&S

Lorazepam

(lor-**AYZ**-eh-pam)
Pregnancy Category: D
Apo-Lorazepam ✱, Ativan, Lorazepam Intensol, Novo-Lorazem ✱, Nu-Loraz ✱, PMS-Lorazepam ✱, Pro-Lorazepam ✱ **(C-IV) (Rx)**
Classification: Antianxiety agent, benzodiazepine

See also *Tranquilizers, Antimanic Drugs, and Hypnotics.*
Action/Kinetics: Absorbed and eliminated faster than other benzodiazepines. **Peak plasma levels: PO,** 1–6 hr; **IM,** 1–1.5 hr. **t½:** 10–20 hr. Metabolized to inactive compounds, which are excreted through the kidneys.
Uses: PO: Anxiety, tension, anxiety with depression, insomnia, acute alcohol withdrawal symptoms. **Parenteral:** Amnesic agent, anticonvulsant, antitremor drug, adjunct to skeletal muscle relaxants, preanesthetic medication, adjunct prior to endoscopic procedures, treatment of status epilepticus, relief of acute alcohol withdrawal symptoms. *Investigational:* Antiemetic in cancer chemotherapy.
Additional Contraindications: Narrow-angle glaucoma. Parenterally in children less than 18 years.
Special Concerns: PO dosage has not been established in children less than 12 years of age and IV dosage has not been established in children less than 18 years of age. Use cautiously in presence of renal and hepatic disease.
Additional Drug Interactions: With parenteral lorazepam, scopolamine → sedation, hallucinations, and behavioral abnormalities.
How Supplied: *Concentrate:* 2 mg/mL; *Injection:* 2 mg/mL, 4 mg/mL; *Tablet:* 0.5 mg, 1 mg, 2 mg

Dosage

- **Tablets, Concentrate**

  Anxiety.

Adults: 1–3 mg b.i.d.–t.i.d.

Hypnotic.

Adults: 2–4 mg at bedtime. **Geriatric/debilitated clients, initial:** 0.5–2 mg/day in divided doses. Dose can be adjusted as required.

- **IM**

Preoperatively.

Adults: 0.05 mg/kg up to maximum of 4 mg 2 hr before surgery for maximum amnesic effect.

- **IV**

Preoperatively.

Adults, initial: 0.044 mg/kg or a total dose of 2 mg, whichever is less.

Amnesic effect.

Adults: 0.05 mg/kg up to a maximum of 4 mg administered 15–20 min prior to surgery.

Antiemetic in cancer chemotherapy.

Initial: 2 mg 30 min before beginning chemotherapy; **then,** 2 mg q 4 hr as needed.

HEALTH CARE CONSIDERATIONS

See also *Health Care Considerations* for *Tranquilizers, Antimanic Drugs, and Hypnotics.*

Administration/Storage

1. If higher doses are required, increase the evening dose before the daytime doses.

IV 2. For IV use, dilute just before use with equal amounts of either sterile water for injection, NaCl injection, or 5% dextrose injection.

3. Do not exceed an IV rate of 2 mg/min.

4. Do not use if solution is discolored or contains a precipitate.

Assessment

1. Record indications for therapy, onset, and duration of symptoms. Assess mental status; describe characteristics of anxiety.

2. List other agents used to treat this condition and the outcome.

Client/Family Teaching

1. Take only as directed; report loss of effectiveness.

2. Drug may cause dizziness and drowsiness; use with caution until drug effects realized.

3. Report immediately any increased depression or suicidal ideations.

4. Avoid alcohol and any other CNS depressants.

5. With long-term therapy, do not stop suddenly. Drug should be tapered by provider to prevent withdrawal symptoms.

Outcome/Evaluate

- ↓ Levels of anxiety, tension, and depression
- Control of alcohol withdrawal
- Muscle relaxation/amnesia

Losartan potassium

(loh-SAR-tan)

Pregnancy Category: C (first trimester), D (second and third trimesters)

Cozaar **(Rx)**

Classification: Antihypertensive, angiotensin II receptor antagonist

See also *Antihypertensive Agents.*

Action/Kinetics: Angiotensin II, a potent vasoconstrictor, is the primary vasoactive hormone of the renin-angiotensin system; it is involved in the pathophysiology of hypertension. Angiotensin II increases systemic vascular resistance, causes sodium and water retention, and leads to increased heart rate and vasoconstriction. Losartan competitively blocks the angiotensin AT_1 receptor located in vascular smooth muscle and the adrenal glands, which is involved in mediating the effects of angiotensin II. Thus, BP is reduced. No significant effects on heart rate, has minimal orthostatic effects, and does not affect potassium levels significantly. Also, losartan does act on the AT_2 receptor. Undergoes significant first-pass metabolism in the liver, where it is converted to an active carboxylic acid metabolite that is responsible for most of the angiotensin receptor blockade. Rapidly absorbed after PO administration, although food slows absorption. **Peak plasma levels of losartan and metabolite:** 1 hr and 3–4 hr, respectively. **t½, losartan:** 2 hr; **t½, metabolite:** 6–9 hr. The drug and metabolite are highly bound to plasma proteins. Maximum effects are usually seen within 1 week, although from 3 to 6 weeks may be required in some clients. Drug and metabolites are excreted through both the urine (35%) and feces (60%).

Uses: Treatment of hypertension, alone or in combination with other antihypertensive agents. *Investigational:* Treatment of heart failure.

Contraindications: Lactation. Use after pregnancy is discouraged.

Special Concerns: When used alone, the effect to decease BP in blacks was less than in non-blacks. Dosage adjustments are not required in clients with renal impairment, unless they are volume depleted. In clients with severe CHF, there is a risk of oliguria and/or progressive azotemia with acute renal failure and/or death (which are rare). In those with unilateral or bilateral renal artery stenosis, there is a risk of increased serum creatinine or BUN. Lower doses are recommended in those with hepatic insufficiency. Safety and efficacy have not been determined in children less than 18 years of age.

Side Effects: *GI:* Diarrhea, dyspepsia, anorexia, constipation, dental pain, dry mouth, flatulence, gastritis, vomiting, taste perversion. *CV:* Angina pectoris, second-degree AV block, ***CVA, MI, ventricular tachycardia, ventricular fibrillation,*** hypotension, palpitation, sinus bradycardia, tachycardia, orthostatic effects. *CNS:* Dizziness, insomnia, anxiety, anxiety disorder, ataxia, confusion, depression, abnormal dreams, hypesthesia, decreased libido, impaired memory, migraine, nervousness, paresthesia, peripheral neuropathy, panic disorder, sleep disorder, somnolence, tremor, vertigo. *Respiratory:* URI, cough, nasal congestion, sinus disorder, sinusitis, dyspnea, bronchitis, pharyngeal discomfort, epistaxis, rhinitis, respiratory congestion. *Musculoskeletal:* Muscle cramps, myalgia, joint swelling, musculoskeletal pain, stiffness, arthralgia, arthritis, fibromyalgia, muscle weakness; pain in the back, legs, arms, hips, knees, shoulders. *Dermatologic:* Alopecia, dermatitis, dry skin, ecchymosis, erythema, flushing, photosensitivity, pruritus, rash, sweating, urticaria. *GU:* Impotence, nocturia, urinary frequency, UTI. *Ophthalmologic:* Blurred vision, burning/stinging in the eye, conjunctivitis, decrease in visual acuity. *Miscellaneous:* Gout, anemia, tinnitus, facial edema, fever, syncope.

Laboratory Test Considerations: Minor ↑ BUN, serum creatinine. Occasional ↑ liver enzymes and/or serum bilirubin. Small ↓ H&H.

OD **Management of Overdose:** *Symptoms:* Hypotension, tachycardia, bradycardia (due to vagal stimulation). *Treatment:* Supportive treatment. Hemodialysis is not indicated.

Drug Interactions: Administration of losartan and phenobarbital resulted in a decreased plasma level (20%) of losartan.

How Supplied: *Tablet:* 25 mg, 50 mg

Dosage

- **Tablets**

Hypertension.

Adults: 50 mg once daily with or without food. Total daily doses range from 25 to 100 mg. In those with possible depletion of intravascular volume (e.g., clients treated with a diuretic), use 25 mg once daily. If the antihypertensive effect (measured at trough) is inadequate, a twice-a-day regimen, using the same dose, may be tried; or an increase in dose may give a more satisfactory result. If BP is not controlled by losartan alone, a diuretic (e.g., hydrochlorothiazide) may be added.

HEALTH CARE CONSIDERATIONS

See also *Health Care Considerations* for *Antihypertensive Agents.*

Administration/Storage: May be given with other antihypertensive drugs.

Assessment

1. Record indications for therapy, onset and duration of disease, previous agents used and the outcome.
2. Monitor CBC, liver and renal function studies. Correct any volume depletion prior to using to prevent sympathomimetic hypotension. Reduce starting dose with volume depletion or hepatic impairment. Observe for S&S of fluid or electrolyte imbalance.

Client/Family Teaching

1. Take only as directed with or without food.
2. Regular exercise, proper low-salt diet, and life-style changes (i.e., no smoking, low alcohol, low-fat diet, low stress, adequate rest) may also contribute to enhanced BP control.
3. Do not change positions suddenly, dangle before rising, and rest until symptoms subside to prevent postural symptoms.
4. Avoid any OTC agents.
5. May cause photosensitivity reaction; use precautions.
6. Use effective contraception; report immediately if pregnancy is suspected because drug during second and third trimesters is associated with fetal injury and morbidity.

Outcome/Evaluate: Desired level of BP control

COMBINATION DRUG

Losartan potassium and Hydrochlorothiazide

(loh-**SAR**-tan, **hy**-droh-klor-oh- **THIGH**-ah-zyd)

Pregnancy Category: C (first trimester), D (second and third trimesters)

Hyzaar **(Rx)**

Classification: Antihypertensive

See also *Losartan potassium, Hydrochlorothiazide,* and *Diuretics, Thiazide.*

Content: Each tablet contains *Antihypertensive:* Losartan potassium, 50 mg, and *Diuretic:* Hydrochlorothiazide, 12.5 mg.

Action/Kinetics: Losartan undergoes significant first-pass metabolism in the liver, where it is converted to an active carboxylic acid metabolite that is responsible for most of the angiotensin receptor blockade. The drug is rapidly absorbed after PO administration, although food does slows absorption. **Peak plasma levels of losartan and metabolite:** 1 hr and 3–4 hr, respectively. **t½, losartan:** 2 hr; **t½, metabolite:** 6–9 hr. Losartan and its active metabolite are highly bound to plasma proteins. Maximum effects are usually seen within 1 week, although from 3 to 6 weeks may be required in some clients. The drug and metabolites are excreted through both the urine (35%) and feces (60%).

Peak effects, hydrochlorothiazide: 4 hr; **duration:** 6–12 hr. **Hydrochlorothiazide t½, plasma:** 5.6–14.8 hr. Most of an oral dose is excreted unchanged.

Uses: Treatment of hypertension. Not indicated for initial therapy. Use the combination of losartan potassium and hydrochlorothiazide when BP is not controlled adequately with losartan potassium alone. Also used for clients whose BP is inadequately controlled by 25 mg/day of hydrochlorothiazide or is controlled but experiences hypokalemia.

Contraindications: Use in pregnancy, especially during the second and third trimesters. In those with anuria or hypersensitivity to sulfonamide-derived drugs (e.g., hydrochlorothiazide). In severe renal impairment. Lactation.

Special Concerns: Use with caution in clients with impaired hepatic function or progressive liver disease. Hypersensitivity reactions to hydrochlorothiazide may occur in those with or without a history of allergy or bronchial asthma, although such reactions are more likely in these clients. Thiazides may worsen or activate systemic lupus erythematosus. Safety and efficacy have not been determined in children.

Side Effects: See individual drug entries.

Drug Interactions: See individual drug entries.

How Supplied: See Content

Dosage

- **Tablets**

Hypertension.

Adults: One tablet (losartan, 50 mg, and hydrochlorothiazide, 12.5 mg) daily. If BP is not controlled after approximately 3 weeks of therapy, the dose may be increased to 2 tablets daily. The total daily dose should not exceed 2 tablets.

HEALTH CARE CONSIDERATIONS

See also *Health Care Considerations* for *Losartan potassium* and *Antihypertensive Agents.*

Administration/Storage: May be administered with other antihypertensive drugs.

Assessment

1. Record duration of disease, previous agents used and the outcome.
2. Monitor CBC, renal and LFTs; report any dysfunction.
3. With renal impairment, determine that C_{CR} > 30 mL/min (if below 30 mL/min loop diuretics are preferable to thiazides).
4. Determine any sensitivity to sulfonamides, allergy, or bronchial asthma; may exhibit a hypersensitive reaction to hydrochlorothiazide.

Client/Family Teaching

1. Take only as directed at the same time(s) each day with or without food.
2. Regular exercise, low-salt diet, and life-style changes (i.e., no smoking, low alcohol, low-fat diet, low stress, adequate rest) contribute to enhanced BP control.
3. Do not change positions suddenly, dangle before rising, and rest until postural symptoms subside.
4. Avoid any OTC agents.
5. May cause photosensitivity.
6. Use effective contraception; report pregnancy as drug during second and third trimesters associated with fetal injury and morbidity.

Outcome/Evaluate: Control of BP

Loteprednol etabonate

(loh-teh-PRED-nohl)

Pregnancy Category: C

Alrex, Lotemax **(Rx)**

Classification: Corticosteroid, ophthalmic

See also *Corticosteroids.*

Action/Kinetics: Rapidly metabolized to inactive compounds by eye esterases. After ocular use, minimal amounts are absorbed.

Uses: 0.2% Suspension: Treat seasonal allergic conjunctivitis. **0.5% Suspension:** Treat steroid-responsive inflammatory conditions of the conjunctiva.

Contraindications: Bacterial, fungal, or viral eye infection.

Special Concerns: Use with caution with cataracts, diabetes mellitus, glaucoma, intraocular hypertension, use beyond 10 days. Safety and efficacy have not been determined in children.

Side Effects: *Ophthalmic:* Increased IOP, thinning of sclera or cornea, blurred vision, discharge, dry eyes, burning on instillation.

How Supplied: *Ophthalmic Suspension:* 0.2%, 0.5%

Dosage

- **Suspension, 0.2%**

Seasonal allergic conjunctivitis.
1 gtt in the affected eye(s) q.i.d.
- **Suspension, 0.5%**

Conjunctivitis, steroid-responsive.
1–2 gtt into the conjunctival sac of the affected eye q.i.d. For the first week, dose may be increased to 1 gtt every hour.

Conjunctivitis, postoperative.
1–2 gtt into the conjunctival sac of the affected eye q.i.d. beginning 24 hr after surgery and continuing for 2 weeks.

Contact lens-associated giant papillary conjunctivitis.
1 gtt q.i.d.

HEALTH CARE CONSIDERATIONS

See also *Health Care Considerations* for *Corticosteroids*.

Administration/Storage: Re-evaluate if symptoms do not improve after 2 days of treatment.

Assessment: Record indications for therapy, type, and onset of symptoms.

Client/Family Teaching

1. Shake well before use. Instill as directed.
2. Contact lenses may continue to be worn if the drug is used to treat lens-associated giant papillary conjunctivitis. Remove lens prior to each instillation; reinsert 10–15 min later.
3. Report if symptoms do not improve after 2 days of treatment.

Outcome/Evaluate: ↓ Eye irritation, inflammation, and allergic S&S

Lovastatin (Mevinolin)

(**LOW**-vah-**STAT**-in, me-**VIN**-oh-lin)
Pregnancy Category: X
Apo-Lovastatin ✱, Mevacor **(Rx)**
Classification: Antihyperlipidemic

See also *Antihyperlipidemic Agents—HMG-CoA Reductase Inhibitors*.

Action/Kinetics: Isolated from a strain of *Aspergillus terreus*. Approximately 35% of a dose is absorbed. Extensive first-pass effect—less than 5% reaches the general circulation. Absorption is decreased by about one-third if the drug is given on an empty stomach rather than with food. **Onset:** within 2 weeks using multiple doses. **Time to peak plasma levels:** 2–4 hr. **Time to peak effect:** 4–6 weeks using multiple doses. **Duration:** 4–6 weeks after termination of therapy. Over 95% is bound to plasma proteins. Metabolized in the liver (its main site of action) to active metabolites. Over 80% of a PO dose is excreted in the feces, via the bile, and approximately 10% is excreted through the urine.

Uses: As an adjunct to diet in primary hypercholesterolemia (types IIa and IIb) in clients with a significant risk of CAD and who have not responded to diet or other measures. May also be useful in clients with combined hypercholesterolemia and hypertriglyceridemia. To slow the progression of coronary atherosclerosis in clients with CAD in order to lower total and LDL cholesterol levels. *Investigational:* Diabetic dyslipidemia, nephrotic hyperlipidemia, familial dysbetalipoproteinemia, and familial combined hyperlipidemia.

Contraindications: During pregnancy and lactation, active liver disease, persistent unexplained elevations of serum transaminases. Use in children less than 18 years of age. Use with mibefradil (Posicor).

Special Concerns: Use with caution in clients who have a history of liver disease or who are known heavy consumers of alcohol. Carefully monitor clients with impaired renal function.

Side Effects: See Antihyperlipidemic Agents—HMG-CoA Reductase Inhibitors. *CNS:* Headache, dizziness, insomnia, paresthesia. *GI:* Flatus (most common), abdominal pain, cramps, diarrhea, constipation, dyspepsia, N&V, heartburn, dysgeusia, acid regurgitation, dry mouth. *Musculoskeletal:* Myalgia, muscle cramps, pain, arthralgia, leg pain, shoulder pain, localized pain. *Miscellaneous:* Blurred vision, eye irritation, rash, pruritus, chest pain, alopecia.

Additional Drug Interactions
Isradipine / ↑ Clearance of lovastatin
Niacin / ↑ Risk of rhabdomyolysis or severe myopathy

How Supplied: *Tablet:* 10 mg, 20 mg, 40 mg

Dosage

- **Tablets**

Adults/adolescents, initial: 20 mg once daily with the evening meal. Initiate at 10 mg/day in clients on immunosuppressants. Dose range: 10–80 mg/day in single or two divided doses, not to exceed 20 mg/day if given with immunosuppressants. Adjust dose at intervals of every 4 weeks, if necessary. If C_{CR} is less than 30 mL/min, use doses greater than 20 mg/day with caution.

L

HEALTH CARE CONSIDERATIONS

See also *Health Care Considerations* for *Antihyperlipidemic Agents—HMG-CoA Reductase Inhibitors*.

Administration/Storage

1. Place on standard cholesterol-lowering diet before starting lovastatin; continue during therapy.
2. Dosage modification is not necessary with renal insufficiency.

Assessment

1. Record serum cholesterol profile, other therapies and the outcome.
2. Note hepatic disease and any heavy consumption of alcohol.
3. Determine if pregnant.
4. Request recent eye exam; slight changes have been noted in the lenses of some clients.
5. Assess LFTs q 4–6 weeks for the first 15 mo of therapy. A threefold increase in serum transaminase or new-onset abnormal liver function is an indication to discontinue therapy.
6. Assess life-style, including diet (intake of fats, CHOs, and proteins), activity (regular exercise), alcohol consumption, and smoking history. Identify areas that may contribute to increased cholesterol levels.

Client/Family Teaching

1. Take with meals. Avoid coadministration with grapefruit juice due to increased serum levels of lovastatin. Continue cholesterol-lowering diet and exercise program as prescribed. Cholesterol production by the liver is highest in the evening; drug usually taken with the evening meal.
2. Adhere to dietary restrictions, daily exercise, and weight loss in the overall management and control of hypercholesterolemia/hyperlipidemia.
3. Practice reliable birth control; drug is pregnancy category X.
4. Report malaise, muscle spasms, or fever. These may be mistaken for the flu, but could be serious side effects of drug therapy.
5. Any RUQ abdominal pain or change in color and consistency of stools should be reported.
6. Periodic LFTs and eye exams are mandatory; report any early visual disturbances.

Outcome/Evaluate

- ↓ Cholesterol/triglyceride levels
- ↓ progression of coronary atherosclerosis

Loxapine hydrochloride

(LOX-ah-peen)
Pregnancy Category: C
Loxapac ✦, Loxitane C, Loxitane IM **(Rx)**

Loxapine succinate

(LOX-ah-peen)
Pregnancy Category: C
Loxapac ✦, Loxitane **(Rx)**
Classification: Antipsychotic, tricyclic

See also *Antipsychotic Agents, Phenothiazines*.

Action/Kinetics: Thought to act by blocking dopamine at postsynaptic brain receptors. Causes significant extrapyramidal symptoms, moderate sedative effects, and a low incidence of anticholinergic effects, as well as orthostatic hypotension. **Onset:** 20–30 min. **Peak effects:** 1.5–3 hr. **Duration:** about 12 hr. **t½:** 3–4 hr. Partially metabolized in the liver; excreted in urine, and unchanged in feces.

Uses: Psychotic disorders. *Investigational:* Anxiety neurosis with depression.

Additional Contraindications: History of convulsive disorders.

Special Concerns: Use with caution in clients with CV disease. Use during lactation only if benefits outweigh risks. Dosage has not been established in children less than 16 years of age. Geriatric clients may be more prone to developing orthostatic hypotension, anticholinergic, sedative, and extrapyramidal side effects.

Additional Side Effects: Tachycardia, hypertension, hypotension, lightheadedness, and syncope.

How Supplied: Loxapine hydrochloride: *Concentrate:* 25 mg/mL; *Injection:* 50 mg/mL. Loxapine succinate: *Capsule:* 5 mg, 10 mg, 25 mg, 50 mg

Dosage

- **Capsules, Oral Solution**

  Psychoses.

Adults, initial: 10 mg (of the base) b.i.d. For severe cases, up to 50 mg/day may be required. Increase dosage rapidly over 7–10 days until symptoms are controlled. **Range:** 60–100 mg up to 250 mg/day. **Maintenance:** If possible reduce dosage to 20–60 mg/day.

- **IM**

  Psychoses.

Adults: 12.5–50 mg (of the base) q 4–6 hr; once adequate control has been established, switch to PO medication after control achieved (usually within 5 days).

HEALTH CARE CONSIDERATIONS

See also *Health Care Considerations* for *Antipsychotic Agents, Phenothiazines*.

Administration/Storage

1. Measure the concentrate dosage *only* with the enclosed calibrated dropper.

2. Mix oral concentrate with orange or grapefruit juice immediately before administration to disguise unpleasant taste.

Assessment

1. Note indications for therapy, type, onset, and characteristics of symptoms.
2. List agents used previously and the outcome.
3. Record/document mental status and behavioral manifestations.

Client/Family Teaching

1. Drug may cause orthostatic effects.
2. Do not stop abruptly. Attend therapy and keep scheduled visits for evaluation of condition and effectiveness of drug therapy.
3. Caution, may cause photosensitivity.

Outcome/Evaluate: ↓ Agitated/hyperactive behaviors

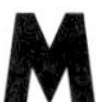

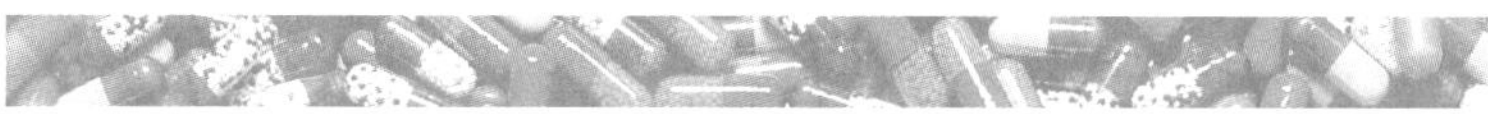

Mafenide acetate

(MAH-fen-eyed)
Pregnancy Category: C
Sulfamylon **(Rx)**
Classification: Sulfonamide, topical

See also *Sulfonamides.*

Action/Kinetics: Active against many gram-positive and gram-negative organisms and in the presence of serum and pus. When applied topically, it diffuses through devascularized areas, is absorbed, and is rapidly metabolized.

Uses: Topical application to prevent infections in second- and third-degree burns. To control bacterial infections when used under moist dressing over meshed autografts on excised burn wounds.

Contraindications: Use for established infections or in infants less than 1 month of age.

Special Concerns: Use with caution during lactation and in those with acute renal failure.

Side Effects: *Allergic:* Rash, itching, swelling, hives, blisters, facial edema, erythema, eosinophilia. *Dermatologic:* Pain or burning (common) on application; excoriation of new skin, bleeding (rare). *Respiratory:* Hyperventilation or tachypnea, decrease in arterial pCO_2. *Metabolic:* Acidosis, increase in serum chloride. *Miscellaneous:* ***Fatal hemolytic anemia with DIC,*** diarrhea.

How Supplied: *Cream:* 85 mg(as acetate)/g; *Topical Solution:* 5% as acetate

Dosage

• **Cream**

1/16-in.-thick film applied over entire surface of burn with gloves once or twice daily until healing is progressing satisfactorily or until site is ready for grafting.

HEALTH CARE CONSIDERATIONS

See also *General Health Care Considerations for All Anti-Infectives* and *Sulfonamides.*

Administration/Storage

1. Continue until healing is progressing well or until the burn site is ready for grafting. Do not withdraw if there is still possibility of infections.
2. Avoid exposure to excessive heat.

Client/Family Teaching

1. Apply cream aseptically to a cleansed, debrided, burn site using a gloved hand.
2. Undertake daily bathing to assist in wound debridement.
3. Cover treated burns with only a thin dressing.
4. Causes pain on application; use analgesics as prescribed.
5. Report any abnormal odor or drainage or unusual reactions including rashes, bruising, bleeding, swelling, or breathing difficulty.

Outcome/Evaluate: Readiness for grafting at burn site; infection prophylaxis

Masoprocol

(mah-SOH-proh-kol)
Pregnancy Category: B
Actinex **(Rx)**
Classification: Dermatologic agent

Action/Kinetics: Mechanism of action is unknown. Less than 1%–2% is absorbed through the skin over a 4-day period following application.

Uses: Actinic (solar) keratoses.

Contraindications: Hypersensitivity to masoprocol or other ingredients in the formulation. Use with an occlusive dressing.

Special Concerns: Use with caution during lactation. Safety and efficacy have not been

M

determined in children. The presence or absence of local skin reactions does not correlate with effectiveness of the drug.
Side Effects: *Dermatologic:* Commonly, erythema, flaking, itching, dryness, edema, burning, soreness, allergic contact dermatitis. Also, bleeding, crusting, eye irritation, oozing, rash, soreness, skin irritation, stinging, tightness, tingling, blistering, eczema, fissuring, leathery feeling to the skin, skin roughness, wrinkling, excoriation.
How Supplied: *Cream:* 10%

Dosage

• **Cream**

Following washing and drying areas where actinic keratoses are located, the drug should be gently massaged into the area, until it is evenly distributed, morning and evening for 28 days.

HEALTH CARE CONSIDERATIONS

Administration/Storage: For external use only.

Assessment

1. Note sulfite sensitivity; may cause allergic-type reactions, esp. in asthmatics or atopic nonasthmatics.
2. Record symptoms and onset of skin disorder; list other treatments used and the outcome.
3. Assess carefully and describe characteristics (including location and size) of lesions to be treated.

Client/Family Teaching

1. Administer using the following guidelines:
• Wash hands.
• Wash and dry involved area thoroughly.
• Apply cream evenly and gently; massage into actinic lesion.
• Wash hands immediately after application.
• Exercise special care if drug must be applied near the eyes, nose, or mouth. If contact with eyes, wash promptly with water.
• Apply each morning and evening for 28 days as directed.
• Do not cover treated areas with any type of occlusive dressing.
• Protect linens, fabrics, and clothing as cream may stain.
• Avoid all other skin products and makeup during therapy.
2. A local transient burning sensation may be felt immediately after applying.
3. Local skin reactions are frequent (bright-red skin, inflamed) and usually resolve within 2 weeks of discontinuing therapy. Stop drug and report any evidence of severe reaction characterized by blistering or oozing lesions.
4. Avoid undue sun exposure, especially since solar keratoses may be sun induced.

Outcome/Evaluate: ↓ Number and size of actinic lesions

Mazindol

(MAYZ-in-dohl)
Pregnancy Category: C
Mazanor, Sanorex **(C-IV) (Rx)**
Classification: Anorexiant

See also *Amphetamines and Derivatives.*
Action/Kinetics: Onset: 30–60 min; **duration:** 8–15 hr. **t½:** Less than 24 hr. **Therapeutic blood levels:** 0.003–0.012 mcg/mL. Excreted in urine partially unchanged.
Uses: Short-term (8–12 weeks) treatment of exogenous obesity in conjunction with a weight reduction program including exercise, reduced caloric intake, and behavior modification.
Additional Side Effects: Testicular pain.
How Supplied: *Tablet:* 1 mg, 2 mg

Dosage

• **Tablets**

Adults, initial: 1 mg once daily 1 hr before the first meal of the day; **then,** dose can be increased to 1 mg t.i.d. before meals or 2 mg once daily 1 hr before lunch.

HEALTH CARE CONSIDERATIONS

See also *Health Care Considerations* for *Amphetamines and Derivatives.*

Client/Family Teaching

1. Review goals and time frame for achieving. Identify importance of diet, regular exercise, and reduced caloric intake in the overall management of obesity.
2. Take with meals if GI distress occurs.
3. Attend diet counseling and support groups.

Outcome/Evaluate: Weight reduction

Mebendazole

(meh-BEN-dah-zohl)
Pregnancy Category: C
Vermox **(Rx)**
Classification: Anthelmintic

See also *Anthelmintics.*
Action/Kinetics: Anthelmintic effect occurs by blocking the glucose uptake of the organisms, thereby reducing their energy until death results. It also inhibits the formation of microtubules in the helminth. **Peak plasma levels:** 2–4 hr. Poorly absorbed from the GI tract. Excreted in feces as unchanged drug or metabolites.

Uses: Whipworm, pinworm, roundworm, common and American hookworm infections; in single or mixed infections. Mebendazole is not effective for hydatid disease.
Contraindications: Hypersensitivity to mebendazole.
Special Concerns: Use with caution in children under 2 years of age and during lactation.
Side Effects: *GI:* Transient abdominal pain and diarrhea. *Hematologic:* Reversible neutropenia. *Miscellaneous:* Fever.
Drug Interactions: Carbamazepine and hydantoin may ↓ effect due to ↓ plasma levels of mebendazole.
How Supplied: *Chew Tablet:* 100 mg

Dosage

- **Tablets, Chewable**

Whipworm, roundworm, and hookworm.
Adults and children: 1 tablet morning and evening on 3 consecutive days.
Pinworms.
1 tablet, one time. All treatments can be repeated after 3 weeks if the client is not cured.

HEALTH CARE CONSIDERATIONS

See also *Health Care Considerations* for *Anthelmintics.*

Client/Family Teaching

1. Tablets may be chewed, swallowed, or crushed and mixed with food. Fasting or purging are not required.
2. Pinworms may be highly contagious:
- Carefully wash hands with soap and water before and after eating and toileting; clean nails and keep out of mouth.
- Advise school nurse of treatment.
- Do not share washcloths and towels. Wear tight underpants; change daily. Sleep alone; wear shoes during waking hours.
- Do not shake or share linens/clothing; wash in hot water.
- Clean toilet and seats with disinfectant daily; vacuum or wet mop bedroom floors daily.

3. Wash all fruits and vegetables. Thoroughly cook all meats and vegetables.
4. Immobilization followed by death of parasites is slow. Complete clearance from the GI tract may take up to 3 days after initiation of treatment.

Outcome/Evaluate

- Three consecutive negative stool and/or perianal swabs
- Organism expulsion/destruction

Meclizine hydrochloride

(MEK-lih-zeen)
Pregnancy Category: B
Antivert, Antivert/25 and /50, Antivert/25 Chewable, Antrizine, Bonamine ✦, Bonine, Dizmiss, Dramamine II, Meni-D, Ru-Vert-M **(OTC and Rx)**
Classification: Antihistamine (piperidine-type), antiemetic, antimotion sickness

See also *Antihistamines* and *Antiemetics.*
Action/Kinetics: Mechanism for the antiemetic effect may be due to a central anticholinergic effect to decrease vestibular stimulation and depress labyrinthine activity. May also act on the CTZ to decrease vomiting. **Onset:** 30–60 min; **Duration:** 8–24 hr. **t½:** 6 hr.
Uses: Nausea and vomiting, dizziness of motion sickness, vertigo associated with diseases of the vestibular system.
Special Concerns: Safety for use during lactation and in children less than 12 years of age has not been determined. Pediatric and geriatric clients may be more sensitive to the anticholinergic effects of meclizine.
Side Effects: *CNS:* Drowsiness, excitation, nervousness, restlessness, insomnia, euphoria, vertigo, hallucinations (auditory or visual). *GI:* N&V, diarrhea, constipation, anorexia. *GU:* Urinary frequency or retention; difficulty in urination. *CV:* Hypotension, tachycardia, palpitations. *Miscellaneous:* Dry nose and throat, blurred or double vision, tinnitus, rash, urticaria.
How Supplied: *Capsule:* 25 mg, 30 mg; *Chew Tablet:* 25 mg; *Tablet:* 12.5 mg, 25 mg, 50 mg

Dosage

- **Capsules, Tablets, Chewable Tablets**

Motion sickness.
Adults: 25–50 mg 1 hr before travel; may be repeated q 24 hr during travel.
Vertigo.
Adults: 25–100 mg/day in divided doses.

HEALTH CARE CONSIDERATIONS

See also *Health Care Considerations* for *Antihistamines* and *Antiemetics.*

Assessment

1. Record onset, duration, and characteristics of symptoms.
2. Assess for other adverse symptoms; drug may mask signs of drug overdose or pathology such as increased ICP or intestinal obstruction.

M

Client/Family Teaching
1. Take only as directed and report if condition does not improve.
2. Antiemetics tend to cause drowsiness and dizziness. Do not drive or perform other hazardous tasks until drug response evident.

Outcome/Evaluate
- Prevention of motion sickness
- Control of vertigo

Meclofenamate sodium

(me-kloh-fen-**AM**-ayt)
Meclomen **(Rx)**
Classification: Nonsteroidal anti-inflammatory drug

See also *Nonsteroidal Anti-Inflammatory Drugs.*

Action/Kinetics: Peak plasma levels: 30–60 min. **t½:** 2–3.3 hr. Peak anti-inflammatory activity may not be observed for 2–3 weeks. Excreted through urine and feces.

Uses: Acute and chronic rheumatoid arthritis and osteoarthritis. Not indicated as the initial drug for rheumatoid arthritis due to GI side effects. Has been used in combination with gold salts or corticosteroids. Mild to moderate pain. Primary dysmenorrhea, excessive menstrual blood loss. *Investigational:* Sunburn, prophylaxis of migraine, migraine due to menses.

Additional Contraindications: Use during pregnancy, lactation, or in children less than 14 years of age.

Special Concerns: Safe use during lactation not established. Safety and efficacy not established in functional class IV rheumatoid arthritis.

Laboratory Test Considerations: ↑ Serum transaminase, alkaline phosphatase; rarely, ↑ serum creatinine or BUN.

Additional Side Effects: Severe diarrhea, nausea, headache, rash, dermatitis, abdominal pain, pyrosis, flatulence, malaise, fatigue, paresthesia, insomnia, depression, taste disturbances, nocturia, blood loss (through feces: 2 mL/day).

Drug Interactions
Aspirin / ↓ Plasma levels of meclofenamate
Warfarin / ↑ Effect of warfarin

How Supplied: *Capsule:* 50 mg, 100 mg

Dosage
- **Capsules**

Rheumatoid arthritis, osteoarthritis.

Adults, usual: 200–400 mg/day in three to four equal doses. Initiate at lower dose and increase to maximum of 400 mg/day if necessary. After initial satisfactory response, lower dosage to decrease severity of side effects.

Mild to moderate pain.

Adults: 50 mg q 4–6 hr (100 mg may be required in some clients), not to exceed 400 mg/day.

Excessive menstrual blood loss and primary dysmenorrhea.

Adults: 100 mg t.i.d. for up to 6 days, starting at the onset of menses.

HEALTH CARE CONSIDERATIONS

See also *Health Care Considerations* for *Nonsteroidal Anti-Inflammatory Drugs.*

Administration/Storage
1. Lower doses may be effective for chronic use.
2. Reduce dose or discontinue temporarily if diarrhea occurs.

Client/Family Teaching
1. May take with food or milk to diminish GI upset.
2. Report any changes in stool color or diarrhea.
3. Take as ordered and do not become discouraged; may take 2–3 weeks to see improvement in arthritic conditions.

Outcome/Evaluate
- Improvement in joint pain and mobility with ↓ inflammation
- Relief of pain and dysmenorrhea

Medroxyprogesterone acetate

(meh-**drox**-see-proh-**JESS**-ter-ohn)
Pregnancy Category: X
Alti-MPA ✱, Amen, Curretab, Cycrin, Depo-Provera, Depo-Provera C-150, Gen-Medroxy ✱, Novo-Medrone ✱, Provera **(Rx)**
Classification: Progestational hormone, synthetic

See also *Progesterone and Progestins* and *Antineoplastic Agents.*

Action/Kinetics: Synthetic progestin devoid of estrogenic and androgenic activity. Prevents stimulation of endometrium by pituitary gonadotropins. Priming with estrogen is necessary before response is noted. Rapidly absorbed from GI tract. **Maximum levels:** 1–2 hr. **t½, after PO:** 2–3 hr for first 6 hr; then, 8–9 hr. **t½, long-acting forms IM:** About 10 weeks with maximum levels within 24 hr.

Uses: Secondary amenorrhea, abnormal uterine bleeding due to hormonal imbalance (no organic pathology). Adjunct in palliative treatment of inoperable, recurrent, or metastatic endometrial or renal carcinoma. Long-acting contraceptive (injectable form). Reduce endometrial hyperplasia in postmenopausal women receiving 0.625 mg conjugated estrogen for 12 to 14 days/month; can begin on the 1st or 16th day of the cycle. *Investigational:* Polycystic ovary syndrome, precocious puberty. With estrogen to treat menopausal symptoms and hypermenorrhea. To stimulate respiration in obesity-hypoventilation syndrome (oral).

Contraindications: Clients with or a history of thrombophlebitis, thromboembolic disease, cerebral apoplexy. Liver dysfunction. Known or suspected malignancy of the breasts or genital organs. Missed abortion; as a diagnostic for pregnancy. Undiagnosed vaginal bleeding. Use during the first 4 months of pregnancy.

Special Concerns: The overall risk of breast, liver, ovarian, endometrial, and cervical cancer is not thought to increase with use of the injectable long-acting contraceptive preparation. Possibility of ectopic pregnancy. Use with caution in clients with a history of depression. Due to the possibility of fluid retention, use with caution in clients with epilepsy, migraine, asthma, or cardiac or renal dysfunction.

Side Effects: *GU:* Amenorrhea or infertility for up to 18 months. *CV:* Thrombophlebitis, ***pulmonary embolism.*** *GI:* Nausea (rare), jaundice. *CNS:* Nervousness, drowsiness, insomnia, fatigue, dizziness, headache (rare). *Dermatologic:* Pruritus, urticaria, rash, acne, hirsutism, alopecia, angioneurotic edema. *Miscellaneous:* ***Hyperpyrexia, anaphylaxis,*** decrease in glucose tolerance, weight gain, fluid retention.

Drug Interactions: Aminoglutethimide may ↑ metabolism of medroxyprogesterone → ↓ effect.

How Supplied: *Injection:* 150 mg/mL, 400 mg/mL; *Tablet:* 2.5 mg, 5 mg, 10 mg

Dosage

• **Tablets**

Secondary amenorrhea.

5–10 mg/day for 5–10 days, with therapy beginning at any time during the menstrual cycle. If endometrium has been estrogen primed: 10 mg medroxyprogesterone/day for 10 days beginning any time.

Abnormal uterine bleeding with no pathology.

5–10 mg/day for 5–10 days, with therapy beginning on day 16 or 21 of the menstrual cycle. If endometrium has been estrogen primed: 10 mg/day for 10 days, beginning on day 16 of the menstrual cycle. Bleeding usually begins within 3–7 days.

• **IM**

Endometrial or renal carcinoma.

Initial: 400–1,000 mg/week; **then, if improvement noted,** 400 mg/month. Medroxyprogesterone is not intended to be the primary therapy.

Long-acting contraceptive.

150 mg of depot form q 3 months by deep IM injection given only during the first 5 days after the onset of a normal menstrual period, within 5 days postpartum if not breastfeeding, or 6 weeks postpartum if breastfeeding.

HEALTH CARE CONSIDERATIONS

See also *Health Care Considerations* for *Antineoplastic Agents* and *Progesterone and Progestins.*

Assessment

1. Record type, onset, and duration of symptoms.
2. Note thromboembolic disease.
3. Monitor calcium levels and LFTs. With severe hypercalcemia, have IV fluids, diuretics, corticosteroids, and phosphate supplements available; monitor closely once corrected.

Client/Family Teaching

1. With cancer therapy, the combined effect of the drug and osteolytic metastases may result in hypercalcemia. Report insomnia, lethargy, anorexia, and N&V. Increase fluids to minimize hypercalcemia.
2. Keep scheduled appointments for contraceptive evaluation and regular GYN exams. Additional barrier protection is necessary to prevent STDs and HIV transmission.

Outcome/Evaluate

- Prevention of pregnancy
- Control of tumor size and spread
- Regular menses; normal hormone levels
- ↓ endometrial hyperplasia in postmenopausal women receiving estrogen

Mefenamic acid

(meh-fen-**NAM**-ick **AH**-sid)

Pregnancy Category: C

Apo-Mefenamic ✱, Nu-Mefenamic ✱, PMS-Mefenamic Acid ✱, Ponstan ✱, Ponstel **(Rx)**

Classification: Nonsteroidal, anti-inflammatory drug

See also *Nonsteroidal Anti-Inflammatory Drugs.*

Action/Kinetics: Inhibits prostaglandin synthesis. Is an anti-inflammatory, antipyretic, and analgesic. **Peak plasma levels:** 2–4 hr; **t½:** 2–4 hr; **duration:** 4–6 hr. Slowly absorbed from the GI tract, metabolized by the liver, and excreted in the urine and feces.

Uses: Short-term relief (< 1 week) of mild to moderate pain (e.g., pain associated with tooth extraction and musculoskeletal disorders). Primary dysmenorrhea. *Investigational:* PMS, sunburn.

Contraindications: Ulceration or chronic inflammation of the GI tract, pregnancy or possibility thereof, children under 14, and hypersensitivity to the drug.

Special Concerns: Dosage has not been established in children less than 14 years of age. Use with caution in clients with impaired renal or hepatic function, asthma, or clients on anticoagulant therapy.

Laboratory Test Considerations: False + test for urinary bile using diazo tablets.

Additional Side Effects: ***Autoimmune hemolytic anemia if used more than 12 months.*** Diarrhea may be significant. Rash (maculopapular type).

Drug Interactions

Anticoagulants / ↑ Hypoprothrombinemia due to ↓ plasma protein binding
Insulin / ↑ Insulin requirement
Lithium / ↑ Plasma levels of lithium

How Supplied: *Capsule:* 250 mg

M

Dosage

- **Capsules**

Analgesia, primary dysmenorrhea.

Adults and children over 14 years of age, initial: 500 mg; **then,** 250 mg q 6 hr.

HEALTH CARE CONSIDERATIONS

See also *Health Care Considerations* for *Nonsteroidal Anti-inflammatory Drugs.*

Administration/Storage: Do not use for more than a week at a time.

Client/Family Teaching

1. Take with food to minimize GI upset.
2. Use caution when driving or operating machinery; drug may cause dizziness or confusion.
3. Report any unusual bleeding, rashes, itching, diarrhea, lightheadedness, or increased sweating.

Outcome/Evaluate

- Relief of pain
- Control of uterine cramping

Megestrol acetate

(meh-**JESS**-trohl)

Pregnancy Category: D

Apo-Megestrol ✷, Linmegestrol ✷, Megace, Megace OS ✷, Nu-Megestrol ✷ **(Rx)**

Classification: Synthetic progestin

See also *Progesterone and Progestins* and *Antineoplastic Agents.*

Action/Kinetics: Antineoplastic activity is due to suppression of gonadotropins (antiluteinizing effect). Has appetite-enhancing properties (mechanism unknown). Contains tartrazine, which can cause allergic-type reactions, including asthma, often occurring in aspirin sensitivity.

Uses: Tablets: Palliative treatment of advanced endometrial or breast cancer. Should not be used instead of chemotherapy, radiation, or surgery. **Oral suspension:** Treatment of anorexia, cachexia, or an unexplained, significant weight loss in clients with a diagnosis of AIDS.

Contraindications: Use as a diagnostic aid test for pregnancy, in known or suspected pregnancy, or for prophylaxis to avoid weight loss. Use during the first 4 months of pregnancy.

Special Concerns: Use with caution in clients with a history of thromboembolic disease. Use in HIV-infected women with endometrial or breast cancer has not been widely studied. Long-term use may increase the risk of respiratory infections and may cause secondary adrenal suppression. Safety and efficacy in children have not been determined.

Side Effects: *GI:* Diarrhea, flatulence, nausea, dyspepsia, vomiting, constipation, dry mouth, hepatomegaly, increased salivation, abdominal pain, oral moniliasis. *CV:* Hypertension, ***cardiomyopathy,*** palpitation. *CNS:* Insomnia, headache, paresthesia, confusion, ***seizures,*** depression, neuropathy, hypesthesia, abnormal thought process. *Respiratory:* Pneumonia, dyspnea, cough, pharyngitis, chest pain, lung disorder, increased risk of respiratory infection with chronic use. *Dermatologic:* Rash, alopecia, herpes, pruritus, vesiculobullous rash, sweating, skin disorder. *GU:* Impotence, decreased libido, urinary frequency, albuminuria, urinary incontinence, UTI, gynecomastia. *Body as a whole:* Asthenia, anemia, fever, pain, moniliasis, infection, sarcoma. *Miscellaneous:* Leukopenia, edema, peripheral edema, amblyopia.

Laboratory Test Considerations: Hyperglycemia, ↑ LDH.

How Supplied: *Suspension:* 40 mg/mL; *Tablet:* 20 mg, 40 mg

Dosage

- **Oral Suspension**

Appetite stimulant in AIDS clients.

Adults, initial: 800 mg/day (20 mL/day). The dose should be adjusted to 400 mg/day (10 mL/day) after 1 month.

- **Tablets**

Breast cancer.

40 mg q.i.d.

Endometrial cancer.

40–320 mg/day in divided doses. To determine efficacy, treatment should be continued for at least 2 months.

HEALTH CARE CONSIDERATIONS

See also *Health Care Considerations* for *Antineoplastic Agents*, *Progesterone and Progestins*, and *Medroxyprogesterone Acetate*.

Administration/Storage: The oral suspension is available in a lemon-lime flavor that contains 40 mg of micronized megestrol acetate/mL; shake well before using.

Assessment

1. Record indications for therapy, type and duration of symptoms.
2. Note thromboembolic disease.
3. Determine if pregnant.
4. Note sensitivity to tartrazines.
5. With long-term therapy, assess for respiratory infections and adrenal suppression.

Client/Family Teaching

1. Take exactly as prescribed; do not skip or double up doses. May take with meals if GI upset occurs.
2. Report vaginal bleeding, edema, swelling or pain in leg veins, pain/weakness in thumb (CTS).
3. Practice reliable birth control.

Outcome/Evaluate

- ↓ Tumor size and spread
- Prevention of further weight loss

Meloxicam

(meh-**LOX**-ih-kam)

Pregnancy Category: C (D 3rd trimester)

Mobic **(Rx)**

Classification: Nonsteroidal anti-inflammatory agent (NSAID)

Action/Kinetics: Inhibits prostaglandin synthesis by decreasing the activity of the enzyme, cyclo-oxygenase, which results in decreased formation of prostaglandin precursors. **t½:** 15-20 hours. **Peak:** 5-10 hours. **Elimination:** urine & feces.

Uses: Relief of signs and symptoms of osteoarthritis.

Contraindications: Hypersensitivity to meloxicam or any component, aspirin, or other nonsteroidal anti-inflammatory drugs.

Special Concerns: Gastrointestinal irritation, ulceration, bleeding, and perforation may occur with NSAIDs. Use with caution in persons with prior history or symptoms of GI disease, congestive heart failure, dehydration, hypertension or asthma. May alter platelet function; use with caution in persons receiving anticoagulants or with hemostatic disorders.

Side Effects: *GI:* Diarrhea, dyspepsia, nausea, flatulence, abdominal pain. *Miscellaneous:* Occasionally, anaphylactoid reactions may occur, even with no prior use of meloxicam.

Laboratory Test Considerations: May increase warfarin INR; monitor closely.

Drug Interactions: ACE inhibitors, anticoagulants, antiplatelet drugs, aspirin, cholestyramine, corticosteroids, cyclosporine, hydralazine, lithium, loop diuretics, thiazide diuretics.

How Supplied: *Tablet:* 7.5 mg

Dosage

- **Tablets**

  Osteoarthritis

7.5 mg once daily. Some may gain additional benefit from 15 mg once daily. Maximum recommended daily dose: 15 mg.

HEALTH CARE CONSIDERATIONS

See also *Health Care Considerations* for *Nonsteroidal Anti-Inflammatory Drugs*.

Assessment

1. Record indication for use of the medication, symptoms, and other medicine being taken.
2. Assess and record involved joints, limitations in ROM, erythema, swelling, pain, and warmth.

Client/Family Teaching

1. Use exactly as ordered as adverse reactions may occur with overuse.
2. Take with food or milk and drink increased fluids unless instructed otherwise.
3. While taking this medication, do not use alcohol, excessive amounts of vitamin C, salicylate-containing prescription or OTC medications containing aspirin or salicylate, or other NSAIDs without consulting your health care provider.
4. GI bleeding, ulceration, or perforation can occur with or without pain. Report to your health care provider any persistent cramping or pain in stomach, persistent nausea or vomiting, ringing in the ears, difficulty breathing, shortness of breath, unusual bruising or bleeding. Stop the medication.

Outcome/Evaluate: ↓ Joint pain and inflammation with improved mobility.

Menotropins

(men-oh-**TROH**-pinz)

Pregnancy Category: X

Humegon, Pergonal, Repronex **(Rx)**

Classification: Ovarian stimulant

Action/Kinetics: Menotropins are a mixture of FSH and LH extracted from the urine of postmenopausal women. Causes growth and maturation of ovarian follicles. For ovulation to occur, HCG is administered the day following menotropins. **Time to peak effect, females:** 18 hr. In men, menotropins with HCG given for a minimum of 3 months induce spermatogenesis. Eliminated through the kidneys.

Uses: Females: In combination with HCG to induce ovulation in clients with anovulatory cycles not due to primary ovarian failure. **Males:** In combination with HCG to induce spermatogenesis in clients with primary or secondary hypogonadotrophic hypogonadism.

Contraindications: *Women:* Pregnancy. Primary ovarian failure as indicated by high levels of urinary gonadotropins, ovarian cysts, intracranial lesions, including pituitary tumors. Overt thyroid and adrenal dysfunction. Any cause of infertility other than anovulation. Abnormal bleeding of undetermined origin. Ovarian cysts or enlargement of the ovaries not due to polycystic ovarian syndrome. *Men:* Normal gonadotropin levels, primary testicular failure, disorders of fertility other than hypogonadotrophic hypogonadism. Thyroid or adrenal dysfunction. Absence of neoplastic disease should be established before treatment is initiated.

M

Side Effects: *Women. GU:* Ovarian overstimulation, hyperstimulation syndrome (maximal 7–10 days after discontinuation of drug), ovarian enlargement (20% of clients), adnexal torsion, ***ruptured ovarian cysts, ectopic pregnancy,*** multiple births (20%). *CV:* ***Hemoperitoneum, thromboembolism,*** tachycardia, pulmonary and vascular complications. *Hypersentivity:* Generalized urticaria, angioneurotic edema, facial edema, ***dysnpea indicating laryngeal edema.*** *CNS:* Headaches, malaise, dizziness. *GI:*N&V, abdominal pain, diarrhea, abdominal cramps, bloating. *At injection site:* Pain, rash, swelling, irritation. *Miscellaneous:* Fever, chills, musculoskeletal aches, joint pains, body rashes, dyspnea, tachypnea.

Men. Gynecomastia, breast pain, mastitis, nausea, abnormal lipoprotein fraction, abnormal AST and ALT.

How Supplied: *Powder for injection, lyophilized:* 75 IU FSH/75 IU LH, 150 IU FSH/ 150 IU LH

Dosage

- **IM**

Induction of ovulation.

Individualized, initial: 75 IU of FSH and 75 IU of LH for 7–12 days (maximum), followed by 10,000 USP units of HCG 1 day after last dose of menotropins. **Subsequent courses:** Same dosage schedule for two more courses, if ovulation has occurred. **Then,** dose may be increased to 150 IU of FSH and 150 IU of LH for 7–12 days, followed by HCG as in the preceding for two or more courses.

Induction of spermatogenesis.

It may be necessary to give HCG alone, 5,000 IU 3 times/week, for 4–6 months prior to menotropins; **then,** 75 IU FSH and 75 IU LH IM 3 times/week and HCG 2,000 IU 2 times/week for at least 4 months. If no response after 4 months, double each dose of menotropins with the HCG dose unchanged.

HEALTH CARE CONSIDERATIONS

Administration/Storage

1. Administer parenterally; menotropins are destroyed in the GI tract.
2. To prepare solution, dissolve the contents of one ampule in 1–2 mL sterile saline. Reconstituted solutions must be used immediately; discard any unused portions.
3. Store the lyophilized powder at room temperature or in the refrigerator (3°C–25°C, or 37°F–77°F).

Assessment

1. Record indications for therapy and other therapy or drugs used.
2. Assess for high levels of urinary gonadotropins or presence of ovarian cysts; drug contraindicated.
3. Obtain CBC, electrolytes, urinary gonadotropin levels, thyroid and adrenal function studies; assess neuro status, check peripheral pulses.

Interventions

1. If urinary estrogen excretion levels greater than 100 mcg or if daily estriol excretion exceeds 50 mcg, *withhold HCG* and report; these signal impending hyperstimulation syndrome.
2. If hospitalized for hyperstimulation, perform the following:
   - Place client on bed rest.
   - Monitor I&O; weigh daily.
   - Monitor urine sp. gravity, serum and urine lytes.
   - Assess for hemoconcentration; heparin may prevent hypercoagulability.
   - Increase fluid intake; replace electrolytes.
   - Provide analgesics for comfort.
3. Monitor CBC; an occasional client will develop erythrocytosis.

Client/Family Teaching

1. Report any pain, coolness, or pale bluish color of an extremity (signs of arterial bloodclot).

2. Report any fevers or abdominal pain. Fever or lower abdominal pain may be the result of overstimulation of the ovaries that has caused cysts to form, a loss of fluid into the peritoneum, or bleeding. Need exam every other day with this during drug therapy and for 2 weeks thereafter; hospitalization may be necessary.
3. Deliver a 24-hr urine daily for estrogen to lab facility.
4. Graph basal body temperature.
5. Signs of ovulation include an increase in the basal body temperature, and an increase in the appearance and volume of cervical mucus.
6. Engage in daily intercourse from the day before administration until ovulation occurs.
7. If symptoms indicate overstimulation of the ovaries, a significant ovarian enlargement may have occurred. Report and abstain from intercourse because of increased risk of ovarian cyst rupture.
8. Pregnancy usually occurs 4–6 weeks after completion of therapy. Multiple births may occur.

Outcome/Evaluate

- Ovulation evidenced by ↑ estrogen levels and desired pregnancy
- Male spermatogenesis evidenced by ↑ testosterone levels

Meperidine hydrochloride (Pethidine hydrochloride)

(meh-**PER**-ih-deen)

Pregnancy Category: C

Demerol Hydrochloride **(C-II) (Rx)**

Classification: Narcotic analgesic, synthetic

See also *Narcotic Analgesics.*

Action/Kinetics: Only one-tenth as potent an analgesic as morphine. Its analgesic effect is only one-half when given PO rather than parenterally. Has no antitussive effects and does not produce miosis. Produces moderate spasmogenic effects on smooth muscle. **Duration:** Less than that of most opiates; keep in mind when establishing a dosing schedule. Produces both psychologic and physical dependence; overdosage causes severe respiratory depression (see *Narcotic Overdose*). **Onset:** 10–45 min. **Peak effect:** 30–60 min. **Duration:** 2–4 hr. **t½:** 3–4 hr.

Uses: Analgesic for severe pain, hepatic and renal colic, obstetrics, preanesthetic medication, adjunct to anesthesia. Particularly useful for minor surgery, as in orthopedics, ophthalmology, rhinology, laryngology, and dentistry, and for diagnostic procedures such as cystoscopy, retrograde pyelography, and gastroscopy. Spasms of GI tract, uterus, urinary bladder. Anginal syndrome and distress of CHF.

Additional Contraindications: Hypersensitivity to drug, convulsive states as in epilepsy, tetanus and strychnine poisoning, children under 6 months, diabetic acidosis, head injuries, shock, liver disease, respiratory depression, increased cranial pressure, and before labor during pregnancy.

Special Concerns: Use with caution during lactation and in older or debilitated clients. Use with extreme caution in clients with asthma. Atropine-like effects may aggravate glaucoma, especially when given with other drugs which should be used with caution in glaucoma.

Additional Side Effects: Transient hallucinations, transient hypotension (high doses), visual disturbances. Meperidine may accumulate in clients with renal dysfunction, leading to an increased risk of CNS toxicity.

OD **Management of Overdose:** *Symptoms:* Severe respiratory depression. See *Narcotic Analgesics. Treatment:* Naloxone 0.4 mg IV is effective in the treatment of acute overdosage. In PO overdose, gastric lavage and induced emesis are indicated. Treatment, however, is aimed at combating the progressive respiratory depression usually through artificial ventilation.

Additional Drug Interactions

Antidepressants, tricyclic / Additive anticholinergic side effects

Hydantoins / ↓ Effect of meperidine due to ↑ breakdown by liver

MAO inhibitors / ↑ Risk of severe symptoms including hyperpyrexia, restlessness, hyper- or hypotension, convulsions, or coma

How Supplied: *Injection:* 10 mg/mL, 25 mg/mL, 50 mg/mL, 75mg/mL, 100 mg/mL; *Syrup:* 50 mg/5 mL; *Tablet:* 50 mg, 100 mg

Dosage

- **Tablets, Syrup, IM, SC**

Analgesic.

Adults: 50–100 mg q 3–4 hr as needed; **pediatric:** 1.1–1.8 mg/kg, up to adult dosage, q 3–4 hr as needed.

Preoperatively.

Adults, IM, SC: 50–100 mg 30–90 min before anesthesia; **pediatric, IM, SC:** 1–2 mg/kg 30–90 min before anesthesia.

Obstetrics.

Adults, IM, SC: 50–100 mg q 1–3 hr.

- **IV**

Support of anesthesia.

M

IV infusion: 1 mg/mL or **slow IV injection:** 10 mg/mL until client needs met.

HEALTH CARE CONSIDERATIONS

See also *Health Care Considerations* for *Narcotic Analgesics*.

Administration/Storage

1. For repeated doses, IM administration is preferred over SC use.
2. More effective when given parenterally than when given PO.
3. Take the syrup with ½ glass of water to minimize anesthetic effect on mucous membranes.
4. If used concomitantly with phenothiazines or antianxiety agents, reduce the dose by 25%–50%.

IV 5. Meperidine for IV use is incompatible with the following drugs: aminophylline, barbiturates, heparin, iodide, methicillin, morphine sulfate, phenytoin, sodium bicarbonate, sulfadiazine, and sulfisoxazole.

Assessment

1. Record intensity, location, onset, duration, and level of pain (use a rating scale).
2. Note any head injury, seizure disorder, or conditions that compromise respirations.
3. Assess renal function; note any glaucoma.

Client/Family Teaching

1. Use pain rating scale to evaluate drug effectiveness.
2. Drug causes dizziness and drowsiness; do not engage in activities that require mental alertness.
3. Rise slowly, do not to change positions abruptly due to postural effect.
4. Store safely away from bedside; record dose and time of administration. Drug causes dependence.

Outcome/Evaluate: Desired level of analgesia

Meprobamate

(meh-proh-**BAM**-ayt)

Apo-Meprobamate ✱, Equanil, Equanil Wyseals, Meprospan 200 and 400, Miltown 200, 400 and 600, Neuramate, Novo-Mepro ✱ **(C-IV) (Rx)**

Classification: Nonbenzodiazepine antianxiety agent

See also *Tranquilizers/Antimanic Drugs/Hypnotics*.

Action/Kinetics: Also possesses muscle relaxant and anticonvulsant effects. Acts on the limbic system and the thalamus, as well as inhibits polysynaptic spinal reflexes. **Onset:** 1 hr. **Blood levels, chronic therapy:** 5–20 mcg/mL. **t½:** 6–24 hr. Extensively metabolized in liver and inactive metabolites and some unchanged drug (8%–19%) are excreted in the urine.

Uses: Short-term treatment (no more than 4 months) of anxiety.

Contraindications: Hypersensitivity to meprobamate or carisoprodol. Porphyria. Children less than 6 years of age.

Special Concerns: Use with caution in pregnancy, lactation, epilepsy, liver and kidney disease. Geriatric clients may be more sensitive to the depressant effects of meprobamate; also, due to age-related impaired renal function, the dose of meprobamate may have to be reduced.

Side Effects: *CNS:* Ataxia, drowsiness, dizziness, weakness headache, paradoxical excitement, euphoria, slurred speech, vertigo. *GI:* N&V, diarrhea. *Miscellaneous:* Visual disturbances, allergic reactions including hematologic and dermatologic symptoms, paresthesias.

Laboratory Test Considerations: *With test methods:* ↑ 17-Hydroxycorticosteroids, 17-ketogenic steroids, and 17-ketosteroids. *Pharmacologic effects:* ↑ Alkaline phosphatase, bilirubin, serum transaminase, urinary estriol (calorimetric tests), porphobilinogen. ↓ PT in clients on Coumarin.

OD **Management of Overdose:** *Symptoms:* Drowsiness, stupor, lethargy, ataxia, ***shock, coma, respiratory collapse, death.*** Also, arrhythmias, tachycardia or bradycardia, reduced venous return, ***profound hypotension, CV collapse.*** Excessive oronasal secretions, ***relaxation of pharyngeal wall leading to obstruction of airway.*** *Treatment:* Induction of vomiting or gastric lavage if detected shortly after ingestion. It is imperative that gastric lavage be continued or gastroscopy be performed as incomplete gastric emptying can cause relapse and death.

- Give fluids to treat hypotension. Avoid fluid overload.
- Institute artificial respiration.
- Use care in treating seizures due to combined CNS depressant effects.
- Use forced diuresis and vasopressors followed by hemodialysis or hemoperfusion if condition deteriorates.

Drug Interactions: Additive depressant effects when used with CNS depressants, MAO inhibitors, and tricyclic antidepressants.

How Supplied: *Tablet:* 200 mg, 400 mg, 600 mg

Dosage

- **Tablets**

  Anxiety.

Adults, initial: 400 mg t.i.d.–q.i.d. (or 600 mg b.i.d.). May be increased, if necessary, up to maximum of 2.4 g/day. **Pediatric, 6–12 years of age:** 100–200 mg b.i.d.–t.i.d. (the 600-mg tablet is not recommended for use in children).

HEALTH CARE CONSIDERATIONS

See also *Healtlh Care Considerations* for *Tranquilizers Antimanic Drugs Hypnotics.*

Administration/Storage: Do not crush or chew tablets.

Assessment

1. Record onset and duration of symptoms; identify causes.
2. Assess mental status and note behavioral manifestations.

Outcome/Evaluate: ↓ Symptoms of anxiety

Mercaptopurine (6-Mercaptopurine)

(mer-kap-toe-**PYOUR**-een)

Pregnancy Category: D

Purinethol (Abbreviation: 6-MP) **(Rx)**

Classification: Antineoplastic, antimetabolite (purine analog)

See also *Antineoplastic Agents.*

Action/Kinetics: Cell-cycle specific for the S phase of cell division. Converted to thioinosinic acid by the enzyme hypoxanthine-guanine phosphoribosyltransferase. Thioinosinic acid then inhibits reactions involving inosinic acid. Also, both thioinosinic acid and 6-methylthioinosinate (also formed from mercaptopurine) inhibit RNA synthesis. About 50% absorbed from GI tract. **Plasma t½:** 47 min in adults and 21 min in children. Metabolites are excreted in urine with up to 39% excreted unchanged. Cross-resistance with thioguanine has been observed.

Uses: Acute lymphocytic or myelocytic leukemia. Lymphoblastic leukemia, especially in children. Acute myelogenous and myelomonocytic leukemia. Effectiveness varies depending on use. The drug is not effective for leukemia of the CNS, solid tumors, lymphomas, or chronic lymphatic leukemia. *Investigational:* Inflammatory bowel disease, chronic myelocytic leukemia, polycythemia vera, non-Hodgkin's lymphoma, psoriatic arthritis.

Contraindications: Use in resistance to mercaptopurine or thioguanine. To treat CNS leukemia, chronic lymphatic leukemia, lymphomas (including Hodgkin's disease), solid tumors. Lactation.

Special Concerns: Use with caution in clients with impaired renal function. Use during lactation only if benefits clearly outweigh risks. Severe bone marrow depression (anemia, leukopenia, thrombocytopenia) may occur. There is an increased risk of pancreatitis when used for inflammatory bowel disease.

Additional Side Effects: Hepatotoxicity, oral lesions, drug fever, hyperuricemia. Produces less GI toxicity than folic acid antagonists, and side effects are less frequent in children than in adults. Pancreatitis (when used for inflammatory bowel disease).

OD **Management of Overdose:** *Symptoms:* Immediate symptoms include N&V, diarrhea, and anorexia while delayed symptoms include myelosuppression, gastroenteritis, and liver dysfunction. *Treatment:* Induction of emesis if detected soon after ingestion. Supportive measures.

Drug Interactions

Allopurinol / ↑ Effect of methotrexate due to ↓ breakdown by liver (reduce dose of methotrexate by 25%–33%)

Trimethoprim–Sulfamethoxazole / ↑ Risk of bone marrow suppression

How Supplied: *Tablet:* 50 mg

Dosage

- **Tablets**

Highly individualized: 2.5 mg/kg/day. **Adults, usual:** 100–200 mg; **pediatric:** 50 mg. Dosage may be increased to 5 mg/kg/day after 4 weeks if beneficial effects are not noted. Dosage is increased until symptoms of toxicity appear. **Maintenance after remission:** 1.5–2.5 mg/kg/day.

HEALTH CARE CONSIDERATIONS

See also *Health Care Considerations* for *Antineoplastic Agents.*

Administration/Storage: Since the maximum effect on the blood count may be delayed and the count may drop for several days after drug has been discontinued, stop therapy at first sign of abnormally large drop in leukocyte count. Nadir: 14 days.

Assessment

1. Record indications for therapy, onset of symptoms, and other treatments prescribed.
2. Obtain liver and renal function studies, uric acid, and hematologic profile. Drug causes granulocyte and platelet suppression. Nadir: 10–14 days; recovery: 21–28 days.

Client/Family Teaching

1. Take drug in one dose daily at any convenient time.

M

2. Avoid alcoholic beverages.

Outcome/Evaluate

- Improved hematologic profile
- ↓ Malignant cell proliferation
- Symptoms of disease remission

Mesalamine (5-aminosalicylic acid)

(mes-AL-ah-meen)

Pregnancy Category: B

Asacol, Mesasal, Novo-5 ASA ✱, Pentasa, Quintasa ✱, Rowasa, Salofalk ✱ **(Rx)**

Classification: Anti-inflammatory agent

Action/Kinetics: Chemically related to acetylsalicylic acid. Acts locally in the colon to inhibit cyclo-oxygenase and therefore prostaglandin synthesis, resulting in a reduction of inflammation of colitis. Following PR administration, between 10% and 30% is absorbed and is excreted through the urine as the N-acetyl-5-aminosalicylic acid metabolite; the remainder is excreted in the feces. PO tablets are coated with an acrylic-based resin that prevents release of mesalamine until it reaches the terminal ileum and beyond. Approximately 28% of the drug found in tablets is absorbed with the remaining drug available for action in the colon. Capsules are ethylcellulose coated, controlled release designed to release the drug throughout the GI tract; from 20% to 30% is absorbed. **t½, mesalamine:** 0.5–1.5 hr; **t½, N-acetyl mesalamine:** 5–10 hr. **Time to reach maximum plasma levels:** 4–12 hr for both mesalamine and metabolite. Excreted mainly through the kidneys.

Uses: PO: Maintaining remission and treatment of mild to moderate active ulcerative colitis. **Rectal:** Treatment of active mild to moderate distal ulcerative colitis, proctosigmoiditis, or proctitis.

Contraindications: Hypersensitivity to salicylates.

Special Concerns: Use with caution in clients with sulfasalazine sensitivity, in those with impaired renal function, and during lactation. Safety and efficacy have not been established in children. Pyloric stenosis may delay the drug in reaching the colon.

Side Effects: *Sulfite sensitivity:* Hives, wheezing, itching, ***anaphylaxis.*** *Intolerance syndrome:* Acute abdominal pain, cramping, bloody diarrhea, rash, fever, headache. *GI:* Abdominal pain or discomfort, flatulence, cramps, dyspepsia, nausea, diarrhea, hemorrhoids, rectal pain or burning, rectal urgency, constipation, bloating, worsening of colitis, eructation, pain following insertion of enema, vomiting (after PO use). *CNS:* Headache, dizziness, insomnia, fatigue, malaise, chills, fever, asthenia. *Respiratory:* Cold, sore throat; increased cough, pharyngitis, rhinitis following PO use. *Dermatologic:* Acne, pruritus, itching, rash. *Musculoskeletal:* Back pain, hypertonia, arthralgia, myalgia, leg and joint pain, arthritis. *Miscellaneous:* Flu-like symptoms, hair loss, anorexia, peripheral edema, urinary burning, sweating, pain, chest pain, conjunctivitis, dysmenorrhea, pancreatitis.

In addition to the preceding, PO use may result in the following side effects. *GI:* Anorexia, gastritis, gastroenteritis, cholecystitis, dry mouth, increased appetite, oral ulcers, tenesmus, perforated peptic ulcer, bloody diarrhea, duodenal ulcer, dysphagia, esophageal ulcer, fecal incontinence, GI bleeding, oral moniliasis, rectal bleeding, abnormal stool color and texture. *CNS:* Anxiety, depression, hyperesthesia, nervousness, confusion, peripheral neuropathy, somnolence, emotional lability, vertigo, paresthesia, migraine, tremor, transverse myelitis, Guillain-Barré syndrome. *Dermatologic:* Dry skin, psoriasis, pyoderma gangrenosum, urticaria, erythema nodosum, eczema, photosensitivity, lichen planus, nail disorder. *CV:* Pericarditis, myocarditis, vasodilation, palpitations, ***fatal myocarditis,*** chest pain, T-wave abnormalities. *GU:* Nephropathy, interstitial nephritis, urinary urgency, dysuria, hematuria, menorrhagia, epididymitis, amenorrhea, hypomenorrhea, metrorrhagia, nephrotic syndrome, urinary frequency, albuminuria, nephrotoxicity. *Hematologic:* ***Agranulocytosis,*** anemia, eosinophilia, leukopenia, thrombocytopenia, lymphadenopathy, thrombocythemia, ecchymosis. *Respiratory:* Worsening of asthma, sinusitis, interstitial pneumonitis, pulmonary infiltrates, fibrosing alveolitis. *Ophthalmologic:* Eye pain, blurred vision. *Miscellaneous:* Ear pain, tinnitus, taste perversion, neck pain, enlargement of abdomen, facial edema, gout, hypersensitivity pneumonitis, breast pain, Kawasaki-like syndrome.

Laboratory Test Considerations: ↑ AST, ALT, BUN, LDH, alkaline phosphatase, serum creatinine, amylase, lipase, GTTP.

OD **Management of Overdose:** *Symptoms:* Salicylate toxicity manifested by tinnitus, vertigo, headache, confusion, drowsiness, sweating, hyperventilation, vomiting, and diarrhea. Severe toxicity results in disruption of electrolyte balance and blood pH, ***hyperthermia, and dehydration.*** *Treatment:* Therapy to treat salicylate toxicity, including emesis, gastric lavage, fluid and electrolyte replacement (if necessary), maintenance of adequate renal function.

How Supplied: *Capsule, Extended Release:* 250 mg; *Rectal Suspension:* 4 g/60 mL; *Sup-*

pository: 500 mg; *Tablet, Delayed Release:* 400 mg

Dosage

- **Suppository**

One suppository (500 mg) b.i.d.

- **Rectal Suspension Enema**

4 g in 60 mL once daily for 3–6 weeks, usually given at bedtime. For maintenance, the drug can be given every other day or every third day at doses of 1–2 g.

- **Capsules, Extended-Release**

1 g (4 capsules) q.i.d. for a total daily dose of 4 g for up to 8 weeks.

- **Tablets, Enteric-Coated**

800 mg t.i.d. for a total dose of 2.4 g/day for 6 weeks.

HEALTH CARE CONSIDERATIONS

Administration/Storage

1. Shake the bottle well to ensure suspension is homogeneous.
2. Beneficial effects using the suppository or enema may be seen within 3–21 days, with a full course of therapy lasting up to 6 weeks.

Assessment

1. Determine any sulfite sensitivity.
2. Record character/frequency of stools. Assess abdomen for bowel sounds, distension, pain/tenderness.
3. Monitor chemistries, liver and renal function studies, and abdominal films.

Client/Family Teaching

1. Take tablets whole, being careful not to break the outer coating.
2. Review technique for enema/suppository administration.

- Prior to use, shake bottle until all contents are thoroughly mixed. Remove cap, insert tip into rectum, and squeeze steadily to completely discharge contents.
- Lie on the left side with the lower leg extended and the upper right leg flexed forward. The knee-chest position may also be used for suppository administration.
- Retain the enema for 8 hr to ensure proper absorption; may best be accomplished by administering at bedtime, after bowel movement, and retaining throughout the sleep cycle.
- For maximal effect, retain suppository for 1–3 hr or more.
- Protect bed linens with towels or rubber pads.

3. Hold drug and report severe abdominal pain, cramping, bloody diarrhea, rash, fever, or headache.
4. Avoid smoking and cold foods; increases bowel motility.
5. The therapy may last 3–6 weeks; follow as prescribed.

Outcome/Evaluate

- Relief of pain and diarrhea
- Normalization of bowel patterns

Mesoridazine besylate

(mez-oh-**RID**-ah-zeen)

Serentil **(Rx)**

Classification: Antipsychotic, piperidine-type phenothiazine

See also *Antipsychotic Agents, Phenothiazines.*

Action/Kinetics: Pronounced sedative and hypotensive effects, moderate anticholinergic effects, and a low incidence of extrapyramidal symptoms and antiemetic effects.

Uses: Schizophrenia, acute and chronic alcoholism, behavior problems in clients with mental deficiency and chronic brain syndrome, psychoneurosis.

Special Concerns: Use during pregnancy only if benefits clearly outweigh risks. Dosage has not been established in children less than 12 years of age. Geriatric, debilitated, and emaciated clients require a lower initial dose.

How Supplied: *Concentrate:* 25 mg/mL; *Injection:* 25 mg/mL; *Tablet:* 10 mg, 25 mg, 50 mg, 100 mg

Dosage

- **Oral Solution, Tablets**

Psychotic disorders.

Adults and adolescents, initial: 50 mg t.i.d.; **optimum total dose:** 100–400 mg/day.

Alcoholism.

Adults, initial: 25 mg b.i.d.; **optimum total dose:** 50–200 mg/day.

Behavior problems in mental deficiency and chronic brain syndrome.

Adults, initial: 25 mg b.i.d.; **optimum total dose:** 75–300 mg/day.

Psychoneurotic manifestations.

Adults, initial: 10 mg t.i.d.; **optimum total dose:** 30–150 mg/day.

- **IM**

Psychotic disorders.

Adults and adolescents, initial: 25 mg (base); **then,** repeat the dose in 30–60 min as needed. **Optimum total dose:** 25–200 mg/day.

HEALTH CARE CONSIDERATIONS

See also *Health Care Considerations* for *Antipsychotic Agents, Phenothiazines.*

Administration/Storage

1. Acidified tap or distilled water, orange

M

juice, or grape juice may be used to dilute the concentrate prior to use.
2. Do not prepare or store bulk dilutions.

Assessment

1. Record onset, duration, and characteristics of symptoms; describe behavioral manifestations.
2. List other agents trialed and the outcome.
3. Observe for increased sedation, orthostatic and cholinergic effects. Keep supine for at least 30 min after parenteral administration to minimize orthostatic effect.

Outcome/Evaluate: Improved patterns of behavior with ↓ agitation, ↓ hyperactivity, and reality orientation

Metaproterenol sulfate (Orciprenaline sulfate)

(met-ah-proh-**TER**-ih-nohl)

Pregnancy Category: C

Alti-Orciprenaline ✤, Alupent, Arm-A-Med Metaproterenol Sulfate, Metaprel, Orcipren ✤, Tanta Orciprenaline ✤ **(Rx)**

Classification: Adrenergic agent, direct-acting; bronchodilator

M

See also *Sympathomimetic Drugs*.

Action/Kinetics: Markedly stimulates beta-2 receptors, resulting in relaxation of smooth muscles of the bronchial tree, as well as peripheral vasodilation. Minimal effects on beta-1 receptors. Similar to isoproterenol but with a longer duration of action and fewer side effects. **Onset: Inhalation aerosol,** within 1 min; **peak effect:** 1 hr; **duration:** 1–5 hr. **Onset, hand bulb nebulizer or IPPB:** 5–30 min; **duration:** 4–6 hr after repeated doses. **PO: Onset,** 15–30 min; **peak effect:** 1 hr. **Duration:** 4 hr. Marked first-pass effect after PO use. Metabolized in the liver and excreted through the kidney.

Uses: Bronchodilator in asthma, bronchitis, emphysema, and other conditions associated with reversible bronchospasms. Treatment of acute asthmatic attacks in children over 6 years of age.

Special Concerns: Dosage of syrup or tablets not determined in children less than 6 years of age.

Additional Side Effects: *GI:* Diarrhea, bad taste or taste changes. *Respiratory:* Worsening of asthma, nasal congestion, hoarseness. *Miscellaneous:* Hypersensitivity reactions, rash, fatigue, backache, skin reactions.

Drug Interactions: Possible potentiation of adrenergic effects if used before or after other sympathomimetic bronchodilators.

How Supplied: *Metered dose inhaler (aerosol):* 0.65 mg/inh; *Solution for Inhalation:* 0.4%, 0.6%, 5%; *Syrup:* 10 mg/5 mL; *Tablet:* 10 mg, 20 mg

Dosage

- **Syrup, Tablets**

  Bronchodilation.

Adults and children over 27.2 kg or 9 years: 20 mg t.i.d.–q.i.d.; **children under 27.2 kg or 6–9 years of age:** 10 mg t.i.d.–q.i.d.; **children less than 6 years of age:** 1.3–2.6 mg/kg/day of the syrup has been studied.

- **Inhalation. Hand Nebulizer**

  Bronchodilation.

Usual dose is 10 inhalations (range: 5–15 inhalations) of undiluted 5% solution.

- **IPPB**

  Bronchodilation.

0.3 mL (range: 0.2–0.3 mL) of 5% solution diluted to 2.5 mL saline or other diluent.

- **MDI**

  Bronchodilation.

2–3 inhalations (1.30–2.25 mg) q 3–4 hr. Do not exceed a total daily dose of 12 inhalations (9 mg).

HEALTH CARE CONSIDERATIONS

See also *Special Health Care Considerations for Adrenergic Bronchodilators* under *Sympathomimetic Drugs*.

Administration/Storage: Refrigerate unit dose vials at 2°C–8°C (35°F–46°F).

Client/Family Teaching

1. Review appropriate method for administration. Shake container before each use.
2. Report loss of effectiveness with prescribed dosage and frequency.
3. Store the inhalant solution at room temperature, but avoid excessive heat and light.
4. Do not use the solution if it is brown or shows a precipitate.
5. Do not use inhalant solutions more often than q 4 hr to relieve acute bronchospasms. In chronic bronchospastic disease, the dose can be given t.i.d.–q.i.d. A single dose of nebulized drug may not completely abort acute asthma attack.
6. Stop smoking to help preserve lung function.

Outcome/Evaluate

- Improved airway exchange; ↑ oxygen saturation levels
- Relief of respiratory distress

Metformin and Glyburide

(met-**FOR**-min/**GLYE**-byou-ryd)

Pregnancy Category: B

Glucovance **(Rx)**

Classification: Oral Antidiabetic

See also *Metformin* and *Glyburide*.
Content: *Sulfonylurea:* Glyburide 1.25 mg, 2.5 mg or 5 mg. *Oral antidiabetic, biguanide:* Metformin 250mg, 500 mg.
Action/Kinetics: See also glyburide and metformin. Combines glyburide and metformin HCl, two antihyperglycemic agents with complementary mechanisms of action, to improve glycemic control in persons with type 2 diabetes.
Uses: As combination therapy for persons with type 2 diabetes with a HbA1c >8.
Contraindications: See also Metformin. Renal disease or dysfunction (serum creatinine levels >1.5 mg/dL in males and >1.4 mg/dL in females) or abnormal C_{CR}. Persons with impaired liver function, dehydration, congestive heart failure, or other conditions of hypoperfusion.
Special Concerns: See also Metformin. **Lactic acidosis** is a rare, but serious, metabolic complication that can occur due to metformin accumulation during treatment with this medication; when it occurs it is **fatal** in approximately 50% of cases. Metformin should not be used in clients with significant renal dysfunction. Caution should be excercised in persons >80 yr., those having congestive heart failure or other conditions where there is possibility of hypoperfusion. Because the liver is responsible for the clearance of lactic acid, persons with impaired liver function should not take metformin. Lactic acidosis onset is subtle. Signs and symptoms include general maliase, unusual muscle pain, difficulty breathing, unusual abdominal discomfort, coldness, dizziness, suddenly developing a slow or irregular heartbeat.
Side Effects: GI upset, hypoglycemia.
How Supplied: *Tablet:* Glyburide 1.25 mg/Metformin 250 mg; Glyburide 2.5 mg/Metformin 500 mg; Glyburide 5 mg/Metformin 500 mg.

Dosage

- **Tablets**

Initial: *Newly diagnosed clients with type 2 diabetes*

HbA1c<9%: 1.25 mg/250 mg daily with a meal; *HbA1c >9%:* 1.25 mg/250 mg bid with meals.

Replacement: *Clients not adequately controlled on either glyburide (or another sulfonylurea or metformin alone) HbA1c> 7%:* 2.5 mg/500 mg bid with meals;

Clients: previously treated with combination therapy with a sulfonylurea and metformin

Switch: 2.5 mg/ 500 mg with meals; or 5 mg/500 mg with meals; **not** to exceed total daily doses already being taken. Clients should be monitored closely for signs and symptoms of hypoglycemia following such a switch. **Titrate as needed to maximum dose of 10 mg/2000 mg or 20 mg/2000 mg.** Glucovance 5 mg/500 mg should not be used as initial therapy, due to an increased risk of hypoglycemia. Dosage increases should be made in increments of 1.25 mg/250 mg per day every 2 weeks up to the minimum effective dose necessary to achieve adequate control of blood glucose. In order to avoid hypoglycemia, the starting dose of glucovance should not exceed the daily dose of glyburide (or equivalent dose of another sulfonylurea) and metformin already being taken. The daily dose should be titrated in increments of no more than 5 mg/500 mg up to the minimum effective dose necessary to achieve adequate control of blood glucose.

HEALTH CARE CONSIDERATIONS

See *Health Care Considerations* for *Metformin* and *Glyburide*.
Administration/Storage: Taking with food may decrease stomach upset.
Client/Family Teaching: See individual components.
Outcome/Evaluate: Control of BS; prevention of microvascular complications, HbA1c<7.
Treatment of Overdose: Supportive treatment measure; dialysis is effective in removing metformin accumulation and may reverse developing lactic acidosis.
Laboratory Tests: Monitor LFTs, renal function, BS and HbA1c.

M

Metformin hydrochloride

(met-**FOR**-min)
Pregnancy Category: B
Apo-Metformin ✦, Gen-Metformin ✦, Glucophage, Glucophage XR, Glycon ✦, Novo-Metformin ✦, Nu-Metformin ✦, PMS-Metformin ✦ **(Rx)**
Classification: Oral antidiabetic

Action/Kinetics: Decreases hepatic glucose production, decreases intestinal absorption of glucose, and increases peripheral uptake and utilization of glucose. Does not cause hypoglycemia in either diabetic or nondiabetic clients, and it does not cause hyperinsulinemia. Insulin secretion remains unchanged, while fasting insulin levels and day-long plasma insulin response may decrease. In contrast to sulfonylureas, the body weight of clients treated with metformin

remains stable or may decrease somewhat. Food decreases and slightly delays the absorption of metformin. Negligibly bound to plasma protein; steady-state plasma levels (less than 1 mcg/mL) are reached within 24–48 hr. Excreted unchanged in the urine; no biliary excretion. **t½, plasma elimination:** 6.2 hr. The plasma and blood half-lives are prolonged in decreased renal function.
Uses: Alone as an adjunct to diet to lower blood glucose in clients having NIDDM whose blood glucose cannot be managed satisfactorily via diet alone. Also, metformin may be used concomitantly with a sulfonylurea when diet and metformin or a sulfonylurea alone do not result in adequate control of blood glucose.
Contraindications: Renal disease or dysfunction (serum creatinine levels greater than 1.5 mg/dL in males and greater than 1.4 mg/dL in females) or abnormal C_{CR} due to cardiovascular collapse, acute MI, or septicemia. In clients undergoing radiologic studies using iodinated contrast media, because use of such products may cause alteration of renal function, leading to acute renal failure and lactic acidosis. Acute or chronic metabolic acidosis, including diabetic ketoacidosis, with or without coma. Lactation.
Special Concerns: Cardiovascular collapse, acute CHF, acute MI, and other conditions characterized by hypoxia have been associated with lactic acidosis, which may also be caused by metformin. Use of oral hypoglycemic agents may increase the risk of cardiovascular mortality. Although hypoglycemia does not usually occur with metformin, it may result with deficient caloric intake, with strenuous exercise not supplemented by increased intake of calories, or when metformin is taken with sulfonylureas or alcohol. Because of age-related decreases in renal function, use with caution as age increases. Safety and efficacy have not been determined in children.
Side Effects: *Metabolic:* Lactic acidosis (fatal in approximately 50% of cases). *GI:* Diarrhea, N&V, abdominal bloating, flatulence, anorexia, unpleasant or metallic taste. *Hematologic:* Asymptomatic subnormal serum vitamin B_{12} levels.
OD **Management of Overdose:** *Symptoms:* Lactic acidosis.
Drug Interactions
Alcohol / Alcohol ↑ the effect of metformin on lactate metabolism
Cimetidine / Cimetidine ↑ (by 60%) peak metformin plasma and whole blood levels
Furosemide / Furosemide ↑ metformin plasma and blood levels; also, metformin ↓ the half-life of furosemide
Iodinated contrast media / ↑ Risk of acute renal failure and lactic acidosis
Nifedipine / Nifedipine ↑ the absorption of metformin, leading to ↑ plasma metformin levels
How Supplied: *Tablet:* 500 mg, 850 mg, 1000 mg; *Tablet, Extended Release:* 500 mg

Dosage
- **Tablets**

NIDDM.

Adults, using 500-mg tablet: Starting dose is one 500-mg tablet b.i.d. given with the morning and evening meals. Dosage increases may be made in increments of 500 mg every week, given in divided doses, up to a maximum of 2,500 mg/day. If a 2,500-mg daily dose is required, it may be better tolerated when given in divided doses t.i.d. with meals. **Adults, using 850-mg tablet:** Starting dose is 850 mg once daily given with the morning meal. Dosage increases may be made in increments of 850 mg every other week, given in divided doses, up to a maximum of 2,550 mg/day. **Usual maintenance dose:** 850 mg b.i.d. with the morning and evening meals. However, some clients may require 850 mg t.i.d. with meals.
- **Tablets, extended release:**

Initial: 500 mg once daily (with the evening meal); dosage may be increased by 500 mg weekly; maximum dose: 2000 mg once daily. If glycemic control is not achieved at maximum dose, may divide dose to 1000 mg twice daily; if doses >2000 mg/day are needed, switch to regular release tablets and titrate to maximum dose of 2550 mg/day

HEALTH CARE CONSIDERATIONS
Administration/Storage
1. Individualize dosage based on tolerance and effectiveness.
2. Give with meals starting at a low dose with gradual escalation. This will reduce GI side effects and allow determination of the minimal dose necessary for adequate control of blood glucose.
3. No transition period is required when transferring from standard oral hypoglycemic drugs (other than chlorpropamide) to metformin. When transferring from chlorpropamide, exercise caution during the first 2 weeks because of chlorpropamide's long duration of action.
4. If the maximum dose of metformin for 4 weeks does not provide adequate control of blood glucose, gradual addition of an oral sulfonylurea (data are available for glyburide, chlorpropamide, tolbutamide, and glipizide) may be considered, while maintaining the

maximum dose of metformin. The desired control of blood glucose may be attained by adjusting the dose of each drug.
5. If no response to 1–3 months of concomitant metformin and oral sulfonylurea therapy, consider initiating insulin therapy and discontinuing the oral agents.
6. The initial and maintenance doses of metformin in geriatric and debilitated clients should be conservative because of the potential for decreased renal function. Do not titrate these clients to the maximum dose.

Assessment

1. Record age at diabetes onset, previous therapies utilized, and the outcome.
2. Monitor CBC, BS, electrolytes, HbA1c, urinalysis, liver and renal function studies. Assess for liver or renal failure; may precipitate lactic acidosis (i.e., serum lactate levels greater than 5 mmol/L, decreased blood pH, increased anion gap).
3. Hold drug for procedures utilizing iodinated contrast agents.
4. If anemia develops, exclude vitamin B_{12} deficiency; may interfere with B_{12} absorption.
5. For surgery, withhold and do not administer until normal diet resumed.
6. A small dose with insulin therapy may enhance glucose control.

Client/Family Teaching

1. Take with food to diminish GI upset.
2. May cause a metallic taste; should subside.
3. Regular exercise, decreased caloric intake, and weight loss are required to reduce blood glucose levels; medication neither replaces nor excuses compliance with these modalities.
4. Inadequate caloric intake or strenuous exercise without caloric replacement may precipitate hypoglycemia.
5. Do regular blood sugar monitoring (fingersticks) and maintain record for provider review.
6. Avoid alcohol and any situations that may precipitate dehydration.
7. Consume plenty of fluids; report when illnesses with fever, vomiting, and diarrhea are persistent/severe.
8. Stop drug and immediately report any symptoms of difficulty breathing, severe weakness, muscle pain, increased sleepiness, or sudden increased abdominal distress.
9. Extended release tablets: Inert componets of the tablet may be excreted in the stool.

Outcome/Evaluate

- Control of BS; prevention of microvascular complications
- HbA1c <8%)

Methadone hydrochloride

(METH-ah-dohn)

Pregnancy Category: C

Dolophine, Methadose **(C-II) (Rx)**

Classification: Narcotic analgesic, morphine type

See also *Narcotic Analgesics*.

Action/Kinetics: Produces only mild euphoria, which is the reason it is used as a heroin withdrawal substitute and for maintenance programs. Produces physical dependence; withdrawal symptoms develop more slowly and are less intense but more prolonged than those associated with morphine. Does not produce sedation or narcosis. Not effective for preoperative or obstetric anesthesia. Only one-half as potent PO as when given parenterally. **Onset:** 30–60 min. **Peak effects:** 30–60 min. **Duration:** 4–6 hr. **t½:** 15–30 hr. Both the duration and half-life increase with repeated use due to cumulative effects.

Uses: Severe pain. Drug withdrawal and maintenance of narcotic dependence.

Additional Contraindications: IV use, liver disease, during pregnancy, in children, or in obstetrics (due to long duration of action and chance of respiratory depression in the neonate).

Special Concerns: Use with caution during lactation.

Laboratory Test Considerations: ↑ Immunoglobulin G.

Additional Side Effects: Marked constipation, excessive sweating, pulmonary edema, choreic movements.

Drug Interactions: Rifampin and phenytoin ↓ plasma methadone levels by ↑ breakdown by liver; thus, possible symptoms of narcotic withdrawal may develop.

How Supplied: *Oral Concentrate:* 10 mg/mL; *Oral Solution:* 5 mg/5 mL, 10 mg/5 mL; *Tablet:* 5 mg, 10 mg, 40 mg; *Tablet, Dispersable:* 40 mg

Dosage

- **Tablets, Oral Solution, Oral Concentrate**

Analgesia.

Adults, individualized: 2.5–10 mg q 3–4 hr, although higher doses may be necessary for severe pain or due to development of tolerance.

Narcotic withdrawal.

Initial: 15–20 mg/day PO (some may require 40 mg/day); **then,** depending on need of the client, slowly decrease dosage.

Maintenance following narcotic withdrawal.

M

Adults, individualized, initial: 20–40 mg PO 4–8 hr after heroin is stopped; **then,** adjust dosage as required up to 120 mg/day.

HEALTH CARE CONSIDERATIONS

See also *Health Care Considerations* for *Narcotic Analgesics.*

Administration/Storage

1. Dilute solution in at least 90 mL of water prior to administration.
2. If taking dispersible tablets, dilute in 120 mL of water, orange juice, citrus-flavored drink, or other acidic fruit drink. Allow at least 1 min for complete drug dispersion.
3. For repeated analgesic doses, IM administration is preferred over SC administration; Inspect sites for signs of irritation.
4. Duration of treatment for detoxification purposes is no longer than 21 days. Do not repeat treatment for 4 weeks.

Client/Family Teaching

1. If ambulatory and not suffering acute pain, side effects may be more pronounced.
2. Report N&V; a lower drug dose may relieve symptoms.
3. To minimize constipation, exercise regularly and increase intake of fluids, fruit, and bulk.
4. For clients on narcotic withdrawal therapy, store drug out of the reach of children.
5. Continue to attend group therapy as with Narcotics Anonymous. Identify social service groups for assistance in child care, food and living arrangements, and expenses.

Outcome/Evaluate

- Control of severe pain
- Detoxification and maintenance in narcotic-dependent individual

M

Methamphetamine hydrochloride

(meth-am-**FET**-ah-meen)

Pregnancy Category: C

Desoxyn **(C-II) (Rx)**

Classification: Central nervous system stimulant, amphetamine-type

See also *Amphetamines and Derivatives.*

Action/Kinetics: t½: 4–5 hr, depending on urinary pH.

Uses: Attention-deficit disorders in children over 6 years of age. Obesity (use controversial and often not recommended).

Contraindications: Use for obesity. Attention-deficit disorders in children less than 6 years of age.

How Supplied: *Tablet:* 5 mg; *Tablet, Extended Release:* 5 mg, 10 mg, 15 mg

Dosage

- **Tablets**

ADD in children 6 years and older.

Initial: 5 mg 1–2 times/day; increase in increments of 5 mg/day at weekly intervals until optimum dose is reached (usually 20–25 mg/day).

- **Extended-Release Tablets**

ADD in children 6 years and older, maintenance.

20–25 mg once daily.

Obesity.

Either one 5-mg tablet 30 min before each meal or 10–15 mg of the long-acting form in the morning. Do not exceed more than a few weeks of treatment.

HEALTH CARE CONSIDERATIONS

See also *Health Care Considerations* for *Amphetamines and Derivatives.*

Administration/Storage

1. When used to facilitate verbalization during psychotherapeutic interview, give second dose only if the first dose has proven effective.
2. When used for attention-deficit disorders, the total daily dose can be given in two divided doses or once a day using the long-acting product. Do not use the long-acting product to initiate therapy. Evaluate client progress periodically to determine the need for continued treatment.

Assessment

1. Record indications for therapy, type, onset, and duration of symptoms. List other agents prescribed and the outcome.
2. Assess mental status and note behavioral manifestations.

Outcome/Evaluate: ↑ Attention span; ability to sit quietly and concentrate

Methazolamide

(meth-ah-**ZOH**-lah-myd)

Pregnancy Category: C

Glauctabs, Neptazane **(Rx)**

Classification: Antiglaucoma drug

Action/Kinetics: Inhibition of carbonic anhdyrase decreases the secretion of aqueous humor resulting in a decrease in intraocular pressure. Has weak diuretic effects and, due to inhibition of carbonic anhydrase, produces an alkaline urine. Excretion of both urinary citrate and uric acid is decreased. Distributed to the plasma, CSF, aqueous humor of the eye, red blood cells, bile, and extracellular fluid. **Onset:** 2–4 hr. **Peak effect:** 6–8 hr. **Duration:** 10–18 hr. **t½, elimination:** 14 hr. About 25% excreted unchanged in the urine.

Uses: Treatment of chronic open-angle glaucoma, secondary glaucoma. Preoperatively in acute angle-closure glaucoma to lower IOP prior to surgery.
Contraindications: Use in marked kidney or liver disease or dysfunction, in adrenal gland failure, and in hyperchloremic acidosis. Long-term use in clients with angle-closure glaucoma, since organic closure of the angle may occur even if IOP is lowered. Lactation.
Special Concerns: Use with caution in those with pulmonary obstruction or emphysema as acidosis may be aggravated or precipitated. Use with caution in those with cirrhosis or hepatic insufficiency due to the possibility of hepatic coma. The safety and efficacy have not been determined for use in children.
Side Effects: *GI:* Taste alteration, N&V, diarrhea, melena. *CNS:* Paresthesias (especially a "tingling" feeling in the extremities), fatigue, malaise, loss of appetite, drowsiness, confusion, ***convulsions.*** *Metabolic:* Metabolic acidosis, electrolyte imbalance. *GU:* Polyuria, hematuria, glycosuria. Rarely, crystalluria and renal calculi. *Dermatologic:* Urticaria, photosensitivity. *Miscellaneous:* Hearing dysfunction or tinnitus, transient myopia, hepatic insufficiency, flaccid paralysis.

NOTE: Side effects may be observed that are due to the sulfonamide. See *Sulfonamides.*

Drug Interactions
Aspirin (high doses) / Symptoms of anorexia, tachypnea, lethargy, coma, and death are possible
Corticosteroids / ↑ Risk of hypokalemia
How Supplied: *Tablets:* 25 mg, 50 mg

Dosage
- **Tablets**
  Glaucoma.
  50–100 mg b.i.d.–t.i.d.

HEALTH CARE CONSIDERATIONS

Administration/Storage
1. May be used with a miotic and osmotic agent.
2. Store at controlled room temperatures of 15°C–30°C (59°F–86°F).

Assessment
1. Record indications for therapy; note sulfonamide sensitivity.
2. List drugs currently prescribed to ensure none interact unfavorably.
3. Obtain baseline CBC, electrolytes, and LFTs.

Client/Family Teaching
1. Take as directed; do not exceed prescribed dosage.
2. Report for eye evaluations and electrolyte determinations.
3. Report any unusual fever, bleeding, rash, or fatigue.

Outcome/Evaluate: ↓ IOP

Methenamine hippurate
(meh-**THEEN**-ah-meen)
Pregnancy Category: C
Hip-Rex ✦, Hiprex, Urex **(Rx)**

Methenamine mandelate
(meh-**THEEN**-ah-meen)
Pregnancy Category: C
Mandelamine ✦ **(Rx)**
Classification: Urinary tract anti-infective

Action/Kinetics: Converted in an acid medium into ammonia and formaldehyde (the active principle), which denatures protein. Formaldehyde levels in the urine may be bacteriostatic or bactericidal, depending on the pH; it is most effective when the urine has a pH value of 5.5 or less, which is maintained by using the hippurate or mandelate salt. Readily absorbed from GI tract, but up to 60% may be hydrolyzed by gastric acid if tablets are not enteric-coated. To be effective, urinary formaldehyde concentration must be greater than 25 mcg/mL. **Peak levels of formaldehyde:** 2 hr if using hippurate and 3–8 hr if using mandelate (if urinary pH is 5.5 or less) **t½:** 3–6 hr. Seventy to 90% of drug and metabolites excreted in urine within 24 hr.
Uses: Acute, chronic, and recurrent UTIs by susceptible organisms, especially gram-negative organisms including *Escherichia coli.* As a prophylactic before urinary tract instrumentation. Never used as sole agent in the treatment of acute infections.
Contraindications: Renal insufficiency, severe liver damage, severe dehydration. Concurrent use of sulfonamides as an insoluble precipitate may form with formaldehyde.
Special Concerns: Use with caution in gout (methenamine may cause urate crystals to precipitate in the urine).
Side Effects: *GI:* N&V, diarrhea, anorexia, cramps, stomatitis. *GU:* Hematuria, albuminuria, crystalluria, dysuria, urinary frequency or urgency, bladder irritation. *Dermatologic:* Skin rashes, urticaria, pruritus, erythematous eruptions. *Other:* Headache, dyspnea, edema, lipoid pneumonitis.

Laboratory Test Considerations: False + urinary glucose with Benedict's solution. Drug interferes with determination of urinary catecholamines and estriol levels by acid hydrolysis technique (enzymatic techniques not affected). False + catecholamines, hydroxycorticosteroids, vanillylmandelic acid; false – 5-hydroxyindoleacetic acid.

OD **Management of Overdose:** *Treatment:* Absorption following overdose may be minimized by inducing vomiting or by gastric lavage, followed by activated charcoal. Fluids should be forced.

Drug Interactions

Acetazolamide / ↓ Effect of methenamine due to inhibition of conversion to formaldehyde

Sodium bicarbonate / ↓ Effect of methenamine due to inhibition of conversion to formaldehyde

Sulfonamides / ↑ Chance of sulfonamide crystalluria due to acid urine produced by methenamine

Thiazide diuretics / ↓ Effect of methenamine due to ↑ alkalinity of urine produced by thiazides

How Supplied: Methenanamine hippurate: *Tablet:* 1 g Methenamine mandelate: *Tablet, Enteric coated:* 0.5 g, 1 g; *Suspension:* 0.5 g/5 mL

Dosage

- **Tablets**

Hippurate: **Adults and children over 12 years:** 1 g b.i.d. in the morning and evening; **children, 6–12 years:** 0.5 g b.i.d.

- **Oral Suspension, Enteric-Coated Tablets**

Mandelate: **Adults:** 1 g q.i.d. after meals and at bedtime; **children 6–12 years:** 0.5 g q.i.d.; **children under 6 years:** 0.25 g/13.6 kg q.i.d.

HEALTH CARE CONSIDERATIONS

See also *General Health Care Considerations for All Anti-Infectives.*

Assessment

1. Record indications for therapy, onset and duration of symptoms.
2. Note any history of gout.
3. List other agents prescribed. Urine may become turbid and full of sediment when methenamine is administered with sulfamethizole.
4. Obtain baseline C&S. Monitor urine for evidence of hematuria and/or albuminuria.
5. Maintain acidic urine when treating *Proteus* or *Pseudomonas* infections.
6. Oral suspensions have a vegetable oil base; take particular care with the elderly or debilitated to prevent lipid pneumonia.

Client/Family Teaching

1. May take with food if GI upset occurs.
2. Consume 1.5–2 L/day of fluids.
3. To maintain an acidic urine, alkalizing foods (e.g., milk products) or medication (e.g., acetazolamide, bicarbonate) should be avoided.
4. Foods (such as prunes, plums, and cranberry juice) may help maintain acid urine. Drugs such as ascorbic acid, methionine, ammonium chloride, or sodium diphosphate may additionally be required.
5. Use Labstix or Nitrazine paper to test pH of urine to ensure 5.5 or lower.
6. With high dosage, report any evidence of bladder irritation or painful and frequent micturition.
7. Report adverse effects of N&V, skin rash, tinnitus, and muscle cramps as these may require termination of drug therapy.

Outcome/Evaluate

- Resolution of UTI
- Negative urine C&S results

Methimazole (Thiamazole)

(meth-**IM**-ah-zohl)

Pregnancy Category: D

Tapazole **(Rx)**

Classification: Antithyroid drug

See also *Antithyroid Drugs.*

Action/Kinetics: Onset is more rapid but effect is less consistent than that of propylthiouracil. Bioavailability may be affected by food. **t½:** 4–14 hr. **Onset:** 10–20 days. **Time to peak effect:** 2–10 weeks. **t½:** 6–13 hr. Crosses the placenta; high levels appear in breast milk. Metabolized in the liver and excreted through the kidneys (7% unchanged).

Special Concerns: Incidence of hepatic toxicity may be greater than for propylthiouracil.

How Supplied: *Tablet:* 5 mg, 10 mg

Dosage

- **Tablets**

Mild hyperthyroidism.

Adults, initial: 15 mg/day.

Moderately severe hyperthyroidism.

Adults, initial: 30–40 mg/day.

Severe hyperthyroidism.

Adults, initial: 60 mg/day. For hyperthyroidism, the daily dose is usually given in three equal doses 8 hr apart. **Maintenance:** 5–15 mg/day as a single dose or divided into two doses. **Pediatric:** 0.4 mg/kg given once daily or divided into two doses; **maintenance:** 0.2 mg/kg. Alternatively, **initial:** 0.5–0.7 mg/kg/day (15–20 mg/m^2/day in three divided doses); **maintenance:** ⅓–⅔ initial dose when client is euthyroid up to a maximum of 30 mg/day.

Thyrotoxic crisis.

Adults: 15–20 mg/4 hr during the first day as an adjunct to other treatments.

HEALTH CARE CONSIDERATIONS

See also *Health Care Considerations* for *Antithyroid Drugs.*

Assessment

1. Record indications for therapy, type and onset of symptoms.
2. Monitor CBC, thyroid function/scan, height, weight, and VS.
3. Assess for changes in extremity sensation; may develop paresthesias.

Client/Family Teaching

1. May take with a snack to reduce gastric irritation. Report if GI upset persists.
2. Take as prescribed at evenly spaced intervals and with evenly spaced doses throughout the day.
3. Report any unexpected symptoms immediately. Desired effects may not be evident for weeks; dosage may require adjustment.
4. Report any sore throats, fever, chills, and unexplained bleeding (S&S of agranulocytosis).
5. Report hair loss.
6. Drug is usually administered until client becomes euthyroid or for a year; then if more treatment is necessary, radiopharmaceuticals (I-131) may be considered.

Outcome/Evaluate

- Promotion of normal metabolism
- Serum thyroid function levels within desired range; ↓ T_4 ↑ TSH

Methocarbamol

(meth-oh-**KAR**-bah-mohl)

Robaxin, Robaxin Injectable ✱, Robaxin-750

(Rx)

Classification: Centrally acting muscle relaxant

See also *Skeletal Muscle Relaxants, Centrally Acting.*

Action/Kinetics: Beneficial effect may be related to the sedative properties of the drug. Has no direct effect on the contractile mechanism of striated muscle, the motor endplate, or the nerve fiber and it does not directly relax tense skeletal muscles. Of limited usefulness. May be given IM or IV in polyethylene glycol 300 (50% solution). PO therapy should be initiated as soon as possible. **Onset:** 30 min. **Peak plasma levels:** 2 hr after 2 g. **t½:** 1–2 hr. Inactive metabolites are excreted in the urine.

Uses: Adjunct for the relief of acute, painful musculoskeletal conditions (e.g., sprains, strains). Adjunct in tetanus.

Contraindications: Hypersensitivity, when muscle spasticity is required to maintain upright position, seizure disorders, pregnancy, lactation, children under 12 years. Renal disease (parenteral dosage form only since it contains polyethylene glycol 300).

Special Concerns: Use with caution in epilepsy and during lactation. Use the injectable form with caution in suspected or known epileptics.

Side Effects: *Following PO use. CNS:* Dizziness, drowsiness, lightheadedness, vertigo, lassitude, headache. *GI:* Nausea. *Miscellaneous:* Allergic symptoms including rash, urticaria, pruritus, conjunctivitis, nasal congestion, blurred vision, fever. *Following IV use (in addition to the preceding). CV:* Hypotension, bradycardia, syncope. *CNS:* Fainting, mild muscle incoordination. *Miscellaneous:* Metallic taste, GI upset, flushing, nystagmus, double vision, thrombophlebitis, sloughing or pain at injection site, ***anaphylaxis.***

M

Laboratory Test Considerations: Color interference in 5-HIAA and VMA.

OD **Management of Overdose:** *Symptoms:* CNS depression, including coma, is often seen when methocarbamol is used with alcohol or other CNS depressants. *Treatment:* Supportive, depending on the symptoms.

Drug Interactions: Central nervous system depressants (including alcohol) may ↑ the effect of methocarbamol.

How Supplied: *Injection:* 100 mg/mL; *Tablet:* 500 mg, 750 mg

Dosage

- **Tablets**

Skeletal muscle disorders.

Adults, initial: 1.5 g q.i.d. for the first 2–3 days (for severe conditions, 8 g/day may be given); **maintenance:** 1 g q.i.d., 0.75 g q 4 hr, or 1.5 g t.i.d.

- **IM, IV**

Skeletal muscle disorders.

Adults, usual initial: 1 g; in severe cases, up to 2–3 g may be necessary. **IV administration should not exceed 3 days.**

Tetanus.

Adults: 1–2 g IV, initially, into tube of previously inserted indwelling needle. An additional 1–2 g may be added to the infusion for a total initial dose of 3 g. May be given q 6 hr (up to 24 g/day may be needed) until PO administration is feasible. **Pediatric, initial:** 15 mg/kg given into tube of previously inserted indwelling needle. Dose may be repeated q 6 hr.

HEALTH CARE CONSIDERATIONS

See also *Health Care Considerations* for *Skeletal Muscle Relaxants.*

Administration/Storage

1. If administered IM, inject no more than 5 mL into each gluteal region.
2. When administering IM to a child, use the vastus lateralis; with adults, select a large muscle mass. Document and rotate sites.
IV 3. If administered IV, do not exceed a rate of 3 mL/min.
4. For IV drip, one ampule may be added to no more than 250 mL of NaCl or D5W.
5. With IV, check frequently for infiltration. Extravasation of fluid may cause sloughing/thrombophlebitis.
6. Before removing IV, clamp off the tubing to prevent extravasation of the hypertonic solution, which may cause thrombophlebitis.

Interventions

1. Monitor VS. Maintain a recumbent position during IV administration for 10–15 min after injection to minimize side effects of postural hypotension.
2. Keep side rails up and supervise ambulation of elderly clients or those who have been immobilized prior to drug therapy.
3. Observe seizure precautions.

Client/Family Teaching

1. Drug causes drowsiness; do not operate dangerous machinery and equipment or drive a car.
2. Rise slowly from a recumbent position and dangle legs before standing up to minimize hypotensive effects.
3. Diplopia, blurred vision, and nystagmus may occur; report if persistent.
4. Report any skin eruptions/rash, or itching; allergic responses which may require drug withdrawal.
5. Nausea, anorexia, and a metallic taste may occur; report if severe or interferes with nutrition.
6. Avoid alcohol and CNS depressants.
7. Urine may turn black, brown, or green; will resolve once drug stopped.

Outcome/Evaluate

- Improvement in muscle spasticity, pain, and mobility
- Control of tetanus-induced neuromuscular manifestations

M

Methotrexate, Methotrexate sodium

(meth-oh-**TREKS**-ayt)
Pregnancy Category: D (X for pregnant psoriatic or rheumatoid arthritis clients)
Amethopterin, Folex PFS, Rheumatrex Dose Pack (Abbreviation: MTX) **(Rx)**
Classification: Antineoplastic, antimetabolite (folic acid analog)

See also *Antineoplastic Agents.*

Action/Kinetics: Cell-cycle specific for the S phase of cell division. Acts by inhibiting dihydrofolate reductase, which prevents reduction of dihydrofolate to tetrahydrofolate; this results in decreased synthesis of purines and consequently DNA. The most sensitive cells are bone marrow, fetal cells, dermal epithelium, urinary bladder, buccal mucosa, intestinal mucosa, and malignant cells. When used for rheumatoid arthritis it may affect immune function. Variable absorption from GI tract. **Peak serum levels, IM:** 30–60 min; **PO:** 1–2 hr. **$t^{1/2}$:** initial, 1 hr; intermediate, 2–3 hr; final, 8–12 hr. May accumulate in the body. Excreted by kidney (55%–92% in 24 hr). Renal function tests are recommended before initiation of therapy; perform daily leukocyte counts during therapy.

Uses: Uterine choriocarcinoma (curative), chorioadenoma destruens, hydatidiform mole, acute lymphocytic and lymphoblastic leukemia, lymphosarcoma, and other disseminated neoplasms in children; meningeal leukemia, some beneficial effect in regional chemotherapy of head and neck tumors, breast tumors, and lung cancer. In combination for advanced stage non-Hodgkin's lymphoma. Advanced mycosis fungoides. High doses followed by leucovorin rescue in combination with other drugs for prolonging relapse-free survival in nonmetastatic osteosarcoma in individuals who have had surgical resection or amputation for the primary tumor. Severe, recalcitrant, disabling psoriasis. Rheumatoid arthritis (severe, active, classical, or definite) in clients who have had inadequate response to NSAIDs and at least one or more antirheumatic drugs (disease modifying). *Investigational:* Severe corticosteroid-dependent asthma to reduce corticosteroid dosage; adjunct to treat osteosarcoma. Psoriatic arthritis and Reiter's disease.

Contraindications: Psoriasis clients with kidney or liver disease; blood dyscrasias as hypoplasia, thrombocytopenia, anemia, or leukopenia. Alcoholism, alcoholic liver disease, or other chronic liver disease. Immunodeficiency syndromes. Pregnancy and lactation.

Special Concerns: Use with caution in impaired renal function and elderly clients. Use with extreme caution in the presence of active infection and in debilitated clients. Safety and efficacy have not been established for juvenile rheumatoid arthritis.

Additional Side Effects: ***Severe bone marrow depression.*** Hepatotoxicity, fibrosis, cirrhosis. ***Hemorrhagic enteritis, intestinal ulceration or perforation,*** acne, ecchymosis, hematemesis, melena, increased pigmentation, diabetes, leukoencephalopathy, chronic interstitial obstructive pulmonary disease, acute renal failure. Intrathecal use may result in chemical arachnoiditis, transient paresis, or ***seizures.*** Concomitant exposure to sunlight may aggravate psoriasis.

OD **Management of Overdose:** *Symptoms:* See *Antineoplastic Agents,* Chapter 2. *Treatment:* Leucovorin, given as soon as possible, may decrease toxic effects. The dose used is 10 mg/m² PO or parenterally followed by 10 mg/m² PO q 6 hr for 72 hr. Charcoal hemoperfusion will reduce serum levels. In massive overdosage, hydration and urinary alkalinization are needed to prevent precipitation of methotrexate and metabolites in the renal tubules.

Drug Interactions

Alcohol, ethyl / Additive hepatotoxicity; combination can result in coma
Aminoglycosides, oral / ↓ Absorption of PO methotrexate
Anticoagulants, oral / Additive hypoprothrombinemia
Chloramphenicol / ↑ Effect of methotrexate by ↓ plasma protein binding
Etretinate / Possible hepatotoxicity if used together for psoriasis
Folic acid–containing vitamin preparations / ↓ Response to methotrexate
Ibuprofen / ↑ Effect of methotrexate by ↓ renal secretion
NSAIDs / Possible fatal interaction
PABA / ↑ Effect of methotrexate by ↓ plasma protein binding
Phenylbutazone / ↑ Effect of methotrexate by ↓ renal secretion
Phenytoin / ↑ Effect of methotrexate by ↓ plasma protein binding
Probenecid / ↑ Effect of methotrexate by ↓ renal clearance
Procarbazine / Possible ↑ nephrotoxicity
Pyrimethamine / ↑ Methotrexate toxicity
Salicylates (aspirin) / ↑ Effect of methotrexate by ↓ plasma protein binding; also, salicylates ↓ renal excretion of methotrexate
Smallpox vaccination / Methotrexate impairs immunologic response to smallpox vaccine
Sulfonamides / ↑ Effect of methotrexate by ↓ plasma protein binding
Tetracyclines / ↑ Effect of methotrexate by ↓ plasma protein binding
Thiopurines / ↑ Plasma levels of thiopurines

How Supplied: *Injection:* 2.5mg/mL, 25 mg/mL; *Powder for injection, lyophilized:* 20 mg/vial, 50 mg/vial, 1 g/vial; *Tablet:* 2.5 mg

Dosage

• **Tablets (Methotrexate). IM, IV, IA, Intrathecal (Methotrexate Sodium)**

Choriocarcinoma and similar trophoblastic diseases.

Dose individualized. PO, IM: 15–30 mg/day for 5 days. May be repeated 3–5 times with 1-week rest period between courses.

Acute lymphatic (lymphoblastic) leukemia.

Initial: 3.3 mg/m² (with 60 mg/m² prednisone daily); **maintenance: PO, IM,** 30 mg/m² 2 times/week or **IV,** 2.5 mg/kg q 14 days.

Meningeal leukemia.

Intrathecal: 12 mg/m² q 2–5 days until cell count returns to normal.

Lymphomas.

PO: 10–25 mg/day for 4–8 days for several courses of treatment with 7- to 10-day rest periods between courses.

Mycosis fungoides.

PO: 2.5–10 mg/day for several weeks or months; **alternatively, IM:** 50 mg once weekly or 25 mg twice weekly.

Lymphosarcoma.

0.625–2.5 mg/kg/day in combination with other drugs.

Osteosarcoma.

Used in combination with other drugs, including doxorubicin, cisplatin, bleomycin, cyclophosphamide, and dactinomycin. **Usual IV starting dose for methotrexate:** 12 g/m²; dose may be increased to 15 g/m² to achieve a peak serum level of 10^{-3} mol/L at the end of the methotrexate infusion.

Psoriasis.

Adults, usual: PO, IM, IV, 10–25 mg/week, continued until beneficial response observed. Weekly dose should not exceed 50 mg. **Alternate regimens: PO,** 2.5 mg q 12 hr for three doses or q 8 hr for four doses each week (not to exceed 30 mg/week); **or PO,** 2.5 mg daily for 5 days followed by 2 days of rest (dose should not exceed 6.25 mg/day). Once beneficial effects are noted, reduce

M

dose to lowest possible level with longest rest periods between doses.

Rheumatoid arthritis.

Initial: Single PO doses of 7.5 mg/week or divided PO doses of 2.5 mg at 12-hr intervals for three doses given once a week; **then,** adjust dosage to achieve optimum response, not to exceed a total weekly dose of 20 mg. Once response has been reached, reduce the dose to the lowest possible effective dose.

HEALTH CARE CONSIDERATIONS

See also *Health Care Considerations* for *Antineoplastic Agents.*

Administration/Storage

1. Use only sterile, preservative-free NaCl injection to reconstitute powder for intrathecal administration.
2. Prevent inhalation of medication particles and skin exposure.
3. When used for rheumatoid arthritis, improvement is thought to be maintained for up to 2 years with continuous therapy. When discontinued, the arthritis usually worsens within 3–6 weeks.

M

IV 4. Six hours prior to initiation of a methotrexate infusion, hydrate with 1 L/m² of IV fluid. Continue hydration at 125 mL/m²/hr during the methotrexate infusion and for 2 days after infusion completed.
5. Alkalinize urine (see *Sodium Bicarbonate*) to a pH > 7 during infusion.
6. Follow guidelines provided for leucovorin rescue schedule following high doses of methotrexate.

Assessment

1. List drugs client currently prescribed. Determine if receiving other organic acids, such as aspirin, phenylbutazone, probenecid, and/or sulfa drugs; these affect renal clearance of methotrexate and increase thrombocytopenia and GI side effects. Note any acute infections.
2. Monitor CBC, uric acid, liver and renal function studies; report oliguria. Drug causes granulocyte and platelet suppression. Nadir: 10 days; recovery: 14 days.
3. Have calcium leucovorin—a potent antidote for folic acid antagonists—readily available in case of overdosage. Antidotes are ineffective if not administered within 4 hr of overdosage; may give corticosteroids concomitantly with initial dose of methotrexate.

Client/Family Teaching

1. Take tablets at bedtime with an antacid to minimize GI upset.
2. Avoid salicylates and alcohol as liver toxicity and bleeding may result.
3. Report oral ulcerations, one of the first signs of toxicity.
4. Avoid vaccinations (especially for smallpox) because the impaired immunologic response may result in vaccinia.
5. Consume 2–3 L/day of fluids to prevent renal damage and facilitate drug excretion.
6. Test urine pH and report if less than 6.5; bicarbonate tablets may be prescribed to assist in alkalizing the urine.
7. Allopurinol may be prescribed to reduce uric acid levels.
8. Avoid sun exposure and use sunscreens, sunglasses, and appropriate clothing when necessary.

Outcome/Evaluate

- Suppression of malignant cell proliferation, ↓ tumor size/spread
- Improvement in skin lesions
- ↓ Joint swelling/pain; ↑ mobility

Methsuximide

(meth-**SUCKS**-ih-myd)

Celontin **(Rx)**

Classification: Anticonvulsant, succinimide type

See also *Anticonvulsants* and *Succinimides.*

Action/Kinetics: Peak levels: 1–4 hr. **t½:** 1–3 hr for methsuximide and 36–45 hr for the active metabolite. **Therapeutic serum levels:** 10–40 mcg/mL.

Uses: Treat absence seizures refractory to other drugs. May be given with other anticonvulsants when absence seizures coexist with other types of epilepsy.

Additional Side Effects: Most common are ataxia, dizziness, and drowsiness.

Additional Drug Interactions: Methsuximide may ↑ the effect of primidone.

How Supplied: *Capsule:* 150 mg, 300 mg

Dosage

- **Capsules**

Absence seizures.

Adults and children, initial: 300 mg/day for first week; **then,** if necessary, increase dosage by 300 mg/day at weekly intervals until control established. **Maximum daily dose:** 1.2 g in divided doses.

HEALTH CARE CONSIDERATIONS

See also *Health Care Considerations* for *Anticonvulsants* and *Succinimides.*

Administration/Storage: The 150-mg dosage form can be used for children.

Assessment

1. Record type and frequency of seizures,

noting characteristics, other drugs prescribed, and the outcome.
2. Note baseline level of consciousness and balance; drug may impair.

Outcome/Evaluate
- Control of seizures
- Therapeutic drug levels (10–40 mcg/mL)

Methyldopa

(meth-ill-**DOH**-pah)

Pregnancy Category: B (PO)

Aldomet, Apo-Methyldopa ✦, Dopamet ✦, Novo-Medopa ✦, Nu-Medopa ✦ **(Rx)**

Methyldopate hydrochloride

(meth-ill-**DOH**-payt)

Pregnancy Category: B (PO), C (IV)

Aldomet Hydrochloride **(Rx)**

Classification: Antihypertensive, centrally acting antiadrenergic

---

See also *Antihypertensive Agents.*

Action/Kinetics: The active metabolite, alpha-methylnorepinephrine, lowers BP by stimulating central inhibitory alpha-adrenergic receptors, false neurotransmission, and/or reduction of plasma renin. Little change in CO. **PO: Onset:** 7–12 hr. **Duration:** 12–24 hr. All effects terminated within 48 hr. Absorption is variable. **IV: Onset:** 4–6 hr. **Duration:** 10–16 hr. Seventy percent of drug excreted in urine. **Full therapeutic effect:** 1–4 days. **t½:** 1.7 hr. Metabolites excreted in the urine.

Uses: Moderate to severe hypertension. Particularly useful for clients with impaired renal function, renal hypertension, resistant cases of hypertension complicated by stroke, CAD, or nitrogen retention, and for hypertensive crisis (parenterally).

Contraindications: Sensitivity to drug (including sulfites), labile and mild hypertension, pregnancy, active hepatic disease, use with MAO inhibitors, or pheochromocytoma.

Special Concerns: Use with caution in clients with a history of liver or kidney disease. A decrease in dose in geriatric clients may prevent syncope.

Side Effects: *CNS:* Sedation (transient), weakness, headache, asthenia, dizziness, paresthesias, Parkinson-like symptoms, psychic disturbances, symptoms of CV impairment, choreoathetotic movements, Bell's palsy, decreased mental acuity, verbal memory impairment. *CV:* Bradycardia, orthostatic hypotension, hypersensitivity of carotid sinus, worsening of angina, paradoxical hypertensive response (after IV), myocarditis, CHF, pericarditis, vasculitis. *GI:* N&V, abdominal distention, diarrhea or constipation, flatus, colitis, dry mouth, sore or "black tongue," pancreatitis, sialoadenitis. *Hematologic:* ***Hemolytic anemia,*** leukopenia, granulocytopenia, thrombocytopenia, ***bone marrow depression.*** *Endocrine:* Gynecomastia, amenorrhea, galactorrhea, lactation, hyperprolactinemia. *GU:* Impotence, failure to ejaculate, decreased libido. *Dermatologic:* Rash, ***toxic epidermal necrolysis.*** *Hepatic:* Jaundice, hepatitis, liver disorders, abnormal liver function tests. *Miscellaneous:* Edema, fever, lupus-like symptoms, nasal stuffiness, arthralgia, myalgia, ***septic shock-like syndrome.***

Laboratory Test Considerations: False + or ↑ : Alkaline phosphatase, bilirubin, BUN, BSP, cephalin flocculation, creatinine, AST, ALT, uric acid, Coombs' test, PT. Positive lupus erythematosus cell preparation and antinuclear antibodies.

OD **Management of Overdose:** *Symptoms:* CNS, GI, and CV effects including sedation, weakness, lightheadedness, dizziness, coma, bradycardia, acute hypotension, impairment of AV conduction, constipation, diarrhea, distention, flatus, N&V. *Treatment:* Induction of vomiting or gastric lavage if detected early. General supportive treatment with special attention to HR, CO, blood volume, urinary function, electrolyte imbalance, paralytic ileus, and CNS activity. In severe cases, hemodialysis is effective.

Drug Interactions

Anesthetics, general / Additive hypotension
Antidepressants, tricyclic / Tricyclic antidepressants may block hypotensive effect of methyldopa
Haloperidol / Methyldopa ↑ toxic effects of haloperidol
Levodopa / ↑ Effect of both drugs
Lithium / ↑ Possibility of lithium toxicity
MAO inhibitors / Metabolites of methyldopa, usually metabolized by MAO inhibitors, may → excessive sympathetic stimulation
Methotrimeprazine / Additive hypotensive effect
Phenothiazines / ↑ Risk of serious ↑ BP
Propranolol / Paradoxical hypertension
Sympathomimetics / Potentiation of hypertensive effect of sympathomimetics
Thiazide diuretics / Additive hypotensive effect
Thioxanthenes / Additive hypotensive effect
Tolbutamide / ↑ Hypoglycemia due to ↓ breakdown by liver
Tricyclic antidepressants / ↓ Effect of methyldopa

M

Vasodilator drugs / Additive hypotensive effect
Verapamil / ↑ Effect of methyldopa
How Supplied: Methyldopa: *Oral Suspension:* 50 mg/mL; *Tablet:* 125 mg, 250 mg, 500 mg. Methyldopate hydrochloride: *Injection:* 50 mg/mL

Dosage

- **Methyldopa. Tablets**
  Hypertension.

Initial: 250 mg b.i.d.–t.i.d. for 2 days. Adjust dose q 2 days. If increased, start with evening dose. **Usual maintenance:** 0.5–3.0 g/day in two to four divided doses; **maximum:** 3 g/day. Gradually transfer to and from other antihypertensive agents, with initial dose of methyldopa not exceeding 500 mg. *NOTE:* Do not use combination medication to initiate therapy. **Pediatric, initial:** 10 mg/kg/day in two to four divided doses, adjusting maintenance to a maximum of 65 mg/kg/day (or 3 g/day, whichever is less).

- **Methyldopate HCl. IV Infusion**
  Hypertension.

Adults: 250–500 mg q 6 hr; **maximum:** 1 g q 6 hr for hypertensive crisis.

Switch to PO methyldopa, at same dosage level, when BP is brought under control. **Pediatric:** 20–40 mg/kg/day in divided doses q 6 hr; **maximum:** 65 mg/kg/day (or 3 g/day, whichever is less).

HEALTH CARE CONSIDERATIONS

See also *Health Care Considerations* for *Antihypertensive Agents.*

Administration/Storage

1. Tolerance may occur following 2–3 months of therapy. Increasing the dose or adding a diuretic often restores effect on BP.
IV 2. For IV, mix with 100 mL of D5W or administer in D5W at a concentration of 10 mg/mL. Infuse over 30–60 min.

Assessment

1. Record indications for therapy, onset of symptoms, other agents prescribed and the outcome.
2. Monitor CBC, LFTs, and Coombs' test. If blood transfusion required, obtain both direct and indirect Coombs' tests; if positive, consult hematologist.
3. Note any jaundice; contraindicated with active hepatic disease.
4. Assess for drug tolerance; may occur during the second or third month of therapy.

Client/Family Teaching

1. To prevent dizziness and fainting, rise to a sitting position slowly and dangle legs over the edge of the bed.
2. Sedation may occur initially; should disappear once maintenance dose established.
3. In rare cases, may darken or turn urine blue; not harmful.
4. Withhold and report any of the following symptoms: tiredness, fever, or yellowing of skin/sclera.
5. Continue to follow prescribed diet and exercise program in the overall goal of BP control.
6. Do not take any other medications or remedies unless appoved.

Outcome/Evaluate: ↓ BP

COMBINATION DRUG

Methyldopa and Hydrochlorothiazide

(meth-ill-**DOH**-pah, hy-droh-klor-oh-**THIGH**-ah-zyd)
Pregnancy Category: C
Aldoril 15, Aldoril 25, Aldoril D30, Aldoril D50, Apo-Methazide ✦, Novo-Doparil ✦, PMS-Dopazide ✦ **(Rx)**
Classification: Antihypertensive

See also *Methyldopa* and *Hydrochlorothiazide.*
Content: *Antihypertensive:* Methyldopa, 250 or 500 mg. *Diuretic/antihypertensive:* Hydrochlorothiazide, 15–50 mg.
Uses: Hypertension (not for initial treatment).
Contraindications: Active hepatic disease.
Special Concerns: Use in pregnancy only if benefits outweigh risks.
How Supplied: See Content

Dosage

- **Tablets**

Adults: 1 tablet b.i.d.–t.i.d. for first 48 hr; **then,** increase or decrease dose, depending on response, in intervals of not less than 2 days. Maximum daily dosage: methyldopa, 3.0 g; hydrochlorothiazide, 100–200 mg.

HEALTH CARE CONSIDERATIONS

See also *Health Care Considerations* for *Antihypertensive Agents* and individual agents.

Administration/Storage

1. If Aldoril is given together with antihypertensives other than thiazides, do not exceed the initial dose of 500 mg/day of methyldopa in divided doses.
2. Additional methyldopa may be given separately if Aldoril alone does not control BP adequately.
3. If tolerance is observed after 2–3 months of therapy, the dose of either methyldopa

and/or hydrochlorothiazide may be increased to restore control.
Outcome/Evaluate: Control of hypertension

Methylergonovine maleate

(meth-ill-er-**GON**-oh-veen)
Pregnancy Category: C
Methergine **(Rx)**
Classification: Oxytocic agent

Action/Kinetics: Synthetic drug related to ergonovine. Methylergonovine stimulates the rate, tone, and amplitude of uterine contractions. The uterus becomes more sensitive to the drug toward the end of pregnancy. **Onset** (uterine contractions): **PO,** 5–10 min; **IM,** 2–5 min; **IV,** immediate. **t½, IV:** 2–3 min (initial) and 20–30 min (final). **Duration, PO, IM:** 3 hr; **IV:** 45 min.
Uses: Management and prevention of postpartum and postabortal hemorrhage by producing firm uterine contractions and decreasing uterine bleeding. During the second stage of labor following delivery of the anterior shoulder, but only under full obstetric supervision. *Investigational:* Ergonovine has been used to diagnose Prinzmetal's angina (variant angina).
Contraindications: Pregnancy, toxemia, hypertension. Ergot hypersensitivity. To induce labor or threatened spontaneous abortions. Administration before delivery of the placenta.
Special Concerns: Use with caution in sepsis, obliterative vascular disease, impaired renal or hepatic function, and during lactation.
Side Effects: *CV:* Hypertension that may be associated with seizure or headache; hypotension, thrombophlebitis, palpitation. *GI:* N&V, diarrhea, foul taste. *CNS:* Dizziness, headache, tinnitus, hallucinations. *Miscellaneous:* Sweating, chest pain, dyspnea, hematuria, water intoxication, leg cramps, nasal congestion.

NOTE: ***Use of methylergonovine during labor may result in uterine tetany with rupture, cervical and perineal lacerations, embolism of amniotic fluid as well as hypoxia and intracranial hemorrhage in the infant.***

OD **Management of Overdose:** *Symptoms:* Initially, N&V, abdominal pain, increase in BP, tingling of extremities, numbness. Symptoms of severe overdose include hypotension, hypothermia, ***respiratory depression, seizures, coma.*** *Treatment:* Induce vomiting or perform gastric lavage. Administer a cathartic; institute diuresis. Maintain respiration, especially if seizures or coma occur. Treat seizures with anticonvulsant drugs. Warm extremities to control peripheral vasospasm.
Drug Interactions: Hypertension may occur if methylergonovine is used with vasoconstrictors.
How Supplied: *Injection:* 0.2 mg /mL; *Tablet:* 0.2 mg

Dosage

- **IM, IV (Emergencies Only)**

0.2 mg q 2–4 hr following delivery of placenta, of the anterior shoulder, or during the puerperium.

- **Tablets**

0.2 mg t.i.d.–q.i.d. until danger of hemorrhage and uterine atony is over (usually within 2 days, but no more than 1 week).

HEALTH CARE CONSIDERATIONS

Administration/Storage

IV 1. Administer slowly over 1 min; check VS for evidence of shock or hypertension after IV administration. Have emergency drugs available.
2. Discard ampules if discolored.

Assessment

1. Record indications for therapy, onset and duration of symptoms.
2. Record fundal tone and nonphasic contractures; massage to check for relaxation or severe cramping.
3. Monitor baseline calcium; correct if low to improve drug effectiveness. Monitor prolactin levels; assess for decreased milk production.

Client/Family Teaching

1. Take only as directed; do not exceed dosage.
2. Avoid smoking; nicotine constricts blood vessels.
3. Report any S&S of ergotism (cold/numb fingers/toes, N&V, headache, muscle or chest pain, weakness).
4. Abdominal cramps may be experienced; report any severe cramping or increased bleeding.

Outcome/Evaluate: Improved uterine tone; control of postpartum hemorrhage

Methylphenidate hydrochloride

(meth-ill-**FEN**-ih-dayt)
Pregnancy Category: C
PMS-Methylphenidate ✦, Riphenidate ✦, Ritalin, Ritalin-SR **(C-II) (Rx)**
Classification: Central nervous system stimulant

M

Action/Kinetics: May act by blocking the reuptake mechanism of dopaminergic neurons. In children with attention-deficit disorders, methylphenidate causes decreases in motor restlessness with an increased attention span. In narcolepsy the drug acts on the cerebral cortex and subcortical structures (e.g., thalamus) to increase motor activity and mental alertness and decrease fatigue. **Peak blood levels, children:** 1.9 hr for tablets and 4.7 hr for extended-release tablets. **Duration:** 4–6 hr. **t½:** 1–3 hr. Metabolized by the liver and excreted by the kidney.

Uses: Attention-deficit disorders in children as part of overall treatment regimen. Narcolepsy. *Investigational:* Depression in elderly, cancer, and poststroke clients. Anesthesia-related hiccups.

Contraindications: Marked anxiety, tension and agitation, glaucoma. Severe depression, to prevent normal fatigue, diagnosis of Tourette's syndrome, motor tics. In children who manifest symptoms of primary psychiatric disorders (psychoses) or acute stress.

Special Concerns: Use with caution during lactation. Use with great caution in clients with history of hypertension or convulsive disease. Safety and efficacy in children less than 6 years of age have not been established.

Side Effects: *CNS:* Nervousness, insomnia, headaches, dizziness, drowsiness, chorea, depressed mood (transient). Toxic psychoses, dyskinesia, Tourette's syndrome. Psychologic dependence. *CV:* Palpitations, tachycardia, angina, arrhythmias, hyper- or hypotension, cerebral arteritis or occlusion. *GI:* Nausea, anorexia, abdominal pain, weight loss (chronic use). *Allergic:* Skin rashes, fever, urticaria, arthralgia, exfoliative dermatitis, erythema multiforme with necrotizing vasculitis, erythema. *Hematologic:* Thrombocytopenic purpura, leukopenia, anemia. *Miscellaneous:* Hair loss, abnormal liver function.

In children, the following side effects are more common: anorexia, abdominal pain, weight loss (chronic use), tachycardia, insomnia.

Laboratory Test Considerations: ↑ Urinary excretion of epinephrine.

OD **Management of Overdose:** *Symptoms:* Characterized by CV symptoms (hypertension, cardiac arrhythmias, tachycardia), mental disturbances, agitation, headaches, vomiting, hyperreflexia, ***hyperpyrexia, convulsions, and coma.*** *Treatment:* Symptomatic. Treat excess CNS stimulation by keeping the client in quiet, dim surroundings to reduce external stimuli. Protect the client from self-injury. A short-acting barbiturate may be used. Undertake emesis or gastric lavage if the client is conscious. Adequate circulatory and respiratory function must be maintained. Hyperpyrexia may be treated by cooling the client (e.g., cool bath, hypothermia blanket).

Drug Interactions

Anticoagulants, oral / ↑ Effect of anticoagulants due to ↓ breakdown by liver

Anticonvulsants (phenobarbital, phenytoin, primidone) / ↑ Effect of anticonvulsants due to ↓ breakdown by liver

Guanethidine / ↓ Effect of guanethidine by displacement from its site of action

MAO inhibitors / Possibility of hypertensive crisis, hyperthermia, convulsions, coma

Tricyclic antidepressants / ↑ Effect of antidepressants due to ↓ breakdown by liver

How Supplied: *Tablet:* 5 mg, 10 mg, 20 mg; *Tablet, Extended Release:* 20 mg

Dosage

- **Tablets**

Narcolepsy.

Adults: 5–20 mg b.i.d.–t.i.d. preferably 30–45 min before meals.

Attention-deficit disorders.

Pediatric, 6 years and older, initial: 5 mg b.i.d. before breakfast and lunch; **then,** increase by 5–10 mg/week to a maximum of 60 mg/day.

- **Extended-Release Tablets**

Narcolepsy.

Adults: 20 mg 1–3 times/day q 8 hr, preferably on an empty stomach.

Attention-deficit disorders.

Pediatric, 6 years and older: 20 mg 1–3 times/day.

HEALTH CARE CONSIDERATIONS

See also *Health Care Considerations* for *Pemoline.*

Administration/Storage

1. If receiving for ADD and no improvement is noticed in 1 mo, or if stimulation occurs, discontinue drug.
2. Discontinue periodically to assess condition as drug therapy is not indefinite; discontinue at puberty.
3. Sustained-release tablets are effective for 8 hr and may be substituted for regular-release tablets if the 8-hr dosage of the sustained-release tablets is the same as the titrated 8-hr dosage of regular tablets.

Assessment

1. Record indications for therapy, type and onset of symptoms. Note other drugs prescribed that may interact unfavorably.
2. Ensure psychologic evaluations show no evidence of psychotic disorder or severe stress.

3. Obtain baseline CBC, CNS evaluation, and ECG.

Client/Family Teaching

1. Take before breakfast and lunch to avoid interference with sleep.
2. Use caution when driving or operating hazardous machinery as drug may mask fatigue and/or cause physical incoordination, dizziness, or drowsiness.
3. Record weight 2 times/week and report any significant loss as weight loss may occur.
4. Report any overt changes in client mood or attention span.
5. Skin rashes, fever, or pain in the joints should be reported immediately.
6. Therapy may be interrupted every few months ("drug holiday") to determine if still necessary in those responsive to therapy.
7. Avoid caffeine in any form.

Outcome/Evaluate

- ↑ Ability to sit quietly/concentrate
- ↓ Daytime sleeping

Methylprednisolone

(meth-ill-pred-**NISS**-oh-lohn)

Pregnancy Category: C

Tablets: Medrol, Meprolone **(Rx)**

Methylprednisolone acetate

(meth-ill-pred-**NISS**-oh-lohn)

Pregnancy Category: C

Cream: Medrol Veriderm Cream ✱. **Enema:** Medrol Enpak **(Rx)**. **Parenteral:** depMedalone-40 and -80, Depoject 40 and 80, Depo-Medrol, D-Med 80, Duralone-40 and -80, Medralone-40 and -80, M-Prednisol-40 and -80 **(Rx)**

Methylprednisolone sodium succinate

(meth-ill-pred-**NISS**-oh-lohn)

Pregnancy Category: C

Parenteral: A-methaPred, Solu-Medrol **(Rx)**

Classification: Glucocorticoid

See also *Corticosteroids*.

Action/Kinetics: Low incidence of increased appetite, peptic ulcer, psychic stimulation, and sodium and water retention. May mask negative nitrogen balance. **Onset:** Slow, 12–24 hr. **t½, plasma:** 78–188 min. **Duration:** Long, up to 1 week. Rapid onset of sodium succinate by both IV and IM routes. Long duration of action of the acetate.

Additional Uses: Severe hepatitis due to alcoholism. Within 8 hr of severe spinal cord injury (to improve neurologic function). Septic shock (controversial).

Special Concerns: Use during pregnancy only if benefits outweigh risks.

Laboratory Test Considerations: ↓ Immunoglobulins A, G, M.

Additional Drug Interactions

Erythromycin / ↑ Effect of methylprednisolone due to ↓ breakdown by liver

Troleandomycin / ↑ Effect of methylprednisolone due to ↓ breakdown by liver

How Supplied: Methylprednisolone: *Tablet:* 2 mg, 4 mg, 8 mg, 16 mg, 24 mg, 32 mg. Methylprednisolone acetate: *Injection:* 20 mg/mL, 40 mg/mL, 80 mg/mL. Methylprednisolone sodium succinate: *Powder for injection:* 40 mg, 125 mg, 500 mg, 1 g, 2 g

Dosage

METHYLPREDNISOLONE

- **Tablets**

Rheumatoid arthritis.

Adults: 6–16 mg/day. Decrease gradually when condition is under control. **Pediatric:** 6–10 mg/day.

SLE.

Adults, acute: 20–96 mg/day; **maintenance:** 8–20 mg/day.

Acute rheumatic fever.

1 mg/kg body weight daily. Drug is always given in four equally divided doses after meals and at bedtime.

METHYLPREDNISOLONE ACETATE

- **IM**

Adrenogenital syndrome.

40 mg q 2 weeks.

Rheumatoid arthritis.

40–120 mg/week.

Dermatologic lesions, dermatitis.

40–120 mg/week for 1–4 weeks; for severe cases, a single dose of 80–120 mg should provide relief.

Seborrheic dermatitis.

80 mg/week.

Asthma, rhinitis.

80–120 mg.

- **Intra-articular, Soft Tissue and Intralesional Injection**

4–80 mg, depending on site.

- **Retention Enema**

40 mg 3–7 times/week for 2 or more weeks.

METHYLPREDNISOLONE SODIUM SUCCINATE

- **IM, IV**

Most conditions.

Adults, initial: 10–40 mg, depending on the disease; **then,** adjust dose depending on response, with subsequent doses given either **IM, IV.**

Severe conditions.

Adults: 30 mg/kg infused IV over 10–20 min; may be repeated q 4–6 hr for 2–3 days

M

only. **Pediatric:** not less than 0.5 mg/kg/day.

HEALTH CARE CONSIDERATIONS

See also *Health Care Considerations* for *Corticosteroids*.

Administration/Storage

1. Dosage must be individualized.
2. Methylprednisolone acetate is not for IV use.
3. Use sodium succinate solutions within 48 hr after preparation.
4. For alternate day therapy, twice the usual PO dose is given every other morning (client receives beneficial effect while minimizing side effects).

Assessment

1. Record indications for treatment; describe clinical presentation.
2. Monitor CBC, HbA1C, glucose, and electrolytes.

Outcome/Evaluate

- Relief of allergic manifestations
- ↓ Pain/inflammation; ↑ mobility
- ↓ Nerve fiber destruction in spinal cord injury (SCI)

M

Methysergide maleate

(meth-ih-**SIR**-jyd)

Pregnancy Category: X

Sansert **(Rx)**

Classification: Prophylactic for vascular headaches

Action/Kinetics: Semisynthetic ergot alkaloid derivative. May act by directly stimulating smooth muscle leading to vasoconstriction. Blocks the effects of serotonin, a powerful vasodilator believed to play a role in vascular headaches; it also inhibits the release of histamine from mast cells and prevents the release of serotonin from platelets. Has weak emetic and oxytocic activity. **Onset:** 1–2 days. **Peak plasma levels:** 60 ng/mL. **Duration:** 1–2 days. Excreted through the urine as unchanged drugs and metabolites.

Uses: Prevention or reduction of the intensity and frequency of vascular headache (in clients having one or more per week or in cases where headaches are so severe preventive therapy is indicated). Prophylaxis of vascular headache.

Contraindications: Severe renal or hepatic disease, severe hypertension, CAD, peripheral vascular disease, tendency toward thromboembolic disease, cachexia (profound ill health or malnutrition), severe arteriosclerosis, pulmonary disease, phlebitis or cellulitis of lower limbs, collagen diseases or fibrotic processs, debilitated states, valvular heart disease, infectious disease, or peptic ulcer. Use to terminate acute attacks. Pregnancy, lactation, use in children.

Special Concerns: Geriatric clients may be more affected by peripheral vasoconstriction leading to the possibility of hypothermia.

Side Effects: The drug is associated with a high incidence of side effects. *Fibrosis:* ***Retroperitoneal fibrosis, cardiac fibrosis, pleuropulmonary fibrosis,*** Peyronie's-like disease. The fibrotic condition may result in vascular insufficiency in the lower legs. *CV:* Vasoconstriction of arteries leading to paresthesia, chest pain, abdominal pain, or extremities that are cold, numb, or painful. Tachycardia, postural hypotension. *CNS:* Dizziness, ataxia, drowsiness, vertigo, insomnia, euphoria, lightheadedness, and psychic reactions such as depersonalization, depression, and hallucinations. *GI:* N&V, diarrhea, heartburn, abdominal pain, increased gastric acid, constipation. *Hematologic:* Eosinophilia, neutropenia. *Other:* Peripheral edema, flushing of face, skin rashes, transient alopecia, myalgia, arthralgia, weakness, weight gain, telangiectasia.

Drug Interactions: Narcotic analgesics are inhibited by methysergide.

How Supplied: *Tablet:* 2 mg

Dosage

- **Tablets**

Adults: Administer 4–8 mg/day in divided doses. Continuous administration should not exceed 6 months. May be readministered after a 3- to 4-week rest period.

HEALTH CARE CONSIDERATIONS

Administration/Storage: If drug is not effective after 3 weeks, it is not likely to be beneficial and should be discontinued.

Assessment

1. Record frequency and severity of headaches and efforts made in the past to control or prevent them.
2. Obtain CBC, liver and renal function studies; assess for dysfunction.
3. Determine behavior prior to therapy. Review diet (tyramine foods, additives, preservatives, colorings), activity, substance use (including caffeine and nicotine), OTC medications, and stress levels; may have precipitated event.

Client/Family Teaching

1. Take with meals or milk to minimize GI irritation R/T increased hydrochloric acid production.
2. Discontinue gradually to avoid migraine headache rebound.
3. Report symptoms of nervousness, weak-

ness, insomnia, rashes, alopecia, or peripheral edema.
4. Report any unusual weight gain; check extremities for swelling. If weight gain excessive, adjust caloric intake; maintain a low-salt diet.
5. Keep a diary noting any events, foods, or activities that may relate to the onset of headaches.
6. Administration should not be continued on a regular basis for longer than 6 months without a 3- to 4-week rest.
7. General malaise, fatigue, weight loss, low-grade fever, or urinary tract problems may be symptoms of fibrosis (cardiac or pleuropulmonary); report immediately.
8. Do not drive or engage in other hazardous tasks until drug effects are realized; may cause drowsiness.
9. If dizziness or lightheadedness occurs upon arising, rise slowly from a supine position and dangle legs for a few minutes before standing erect. If feeling faint, lie down with the legs elevated.
10. Avoid alcohol, caffeine, nicotine, and cannabis, as these may precipitate vascular headaches.
11. Report if psychologic changes occur, especially hallucinations.

Outcome/Evaluate: ↓ Frequency/intensity of vascular headaches; Headache prophylaxis

Metipranolol hydrochloride

(met-ih-**PRAN**-oh-lohl)
Pregnancy Category: C
OptiPranolol **(Rx)**
Classification: Beta-adrenergic blocking agent

See also *Beta-Adrenergic Blocking Agents.*
Action/Kinetics: Blocks both beta-1- and beta-2-adrenergic receptors. Reduction in intraocular pressure may be related to a decrease in production of aqueous humor and a slight increase in the outflow of aqueous humor. A decrease from 20% to 26% in intraocular pressure may be seen if the intraocular pressure is greater than 24 mm Hg at baseline. May be absorbed and exert systemic effects. When used topically, has no local anesthetic effect and exerts no action on pupil size or accommodation. **Onset:** 30 min. **Maximum effect:** 1–2 hr. **Duration:** 12–24 hr.
Uses: To reduce IOP in clients with ocular hypertension and chronic open-angle glaucoma.
Special Concerns: Use with caution during lactation. Safety and effectiveness have not been determined in children.
Side Effects: *Ophthalmologic:* Local discomfort, dermatitis of the eyelid, blepharitis, conjunctivitis, browache, tearing, blurred vision, abnormal vision, photophobia, edema. Due to absorption, the following systemic side effects have been reported. *CV:* Hypertension, MI, atrial fibrillation, angina, bradycardia, palpitation. *CNS:* Headache, dizziness, anxiety, depression, somnolence, nervousness. *Respiratory:* Dyspnea, rhinitis, bronchitis, coughing. *Miscellaneous:* Allergic reaction, asthenia, nausea, epistaxis, arthritis, myalgia, rash.
How Supplied: *Ophthalmic solution:* 0.3%

Dosage

- **Ophthalmic Solution (0.3%)**

Adults: 1 gtt in the affected eye(s) b.i.d. Increasing the dose or more frequent administration does not increase the beneficial effect.

HEALTH CARE CONSIDERATIONS

See also *Health Care Considerations* for *Beta-Adrenergic Blocking Agents.*

Administration/Storage
1. May be used concomitantly with other drugs to lower intraocular pressure.
2. Due to diurnal variation in response, measure IOP at different times during the day.

Assessment
1. Note ocular condition and record pretreatment pressures.
2. Record baseline ECG and VS.

Client/Family Teaching
1. Transient burning or stinging is common during administration; report if severe.
2. Take only as directed; report any persistent bothersome side effects or symptoms of intolerance.
3. Report for F/U visits to assess for systemic effects, measure intraocular pressures, and determine drug effectiveness.

Outcome/Evaluate: ↓ IOP

Metoclopramide

(meh-toe-kloh-**PRAH**-myd)
Pregnancy Category: B
Apo-Metoclop ✱, Maxeran ✱, Maxolon, Nu-Metoclopramide ✱, Octamide PFS, PMS-Metoclopramide ✱, Reglan **(Rx)**
Classification: Gastrointestinal stimulant

Action/Kinetics: Dopamine antagonist that acts by increasing sensitivity to acetylcholine; results in increased motility of the upper GI tract and relaxation of the pyloric sphincter and duodenal bulb. Gastric emptying

M

time and GI transit time are shortened. No effect on gastric, biliary, or pancreatic secretions. Facilitates intubation of the small bowel and speeds transit of a barium meal. Produces sedation, induces release of prolactin, increases circulating aldosterone levels (is transient), and is an antiemetic. **Onset, IV:** 1–3 min; **IM,** 10–15 min; **PO,** 30–60 min. **Duration:** 1–2 hr. **t½:** 5–6 hr. Significant first-pass effect following PO use; unchanged drug and metabolites excreted in urine. Renal impairment decreases clearance of the drug.

Uses: PO: Acute and recurrent diabetic gastroparesis, gastroesophageal reflux. **Parenteral:** Facilitate small bowel intubation, stimulate gastric emptying, and increase intestinal transit of barium to aid in radiologic examination of stomach and small intestine. Prophylaxis of N&V in cancer chemotherapy and following surgery (when nasogastric suction is not desired). *Investigational:* To improve lactation. N&V due to various causes, including vomiting during pregnancy and labor, gastric ulcer, anorexia nervosa. Improve client response to ergotamine, analgesics, and sedatives when used to treat migraine (may increase absorption). Postoperative gastric bezoars. Atonic bladder. Esophageal variceal bleeding.

M

Contraindications: Gastrointestinal hemorrhage, obstruction, or perforation; epilepsy; clients taking drugs likely to cause extrapyramidal symptoms, such as phenothiazines. Pheochromocytoma.

Special Concerns: Use with caution during lactation and in hypertension. Extrapyramidal effects are more likely to occur in children and geriatric clients.

Side Effects: *CNS:* Restlessness, drowsiness, fatigue, lassitude, akathisia, anxiety, insomnia, confusion. Headaches, dizziness, extrapyramidal symptoms (especially acute dystonic reactions), Parkinson-like symptoms (including cogwheel rigidity, mask-like facies, bradykinesia, tremor), dystonia, myoclonus, ***depression (with suicidal ideation),*** tardive dyskinesia (including involuntary movements of the tongue, face, mouth, or jaw), seizures, hallucinations. *GI:* Nausea, bowel disturbances (usually diarrhea). *CV:* Hypertension (transient), hypotension, SVT, bradycardia. *Hematologic:* ***Agranulocytosis,*** leukopenia, neutropenia. Methemoglobinemia in premature and full-term infants at doses of 1–4 mg/kg/day IM, IV, or PO for 1–3 or more days. *Endocrine:* Galactorrhea, amenorrhea, gynecomastia, impotence (due to hyperprolactinemia), fluid retention (due to transient elevation of aldosterone). ***Neuroleptic malignant syndrome: Hyperthermia, altered consciousness, autonomic dysfunction, muscle rigidity, death.*** *Miscellaneous:* Incontinence, urinary frequency, porphyria, visual disturbances, flushing of the face and upper body, hepatotoxicity.

OD **Management of Overdose:** *Symptoms:* Agitation, irritability, hypertonia of muscles, drowsiness, disorientation, extrapyramidal symptoms. *Treatment:* Treat extrapyramidal effects by giving anticholinergic drugs, anti-Parkinson drugs, or antihistamines with anticholinergic effects. General supportive treatment. Reverse methemoglobinemia by giving methylene blue.

Drug Interactions

Acetaminophen / ↑ GI absorption of acetaminophen
Anticholinergics / ↓ Effect of metoclopramide
Cimetidine / ↓ Effect of cimetidine due to ↓ absorption from GI tract
CNS depressants / Additive sedative effects
Cyclosporine / ↓ Absorption of cyclosporine → ↑ immunosuppressive and toxic effects
Digoxin / ↓ Effect of digoxin due to ↓ absorption from GI tract
Ethanol / ↑ GI absorption of ethanol
Levodopa / ↑ GI absorption of levodopa and levodopa ↓ effects of metoclopramide on gastric emptying and lower esophageal pressure
MAO inhibitors / ↑ Release of catecholamines → toxicity
Narcotic analgesics / ↓ Effect of metoclopramide
Succinylcholine / ↑ Effect of succinylcholine due to inhibition of plasma cholinesterase
Tetracyclines / ↑ GI absorption of tetracyclines

How Supplied: *Concentrate:* 10 mg/mL; *Injection:* 5 mg/mL; *Tablet:* 5 mg, 10 mg

Dosage

- **Tablets, Syrup, Concentrate**

Diabetic gastroparesis.

Adults: 10 mg 30 min before meals and at bedtime for 2–8 weeks (therapy should be reinstituted if symptoms recur).

Gastroesophageal reflux.

Adults: 10–15 mg q.i.d. 30 min before meals and at bedtime. If symptoms occur only intermittently, single doses up to 20 mg prior to the provoking situation may be used.

To enhance lactation.

Adults: 30–45 mg/day.

- **IM, IV**

Prophylaxis of vomiting due to chemotherapy.

Initial: 1–2 mg/kg IV q 2 hr for two doses, with the first dose 30 min before chemotherapy; **then,** 10 mg or more q 3 hr for three doses. Inject slowly IV over 15 min.

Prophylaxis of postoperative N&V.

Adults: 10–20 mg IM near the end of surgery.

Facilitate small bowel intubation.

Adults: 10 mg given over 1–2 min; **pediatric, 6–14 years:** 2.5–5 mg; **pediatric, less than 6 years:** 0.1 mg/kg.

Radiologic examinations to increase intestinal transit time.

Adults: 10 mg as a single dose given IV over 1–2 min.

HEALTH CARE CONSIDERATIONS

Administration/Storage

1. After PO use, absorption of certain drugs from the GI tract may be affected (see *Drug Interactions*).

IV 2. Inject slowly IV over 1–2 min to prevent transient feelings of anxiety and restlessness.

3. Metoclopramide is physically and/or chemically incompatible with a number of drugs; check package insert if drug is to be admixed.

4. For IV use, dilute doses greater than 10 mg in 50 mL of D5W, D5/0.45% NaCl, RL injection, Ringer's injection, or NaCl injection; infuse over 15 min.

Assessment

1. Record indications for therapy, type and onset of symptoms. List drugs prescribed, ensuring none interact unfavorably.

2. Assess abdomen for bowel sounds and distention; note any N&V.

Client/Family Teaching

1. Do not operate a car or hazardous machinery until drug effects realized; drug has a sedative effect.

2. Report any persistent side effects so they can be properly evaluated and counteracted.

3. Avoid alcohol and any other CNS depressants.

4. Extrapyramidal effects (trembling hands, facial grimacing) should be reported; may be treated with IM diphenhydramine.

Outcome/Evaluate

- Prevention of N&V
- Enhanced gastric motility
- Promotion of gastric emptying
- Prophylaxis of gastric bezoars

Metolazone

(meh-**TOH**-lah-zohn)

Pregnancy Category: B

Mykrox, Zaroxolyn **(Rx)**

Classification: Diuretic, thiazide

See also *Diuretics, Thiazide.*

Action/Kinetics: Onset: 1 hr. **Peak blood levels, rapid availability tablets:** 2–4 hr; **t½, elimination:** About 14 hr. **Peak blood levels, slow availability tablets:** 8 hr. **Duration, rapid or slow availablity tablets:** 24 hr or more. Most excreted unchanged through the urine.

Uses: Slow availability tablets: Edema accompanying CHF; edema accompanying renal diseases, including nephrotic syndrome and conditions of reduced renal function. Alone or in combination with other drugs for the treatment of hypertension.

Rapid availability tablets: Treatment of newly diagnosed mild to moderate hypertension alone or in combination with other drugs. The rapid availability tablets are not to be used to produce diuresis.

Investigational: Alone or as an adjunct to treat calcium nephrolithiasis, premanagement of menstrual syndrome, and adjunct treatment of renal failure.

Contraindications: Anuria, prehepatic and hepatic coma, allergy or hypersensitivity to metolazone. Routine use during pregnancy. Lactation.

Special Concerns: Use with caution in those with severely impaired renal function. Safety and effectiveness have not been determined in children.

Side Effects: See *Diuretics, Thiazide.* The most commonly reported side effects are dizziness, headache, muscle cramps, malaise, lethargy, lassitude, joint pain/swelling, and chest pain.

Additional Drug Interactions

Alcohol / ↑ Hypotensive effect
Barbiturates / Hypotensive effect
Narcotics / Hypotensive effect
NSAIDs / ↓ Hypotensive effect of metolazone
Salicylates / Hypotensive effect of metolazone

How Supplied: *Tablets:* 0.5 mg, 2.5 mg, 5 mg, 10 mg.

Dosage

- **Slow Availability Tablets**

Edema due to cardiac failure or renal disease.

Adults: 5–20 mg once daily. For those who experience paroxysmal nocturnal dyspnea, a larger dose may be required to ensure prolonged diuresis and saluresis for a 24-hr period.

Mild to moderate essential hypertension.

Adults: 2.5–5 mg once daily.

- **Rapid Availability Tablets**

Mild to moderate essential hypertension.

Adults, initial: 0.5 mg once daily, usually in the morning. If inadequately controlled, the dose may be increased to 1 mg once a day. Increasing the dose higher than 1 mg does not increase the effect.

HEALTH CARE CONSIDERATIONS

See also *Health Care Considerations* for *Diuretics, Thiazide.*

Administration/Storage

1. Formulations of slow availability tablets should not be interchanged with formulations of rapid availability tablets as they are not therapeutically equivalent.
2. The antihypertensive effect may be observed from 3 to 4 days to 3 to 6 weeks.
3. If BP is not controlled with 1 mg of the rapid availability tablets, add another antihypertensive drug, with a different mechanism of action, to the therapy.
4. Store tablets at room temperature in a tight, light-resistant container.

M

Assessment

1. Record indications for therapy, noting onset, duration, and clinical characteristics.
2. Monitor BP, ECG, CBC, electrolytes, liver and renal function studies; assess for symptoms of electrolyte imbalance (i.e., ↓ Na, ↓ K, ↓ Mg and hypochloremic alkalosis).

Client/Family Teaching

1. Take exactly as directed.
2. May cause orthostatic hypotension and syncope; use caution.
3. Weigh self regularly; report increases of more than 3 lb/day.

Outcome/Evaluate: ↓ Edema; ↓ BP

Metoprolol succinate

(me-toe-**PROH**-lohl)

Pregnancy Category: C

Toprol XL **(Rx)**

Metoprolol tartrate

(me-toe-**PROH**-lohl)

Pregnancy Category: B

Apo-Metoprolol ✦, Apo-Metoprolol (Type L) ✦, Betaloc ✦, Betaloc Durules ✦, Gen-Metoprolol ✦, Lopressor, Novo-Metoprol ✦, Nu-Metop ✦, PMS-Metoprolol-B ✦ **(Rx)**

Classification: Beta-adrenergic blocking agent

See also *Beta-Adrenergic Blocking Agents.*

Action/Kinetics: Exerts mainly beta-1-adrenergic blocking activity although beta-2 receptors are blocked at high doses. Has no membrane stabilizing or intrinsic sympathomimetic effects. Moderate lipid solubility. **Onset:** 15 min. **Peak plasma levels:** 90 min. **t½:** 3–7 hr. Effect of drug is cumulative. Food increases bioavailability. Exhibits significant first-pass effect. Metabolized in liver and excreted in urine.

Uses: Metoprolol Succinate: Alone or with other drugs to treat hypertension. Chronic management of angina pectoris.

Metoprolol Tartrate: Hypertension (either alone or with other antihypertensive agents, such as thiazide diuretics). Acute MI in hemodynamically stable clients. Angina pectoris. *Investigational:* IV to suppress atrial ectopy in COPD, aggressive behavior, prophylaxis of migraine, ventricular arrhythmias, enhancement of cognitive performance in geriatric clients, essential tremors.

Additional Contraindications: Myocardial infarction in clients with a HR of less than 45 beats/min, in second- or third-degree heart block, or if SBP is less than 100 mm Hg. Moderate to severe cardiac failure.

Special Concerns: Safety and effectiveness have not been established in children. Use with caution in impaired hepatic function and during lactation.

Laboratory Test Considerations: ↑ Serum transaminase, LDH, alkaline phosphatase.

Additional Drug Interactions

Cimetidine / May ↑ plasma levels of metoprolol
Contraceptives, oral / May ↑ effects of metoprolol
Methimazole / May ↓ effects of metoprolol
Phenobarbital / ↓ Effect of metoprolol due to ↑ breakdown by liver
Propylthiouracil / May ↓ the effects of metoprolol
Quinidine / May ↑ effects of metoprolol
Rifampin / ↓ Effect of metoprolol due to ↑ breakdown by liver

How Supplied: Metoprolol succinate: *Tablet, Extended Release:* 50 mg, 100 mg, 200 mg. Metoprolol tartrate: *Injection:* 1 mg/mL; *Tablet:* 50 mg, 100 mg

Dosage

- **Metoprolol Succinate Tablets**

Angina pectoris.

Individualized. Initial: 100 mg/day in a single dose. Dose may be increased slowly, at weekly intervals, until optimum effect is reached or there is a pronounced slowing of HR. Doses above 400 mg/day have not been studied.

Hypertension.

Initial: 50–100 mg/day in a single dose with or without a diuretic. Dosage may be increased in weekly intervals until maximum effect is reached. Doses above 400 mg/day have not been studied.

• **Metoprolol Tartrate Tablets**

Hypertension.

Initial: 100 mg/day in single or divided doses; **then,** dose may be increased weekly to maintenance level of 100–450 mg/day. A diuretic may also be used.

Aggressive behavior.

200–300 mg/day.

Essential tremors.

50–300 mg/day.

Prophylaxis of migraine.

50–100 mg b.i.d.

Ventricular arrhythmias.

200 mg/day.

• **Metoprolol Tartrate Injection (IV) and Tablets**

Early treatment of MI.

3 IV bolus injections of 5 mg each at approximately 2-min intervals. If clients tolerate the full IV dose, give 50 mg q 6 hr PO beginning 15 min after the last IV dose (or as soon as client's condition allows). This dose is continued for 48 hr followed by **late treatment:** 100 mg b.i.d. as soon as feasible; continue for 1–3 months (although data suggest treatment should be continued for 1–3 years). In clients who do not tolerate the full IV dose, begin with 25–50 mg q 6 hr PO beginning 15 min after the last IV dose or as soon as the condition allows.

HEALTH CARE CONSIDERATIONS

See also *Health Care Considerations* for *Beta-Adrenergic Blocking Agents* and *Antihypertensive Agents.*

Assessment

1. Record indications for therapy; note any cardiac disease.
2. Monitor liver and renal function studies, ECG, and VS.

Client/Family Teaching

1. Take doses at the same time each day.
2. Continue with diet, regular exercise, and weight loss in the overall plan to control BP.
3. Report any symptoms of fluid overload such as sudden weight gain, edema, or dyspnea.
4. Dress appropriately; may cause an increased sensitivity to cold.

Outcome/Evaluate

- ↓ BP; ↓ anginal attacks
- Prevention of myocardial reinfarction and associated mortality

Metronidazole

(meh-troh-**NYE**-dah-zohl)

Pregnancy Category: B

Apo-Metronidazole ✱, Femazole, Flagyl, Flagyl 500 Injection ✱, Flagyl ER, Flagyl I.V., Flagyl I.V. RTU, Metric 21, Metro-Cream Topical, MetroGel Topical, MetroGel-Vaginal, Metro I.V., Metryl, Metryl-500, Metryl I.V., NidaGel ✱, Noritate Cream 1%, Novo-Nidazol ✱, PMS-Metronidazole ✱, Protostat, Satric, Satric 500, Trikacide ✱ **(Rx)**

Classification: Systemic trichomonacide, amebicide

See also *Anti-Infectives.*

Action/Kinetics: Effective against anaerobic bacteria and protozoa. Specifically inhibits growth of trichomonae and amoebae by binding to DNA, resulting in loss of helical structure, strand breakage, inhibition of nucleic acid synthesis, and cell death. Well absorbed from GI tract and widely distributed in body tissues. **Peak serum concentration: PO,** 6–40 mcg/mL, depending on the dose, after 1–2 hr. **t½: PO,** 6–12 hr average: 8 hr. Eliminated primarily in urine (20% unchanged), which may be red-brown in color following either PO or IV use. The mechanism for its effectiveness in reducing the inflammatory lesions of acne rosacea is not known.

Uses: Systemic: Amebiasis. Symptomatic and asymptomatic trichomoniasis; to treat asymptomatic partner. Amebic dysentery and amebic liver abscess. To reduce postoperative anaerobic infection following colorectal surgery, elective hysterectomy, and emergency appendectomy. Anaerobic bacterial infections of the abdomen, female genital system, skin or skin structures, bones and joints, lower respiratory tract, and CNS. Also, septicemia, endocarditis, hepatic encephalopathy. PO for Crohn's disease and pseudomembranous colitis. *Investigational:* giardiasis, *Gardnerella vaginalis.*

Topical: Inflammatory papules, pustules, and erythema of rosacea. *Investigational:* Infected decubitus ulcers (use 1% solution prepared from oral tablets).

Vaginal: Bacterial vaginosis.

Contraindications: Blood dyscrasias, active organic disease of the CNS, trichomoniasis during the first trimester of pregnancy, lactation. Topical use if hypersensitive to parabens or other ingredients of the formulation. Consumption of alcohol during use.

Special Concerns: Safety and efficacy have not been established in children.

Side Effects: Systemic Use. G*I:* Nausea, dry mouth, metallic taste, vomiting, diar-

M

rhea, abdominal discomfort, constipation. *CNS:* Headache, dizziness, vertigo, incoordination, ataxia, confusion, irritability, depression, weakness, insomnia, syncope, seizures, peripheral neuropathy including paresthesias. *Hematologic:* Leukopenia, ***bone marrow aplasia.*** *GU:* Burning, dysuria, cystitis, polyuria, incontinence, dryness of vagina or vulva, dyspareunia, decreased libido. *Allergic:* Urticaria, pruritus, erythematous rash, flushing, nasal congestion, fever, joint pain. *Miscellaneous:* Furry tongue, glossitis, stomatitis (due to overgrowth of *Candida*) ECG abnormalities, thrombophlebitis.

Topical Use: Watery eyes if gel applied too closely to this area; transient redness; mild burning, dryness, and skin irritation.

Vaginal Use: Symptomatic candida vaginitis, N&V.

OD **Management of Overdose:** *Symptoms:* Ataxia, N&V, peripheral neuropathy, ***seizures*** up to 5–7 days. *Treatment:* Supportive treatment.

Drug Interactions

Barbiturates / Possible therapeutic failure of metronidazole

Cimetidine / ↑ Serum levels of metronidazole due to ↓ clearance

Disulfiram / Concurrent use may cause confusion or acute psychosis

Ethanol / Possible disulfiram-like reaction, including flushing, palpitations, tachycardia, and N&V

Hydantoins / ↑ Effect of hydantoins due to ↓ clearance

Lithium / ↑ Lithium toxicity

Warfarin / ↑ Anticoagulant effect

How Supplied: *Capsule:* 375 mg; *Cream:* 0.75%, 1%; *Gel/jelly:* 0.75%; *Injection:* 500 mg/100 mL; *Tablet:* 250 mg, 500 mg; *Tablet, Extended-Release:* 750 mg

Dosage

- **Capsules, Tablets**

Amebiasis: Acute amebic dysentery or amebic liver abscess.

Adult: 500–750 mg t.i.d. for 5–10 days; **pediatric:** 35–50 mg/kg/day in three divided doses for 10 days.

Trichomoniasis, female.

250 mg t.i.d. for 7 days, 2 g given on 1 day in single or divided doses, or 375 mg b.i.d. for 7 days. **Pediatric:** 5 mg/kg t.i.d. for 7 days. An interval of 4–6 weeks should elapse between courses of therapy. *NOTE:* Do not treat pregnant women during the first trimester. *Male:* Individualize dosage; usual, 250 mg t.i.d. for 7 days.

Giardiasis.

250 mg t.i.d. for 7 days.

G. vaginalis.

500 mg b.i.d. for 7 days.

- **Tablets, Extended-Release**

Bacterial vaginosis.

One 750-mg tablet per day for 7 days.

- **IV**

Anaerobic bacterial infections.

Adults, initially: 15 mg/kg infused over 1 hr; **then,** after 6 hr, 7.5 mg/kg q 6 hr for 7–10 days (daily dose should not exceed 4 g). Treatment may be necessary for 2–3 weeks, although PO therapy should be initiated as soon as possible.

Prophylaxis of anaerobic infection during surgery.

Adults: 15 mg/kg given over a 30- to 60-min period, with completion 1 hr prior to surgery and 7.5 mg/kg infused over 30–60 min 6 and 12 hr after the initial dose.

- **Topical (0.75%, 1%)**

Rosacea.

After washing, apply a thin film and rub in well either once daily or b.i.d. in the morning and evening for 4–9 weeks.

- **Vaginal (0.75%)**

Bacterial vaginosis.

One applicatorful (5 g) in the morning and evening for 5 days. Metro-Gel Vaginal allows for once-daily dosing at bedtime.

HEALTH CARE CONSIDERATIONS

See also *General Health Care Considerations for All Anti-Infectives.*

Administration/Storage

1. For topical use, therapeutic results should be seen within 3 weeks with continuing improvement through 9 weeks of therapy.
2. Cosmetics may be used after application of topical metronidazole.

IV 3. Do not give by IV bolus. Administer each single dose over 1 hr.

4. Do not use syringes with aluminum needles or hubs.
5. Discontinue primary IV infusion during infusion of metronidazole.
6. The order of mixing to prepare the powder for injection is important:

- Reconstitute.
- Dilute in IV solutions in glass or plastic containers.
- Neutralize pH with $NaHCO_3$ solution. Do not refrigerate neutralized solutions.

7. Premixed, ready to use Flagyl comes 5 mg/mL (500 mg metronidazole in 100 mL of solution) in plastic bags; administer over 1 hr.
8. Drug has a high sodium content.

Assessment

1. Record indications for therapy and symptom characteristics.
2. Monitor CBC and cultures.

Client/Family Teaching

1. Take with food or milk to reduce GI upset; may cause a metallic taste.
2. Report any symptoms of CNS toxicity, such as ataxia or tremor and any unusual bruising or bleeding.
3. Do not perform tasks that require mental alertness until drug effects are realized; dizziness may occur.
4. During treatment for trichomoniasis, partner should also have therapy since organisms may be located in the male urogenital tract and reinfect partner. Use a condom to prevent reinfections.
5. Do not engage in intercourse while using the vaginal gel.
6. Drug may turn urine brown; do not be alarmed.
7. No alcohol; a disulfiram-like reaction may occur. Symptoms include abdominal cramps, vomiting, flushing, and headache.

Outcome/Evaluate

- Symptomatic improvement
- Negative culture reports

Mexiletine hydrochloride

(mex-**ILL**-eh-teen)

Pregnancy Category: C

Mexitil, Novo-Mexiletine ✱ **(Rx)**

Classification: Antiarrhythmic, class IB

See also *Antiarrhythmic Drugs*.

Action/Kinetics: Similar to lidocaine but is effective PO. Inhibits the flow of sodium into the cell, thereby reducing the rate of rise of the action potential. The drug decreases the effective refractory period in Purkinje fibers. BP and pulse rate are not affected following use, but there may be a small decrease in CO and an increase in peripheral vascular resistance. Also has both local anesthetic and anticonvulsant effects. **Onset:** 30–120 min. **Peak blood levels:** 2–3 hr. **Therapeutic plasma levels:** 0.5–2 mcg/mL. **Plasma t½:** 10–12 hr. Approximately 10% excreted unchanged in the urine; acidification of the urine enhances excretion, whereas alkalinization decreases excretion.

Uses: Documented life-threatening ventricular arrhythmias (such as ventricular tachycardia). *Investigational:* Prophylactically to decrease the incidence of ventricular tachycardia and other ventricular arrhythmias in the acute phase of MI. To reduce pain, dysesthesia, and paresthesia associated with diabetic neuropathy.

Contraindications: Cardiogenic shock, preexisting second- or third-degree AV block (if no pacemaker is present). Use with lesser arrhythmias. Lactation.

Special Concerns: There is the possibility of increased risk of death when used in clients with non-life-threatening cardiac arrhythmias. Use with caution in hypotension, severe CHF, or known seizure disorders. Dosage has not been established in children.

Side Effects: *CV:* ***Worsening of arrhythmias,*** palpitations, chest pain, increased ventricular arrhythmias (PVCs), CHF, angina or angina-like pain, hypotension, bradycardia, syncope, ***AV block or conduction disturbances,*** atrial arrhythmias, hypertension, ***cardiogenic shock,*** hot flashes, edema. *GI:* High incidence of upper GI distress, N&V, heartburn. Also, diarrhea or constipation, changes in appetite, dry mouth, abdominal cramps or pain, abdominal discomfort, salivary changes, dysphagia, altered taste, pharyngitis, changes in oral mucous membranes, upper GI bleeding, peptic ulcer, esophageal ulceration. *CNS:* High incidence of lightheadedness, dizziness, tremor, coordination difficulties, and nervousness. Also, changes in sleep habits, headache, fatigue, weakness, tinnitus, paresthesias, numbness, depression, confusion, difficulty with speech, short-term memory loss, hallucinations, malaise, psychosis, ***seizures,*** loss of consciousness. *Hematologic:* Leukopenia, neutropenia, agranulocytosis, thrombocytopenia. *GU:* Decreased libido, impotence, urinary hesitancy or retention. *Dermatologic:* Rash, dry skin. Rarely, exfoliative dermatitis, and ***Stevens-Johnson syndrome.*** *Miscellaneous:* Blurred vision, visual disturbances, dyspnea, arthralgia, fever, diaphoresis, loss of hair, hiccoughs, laryngeal or pharyngeal changes, syndrome of SLE, myelofibrosis.

Laboratory Test Considerations: ↑ AST. Positive ANA. Abnormal LFTs.

OD **Management of Overdose:** *Symptoms:* Nausea. CNS symptoms (dizziness, drowsiness, paresthesias, seizures) usually precede CV symptoms (hypotension, sinus bradycardia, intermittent left bundle branch block (LBBB), ***temporary asystole). Massive overdoses cause coma and respiratory arrest.*** *Treatment:* General supportive treatment. Give atropine to treat hypotension or bradycardia. Acidification of the urine may increase rate of excretion.

Drug Interactions

Aluminum hydroxide / ↓ Absorption of mexiletine

M

Atropine / ↓ Absorption of mexiletine
Caffeine / ↓ Clearance of caffeine (50%)
Cimetidine / ↑ or ↓ Plasma levels of mexiletine
Magnesium hydroxide / ↓ Absorption of mexiletine
Metoclopramide / ↑ Absorption of mexiletine
Narcotics / ↓ Absorption of mexiletine
Phenobarbital / ↓ Plasma levels of mexiletine
Phenytoin / ↑ Clearance → ↓ plasma levels of mexiletine
Rifampin / ↑ Clearance → ↓ plasma levels of mexiletine
Theophylline / ↑ Effect of theophylline due to ↑ serum levels
Urinary acidifiers / ↑ Rate of excretion of mexiletine
Urinary alkalinizers / ↓ Rate of excretion of mexiletine
How Supplied: *Capsule:* 150 mg, 200 mg, 250 mg

Dosage

- **Capsules**

Antiarrhythmic.

Adults, individualized, initial: 200 mg q 8 hr if rapid control of arrhythmia not required; dosage adjustment may be made in 50- or 100-mg increments q 2–3 days, if required. **Maintenance:** 200–300 mg q 8 hr, depending on response and tolerance of client. If adequate response is not achieved with 300 mg or less q 8 hr, 400 mg q 8 hr may be tried although the incidence of CNS side effects increases. If the drug is effective at doses of 300 mg or less q 8 hr, the same total daily dose may be given in divided doses q 12 hr (e.g., 450 mg q 12 hr). Maximum total daily dose: 1,200 mg.

Rapid control of arrhythmias.

Initial loading dose: 400 mg followed by a 200-mg dose in 8 hr.

Diabetic neuropathy.

Initial: 150 mg/day for 3 days; **then,** 300 mg/day for 3 days. **Maintenance:** 10 mg/kg/day.

HEALTH CARE CONSIDERATIONS

See also *Health Care Considerations* for *Antiarrhythmic Drugs.*

Administration/Storage

1. Reduce dose with severe liver disease and marked right-sided CHF.
2. If transferring to mexiletine from other class I antiarrhythmics, initiate mexiletine at a dose of 200 mg and then titrate according to the response at the following times: 6–12 hr after the last dose of quinidine sulfate, 3–6 hr after the last dose of procainamide, 6–12 hr after the last dose of disopyramide, or 8–12 hr after the last dose of tocainide.
3. Hospitalize client when transferring to mexiletine if there is a chance that withdrawal of the previous antiarrhythmic may produce life-threatening arrhythmias.

Assessment

1. Record indications for therapy; list any other agents trialed and the outcome.
2. Note evidence of CHF; assess ECG for AV block.
3. Record pulmonary assessment findings; note SaO_2/PO_2.
4. Monitor ECG, CXR, CBC, electrolytes, renal and LFTs.
5. Assess urinary pH; alkalinity decreases and acidity increases renal drug excretion.

Client/Family Teaching

1. Take with food or an antacid to ↓ GI upset.
2. Report any bruising, bleeding, fevers, or sore throat or adverse CNS effects such as dizziness, tremor, impaired coordination, N&V.
3. Immediately report any increase in heart palpitations, irregularity, or rate less than 50 beats/min.
4. Do not perform tasks that require mental alertness until drug effects are realized.
5. Carry identification that lists drugs currently prescribed.

Outcome/Evaluate

- Control of ventricular arrhythmias
- Therapeutic drug levels (0.5–2 mcg/mL)
- ↓ S&S of diabetic neuropathy

Miconazole

(my-**KON**-ah-zohl)
Pregnancy Category: C
Topical: Micatin, Monistat-Derm. **Vaginal:** Micozole ♣, Monazole ♣, Monistat 3, Monistat 7, M-Zole 3 Combination Pack **(Rx) (OTC)**
Classification: Antifungal agent

See also *Anti-Infectives.*

Action/Kinetics: Broad-spectrum fungicide that alters the permeability of the fungal membrane by inhibiting synthesis of sterols; thus, essential intracellular materials are lost. The drug also inhibits biosynthesis of triglycerides and phospholipids and also inhibits oxidative and peroxidative enzyme activity. May be fungistatic or fungicidal, depending on the concentration.

Uses: Topical, Vaginal: Tinea pedis, tinea cruris, tinea corporis caused by *Trichophyton rubrum, T. mentagrophytes,* and *Epidermophyton floccosum* (both OTC and Rx). Moniliasis and tinea versicolor (Rx only).

Contraindications: Hypersensitivity. Use of topical products in or around the eyes.
Special Concerns: Safe use in children less than 1 year of age has not been established.
Side Effects: Following systemic use. *GI:* N&V, diarrhea, anorexia. *Hematologic:* Thrombocytopenia, aggregation of erythrocytes, rouleaux formation on blood smears. Transient decrease in hematocrit. *Dermatologic:* Pruritus, rash, flushing, phlebitis at injection site. *CV:* Transient tachycardia or arrhythmias following rapid injection of undiluted drug. *Miscellaneous:* Fever, chills, drowsiness, transient decrease in serum sodium values. Hyperlipemia due to the vehicle (polyethylene glycol 40 and castor oil). **Following topical use:** Vulvovaginal burning, pelvic cramps, hives, skin rash, headache, itching, irritation, maceration, and allergic contact dermatitis.
Drug Interactions
Amphotericin B / ↓ Activity of miconazole of each drug
Coumarin anticoagulants / Miconazole ↑ anticoagulant effect
How Supplied: *Topical Cream:* 2%; *Powder:* 2%; *Spray:* 2%; *Vaginal Cream:* 2%; *Suppository:* 100 mg, 200 mg; *Combination Pack:* Suppositories, 200 mg and Cream, 2%

Dosage

- **Topical, Aerosol Powder, Aerosol Solution, Cream, Lotion, Powder**

Apply to cover affected areas in morning and evening (once daily for tinea versicolor) for 7 days.

- **Vaginal Cream or Suppository**

Monistat 3: One suppository daily at bedtime for 7 days (100-mg suppositories) or 3 consecutive days (200-mg suppositories).
Monistat 7: One applicator full of cream or one suppository at bedtime daily for 7 days. Course may be repeated after presence of other pathogens has been ruled out.

- **Combination Pack**

Vaginal yeast infections, relief of external vulval itching and irritation due to yeast infection.
Three day treatment consisting of miconizole suppositories, 200 mg and miconazole nitrate cream, 2%.

HEALTH CARE CONSIDERATIONS

See also *General Health Care Considerations for All Anti-Infectives.*

Administration/Storage

1. The lotion is preferred for intertriginous areas.
2. To reduce recurrence of symptoms, tinea cruris, tinea corporis, and candida should be treated for 2 weeks; tinea pedis should be treated for 1 month.
3. Refrigerate vaginal products below 15°C–30°C (59°F–86°F).

Assessment

1. Determine any previous experience with this drug, any sensitivity, and response obtained.
2. Monitor cultures, CBC, electrolytes, and LFTs.
3. Record clinical presentation, noting size, number, and extent of lesions.

Client/Family Teaching

1. Review technique for administration; use only as directed.
2. Use sanitary pads to protect clothing and linens when using cream or suppositories.
3. When used for vaginal infections, refrain from intercourse or use a condom to prevent reinfection.
4. When used vaginally, continue treatment during menses.
5. Report if exposed to HIV and recurrent vaginal infections occur.
6. Report persistent N&V, diarrhea, dizziness, and pruritus.

Outcome/Evaluate

- Negative culture reports
- Resolution of vaginitis evidenced by ↓ in itching/burning; ↓ discharge
- ↓ Size and number of lesions

Midazolam hydrochloride

(my-**DAYZ**-oh-lam)
Pregnancy Category: D
Versed **(C-IV) (Rx)**
Classification: Benzodiazepine sedative; adjunct to general anesthesia

See also *Tranquilizers/Antimanic Drugs/Hypnotics.*
Action/Kinetics: Short-acting benzodiazepine with sedative–general anesthetic properties. Depresses the response of the respiratory system to carbon dioxide stimulation, which is more pronounced in clients with COPD. Possible mild to moderate decreases in CO, mean arterial BP, SV, and systemic vascular resistance. HR may rise somewhat in those with slow HRs (< 65/min) and decrease in others (especially those with HRs more than 85/min). **Onset, IM:** 15 min; **IV:** 2–2.5 min for induction (if combined with a preanesthetic narcotic, induction is about 1.5 min). If preanesthetic medication (morphine) is given, the **Peak plasma levels, IM:** 45 min. **Maximum effect:** 30–60 min.

Time to recovery: Usually within 2 hr, although up to 6 hr may be required. About 97% bound to plasma protein. **t½, elimination:** 1.2–12.3 hr. Rapidly metabolized in the liver to inactive compounds; excreted through the urine.

Uses: IV, IM: Preoperative sedation, anxiolysis, and amnesia. **IV:** Sedation, anxiolysis, and amnesia prior to or during short diagnostic, therapeutic, or endoscopic procedures (either alone or with other CNS depressants). Induction of general anesthesia before administration of other anesthetics. Supplement to nitrous oxide and oxygen in balanced anesthesia. Sedation of intubated and mechanically ventilated clients as a component of anesthesia or during treatment in a critical care setting. *Investigational:* Treat epileptic seizures. Alternative to terminate refractory status epilepticus.

Contraindications: Hypersensitivity to benzodiazepines. Acute narrow-angle glaucoma. Use in obstetrics, coma, shock, or acute alcohol intoxication where VS are depressed. IA injection.

Special Concerns: Use with caution during lactation. Pediatric clients may require higher doses than adults. Hypotension may be more common in conscious sedated clients who have received a preanesthetic narcotic. Geriatric and debilitated clients require lower doses to induce anesthesia and they are more prone to side effects. Use IV with extreme caution in severe fluid or electrolyte disturbances.

Side Effects: Fluctuations in VS, including decreased respiratory rate and tidal volume, apnea, variations in BP and pulse rate are common. The following are general side effects regardless of the route of administration. *CV:* Hypotension, cardiac arrest. *CNS:* Oversedation, headache, drowsiness, grogginess, confusion, retrograde amnesia, euphoria, nervousness, agitation, anxiety, argumentativeness, restlessness, emergence delirium, increased time for emergence, dreaming during emergence, nightmares, insomnia, tonic-clonic movements, ataxia, muscle tremor, involuntary or athetoid movements, dizziness, dysphoria, dysphonia, slurred speech, paresthesia. *GI:* Hiccoughs, N&V, acid taste, retching, excessive salivation. *Ophthalmologic:* Double vision, blurred vision, nystagmus, pinpoint pupils, visual disturbances, cyclic eyelid movements, difficulty in focusing. *Dermatologic:* Hives, swelling or feeling of burning, warmth or cold feeling at injection site, hive-like wheal at injection site, pruritus, rash. *Miscellaneous:* Blocked ears, loss of balance, chills, weakness, faint feeling, lethargy, yawning, toothache, hematoma.

More common following IM use: Pain at injection site, headache, induration and redness, muscle stiffness.

More common following IV use: *Respiratory:* ***Bronchospasm,*** coughing, dyspnea, laryngospasm, hyperventilation, shallow respirations, tachypnea, airway obstruction, wheezing, respiratory depression and ***respiratory arrest*** when used for conscious sedation. *CV:* PVCs, bigeminy, bradycardia, tachycardia, vasovagal episode, nodal rhythm.*At injection site:* Tenderness, pain, redness, induration, phlebitis.

Drug Interactions

Alcohol / ↑ Risk of apnea, airway obstruction, desaturation or hypoventilation
Anesthetics, inhalation / ↓ Dose if midazolam used as an induction agent
CNS Depressants / ↑ Risk of apnea, airway obstruction, desaturation or hypoventilation
Droperidol / ↑ Hypnotic effect of midazolam when used as a premedication
Fentanyl / ↑ Hypnotic effect of midazolam when used as a premedication
Indinavir / Possible prolonged sedation and respiratory depression
Meperidine / See *Narcotics;* also, ↑ Risk of hypotension
Narcotics / ↑ Hypnotic effect of midazolam when used as premedications
Propofol / ↑ Effect of propofol
Ritonavir / Possible prolonged sedation and respiratory depression
Thiopental / ↓ Dose if midazolam used as an induction agent

How Supplied: *Injection:* 1 mg/mL, 5 mg/mL; *Syrup:* 2 mg/mL

Dosage

• **IM**

Preoperative sedation, anxiolysis, amnesia.

Adults: 0.07–0.08 mg/kg IM (average: 5 mg) 1 hr before surgery. **Children:** 0.1–0.15 mg/kg (up to 0.5 mg/kg may be needed for more anxious clients).

• **IV**

Conscious sedation, anxiolysis, amnesia for endoscopic or CV procedures in healthy adults less than 60 years of age.

Using the 1 mg/mL (can be diluted with 0.9% sodium chloride or D5W) product, titrate slowly to the desired effect (usually slurred speech); initial dose should be no higher than 2.5 mg IV (may be as low as 1 mg IV) within a 2-min period; wait an additional 2 min to evaluate the sedative effect. If additional sedation is necessary, give small increments waiting an additional 2 min or more after each increment to evaluate the effect. Total doses greater than 5 mg are usually not required. **Children:** Dosage must be individualized by the physician.

Conscious sedation for endoscopic or CV procedures in debilitated or chronically ill clients or clients aged 60 or over.
Slowly titrate to the desired effect using no more than 1.5 mg initially IV (may be as little as 1 mg IV) given over a 2-min period; wait an additional 2 min or more to evaluate the effect. If additional sedation is needed, no more than 1 mg should be given over 2 min; wait an additional 2 min or more after each increment in dose. Total doses greater than 3.5 mg are usually not needed.

Induction of general anesthesia, before use of other general anesthetics, in unmedicated clients.
Adults, unmedicated clients up to 55 years of age, IV, initial: 0.3–0.35 mg/kg given over 20–30 sec, waiting 2 min for effects to occur. If needed, increments of about 25% of the initial dose can be used to complete induction; or, induction can be completed using a volatile liquid anesthetic. Up to 0.6 mg/kg may be used but recovery will be prolonged. **Adults, unmedicated clients over 55 years of age who are good risk surgical clients, initial IV:** 0.15–0.3 mg/kg given over 20–30 sec. **Adults, unmedicated clients over 55 years of age with severe systemic disease or debilitation, initial IV:** 0.15–0.25 mg/kg given over 20–30 sec. **Pediatric:** 0.05–0.2 mg/kg IV.

Induction of general anesthesia, before use of other general anesthetics, in medicated clients.
Adults, premedicated clients up to 55 years of age, IV, initial: 0.15–0.35 mg/kg. If less than 55 years of age, 0.25 mg/kg may be given over 20–30 sec, allowing 2 min for effect. **Adults, premedicated clients over 55 years of age who are good risk surgical clients, initial, IV:** 0.2 mg/kg. **Adults, premedicated clients over 55 years of age with severe systemic disease or debilitation, initial, IV:** 0.15 mg/kg may be sufficient.

Maintenance of balanced anesthesia for short surgical procedures.
IV: Incremental injections about 25% of the dose used for induction when signs indicate anesthesia is lightening.

NOTE: Narcotic preanesthetic medication may include fentanyl, 1.5–2 mcg/kg IV 5 min before induction; morphine, up to 0.15 mg/kg IM; meperidine, up to 1 mg/kg IM; or, Innovar, 0.02 mL/kg IM. Sedative preanesthetic medication may include secobarbital sodium, 200 mg PO or hydroxyzine pamoate, 100 mg PO. Except for fentanyl, give all preanesthetic medications 1 hr prior to midazolam. Always individualize doses.

HEALTH CARE CONSIDERATIONS

See also *Health Considerations* for *Tranquilizers/Antimanic Drugs/Hypnotics*.

Administration/Storage

1. When used for procedures via the mouth, use a topical anesthetic.
2. Give IM doses in a large muscle mass.
IV 3. When used for conscious sedation, do not give by rapid or single bolus IV.
4. When used for induction of general anesthesia, give the initial dose over 20–30 sec.
5. If preanesthetic medications with a depressant component are given (e.g., narcotic analgesics or CNS depressants), reduce the midazolam dosage by 50% compared with healthy, young unmedicated clients.
6. Give maintenance doses to all clients in increments of 25% of the dose first required to achieve the sedative endpoint.
7. Give a narcotic preanesthetic for bronchoscopic procedures.
8. Carefully monitor all IV doses with the immediate availability of oxygen, resuscitative equipment, and personnel who are skilled in maintaining a patent airway and for support of ventilation; continue monitoring during recovery period.
9. May be mixed in the same syringe with atropine, meperidine, morphine, or scopolamine
10. At a concentration of 0.5 mg/mL midazolam is compatible with D5W and 0.9% NaCl for up to 24 hr and with RL solution for up to 4 hr.

Client/Family Teaching

1. Drug may cause dizziness and drowsiness. Avoid alcohol, CNS depressants, and activities that require mental alertness for 24 hr following drug administration.
2. Repeat postprocedure instructions and obtain in writing as may not fully recall instructions; transient amnesia is normal and memory of procedure may be minimal.

Outcome/Evaluate: Desired level of sedation and amnesia; ↓ anxiety

M

Midodrine hydrochloride

(MIH-doh-dreen)
Pregnancy Category: C
Amatine ✦, ProAmatine **(Rx)**
Classification: Treat orthostatic hypotension

Action/Kinetics: Midodrine, a prodrug, is converted to an active metabolite—desglymidodrine—that is an alpha-1 agonist. Desglymidodrine produces an increase in vascular tone and elevation of BP by activating alpha-adrenergic receptors of the arteriolar and venous vasculature. No effect on cardiac beta-adrenergic receptors. The active metabolite does not cross the blood-brain barrier; thus, there are no CNS effects. Standing systolic BP is increased by approximately 15–30 mm Hg at 1 hr after a 10-mg dose; duration: 2–3 hr. Rapidly absorbed from the GI tract. **Peak plasma levels, midodrine:** 30 min; **t½:** 25 min. **Peak plasma levels, desglymidodrine:** 1–2hr; **t½:** 3–4 hr. The bioavailability of the active metabolite is not affected by food. Desglymidodrine is eliminated in the urine.

Uses: Orthostatic hypotension in those whose lives are significantly impaired despite standard clinical care. *Investigational:* Management of urinary incontinence.

Contraindications: Use in severe organic heart disease, acute renal disease, urinary retention, pheochromocytoma, thyrotoxicosis, persistent and excessive supine hypertension.

Special Concerns: Use with caution in impaired renal or hepatic function, during lactation, in orthostatic hypotensive clients who are also diabetic, or in those with a history of visual problems or who are also taking fludrocortisone acetate. Safety and efficacy have not been determined in children.

Side Effects: *CNS:* Paresthesia, pain, headache, feeling of pressure or fullness in the head, confusion, abnormal thinking, nervousness, anxiety. Rarely, dizziness, insomnia, somnolence. *GI:* Dry mouth. Rarely, canker sore, nausea, GI distress, flatulence. *Dermatologic:* Piloerection, pruritus, rash, vasodilation, flushed face. Rarely, erythema multiforme, dry skin. *Miscellaneous:* Dysuria, supine hypertension. Rarely, visual field defect, skin hyperesthesia, impaired urination, asthenia, backache, pyrosis, leg cramps.

OD **Management of Overdose:** *Symptoms:* Hypertension, piloerection, sensation of coldness, urinary retention. *Treatment*: Emesis and administration of an alpha-adrenergic blocking agent (e.g., phentolamine).

Drug Interactions

Alpha-adrenergic agonists / ↑ Pressor effects of midodrine

Alpha-adrenergic antagonists / Antagonism of the effects of midodrine

Beta-adrenergic blockers / ↑ Risk of bradycardia, AV block, or arrhythmias

Cardiac glycosides / ↑ Risk of bradycardia, AV block, or arrhythmias

Fludrocortisone / ↑ Intraocular pressure and glaucoma

Psychopharmacologic drugs / ↑ Risk of bradycardia, AV block, or arrhythmias

How Supplied: *Tablet:* 2.5 mg, 5 mg

Dosage

- **Tablets**

Orthostatic hypotension.

10 mg t.i.d. given during the daytime hours when the client is upright and pursuing daily activities (e.g., shortly before or upon arising in the morning, midday, and late afternoon–not later than 6:00 p.m.). To control symptoms, dosing may be q 3 hr. Initial dose in impaired renal function: 2.5 mg t.i.d.

Urinary incontinence.

2.5–5 mg b.i.d.–t.i.d.

HEALTH CARE CONSIDERATIONS

Assessment

1. Record onset, duration, and characteristics of symptoms. Note other nonpharmacologic treatments (i.e., support stockings, increased salt in diet, fluid expansion, sleeping with head of bed raised) trialed.
2. Orthostatic hypotension is defined as SBP reductions > 20 mm Hg or DBP of over 10 mm Hg reduction within 3 min of standing; assess carefully on several occasions.
3. Record any acute renal disease, urinary retention, pheochromocytoma, severe organic heart disease, or thyrotoxicosis, as these preclude drug therapy. Assess for liver and renal dysfunction.

Client/Family Teaching

1. Do not take after the evening meal or within 4 hr of bedtime.
2. Use OTC products containing phenylephrine or phenylpropanolamine (e.g.; cold remedies/diet aids) cautiously; may increase supine BP.
3. May experience supine hypertension; check BP regularly while lying and sitting and keep a record.
4. Stop drug and report blurred vision, pounding in ears, headache, cardiac awareness, increased dizziness/syncope.

Outcome/Evaluate: Relief of symptomatic orthostatic hypotension: ↓ dizziness, ↓ lightheadedness, ↓ unsteadiness

Miglitol

(MIG-lih-tohl)

Pregnancy Category: B

Glyset **(Rx)**

Classification: Antidiabetic, oral

See also *Antidiabetic Agents*.

Action/Kinetics: Acts by delaying digestion of ingested carbohydrates resulting in smaller rise in blood glucose levels after meals. Effect is due to reversible inhibition of membrane-bound intestinal glucoside hydrolase enzymes which hydrolyze oligosaccharides and disaccharides to glucose and other monosaccharides. Reduces levels of glycosylated hemoglobin in type II diabetes. Does not enhance insulin secretion or increase insulin sensitivity. Does not cause hypoglycemia when given in fasted state. Absorption is saturable at high doses (i.e., only 50% to 70% of 100 mg dose is absorbed while 25 mg dose is 100% absorbed). **Peak levels:** 2–3 hr. Drug is not metabolized and is eliminated unchanged in urine. Reduce dose in impaired renal function.
Uses: Alone as adjunct to diet to treat non-insulin-dependent diabetes. With sulfonylurea when diet plus either miglitol or a sulfonylurea alone do not result in adequate control (effects of sulfonylurea and miglitol are additive).
Contraindications: Lactation, diabetic ketoacidosis, inflammatory bowel disease, colonic ulceration, partial intestinal obstruction, those predisposed to intestinal obstruction, chronic intestinal diseases associated with marked disorders of digestion or absorption, conditions that may deteriorate due to increased gas formation in the intestine, hypersensitivity to drug.
Special Concerns: When given with sulfonylurea or insulin, miglitol causes further decrease in blood sugar and increased risk of hypoglycemia. Safety and efficacy have not been determined in children.
Side Effects: *GI:* Flatulence, diarrhea, abdominal pain, soft stools, abdominal discomfort. *Dermatologic:* Skin rash (transient).

Drug Interactions

Amylase / ↓ Effect of miglitol
Charcoal / Adsorbent effect ↓ effect of miglitol
Digoxin / May ↓ plasma levels of digoxin
Pancreatin / ↓ Effect of miglitol
Propranolol / Significant ↓ bioavailability of propranolol
Ranitidine / Significant ↓ bioavailability of ranitidine

How Supplied: *Tablets:* 25 mg, 50 mg, 100 mg

Dosage

- **Tablets**

  Type II diabetes.

Individualize dosage. **Initial:** 25 mg t.i.d. with first bite of each main meal (some may benefit from starting with 25 mg once daily to minimize GI side effects). After 4 to 8 weeks of 25 mg t.i.d. dose, increase dosage to 50 mg t.i.d. for about 3 months. Measure glycosylated hemoglobin; if not satisfactory, increase dose to 100 mg t.i.d. **Maintenance:** 50 mg t.i.d., up to 100 mg t.i.d. (maximum).

HEALTH CARE CONSIDERATIONS

See also *Health Care Considerations* for *Antidiabetic Agents.*

Assessment

1. Record indications, other agents trialed, and outcome.
2. Determine any IBD, colonic ulceration, intestinal obstruction, or severe digestion/absorption problems.
3. Monitor BS, HbA1-C, and renal function; reduce dose with impaired function and avoid if creatinine > 2 mg/dL.

Client/Family Teaching

1. Take with first bite of each meal.
2. May experience abdominal pain and diarrhea which should diminish with continued treatment.
3. Any stress, fever, trauma, infection, or surgery may alter glucose control; monitor FS regularly.
4. Drug inhibits breakdown of table sugar; have glucose available for episodes of marked hypoglycemia.
5. Continue prescribed diet and regular exercise. Report for F/U as scheduled.

Outcome/Evaluate: ↓ BS; HbA1-C < 8

M

Minocycline hydrochloride

(mih-no-**SYE**-kleen)
Pregnancy Category: D
Alti-Minocycline ✱, Apo-Minocycline ✱, Gen-Minocycline ✱, Dynacin, Minocin, Novo-Minocycline ✱, Vectrin **(Rx)**
Classification: Antibiotic, tetracycline

See also *Anti-Infectives* and *Tetracyclines.*
Action/Kinetics: In fasting adults, 90% to 100% of an oral dose is absorbed. **Peak plasma levels:** 1–4 hr. Absorption is less affected by milk or food than for other tetracyclines. **$t^{1/2}$, elimination:** 11–26 hr. Metabolized in the liver.
Uses: See also *Tetracyclines.* To eliminate meningococci from the nasopharynx of asymptomatic *Neisseria meningitidis* carriers in which the risk of meningococcal meningitis is high. *Note:* Due to adverse CNS effects, use rifampin to treat meningococcus carriers when the drug susceptibility is not known or when the organism is sulfa-resistant. Use mi-

nocycline only when rifampin is contraindicated.

(1) Granulomas of the skin caused by *Mycobacterium marinum*. (2) In combination with gonococcal regimens for presumptive treatment of coexisting chlamydial infections. (3) Uncomplicated gonogoccal urethritis in adult males. (4) Treatment of uncomplicated urethral, endocervical, or rectal infections caused by *Chlamydia trachomatis* or *Ureaplasma urealyticum* in adults. (5) Intrapleurally as a sclerosing agent to control pleural effusions assocated with metastatic tumors. (6) Treatment of cholera and nocardiosis. (7) Adjunctive treatment of inflammatory acne unresponsive to oral tetracycline HCl or oral erythromycin.

Additional Side Effects: Blue-gray pigmentation areas of cutaneous inflammation, vertigo, ataxia, drowsiness, ***Stevens-Johnson syndrome*** (rare).

How Supplied: *Capsules:* 50 mg, 100 mg; *Powder for Injection:* 100 mg; *Syrup:* 50 mg/5 mL; *Tablets:* 100 mg.

Dosage

M

- **Capsules, Injection, Suspension, Tablets**

Infections against which effective, including asymptomatic meningococcus carriers.

Adults, initial: 200 mg; **then,** 100 mg q 12 hr. An alternative regimen is 100–200 mg initially followed by 50 mg q 6 hr. The length of treatment is 5 days for meningococcus carriers. **Children over 8 years of age, initial:** 4 mg/kg; **then,** 2 mg/kg q 12 hr.

Mycobacterial infections.

100 mg PO b.i.d. for 6–8 weeks.

Uncomplicated gongococcal urethritis in adult males.

100 mg b.i.d. for 5 days.

Uncomplicated urethral, endocervical, or rectal infections due to Chlamydia trachomatis *or* Ureaplasma urealyticum.

100 mg PO b.i.d. for at least 7 days.

Nongonococcal urethritis caused by C. trachomatis or Mycoplasma.

100/day PO in 1 or 2 divided doses for 1 to 3 weeks.

Sclerosing agent to control pleural effusions associated with metastatic cancer.

300 mg diluted with 40–50 mL of 0.9% NaCl injection and instilled into the pleural space through a thoracostomy tube.

Cholera in conjunction with fluid and electrolyte replacement.

Initial: 200 mg PO; **then,** 100 mg PO 12 hr for 48–72 hr.

Adjunct to treat inflammatory acne unresponsive to PO tetracycline HCl or erythromycin.

50 mg PO 1–3 times/day.

HEALTH CARE CONSIDERATIONS

See also *Health Care Considerations* for *Anti-Infectives* and *Tetracyclines*.

Administration/Storage

IV 1. Do not dissolve in solutions containing calcium; forms a precipitate.
2. After dissolving medication in the vial, further dilute to 500–1,000 mL with any of the following: dextrose, dextrose and NaCl injection, NaCl injection, Ringer's injection, RL injection.
3. Start administration of the final dilution immediately.
4. Discard reconstituted solutions after 24 hr at room temperature.

Assessment

1. Record onset, duration, location, and characteristics of symptoms.
2. Monitor cultures and CBC; identify contacts when treating a contagious disease.

Client/Family Teaching

1. Take complete prescription; may take with meals if GI upset occurs.
2. With STDs, use condoms during therapy to prevent reinfections and obtain periodic cultures.
3. Practice reliable birth control; may cause fetal harm.
4. Report any unusual bruising or bleeding, severe rash or diarrhea and lack of improvement after 72 hr.

Outcome/Evaluate: Symptomatic improvement; resolution of infection

Minoxidil, oral

(mih-**NOX**-ih-dil)
Pregnancy Category: C
Loniten **(Rx)**
Classification: Antihypertensive, depresses sympathetic nervous system

See also *Antihypertensive Agents*.

Action/Kinetics: Decreases elevated BP by decreasing peripheral resistance by a direct effect. Causes increase in renin secretion, increase in cardiac rate and output, and salt/water retention. Does not cause orthostatic hypotension. **Onset:** 30 min. **Peak plasma levels:** reached within 60 min; **plasma t½:** 4.2 hr. **Duration:** 24–48 hr. Ninety percent absorbed from GI tract; excretion: renal (90% metabolites). The time needed to reach the maximum effect is inversely related to the dose.

Uses: Severe hypertension not controllable by the use of a diuretic plus two other antihypertensive drugs. Usually taken with at least two other antihypertensive drugs (a diuretic and a drug to minimize tachycardia such as

a beta-adrenergic blocking agent). Can produce severe side effects; reserve for resistant cases of hypertension. Close medical supervision required, including possible hospitalization during initial administration. Topically to promote hair growth in balding men.
Contraindications: Pheochromocytoma. Within 1 month after a MI. Dissecting aortic aneurysm.
Special Concerns: Safe use during lactation not established. Use with caution and at reduced dosage in impaired renal function. Geriatric clients may be more sensitive to the hypotensive and hypothermic effects of minoxidil; also, may be necessary to decrease the dose due to age-related decreases in renal function. BP controlled too rapidly may cause syncope, stroke, MI, and ischemia of affected organs. Experience with use in children is limited.
Side Effects: *CV:* Edema, ***pericardial effusion that may progress to tamponade*** (acute compression of heart caused by fluid or blood in pericardium), CHF, angina pectoris, changes in direction of T waves, increased HR. In children, rebound hypertension following slow withdrawal. *GI:* N&V. *CNS:* Headache, fatigue. *Hypersensitivity:* Rashes, including bullous eruptions and ***Stevens-Johnson syndrome.*** *Hematologic:* Initially, decrease in hematocrit, hemoglobin, and erythrocyte count but all return to normal. Rarely, thrombocytopenia and leukopenia. *Other:* Hypertrichosis (enhanced hair growth, pigmentation and thickening of fine body hair 3–6 weeks after initiation of therapy), breast tenderness, darkening of skin.
Laboratory Test Considerations: Nonspecific changes in ECG. ↑ Alkaline phosphatase, serum creatinine, and BUN.
OD **Management of Overdose:** *Symptoms:* Excessive hypotension. *Treatment:* Give NSS IV (to maintain BP and urine output). Vasopressors, such as phenylephrine and dopamine, can be used but only in underperfusion of a vital organ.
Drug Interactions: Concomitant use with guanethidine may result in severe hypotension.
How Supplied: *Tablet:* 2.5 mg, 10 mg

Dosage

- **Tablets**

Hypertension.

Adults and children over 12 years, Initial: 5 mg/day. For optimum control, dose can be increased to 10, 20, and then 40 mg in single or divided doses/day. Do not exceed 100 mg/day. **Children under 12 years: Initial,** 0.2 mg/kg/day. Effective dose range: 0.25–1.0 mg/kg/day. Dosage must be titrated to individual response. Do not exceed 50 mg/day.

HEALTH CARE CONSIDERATIONS

See also *Health Care Considerations* for *Antihypertensive Agents.*

Administration/Storage

1. Give once daily if supine DBP has been reduced less than 30 mm Hg and twice daily (in two equal doses) if it has been reduced more than 30 mm Hg.
2. Wait at least 3 days between dosage adjustments as the full response is not obtained until then. However, if more rapid control is required, may adjust q 6 hr but with careful monitoring.

Assessment

1. Anticipate BP decreases within 30 min.
2. List other agents trialed and the outcome. Note if diruetic prescribed.
3. Assess cardiopulmonary status.
4. Monitor CBC, glucose, electrolytes, and renal function studies.

Client/Family Teaching

1. Can be taken with fluids and without regard to meals.
2. Record weight daily; report any S&S of fluid overload (gain of 6 lb/week; edema of extremities, face, and abdomen; or dyspnea).
3. Report any symptoms of angina, fainting, dizziness, or dyspnea that occurs, especially when lying down.
4. Drug may cause elongation, thickening, and increased pigmentation of body hair; should resolve once discontinued.

Outcome/Evaluate: ↓ BP; control of hypertension

Minoxidil, topical solution

(mih-**NOX**-ih-dill)
Pregnancy Category: C
Apo-Gain ♣, Gen-Minoxidil ♣, Minoxigaine ♣, Minox ♣, Rogaine, Rogaine Extra Strength for Men **(Rx) (OTC)**
Classification: Hair growth stimulant

Action/Kinetics: The topical solution stimulates vertex hair growth in clients with male pattern baldness or in women with androgenetic alopecia. Mechanism may be related to dilation of arterioles and stimulation of resting hair follicles into active growth. Following topical administration, approximately 1.4% is absorbed into the systemic circulation. **Onset:** 4 months but is variable.

Duration: New hair growth may be lost 3–4 months after withdrawal of therapy. Minoxidil and its inactive metabolites are excreted in the urine. Also, see *Minoxidil, oral.*

Uses: To treat male and female pattern baldness (alopecia androgenetica). Extra Strength (5%) is only for treatment of hereditary male pattern baldness. *Investigational:* Alopecia areata.

Contraindications: Lactation. Use of 5% solution in women.

Special Concerns: Use with caution in clients with hypertension, coronary heart disease, or predisposition to heart failure. Safety and efficacy in clients under 18 years of age have not been determined. Increased systemic absorption may occur if the scalp is irritated or there are abrasions.

Side Effects: *Dermatologic:* Allergic contact dermatitis, irritant dermatitis, pruritus, dry skin, flaking of scalp, alopecia, hypertrichosis, erythema, worsening of hair loss. *Allergic:* Hives, facial swelling, allergic rhinitis. *CNS:* Dizziness, lightheadedness, headache, faintness, anxiety, depression, fatigue. *Respiratory:* Sinusitis, bronchitis, respiratory infection. *Miscellaneous:* Conjunctivitis, decreased visual acuity, vertigo. *NOTE:* The incidence of side effects due to placebos is often similar to the incidence of side effects due to the drug itself.

M

Drug Interactions

Corticosteroids, topical / Enhance absorption of topical minoxidil

Guanethidine / Possible ↑ risk of orthostatic hypotension

Petrolatum / Enhances absorption of topical minoxidil

Retinoids / Enhance absorption of topical minoxidil

How Supplied: *Solution:* 2%, 5%

Dosage

- **Topical Solution: 2%, 5%**

  Stimulate hair growth.

Adults: Apply 1 mL b.i.d. directly onto the scalp in the hair loss area. 5% solution not to be used on women.

HEALTH CARE CONSIDERATIONS

Administration/Storage

1. Use only in clients with normal, healthy scalps. Dermatitis, scalp abrasions, scalp psoriasis, or severe sunburn may increase the absorption of topical minoxidil and lead to systemic side effects (See *Minoxidil, oral*).
2. Hair may be shampooed before treatment, but dry the hair and scalp prior to topical application.
3. The product comes with a metered spray attachment (for application to large areas of the scalp), extender spray attachment (for application to small scalp areas or under the hair), and a rub-on applicator tip (to spread the solution on the scalp). Follow the directions on the package insert carefully for each of these methods of application.
4. If the fingertips are used to apply the drug, wash the hands thoroughly after application.
5. At least 4 months of continuous therapy is necessary before evidence of hair growth can be expected. Further hair growth continues through 1 year of treatment.
6. The alcohol base in topical minoxidil will cause irritation and burning of the eyes, abraded skin, or mucous membranes. If contact with any of these areas, wash the site with copious amounts of water.
7. Avoid inhaling the spray mist.

Client/Family Teaching

1. Review appropriate method and frequency for application; solution may dry and leave a residue on the hair, this is harmless.
2. More frequent than prescribed applications will not enhance hair growth but will increase systemic side effects. Review info booklet.
3. New hair growth will be soft and hard to see and is not permanent. Drug is a treatment, not a cure; cessation of therapy will lead to hair loss within a few months. Topical minoxidil must be used indefinitely to sustain the effect.
4. Treatment has positive benefits for only approximately one-half the population. May take up to 4 months of continuous therapy before any response is noted.
5. Report any evidence of irritation or rash.
6. Do not apply any other topical products to the scalp without approval.
7. Consult provider before using if no family history of gradual hair loss, if hair loss is sudden or patchy, if hair loss is accompanied by other symptoms, or if the reasons for hair loss are not clear.

Outcome/Evaluate: Stimulation of hair growth

Mirtazapine

(mir-**TAZ**-ah-peen)

Pregnancy Category: C

Remeron **(Rx)**

Classification: Antidepressant, tetracyclic

See also *Antidepressants.*

Action/Kinetics: Enhances central noradrenergic and serotonergic activity, perhaps by antagonism at central presynaptic alpha-

2 adrenergic inhibitory autoreceptors and heteroreceptors. Also a potent antagonist of 5-HT_2, 5-HT_3, and histamine H_1 receptors. Moderate antagonist of peripheral alpha-1 adrenergic receptors and muscarinic receptors. Rapidly and completely absorbed from the GI tract. **Peak plasma levels:** Within 2 hr. **t½:** 20–40 hr. Extensively metabolized in the liver and excreted in both the urine (75%) and feces (15%). Females exhibit significantly longer elimination half-lives than males.

Uses: Treatment of depression.

Contraindications: Use in combination with a MAO inhibitor or within 14 days of initiating or discontinuing therapy with a MAO inhibitor.

Special Concerns: Use with caution in those with impaired renal or hepatic disease, in geriatric clients, during lactation, in CV or cerebrovascular disease that can be exacerbated by hypotension (e.g., history of MI, angina, ischemic stroke), and in conditions that would predispose to hypotension (e.g., dehydration, hypovolemia, treatment with antihypertensive medications). The effect of mirtazapine for longer than 6 weeks has not been evaluated, although treatment is indicated for 6 months or longer. Safety and efficacy have not been determined in children.

Side Effects: Side effects with an incidence of 0.1% or greater are listed. *CNS:* Somnolence, dizziness, activation of mania or hypomania, suicidal ideation, sedation, drowsiness, abnormal dreams, abnormal thinking, tremor, confusion, hypesthesia, apathy, depression, hypokinesia, vertigo, twitching, agitation, anxiety, amnesia, hyperkinesia, paresthesia, ataxia, delirium, delusions, depersonalization, dyskinesia, extrapyramidal syndrome, increased libido, abnormal coordination, dysarthria, hallucinations, neurosis, dystonia, hostility, increased reflexes, emotional lability, euphoria, paranoid reaction. *GI:* N&V, anorexia, dry mouth, constipation, ulcer, eructation, glossitis, cholecystitis, gum hemorrhage, stomatitis, colitis, abnormal liver function tests. *CV:* Hypertension, vasodilation, angina pectoris, ***MI,*** bradycardia, ventricular extrasystoles, syncope, migraine, hypotension. *Hematologic:* Agranulocytosis. *Body as a whole:* Asthenia, flu syndrome, back pain, malaise, abdominal pain, acute abdominal syndrome, chills, fever, facial edema, photosensitivity reaction, neck rigidity, neck pain, enlarged abdomen. *Respiratory:* Dyspnea, increased cough, sinusitis, epistaxis, bronchitis, asthma, pneumonia. *GU:* Urinary frequency, UTI, kidney calculus, cystitis, dysuria, urinary incontinence, urinary retention, vaginitis, hematuria, breast pain, amenorrhea, dysmenorrhea, leukorrhea, impotence. *Musculoskeletal:* Myalgia, myasthenia, arthralgia, arthritis, tenosynovitis. *Dermatologic:* Pruritus, rash, acne, exfoliative dermatitis, dry skin, herpes simplex, alopecia. *Metabolic/nutritional:* Increased appetite, weight gain, peripheral edema, edema, thirst, dehydration, weight loss. *Ophthalmic:* Eye pain, abnormal accommodation, conjunctivitis, keratoconjunctivitis, lacrimation disorder, glaucoma. *Miscellaneous:* Deafness, hyperacusis, ear pain.

Laboratory Test Considerations: ↑ ALT and nonfasting cholesterol and triglycerides.

OD **Management of Overdose:** *Symptoms:* Disorientation, drowsiness, impaired memory, tachycardia. *Treatment:* General supportive measures. If the client is unconscious, establish and maintain an airway. Consider induction of emesis or gastric lavage and administration of activated charcoal. Monitor cardiac and vital signs.

Drug Interactions

Alcohol / Additive impairment of motor skills

Diazepam / Additive impairment of motor skills

How Supplied: *Tablet:* 15 mg, 30 mg

Dosage

- **Tablets**

Treatment of depression.

Initial: 15 mg/day given as a single dose, preferably in the evening before sleep. Those not responding to the 15-mg dose may respond to doses up to a maximum of 45 mg/day. Do not make dose changes at intervals of less than 1 to 2 weeks. Consider treatment for up to 6 months.

HEALTH CARE CONSIDERATIONS

See also *Health Care Considerations* for *Antidepressants.*

Assessment

1. Record indications, onset, duration, and symptom characteristics.
2. Note precipitating events that may relate to depression, i.e., death, divorce, illness, or job loss.
3. List drugs currently and previously prescribed to ensure no MAO inhibitor use within past 2 weeks.
4. Monitor ECG, CBC, LFTs, cholesterol, and triglyceride levels.

Client/Family Teaching

1. Take as directed; do not exceed prescribed dosing schedule.

M

2. Report any S&S of infection or flu (fever, sore throat, stomatitis, etc.); drug may cause agranulocytosis.
3. Do not engage in activities that require mental alertness until drug effects realized; dizziness and drowsiness may occur.
4. Avoid alcohol and OTC agents; may potentiate drug's cognitive and motor skill impairment.
5. Report as scheduled for follow-up labs and evaluation of clinical response to drug therapy.

Outcome/Evaluate: Improved sleeping and eating patterns; improved mood, ↑ interest in social activities

Misoprostol

(my-soh-**PROST**-ohl)

Pregnancy Category: X

Cytotec **(Rx)**

Classification: Prostaglandin

Action/Kinetics: Synthetic prostaglandin E_1 analog that inhibits gastric acid secretion, protects the gastric mucosa by increasing bicarbonate and mucous production, and decreases pepsin levels during basal conditions. May also stimulate uterine contractions that may endanger pregnancy. Rapidly converted to the active misoprostol acid. **Time for peak levels of misoprostol acid:** 12 min. **t½, misoprostol acid:** 20–40 min. Misoprostol acid is less than 90% bound to plasma protein. *NOTE:* Misoprostol does not prevent development of duodenal ulcers in clients on NSAIDs.

Uses: Prevention of aspirin and other nonsteroidal anti-inflammatory-induced gastric ulcers in clients with a high risk of gastric ulcer complications (e.g., geriatric clients with debilitating disease) or in those with a history of ulcer. *Investigational:* Treat duodenal ulcers including those unresponsive to histamine H_2 antagonists. With cyclosporine and prednisone to decrease the incidence of acute graft rejection in renal transplant clients (the drug improves renal function). With methotrexate to induce abortion.

Contraindications: Allergy to prostaglandins, pregnancy, during lactation (may cause diarrhea in nursing infants).

Special Concerns: Use with caution in clients with renal impairment and in clients older than 64 years of age. Safety and efficacy have not been established in children less than 18 years of age. May cause miscarriage with potentially serious bleeding.

Side Effects: *GI:* Diarrhea, abdominal pain, nausea, dyspepsia, flatulence, vomiting, constipation. *Gynecologic:* Spotting, cramps, dysmenorrhea, hypermenorrhea, menstrual disorders, postmenopausal vaginal bleeding. *Miscellaneous:* Headache.

OD Management of Overdose: *Symptoms:* Abdominal pain, diarrhea, dyspnea, sedation, tremor, fever, palpitations, bradycardia, hypotension, ***seizures.*** *Treatment:* Use supportive therapy.

How Supplied: *Tablet:* 100 mcg, 200 mcg

Dosage

- **Tablets**

Adults: 200 mcg q.i.d. with food. Dose can be reduced to 100 mcg if the larger dose cannot be tolerated. In renal impairment, the 200-mcg dose can be reduced if necessary.

HEALTH CARE CONSIDERATIONS

Administration/Storage

1. Reduce diarrhea by giving after meals and at bedtime; avoid magnesium-containing antacids. Diarrhea is usually self-limiting.
2. Maximum plasma levels are decreased if drug is taken with food.
3. Take for the duration of NSAID therapy.
4. Drug may increase gastric bicarbonate and mucous production.

Assessment

1. Record any ulcer disease; assess GI symptoms, clinical presentation and indications.
2. Obtain a negative pregnancy test unless being used with methotrexate to induce abortion.

Client/Family Teaching

1. Do not share medications.
2. Avoid foods/spices that may aggravate condition: caffeine, alcohol, and black pepper.
3. Take misoprostol exactly as prescribed for the duration of aspirin or NSAID therapy.
4. May experience abdominal discomfort and/or diarrhea; take misoprostol after meals and at bedtime to minimize these side effects. Avoid magnesium-containing antacids.
5. Report persistent diarrhea or increased menstrual bleeding.
6. All women of childbearing age must practice effective contraceptive measures; drug has abortifacient properties.
7. With abortion, report any increased bleeding, pain, or fever.

Outcome/Evaluate: Prevention of drug-induced gastric ulcers

Moexipril hydrochloride

(moh-**EX**-ih-prill)

Pregnancy Category: C (first trimester), D (second and third trimesters)

Univasc **(Rx)**
Classification: Angiotensin-converting enzyme inhibitor

See also *Angiotensin-Converting Enzyme Inhibitors.*
Action/Kinetics: Converted in the liver to the active moexiprilat. **Onset:** 1–2 hr. **Peak effect:** 3–6 hr. **Duration:** 24 hr. Food decreases absorption of the drug. **t½, moexiprilat:** 2–9 hr. About 50% is bound to plasma protein. Active metabolite is excreted through both the urine and feces.
Uses: Treatment of hypertension alone or in combination with thiazide diuretics.
Contraindications: In those with a history of angioedema as a result of previous treatment with ACE inhibitors.
Special Concerns: Use with caution during lactation, in clients with impaired renal function or renal artery stenosis, hyperkalemia, CHF, severe hepatic impairment, and volume depletion. Those who are salt or volume depleted are at a greater risk of developing hypotension. Safety and efficacy have not been determined in children.
Side Effects: *GI:* Abdominal pain, N&V, diarrhea, dysgeusia, constipation, dry mouth, dyspepsia, pancreatitis, hepatitis, changes in appetite, weight changes. *CNS:* Insomnia, sleep disturbances, headache, dizziness, fatigue, drowsiness/sleepiness, malaise, nervousness, anxiety, mood changes. *CV:* Chest pain, hypotension, palpitations, angina pectoris, ***CVA, MI,*** orthostatic hypotension, rhythm disturbances, peripheral edema. *Respiratory:* Cough, bronchospasm, dyspnea, URI, pharyngitis, rhinitis. *GU:* Oliguria, urinary frequency, renal insufficiency. *Dermatologic:* Flushing, rash, diaphoresis, photosensitivity, pruritus, urticaria, pemphigus. *Musculoskeletal:* Myalgia, arthralgia. *Miscellaneous:* Angioedema, neutropenia, syncope, anemia, tinnitus, flu syndrome, pain.
Drug Interactions
Diuretics / Excessive hypotension
Lithium / Moexipril ↑ serum levels of lithium → lithium toxicity
Potassium-sparing diuretics / ↑ Hyperkalemic effect of moexipril
Potassium supplements / ↑ Hyperkalemic effect of moexipril
How Supplied: *Tablet:* 7.5 mg, 15 mg

Dosage
- **Tablets**

Hypertension.
Initial, adults not receiving diuretics: 7.5 mg 1 hr before meals once daily. Dose is adjusted depending on response. **Maintenance:** 7.5–30 mg daily in one or two divided doses 1 hr before meals. **Initial, adults receiving diuretics:** Discontinue diuretic 2–3 days before beginning moexipril at a dose of 7.5 mg. If BP is not controlled, diuretic therapy can be resumed. If diuretic cannot be discontinued, give moexipril in an initial dose of 3.75 mg once daily 1 hr before meals. In those with impaired renal function, start with 3.75 mg once daily if C_{CR} is less than 40 mL/min/1.73 m^2. The dose may be increased to a maximum of 15 mg/day.

HEALTH CARE CONSIDERATIONS

See also *Health Care Considerations* for *Angiotensin-Converting Enzyme Inhibitors.*
Assessment
1. Record indications for therapy, onset of disease, other agents trialed and the outcome.
2. Assess for dehydration, CHF, or hyperkalemia. Monitor ECG, electrolytes, renal and LFTs; reduce dose with renal impairment.

Client/Family Teaching
1. Take on an empty stomach 1 hr before meals.
2. Rise slowly from a sitting or lying position; report persistent dizziness/lightheadedness, or fainting.
3. Seek help if angioedema (respiratory difficulty or swelling of lips, eyes, tongue, face) or neutropenia (fever, sore throat) occurs.
4. Use reliable contraception; stop drug and report if pregnancy is suspected, as drug is harmful to fetus.
5. Do not take potassium supplements or potassium-containing salt substitutes; drug may increase potassium levels.

Outcome/Evaluate: ↓ BP

M

Mometasone furoate monohyrate

(moh-MET-ah-sohn)
Pregnancy Category: C
Nasonex **(Rx)**
Classification: Corticosteroid, nasal

See also *Corticosteroids.*
Action/Kinetics: Anti-inflammatory corticosteroid. Undetected in plasma although some may be swallowed after use. No effect on adrenal function.
Uses: Prophylaxis and treatment of the nasal symptoms of seasonal allergic rhinitis and perennial allergic rhinitis.

Contraindications: Use in those with recent nasal septum ulcers, nasal surgery, or nasal trauma until healing has occurred.
Special Concerns: Use with caution, if at all, in those with active or quiescent tuberculosis infection of the respiratory tract, or in untreated fungal, bacterial, systemic viral infections, or ocular herpes simplex. Use with caution during lactation. Safety and efficacy have not been determined in children less than 12 years of age.
Side Effects: *Respiratory:* Pharyngitis, epistaxis, blood-tinged mucus, coughing, URI, sinusitis, rhinitis, asthma, bronchitis. Rarely, nasal ulcers and nasal and oral candidiasis. *GI:* Diarrhea, dyspepsia, nausea. *Miscellaneous:* Headache, viral infection, dysmenorrhea, musculoskeletal pain, arthralgia, chest pain, conjunctivitis, earache, flu-like symptoms, myalgia, increased IOP.
How Supplied: *Nasal spray:* 50 mcg/actuation

Dosage

- **Nasal Spray**

Seasonal/perennial allergic rhinitis.

Adults and children over 12 years: 2 sprays (50 mcg in each spray) in each nostril once daily (i.e., total daily dose: 200 mcg). In those with a known seasonal allergen that precipitates seasonal allergic rhinitis, give prophylactically, 200 mcg/day, 2 to 4 weeks prior to the anticipated start of the pollen season.

M

HEALTH CARE CONSIDERATIONS

See also *Health Care Considerations* for *Corticosteroids.*
Administration/Storage: Improvement is usually seen within 2 days after the first dose. Maximum benefit: within 1 to 2 weeks.
Assessment: Record onset, duration, and characteristics of symptoms.
Client/Family Teaching
1. Review enclosed instructions to ensure proper use.
2. Prior to initial use, prime the pump by actuating ten times or until a fine spray appears.
3. The pump may be stored, unused, for up to 1 week without repriming. If more than one week has elasped between use, reprime by actuating 2 times, or until a fine spray appears.
4. Use regularly as directed. Do not increase dose or use as this does not increase effectiveness.
5. Identify triggers and practice avoidance.
6. Report if condition does not improve or worsens after 3-5 days of therapy.
Outcome/Evaluate: Relief of allergic rhinitis

Montelukast sodium

(mon-teh-**LOO**-kast)
Pregnancy Category: B
Singulair **(Rx)**
Classification: Antiasthmatic

Action/Kinetics: Cysteinyl leukotrienes and leukotriene receptor occupation are associated with symptoms of asthma, including airway edema, smooth muscle contraction, and inflammation. Montelukast binds with cysteinyl leukotriene receptors thus preventing the action of cysteinyl leukotrienes. Rapidly absorbed after PO use. **Time to peak levels:** 3–4 hr for 10 mg tablet and 2–2.5 hr for 5 mg tablet. Metabolized in liver and mainly excreted in feces. **t½:** 2.7–5.5 hr.
Uses: Prophylaxis and chronic treatment of asthma in adults and children aged 6 years of age and older. *Investigational:* With loratidine for hayfever.
Contraindications: Use to reverse bronchospasm in acute asthma attacks, including status asthmaticus. Use to abruptly substitute for inhaled or oral corticosteroids. Use as monotherapy to treat and manage exercise-induced bronchospasm. Use with known aspirin or NSAID sensitivity.
Special Concerns: Use with caution during lactation. Safety and efficacy have not been determined for children less than 6 years of age.
Side Effects: *Adolescents and adults aged 15 and older. GI:* Dyspepsia, infectious gastroenteritis, abdominal pain, dental pain. *CNS:* Headache, dizziness. *Body as a whole:* Asthenia, fatigue, trauma. *Respiratory:* Influenza, cough, nasal congestion. *Dermatologic:* Rash. *Miscellaneous:* Pyuria.
Children, aged 6 to 14 years. GI: Nausea, diarrhea. *Respiratory:* Pharyngitis, laryngitis, otitis, sinusitus. *Miscellaneous:* Viral infection.
Laboratory Test Considerations: ↑ ALT, AST.
How Supplied: *Tablets:* 10 mg. *Chewable Tablets:* 5 mg.

Dosage

- **Tablets**

Asthma.

Adolescents and adults age 15 years and older: 10 mg once daily taken in evening.

- **Chewable tablets**

Asthma.

Pediatric clients aged 6 to 14 years: 5 mg chewable tablet once daily taken in evening.

HEALTH CARE CONSIDERATIONS

Administration/Storage: Take daily as prescribed, even when client is asymptomatic. Contact provider if asthma is not well controlled.

Assessment

1. Record indications for therapy, onset, triggers, and characteristics of disease. List other agents trialed and outcome.
2. Note other agents prescribed for asthma and reinforce which should be continued.
3. Record pulmonary assessments, PFTs, and x-rays when indicated.
4. Chewable 5 mg tablet contains 0.842 mg of phenylalanine and should not be used with phenylketonurics.
5. Assist to identify and eliminate/minimize triggers.

Client/Family Teaching

1. Take once daily in evening as directed.
2. Drug should be continued during acute attacks as well as during symptom free periods.
3. Use short-acting prescribed β-agonist inhalers to treat acute asthma attacks. Report if increased use and frequency of inhalers is needed for symptom control.
4. Continue other prescribed antiasthma meds during this therapy.
5. With exercise-induced asthma, must continue to use prescribed inhaler for prophylaxis unless otherwise instructed.
6. Report any unusual side effects, changes in disease, or significant drop in peak flow readings.
7. Notify provider if pregnancy suspected or planned.
8. Ensure that environment is assessed for triggers and that appropriate steps are taken to minimize or avoid exposures.

Outcome/Evaluate: Prophylaxis of asthma attack; asthma control; ↑ FEV1

Moricizine hydrochloride

(mor-**IS**-ih-zeen)

Pregnancy Category: B

Ethmozine **(Rx)**

Classification: Antiarrhythmic, class I

See also *Antiarrhythmic Agents.*

Action/Kinetics: Causes a stabilizing effect on the myocardial membranes as well as local anesthetic activity. Shortens phase II and III repolarization leading to a decreased duration of the action potential and an effective refractory period. Also, there is a decrease in the maximum rate of phase O depolarization and a prolongation of AV conduction in clients with ventricular tachycardia. Whether the client is at rest or is exercising, has minimal effects on cardiac index, stroke index volume, systemic or pulmonary vascular resistance or ejection fraction, and pulmonary capillary wedge pressure. There is a small increase in resting BP and HR. The time, course, and intensity of antiarrhythmic and electrophysiologic effects are not related to plasma levels of the drug. **Onset:** 2 hr. **Peak plasma levels:** 30–120 min. **t½:** 1.5–3.5 hr (reduced after multiple dosing). **Duration:** 10–24 hr. 95% is protein bound. Significant first-pass effect. Metabolized almost completely by the liver with metabolites excreted through both the urine and feces; the drug induces its own metabolism. Food delays the rate of absorption resulting in lower peak plasma levels; however, the total amount absorbed is not changed.

Uses: Documented life-threatening ventricular arrhythmias (e.g., sustained VT) where benefits of the drug are determined to outweigh the risks. *Investigational:* Ventricular premature contractions, couplets, and nonsustained VT.

Contraindications: Preexisting second- or third-degree block, right bundle branch block when associated with bifascicular block (unless the client has a pacemaker), cardiogenic shock. Lactation.

Special Concerns: There is the possibility of increased risk of death when used in clients with non-life-threatening cardiac arrhythmias. Safety and effectiveness in children less than 18 years of age have not been determined. Geriatric clients have a higher rate of side effects. Increased survival rates following use of antiarrhythmic drugs have not been proven in clients with ventricular arrhythmias. Use with caution in clients with sick sinus syndrome due to the possibility of sinus bradycardia, sinus pause, or sinus arrest. Use with caution in clients with CHF.

Side Effects: *CV:* ***Proarrhythmias, including new rhythm disturbances or worsening of existing arrhythmias;*** ECG abnormalities, including conduction defects, sinus pause, junctional rhythm, AV block; palpitations, ***sustained VT,*** cardiac chest pain, CHF, ***cardiac death,*** hypotension, hypertension, atrial fibrillation, atrial flutter, syncope, bradycardia, ***cardiac arrest, MI, pulmonary embolism,*** vasodilation, thrombophlebitis, ***cerebrovascular events.*** *CNS:* Dizziness (common), anxiety, headache, fatigue, nervousness, paresthesias, sleep disorders, tremor, anxiety, hypoesthesias, depression, euphoria, somnolence, agitation, confusion, ***seizures,*** hallucinations, loss of memory, vertigo, coma. *GI:* Nausea, dry mouth, abdominal pain, vomiting, diarrhea, dyspepsia, anorexia, ileus, flatulence, dysphagia, bitter taste. *Musculoskeletal:* Asthe-

M

nia, abnormal gait, akathisia, ataxia, abnormal coordination, dyskinesia, pain. *GU:* Urinary retention, dysuria, urinary incontinence, urinary frequency, impotence, kidney pain, decreased libido. *Respiratory:* Dyspnea, apnea, asthma, hyperventilation, pharyngitis, cough, sinusitis. *Ophthalmologic:* Nystagmus, diplopia, blurred vision, eye pain, periorbital edema. *Dermatologic:* Rash, pruritus, dry skin, urticaria. *Miscellaneous:* Sweating, drug fever, hypothermia, temperature intolerance, swelling of the lips and tongue, speech disorder, tinnitus, jaundice.

Laboratory Test Considerations: ↑ Bilirubin and liver transaminases.

OD **Management of Overdose:** *Symptoms:* Vomiting, hypotension, lethargy, worsening of CHF, ***MI, conduction disturbances, arrhythmias (e.g., junctional bradycardia, VT, ventricular fibrillation, asystole), sinus arrest, respiratory failure.*** *Treatment:* In acute overdose, induce vomiting, taking care to prevent aspiration. Hospitalize and closely monitor for cardiac, respiratory, and CNS changes. Provide life support, including an intracardiac pacing catheter, if necessary.

M

Drug Interactions

Cimetidine / ↑ Plasma levels of moricizine due to ↓ excretion

Digoxin / Additive prolongation of the PR interval (but no significant increase in the rate of second- or third-degree AV block)

Propranolol / Additive prolongation of the PR interval

Theophylline / ↓ Plasma levels of theophylline due to ↑ rate of clearance

How Supplied: *Tablet:* 200 mg, 250 mg, 300 mg

Dosage

• **Tablets**

Antiarrhythmic.

Adults: 600–900 mg/day in equally divided doses q 8 hr. If needed, the dose can be increased in increments of 150 mg/day at 3-day intervals until the desired effect is obtained. In clients with hepatic or renal impairment, the initial dose should be 600 mg or less with close monitoring and dosage adjustment.

HEALTH CARE CONSIDERATIONS

See also *Health Care Considerations* for *Antiarrhythmic Agents.*

Administration/Storage

1. When transferring clients from other antiarrhythmics to moricizine, withdraw the previous drug for one to two plasma half-lives before starting moricizine. For example, when transferring from quinidine or disopyramide, moricizine can be started 6–12 hr after the last dose; when transferring from procainamide, moricizine can be initiated 3–6 hr after the last dose; when transferring from mexiletine, propafenone, or tocainide, moricizine can be started 8–12 hr after the last dose; and, when transferring from flecainide, moricizine can be started 12–24 hr after the last dose.
2. If clients are well controlled on an 8-hr regimen, they might be given the same total daily dose q 12 hr to increase compliance.

Assessment

1. Record cardiac history, note preexisting conditions and ECG abnormalities.
2. Monitor ECG, electrolytes, CXR, PFTs, liver and renal function studies; correct any electrolyte disturbance and reduce dose with liver or renal dysfunction.
3. Monitor cardiac rhythm closely to observe for drug-induced rhythm disturbances.
4. Hospitalize clients for initial dosing. Antiarrhythmic response may be determined by ECG, exercise testing, or programmed electrical stimulation testing.
5. Assess pacing parameters with pacemakers.
6. Monitor VS and report any persistent temperature elevations.

Client/Family Teaching

1. Take before meals; food delays rate of absorption.
2. Drug may cause dizziness. Use care when rising from a lying or sitting position.
3. Advise family member or significant other to learn CPR.

Outcome/Evaluate: Termination of life-threatening ventricular arrhythmias

Morphine hydrochloride

(MOR-feen)

Pregnancy Category: C

Morphitec-1, -5, -10, -20 ✦, M.O.S. ✦, M.O.S.-S.R. ✦ **(Rx)**

Morphine sulfate

(MOR-feen SUL-fayt)

Pregnancy Category: C

Astramorph PF, Duramorph, Infumorph, Kadian, M-Eslon ✦, M.O.S.-Sulfate ✦, MS Contin, MS-IR, MSIR Capsules, Oramorph SR, RMS, RMS Rectal Suppositories, Roxanol, Roxanol 100, Roxanol Rescudose, Roxanol-T, Roxanol UD, Statex ✦ **(C-II) (Rx)**

Classification: Narcotic analgesic, morphine type

See also *Narcotic Analgesics.*

Action/Kinetics: Morphine is the prototype for opiate analgesics. **Onset:** approximately 15–60 min, based on epidural or intrathecal use. **Peak effect:** 30–60 min. **Du-**

ration: 3–7 hr. **t½:** 1.5–2 hr. Oral morphine is only one-third to one-sixth as effective as parenteral products.
Uses: Intrathecally, epidurally, PO (including sustained-release products), or by continuous IV infusion for acute or chronic pain. In low doses, morphine is more effective against dull, continuous pain than against intermittent, sharp pain. Large doses, however, will dull almost any kind of pain. Preoperative medication. To facilitate induction of anesthesia and reduce dose of anesthetic. *Investigational:* Acute LV failure (for dyspneic seizures) and pulmonary edema. Morphine should not be used with papaverine for analgesia in biliary spasms but may be used with papaverine in acute vascular occlusions.
Additional Contraindications: Epidural or intrathecal morphine if infection is present at injection site, in clients on anticoagulant therapy, bleeding diathesis, if client has received parenteral corticosteroids within the past 2 weeks.
Special Concerns: May increase the length of labor. Clients with known seizure disorders may be at greater risk for morphine-induced seizure activity.
How Supplied: Morphine hydrochloride: *Syrup:* 1 mg/mL, 5 mg/mL, 10 mg/mL, 20 mg/mL; *Concentrate:* 20 mg/mL, 50 mg/mL; *Suppository:* 10 mg, 20 mg, 30 mg; *Tablets:* 10 mg, 20 mg, 40 mg, 60 mg; *Slow-release tablets:* 30 mg, 60 mg. Morphine sulfate: *Capsule:* 15 mg, 30 mg; *Capsule, Extended Release:* 20 mg, 50 mg, 100 mg; *Oral Concentrate:* 20 mg/mL; *Injection:* 0.5 mg/mL, 1 mg/mL, 2 mg/mL, 4 mg/mL, 5 mg/mL, 8 mg/mL, 10 mg/mL, 15 mg/mL, 25 mg/mL, 50 mg/mL; *Solution:* 10 mg/5 mL, 20 mg/5 mL; *Suppository:* 5 mg, 10 mg, 20 mg, 30 mg; *Tablet:* 10 mg, 15 mg, 30 mg; *Tablet, Extended Release:* 15 mg, 30 mg, 60 mg, 100 mg, 200 mg

Dosage

- **Capsules, Tablets, Oral Solution, Soluble Tablets, Syrup**

Analgesia.
5–30 mg q 4 hr.

- **Sustained-Release Tablets**

Analgesia.
30 mg q 8–12 hr, depending on client needs and response. Kadian is indicated for once-daily dosing at doses of 20, 50, or 100 mg where analgesia is indicated for just a few days.

- **IM, SC**

Analgesia.
Adults: 5–20 mg/70 kg q 4 hr as needed; **pediatric:** 100–200 mcg/kg up to a maximum of 15 mg.

- **IV Infusion**

Analgesia.
Adults: 2.5–15 mg/70 kg in 4–5 mL of water for injection (should be administered slowly over 4–5 min).

- **IV Infusion, Continuous**

Analgesia.
Adults: 0.1–1 mg/mL in D5W by a controlled-infusion pump.

- **Rectal Suppositories**

Adults: 10–30 mg q 4 hr.

- **Intrathecal**

Adults: 0.2–1 mg as a single daily injection.

- **Epidural**

Initial: 5 mg/day in the lumbar region; if analgesia is not manifested in 1 hr, increasing doses of 1–2 mg can be given, not to exceed 10 mg/day. For continuous infusion, 2–4 mg/day with additional doses of 1–2 mg if analgesia is not satisfactory.

HEALTH CARE CONSIDERATIONS

M

See also *Health Care Considerations* for *Narcotic Analgesics.*

Administration/Storage

1. The contents of the immediate release capsule may be delivered through a NG or a gastric tube.
2. For intrathecal use, do not give more than 2 mL of the 5-mg/10-mL preparation or 1 mL of the 10-mg/10-mL product.
3. Give intrathecally only in the lumbar region; repeated injections are not recommended.
4. To reduce the chance of side effects with intrathecal administration, a constant IV infusion of naloxone (0.6 mg/hr for 24 hr after intrathecal injection) is recommended.
5. In certain circumstances (e.g., tolerance, severe pain), the physician may prescribe doses higher than those listed under *Dosage.* Dose may be lower in geriatric clients or those with respiratory disease.
IV 6. For IV use, dilute 2–10 mg with at least 5 mL sterile water or NSS and administer over 4–5 min. For continous infusions, reconstitute to a concentration of 0.1–1 mg/mL and administer as prescribed to control symptoms.
7. Rapid IV administration increases the risk of adverse effects; have a narcotic antagonist (e.g., naloxone) available.

Assessment

1. Record location and characteristics of pain. Rate utilizing a pain-rating scale.

2. List other agents prescribed and the outcome.
3. Note any seizure disorder.

Client/Family Teaching

1. May be administered with food to diminish GI upset. Do not crush or chew controlled-release tablets.
2. Immediate-release capsules may be swallowed intact or the contents of the capsule may be sprinkled on food or stirred in juice to avoid the bitter taste.
3. Drug may cause dizziness and drowsiness; avoid activities that require mental alertness.
4. Practice cough and deep-breathing exercises or incentive spirometry to minimize the development of atelectasis.
5. Record drug use for breakthrough pain when SR therapy prescribed, to ensure adequate dosage.
6. Avoid alcohol and CNS depressants.

Outcome/Evaluate

- Relief of pain
- Control of respirations during mechanical ventilation

M

Moxifloxacin hydrochloride

(mox-ee-FLOX-ah-sin)
Pregnancy Category: C
Avelox **(Rx)**
Classification: Antibiotic, fluoroquinolone

See also *Fluoroquinolones.*

Action/Kinetics: Well absorbed from the GI tract (about 90% bioavailable). A high fat meal does not affect absorption. **t½, elimination:** About 12 hr. Steady state is reached in 3 days (400 mg/day). Widely distributed in the body. Metabolized in the liver; metabolites and unchanged drug are excreted in the feces and urine.

Uses: (1) Acute bacterial sinusitis due to *Streptococcus pneumoniae, Haemophilus influenzae,* or *Moraxella catarrhalis.* (2) Acute bacterial exacerbation of chronic bronchitis due to *S. pneumoniae, H. influenzae, Haemophilus parainfluenzae, Klebsiella pneumoniae, Staphylococcus aureus,* or *M. catarrhalis.* (3) Mild to moderate community acquired pneumonia due to *S. pneumoniae, H. influenzae, Mycoplasma pneumoniae, Chlamydia pneumoniae,* or *M. catarrhalis.*

Contraindications: Hypersensitivitiy to moxifloxacin or any quinolone antibiotic. Use with moderate to severe hepatic insufficiency. Use in clients with known prolongation of the QT interval (the drug prolongs the QT interval in some), with uncorrected hypokalemia, and in those receiving class IA (e.g., quinidine, procainamide) or Class III (e.g., amiodarone, sotalol) antiarrhythmic drugs. Lactation.

Special Concerns: Use with caution in those with clinically significant bradycardia or acute myocardial ischemia, in clients with known or suspected CNS disorders (e.g., severe cerebral arteriosclerosis, epilepsy), or in the presence of risk factors that predispose to seizures or lower the seizure threshold. Safety and efficacy have not been determined in children, adolescents less than 18 years of age, in pregnancy, and during lactation.

Side Effects: *Hypersensitivity:* ***Anaphylaxis after the first dose, CV collapse,*** loss of consciousness, tingling, pharyngeal or facial edema, dyspnea, urticaria, itching. *CNS:* Dizziness, headache, convulsions, confusion, tremors, hallucinations, depression, insomnia, nervousness, anxiety, depersonalization, hypertonia, incoordination, somnolence, vertigo, paresthesia, suicidal thoughts/acts (rare). *GI:* N&V, diarrhea, abdominal pain, taste perversion, dyspepsia, dry mouth, constipation, oral moniliasis, anorexia, stomatitis, gastritis, glossitis, GI disorder, pseudomembranous colitis, cholestatic jaundice. *CV:* Palpitation, vasodilatation, tachycardia, hypertension, peripheral edema, hypotension. *Body as a whole:* Asthenia, moniliasis, pain, malaise, allergic reaction, leg pain, pelvic pain, back pain, chills, infection, chest pain, hand pain. *Hematologic:* Thrombocytopenia, thrombocythemia, eosinophilia, leukopenia. *Respiratory:* Asthma, dyspnea, increased cough, pneumonia, pharyngitis, rhinitis, sinusitis. *Musculoskeletal:* Arthralgia, myalgia. *Dermatologic:* Rash, pruritus, sweating, urticaria, dry skin. *GU:* Vaginal moniliasis, vaginitis, cystitis. *Miscellaneous:* Tinnitus, amblyopia.

Laboratory Test Considerations: ↑ GGTP, lactic dehydrogenase, MCH, WBCs, PT ratio, ionized calcium, chloride, albumin, globulin, bilirubin. ↓ Hemoglobin, RBCs, eosinophils, basophils, glucose, pO_2. Either ↑ or ↓ Amylase, PT, bilirubin, neutrophils. Hyperglycemia, hyperlipidemia. Abnormal LFTs and kidney function.

Drug Interactions

Antacids / Significant ↓ bioavailability of moxifloxacin
Antidepressants, tricyclic / Potential to add to the QTC prolonging effect of moxifloxacin
Antipsychotics / Potential to add to the QTC prolonging effect of moxifloxacin
Cisapride / Potential to add to the QTC prolonging effect of moxifloxacin
Didanosine / ↓ Absorption of moxifloxacin

Erythromycin / Potential to add to the QTC prolonging effect of moxifloxacin
Iron products / Significant ↓ bioavailabilitiy of moxifloxaicn
NSAIDs / ↑ Risk of CNS stimulation and convulsions
Sucralfate / ↓ Absorption of moxifloxacin
How Supplied: *Tablets:* 400 mg

Dosage

- **Tablets**

Acute bacterial sinusitis, community acquired pneumonia.
Adults: 400 mg q 24 hr for 10 days.
Acute bacterial exacerbation of chronic bronchitis.
Adults: 400 mg q 24 hr for 5 days.

HEALTH CARE CONSIDERATIONS

Assessment

1. Determine onset, location, and characteristics of symptoms.
2. List drugs prescribed to ensure none interact.
3. Avoid with uncorrected hypokalemia, prolonged QT intervals and if receiving class 1A or III antiarrhythmic agents.
4. Monitor electrolytes, CBC, renal and LFTs; avoid with moderate-severe liver dysfunction.

Client/Family Teaching

1. Take once a day at the same time, as directed.
2. May take with or without meals. Drink fluids liberally.
3. Take at least 4 hr before or 8 hr after multivitamins containing iron or zinc, antacids containing magnesium/calcium/aluminum, sucralfate, or didanosine (chewable/ buffered tablets or the pediatric powder for PO solution).
4. Do not perform activities that require mental alertness until drug effects realized.
5. May cause GI upset, dizziness, and headaches.
6. Stop drug and report any skin rash immediately.
7. Report any adverse effects, lack of effectiveness or worsening of condition.

Outcome/Evaluate: Resolution of infection; symptomatic improvement

Mupirocin

(myou-**PEER**-oh-sin)
Pregnancy Category: B
Bactroban **(Rx)**

Mupirocin calcium

Pregnancy Category: B
Bactroban Cream, Bactroban Nasal **(Rx)**
Classification: Anti-infective, topical

Action/Kinetics: Binds to bacterial isoleucyl transfer RNA synthetase, which results in inhibition of protein synthesis by the organism. Not absorbed into the systemic circulation. Serum present in exudative wounds decreases the antibacterial activity. Metabolized to the inactive monic acid in the skin which is removed by normal skin desquamation. No cross resistance with other antibiotics such as chloramphenicol, erythromycin, gentamicin, lincomycin, methicillin, neomycin, novobiocin, penicillin, streptomycin, or tetracyclines.
Uses: Topical: To treat impetigo and secondarily infected traumatic skin lesions due to *Staphylococcus aureus, Streptococcus pyogenes,* and beta-hemolytic streptococcus. **Nasal:** Eradication of nasal colonization with methicillin-resistant *S. aureus* in adult clients and health care workers.
Contraindications: Ophthalmic use. Lactation. Use if absorption of large quantities of polyethylene glycol is possible (i.e., large, open wounds). Use with other nasal products.
Special Concerns: Superinfection may result from chronic use. Safety and efficacy have not been established in children for mupirocin nasal.
Side Effects: Topical use: Superinfection, rash, burning, stinging, pain, nausea, tenderness, erythema, swelling, dry skin, contact dermatitis, and increased exudate.
Nasal use: Headache, rhinitis, respiratory disorder (including upper respiratory tract congestion), pharyngitis, taste perversion, burning, stinging, cough, pruritus, blepharitis, diarrhea, dry mouth, ear pain, epistaxis, nausea, rash.
How Supplied: *Nasal Ointment:* 2%; *Ointment:* 2%; *Topical Cream:* 2%

Dosage

- **Topical Cream**

Apply to affected area t.i.d. for 10 days.

- **Topical Ointment**

A small amount of ointment is applied to the affected area t.i.d. If no response is seen after 3–5 days, the client should be reevaluated.

- **Nasal Ointment**

Divide about one-half of the ointment from the single-use tube between the nostrils and apply in the morning and evening for 5 days.

HEALTH CARE CONSIDERATIONS

Administration/Storage

1. A gauze dressing may be used if desired.
2. After application in the nose, close the nostrils by pressing them together for about 1 min.
3. Store the topical ointment between 15°C–30°C (59°F–86°F); store the nasal ointment below 25°C (77°F).

Assessment: Record type, onset, duration, and characteristics of symptoms.

Client/Family Teaching

1. Review technique for administering topical and/or nasal medications; use aseptic measures and hand washing before and after therapy to prevent contamination.
2. Report any symptoms of chemical irritation or hypersensitivity such as increased rash, itching, pain at site, or lack of healing.
3. Do not use other nasal products during nasal therapy.
4. Report if no improvement in skin infection after 3–5 days.
5. Notify school nurse to ensure appropriate screening is performed when treating school-aged children with impetigo.

Outcome/Evaluate: Healing of skin lesions; symptomatic improvement

M

Mycophenolate mofetil

(my-koh-FEN-oh-layt)
Pregnancy Category: C
CellCept, CellCept IV **(Rx)**
Classification: Immunosuppressant

Action/Kinetics: Rapidly absorbed after PO administration and hydrolyzed to the active mycophenolic acid (MPA). MPA has potent cytostatic effects on lymphocytes. Inhibits proliferative responses of T- and B-lymphocytes to both mitogenic and allospecific stimulation. MPA also suppresses antibody formation of B-lymphocytes. MPA and additional metabolites are excreted in the urine. **t½:** 17.9 hr.

Uses: With cyclosporine and corticosteroids to prevent organ rejection in those receiving allogeneic renal transplants or undergoing heart transplants.

Contraindications: Hypersensitivity to mycophenolate or MPA. Lactation.

Special Concerns: Clients receiving immunosuppressant drugs are at a higher risk of developing lymphomas and other malignancies, especially of the skin. Higher blood levels are seen in those with severe impaired renal function. Use with caution in active serious digestive system disease. Safety and efficacy have not been determined in children.

Side Effects: *Hematologic:* Severe neutropenia, anemia, leukopenia, thrombocytopenia, hypochromic anemia, leukocytosis. *GI:* ***GI tract hemorrhage/perforations,*** GI tract ulceration, diarrhea, constipation, nausea, dyspepsia, vomiting, oral moniliasis, anorexia, esophagitis, flatulence, gastritis, gastroenteritis, GI moniliasis, gingivitis, gum hyperplasia, hepatitis, ileus, infection, mouth ulceration, rectal disorder. *CNS:* Tremor, insomnia, dizziness, anxiety, depression, hypertonia, paresthesia, somnolence. *GU:* UTI, hematuria, kidney tubular necrosis, urinary tract disorder, albuminuria, dysuria, hydronephrosis, impotence, pain, pyelonephritis, urinary frequency. *CV:* Hypertension, angina pectoris, atrial fibrillation, cardiovascular disorder, hypotension, palpitation, peripheral vascular disorder, postural hypotension, tachycardia, thrombosis, vasodilation. *Respiratory:* Infection, dyspnea, increased cough, pharyngitis, bronchitis, pneumonia, asthma, lung disorder, lung edema, pleural effusion, rhinitis, sinusitis. *Dermatologic:* Acne, rash, alopecia, fungal dermatitis, hirsutism, pruritus, benign skin neoplasm, skin disorder, skin hypertrophy, skin ulcer, sweating. *Metabolic/Endocrine:* Peripheral edema, dehydration, hypercholesterolemia, hypophosphatemia, edema, hypokalemia, hyperkalemia, hyperglycemia, diabetes mellitus, parathyroid disorder. *Musculoskeletal:* Arthralgia, joint disorder, leg cramps, myalgia, myasthenia. *Ophthalmologic:* Amblyopia, cataract, conjunctivitis. *Body as a whole:* Pain, abdominal pain, fever, chills, headache, infection, malaise, ***sepsis,*** asthenia, chest pain, back pain. *Miscellaneous:* Increased incidence of lymphoma/lymphoproliferative disease, nonmelanoma skin carcinoma, and other malignancies. Increased incidence of opportunistic infections, including herpes simplex, CMV, herpes zoster, *Candida, Aspergillus/Mucor* invasive disease, and *Pneumocystis carinii*. Enlarged abdomen, accidental injury, cyst, facial edema, flu syndrome, ***hemorrhage,*** hernia, weight gain, pelvic pain, ecchymosis, polycythemia.

Laboratory Test Considerations: ↑ Alkaline phosphatase, creatinine, gamma glutamyl transpeptidase, LDH, AST, ALT. Also, hypercalcemia, hyperlipemia, hyperuricemia, hypervolemia, hypocalcemia, hypoglycemia, hypoproteinemia, acidosis.

OD Management of Overdose: *Symptoms:* Nausea, vomiting, diarrhea, hematologic abnormalities, especially neutropenia. *Treatment:* Reduce dose of the drug. Removal of MPA by bile acid sequestrants (e.g., cholestyramine).

Drug Interactions
Acyclovir / ↑ Plasma levels of both drugs due to competition for renal tubular excretion
Antacids containing aluminum/magnesium / ↓ Absorption of mycophenolate
Cholestyramine / ↓ Absorption of mycophenolate
Ganciclovir / ↑ Plasma levels of both drugs due to competition for renal tubular excretion
Phenytoin / ↓ Plasma protein binding of phenytoin
Probenecid / Significant ↑ plasma levels of MPA
Salicylates / ↑ Free fraction of MPA
Theophylline / ↓ Plasma protein binding of theophylline
How Supplied: *Capsules:* 250 mg; *Powder for Injection:* 500 mg; *Tablets:* 500 mg

Dosage
- **Capsules**

Prevent rejection following allogeneic renal transplantation and heart transplants.
Adults: 1 g b.i.d. in combination with corticosteroids and cyclosporine.

HEALTH CARE CONSIDERATIONS

Administration/Storage
1. Start therapy within 72 hr following transplantation.
2. Give on an empty stomach.
3. Avoid doses of 1 g b.i.d. in CRF (i.e., GFR less than 25 mL/min/1.73 m^2) outside the immediate posttreatment period.
4. Mycophenolate is teratogenic; do not open or crush capsules. Avoid inhalation or direct contact with the skin or mucous membranes; wash the area thoroughly with soap and water if contact occurs. Rinse the eyes with plain water.
5. Dispense tablets in light-resistant containers, i.e., manufacturer's original container.

Assessment
1. Note date of transplant, other agents used and the outcome.
2. Record a negative pregnancy test 1 week prior to initiating therapy in all women of childbearing age.
3. Monitor renal and LFTs, and hematologic profiles and observe closely for severe neutropenia (day 31 to day 180) posttransplant. If ANC is less than 1.3×10^3, then drug therapy must be interrupted or decreased.

Client/Family Teaching
1. Take exactly as directed on an empty stomach twice a day; taken with cyclosporine and steroids.
2. Do not remove from manufacturer's original container.
3. With increased immunosuppression the susceptibility to infection and the risk of lymphoproliferative disease and other malignancies may be increased.
4. Practice two reliable forms of contraception simultaneously before, during, and for 6 weeks following therapy.
5. Report for all scheduled lab studies to evaluate response to therapy and to identify any potential problems. Need CBC weekly during first month, twice monthly for the second and third months, and then monthly thereafter for the first year.

Outcome/Evaluate: Prevention of transplant rejection; improved organ function

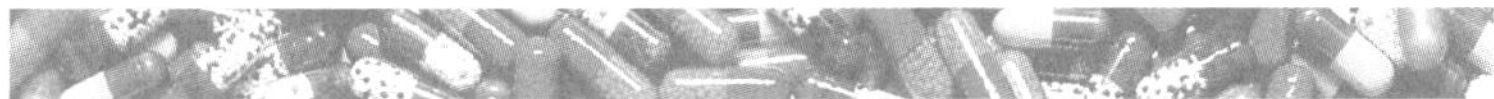

Nabumetone
(nah-**BYOU**-meh-tohn)
Pregnancy Category: B
Relafen **(Rx)**
Classification: Nonsteroidal anti-inflammatory agent

See also *Nonsteroidal Anti-Inflammatory Drugs.*
Action/Kinetics: Time to peak plasma levels: 2.5–4 hr. **t½ of active metabolite:** 22.5–30 hr.
Uses: Acute and chronic treatment of osteoarthritis and rheumatoid arthritis. Has also been used to treat mild to moderate pain including postextraction dental pain, postsurgical episiotomy pain, and soft tissue athletic injuries.
Contraindications: Lactation.
Special Concerns: Safety and efficacy have not been determined in children.
How Supplied: *Tablet:* 500 mg, 750 mg

Dosage
- **Tablets**

Osteoarthritis, rheumatoid arthritis.
Adults, initial: 1,000 mg as a single dose; **maintenance:** 1,500–2,000 mg/day. Doses greater than 2,000 mg/day have not been studied.

HEALTH CARE CONSIDERATIONS

See also *Health Care Considerations* for *Nonsteroidal Anti-Inflammatory Drugs.*

Administration/Storage

1. May be taken with or without food.
2. The total daily dose may be given either once or in two divided doses.
3. Use the lowest effective dose for chronic treatment.

Assessment

1. Record type, onset, and characteristics of symptoms. List any other drugs used and the outcome.
2. Note any swelling, pain, inflammation, trauma, or decreased ROM.
3. Monitor CBC, liver and renal function studies with chronic therapy.

Client/Family Teaching

1. Take as directed; may take with food to decrease GI upset.
2. Review side effects that require immediate reporting: persistent headaches, altered vision, rash, swelling of extremities, blood in stools.
3. Avoid tasks that require mental alertness until drug effects realized.
4. Avoid alcohol and aspirin-containing products.

Outcome/Evaluate

- Relief of pain
- Improved mobility; ↑ ROM

N

Nadolol

(NAY-doh-lohl)

Pregnancy Category: C

Alti-Nadolol ✦, Apo-Nadol ✦, Corgard, Novo-Nadolol ✦ **(Rx)**

Classification: Beta-adrenergic blocking agent

See also *Beta-Adrenergic Blocking Agents.*

Action/Kinetics: Manifests both beta-1- and beta-2-adrenergic blocking activity. Has no membrane stabilizing or intrinsic sympathomimetic activity. Low lipid solubility. **Peak serum concentration:** 3–4 hr. **t½:** 20–24 hr (permits once-daily dosage). **Duration:** 17–24 hr. Absorption variable, averaging 30%; steady plasma level achieved after 6–9 days of administration. Excreted unchanged by the kidney.

Uses: Hypertension, either alone or with other drugs (e.g., thiazide diuretic). Angina pectoris. *Investigational:* Prophylaxis of migraine, ventricular arrhythmias, aggressive behavior, essential tremor, tremors associated with lithium or parkinsonism, antipsychotic-induced akathisia, rebleeding of esophageal varices, situational anxiety, reduce intraocular pressure.

Contraindications: Use in bronchial asthma or bronchospasm, including severe COPD.

Special Concerns: Dosage has not been established in children.

How Supplied: *Tablet:* 20 mg, 40 mg, 80 mg, 120 mg, 160 mg

Dosage

- **Tablets**

Hypertension.

Initial: 40 mg/day; **then,** may be increased in 40- to 80-mg increments until optimum response obtained. **Maintenance:** 40–80 mg/day although up to 240–320 mg/day may be needed.

Angina.

Initial: 40 mg/day; **then,** increase dose in 40- to 80-mg increments q 3–7 days until optimum response obtained. **Maintenance:** 40–80 mg/day, although up to 160–240 mg/day may be needed.

Aggressive behavior.

40–160 mg/day.

Antipsychotic-induced akathisia.

40–80 mg/day.

Essential tremor.

120–240 mg/day.

Lithium-induced tremors.

20–40 mg/day.

Tremors associated with parkinsonism.

80–320 mg/day.

Prophylaxis of migraine.

40–80 mg/day.

Rebleeding from esophageal varices.

40–160 mg/day.

Situational anxiety.

20 mg.

Ventricular arrhythmias.

10–640 mg/day.

Reduction of intraocular pressure.

10–20 mg b.i.d.

NOTE: For all uses decrease dose in clients with renal failure.

HEALTH CARE CONSIDERATIONS

See also *Health Care Considerations* for *Beta-Adrenergic Blocking Agents* and *Antihypertensive Agents.*

Client/Family Teaching

1. Report any rapid weight gain, increased SOB, or extremity swelling.
2. Do not perform tasks that require mental alertness until drug effects realized; may cause dizziness.
3. May cause increased sensitivity to cold; dress appropriately.

Outcome/Evaluate

- ↓ BP, ↓ HR
- ↓ Frequency/intensity of angina

Nafarelin acetate

(NAF-ah-rel-in)
Pregnancy Category: X
Synarel **(Rx)**
Classification: Gonadotropin-releasing hormone

Action/Kinetics: Produced through biotechnology; differs by only one amino acid from naturally occurring GnRH. Stimulates the release of LH and FSH from the adenohypophysis. Causes estrogen and progesterone synthesis in the ovary, resulting in the maturation and subsequent release of an ovum. With repeated use of the drug, however, the pituitary becomes desensitized and no longer produces endogenous LH and FSH; thus endogenous estrogen is not produced, leading to a regression of endometrial tissue, cessation of menstruation, and a menopausal-like state. Broken down by the enzyme peptidase. **Peak serum levels:** 10–40 min. **t¹/₂:** 3 hr; 80% is bound to plasma proteins.
Uses: Endometriosis (including reduction of endometriotic lesions) in clients aged 18 or older. Central precocious puberty in children of both sexes.
Contraindications: Hypersensitivity to GnRH or analogs. Abnormal vaginal bleeding of unknown origin. Pregnancy or possibility of becoming pregnant. Lactation.
Special Concerns: Rule out pregnancy before initiating therapy. Safety and effectiveness have not been established in children.
Side Effects: *Due to hypoestrogenic effects:* Hot flashes (common), decreased libido, vaginal dryness, headaches, emotional lability, insomnia. *Due to androgenic effects:* Acne, myalgia, reduced breast size, edema, seborrhea, weight gain, increased libido, hirsutism. *Musculoskeletal:* Decrease in vertebral trabecular bone density and total vertebral bone mass. *Miscellaneous:* Nasal irritation, depression, weight loss.
Laboratory Test Considerations: ↑ Cholesterol and triglyceride levels, plasma phosphorus, eosinophils. ↓ Serum calcium, WBCs.
How Supplied: *Spray:* 0.2 mg/inh

Dosage

- **Nasal Spray**

Endometriosis.

200 mcg into one nostril in the morning and 200 mcg into the other nostril at night (400 mcg b.i.d. may be required by some women).

Central precocious puberty.

400 mcg (2 sprays) into each nostril in the morning (i.e., 4 sprays) and in the evening (total of 8 sprays/day). If adequate suppression is not achieved, 3 sprays (600 mcg) into alternating nostrils t.i.d. (i.e., a total of 9 sprays/day).

HEALTH CARE CONSIDERATIONS

Administration/Storage

1. Initiate therapy between days 2 and 4 of the menstrual cycle.
2. Use for longer than 6 months is not recommended due to the lack of safety data.
3. Store at room temperature in an upright position protected from light.

Assessment

1. Perform a complete history, recording any osteoporosis, alcohol, tobacco, or corticosteroid use; major risk factors for bone mineral loss that would preclude any repeated courses.
2. Record description of menstrual cycles and any abnormal vaginal bleeding of unknown origin; drug is contraindicated. Record abdominal/vaginal assessments and ultrasound findings.
3. Determine if pregnant; drug is teratogenic.

Client/Family Teaching

1. Begin treatment between the second and fourth day of the menstrual cycle. Keep accurate records of menstrual patterns and cycles.
2. Use the spray upon arising and just before bedtime, alternating nostrils to decrease mucosal irritation.
3. Menses should cease while on therapy; report if regular menses continues.
4. Breakthrough bleeding may occur if successive doses are missed.
5. Use nonhormonal contraception; drug may cause fetal harm.
6. If a topical nasal decongestant is required during treatment, use at least 30 min after nafarelin to prevent interference with drug absorption.
7. Drug may cause hypoestrogenic and androgenic side effects; report if evident as a change in drug dosage or therapy may be indicated.

Outcome/Evaluate

- Restoration of pituitary-gonadal function in 4–8 weeks
- ↓ Number/size of endometriotic lesions

N

Naftifine hydrochloride

(NAF-tih-feen)
Pregnancy Category: B
Naftin **(Rx)**
Classification: Antifungal agent

See also *Anti-Infectives*.
Action/Kinetics: Synthetic antifungal agent with a broad spectrum of activity. Thought to inhibit squalene 2,3-epoxidase, which is responsible for synthesis of sterols. The decreased levels of sterols (especially ergosterol) and the accumulation of squalene in cells result in fungicidal activity. Although used topically, approximately 6% of the drug is absorbed. Naftifine and its metabolites are excreted via the feces and urine. **t½:** 2–3 days.
Uses: To treat tinea cruris, tinea pedis, and tinea corporis caused by *Candida albicans, Epidermophyton floccosum, Microsporum canis, M. audouinii, M. gypseum, Trichophyton rubrum, T. mentagrophytes,* and *T. tonsurans.*
Contraindications: Ophthalmic use.
Special Concerns: Discontinue nursing while using naftifine and for several days after the last application. Safety and efficacy in children have not been determined.
Side Effects: *Topical cream:* Burning, stinging, dryness, itching, local irritation, erythema. *Topical gel:* Burning, stinging, itching, rash, tenderness, erythema.
How Supplied: *Cream:* 1%; *Gel/jelly:* 1%

Dosage

- **Topical Cream (1%), Topical Gel (1%)**

Massage into affected area and surrounding skin once daily if using the cream and twice daily (morning and evening) if using the gel.

HEALTH CARE CONSIDERATIONS

See also *General Health Care Considerations for All Anti-Infectives.*

Client/Family Teaching

1. Wash hands before and after use.
2. Avoid contact with eyes, nose, mouth, or other mucous membranes; for external use only.
3. Occlusive dressings, diapers, or wrappings should not be used; do not cover area.
4. Report any excessive itching or burning.
5. Beneficial effects are usually observed within 1 week; treatment should be continued for 1–2 weeks after symptoms diminish. If no beneficial effects after 4 weeks of treatment, seek reevaluation.

Outcome/Evaluate: Negative cultures; clinical improvement

Nalidixic acid

(nah-lih-DICKS-ick AH-sid)
Pregnancy Category: B
NegGram **(Rx)**
Classification: Urinary germicide

Action/Kinetics: Thought to inhibit the DNA synthesis, probably by interfering with DNA polymerization. Is either bacteriostatic or bactericidal. Rapidly absorbed from the GI tract. **Peak plasma concentration:** 20–40 mcg/mL after 1–2 hr; **peak urine levels:** 150–200 mcg/mL after 3–4 hr. **t½, plasma:** 1.5 hr (increased to 21 hr in anuric clients); **t½, urine:** 6 hr. Metabolized in the liver to hydroxynalidixic acid (comparable activity to nalidixic acid) and inactive compounds which are rapidly excreted. Extensively protein bound.

Sensitivity determinations are recommended before and periodically during prolonged administration of nalidixic acid. Renal and liver function tests are advisable if course of therapy exceeds 2 weeks.
Uses: Acute and chronic UTIs caused by susceptible gram-negative organisms, including *Escherichia coli, Proteus, Enterobacter,* and *Klebsiella.*
Contraindications: Lactation. Use in infants less than 3 months of age.
Special Concerns: Use with caution in prepubertal children, clients with liver disease, severely impaired kidney function, epilepsy, and severe cerebral arteriosclerosis.
Side Effects: *GI:* N&V, diarrhea, abdominal pain. *CNS:* Drowsiness, headache, dizziness, weakness, vertigo, toxic psychoses, intracranial hypertension, ***seizures (rare)***. Also, increased intracranial pressure with bulging anterior fontanel, papilledema, and headache; sixth cranial nerve palsy in children and infants. *Allergic:* Photosensitivity (e.g., erythema, painful bullae on exposed skin), skin rashes, arthralgia (joint swelling and stiffness), pruritus, urticaria, angioedema, eosinophilia, anaphylaxis (rare). *Hematologic:* Leukopenia, thrombocytopenia, ***hemolytic anemia*** (especially in clients with G6PD deficiency). *Ophthalmic:* Reversible subjective visual disturbances, including overbrightness of lights, difficulty in focusing, changes in color perception, double vision, decreased visual acuity. *Other:* Metabolic acidosis, cholestatic jaundice, cholestasis, paresthesia.
Laboratory Test Considerations: False + for urinary glucose with Benedict's solution, Fehling's solution, or Clinitest Reagent tablets. Falsely elevated 17-ketosteroids.
OD **Management of Overdose:** *Symptoms:* Toxic psychoses, convulsions, in-

creased intracranial pressure, nausea, vomiting, lethargy, metabolic acidosis. *Treatment:* Gastric lavage if the overdose is identified early. If absorption has occurred, fluid administration is increased with supportive measures. In severe cases, use of anticonvulsants may be necessary.

Drug Interactions

Antacids, oral / ↓ Effect of nalidixic acid due to ↓ absorption from GI tract
Anticoagulants, oral / ↑ Effect of anticoagulants due to ↓ plasma protein binding
Nitrofurantoin / ↓ Effect of nalidixic acid

How Supplied: *Suspension:* 250 mg/5 mL; *Tablet:* 250 mg, 500 mg, 1 g

Dosage

- **Oral Suspension, Tablets**

Adults: initially, 1 g q.i.d. for 1–2 weeks; **maintenance,** if necessary, 0.5 g q 6 hr. Maximum daily dose: 4 g. **Children, 3 months to 12 years, initial:** 55 mg/kg/day in four equally divided doses; **maintenance:** 33 mg/kg/day.

HEALTH CARE CONSIDERATIONS

See also *General Health Care Considerations for All Anti-Infectives.*

Administration/Storage: Underdosage (less than 4 g/day) may lead to emergence of bacterial resistance.

Assessment

1. Obtain CBC, urine culture, liver and renal function studies; note any dysfunction.
2. Assess for any adverse CNS effects (seizures, psychosis, severe headaches, or ↑ ICP); withhold drug.

Client/Family Teaching

1. Take 1 hr before meals, on an empty stomach. If GI upset occurs, may be taken with food. Drink at least 2–3 L/day of water.
2. Do not perform tasks that require mental alertness; may cause drowsiness, confusion, blurred vision, and dizziness.
3. Avoid prolonged exposure to sunlight or ultraviolet light; wear protective clothing and sunscreen if exposed. Photosensitivity may remain for 3 months following therapy.

Outcome/Evaluate: Negative urine cultures; symptomatic improvement (↓ dysuria, ↓ frequency)

Nalmefene hydrochloride

(NAL-meh-feen)
Pregnancy Category: B
Revex **(Rx)**
Classification: Narcotic antagonist

See also *Narcotic Antagonists.*

Action/Kinetics: Prevents or reverses respiratory depression, sedation, and hypotension due to opioids, including propoxyphene, nalbuphine, pentazocine, and butorphanol. Has a significantly longer duration of action than naloxone. Does not produce respiratory depression, psychotomimetic effects, or pupillary constriction (i.e., it has no intrinsic activity). Also, tolerance, physical dependence, or abuse potential have not been noted. **Onset, after IV:** 2 min. **Duration:** Up to 8 hr. **t½:** 10.8 hr. Metabolized by the liver and excreted in the urine.

Uses: For complete or partial reversal of the effects of opioid drugs postoperatively. Management of known or suspected overdose of opiates.

Special Concerns: Will precipitate acute withdrawal symptoms in those who have some degree of tolerance and dependence on opioids. Use with caution during lactation, in high CV risk clients, or in those who have received potentially cardiotoxic drugs. Reversal of buprenorphine- induced respiratory depression may be incomplete; therefore artificial respiration may be necessary. Safety and effectiveness have not been determined in children.

N

Side Effects: *CV:* Tachycardia, hypertension, hypotension, vasodilation, bradycardia, arrhythmia. *GI:* N&V, diarrhea, dry mouth. *CNS:* Dizziness, somnolence, depression, agitation, nervousness, tremor, confusion, withdrawal syndrome, myoclonus. *Body as a whole:* Fever, headache, chills, postoperative pain. *Miscellaneous:* Pharyngitis, pruritus, urinary retention.

Laboratory Test Considerations: ↑ AST.

How Supplied: *Injection:* 1 mg/mL, 100 mcg/mL

Dosage

- **IV**

Reversal of postoperative depression due to opiates.

Adults: Titrate in 0.25-mcg/kg incremental doses at 2–5-min intervals until the desired degree of reversal is achieved (i.e., adequate ventilation and alertness without significant pain or discomfort). If client is an increased CV risk, use an incremental dose of 0.1 mcg/kg (the drug may be diluted 1:1 with saline or sterile water). A total dose greater than 1 mcg/kg does not provide additional effects.

Management of known or suspected overdose of opiates.

Adults, initial: 0.5 mg/70 kg; **then,** 1 mg/70 kg 2–5 min later, if needed. Doses greater than 1.5 mg/70 kg do not increase the beneficial effect. If there is a reasonable suspicion of dependence on opiates, give a challenge dose of 0.1 mg/70 kg first; if there is no evidence of withdrawal in 2 min, give the recommended dose.

HEALTH CARE CONSIDERATIONS

See also *Health Care Considerations* for *Narcotic Antagonists.*

Administration/Storage

1. Give SC or IM at doses of 1 mg if IV access is lost or not readily obtainable. This dose is effective in 5–15 min.

IV 2. Treatment should follow, not precede, establishment of a patent airway, ventilatory assistance, oxygen, and circulatory access.

3. Nalmefene is supplied in two concentrations—ampules containing 1 mL (blue label) at a concentration suitable for postoperative use (100 mcg) and ampules containing 2 mL (green label) suitable for management of overdose (1 mg/mL), i.e., **10 times as concentrated.** Follow specific guidelines, as indicated.

N

Assessment

1. Record type and amount of agent used and when administered/ingested.

2. Note any opioid dependence; may induce acute withdrawal symptoms.

3. Identify high CV risk or if received cardiotoxic drugs; increases risk for cardiac complications.

4. Observe carefully for recurrent respiratory depression. Compared to naloxone (1.1 hr) the half-life of nalmefene is much longer (10.8 hr). Overdose with long-acting opiates (e.g., methadone, LAAM) may cause recurrence of respiratory depression.

5. With renal failure, if more than one dose required, administer incremental doses slowly (over 60 sec) to prevent dizziness and hypertension.

6. Client may experience N&V, fever, headaches, chills, pain, dizziness, and tachycardia.

Outcome/Evaluate: Reversal of opioid-induced drug effects; ↓ risk of renarcotization

Naloxone hydrochloride

(nal-**OX**-ohn)

Pregnancy Category: B

Narcan **(Rx)**

Classification: Narcotic antagonist

See also *Narcotic Antagonists.*

Action/Kinetics: Combines competitively with opiate receptors and blocks or reverses the action of narcotic analgesics. Since the duration of action of naloxone is shorter than that of the narcotic analgesics, the respiratory depression may return when the narcotic antagonist has worn off. **Onset: IV,** 2 min; **SC, IM:** <5 min. **Time to peak effect:** 5–15 min. **Duration:** Dependent on dose and route of administration but may be as short as 45 min. **t½:** 60–100 min. Metabolized in the liver to inactive products; eliminated through the kidneys.

Uses: Respiratory depression induced by natural and synthetic narcotics, including butorphanol, methadone, nalbuphine, pentazocine, and propoxyphene. Drug of choice when nature of depressant drug is not known. Diagnosis of acute opiate overdosage. Not effective when respiratory depression is induced by hypnotics, sedatives, or anesthetics and other nonnarcotic CNS depressants. Adjunct to increase BP in septic shock. *Investigational:* Treatment of Alzheimer's dementia, alcoholic coma, and schizophrenia.

Contraindications: Sensitivity to drug. Narcotic addicts (drug may cause severe withdrawal symptoms). Use in neonates.

Special Concerns: Safe use during lactation and in children is not established.

Side Effects: N&V, sweating, hypertension, tremors, sweating due to reversal of narcotic depression. If used postoperatively, excessive doses may cause ***VT and fibrillation,*** hypo- or hypertension, pulmonary edema, and ***seizures (infrequent)***.

How Supplied: *Injection:* 0.02 mg/mL, 0.4 mg/mL, 1 mg/mL

Dosage

- **IV, IM, SC**

Narcotic overdose.

Initial: 0.4–2 mg IV; if necessary, additional IV doses may be repeated at 2- to 3-min intervals. If no response after 10 mg, reevaluate diagnosis. **Pediatric, initial:** 0.01 mg/kg IV; **then,** 0.1 mg/kg IV, if needed. The SC or IM route may be used if an IV route is not available.

To reverse postoperative narcotic depression.

Adults: IV, initial, 0.1- to 0.2-mg increments at 2- to 3-min intervals; **then,** repeat at 1- to 2-hr intervals if necessary. Supplemental IM dosage increases the duration of reversal. **Children: Initial,** 0.005–0.01 mg IV at 2- to 3-min intervals until desired response is obtained.

Reverse narcotic-induced depression in neonates.

Initial: 0.01 mg/kg IV, IM, or SC. May be repeated using adult administration guidelines.

HEALTH CARE CONSIDERATIONS

See also *Health Care Considerations* for *Narcotic Antagonists.*

Administration/Storage

IV 1. May administer undiluted at a rate of 0.4 mg over 15 sec with narcotic overdosage. May reconstitute 2 mg in 500 mL of NSS or D5W to provide a 4 mcg/mL or 0.004 mg/mL concentration. Administration rate varies with client response.

2. Do not mix with preparations containing bisulfite, metabisulfite, long-chain or high molecular weight anions, or alkaline pH solutions.

3. When mixed with other solutions, use within 24 hr.

Assessment

1. Identify any evidence of narcotic addiction. Note agent and half-life.

2. Record cardiopulmonary and neurologic assessments.

Interventions

1. The duration of the narcotic may exceed naloxone (the antagonist). Therefore, more than one dose may be necessary to counteract the effects of the narcotic.

2. Monitor VS at 5-min intervals, then every 30 min once stabilized.

3. Titrate to avoid interfering with pain control or readminister narcotic at a lower dosage to maintain pain control.

Outcome/Evaluate: Reversal of narcotic-induced respiratory depression

Naltrexone

(nal-**TREX**-ohn)

Pregnancy Category: C

ReVia **(Rx)**

Classification: Narcotic antagonist

See also *Narcotic Antagonists.*

Action/Kinetics: Competitively binds to opiate receptors, thereby reversing or preventing the effects of narcotics. **Peak plasma levels:** 1 hr. **Duration:** 24–72 hr. Metabolized in the liver; a major metabolite—6-beta-naltrexol—is active. **Peak serum levels, after 50 mg: naltrexone,** 8.6 ng/mL; **6-beta-naltrexol,** 99.3 ng/mL. **t½: naltrexone,** approximately 4 hr; **6-beta-naltrexol,** 13 hr. Naltrexone and its metabolites are excreted in the urine.

Uses: To prevent narcotic use in former narcotic addicts. Adjunct to the psychosocial treatment for alcoholism. *Investigational:* To treat eating disorders and postconcussional syndrome not responding to other approaches.

Contraindications: Those taking narcotic analgesics, dependent on narcotics, or in acute withdrawal from narcotics. Liver failure, acute hepatitis.

Special Concerns: Use with caution during lactation. Safety in children under 18 years of age has not been established.

Side Effects: *CNS:* Headache, anxiety, nervousness, sleep disorders, dizziness, change in energy level, depression, confusion, restlessness, disorientation, hallucinations, nightmares, bad dreams, paranoia, fatigue, drowsiness. *GI:* N&V, diarrhea, constipation, anorexia, abdominal pain or cramps, flatulence, ulcers, increased appetite, weight gain or loss, increased thirst, xerostomia, hemorrhoids. *CV:* Phlebitis, edema, increased BP, changes in ECG, palpitations, epistaxis, tachycardia. *GU:* Delayed ejaculation, increased urinary frequency or urinary discomfort, increased or decreased interest in sex. *Respiratory:* Cough, sore throat, nasal congestion, rhinorrhea, sneezing, excess secretions, hoarseness, SOB, heaving breathing, sinus trouble. *Dermatologic:* Rash, oily skin, itching, pruritus, acne, cold sores, alopecia, athlete's foot. *Musculoskeletal:* Joint/muscle pain, muscle twitches, tremors, pain in legs, knees, or shoulders. *Ophthalmologic:* Blurred vision, aching or strained eyes, burning eyes, light-sensitive eyes, swollen eyes. *Other:* Hepatotoxicity, tinnitus, painful or clogged ears, chills, swollen glands, inguinal pain, cold feet, "hot" spells, "pounding" head, fever, yawning, side pains.

A severe narcotic withdrawal syndrome may be precipitated if naltrexone is administered to a dependent individual. The syndrome may begin within 5 min and may last for up to 2 days.

How Supplied: *Tablet:* 50 mg

Dosage

- **Tablets**

To produce blockade of opiate actions.

Initial: 25 mg followed by an additional 25 mg in 1 hr if no withdrawal symptoms occur.

Maintenance: 50 mg/day.

Alternate dosing schedule for blockade of opiate actions.

The weekly dose of 350 mg may be given as: (a) 50 mg/day on weekdays and 100 mg on Saturday; (b) 100 mg/48 hr; (c) 100 mg eve-

N

ry Monday and Wednesday and 150 mg on Friday; or, (d) 150 mg q 72 hr.

Alcoholism.

50 mg once daily for up to 12 weeks. Treatment for longer than 12 weeks has not been studied.

HEALTH CARE CONSIDERATIONS

See also *Health Care Considerations* for *Narcotic Antagonists.*

Administration/Storage

1. *Never* initiate therapy until determined that client is not dependent on narcotics (i.e., a naloxone challenge test should be completed).
2. Client should be opiate free for at least 7–10 days before beginning therapy.
3. When initiating therapy, begin with 25 mg and observe for 1 hr for any signs of narcotic withdrawal.
4. The blockade produced by naltrexone may be overcome by taking large doses of narcotics; such doses may be fatal.
5. Clients taking naltrexone may not respond to preparations containing narcotics for use in coughs, diarrhea, or pain.

Assessment

1. Determine if opiate addicted and when last dose was ingested; must be opiate free for 7–10 days before initiating therapy. Check urinalysis to confirm absence of opiates; note naloxone challenge test results.
2. Monitor ECG and VS. Report if respirations severely lowered or difficulty breathing evident.
3. Obtain LFTs; monitor monthly during the first 6 months of therapy.

Client/Family Teaching

1. May take with food or milk to diminish GI upset.
2. Headaches, restlessness, and irritability may be caused by naltrexone.
3. Report loss of appetite, unusual fatigue, yellowing of skin or sclera, or itching. Abdominal pain or difficulty with bowel function may warrant a dosage reduction.
4. Remain drug free; identify individuals, agencies, and support groups that may assist in remaining drug free.
5. Attend support groups and behavioral therapy sessions.

Outcome/Evaluate: Maintenance of narcotic-free state in detoxified addicts

Naproxen

(nah-**PROX**-en)

Pregnancy Category: B

Apo-Naproxen ✱, EC-Naprosyn, Naprosyn, Napron X, Naxen ✱, Novo-Naprox ✱, Nu-Naprox ✱, PMS-Naproxen ✱ **(Rx)**

Naproxen sodium

(nah-**PROX**-en)

Pregnancy Category: B

Anaprox, Anaprox DS, Apo-Napro-Na ✱, Apo-Napro-Na DS ✱, Naprelan, Novo-Naprox Sodium ✱, Novo-Naprox Sodium DS ✱, Synflex ✱, Synflex DS ✱ **(Rx)**, Aleve **(OTC)**

Classification: Nonsteroidal, anti-inflammatory analgesic

See also *Nonsteroidal Anti-Inflammatory Drugs.*

Action/Kinetics: Peak serum levels of naproxen: 2–4 hr; **for sodium salt:** 1–2 hr. **t½ for naproxen:** 12–15 hr; **for sodium salt:** 12–13 hr. **Onset, immediate release for analgesia:** 1–2 hr. **Duration, analgesia:** Approximately 7 hr. **Onset,** 24 hr **(both immediate and delayed release):** 30 min; **duration:** 24 hr. **Onset, anti-inflammatory effects:** Up to 2 weeks; **duration:** 2–4 weeks. More than 90% bound to plasma protein. Food delays the rate but not the amount of drug absorbed.

Uses: Rx. Mild to moderate pain. Musculoskeletal and soft tissue inflammation including rheumatoid arthritis, osteoarthritis, bursitis, tendinitis, ankylosing spondylitis. Primary dysmenorrhea, acute gout. Juvenile rheumatoid arthritis (naproxen only). *NOTE:* The delayed-release or enteric-coated products are not recommended for initial treatment of pain because, compared to other naproxen products, absorption is delayed. *Investigational:* Antipyretic in cancer clients, sunburn, acute migraine (sodium salt only), prophylaxis of migraine, migraine due to menses, PMS (sodium salt only). **OTC.** Relief of minor aches and pains due to the common cold, headache, toothache, muscular aches, backache, minor arthritis pain, pain due to menstrual cramps. Decrease fever.

Contraindications: Simultaneous use of naproxen and naproxen sodium. Lactation. Use of delayed-release product for initial treatment of acute pain.

Special Concerns: Safety and effectiveness of naproxen have not been determined in children less than 2 years of age; the safety and effectiveness of naproxen sodium have not been established in children. Geriatric clients may manifest increased total plasma levels of naproxen.

Laboratory Test Considerations: Naproxen may increase urinary 17-ketosteroid values. Both forms may interfere with urinary assays for 5-HIAA.

Drug Interactions
Methotrexate / Possibility of a fatal interaction
Probenecid / ↓ Plasma clearance of naproxen
How Supplied: Naproxen: *Enteric Coated Tablet:* 375 mg, 500 mg; *Suspension:* 25 mg/mL; *Tablet:* 250 mg, 375 mg, 500 mg Naproxen sodium: *Tablet:* 220 mg, 275 mg, 550 mg; *Tablet, Extended Release:* 375 mg, 500 mg

Dosage

NAPROXEN

- **Oral Suspension, Tablets**

Rheumatoid arthritis, osteoarthritis, ankylosing spondylitis, pain, dysmenorrhea, acute tendinitis, bursitis.

Adults, individualized, usual: 250–500 mg b.i.d. May increase to 1.5 g for short periods of time. If no improvement is seen within 2 weeks, consider an additional 2-week course of therapy.

Acute gout.

Adults, initial: 750 mg; **then,** 250 mg naproxen q 8 hr until symptoms subside.

Juvenile rheumatoid arthritis.

Naproxen only, 10 mg/kg/day in two divided doses. If the suspension is used, the following dosage can be used: **13 kg:** 2.5 mL b.i.d.; **25 kg:** 5 mL b.i.d.; **38 kg:** 7.5 mL b.i.d.

- **Delayed Release Tablets**

Rheumatoid arthritis, osteoarthritis, ankylosing spondylitis, pain, dysmenorrhea, acute tendinitis, bursitis.

375–500 mg b.i.d.

NAPROXEN SODIUM

- **Tablets (Rx)**

Rheumatoid arthritis, osteoarthritis, ankylosing spondylitis, pain, dysmenorrhea, acute tendinitis, bursitis.

Adults: 275–550 mg b.i.d. in the morning and evening. May be increased to 1.65 g for short periods of time.

Acute gout.

Adults, initial: 825 mg; **then,** 275 mg q 8 hr until symptoms subside.

Mild to moderate pain, primary dysmenorrhea, acute bursitis and tendinitis.

Adults, initial: 550 mg; **then,** 275 mg q 6–8 hr as needed, not to exceed a total daily dose of 1,375 mg.

- **Controlled Release Tablets**

Rheumatoid arthritis, osteoarthritis, ankylosing spondylitis, pain, dysmenorrhea, acute tendinitis, bursitis.

Adults: 750 mg or 1,000 mg once daily, not to exceed 1,000 mg/day.

Acute gout.

Adults: 1,000 mg once daily. For short periods of time, 1,500 mg may be given.

- **Tablets (OTC)**

Adults: 200 mg q 8–12 hr with a full glass of liquid. For some clients, 400 mg initially followed by 200 mg 12 hr later will provide better relief. Do not exceed 600 mg in a 24-hr period. Do not exceed 200 mg q 12 hr for geriatric clients. Not for use in children less than 12 years of age unless directed by a physician.

HEALTH CARE CONSIDERATIONS

See also *Health Care Considerations* for *Nonsteroidal Anti-Inflammatory Drugs.*

Administration/Storage

1. To be taken in the morning and in the evening. The doses do not have to be equal.
2. Do not give to children.
3. Naproxen suspension can be used to treat children with RA.
4. Delayed-release naproxen is not recommended for acute pain.
5. Do not use the OTC product for more than 10 days for pain or 3 days for fever unless prescribed.

Assessment

1. Note any NSAID hypersensitivity.
2. Record indications for therapy, onset and characteristics of symptoms. With pain, rate using a pain-rating scale and determine if another product should be used initially.
3. Note any joint swelling, pain, trauma, inflammation, or decreased ROM.
4. Determine any GI bleeding or ulcers; use GI protectant if needed. Enteric coated product (EC-Naprosyn) reduces GI side effects.
5. Monitor CBC, liver and renal function studies with chronic therapy.

Client/Family Teaching

1. Take with food to ↓ GI upset; in the morning and evening for optimal effects.
2. Report any lack of response, worsening of symptoms, persistent abdominal pain or dark-colored stools.
3. Avoid all other OTC agents.

Outcome/Evaluate

- Improved joint pain and mobility
- Relief of headaches
- ↓ Uterine cramping

Naratriptan hydrochloride

(NAR-ah-trip-tan)
Pregnancy Category: C
Amerge **(Rx)**
Classification: Antimigraine drug

N

Action/Kinetics: Binds to serotonin 5-HT_{1D} and 5-HT_{1B} receptors. Activation of these receptors located on intracranial blood vessels, including those on arteriovenous anastomoses, leads to vasoconstriction and thus relief of migraine. Another possibility is that activation of these receptors on sensory nerve endings in trigeminal system causes inhibition of pro-inflammatory neuropeptide release. Well absorbed from GI tract. **Peak levels:** 2–3 hr. Unchanged drug and metabolites are primarily eliminated in urine. **t½, elimination:** 6 hr. Excretion is decreased in moderate liver or renal impairment.

Uses: Acute treatment of migraine attacks in adults with or without aura.

Contraindications: Use for prophylaxis of migraine or for management of hemiplegic or basilar migraine. Use in clients with ischemic cardiac, cerebrovascular, or peripheral vascular syndromes; use in uncontrolled hypertension; severe renal impairment (C_{CR} less than 15 mL/min); severe hepatic impairment; within 24 hr of treatment with another 5-HT_1 agonist, dihydroergotamine, or methysergide.

Special Concerns: Safety and efficacy have not been determined for use in cluster headaches or for use in children. Use with caution during lactation and with diseases that may alter the absorption, metabolism, or excretion of drugs, such as impaired renal or hepatic function.

Side Effects: Most common side effects follow. *CNS:* Paresthesia, dizziness, drowsiness, malaise, fatigue. *GI:* Nausea. *Miscellaneous:* Throat and neck symptoms, pain and pressure sensation.

Side effects that occurred in 0.1% to 1% of clients follow. *GI:* Hyposalivation, vomiting, dyspeptic symptoms, diarrhea, GI discomfort and pain, gastroenteritis, constipation. *CNS:* Vertigo, tremors, cognitive function disorders, sleep disorders, disorders of equilibrium, anxiety, depression, detachment. *CV:* Palpitations, increased BP, tachyarrhythmias, syncope, abnormal ECG (PR prolongation, QTc prolongation, ST/T wave abnormalities, premature ventricular contractions, atrial flutter, or atrial fibrillation). *Musculoskeletal:* Muscle pain, arthralgia, articular rheumatism, muscle cramps and spasms, joint and muscle stiffness, tightness, and rigidity. *Dermatologic:* Sweating, skin rashes, pruritus, urticaria. *GU:* Bladder inflammation, polyuria, diuresis. *Body as a whole:* Chills, fever, descriptions of odor or taste, edema and swelling, allergies, allergic reactions, warm/cold temperature sensations, feeling strange, burning/stinging sensation. *Respiratory:* Bronchitis, cough, pneumonia. *Ophthalmic:* Photophobia, blurred vision. *ENT:* Ear, nose, and throat infections; phonophobia, sinusitis, upper respiratory inflammation, tinnitus. *Endocrine/Metabolic:* Thirst, polydipsia, dehydration, fluid retention. *Hematologic:* Increased WBCs.

OD **Management of Overdose:** *Symptoms:* Increased BP, chest pain. *Treatment:* Standard supportive treatment. Possible use of antihypertensive therapy. Monitor ECG if chest pain presents.

Drug Interactions

Dihydroergotamine / Prolonged vasospastic reaction; effects additive

Methysergide / Prolonged vasospastic reaction; effects additive

Oral contraceptives / ↑ Mean plasma levels of naratriptan

Selective serotonin reuptake inhibitors / Possible weakness, hyperreflexia, and incoordination

Serotonin 5-HT_1 agonists / Additive effects

How Supplied: *Tablets:* 1 mg, 2.5 mg

Dosage

- **Tablets**

Migraine headaches.

Adults: Either 1 mg or 2.5 mg taken with fluid. If headache returns or client has had only partial response, dose may be repeated once after 4 hr, for maximum of 5 mg in a 24-hr period.

HEALTH CARE CONSIDERATIONS

Administration/Storage

1. Dose of 2.5 mg is usually more effective but causes more side effects. Choice of dose is made on individual basis, weighing possible benefit of 2.5-mg dose with greater risk for side effects.
2. In mild to moderate renal or hepatic impairment, do not exceed a dose of 2.5 mg over a 24-hr period. Consider a lower initial dose.
3. Safety of treating, on average, more than 4 headaches in 30-day period has not been established.
4. Store medication at controlled room temperature away from light.

Assessment

1. Record onset, frequency, duration, and characteristics of migraines.
2. List all drugs consumed to ensure none interact.
3. Monitor ECG, liver, and renal function studies; assess for dysfunction and dosage adjustment.

Client/Family Teaching

1. Take exactly as directed to relieve headache. Will not reduce or prevent number of attacks experienced.

2. Review patient information brochure.
3. May repeat once every 4 hr if headache returns or if only partial response attained. Do not exceed 5 mg/24 hr.
4. Report any unusual side effects including chest pain, SOB, or palpitations.
5. Practice reliable contraception.
6. Attempt to identify migraine triggers. Keep a headache log for provider review.

Outcome/Evaluate: Relief of migraine headache

Natamycin

(nah-tah-**MY**-sin)
Pregnancy Category: C
Natacyn **(Rx)**
Classification: Antifungal (ophthalmic)

See also *Anti-Infectives.*

Action/Kinetics: Antifungal antibiotic derived from *Streptomyces natalensis*. Binds to the fungal cell membrane, resulting in alteration of permeability and loss of essential intracellular materials. Is fungicidal. After topical administration, therapeutic levels are reached in the corneal stroma but not in the intraocular fluid. Not absorbed systemically.

Uses: For ophthalmic use only. Drug of choice for *Fusarium solanae* keratitis. For treatment of fungal blepharitis, conjunctivitis, and keratitis caused by susceptible organisms. It is active against a variety of yeasts and filamentous fungi including *Candida, Aspergillus, Cephalosporium, Fusarium,* and *Penicillium*. Before initiating therapy, determine the susceptibility of the infectious organism to drug in smears and cultures of corneal scrapings. Effectiveness of natamycin for use as single agent in fungal endophthalmitis not established.

Contraindications: Hypersensitivity to drug.

Special Concerns: Use with caution during lactation. Effectiveness as a single agent to treat fungal endophthalmitis has not been established. Safety and effectiveness have not been determined in children.

Side Effects: Eye irritation, occasional allergies.

How Supplied: *Suspension:* 5%

Dosage

- **Ophthalmic Suspension (5%)**

Fungal keratitis.

Initially, 1 gtt in conjunctival sac q 1–2 hr; can be reduced usually, after 3–4 days to 1 gtt 6–8 times/day. Continue therapy for 14–21 days, during which dosage can be reduced gradually at 4 to 7-day intervals.

Fungal blepharitis/conjunctivitis.

1 gtt 4–6 times/day.

HEALTH CARE CONSIDERATIONS

See also *General Health Care Considerations for All Anti-Infectives.*

Administration/Storage
1. Store at room temperature or in refrigerator avoiding exposure to light and excessive heat. Do not freeze.
2. Shake well before using.
3. Avoid contamination of dropper.
4. Discontinue if toxicity suspected.
5. Review therapy if no improvement noted after 7–10 days.

Assessment: Record indications for therapy and clinical presentation.

Client/Family Teaching
1. Continue for 14–21 days even if condition controlled.
2. Report increased itching, pain, burning, visual difficulty, or stinging.
3. To prevent reinfection, do not share eye makeup, washcloths, towels, or eye medications.

Outcome/Evaluate: Ophthalmic and symptomatic improvement

N

Nedocromil sodium

(neh-**DAH**-kroh-mill)
Pregnancy Category: B
Mireze ✦, Tilade **(Rx)**
Classification: Antiasthmatic

Action/Kinetics: Inhibits the release of various mediators, such as histamine, leukotriene C_4, and prostaglandin D_2, from a variety of cell types associated with asthma. Has no intrinsic bronchodilator, antihistamine, or glucocorticoid activity; also, systemic bioavailability is low. **t½:** 3.3 hr. About 89% bound to plasma protein; excreted unchanged.

Uses: Maintenance therapy in adults and children (age six and older) with mild to moderate bronchial asthma.

Contraindications: Use for the reversal of acute bronchospasms, especially status asthmaticus.

Special Concerns: Use with caution during lactation. Safety and efficacy have not been established in children less than 12 years of age. Has not been shown to be able to substitute for the total dose of corticosteroids.

Side Effects: *Respiratory:* Coughing, pharyngitis, rhinitis, URTI, increased sputum, bronchitis, dyspnea, ***bronchospasm.*** *GI tract:*

N&V, dyspepsia, abdominal pain, dry mouth, diarrhea. *CNS:* Dizziness, dysphonia. *Skin:* Rash, sensation of warmth. *Body as a whole:* Headache, chest pain, fatigue, arthritis. *Miscellaneous:* Viral infection, unpleasant taste.
Laboratory Test Considerations: ↑ ALT.
How Supplied: *Metered dose inhaler:* 1.75 mg/inh

Dosage

- **Metered Dose Inhaler**

Bronchial asthma.

Adults and children over 12 years of age: Two inhalations q.i.d. at regular intervals in order to provide 14 mg/day. If the client is under good control on q.i.d. dosing (i.e., requiring inhaled or oral beta agonist no more than twice a week or no worsening of symptoms occur with respiratory infections), a lower dose can be tried. In such instances, reduce the dose to 10.5 mg/day (i.e., used t.i.d.); then, after several weeks with good control, the dose can be reduced to 7 mg/day (i.e., used b.i.d.).

HEALTH CARE CONSIDERATIONS

Administration/Storage

1. Each actuation releases 1.75 mg.
2. Must be used regularly, even during symptom-free period, in order to achieve beneficial effects.
3. Teach the proper method of use of the drug. An illustrated pamphlet is included in each pack of nedocromil.
4. Add nedocromil to existing treatment (e.g., bronchodilators). When clinical response is seen and if asthma is under good control, a gradual decrease in the concomitant medication can be tried.
5. Store between 2°C–30°C (36°F–86°F) and do not freeze.

Assessment

1. Record symptoms, noting type, onset, and duration. List other agents trialed and the outcome.
2. Assess respiratory status thoroughly; not for use with status asthmaticus or for reversal of acute bronchospasm.
3. Monitor peak flow and vital capacity measurements.
4. Record systemic and inhaled steroid therapy accurately. When a reduction is in progress, nedocromil cannot substitute for total steroid dose/requirements.
5. Review drug usage and time between prescriptions to ensure proper use.

Client/Family Teaching

1. Review correct procedure for administration; use the step-by-step instructions provided with the drug.
2. Beneficial *preventative* effects will not be obtained if incorrectly administered by topical lung application. Drug is an inhaled anti-inflammatory that reduces lung inflammation.
3. Do not stop therapy during symptom-free periods; must be taken at regular intervals. Continue to use with other prescribed therapies.
4. Report any persistent headaches, unpleasant taste in mouth that interferes with nutrition, severe nausea, or chest pain.
5. Report any coughing or bronchospasm following use; drug should be discontinued, lungs assessed, and alternative therapy substituted.

Outcome/Evaluate: ↓ Severity/frequency of asthmatic episodes

Nefazodone hydrochloride

(nih-**FAY**-zoh-dohn)
Pregnancy Category: C
Serzone **(Rx)**
Classification: Antidepressant

Action/Kinetics: Exact antidepressant mechanism not known. Inhibits neuronal uptake of serotonin and norepinephrine and antagonizes central 5-HT_2 receptors and alpha-1-adrenergic receptors (which may cause postural hypotension). Produces none to slight anticholinergic effects, moderate sedation, and slight orthostatic hypotension. **Peak plasma levels:** 1 hr. **t½:** 2–4 hr. **Time to reach steady state:** 4–5 days. Extensively metabolized by the liver with less than 1% excreted unchanged in the urine. Food delays the absorption of nefazodone and decreases the bioavailability by approximately 20%.
Uses: Maintenance treatment of depression and for depression in hospitalized clients.
Contraindications: Use with terfenadine or astemizole; in combination with an MAO inhibitor or within 14 days of discontinuing MAO inhibitor therapy. Clients hypersensitive to nefazodone or other phenylpiperazine antidepressants.
Special Concerns: Use with caution in clients with a recent history of MI, unstable heart disease and taking digoxin, or a history of mania. Use with caution during lactation. Safety and efficacy have not been determined in individuals below 18 years of age. There is a possibility of a suicide attempt in depression that may persist until significant remission occurs.
Side Effects: *CNS:* Dizziness, insomnia, agitation, somnolence, lightheadedness, activation of mania or hypomania, confusion, memory impairment, paresthesia, abnormal dreams, decreased concentration, ataxia, in-

coordination, psychomotor retardation, tremor, hypertonia, decreased libido, vertigo, twitching, depersonalization, hallucinations, ***suicide thoughts/attempt,*** apathy, euphoria, hostility, abnormal gait, abnormal thinking, derealization, paranoid reaction, dysarthria, myoclonus, ***neuroleptic malignant syndrome (rare)***. *CV:* Postural hypotension, hypotension, sinus bradycardia, tachycardia, hypertension, syncope, ventricular extrasystoles, angina pectoris, ***CVA (rare)***. *GI:* Nausea, dry mouth, constipation, dyspepsia, diarrhea, increased appetite, vomiting, eructation, periodontal abscess, gingivitis, colitis, gastritis, mouth ulceration, stomatitis, esophagitis, peptic ulcer, rectal hemorrhage. *Dermatologic:* Pruritus, dry skin, acne, alopecia, urticaria, maculopapular rash, vesiculobullous rash, eczema. *Musculoskeletal:* Asthenia, arthralgia, arthritis, tenosynovitis, muscle stiffness, bursitis. *Respiratory:* Pharyngitis, increased cough, dyspnea, bronchitis, asthma, pneumonia, laryngitis, voice alteration, epistaxis, hiccups. *Hematologic:* Ecchymosis, anemia, leukopenia, lymphadenopathy. *Ophthalmologic:* Blurred vision, abnormal vision, visual field defect, dry eye, eye pain, abnormal accommodation, diplopia, conjunctivitis, mydriasis, keratoconjunctivitis, photophobia, night blindness. *Body as a whole:* Headache, infection, flu syndrome, chills, fever, neck rigidity, allergic reaction, malaise, photosensitivity, facial edema, hangover effect, enlarged abdomen, hernia, pelvic pain, halitosis, cellulitis, weight loss, gout, dehydration. *GU:* Urinary frequency, UTI, urinary retention, vaginitis, breast pain, cystitis, urinary urgency, metrorrhagia, amenorrhea, polyuria, vaginal hemorrhage, breast enlargement, menorrhagia, urinary incontinence, abnormal ejaculation, hematuria, nocturia, kidney calculus. *Miscellaneous:* Peripheral edema, thirst, abnormal LFTs, ear pain, hyperacusis, deafness, taste loss.

Laboratory Test Considerations: ↑ AST, ALT, LDH. ↓ Hematocrit. Hypercholesterolemia, hypoglycemia.

OD **Management of Overdose:** *Symptoms:* N&V, somnolence, increased incidence of severity of any of the reported side effects. *Treatment:* Symptomatic and supportive in the cases of hypotension or excessive sedation. Gastric lavage may be used.

Drug Interactions

Alprazolam / ↑ Plasma levels of alprazolam
Astemizole / ↑ Plasma levels of astemizole resulting in QT prolongation and possible serious CV events, including death due to ventricular tachycardia of the torsades de pointes type
Cisapride / ↑ Risk of serious cardiac arrhythmias
Digoxin / ↑ Plasma levels of digoxin
MAO inhibitors / Serious and possibly fatal reactions including symptoms of hyperthermia, rigidity, myoclonus, autonomic instability with possible rigid fluctuations of VS, and mental status changes that may include extreme agitation progressing to delirium and coma
Propranolol / ↓ Plasma levels of propranolol
Terfenadine / ↑ Plasma levels of terfenadine resulting in QT prolongation and possible serious CV events, including death due to ventricular tachycardia of the torsades de pointes type
Triazolam / ↑ Plasma levels of triazolam

How Supplied: *Tablet:* 100 mg, 150 mg, 200 mg, 250 mg

Dosage

- **Tablets**

Antidepressant.

Adults, initial: 200 mg/day given in two divided doses. Increase dose in increments of 100–200 mg/day at intervals of no less than 1 week. The effective dose range is 300–600 mg/day. The initial dose for elderly or debilitated clients is 100 mg/day given in two divided doses.

N

HEALTH CARE CONSIDERATIONS

Administration/Storage

1. Several weeks may be required for the full beneficial effect to be observed.
2. Although long-term use has not been studied, it is usually recommended that the drug be given for a period of 6 months or longer.
3. At least 14 days should elapse between discontinuation of an MAO inhibitor and initiation of therapy with nefazodone; also, at least 7 days should elapse after stopping nefazodone and before starting an MAO inhibitor.

Assessment

1. Record indications for therapy, onset and duration of symptoms, and any precipitating factors.
2. List drugs currently prescribed to ensure none interact unfavorably.
3. Determine any CAD, recent MI, or conditions requiring digoxin administration.
4. Monitor CBC, ECG, liver and renal function studies.

Client/Family Teaching

1. Take before meals; food may inhibit absorption.
2. Do not perform activities that require mental alertness or coordination until drug effects realized; may cause dizziness, drowsiness, confusion, incoordination, decreased concentration and response time.
3. Avoid all OTC agents, alcohol and any other CNS depressants.
4. May take several weeks (2–4) before any effects are realized; do not become discouraged.
5. Report any unusual sensations or side effects, increased depression, or suicidal thoughts/behavior.
6. Use reliable birth control.

Outcome/Evaluate: Symptomatic improvement; ↓ depression, as evidenced by improved sleeping and eating patterns, ↓ fatigue, and ↑ social interaction

Nelfinavir mesylate

(nel-**FIN**-ah-veer)
Pregnancy Category: B
Viracept **(Rx)**
Classification: Antiviral, protease inhibitor

N

See also *Antiviral Drugs.*

Action/Kinetics: HIV-1 protease inhibitor, resulting in prevention of cleavage of gagpol polyprotein resulting in production of immature, non-infectious viruses. Activity is increased when used with didanosine, lamivudine, stavudine, zalcitabine, or zidovudine. **Peak plasma levels:** 2–4 hr. **Steady-state plasma levels:** 3–4 mcg/mL. Food increases plasma levels 2–3 fold. **t½, terminal:** 3.5–5 hr. Metabolites (one of which is as active as parent compound) and unchanged drug excreted mainly in feces.

Uses: Treat HIV infection when antiretroviral therapy is required.

Contraindications: Administration with astemizole, cisapride, midazolam, rifampin, terfenadine, or triazolam.

Special Concerns: Use with caution with hepatic impairment. Safety and efficacy have not been determined in children less than 2 years of age.

Side Effects: Side effects were determined when used in combination with other antiviral drugs. *GI:* N&V, diarrhea, flatulence, abdominal pain, anorexia, dyspepsia, epigastric pain, GI bleeding, hepatitis, mouth ulcers, pancreatitis. *CNS:* Anxiety, depression, dizziness, emotional lability, hyperkinesia, insomnia, migraine, paresthesia, ***seizures,*** sleep disorder, somnolence, ***suicide ideation.*** *Hematologic:* Anemia, leukopenia, thrombocytopenia. *Respiratory:* Dyspnea, rhinitis, sinusitis, pharyngitis. *GU:* Kidney calculus, sexual dysfunction, urine abnormality. *Ophthalmic:* Eye disorder, acute iritis. *Musculoskeletal:* Arthralgia, arthritis, cramps, myalgia, myasthenia, myopathy. *Dermatologic:* Dermatitis, folliculitis, fungal dermatitis, maculopapular rash, pruritus, urticaria, sweating. *Miscellaneous:* Asthenia, dehydration, allergic reaction, back pain, fever, headache, malaise, pain, accidental injury.

Laboratory Test Considerations: ↑ ALT, AST, creatine phosphokinase, alkaline phosphatase, amylase, lactic dehydrogenase, GGT. Hyperlipidemia, hyperuricemia, hypoglycemia. Abnormal LFTs.

OD **Management of Overdose:** *Symptoms:* See side effects. *Treatment:* Emesis or gastric lavage, followed by activated charcoal.

Drug Interactions

Anticonvulsants / Possible ↓ plasma levels of nelfinavir
Astemizole / Potential for serious and life-threatening cardiac arrhythmias
Didanosine / ↓ Absorption of nelfinavir
Indinavir / Significant ↑ in nelfinavir levels
Oral contraceptives / ↓ Effect of oral contraceptives; use alternative contraceptive measures
Rifabutin / ↑ Levels of rifabutin; reduce dose of rifabutin by one-half
Rifampin / Significant ↓ in nelfinavir levels; do not coadminister
Terfenadine / Potential for serious and life-threatening cardiac arrhythmias

How Supplied: *Powder for Reconstitution:* 50 mg/1 g; *Suspension:* 50 mg/5 mL; *Tablets:* 250 mg

Dosage

- **Powder, Tablets**

HIV.

Adults: 750 mg (i.e., 3-250 mg tablets) t.i.d. in combination with nucleoside analogs. **Children, 2 to 13 years:** 20-30 mg/kg/dose t.i.d.

HEALTH CARE CONSIDERATIONS

See also *Health Care Considerations* for *Antiviral Drugs.*

Assessment

1. Record disease onset, characteristics, and other agents trialed.
2. List drugs prescribed/consumed to ensure none interact unfavorably.
3. Monitor CBC, CD_4 counts, viral load, liver and renal function.

Client/Family Teaching
1. Drug is not cure but helps to manage symptoms.
2. Take as prescribed with snack or light meal to enhance absorption.
3. Do not reconstitute powder with water in its original container. Mix powder with small amount of water, milk, formula, soy formula/milk or dietary supplement. Once mixed, consume entire amount for full dose. Do not mix with acidic foods or juice (e.g., orange or apple juice, apple sauce) due to their bitter taste.
4. Drug is to be taken with nucleoside analogs as prescribed.
5. Report any evidence of increased bruising or bleeding.
6. If diarrhea is bothersome, report as loperamide may be prescribed.
7. Drug does not prevent transmission of disease; practice safe sex.

Outcome/Evaluate: Control of HIV symptoms; ↓ viral load

Neomycin sulfate

(nee-oh-**MY**-sin)
Pregnancy Category: D
Mycifradin Sulfate, Myciguent, Neobiotic **(Rx)**
Classification: Antibiotic, aminoglycoside

See also *Anti-Infectives* and *Aminoglycosides.*

Action/Kinetics: Peak plasma levels: PO, 1–4 hr; **Therapeutic serum level:** 5–10 mcg/mL. **t½:** 2–3 hr.

Uses: PO: Hepatic coma, sterilization of gut prior to surgery, inhibition of ammonia-forming bacteria in GI tract in hepatic encephalopathy. Therapy of intestinal infections due to pathogenic strains of *Escherichia coli,* primarily in children. *Investigational:* Hypercholesterolemia.

Topical: Prophylaxis or treatment of infection in burns, minor cuts, wounds, and skin abrasions. As an aid to healing and for treating superficial skin infections.

Additional Contraindications: Intestinal obstruction (PO). Use of topical products in or around the eyes.

Special Concerns: Safe use during pregnancy has not been determined. Due to the possibility of toxicity, some recommend not to use parenteral neomycin for any purpose. Use with caution in clients with extensive burns, trophic ulceration, or other conditions where significant systemic absorption is possible.

Side Effects: Chronic use of topical neomycin to inflamed skin of those with contact dermatitis and chronic dermatosis increases the chance of hypersensitivity. Ototoxicity, nephrotoxicity. Sprue-like syndrome with steatorrhea, malabsorption, and electrolyte imbalance. Skin rashes after topical or parenteral administration. Chronic use in allergic contact dermatitis and chronic dermatoses increases the risk of sensitization.

Additional Drug Interactions
Digoxin / ↓ Effect of digoxin due to ↓ absorption from GI tract
Penicillin V / ↓ Effect of penicillin due to ↓ absorption from GI tract
Procainamide / ↑ Muscle relaxation produced by neomycin

How Supplied: *Cream:* 5 mg/g; *Ointment:* 5 mg/g; *Solution:* 125 mg/5 mL; *Tablet:* 500 mg

Dosage

- **Oral Solution**

Preoperatively in colorectal surgery.
1 g each of neomycin and erythromycin base for a total of three doses: the first two doses 1 hr apart the afternoon before surgery and the third dose at bedtime the night before surgery.

Hepatic coma, adjunct.
Adults, 4–12 g/day in divided doses for 5–6 days; **children:** 50–100 mg/kg/day in divided doses for 5–6 days.

- **Topical Cream, Ointment**

Neomycin alone or in combination with other antibiotics (bacitracin or gramicidin) and/or an anti-inflammatory agent (corticosteroid). Apply ointment (0.5%) or cream (0.5%) 1–3 times/day to affected area. If necessary, a bandage may be used to cover the area.

HEALTH CARE CONSIDERATIONS

See also *Health Care Considerations* for *Aminoglycosides.*

Administration/Storage: Have available neostigmine to counteract renal failure, respiratory depression and arrest (side effects that may occur when neomycin is administered intraperitoneally).

Assessment
1. Record indications for therapy. Note clinical presentation and symptom characteristics.
2. Describe abdominal assessment findings.
3. Review electrolytes and fluid status.

Client/Family Teaching
1. Consume 2–3 L/day of fluids.

N

2. Carefully follow recommended procedure to prepare the GI tract for surgery.
3. Expect slight laxative effect produced by PO neomycin. Withhold and report with S&S of intestinal obstruction.
4. Anticipate low-residue diet for preoperative disinfection and a laxative immediately preceding PO administration of neomycin sulfate.
5. When used topically, clean the affected area before applying topical ointment or solution; then apply a small amount equal to the surface area of a fingertip.

Outcome/Evaluate

- Improved level of consciousness
- Healing of skin wounds
- Bowel sterilization before surgery

Neostigmine bromide

(nee-oh-STIG-meen)
Pregnancy Category: C
Prostigmin Bromide **(Rx)**

Neostigmine methylsulfate

(nee-oh-STIG-meen)
Pregnancy Category: C
Prostigmin Injection, PMS-Neostigmine Methylsulfate ✱ **(Rx)**
Classification: Indirectly acting cholinergic-acetylcholinesterase inhibitor

N

Action/Kinetics: Acetylcholinesterase inhibitor that causes an increase in the concentration of acetylcholine at the myoneural junction, thus facilitating transmission of impulses across the myoneural junction. In myasthenia gravis, muscle strength is increased. May also act on the autonomic ganglia of the CNS. Prevents or relieves postoperative distention by increasing gastric motility and tone and prevents or relieves urinary retention by increasing the tone of the detrusor muscle of the bladder. Shorter acting than ambenonium chloride and pyridostigmine. Atropine is often given concomitantly to control side effects. **Onset: PO,** 45–75 min; **IM,** 20–30 min; **IV,** 4–8 min. **Time to peak effect, parenteral:** 20–30 min. **Duration:** All routes, 2.5–4 hr. **t½, PO:** 42–60 min; **IM:** 51–90 min; **IV:** 47–60 min. Eliminated through the urine (about 40% unchanged).

Uses: Diagnosis and treatment of myasthenia gravis. Prophylaxis and treatment of postoperative distention or urinary retention. Antidote for tubocurarine and other nondepolarizing drugs.

Contraindications: Hypersensitivity, mechanical obstruction of GI or urinary tract, peritonitis, history of bromide sensitivity. Vesical neck obstruction of urinary bladder. Lactation.

Special Concerns: Safety and effectiveness in children have not been established. Use with caution in clients with bronchial asthma, bradycardia, vagotonia, epilepsy, hyperthyroidism, peptic ulcer, cardiac arrhythmias, or recent coronary occlusion. May cause uterine irritability and premature labor if given IV to pregnant women near term. In geriatric clients, the duration of action may be increased.

Side Effects: *GI:* N&V, diarrhea, abdominal cramps, involuntary defecation, salivation, dysphagia, flatulence, increased gastric and intestinal secretions. *CV:* Bradycardia, tachycardia, hypotension, ECG changes, nodal rhythm, ***cardiac arrest,*** syncope, ***AV block,*** substernal pain, thrombophlebitis after IV use. *CNS:* Headache, ***seizures,*** malaise, weakness, dysarthria, dizziness, drowsiness, loss of consciousness. *Respiratory:* Increased oral, pharyngeal, and bronchial secretions; ***bronchospasms, skeletal muscle paralysis, laryngospasm, central respiratory paralysis, respiratory depression or arrest,*** dyspnea. *Ophthalmologic:* Miosis, double vision, lacrimation, accommodation difficulties, hyperemia of conjunctiva, visual changes. *Musculoskeletal:* Muscle fasciculations or weakness, muscle cramps or spasms, arthralgia. *Other:* Skin rashes, urinary frequency and incontinence, sweating, flushing, allergic reactions, anaphylaxis, urticaria. These effects can usually be reversed by parenteral administration of 0.6 mg of atropine sulfate, which should be readily available.

Cholinergic crisis, due to overdosage, must be distinguished from myasthenic crisis (worsening of the disease), since cholinergic crisis involves removal of drug therapy, while myasthenic crisis involves an increase in anticholinesterase therapy.

OD **Management of Overdose:** *Symptoms:* Abdominal cramps, vomiting, diarrhea, epigastric distress, excessive salivation, cold sweating, pallor, blurred vision, urinary urgency, fasciculation and ***paralysis of voluntary muscles (including the tongue),*** miosis, increased BP (may be accompanied by bradycardia), sensation of internal trembling, panic, severe anxiety. *Treatment:* Discontinue medication temporarily. Give atropine, 0.5–1 mg IV (up to 5–10 or more mg may be needed to get the HR to 80 beats/min). Supportive treatment including artificial respiration and oxygen.

Drug Interactions

Aminoglycosides / ↑ Neuromuscular blockade
Atropine / Atropine suppresses symptoms of excess GI stimulation caused by cholinergic drugs

Corticosteroids / ↓ Effect of neostigmine
Magnesium salts / Antagonize the effects of anticholinesterases
Mecamylamine / Intense hypotensive response
Organophosphate-type insecticides/pesticides / Added systemic effects with cholinesterase inhibitors
Succinylcholine / ↑ Neuromuscular blocking effects

How Supplied: Neostigmine bromide: *Tablet:* 15 mg. Neostigmine methylsulfate: *Injection:* 0.5 mg/mL, 1 mg/mL

Dosage

NEOSTIGMINE BROMIDE

- **Tablets**

Treat myasthenia gravis.

Adults: 15 mg q 3–4 hr; adjust dose and frequency as needed. **Usual maintenance:** 150 mg/day with dosing intervals determined by client response. **Pediatric,** 2 mg/kg (60 mg/m^2) daily in six to eight divided doses.

NEOSTIGMINE METHYLSULFATE

- **IM, IV, SC**

Diagnosis of myasthenia gravis.

Adults, IM, SC: 1.5 mg given with 0.6 mg atropine; **pediatric, IM:** 0.04 mg/kg (1 mg/m^2); or, **IV:** 0.02 mg/kg (0.5 mg/m^2).

Treat myasthenia gravis.

Adults, IM, SC: 0.5 mg. **Pediatric, IM, SC:** 0.01–0.04 mg/kg q 2–3 hr.

Antidote for tubocurarine.

Adults, IV: 0.5–2 mg slowly with 0.6–1.2 mg atropine sulfate. Can repeat if necessary up to total dose of 5 mg. **Pediatric, IV:** 0.04 mg/kg with 0.02 mg/kg atropine sulfate.

Prevention of postoperative GI distention or urinary retention.

Adults, IM, SC: 0.25 mg (1 mL of the 1:4,000 solution) immediately after surgery repeated q 4–6 hr for 2–3 days.

Treatment of postoperative GI distention.

Adults, IM, SC: 0.5 mg (1 mL of the 1:2,000 solution) as required.

Treatment of urinary retention.

Adults, IM, SC: 0.5 mg (1 mL of the 1:2,000 solution). If urination does not occur within 1 hr after 0.5 mg, the client should be catheterized. After the bladder is emptied, 0.5 mg is given q 3 hr for at least five injections.

HEALTH CARE CONSIDERATIONS

Administration/Storage

1. Determine interval doses individually to achieve optimum effects.
2. If greater fatigue occurs at certain times of the day, give a larger part of the daily dose at these times.
3. Do not give if high concentrations of halothane or cyclopropane are present.
4. IV May administer IV form undiluted at a rate of 0.5 mg/min.

Assessment

1. Note any sensitivity to bromide or to drugs in this category.
2. Identify drugs consumed to determine if any interact unfavorably.

Interventions

1. Report symptoms of generalized cholinergic stimulation (evidence of a toxic reaction).
2. Monitor VS for the first hour. Report and hold if HR < 80. If hypotension occurs, keep recumbent until BP stabilizes.
3. When used as an antidote for nondepolarizing drugs, provide ventilatory assistance.

Client/Family Teaching

1. With myasthenia, maintain a written record of periods of muscle strength or weakness so that dosage can be evaluated and adjusted accordingly; space activities to avoid excessive fatigue.
2. Take the dose exactly as prescribed; taking it late may result in myasthenic crisis whereas taking it early may result in cholinergic crisis.
3. If difficulty with coordination or vision avoid use of heavy machinery until effects wear off.
4. If taking for myasthenia gravis, any onset of weakness 1 hr after administration usually indicates overdosage of drug. Weakness 3 hr or more after administration usually indicates underdosage and/or resistance. Report as well as any associated difficulty with respirations or increase in muscle weakness as drug tolerance can develop.
5. Wear and/or carry ID noting therapy with neostigmine and why.

Outcome/Evaluate

- ↑ Muscle strength and function with myasthenia gravis
- Relief of postoperative ileus or urinary retention
- Reversal of respiratory depression R/T nondepolarizing drugs

Nevirapine

(neh-VYE-rah-peen)
Pregnancy Category: C
Viramune **(Rx)**
Classification: Antiviral

See also *Antiviral Drugs*.

N

Action/Kinetics: By binding tightly to reverse transcriptase, nevirapine prevents viral RNA from being converted into DNA. In combination with a nucleoside analogue, it reduces the amount of virus circulating in the body and increases CD4+ cell counts. Readily absorbed, with peak plasma levels occurring 4 hr after a 200-mg dose. Extensively metabolized in the liver. Excreted through both the urine (about 90%) and the feces (about 10%). Induces its own metabolism; following chronic use the half-life decreases from about 45 hr following a single dose to 25 to 30 hr following multiple dosing with 200 or 400 mg daily.
Uses: In combination with nucleoside analogues (e.g., AZT, lamivudine, didanosine, zalcitabine) or protease inhibitors (e.g., saquinavir, indinavir, ritonavir) for the treatment of HIV-1 infections in adults who have experienced clinical and immunologic deterioration. Always use in combination with at least one other antiretroviral agent, as resistant viruses emerge rapidly when nevirapine is used alone.
Contraindications: Lactation.
Special Concerns: The duration of benefit from therapy may be limited. Is not a cure for HIV infections; clients may continue to experience illnesses associated with HIV infections, including opportunistic infections. Has not been shown to reduce the risk of transmitting HIV to others through sexual contact or blood contamination. Use with caution in impaired renal or hepatic function.
Side Effects: *GI:* Nausea, abnormal LFTs, diarrhea, abdominal pain, ulcerative stomatitis, hepatitis. *CNS:* Headache, fatigue, paresthesia. *Hematologic:* Decreased hemoglobin, decreased platelets, decreased neutrophils. *Miscellaneous:* ***Rash (may be severe and life-threatening),*** fever, peripheral neuropathy, myalgia.
Laboratory Test Considerations: ↑ ALT, AST, GGT, total bilirubin.

Drug Interactions

Oral contraceptives / ↓ Plasma levels of oral contraceptives → ↓ effect
Protease inhibitors / ↓ Plasma levels of protease inhibitors
Rifabutin / ↓ Nevirapine trough concentrations
Rifampin / Nevirapine trough concentrations

How Supplied: *Suspension:* 50 mg/5 mL; *Tablet:* 200 mg

Dosage

- **Suspension, Tablets**

  HIV-1 infections.

Initial: 200 mg/day for 14 days. **Maintenance:** 200 mg b.i.d. (e.g., 7:00 a.m. and 7:00 p.m.) in combination with a nucleoside analogue antiretroviral agent.

HEALTH CARE CONSIDERATIONS

See also *Health Care Considerations* for *Antiviral Drugs,* and *Anti-Infectives.*

Administration/Storage

1. Clients who interrupt nevirapine dosing for more than 7 days should restart therapy using one 200-mg tablet for the first 14 days, followed by 200 mg b.i.d. (7 a.m. and 7 p.m.).
2. The suspension is used b.i.d. for children.
3. Store tablets in a tightly closed bottle at 15°C–30°C (59°F–86°F).

Assessment

1. Record disease onset, symptom characteristics, other agents trialed and the outcome.
2. List drugs currently prescribed to ensure none interact unfavorably.
3. Monitor CBC, CD4 counts, viral load, liver and renal function studies.

Client/Family Teaching

1. Drug is not a cure but helps control disease symptoms.
2. Can be taken with or without food.
3. If a dose is skipped, take the next dose as soon as possible; do not double the dose.
4. Take exactly as directed. Should be taken with another antiretroviral agent to prevent emergence of resistant viruses.
5. A rash may occur in the first few weeks of therapy. Notify provider and do not increase dosage until rash subsides.
6. Any severe rash or rash accompanied by flu-like symptoms warrants immediate notification.
7. Drug does not prevent transmission through sexual contact or blood contamination. Practice barrier contraception and nonhormonal form of birth control.

Outcome/Evaluate: Improved CD4 cell counts; ↓ Viral load

Niacin (Nicotinic acid)

(NYE-ah-sin, nih-koh-TIN-ick AH-sid)
Pregnancy Category: C
Nia-Bid, Niaspan, Nico-400, Nicobid, Nicolar, Nicotinex, Slo-Niacin, Span-Niacin, Tega-Span (Rx and OTC)

Niacinamide

(nye-ah-SIN-ah-myd)
Pregnancy Category: C
Papulex ✦ (Rx: Injection; OTC: Tablets)
Classification: Vitamin B complex

Action/Kinetics: Niacin (nicotinic acid) and niacinamide are water-soluble, heat-resistant vitamins prepared synthetically. Niacin (after conversion to the active niacinamide) is a component of the coenzymes nicotinamide-adenine dinucleotide and nicotinamide-adenine dinucleotide phosphate, which are essential for oxidation-reduction reactions involved in lipid metabolism, glycogenolysis, and tissue respiration. Deficiency of niacin results in pellagra, the most common symptoms of which are dermatitis, diarrhea, and dementia. In high doses niacin also produces vasodilation. Reduces serum cholesterol and triglycerides in types II, III, IV, and V hyperlipoproteinemia (mechanism unknown). **Peak serum levels:** 45 min; **t½:** 45 min.
Uses: Prophylaxis and treatment of pellagra; niacin deficiency. Treat hyperlipidemia in clients not responding to either diet or weight loss. Reduce the risk of recurrent nonfatal MI and promote regression of atherosclerosis when combined with bile-binding resins.
Contraindications: Severe hypotension, hemorrhage, arterial bleeding, liver dysfunction, active peptic ulcer. Use of the extended-release tablets and capsules in children.
Special Concerns: Extended-release niacin may be hepatotoxic. Use with caution in diabetics, gall bladder disease, in those who consume a large amount of alcohol, and clients with gout.
Side Effects: *GI:* N&V, diarrhea, peptic ulcer activation, abdominal pain. *Dermatologic:* Flushing, warm feeling, skin rash, pruritus, dry skin, itching and tingling feeling, keratosis nigricans. *Other:* Hypotension, headache, macular cystoid edema, amblyopia. *NOTE:* Megadoses are accompanied by serious toxicity including the symptoms listed in the preceding as well as liver damage, hyperglycemia, hyperuricemia, arrhythmias, tachycardia, and dermatoses.
Drug Interactions
Chenodiol / ↓ Effect of chenodiol
Probenecid / Niacin may ↓ uricosuric effect of probenecid
Sulfinpyrazone / Niacin ↓ uricosuric effect of sulfinpyrazone
Sympathetic blocking agents / Additive vasodilating effects → postural hypotension
How Supplied: Niacin: *Capsule:* 100 mg; *Capsule, Extended Release:* 125 mg, 250 mg, 400 mg, 500 mg, 750 mg; *Elixir:* 50 mg/5 mL; *Tablet:* 50 mg, 100 mg, 250 mg, 500 mg; *Tablet, Extended Release:* 500 mg, 750 mg, 1,000 mg. Niacinamide: *Tablet:* 50 mg, 100 mg, 500 mg

Dosage

NIACIN

• **Extended-Release Capsules, Tablets, Extended-Release Tablets, Capsules, Elixir**

Vitamin.

Adults: Up to 500 mg/day; **pediatric:** Up to 300 mg/day.

Antihyperlipidemic.

Adults, initial: 1 g t.i.d.; **then:** increase dose in increments of 500 mg/day q 2–4 weeks as needed. **Maintenance:** 1–2 g t.i.d. (up to a maximum of 8 g/day). **Niaspan:** Week 1, 375 mg hs; week 2, 500 mg; week 3, 750 mg hs; then, dose may be increased by no more than 500 mg in any 4- week period; do not give doses greater than 2,000 mg/day.

• **IM, IV**

Pellagra.

Adults, IM: 50–100 mg 5 or more times/day. **IV, slow:** 25–100 mg 2 or more times/day. **Pediatric, IV slow:** Up to 300 mg/day.

NIACINAMIDE

• **Tablets**

Vitamin.

Adults: Up to 500 mg/day. **Pediatric:** Up to 300 mg/day. Capsules not recommended for use in children.

HEALTH CARE CONSIDERATIONS

Administration/Storage

IV 1. Other niacins can not be substituted for Niaspan.
2. May administer IV form diluted (to 2 mg/mL solution concentration) at a rate not exceeding 2 mg/min.

Assessment

1. Monitor glucose, HbA1-C, LFTs, and plasma lipid levels periodically throughout therapy.
2. Note any history of PUD or liver or gallbladder dysfunction.
3. Assess diet, exercise, and any life-style changes necessary to decrease coronary risk factors.
4. The extended-release capsules and tablets are not as useful in lowering triglycerides. When using the regular strength tablets for hyperlipidemia, start low and go slow to enhance client tolerance.

Client/Family Teaching

1. Take nicotinic acid PO only with cold water (no hot beverages). Can be taken with meals if GI upset occurs.

N

2. May experience a warm flushing in the face and ears within 2 hr after taking. Take one aspirin to reduce effect. Alcohol may increase these effects.
3. Lie down if feeling weak and dizzy after taking niacin (until this feeling passes) and inform provider.
4. Identify foods sources high in niacin (dairy products, meats, tuna, and eggs); assess consumption.
5. With diabetes, do not take niacin unless specifically ordered and then the BS levels must be closely monitored for hyperglycemia; also monitor for ketonuria and glucosuria. Antidiabetic agents may require a dosage increase.
6. Report any skin color changes or yellowing of the sclera.
7. Clients predisposed to gout may experience flank, joint, or stomach pains; report immediately.
8. If blurred vision or skin lesions occur, remain out of direct sunlight.
9. No unsupervised excessive vitamin ingestion; high doses may impair liver function.

Outcome/Evaluate

- ↓ Cholesterol/triglyceride levels
- Relief of symptoms of pellagra and niacin deficiency

N

Nicardipine hydrochloride

(nye-**KAR**-dih-peen)

Pregnancy Category: C

Cardene, Cardene IV, Cardene SR **(Rx)**

Classification: Calcium channel blocking agent (antianginal, antihypertensive)

See also *Calcium Channel Blocking Agents*.

Action/Kinetics: Moderately increases CO and significantly decreases peripheral vascular resistance. **Onset of action:** 20 min. **Maximum plasma levels:** 30–120 min. Significant first-pass metabolism. Food (especially fats) will decrease the amount of drug absorbed from the GI tract. Steady-state plasma levels are reached after 2–3 days of therapy. **Therapeutic serum levels:** 0.028–0.050 mcg/mL. **t½, at steady state:** 8.6 hr. **Maximum BP-lowering effects, immediate release:** 1–2 hr; **maximum BP-lowering effects, sustained release:** 2–6 hr. **Duration:** 8 hr. Highly bound to plasma protein (> 95%) and metabolized by the liver with excretion through both the urine and feces.

Uses: Immediate release: Chronic stable angina (effort-associated angina) alone or in combination with beta-adrenergic blocking agents.

Immediate and sustained released: Hypertension alone or in combination with other antihypertensive drugs.

IV: Short-term treatment of hypertension when PO therapy is not desired or possible.

Investigational: CHF.

Contraindications: Use in advanced aortic stenosis due to the effect on reducing afterload. During lactation.

Special Concerns: Safety and efficacy in children less than 18 years of age have not been established. Use with caution in clients with CHF, especially in combination with a beta blocker due to the possibility of a negative inotropic effect. Use with caution in clients with impaired liver function, reduced hepatic blood flow, or impaired renal function. Initial increase in frequency, duration, or severity of angina.

Side Effects: *CV:* Pedal edema, flushing, increased angina, palpitations, tachycardia, other edema, abnormal ECG, hypotension, postural hypotension, syncope, ***MI, AV block,*** ventricular extrasystoles, peripheral vascular disease. *CNS:* Dizziness, headache, somnolence, malaise, nervousness, insomnia, abnormal dreams, vertigo, depression, confusion, amnesia, anxiety, weakness, psychoses, hallucinations, paranoia. *GI:* N&V, dyspepsia, dry mouth, constipation, sore throat. *Neuromuscular:* Asthenia, myalgia, paresthesia, hyperkinesia, arthralgia. *Miscellaneous:* Rash, dyspnea, SOB, nocturia, polyuria, allergic reactions, abnormal liver chemistries, hot flashes, impotence, rhinitis, sinusitis, nasal congestion, chest congestion, tinnitus, equilibrium disturbances, abnormal or blurred vision, infection, atypical chest pain.

OD Management of Overdose: *Symptoms:* Marked hypotension, bradycardia, palpitations, flushing, drowsiness, confusion, and slurred speech following PO overdose. Lethal overdose may cause systemic hypotension, bradycardia (following initial tachycardia), and progressive AV block. *Treatment:*

- Treatment is supportive. Monitor cardiac and respiratory function.
- If client is seen soon after ingestion, emetics or gastric lavage should be considered, followed by cathartics.
- *Hypotension:* IV calcium, dopamine, isoproterenol, metaraminol, or norepinephrine. Also, provide IV fluids. Place client in Trendelenburg position.
- *Ventricular tachycardia:* IV procainamide or lidocaine; cardioversion may be necessary. Also, provide slow-drip IV fluids.
- *Bradycardia, asystole, AV block:* IV atropine sulfate (0.6–1 mg), calcium gluconate (10% solution), isoproterenol, norepinephrine; also,

cardiac pacing may be indicated. Provide slow-drip IV fluids.

Drug Interactions

Cimetidine / ↑ Bioavailability of nicardipine → ↑ plasma levels

Cyclosporine / ↑ Plasma levels of cyclosporine possibly leading to renal toxicity

Ranitidine / ↑ Bioavailability of nicardipine

How Supplied: *Capsule:* 20 mg, 30 mg; *Capsule, Extended Release:* 30 mg, 45 mg, 60 mg; *Injection:* 2.5 mg/mL

Dosage

- **Capsules, Immediate Release**

  Angina, hypertension.

Initial, usual: 20 mg t.i.d. (range: 20–40 mg t.i.d.). Wait 3 days before increasing dose to ensure steady-state plasma levels.

- **Capsules, Sustained Release**

  Hypertension.

Initial: 30 mg b.i.d. (range: 30–60 mg b.i.d.).

NOTE: Initial dose in renal impairment: 20 mg t.i.d. Initial dose in hepatic impairment: 20 mg b.i.d.

- **IV**

  Hypertension.

Individualize dose. Initial: 5 mg/hr; the infusion rate may be increased to a maximum of 15 mg/hr (by 2.5-mg/hr increments q 15 min). For a more rapid reduction in BP, initiate at 5 mg/hr but increase the rate q 5 min in 2.5-mg/hr increments until a maximum of 15 mg/hr is reached. **Maintenance:** 3 mg/hr. The IV infusion rate to produce an average plasma level similar to a particular PO dose is as follows: 20 mg q 8 hr is equivalent to 0.5 mg/hr; 30 mg q 8 hr is equivalent to 1.2 mg/hr; and 40 mg q 8 hr is equivalent to 2.2 mg/hr.

HEALTH CARE CONSIDERATIONS

See also *Health Care Considerations* for *Calcium Channel Blocking Agents.*

Administration/Storage

1. When used for treating angina, may be administered safely along with sublingual nitroglycerin, prophylactic nitrates, or beta blockers.
2. When used to treat hypertension, may be administered safely along with diuretics or beta blockers.
3. During initial therapy and when dosage is increased, may experience an increase in the frequency, duration, or severity of angina.
4. If transfer to PO antihypertensives other than nicardipine is planned, initiate therapy after discontinuing infusion. If PO nicardipine is used at a dosage regimen of three times daily, give the first dose 1 hr prior to discontinuing infusion.

IV 5. Ampules must be diluted before infusion. Acceptable diluents are 5% dextrose, D5/0.45% NaCl, D5W with 40 mEq potassium, 0.45% NaCl, and 0.9% NaCl. Nicardipine is incompatible with 5% $NaHCO_3$ and RL solution.

6. The infusion concentration is 0.1 mg/mL. The diluted product is stable at room temperature for 24 hr.
7. Store ampules at room temperature; freezing does not affect the product. Protect ampules from light and elevated temperatures.

Assessment

1. Record indications for therapy. List other agents prescribed and the outcome.
2. Note CHF and if beta blockers prescribed, monitor closely.
3. Monitor ECG, liver and renal function studies; note any dysfunction.
4. Monitor VS. When the immediate-release product is used for hypertension, the maximum lowering of BP occurs 1–2 hr after dosing. Evaluate BP at trough (8 hr after dosing). When the sustained-release product is used, maximum lowering of BP occurs 2–6 hr after dosing.
5. Monitor BP frequently during and following IV infusion. Avoid too rapid or excessive decrease in BP and discontinue infusion if significant hypotension or tachycardia.

Client/Family Teaching

1. Take at the same time each day.
2. Report any persistent and/or bothersome side effects such as dizziness, flushing, increased angina, weight gain or edema.
3. Maintain proper intake of fluids to avoid constipation. Avoid caffeine and alcohol.
4. May experience impotence.
5. Anginal attacks may persist up to 30 min following drug ingestion due to reflex tachycardia; use nitrates as prescribed.
6. Report any change in psychologic state—depression, anxiety, sleep problems, or decreased mental acuity. Particularly important when working with elderly clients since there is a tendency to misdiagnose as senility.

Outcome/Evaluate

- Control of hypertension
- ↓ Frequency/intensity of anginal attacks
- Therapeutic drug levels (0.028–0.050 mcg/mL)

N

Nicotine polacrilex (Nicotine Resin Complex)

(NIK-oh-teen)

Pregnancy Category: X

Nicorette, Nicorette DS, Nicorette Plus ✱

(OTC)

Classification: Smoking deterrent

Action/Kinetics: Following chewing, nicotine is released from an ion exchange resin in the gum product, providing blood nicotine levels approximating those produced by smoking cigarettes. The amount of nicotine released depends on the rate and duration of chewing. Following repeated administration q 30 min, nicotine blood levels reach 25–50 ng/mL. If the gum is swallowed, only a minimum amount of nicotine is released. Metabolized mainly by the liver, with about 10%–20% excreted unchanged in the urine.

Uses: Adjunct with behavioral modification in smokers wishing to give up the smoking habit. Is considered only as an initial aid, with the ultimate goal being abstention from all forms of nicotine. Most likely to benefit are individuals with the following characteristics:

a. smoke brands of cigarettes containing more than 0.9 mg nicotine;

b. smoke more than 15 cigarettes daily;

c. inhale cigarette smoke deeply and frequently;

d. smoke most frequently during the morning;

e. smoke the first cigarette of the day within 30 min of arising;

f. indicate cigarettes smoked in the morning are the most difficult to give up;

g. smoke even if the individual is ill and confined to bed;

h. find it necessary to smoke in places where smoking is not allowed. *NOTE:* Nicotine may be effective in improving the course of difficult-to-treat ulcerative colitis.

Contraindications: Pregnancy, lactation, nonsmokers, serious arrhythmias, angina, vasospastic disease, active temporomandibular joint disease. Use in individuals less than 18 years of age.

Special Concerns: Safety and effectiveness in children and adolescents who smoke have not been determined. Use with caution in hypertension, PUD, oral or pharyngeal inflammation, gastritis, stomatitis, hyperthyroidism, IDDM, and pheochromocytoma.

Side Effects: *CNS:* Dizziness, irritability, headache. *GI:* N&V, indigestion, GI upset, salivation, eructation. *Other:* Sore mouth or throat, hiccoughs, sore jaw muscles.

OD **Management of Overdose:** *Symptoms: GI:* N&V, diarrhea, salivation, abdominal pain. *CNS:* Headache, dizziness, confusion, weakness, fainting, ***seizures.*** *Respiratory:* Labored breathing, ***respiratory paralysis (cause of death).*** *Other:* Cold sweat, disturbed hearing and vision, hypotension, and rapid, weak pulse. *Treatment:* Syrup of ipecac if vomiting has not occurred, saline laxative, gastric lavage followed by activated charcoal (if client is unconscious), maintenance of respiration, maintenance of CV function.

Drug Interactions

Caffeine / Possibly ↓ blood levels of caffeine due to ↑ rate of breakdown by liver

Catecholamines / ↑ Levels of catecholamines

Cortisol / ↑ Levels of cortisol

Furosemide / Possible ↓ diuretic effect of furosemide

Glutethimide / Possible ↓ absorption of glutethimide

Imipramine / Possibly ↓ blood levels of imipramine due to ↑ rate of breakdown by liver

Pentazocine / Possibly ↓ blood levels of pentazocine due to ↑ rate of breakdown by liver

Theophylline / Possibly ↓ blood levels of theophylline due to ↑ rate of breakdown by liver

How Supplied: *Gum:* 2 mg, 4 mg

Dosage

- **Gum**

Initial: One piece of gum chewed whenever the urge to smoke occurs; best results are obtained when the gum is chewed on a fixed schedule, at intervals of 1 to 2 hr, with at least 9 pieces chewed per day. **maintenance:** 9–12 pieces of gum daily during the first month, not to exceed 30 pieces daily of the 2-mg strength and 20 pieces daily of the 4-mg strength.

HEALTH CARE CONSIDERATIONS

Administration/Storage

1. Those who smoke more than 25 cigarettes/day should be started on the 4-mg dose.

2. Evaluate monthly; if client has not smoked for 3 months, slowly withdraw the gum. Do not use for longer than 6 months.

3. Suggested procedures for gradual withdrawal of the gum include:

- Decreasing the total number of pieces/day by one or more pieces q 4–7 days.
- Decreasing the chewing time with each piece from the normal 30 min to 10–15 min

for 4–7 days; then gradually decreasing the number of pieces used per day.

• Increasing the chewing time for more than 30 min and reducing the number of pieces used per day.

• Substituting one or more pieces of sugarless gum for an equal number of pieces of nicotine gum; then, increasing the number of pieces of sugarless gum substituted for nicotine gum q 4–7 days.

• Replacing the 4-mg gum with the 2-mg gum and applying any of the first four procedures listed in the preceding.

Assessment

1. Record nicotine profile: type and brand (cigarettes, chewing tobacco, or cigars), amount used per day, when used, and what increases usage.

2. Note any temporomandibular joint syndrome or cardiac arrhythmia; precludes gum therapy.

Client/Family Teaching

1. Must want to stop smoking and should do so immediately.

2. Use gum only as directed. When client has the urge to smoke, chew one piece slowly for about 30 min. If a slight tingling becomes evident, stop chewing until sensation subsides.

3. Acidic beverages, such as coffee, juices, soft drinks, and wine, interfere with buccal absorption of nicotine; thus, avoid eating and drinking 15 min before and during chewing.

4. Gum will not stick to dentures or appliances.

5. Identify individuals and local support groups that can help with smoking cessation and provide emotional and psychologic support throughout the endeavor. Participate in a formal smoking program.

Outcome/Evaluate: Control of nicotine withdrawal symptoms with smoking cessation

Nicotine transdermal system

(NIK-oh-teen)

Pregnancy Category: D

Habitrol, Prostep **(Rx)**, Nicoderm CQ Step 1, Step 2, or Step 3, Nicotrol **(OTC)**

Classification: Smoking deterrent

Action/Kinetics: Nicotine transdermal system is a multilayered film that provides systemic delivery of varying amounts of nicotine over a 24-hr period after applying to the skin. Nicotine's reinforcing activity is due to stimulation of the cortex (via the locus ceruleus), producing increased alertness and cognitive performance and a "reward" effect due to an action in the limbic system. At low doses the stimulatory effects predominate, whereas at high doses the reward effects predominate. The nicotine transdermal system produces an initial (first day of use) increase in BP, an increase in HR (3%–7%), and a decrease in SV after 10 days. Metabolized in the liver to a large number of metabolites, all of which are less active than nicotine. **t½, following removal of the system from the skin:** 3–4 hr.

Uses: As an aid to stopping smoking for the relief of nicotine withdrawal symptoms. Should be used in conjunction with a comprehensive behavioral smoking cessation program.

Contraindications: Hypersensitivity or allergy to nicotine or any components of the therapeutic system. Use in children and during pregnancy, labor, delivery, and lactation. Use in those with heart disease, hypertension, a recent MI, severe or worsening angina pectoris, those taking certain antidepressants or antiasthmatic drugs, or in severe renal impairment.

Special Concerns: Encourage pregnant smokers to try to stop smoking using educational and behavioral interventions before using the nicotine transdermal system. Use during pregnancy only if the potential benefit outweighs the potential risk of nicotine to the fetus. The use of nicotine transdermal systems for longer than 3 months has not been studied. Before use, screen clients with coronary heart disease (history of MI and/or angina pectoris), serious cardiac arrhythmias, or vasospastic diseases (e.g., Buerger's disease, Prinzmetal's variant angina) carefully. Use with caution in clients with hyperthyroidism, pheochromocytoma, IDDM (nicotine causes the release of catecholamines), in active peptic ulcers, in accelerated hypertension, and during lactation.

Side Effects: *NOTE:* The incidence of side effects is complicated by the fact that clients manifest effects of nicotine withdrawal or by concurrent smoking.

Dermatologic: Erythema, pruritus, or burning at the site of application; cutaneous hypersensitivity, sweating, rash at application site. *Body as a whole:* Allergy, back pain. *GI:* Diarrhea, dyspepsia, dry mouth, abdominal pain, constipation, N&V. *Musculoskeletal:* Arthralgia, myalgia. *CNS:* Abnormal dreams, somnolence, dizziness, impaired concentration, headache, insomnia. *CV:* Tachycardia, hypertension. *Respiratory:* Increased cough, pharyngitis, sinusitis. *GU:* Dysmenorrhea.

N

OD **Management of Overdose:** *Symptoms:* Pallor, cold sweat, N&V, abdominal pain, salivation, diarrhea, headache, dizziness, disturbed hearing and vision, mental confusion, weakness, tremor. Large overdoses may cause prostration, hypotension, ***respiratory failure, seizures, and death.*** *Treatment:* Remove the transdermal system immediately. The surface of the skin may be flushed with water and dried; soap should not be used as it may increase the absorption of nicotine. Diazepam or barbiturates may be used to treat seizures and atropine can be given for excessive bronchial secretions or diarrhea. Respiratory support for respiratory failure and fluid support for hypotension and CV collapse. If transdermal systems are ingested PO, activated charcoal should be given to prevent seizures. If the client is unconscious, the charcoal should be administered by an NGT. A saline cathartic or sorbitol added to the first dose of activated charcoal may hasten GI passage of the system. Doses of activated charcoal should be repeated as long as the system remains in the GI tract as nicotine will continue to be released for many hours.

How Supplied: *Film, Extended Release:* 7 mg/24 hr, 14 mg/24 hr, 15 mg/16 hr, 21 mg/24 hr

N

Dosage

- **Transdermal System**

HABITROL (RX)

Healthy clients, initial: 21 mg/day for 4–8 weeks; **then,** 14 mg/day for 2–4 weeks and 7 mg/day for 2–4 weeks. **Light smokers, those who weigh less than 100 lb or who have CV disease:** 14 mg/day for 4–8 weeks; **then,** 7 mg/day for 2–4 weeks.

PROSTEP (RX)

Clients weighing 100 lb or more: 22 mg/day for 4–8 weeks; **then,** 11 mg/day for 2–4 weeks. **Clients weighing less than 100 lb:** 11 mg/day for 4–8 weeks.

NICODERM CQ (OTC)

Light smokers (10 or less cigarettes/day): One 14-mg/24-hr patch for 16 or 24 hr/day for 6 weeks; **then,** one 7-mg/24-hr patch for 16 or 24 hr/day for 2 weeks. **Heavy smokers (>10 cigarettes/day):** One 21-mg/24-hr patch for 16 or 24 hr/day for 6 weeks; **then,** one 14-mg/24-hr patch for 16 or 24 hr/day for 2 weeks, followed by one 7-mg/24-hr patch for 16 or 24 hr for 2 weeks.

NICOTROL (OTC)

Those who smoke > 10 cigarettes/day: 15 mg/day for 6 weeks. The patch is to be worn for 16 hr and removed at bedtime.

HEALTH CARE CONSIDERATIONS

Administration/Storage

1. There will be differences in the duration and length of therapy, depending on the product prescribed.
2. Apply the transdermal system promptly after its removal from the protective pouch to prevent loss of nicotine due to evaporation. Only use systems where the pouch is intact.
3. Apply system once daily to a nonhairy, clean, and dry site on the trunk or upper, outer arm. After 16 or 24 hr (depending on the regimen established), remove the system. When indicated, apply a new system to an alternate skin site. Do not reuse skin sites for at least a week.
4. When a used system is removed, fold it over and place in the protective pouch that contained the new system. Dispose of the used system to prevent access by children or pets.
5. The goal of therapy with nicotine transdermal systems is complete abstinence. If the client has not stopped smoking by the fourth week of therapy, discontinue treatment.
6. Assess the need for dosage adjustment during the first 2 weeks of therapy.
7. Nicotine will continue to be absorbed from the skin for several hours after removal of the system.
8. Do not store systems above 30°C (86°F); sensitive to heat.

Assessment:

1. Record nicotine profile: type and brand (cigarettes, chewing tobacco, or cigars), amount used per day, when used, and what increases usage.
2. Determine any CAD, liver or renal dysfunction.
3. List meds currently prescribed. Cessation of smoking, with or without nicotine replacement, may alter the response to certain drugs.
4. Record any skin disorders; nicotine transdermal systems may be irritating with skin disorders such as atopic or eczematous dermatitis.

Client/Family Teaching

1. Use extreme caution during application; avoid contact with active systems. If contact occurs, wash area with water only. The eyes should not be touched. These systems can be a dermal irritant and cause contact dermatitis.
2. Report any persistent skin irritations such as erythema, edema, or pruritus at the application site as well as any generalized skin reactions such as hives, urticaria, or a generalized rash and remove the system.
3. Follow manufacturer's guidelines for

proper system application. Review information sheet that comes with the product which contains instructions on how to use and dispose of the transdermal systems.
4. Stop smoking completely. If smoking continues, may experience adverse side effects due to higher nicotine levels in the body.
5. Participate in a formal smoking program. The success or failure of smoking cessation depends on the quality, intensity, and frequency of supportive care.
6. Nicotine in any form can be toxic and addictive; transdermal systems may lead to dependence. To minimize this risk, withdraw system gradually after 4–8 weeks of use.
7. Symptoms of nicotine withdrawal include craving, nervousness, restlessness, irritability, mood lability, anxiety, drowsiness, sleep disturbances, impaired concentration, increased appetite, headache, myalgia, constipation, fatigue, and weight gain; report as dosage may require adjustment.
8. Change site of application daily; do not reuse for 1 week.
9. With Nicotrol, remove patch at bedtime and apply upon arising.
10. Keep all products used and unused away from children and pets; sufficient nicotine is still present in used systems to cause toxicity.
11. If therapy is unsuccessful after 4 weeks, discontinue and identify reasons for failure so that a later attempt may be more successful.

Outcome/Evaluate: Smoking cessation; control of nicotine withdrawal symptoms

Nifedipine

(nye-**FED**-ih-peen)

Pregnancy Category: C

Adalat, Adalat CC, Adalat P.A. 10 and 20 ✱, Adalat XL ✱, Apo-Nifed ✱, Apo-Nifed PA ✱, Gen-Nifedipine ✱, Novo-Nifedin ✱, Nu-Nifed ✱, Procardia, Procardia XL, Taro-Nifedipine ✱ **(Rx)**

Classification: Calcium channel blocking agent (antianginal, antihypertensive)

See also *Calcium Channel Blocking Agents*.

Action/Kinetics: Variable effects on AV node effective and functional refractory periods. CO is moderately increased while peripheral vascular resistance is significantly decreased. **Onset:** 20 min. **Peak plasma levels:** 30 min (up to 4 hr for extended-release). **t½:** 2–5 hr. **Therapeutic serum levels:** 0.025–0.1 mcg/mL. **Duration:** 4–8 hr (12 hr for extended-release). Low-fat meals may slow the rate but not the extent of absorption. Metabolized in the liver to inactive metabolites.

Uses: Vasospastic (Prinzmetal's or variant) angina. Chronic stable angina without vasospasm, including angina due to increased effort (especially in clients who cannot take beta blockers or nitrates or who remain symptomatic following clinical doses of these drugs). Essential hypertension (sustained-release only). *Investigational:* PO, sublingually, or chewed in hypertensive emergencies. Also prophylaxis of migraine headaches, primary pulmonary hypertension, severe pregnancy-associated hypertension, esophageal diseases, Raynaud's phenomenon, CHF, asthma, premature labor, biliary and renal colic, and cardiomyopathy. To prevent strokes and to decrease the risk of CHF in geriatric hypertensives.

Contraindications: Hypersensitivity. Lactation.

Special Concerns: Use with caution in impaired hepatic or renal function and in elderly clients. Initial increase in frequency, duration, or severity of angina (may also be seen in clients being withdrawn from beta blockers and who begin taking nifedipine).

Side Effects: *CV:* Peripheral and pulmonary edema, MI, hypotension, palpitations, syncope, CHF (especially if used with a beta blocker), decreased platelet aggregation, arrhythmias, tachycardia. Increased frequency, length, and duration of angina when beginning nifedipine therapy. *GI:* Nausea, diarrhea, constipation, flatulence, abdominal cramps, dysgeusia, vomiting, dry mouth, eructation, gastroesophageal reflux, melena. *CNS:* Dizziness, lightheadedness, giddiness, nervousness, sleep disturbances, headache, weakness, depression, migraine, psychoses, hallucinations, disturbances in equilibrium, somnolence, insomnia, abnormal dreams, malaise, anxiety. *Dermatologic:* Rash, dermatitis, urticaria, pruritus, photosensitivity, erythema multiforme, ***Stevens-Johnson syndrome.*** *Respiratory:* Dyspnea, cough, wheezing, SOB, respiratory infection, throat, nasal, or chest congestion. *Musculoskeletal:* Muscle cramps or inflammation, joint pain or stiffness, arthritis, ataxia, myoclonic dystonia, hypertonia, asthenia. *Hematologic:* Thrombocytopenia, leukopenia, purpura, anemia. *Other:* Fever, chills, sweating, blurred vision, sexual difficulties, flushing, transient blindness, hyperglycemia, hypokalemia, gingival hyperplasia, allergic hepatitis, hepatitis, tinnitus, gynecomastia, polyuria, nocturia, erythromelalgia, weight gain, epistaxis, facial and peri-

N

orbital edema, hypoesthesia, gout, abnormal lacrimation, breast pain, dysuria, hematuria.
Laboratory Test Considerations: ↑ Alkaline phosphatase, CPK, LDH, AST, ALT. Positive Coombs' test.

Additional Drug Interactions
Anticoagulants, oral / Possibility of ↑ PT
Cimetidine / ↑ Bioavailability of nifedipine
Digoxin / ↑ Effect of digoxin by ↓ excretion by kidney
Magnesium sulfate / ↑ Neuromuscular blockade and hypotension
Quinidine / Possible ↓ effect of quinidine due to ↓ plasma levels; ↑ risk of hypotension, bradycardia, AV block, pulmonary edema, and ventricular tachycardia
Ranitidine / ↑ Bioavailability of nifedipine
Theophylline / Possible ↑ effect of theophylline
How Supplied: *Capsule:* 10 mg, 20 mg; *Tablet, Extended Release:* 30 mg, 60 mg, 90 mg

Dosage

• **Capsules**

Individualized. Initial: 10 mg t.i.d. (range: 10–20 mg t.i.d.); **maintenance:** 10–30 mg t.i.d.–q.i.d. Clients with coronary artery spasm may respond better to 20–30 mg t.i.d.–q.i.d. Doses greater than 120 mg/day are rarely needed while doses greater than 180 mg/day are not recommended.

• **Sustained-Release Tablets**

Initial: 30 or 60 mg once daily for Procardia XL and 30 mg once daily for Adalat CC. Titrate over a 7- to 14-day period. Dosage can be increased as required and as tolerated, to a maximum of 120 mg/day for Procardia XL and 90 mg/day for Adalat CC.

Investigational, hypertensive emergencies. 10–20 mg given PO (capsule is punctured several times and then chewed).

HEALTH CARE CONSIDERATIONS

See also *Health Care Considerations* for *Calcium Channel Blocking Agents.*

Administration/Storage

1. Do not exceed a single dose (other than sustained-released) of 30 mg.
2. Before increasing the dose, carefully monitor BP.
3. Use only the sustained-release tablets to treat hypertension.
4. Sublingual nitroglycerin and long-acting nitrates may be used concomitantly with nifedipine.
5. Concomitant therapy with beta-adrenergic blocking agents may be used. In these cases, note any potential drug interactions.
6. Clients withdrawn from beta blockers may manifest symptoms of increased angina which cannot be prevented by nifedipine; in fact, nifedipine may increase the severity of angina in this situation.
7. Clients with angina may be switched to the sustained-release product at the nearest equivalent total daily dose. Use doses greater than 90 mg/day with caution.
8. Protect capsules from light and moisture and store at room temperature in the original container.
9. During initial therapy and when dosage is increased, may experience an increase in the frequency, duration, or severity of angina.
10. Food may decrease the rate but not the extent of absorption; can be taken without regard to meals.

Assessment

1. Record sensitivity to other CCBs.
2. Note any pulmonary edema, ECG abnormalities, or palpitations. Record cardiopulmonary assessment findings.

Interventions

1. During titration period, note any hypotensive response and increased HR that result from peripheral vasodilation; may precipitate angina.
2. Although beta-blocking drugs may be used concomitantly with chronic stable angina, the combined effects of the drugs cannot be predicted (especially with compromised LV function or cardiac conduction abnormalities). Pronounced hypotension, heart block, and CHF may occur.
3. If therapy with a beta blocker is to be discontinued, gradually decrease dosage to prevent withdrawal syndrome.

Client/Family Teaching

1. May take with or without food. Sustained-release tablets should not be chewed or divided.
2. There is no cause for concern if an empty tablet appears in the stool.
3. Maintain a fluid intake of 2–3 L/day to avoid constipation.
4. Do not use OTC agents unless approved; avoid alcohol and caffeine.
5. Report any symptoms of persistent headache, flushing, nausea, palpitations, weight gain, dizziness, or lightheadedness.
6. Perform daily weights and note any extremity swelling. Peripheral edema may result from arterial vasodilatation precipitated by nifedipine or swelling may indicate increasing ventricular dysfunction and should be reported.
7. If also receiving beta-adrenergic blocking agents, report any evidence of hypotension, exacerbation of angina, or evidence of heart failure.

8. Once beta-blocking agents have been discontinued, report increased anginal pain.

Outcome/Evaluate

- ↓ Frequency and intensity of anginal episodes; ↓ BP
- Improved peripheral circulation
- Prevention of strokes and ↓ risk of CHF in geriatric hypertensives

Nilutamide

((nye-**LOO**-tah-myd))

Pregnancy Category: C

Anadron ✦, Nilandron **(Rx)**

Classification: Antineoplastic, hormone

See also *Antineoplastic Agents.*

Action/Kinetics: Antiandrogen activity with no estrogen, progesterone, mineralocorticoid, or glucocorticoid effects. Binds to the androgen receptor, thus preventing the normal androgenic response. Rapidly and completely absorbed from the GI tract. Extensively metabolized with at least one metabolite showing significant activity. Metabolites excreted through the urine. **t½, elimination:** Approximately 41–49 hr.

Uses: In combination with surgical castration for the treatment of metastatic prostate cancer (stage D_2).

Contraindications: Severe hepatic impairment, severe respiratory insufficiency, hypersensitivity to nilutamide.

Special Concerns: Many clients experience a delay in adaptation to the dark ranging from seconds to a few minutes. Safety and efficacy have not been determined in children.

Side Effects: *GI:* Nausea, constipation, dry mouth, diarrhea, hepatitis, GI disorder, ***GI hemorrhage,*** melena. *CNS:* Dizziness, paresthesia, nervousness. *CV:* Hypertension, ***heart failure,*** angina, syncope. *Respiratory:* Interstitial pneumonitis, dyspnea, lung disorder, increased cough, rhinitis. *Metabolic/nutritional:* Edema, weight loss, intolerance to alcohol. *Ophthalmic:* Cataract, photophobia, impaired adaptation to dark, abnormal vision. *Miscellaneous:* Leukopenia, hot flushes, UTI, malaise, pruritus, arthritis, aplastic anemia (rare).

Laboratory Test Considerations: ↑ AST, ALT, alkaline phosphatase, haptoglobin, BUN, creatinine. Hyperglycemia.

Drug Interactions

Phenytoin / ↓ Metabolism of phenytoin → delayed elimination and ↑ risk of toxicity

Theophylline / Metabolism of theophylline delayed elimination and risk of toxicity

Vitamin K antagonists / Metabolism of vitamin K antagonists delayed elimination and risk of toxicity

How Supplied: *Tablet:* 50 mg

Dosage

- **Tablets**

Metastatic prostate cancer.

300 mg (six 50-mg tablets) once daily for 30 days followed by 150 mg (three 50-mg tablets) once daily.

HEALTH CARE CONSIDERATIONS

See also *Health Care Considerations* for *Antineoplastic Agents.*

Administration/Storage

1. To ensure maximum beneficial effects, initiate treatment on the same day as or the day after surgical castration.
2. Protect from light and store at room temperature at 15°C–30°C (59°F–86°F).

Assessment

1. Note duration of symptoms, previous therapy, and the outcome.
2. Give drug on the day of or the day following surgery for prostate cancer.
3. Obtain CBC, LFTs, and CXR. Assess cardiopulmonary status closely; may cause interstitial pneumonitis.

Client/Family Teaching

1. Review guidelines concerning the dosage and dosing frequency.
2. May take with or without food.
3. Wear tinted glasses to prevent delay in adaptation to the dark. Drive cautiously through tunnels or at night.
4. Immediately report any symptoms of chest pain, cough, or SOB.

Outcome/Evaluate: Control of malignant cell proliferation

Nimodipine

(nye-**MOH**-dih-peen)

Pregnancy Category: C

Nimotop, Nimotop I.V. ✦ **(Rx)**

Classification: Calcium channel blocking agent

See also *Calcium Channel Blocking Agents.*

Action/Kinetics: Has a greater effect on cerebral arteries than arteries elsewhere in the body (probably due to its highly lipophilic properties). Mechanism to reduce neurologic deficits following subarachnoid hemorrhage not known. **Peak plasma levels:** 1 hr. **t½:** 1–2 hr. Significantly bound (over 95%) to plasma protein. Undergoes first-pass metabolism in the liver; metabolites excreted through the urine.

Uses: Improvement of neurologic deficits due to spasm following subarachnoid hemorrhage from ruptured congenital intracranial aneurysms; clients should have Hunt and Hess grades of I–III. *Investigational:* Migraine headaches and cluster headaches.

Contraindications: Lactation.

Special Concerns: Safety and efficacy have not been established in children. Use with caution in clients with impaired hepatic function and reduced hepatic blood flow. The half-life may be increased in geriatric clients.

Side Effects: *CV:* Hypotension, peripheral edema, CHF, ECG abnormalities, tachycardia, bradycardia, palpitations, rebound vasospasm, hypertension, hematoma, ***DIC, DVT.*** *GI:* Nausea, dyspepsia, diarrhea, abdominal discomfort, cramps, ***GI hemorrhage,*** vomiting. *CNS:* Headache, depression, lightheadedness, dizziness. *Hepatic:* Abnormal LFT, hepatitis, jaundice. *Hematologic:* Thrombocytopenia, anemia, purpura, ecchymosis. *Dermatologic:* Rash, dermatitis, pruritus, urticaria. *Miscellaneous:* Dyspnea, muscle pain or cramps, acne, itching, flushing, diaphoresis, wheezing, hyponatremia.

N

Laboratory Test Considerations: ↑ Nonfasting BS, LDH, alkaline phosphatase, ALT. ↓ Platelet count.

How Supplied: *Capsule:* 30 mg

Dosage

- **Capsules**

Adults: 60 mg q 4 hr beginning within 96 hr after subarachnoid hemorrhage and continuing for 21 consecutive days. Reduce the dose to 30 mg q 4 hr in clients with hepatic impairment.

HEALTH CARE CONSIDERATIONS

See also *Health Care Considerations* for *Calcium Channel Blocking Agents.*

Administration/Storage: If unable to swallow capsule (e.g., unconscious or at time of surgery), make a hole in both ends of the capsule (soft gelatin) with an 18-gauge needle and withdraw the contents into a syringe. This may be administered into the NG tube and washed down with 30 mL of NSS.

Assessment

1. Obtain baseline labs; reduce dose with hepatic dysfunction.
2. Determine if pregnant.
3. Perform baseline neurologic scores and thoroughly document deficits. Note VS, I&O, and weights.
4. Initiate therapy within 96 hr of subarachnoid hemorrhage.

Client/Family Teaching

1. Take the drug on time; sleep must be interrupted to give the medication q 4 hr ATC for 21 days.
2. Report any side effects such as nausea, lightheadedness, dizziness, muscle cramps, or muscle pain.
3. Report ↑ SOB, the need to take deep breaths on occasion, or wheezing.

Outcome/Evaluate

- ↓ Neurologic deficits R/T venospasm after subarachnoid hemorrhage
- Termination of migraine and cluster headaches

Nisoldipine

(NYE-sohl-dih-peen)

Pregnancy Category: C

Sular **(Rx)**

Classification: Calcium channel blocking drug

Action/Kinetics: Inhibits the transmembrane influx of calcium into vascular smooth muscle and cardiac muscle, resulting in dilation of arterioles. Has greater potency on vascular smooth muscle than on cardiac muscle. Chronic use results in a sustained decrease in vascular resistance and small increases in SI and LV ejection fraction. Weak diuretic effect and no clinically important chronotropic effects. Well absorbed following PO use; however, absolute bioavailability is low due to presystemic metabolism in the gut wall. Foods high in fat result in a significant increase in peak plasma levels. **Maximum plasma levels:** 6–12 hr. **t½, terminal:** 7–12 hr. Almost completely bound to plasma proteins. Metabolized in the liver and excreted through the urine.

Uses: Treatment of hypertension alone or in combination with other antihypertensive drugs.

Contraindications: Use with grapefruit juice as it interferes with metabolism, resulting in a significant increase in plasma levels of the drug. Use in those with known hypersensitivity to dihydropyridine calcium channel blockers. Lactation.

Special Concerns: Geriatric clients may show a two- to threefold higher plasma concentration; use caution in dosing. Use with caution and at lower doses in those with hepatic insufficiency. Use with caution in clients with CHF or compromised ventricular function, especially in combination with a beta blocker.

Side Effects: *CV:* Increased angina and/or MI in clients with CAD. Initially, excessive hypotension, especially in those taking other antihypertensive drugs. Vasodilation, palpitation, atrial fibrillation, ***CVA, MI,*** CHF, first-degree AV block, hypertension, hypotension, jugular venous distension, migraine, postural hypotension, ventricular extrasystoles, SVT, syncope, systolic ejection murmur, T-wave abnormalities on ECG, venous insufficiency. *Body as a whole:* Peripheral edema, cellulitis, chills, facial edema, fever, flu syndrome, malaise. *GI:* Anorexia, nausea, colitis, diarrhea, dry mouth, dyspepsia, dysphagia, flatulence, gastritis, ***GI hemorrhage,*** gingival hyperplasia, glossitis, hepatomegaly, increased appetite, melena, mouth ulceration. *CNS:* Headache, dizziness, abnormal dreams, abnormal thinking and confusion, amnesia, anxiety, ataxia, cerebral ischemia, decreased libido, depression, hypesthesia, hypertonia, insomnia, nervousness, paresthesia, somnolence, tremor, vertigo. *Musculoskeletal:* Arthralgia, arthritis, leg cramps, myalgia, myasthenia, myositis, tenosynovitis. *Hematologic:* Anemia, ecchymoses, leukopenia, petechiae. *Respiratory:* Pharyngitis, sinusitis, asthma, dyspnea, end-inspiratory wheeze and fine rales, epistaxis, increased cough, laryngitis, pleural effusion, rhinitis. *Dermatologic:* Acne, alopecia, dry skin, exfoliative dermatitis, fungal dermatitis, herpes simplex, herpes zoster, maculopapular rash, pruritus, pustular rash, skin discoloration, skin ulcer, sweating, urticaria. *GU:* Dysuria, hematuria, impotence, nocturia, urinary frequency, vaginal hemorrhage, vaginitis. *Metabolic:* Gout, hypokalemia, weight gain or loss. *Ophthalmic:* Abnormal vision, amblyopia, blepharitis, conjunctivitis, glaucoma, itchy eyes, keratoconjunctivitis, retinal detachment, temporary unilateral loss of vision, vitreous floater, watery eyes. *Miscellaneous:* Diabetes mellitus, thyroiditis, chest pain, ear pain, otitis media, tinnitus, taste disturbance.

Laboratory Test Considerations: ↑ Serum creatine kinase, NPN, BUN, serum creatinine. Abnormal LFTs.

OD Management of Overdose: *Symptoms:* Pronounced hypotension. *Treatment:* Active CV support, including monitoring of CV and respiratory function, elevation of extremities, judicious use of calcium infusion, pressor agents, and fluids. Dialysis is not likely to be beneficial, although plasmapheresis may be helpful.

Drug Interactions: Cimetidine significantly ↑ the plasma levels of nislodipine.

How Supplied: *Extended-Release Tablets:* 10 mg, 20 mg, 30 mg, 40 mg.

Dosage

- **Tablets, Extended-Release**

  Hypertension.

Dose must be adjusted to the needs of each person. **Initial:** 20 mg once daily; **then,** increase by 10 mg/week or longer intervals to reach adequate BP control. **Usual maintenance:** 20–40 mg once daily. Doses beyond 60 mg once daily are not recommended. **Initial dose, clients over 65 years and those with impaired renal function:** 10 mg once daily.

HEALTH CARE CONSIDERATIONS

See also *Health Care Considerations* for *Calcium Channel Blocking Agents.*

Administration/Storage

1. Swallow tablets whole; do not chew, divide, or crush.
2. Do not give tablets with grapefruit juice or a high-fat meal.
3. Closely monitor dosage adjustments in clients over age 65 and those with impaired liver function.

Assessment

1. Record indications for therapy, onset and duration of symptoms, agents trialed, and outcome.
2. Reduce dosage in the elderly and with liver dysfunction.
3. Obtain baseline ECG and note any history or evidence of CHF or compromised LV function.
4. List drugs prescribed to ensure none interact unfavorably.

Client/Family Teaching

1. Take as directed; avoid consumption with high-fat foods or grapefruit juices.
2. Headaches, peripheral edema, and dizziness may occur; report if persistent.
3. Report as scheduled for BP evaluation during titration period. Maintain record of BP.

Outcome/Evaluate: ↓ BP

Nitrofurantoin

(nye-troh-fyour-AN-toyn)

Pregnancy Category: B

Apo-Nitrofurantoin ✱, Furadantin **(Rx)**

Nitrofurantoin macrocrystals

(nye-troh-fyour-AN-toyn)

Pregnancy Category: B

Macrobid, Macrodantin, Nephronex ✦, Novo-Furan ✦ **(Rx)**
Classification: Urinary germicide

See also *Anti-Infectives.*

Action/Kinetics: Interferes with bacterial carbohydrate metabolism by inhibiting acetyl coenzyme A; also interferes with bacterial cell wall synthesis. Bacteriostatic at low concentrations and bactericidal at high concentrations. Tablets are readily absorbed from the GI tract; bioavailability is increased by food. **t½:** 20 min (60 min in anephric clients). **Urine levels:** 50–250 mcg/mL. If the C_{CR} is less than 40 mL/min, urine antibacterial levels are inadequate, with the subsequent higher blood levels increasing the possibility of toxicity. Antibacterial activity is best in an acid urine. From 30% to 50% excreted unchanged in the urine. Nitrofurantoin macrocrystals (Macrodantin) are available; this preparation maintains effectiveness while decreasing GI distress.

Uses: UTIs due to susceptible strains of *Escherichia coli, Staphylococcus aureus* (not for treatment of pyelonephritis or perinephric abscesses), enterococci, and certain strains of *Enterobacter* and *Klebsiella.*

Contraindications: Anuria, oliguria, and clients with impaired renal function (C_{CR} below 40 mL/min); pregnant women, especially near term; infants less than 1 month of age; and lactation.

Special Concerns: Use with extreme caution in anemia, diabetes, electrolyte imbalance, avitaminosis B, or a debilitating disease. Safety during lactation has not been established.

Side Effects: Nitrofurantoin is a potentially toxic drug with many side effects. *GI:* N&V, anorexia, diarrhea, abdominal pain, parotitis, pancreatitis. *CNS:* Headache, dizziness, vertigo, drowsiness, nystagmus, confusion, depression, euphoria, psychotic reactions (rare). *Hematologic:* Leukopenia, thrombocytopenia, eosinophilia, megaloblastic anemia, ***agranulocytosis,*** granulocytopenia, ***hemolytic anemia (especially in clients with G6PD deficiency).*** *Allergic:* Drug fever, skin rashes, pruritus, urticaria, angioedema, exfoliative dermatitis, erythema multiforme ***(rarely, Stevens-Johnson syndrome), anaphylaxis,*** arthralgia, myalgia, chills, sialadenitis, asthma symptoms in susceptible clients; maculopapular, erythematous, or eczematous eruption. *Pulmonary:* Sudden onset of dyspnea, cough, chest pain, fever and chills; pulmonary infiltration with consolidation or pleural effusion on x-ray, elevated ESR, eosinophilia. *After subacute or chronic use:* dyspnea, nonproductive cough, malaise, interstitial pneumonitis. Permanent impairment of pulmonary function with chronic therapy. A lupus-like syndrome associated with pulmonary reactions. *Hepatic:* Hepatitis, cholestatic jaundice, chronic active hepatitis, hepatic necrosis (rare). *CV:* Benign intracranial hypertension, changes in ECG, collapse, cyanosis. *Miscellaneous:* Peripheral neuropathy, asthenia, alopecia, superinfections of the GU tract, muscle pain.

Laboratory Test Considerations: ↑ AST, ALT, serum phosphorus. ↓ Hemoglobin.

OD **Management of Overdose:** *Symptoms:* Vomiting (most common). *Treatment:* Induce emesis. High fluid intake to promote urinary excretion. The drug is dialyzable.

Drug Interactions

Acetazolamide / ↓ Effect of nitrofurantoin due to ↑ alkalinity of urine produced by acetazolamide
Antacids, oral / ↓ Effect of nitrofurantoin due to ↓ absorption from GI tract
Anticholinergic drugs / ↑ Effect of nitrofurantoin due to ↑ absorption from stomach
Magnesium trisilicate / ↓ Absorption of nitrofurantoin from GI tract
Nalidixic acid / Nitrofurantoin ↓ effect of nalidixic acid
Probenecid / High doses ↓ secretion of nitrofurantoin → toxicity
Sodium bicarbonate / ↓ Effect of nitrofurantoin due to ↑ alkalinity of urine produced by sodium bicarbonate

How Supplied: *Capsule:* 25 mg, 50 mg, 100 mg; *Suspension:* 25 mg/5 mL (Nitrofurantoin)

Dosage

- **Capsules, Oral Suspension**

UTIs.

Adults: 50–100 mg q.i.d., not to exceed 600 mg/day. For cystitis, Macrobid is given in doses of 100 mg b.i.d. for 7 days. **Pediatric, 1 month of age and over:** 5–7 mg/kg/day in four equal doses.

Prophylaxis of UTIs.

Adults: 50–100 mg at bedtime. **Pediatric, 1 month of age and over:** 1 mg/kg/day at bedtime or in two divided doses daily.

HEALTH CARE CONSIDERATIONS

See also *General Health Care Considerations for All Anti-Infectives.*

Administration/Storage

1. Administer capsules containing crystals, instead of tablets; crystals cause less GI intolerance.
2. Store PO medications in amber-colored bottles.

3. Continue for at least 3 days after obtaining a negative urine culture.

Assessment

1. Monitor CBC, urine C&S, liver and renal functions; also CXR and PFTs with chronic therapy.
2. Observe for acute or delayed-onset anaphylactic reaction.
3. Drug may alter certain lab results.
4. Monitor for recurrent UTI symptoms; urinary superinfections may occur.
5. Blacks and ethnic groups of Mediterranean and Near Eastern origin should be assessed for symptoms of anemia.

Client/Family Teaching

1. Take with food or milk to minimize gastric irritation and enhance absorption; complete full course of therapy.
2. Increase fluid intake; drink at least 2 qt/day of water. Acidic foods (prunes, cranberry juice, plums) enhance drug action whereas alkaline foods (milk products) minimize drug action.
3. Acid urine enhances antibacterial activity. Drug may turn urine a dark yellow or brown color.
4. Report any persistent or bothersome side effects. Respiratory dysfunction requires immediate intervention.
5. Immediately report any numbness and tingling of extremities or flu-like symptoms; indications for drug withdrawal because condition may worsen and become irreversible.
6. Report persistent N&V and diarrhea as these may be symptoms of a GI superinfection.

Outcome/Evaluate

- Negative urine culture results
- Resolution of infection; symptomatic improvement (↓ dysuria, ↓ frequency)

Nitroglycerin sublingual

(nye-troh-**GLIH**-sir-in)
Pregnancy Category: C
Nitrostat **(Rx)**
Classification: Antianginal agent (coronary vasodilator)

See also *Antianginal Drugs, Nitrates/Nitrites.*

Action/Kinetics: Sublingual. Onset: 1–3 min; **duration:** 30–60 min.

Uses: Agents of choice for prophylaxis and treatment of angina pectoris.

Special Concerns: Dosage has not been established in children.

How Supplied: *Tablet:* 0.3 mg, 0.4 mg, 0.6 mg

Dosage

- **Sublingual Tablets**

150–600 mcg under the tongue or in the buccal pouch at first sign of attack; may be repeated in 5 min if necessary (no more than 3 tablets should be taken within 15 min). For prophylaxis, tablets may be taken 5–10 min prior to activities that may precipitate an attack.

HEALTH CARE CONSIDERATIONS

See also *Health Care Considerations* for *Antianginal Drugs, Nitrates/Nitrites.*

Administration/Storage

1. Place sublingual tablets under the tongue and allow to dissolve; do not swallow.
2. Store in the original container at room temperature protected from moisture. Discard unused tablets if 6 months has elapsed since the original container was opened.

Client/Family Teaching

1. Date sublingual container upon opening (usually only good for 6 months).
2. Let tablet dissolve under the tongue; may sting when it comes in contact with the mucosa.
3. Take *before* stressful activity, i.e., exercise, sex.
4. Report immediately if pain is not controlled with prescribed dosage.

Outcome/Evaluate

- Angina prophylaxis
- Termination of anginal attack

Nitroglycerin sustained-release capsules

(nye-troh-**GLIH**-sir-in)
Pregnancy Category: C
Nitroglyn **(Rx)**

Nitroglycerin sustained-release tablets

(nye-troh-**GLIH**-sir-in)
Pregnancy Category: C
Nitrogard-SR ✱, Nitrong, Nitrong SR ✱ **(Rx)**
Classification: Antianginal agent (coronary vasodilator)

See also *Antianginal Drugs, Nitrates/Nitrites.*

Action/Kinetics: Sustained-release. Onset: 20–45 min; **duration:** 3–8 hr.

Uses: To prevent anginal attacks. "Possibly effective" for the prophylaxis or treatment of anginal attacks.

N

Special Concerns: Dosage has not been established in children.
How Supplied: Nitroclycerin sustained-release capsules: *Capsule, Extended Release:* 2.5 mg, 6.5 mg, 9 mg. Nitroglycerin sustained-release tablets: *Tablet, Extended Release:* 2 mg

Dosage

- **Sustained-Release Capsules**

2.5, 6.5, or 9 mg q 8–12 hr.

- **Sustained-Release Tablets**

1.3, 2.6, or 6.5 mg q 8–12 hr.

HEALTH CARE CONSIDERATIONS

See also *Health Care Considerations* for *Antianginal Drugs, Nitrates/Nitrites.*

Administration/Storage

1. Do not chew sustained-release tablets and capsules; not intended for sublingual use.
2. Give the smallest effective dose 2–4 times/day.
3. Tolerance may develop.

Outcome/Evaluate: Angina prophylaxis

N

Nitroglycerin topical ointment

(nye-troh-**GLIH**-sir-in)
Pregnancy Category: C
Nitro-Bid, Nitrol, Nitrol TSAR Kit ✱, Nitrong ✱ **(Rx)**
Classification: Antianginal agent (coronary vasodilator)

See also *Antianginal Drugs, Nitrates/Nitrites.*
Action/Kinetics: Onset: 30–60 min; **duration:** 2–12 hr (depending on amount used per unit of surface area).
Uses: Prophylaxis and treatment of angina pectoris due to CAD.
Special Concerns: Dosage has not been established in children.
How Supplied: *Ointment:* 2%

Dosage

- **Topical Ointment (2%)**

1–2 in. (15–30 mg) q 8 hr; up to 4–5 in. (60–75 mg) q 4 hr may be necessary. One inch equals approximately 15 mg nitroglycerin. Determine optimum dosage by starting with ½ in. q 8 hr and increasing by ½ in. with each successive dose until headache occurs; then, decrease to largest dose that does not cause headache. When ending treatment, reduce both the dose and frequency of administration over 4–6 weeks to prevent sudden withdrawal reactions.

HEALTH CARE CONSIDERATIONS

See also *Health Care Considerations* for *Antianginal Drugs, Nitrates/Nitrites.*

Client/Family Teaching

1. Squeeze ointment carefully onto dose-measuring application papers, which are packaged with the medicine. Use applicator to spread ointment or fold paper in half and rub back and forth.
2. Use the paper to spread the ointment onto a nonhairy area of skin. Application to the chest may be psychologically helpful, but may be applied to other nonhairy areas.
3. Rotate sites to prevent irritation. Keep a record of areas used to avoid unnecessary repetitive use of sites.
4. Apply ointment in a thin, even layer covering an area of skin 5–6 in. in diameter; remove last dose.
5. Date and tape the application paper over the area, or cover the area with a piece of plastic wrap-type material. A clear plastic cover causes less leakage of ointment, decreases skin irritation, increases the amount absorbed, and prevents clothing stains.
6. Once the dose is established, use the same type of covering to ensure that the same amount of drug is absorbed during each application.
7. Clean around tube opening and tightly cap tube after use.
8. To prevent systemic absorption protect skin from contact with ointment. Wash hands thoroughly after application to avoid headache.
9. Remove at bedtime or as directed to prevent tolerance or loss of drug effect. Remember to reapply upon awakening the next morning.

Outcome/Evaluate: Termination/prevention of anginal episodes

Nitroglycerin transdermal system

(nye-troh-**GLIH**-sir-in)
Pregnancy Category: C
Deponit 0.2 mg/hr and 0.4 mg/hr, Minitran 0.1 mg/hr, 0.2 mg/hr, 0.4 mg/hr, and 0.6 mg/hr, Nitrek 0.2 mg/hr, 0.4 mg/hr, and 0.6 mg/hr, Nitrodisc 0.2 mg/hr, 0.3 mg/hr, and 0.4 mg/hr, Nitro-Dur 0.1 mg/hr, 0.2 mg/hr, 0.3 mg/hr, 0.4 mg/hr, 0.6 mg/hr, and 0.8 mg/hr, Transderm-Nitro 0.1 mg/hr, 0.2 mg/hr, 0.4 mg/hr, and 0.6 mg/hr **(Rx)**
Classification: Antianginal agent (coronary vasodilator)

See also *Antianginal Drugs, Nitrates/Nitrites.*

Action/Kinetics: Onset: 30–60 min; **duration:** 8–24 hr. The amount released each hour is indicated in the name.
Uses: Prophylaxis of angina pectoris due to CAD. *NOTE:* There is some evidence that nitroglycerin patches stop preterm labor.
Special Concerns: Dosage has not been established in children.
How Supplied: *Film, Extended Release:* 0.1 mg/hr, 0.2 mg/hr, 0.3 mg/hr, 0.4 mg/hr, 0.6 mg/hr, 0.8 mg/hr

Dosage

- **Topical Patch**

Initial: 0.2–0.4 mg/hr (initially the smallest available dose in the dosage series) applied each day to skin site free of hair and free of excessive movement (e.g., chest, upper arm). **Maintenance:** Additional systems or strengths may be added depending on the clinical response.

HEALTH CARE CONSIDERATIONS

See also *Health Care Considerations* for *Antianginal Drugs, Nitrates/Nitrites.*
Administration/Storage
1. Follow instructions for specific products on package insert.
2. When terminating therapy, gradually reduce the dose and frequency of application over 4–6 weeks.
3. Tolerance is a significant factor affecting efficacy if the system is used continuously for more than 12 hr/day. Thus, a dosage regimen would include a daily period where the patch is on for 12–14 hr and a period of 10–12 hr when the patch is off (i.e., while asleep).
4. Remove patch before defibrillating as patch may explode.
5. The various products differ in the mechanism for the delivery system; the most important factor is the amount of drug released per hour. A wide range of client variability will be noted. Variables in the rate of absorption include the skin, physical exercise, and elevated ambient temperature.
Client/Family Teaching
1. Apply only as directed. Dry skin completely before applying.
2. Remove old pad and rotate application sites each day to avoid skin irritation. Do not apply to distal extremities.
3. Date patch as a reminder that drug has been administered.
4. Once applied, do not disturb or open patch. Do not stop abruptly.
5. Remove at bedtime or as directed to prevent a diminished response (tolerance) to the drug. Remember to reapply a new system upon awakening the next morning.
6. Bathing or swimming should not interfere with therapy.
Outcome/Evaluate: Control/prevention of anginal episodes

Nitroglycerin translingual spray

(nye-troh-**GLIH**-sir-in)
Pregnancy Category: C
Nitrolingual **(Rx)**
Classification: Antianginal agent (coronary vasodilator)

See also *Antianginal Drugs, Nitrates/Nitrites.*
Action/Kinetics: Onset: 2 min; **duration:** 30–60 min.
Uses: Coronary artery disease to relieve an acute attack or used prophylactically 10–15 min before beginning activities that can cause an acute anginal attack.
Special Concerns: Dosage has not been established in children.
How Supplied: *Spray:* 0.4 mg/Spray

Dosage

- **Spray**

Termination of acute attack.
One to two metered doses (400–800 mcg) on or under the tongue q 5 min as needed; no more than three metered doses should be administered within a 15-min period.
Prophylaxis.
One to two metered doses 5–10 min before beginning activities that might precipitate an acute attack.

HEALTH CARE CONSIDERATIONS

See also *Health Care Considerations* for *Antianginal Drugs, Nitrates/Nitrites.*
Client/Family Teaching
1. Do *not* inhale the spray. Spray under the tongue.
2. Seek immediate medical attention if chest pain persists.
Outcome/Evaluate: Control/prevention of acute anginal episodes

Nizatidine

(nye-**ZAY**-tih-deen)
Pregnancy Category: C
Apo-Nizatidine ✱, Axid **(Rx)**, Axid AR **(OTC)**
Classification: Histamine H_2 receptor antagonist

N

See also *Histamine H_2 Antagonists.*

Action/Kinetics: Decreases gastric acid secretion by blocking the effect of histamine on histamine H_2 receptors. Does not affect the P-450 and P-448 drug metabolizing enzymes. **Onset:** 30 min. **Peak plasma levels:** 0.5–3 hr after a PO dose. **Time to peak effect:** 0.5–3 hr. **Duration, nocturnal:** Up to 12 hr; **basal:** Up to 8 hr. **t½:** 1–2 hr. Approximately 60% of a PO dose is excreted unchanged in the urine. Clients with moderate to severe renal impairment manifest a significant prolongation of t½ with decreased clearance.

Uses: Treatment of acute duodenal ulcer and maintenance following healing of a duodenal ulcer. GERD, including erosive and ulcerative esophagitis. Short-term treatment of benign gastric ulcer. OTC use to prevent meal-induced heartburn.

Contraindications: Hypersensitivity to H_2 receptor antagonists. Cirrhosis of the liver, impaired renal or hepatic function. Lactation.

Special Concerns: Safety and efficacy have not been determined in children.

Side Effects: *CNS:* Headache, fatigue, somnolence, insomnia, dizziness, abnormal dreams, anxiety, nervousness, confusion (rare). *GI:* N&V, diarrhea, pancreatitis, constipation, abdominal discomfort, flatulence, dyspepsia, anorexia, dry mouth. *Dermatologic:* Exfoliative dermatitis, erythroderma, pruritus, urticaria, erythema multiforme. *CV:* Asymptomatic VT; ***rarely, cardiac arrhythmias or arrest following rapid IV use.*** *Respiratory:* Rhinitis, pharyngitis, sinusitis, cough. *Body as a whole:* Asthenia, back pain, chest pain, infection, fever, myalgia. *Miscellaneous:* Impotence, loss of libido, thrombocytopenia, sweating, gynecomastia, hyperuricemia, eosinophilia, gout, and cholestatic or hepatocellular effects (resulting in increased AST, ALT, or alkaline phosphatase).

Laboratory Test Considerations: False + test for urobilinogen.

Drug Interactions

Antacids containing Al and Mg hydroxides / ↓ Nizatidine absorption by about 10%

Aspirin, high doses / ↑ Salicylate serum levels

Simethicone / ↓ Nizatidine absorption by about 10%

How Supplied: *Capsule:* 150 mg, 300 mg; *Tablet:* 75 mg

Dosage

AXID

• **Capsules**

Active duodenal ulcer.

Adults: Either 300 mg once daily at bedtime or 150 mg b.i.d. If the C_{CR} is 20–50 mL/min: 150 mg/day; if C_{CR} is less than 20 mL/min: 150 mg every other day.

Prophylaxis following healing of duodenal ulcer.

Adults: 150 mg/day at bedtime. If C_{CR} is 20–50 mL/min: 150 mg every other day; if C_{CR} is less than 20 mL/min: 150 mg every 3 days.

Treatment of benign gastric ulcer.

Adults: 150 mg b.i.d. or 300 mg at bedtime

GERD, including erosive and ulcerative esophagitis.

Adults: 150 mg b.i.d.

AXID AR

• **Tablets**

Heartburn.

1 tablet b.i.d.

HEALTH CARE CONSIDERATIONS

See also *Health Care Considerations* for *Histamine H_2 Antagonists.*

Administration/Storage

1. Maintain treatment for active duodenal ulcer for up to 8 weeks.
2. Gastric malignancy may be present even though a clinical response to nizatidine has occurred.
3. Doses of 150 and 300 mg can be mixed with commercial juices (apple juice, *Gatorade, Ocean Spray,* and others); such preparations are stable for 48 hr when refrigerated. However, a 10% loss in potency is seen if mixed with *V8* or *Cran-Grape* juices.

Assessment

1. Record type, onset, location, and characteristics of symptoms.
2. Note any allergies to H_2 receptor antagonists.
3. Monitor hepatic and renal function studies; reduce dosage with renal insufficiency.
4. Note *H. pylori* results and diagnostic findings, i.e., radiographic and/or endoscopic.

Client/Family Teaching

1. Take at bedtime due to potential sedative effects.
2. Use caution when performing tasks that require mental alertness until drug effects realized.
3. Continue to take as ordered even if symptoms subside.
4. Report any rashes, flaking of skin, or extreme sleepiness.
5. Avoid alcohol, caffeine, spicy foods, and aspirin-containing products.
6. Do not smoke, as this interferes with drug's effects.

Outcome/Evaluate: Improvement in ulcer pain/irritation; ↓ GERD S&S

Norfloxacin

(nor-**FLOX**-ah-sin)

Pregnancy Category: C

Chibroxin Ophthalmic Solution, Noroxin, Noroxin Ophthalmic Solution ✱ **(Rx)**

Classification: Fluoroquinolone anti-infective

See also *Anti-Infectives* and *Fluoroquinolones.*

Action/Kinetics: Active against gram-positive and gram-negative organisms by inhibiting bacterial DNA synthesis. Not effective against obligate anaerobes. **Peak plasma levels:** 1.4–1.6 mcg/mL after 1–2 hr following a dose of 400 mg and 2.5 mcg/mL 1–2 hr after a dose of 800 mg. **t½:** 3–4.5 hr. Food decreases the absorption of norfloxacin. Approximately 30% excreted unchanged in the urine and 30% through the feces.

Uses: **Systemic:** Uncomplicated UTIs caused by *Escherichia coli, Klebsiella pneumoniae, Enterobacter cloacae, Proteus mirabilis, P. vulgaris, Pseudomonas aeruginosa, Citrobacter freundii, Staphylococcus aureus, S. epidermidis, Enterococcus faecalis, Enterobacter aerogenes, S. saprophyticus,* and *S. agalactiae*. Complicated UTIs caused by *Enterococcus faecalis, E. coli, K. pneumoniae, P. mirabilis, P. aeruginosa,* or *Serratia marcescens*. Urethral gonorrhea and endocervical gonococcal infections due to penicillinase- or non-penicillinase-producing *Neisseria gonorrhoeae*. Prostatitis due to *E. coli*.

Ophthalmic: Superficial ocular infections involving the cornea or conjunctiva due to *Staphylococcus, S. aureus, Streptococcus pneumoniae, E. coli, Haemophilus aegyptius, H. influenzae, Klebsiella pneumoniae, Neisseria gonorrhoeae, Proteus* species, *Enterobacter aerogenes, Serratia marcescens, Pseudomonas aeruginosa,* and *Vibrio* species.

Contraindications: Hypersensitivity to nalidixic acid, cinoxacin, or norfloxacin. Lactation, infants, and children. Ophthalmic use for dendritic keratitis, vaccinia, varicella, mycobacterial infections of the eye, fungal disease of the eye, and use with steroid combinations after uncomplicated removal of a corneal foreign body.

Special Concerns: Use with caution in clients with a history of seizures and in impaired renal function. Geriatric clients eliminate norfloxacin more slowly.

Side Effects: See also *Side Effects* for *Fluoroquinolones.*

GI: N&V, diarrhea, abdominal pain or discomfort, dry/painful mouth, dyspepsia, flatulence, constipation, pseudomembranous colitis, stomatitis. *CNS:* Headache, dizziness, fatigue, malaise, drowsiness, depression, insomnia, confusion, psychoses. *Hematologic:* Decreased hematocrit, eosinophilia, leukopenia, neutropenia, either increased or decreased platelets. *Dermatologic:* Photosensitivity, rash, pruritus, exfoliative dermatitis, ***toxic epidermal necrolysis,*** erythema, erythema multiforme, ***Stevens-Johnson syndrome.*** *Other:* Paresthesia, hypersensitivity, fever, visual disturbances, hearing loss, crystalluria, cylindruria, candiduria, myoclonus (rare), hepatitis, pancreatitis, arthralgia.

Following ophthalmic use: Conjunctival hyperemia, photophobia, chemosis, bitter taste in mouth.

Laboratory Test Considerations: ↑ AST, ALT, alkaline phosphatase, BUN, serum creatinine, and LDH.

Additional Drug Interactions: Nitrofurantoin ↓ antibacterial effect of norfloxacin.

How Supplied: *Ophthalmic solution:* 0.3%; *Tablet:* 400 mg

Dosage

- **Tablets**

Uncomplicated UTIs due to E. coli, K. pneumoniae, or P. mirabilis.

400 mg q 12 hr for 3 days.

Uncomplicated UTIs due to other organisms.

400 mg q 12 hr for 7–10 days.

Complicated UTIs.

400 mg q 12 hr for 10–21 days. Maximum dose for UTIs should not exceed 800 mg/day.

Uncomplicated gonorrhea.

800 mg as a single dose.

Impaired renal function, with C_{CR} equal to or less than 30 mL/min/1.73 m².

400 mg/day for 7–10 days.

Prostatis due to E. coli.

400 mg q 12 hr for 28 days.

- **Ophthalmic Solution**

Acute infections.

Initially, 1–2 gtt q 15–30 min; **then,** reduce frequency as infection is controlled.

Moderate infections.

1–2 gtt 4–6 times/day.

HEALTH CARE CONSIDERATIONS

See also *Health Care Considerations* for *Fluoroquinolones.*

Assessment

1. Record indications for therapy, type, location, and duration of symptoms.
2. Note any seizure disorder or impaired re-

N

nal function; reduce dose with impaired function.
3. Obtain CBC and cultures.
4. Determine if pregnant.

Client/Family Teaching
1. Take 1 hr before or 2 hr after meals, with a glass of water; food decreases drug absorption.
2. Take at evenly spaced intervals, generally every 12 hr.
3. Antacids should not be taken with or for 2 hr after dosing.
4. To prevent crystalluria consume 2–3 L/day of fluids.
5. Use caution if operating equipment or driving a motor vehicle; may cause dizziness.
6. Females of childbearing age should practice contraception.
7. Avoid prolonged sun exposure; wear sunglasses, protective clothing, and a sunscreen to prevent photosensitivity reactions.

Outcome/Evaluate
- Negative culture reports
- Symptomatic improvement (with UTI: ↓ dysuria, hematuria, and frequency; with ophthalmic use: ↓ itching, burning, and discharge).

N

Nortriptyline hydrochloride

(nor-TRIP-tih-leen)

Pregnancy Category: C

Apo-Nortriptyline ✱, Aventyl, Gen-Nortriptyline ✱, Norventyl ✱, Novo-Nortriptyline ✱, Nu-Nortriptyline ✱, PMS-Nortriptyline ✱, Pamelor **(Rx)**

Classification: Antidepressant, tricyclic

See also *Antidepressants, Tricyclic.*

Action/Kinetics: Manifests moderate anticholinergic and sedative effects but slight orthostatic hypotensive effects. **Effective plasma levels:** 50–150 ng/mL. **t½:** 18–44 hr. **Time to reach steady state:** 4–19 days.

Uses: Treatment of symptoms of depression. Chronic, severe neurogenic pain. Dermatologic disorders including chronic urticaria, angioedema, and nocturnal pruritus in atopic eczema.

Contraindications: Use in children (safety and efficacy have not been determined).

Laboratory Test Considerations: ↓ Urinary 5-HIAA.

How Supplied: *Capsule:* 10 mg, 25 mg, 50 mg, 75 mg; *Solution:* 10 mg/5 mL

Dosage

- **Capsules, Oral Solution**

Depression.

Adults: 25 mg t.i.d.–q.i.d. Dose individualized; begin at a low dosage and increase as needed. **Doses above 150 mg/day are not recommended. Elderly clients:** 30–50 mg/day in divided doses.

Dermatologic disorders.

75 mg/day.

HEALTH CARE CONSIDERATIONS

See also *Health Care Considerations* for *Antidepressants, Tricyclic.*

Administration/Storage: Store at controlled room temperatures.

Assessment: Record indications for therapy, type, onset, and characteristics of symptoms. Identify any causative factors.

Client/Family Teaching: Take after meals and at bedtime to minimize GI upset.

Outcome/Evaluate
- Control of symptoms of depression (↓ fatigue, improved sleeping/eating patterns, effective coping)
- ↓ Nocturnal pruritus
- Relief of chronic neurogenic pain

Nystatin

(nye-STAT-in)

Pregnancy Category: C (A for vaginal use)

Tablets: Mycostatin, Nilstat. **Oral Suspension:** Mycostatin, Nadostine ✱, Nilstat, Nystex, PMS Nystatin ✱. **Troches:** Mycostatin Pastilles. **Vaginal Tablets:** Mycostatin, Nadostine ✱, **Topical:** Mycostatin, Nadostine ✱, Nilstat, Nyaderm ✱, Nystex, Nystop, **Topical Powder:** Candistatin ✱, Nystop **(Rx)**

Classification: Antibiotic, antifungal

See also *Anti-Infectives.*

Action/Kinetics: Derived from *Streptomyces noursei*; is both fungistatic and fungicidal against all species of *Candida*. Binds to fungal cell membranes (sterols), resulting in altered cellular permeability and leakage of potassium and other essential intracellular components. Poorly absorbed from the GI tract; unabsorbed nystatin is excreted in the feces.

Uses: *Candida* infections of the skin, mucous membranes, GI tract, vagina, and mouth (thrush). The drug is too toxic for systemic infections although it can be given PO for intestinal moniliasis infections, as it is not absorbed from the GI tract.

Contraindications: Use for systemic mycoses. Use of topical products in or around the eyes.

Special Concerns: Do not use occlusive dressings when treating candidiasis. Do not use lozenges in children less than 5 years of age.

Side Effects: Nystatin has few toxic effects. *GI:* Epigastric distress, N&V, diarrhea. *Other:* Rarely, irritation.

How Supplied: *Capsule:* 500,000 U, 1 million U; *Cream:* 100,000 U/gm; *Lozenge/troche:* 200,000 U; *Ointment:* 100,000 U/gm; *Powder:* 100,000 U/gm; *Suspension:* 100,000 U/mL; *Tablet:* 100,000 U, 500,000 U

Dosage

- **Capsule, Lozenge, Oral Suspension, Tablets**

Intestinal candidiasis.

Tablets, 500,000–1,000,000 units t.i.d.; continue treatment for 48 hr after cure to prevent relapse.

Oral candidiasis.

Oral Suspension, adults and children: 400,000–600,000 units q.i.d. (1/2 dose in each side of mouth, held as long as possible before swallowing); **infants:** 200,000 units q.i.d. (same procedure as with adults); **premature or low birth weight infants:** 100,000 units q.i.d. **Lozenge, adults and children:** 200,000–400,000 units 4–5 times/day, up to 14 days. *NOTE:* Lozenges should not be chewed or swallowed.

- **Vaginal Tablets**

100,000 units (1 tablet) inserted in vagina once each day for 2 weeks.

- **Topical Cream, Ointment, Powder (100,000 units/g each)**

Apply to affected areas b.i.d.–t.i.d., or as indicated, until healing is complete.

HEALTH CARE CONSIDERATIONS

See also *General Health Care Considerations for All Anti-Infectives.*

Administration/Storage

1. A powder for extemporaneous compounding of the oral suspension is available. To reconstitute, add 1/8 tsp of the powder (about 500,000 units) to approximately 1/2–1 cup water and stir well. This product is administered immediately after mixing.
2. Protect drug from heat, light, moisture, and air.
3. The suspension can be stored for 7 days at room temperature or for 10 days in the refrigerator without loss of potency.
4. For *Candida* infections of the feet, the powder can be freely dusted on the feet as well as in socks and shoes.
5. The cream is generally used in *Candida* infections involving intertriginous areas; treat moist lesions with powder.
6. Refrigerate vaginal tablets.

Assessment

1. Record onset, location, duration, and clinical presentation of symptoms.
2. Assess carefully and monitor recovery; severe oral candidiasis especially after XRT may include the esophagus and require systemic therapy as opposed to topical applications.

Client/Family Teaching

1. Review the appropriate method and technique for administration. Use as directed for the amount of time designated to ensure desired results.
2. Do not mix oral suspension in foods because the medication will be inactivated.
3. Drop 1 mL of oral suspension in each side of mouth or apply with a swab to treat oral moniliasis. Swish around and keep in the mouth as long as possible before swallowing.
4. For pediatric use, 250,000 units of cherry flavor nystatin has been frozen in the form of popsicles.
5. Do not use mouthwash with oral candidiasis as this may alter normal flora and promote infections.
6. Vaginal tablets may be administered PO for candidiasis. These should be sucked on as a lozenge and not chewed or swallowed.
7. Insert vaginal tablets high in vagina with applicator.
8. Continue using vaginal tablets even when menstruating; treatment should be continued for 2 weeks. Avoid tampons.
9. Continue vaginal tablets in the gravid client for 3–6 weeks before term to reduce incidence of thrush in the newborn.
10. Discontinue and report if vaginal tablets cause irritation, redness, or swelling.
11. Drug may stain; sanitary pads may help protect clothing and linens.
12. Apply cream or ointment to mycotic lesions with a swab or wear gloves to avoid direct contact with hands as contact dermatitis may ensue.
13. To prevent reinfection, avoid intercourse during therapy or use condoms. Advise partner to seek treatment if symptomatic.
14. Report lack of response, worsening of symptoms or adverse side effects .

Outcome/Evaluate

- Negative culture results
- Improvement in skin and mucous membrane irritation with less discomfort and itching

N

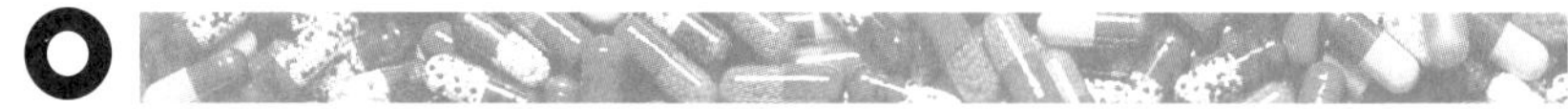

Ofloxacin

(oh-FLOX-ah-zeen)
Pregnancy Category: C
Floxin, Floxin Otic, Ocuflox **(Rx)**
Classification: Antibacterial, fluoroquinolone

See also *Anti-Infectives.*

Action/Kinetics: Effective against a wide range of gram-positive and gram-negative aerobic and anaerobic bacteria. Penicillinase has no effect on the activity of ofloxacin. Widely distributed to body fluids. **Maximum serum levels:** 1–2 hr. **t½, first phase:** 5–7 hr; **second phase:** 20–25 hr. **Peak serum levels at steady state, after PO doses:** 1.5 mcg/mL after 200-mg doses, 2.4 mcg/mL after 300-mg doses, and 2.9 mcg/mL after 400-mg doses. Between 70% and 80% is excreted unchanged in the urine.

Uses: Systemic: Pneumonia or acute bacterial exacerbations of chronic bronchitis or community-acquired pneumonia due to *Haemophilus influenzae* or *Streptococcus pneumoniae*. Not a drug of first choice in the treatment of presumed or confirmed pneumococcal pneumonia. Not effective for syphilis.

Acute, uncomplicated urethral and cervical gonorrhea due to *Neisseria gonorrhoeae;* nongonococcal urethritis, and cervicitis due to *Chlamydia trachomatis*. Mixed infections of the urethra and cervix due to *N. gonorrhoeae* and *C. trachomatis.*

Mild to moderate skin and skin structure infections due to *Staphylococcus aureus, Streptococcus pyogenes,* or *Proteus mirabilis.*

Uncomplicated cystitis due to *Citrobacter diversus, Enterobacter aerogenes, E. coli, Klebsiella pneumoniae, Proteus mirabilis,* or *Pseudomonas aeruginosa*. Complicated UTIs due to *Escherichia coli, K. pneumoniae, P. mirabilis, C. diversus,* or *P. aeruginosa*. Prostatitis due to *E. coli*. Monotherapy for PID.

Ophthalmic: Treatment of conjunctivitis caused by *S. aureus, Staphylococcus epidermidis, S. pneumoniae, Enterobacter cloacae, H. influenzae, P. mirabilis,* and *P. aeruginosa*. Corneal ulcers caused by susceptible organisms.

Otic: Otitis externa due to *S. aureus* and *P. aeruginosa* in clients one year of age and older. Acute otitis media with tympanostomy tubes due to *S. aureus, S. pneumoniae, H. influenzae, Moraxella catarrhalis,* and *P. aeruginosa* (from age one to twelve). Chronic suppurative otitis media due to *S. aureus, P. mirabilis,* and *P. aeruginosa* in those twelve years and older who have perforated tympanic membranes.

Contraindications: Hypersensitivity to quinolone antibacterial agents. Use during lactation. Use for syphilis (ineffective). Ophthalmic use in dendritic keratitis, vaccinia, varicella, mycobacterial infections of the eye, fungal diseases of the eye, and with steroid combinations after uncomplicated removal of a corneal foreign body.

Special Concerns: Safety and effectiveness of the systemic forms have not been established in children, adolescents under the age of 18 years, pregnant women, and lactating women. Safety and effectiveness of the ophthalmic form have not been established in children less than 1 year of age. Use with caution in clients with known or suspected CNS disorders such as severe cerebral atherosclerosis, epilepsy, or factors that predispose to seizures.

Side Effects: See also *Side Effects* for *Fluroquinolones.*

GI: Nausea, diarrhea, vomiting, abdominal pain or discomfort, dry or painful mouth, dyspepsia, flatulence, constipation, pseudomembranous colitis, dysgeusia, decreased appetite. *CNS:* Headache, dizziness, fatigue, malaise, somnolence, depression, insomnia, seizures, sleep disorders, nervousness, anxiety, cognitive change, dream abnormality, euphoria, hallucinations, vertigo. *CV:* Chest pain, edema, hypertension, palpitations, vasodilation. *Hypersensitivity reactions:* Dyspnea, ***anaphylaxis.*** *GU:* External genital pruritus in women, vaginitis, vaginal discharge; burning, irritation, pain, and rash of the female genitalia; glucosuria, proteinuria, hematuria, pyuria, dysmenorrhea, menorrhagia, metrorrhagia, urinary frequency or pain. *Respiratory:* Cough, rhinorrhea. *Dermatologic:* Diaphoresis, vasculitis, photosensitivity, rash, pruritus. *Hematologic:* Leukocytosis, lymphocytopenia, eosinophilia. *Musculoskeletal:* Asthenia, extremity pain, arthralgia, myalgia, possibility of osteochondrosis. *Miscellaneous:* Chills, malaise, syncope, hyperglycemia or hypoglycemia, whole body pain, thirst, weight loss, photophobia, trunk pain, paresthesia, visual disturbances, hypersensitivity, hearing loss, fever.

After ophthalmic use: Transient ocular burning or discomfort, stinging, redness, itching, photophobia, tearing, and dryness.

After otic use: Pruritus, application site re-

action, dizziness, earache, vertigo, taste perversion, paresthesia, rash.
Laboratory Test Considerations: ↑ ALT, AST.
How Supplied: *Ophthalmic solution:* 0.3%; *Otic Solution:* 0.3%; *Tablet:* 200 mg, 300 mg, 400 mg

Dosage

- **Tablets**

Pneumonia, exacerbation of chronic bronchitis.
400 mg q 12 hr for 10 days.
Acute uncomplicated gonorrhea.
One 400-mg dose. The Centers for Disease Control also recommend adding doxycycline.
Cervicitis/urethritis due to C. trachomatis or N. gonorrhoeae.
300 mg q 12 hr for 7 days.
Mild to moderate skin and skin structure infections.
400 mg q 12 hr for 10 days.
Cystitis due to E. coli or K. pneumoniae.
200 mg q 12 hr for 3 days.
Cystitis due to other organisms.
200 mg q 12 hr for 7 days.
Complicated UTIs.
200 mg q 12 hr for 10 days.
Prostatitis.
300 mg q 12 hr for 6 weeks.
Chlamydia.
300 mg PO b.i.d. for 7 days.
Epididymitis.
300 mg PO b.i.d. for 10 days.
PID, outpatient.
400 mg PO b.i.d. for 14 days.
NOTE: The dose should be adjusted in clients with a C_{CR} of 50 mL/min or less. If the C_{CR} is 10–50 mL/min, the dosage interval should be q 24 hr, and if C_{CR} is less than 10 mL/min, the dose should be half the recommended dose given q 24 hr.

- **Ophthalmic Solution (0.3%)**

Conjunctivitis.
Initial: 1–2 gtt in the affected eye(s) q 2–4 hr for the first 2 days; **then,** 1–2 gtt q.i.d. for five additional days.

- **Otic Solution (0.3%)**

Otitis externa, otitis media.
Apply b.i.d.

HEALTH CARE CONSIDERATIONS

See also *Health Care Considerations* for *Fluoroquinolones* and *Anti-Infectives.*

Administration/Storage

1. Do not take with food.
2. Store in tightly closed containers at a temperature below 30°C (86°F).
3. Do not inject the ophthalmic solution subconjunctivally and do not introduce directly into the anterior chamber of the eye.
4. Do not confuse the ophthalmic and otic dosage forms; they are not interchangeable.

Assessment

1. Note any sensitivity to quinolone derivatives.
2. Record indications for therapy, type, onset, and symptom characteristics.
3. Monitor CBC, cultures, liver and renal function studies; reduce dose with altered renal function. Review other prescribed agents; probenecid may block tubular excretion.
4. Assess for any CNS disorders. Report any tremors, restlessness, confusion, and hallucinations; therapy may need to be discontinued.

Client/Family Teaching

1. Do not take with food. Take PO form 1 hr before or 3 hr after meals.
2. Avoid vitamins, iron or mineral combinations, aluminum- or magnesium-based antacids 2 hr before and 2 hr after ingestion of ofloxacin.
3. Do not perform activities that require mental alertness until drug effects are realized; may cause drowsiness and lightheadedness.
4. Avoid contamination of the ophthalmic applicator tip with material from the eye or fingers.
5. Do not confuse the eye and ear dosage forms; they are not interchangeable.
6. May experience burning, stinging, itching, or tearing after eye use; should subside.
7. Drink 2–3 L/day of fluids to assist in drug elimination.
8. Side effects include N&V and diarrhea; report if persistent.
9. Avoid direct sunlight; photosensitivity reaction may occur. If exposed, wear sunglasses, protective clothing, and sunscreen.
10. Clients with diabetes should monitor sugars closely as extreme variations may occur.

Outcome/Evaluate: Negative culture reports; symptomatic improvement

Olanzapine

((oh-**LAN**-zah-peen))
Pregnancy Category: C
Zyprexa **(Rx)**
Classification: Antipsychotic agent, miscellaneous

Action/Kinetics: A thienbenzodiazepine antipsychotic believed to act by antagonizing dopamine D_{1-4} and serotonin ($5HT_2$) receptors. Also binds to muscarinic, histamine H_1 and alpha-1 adrenergic receptors, which can explain many of the side effects. Well absorbed from the GI tract. **Peak plasma levels:** 6 hr after PO dosing. Undergoes significant first-pass metabolism with about 40% metabolized before it reaches the systemic circulation. Food does not affect the rate or extent of absorption. Significantly bound to plasma proteins. Unchanged drug and metabolites are excreted through both the urine and feces.

Uses: Management of psychotic disorders. *Investigational:* Treatment of mania.

Contraindications: Lactation.

Special Concerns: Use with caution in geriatric clients, as the drug may be excreted more slowly in this population. Use with caution in impaired hepatic function and in those where there is a chance of increased core body temperature (e.g., strenuous exercise, exposure to extreme heat, concomitant anticholinergic drug administration, dehydration). Due to anticholinergic side effects, use with caution in clients with significant prostatic hypertrophy, narrow-angle glaucoma, or a history of paralytic ileus. Safety and efficacy have not been determined in children less than 18 years of age.

O

Side Effects: ***Neuroleptic malignant syndrome:*** Hyperpyrexia, muscle rigidity, altered mental status, irregular pulse or BP, tachycardia, diaphoresis, cardiac dysrhythmia, rhabdomyolysis, ***acute renal failure, death.*** *GI:* Dysphagia, constipation, dry mouth, increased appetite, increased salivation, N&V, thirst, aphthous stomatitis, eructation, esophagitis, rectal incontinence, flatulence, gastritis, gastroenteritis, gingivitis, glossitis, hepatitis, melena, mouth ulceration, oral moniliasis, periodontal abscess, ***rectal hemorrhage,*** tongue edema. *CNS:* Tardive dyskinesia, seizures, somnolence, agitation, insomnia, nervousness, hostility, dizziness, anxiety, personality disorder, akathisia, hypertonia, tremor, amnesia, impaired articulation, euphoria, stuttering, ***suicide,*** abnormal gait, alcohol misuse, antisocial reaction, ataxia, CNS stimulation, coma, delirium, depersonalization, hypesthesia, hypotonia, incoordination, decreased libido, obsessive-compulsive symptoms, phobias, somatization, stimulant misuse, stupor, vertigo, withdrawal syndrome. *CV:* Tachycardia, orthostatic/postural hypotension, hypotension, ***CVA, hemorrhage, heart arrest,*** migraine, palpitation, vasodilation, ventricular extrasystoles. *Body as a whole:* Headache, fever, abdominal pain, chest pain, neck rigidity, intentional injury, flu syndrome, chills, facial edema, hangover effect, malaise, moniliasis, neck pain, pelvic pain, photosensitivity. *Respiratory:* Rhinitis, increased cough, pharyngitis, dyspnea, apnea, asthma, epistaxis, hemoptysis, hyperventilation, voice alteration. *GU:* Premenstrual syndrome, hematuria, metrorrhagia, urinary incontinence, UTI, abnormal ejaculation, amenorrhea, breast pain, cystitis, decreased or increased menstruation, dysuria, female lactation, impotence, menorrhagia, polyuria, pyuria, urinary retention, urinary frequency, impaired urination, enlarged uterine fibroids. *Hematologic:* Leukocytosis, lymphadenopathy, thrombocytopenia. *Metabolic/nutritional:* Weight gain or loss, peripheral edema, lower extremity edema, dehydration, hyperglycemia, hyperkalemia, hyperuricemia, hypoglycemia, hypokalemia, hyponatremia, ketosis, water intoxication. *Musculoskeletal:* Joint pain, extremity pain, twitching, arthritis, back and hip pain, bursitis, leg cramps, myasthenia, rheumatoid arthritis. *Dermatologic:* Vesiculobullous rash, alopecia, contact dermatitis, dry skin, eczema, hirsutism, seborrhea, skin ulcer, urticaria. *Ophthalmic:* Amblyopia, blepharitis, corneal lesion, cataract, diplopia, dry eyes, eye hemorrhage, eye inflammation, eye pain, ocular muscle abnormality. *Otic:* Deafness, ear pain, tinnitus. *Miscellaneous:* Diabetes mellitus, goiter, cyanosis, taste perversion.

Laboratory Test Considerations: ↑ ALT, AST, GGT, alkaline phosphatase, serum prolactin, eosinophils, CPK. Hyperprolactinemia.

OD **Management of Overdose:** *Symptoms:* Drowsiness, slurred speech. Possible obtundation, seizures, dystonic reaction of the head and neck. CV symptoms, arrhythmias. *Treatment:* Establish and maintain an airway and ensure adequate oxygenation and ventilation. Gastric lavage followed by activated charcoal and a laxative can be considered, although dystonic reaction may cause aspiration with induced emesis. Begin CV monitoring immediately with continuous ECG monitoring to detect possible arrhythmias. Hypotension and circulatory collapse are treated with IV fluids or sympathomimetic agents. Do not use epinephrine, dopamine, or other sympathomimetics with beta-agonist activity, as beta stimulation may worsen hypotension.

Drug Interactions

Antihypertensive agents / ↑ Effect of antihypertensive agents

Carbamazepine / ↑ Clearance of olanzepine due to ↑ rate of metabolism

CNS depressants / ↑ Effect of CNS depressants

Levodopa and Dopamine agonists / Olanzapine may antagonize the effects of levodopa and dopamine agonists
How Supplied: *Tablet:* 2.5 mg, 5 mg, 7.5 mg, 10 mg

Dosage

- **Tablets**

Psychoses.

Adults, initial: 5–10 mg once daily without regard to meals. Goal is 10 mg daily; increments to reach 10 mg can be in 5-mg amounts but at an interval of 1 week. Doses higher than 10 mg daily are recommended only after clinical assessment and should not be greater than 20 mg/day. The recommended initial dose is 5 mg in those who are debilitated, who have a predisposition to hypotensive reactions, who may have factors that cause a slower metabolism of olanzapine (e.g., nonsmoking female clients over 65 years of age), or who may be more sensitive to the drug. It is recommended that clients who respond to the drug be continued on it at the lowest possible dose to maintain remission with periodic evaluation to determine continued need for the drug.

Mania.

5–20 mg daily.

HEALTH CARE CONSIDERATIONS

Administration/Storage: Protect from light and moisture and store at a controlled room temperature of 20°C–25°C (68°F–77°F).
Assessment
1. Record onset, duration, and characteristics of symptoms; note presenting behaviors. List agents trialed and the outcome.
2. Monitor ECG, CBC, liver and renal function studies.

Client/Family Teaching
1. Take only as directed; do not share medications; do not exceed prescribed dosage.
2. Avoid activities or situations where overheating may occur, e.g., strenuous exercise.
3. Do not drive or perform activities that require mental alertness until drug effects realized.
4. Avoid changing positions suddenly, especially from a lying to a standing position due to orthostatic effects.
5. Report any suicidal ideations, abnormal bleeding, sudden muscle pain or weakness, and irregular heart beat.
6. Avoid alcohol and any other CNS depressants or OTC agents.
7. Practice reliable birth control.
8. Report as scheduled for medication renewals, therapy sessions, and evaluation of drug effectiveness.

Outcome/Evaluate: Improved patterns of behavior with ↓ agitation, ↓ hostility and psychosis, and fewer delusions

Olopatadine hydrochloride

(oh-loh-pah-**TIH**-deen)
Pregnancy Category: C
Patanol **(Rx)**
Classification: Antihistamine, ophthalmic

See also *Antihistamines.*
Action/Kinetics: Selective histamine H-1 receptor antagonist. Little is absorbed into the systemic circulation.
Uses: Prevention of itching in allergic conjunctivitis.
Contraindications: Not to be injected. Not to be instilled while the client is wearing contact lenses.
Special Concerns: Use with caution during lactation. Safety and efficacy have not been determined for children less than 3 years of age.
Side Effects: *Ophthalmic:* Burning or stinging, dry eye, foreign body sensation, hyperemia, keratitis, lid edema, pruritus. Nose/throat: Pharyngitis, rhinitis, sinusitis. *Miscellaneous:* Headache, asthenia, cold syndrome, taste perversion.
How Supplied: *Solution:* 1%

Dosage

- **Solution (0.1%)**

Allergic conjunctivitis.

Adults and children over 3 years of age: 1–2 drops in each affected eye b.i.d. at an interval of 6–8 hr.

HEALTH CARE CONSIDERATIONS

See also *Health Care Considerations* for *Antihistamines.*
Administration/Storage: Store at 4°C–30°C (39°F–86°F).
Assessment: Record indications for therapy; note onset, duration, location, occurrence, and characteristics of symptoms. Identify triggers.
Client/Family Teaching
1. Wash hands before and after administration; do not let the dropper tip touch the eyelids or surrounding areas to prevent contamination.
2. Burning and stinging as well as swelling, redness, and foreign body sensation may occur; report if persistent.

O

3. Remove contact lens before instilling eye drops.
4. Review potential triggers and how to avoid and reduce contact to prevent increased irritation.

Outcome/Evaluate: Relief of allergic ocular manifestations.

Olsalazine sodium

(ohl-**SAL**-ah-zeen)
Pregnancy Category: C
Dipentum **(Rx)**
Classification: Anti-inflammatory drug

Action/Kinetics: A salicylate that is converted by bacteria in the colon to 5-PAS (5-para-aminosalicylate), which exerts an anti-inflammatory effect for the treatment of ulcerative colitis. 5-PAS is slowly absorbed resulting in a high concentration of drug in the colon. The anti-inflammatory activity is likely due to inhibition of synthesis of prostaglandins in the colon. After PO use the drug is only slightly absorbed (2.4%) into systemic circulation where it has a short half-life (< 1 hr) and is more than 99% bound to plasma proteins.
Uses: To maintain remission of ulcerative colitis in clients who cannot take sulfasalazine.
Contraindications: Hypersensitivity to salicylates.
Special Concerns: Use with caution during lactation. Safety and efficacy have not been established in children. May cause worsening of symptoms of colitis.
Side Effects: *GI:* Diarrhea (common), pain or cramps, nausea, dyspepsia, bloating, anorexia, vomiting, stomatitis. *CNS:* Headache, drowsiness, lethargy, fatigue, dizziness, vertigo. *Miscellaneous:* Arthralgia, rash, itching, upper respiratory tract infection. *NOTE:* The following symptoms have been reported on withdrawal of therapy: diarrhea, nausea, abdominal pain, rash, itching, headache, heartburn, insomnia, anorexia, dizziness, lightheadedness, rectal bleeding, depression.
OD **Management of Overdose:** *Symptoms:* Diarrhea, decreased motor activity. *Treatment:* Treat symptoms.
How Supplied: *Capsule:* 250 mg

Dosage

- **Capsules**

Adults: Total of 1 g/day in two divided doses.

HEALTH CARE CONSIDERATIONS

Assessment

1. Note any sensitivity to salicylates and/or intolerance to sulfasalazine.
2. Record indications for therapy, type, onset, and duration of symptoms.
3. With renal disease, monitor urinalysis, BUN, and creatinine. With chronic therapy monitor CBC and renal function studies.
4. Review radiographic/endoscopic findings.

Client/Family Teaching

1. Drug should be taken with food and in evenly divided doses.
2. Report any persistent diarrhea.

Outcome/Evaluate: Symptom remission with ulcerative colitis

Omeprazole

(oh-**MEH**-prah-zohl)
Pregnancy Category: C
Losec ✦, Prilosec **(Rx)**
Classification: Agent to suppress gastric acid secretion

Action/Kinetics: Thought to be a gastric pump inhibitor in that it blocks the final step of acid production by inhibiting the H^+–K^+ ATPase system at the secretory surface of the gastric parietal cell. Both basal and stimulated acid secretions are inhibited. Serum gastrin levels are increased during the first 1 or 2 weeks of therapy and are maintained at such levels during the course of therapy. Because omeprazole is acid-labile, the product contains an enteric-coated granule formulation; however, absorption is rapid. **Peak plasma levels:** 0.5–3.5 hr. **Onset:** Within 1 hr. **t½:** 0.5–1 hr. **Duration:** Up to 72 hr (due to prolonged binding of the drug to the parietal H^+–K^+; ATPase enzyme). Significantly bound (95%) to plasma protein. Metabolized in the liver and inactive metabolites are excreted through the urine. Consider dosage adjustment in Asians.
Uses: Short-term (4 to 8-week) treatment of active duodenal ulcer, active benign gastric ulcer, erosive esophagitis (all grades), and heartburn and other symptoms associated with GERD. In combination with clarithromycin for eradication of *Helicobacter pylori* and treatment of active duodenal ulcer. In combination with clarithromycin and amoxicillin for eradication of *H. pylori* and treatment of active duodenal ulcer. Long-term maintenance therapy for healed erosive esophagitis. Long-term treatment of pathologic hypersecretory conditions such as Zollinger-Ellison syndrome, multiple endocrine adenomas, and systemic mastocytosis. *Investigational:* Posterior laryngitis, enhanced efficacy of pancreatin for treating steatorrhea in cystic fibrosis.
Contraindications: Lactation. Use as maintenance therapy for duodenal ulcer disease.

Special Concerns: Bioavailability may be increased in geriatric clients. Use with caution during lactation. Symptomatic effects with omeprazole do not preclude gastric malignancy. Safety and effectiveness have not been determined in children.

Side Effects: *CNS:* Headache, dizziness. Possibly, anxiety disorders, abnormal dreams, vertigo, insomnia, nervousness, apathy, paresthesia, somnolence, depression, aggression, hallucinations, hemifacial dysesthesia, tremors, confusion. *GI:* Diarrhea, N&V, abdominal pain, abdominal swellling, constipation, flatulence, anorexia, fecal discoloration, esophageal candidiasis, mucosal atrophy of the tongue, dry mouth, irritable colon, gastric fundic gland polyps, gastroduodenal carcinoids. *Hepatic:* ***Pancreatitis.*** Overt liver disease, including hepatocellular, cholestatic, or mixed hepatitis; ***liver necrosis, hepatic failure,*** hepatic encephalopathy. *CV:* Angina, chest pain, tachycardia, bradycardia, palpitation, peripheral edema, elevated BP. *Respiratory:* URI, pharyngeal pain, bronchospasms, cough, epistaxis. *Dermatologic:* Rash, severe generalized skin reaction including ***toxic epidermal necrolysis, Stevens-Johnson syndrome;*** erythema multiforme, skin inflammation, urticaria, pruritus, alopecia, dry skin, hyperhidrosis. *GU:* UTI, acute interstitial nephritis, urinary frequency, hematuria, proteinuria, glycosuria, testicular pain, microscopic pyuria, gynecomastia. *Hematologic:* Pancytopenia, thrombocytopenia, anemia, leukocytosis, neutropenia, hemolytic anemia, ***agranulocytosis***. *Musculoskeletal:* Asthenia, back pain, myalgia, joint pain, muscle cramps, muscle weakness, leg pain. *Miscellaneous:* Rash, angioedema, fever, pain, gout, fatigue, malaise, weight gain, tinnitus, alteration in taste.

When used with clarithromycin the following *additional* side effects were noted: Tongue discoloration, rhinitis, pharyngitis, and flu syndrome.

NOTE: Data are lacking on the effect of long-term hypochlorhydria and hypergastrinemia on the risk of developing tumors.

Laboratory Test Considerations: ↑ AST, ALT, gamma-glutamyl transpeptidase, alkaline phosphatase, bilirubin, serum creatinine. Glycosuria, hyponatremia, hypoglycemia.

OD **Management of Overdose:** *Symptoms:* Confusion, drowsiness, blurred vision, tachycardia, nausea, diaphoresis, flushing, headache, dry mouth. *Treatment:* Symptomatic and supportive. Omeprazole is not readily dialyzable.

Drug Interactions

Ampicillin (esters) / Possible ↓ absorption of ampicillin esters due to ↑ pH of stomach

Clarithromycin / Possible ↑ plasma levels of both drugs

Diazepam / ↑ Plasma levels of diazepam due to ↓ rate of metabolism by the liver

Iron salts / Possible ↓ absorption of iron salts due to ↑ pH of stomach

Ketoconazole / Possible ↓ absorption of ketoconazole due to ↑ pH of stomach

Phenytoin / ↑ Plasma levels of phenytoin due to ↓ rate of metabolism of the liver

Sucralfate / ↓ Absorption of omeprazole; take 30 min before sucralfate

Warfarin / Prolonged rate of elimination of warfarin due to ↓ rate of metabolism by the liver

How Supplied: *Enteric Coated Capsule:* 10 mg, 20 mg, 40 mg

Dosage

- **Capsules, Enteric-Coated**

Active duodenal ulcer.

Adults, 20 mg/day for 4–8 weeks.

Erosive esophagitis, heartburn, symptoms associated with GERD.

Adults: 20 mg/day for 4–8 weeks. **Maintenance of healing erosive esophagitis:** 20 mg daily.

Treatment of H. pylori*, reduction of risk of duodenal ulcer recurrence.*

Days 1–14: Omeprazole, 40 mg daily in the morning, plus clarithromycin, 500 mg t.i.d. **Days 15–28:** Omeprazole, 20 mg daily. Or, omeprazole, 20 mg b.i.d.; clarithromycin, 500 mg b.i.d.; and amoxicillin, 1 g b.i.d. for 10 days. If an ulcer is present, continue omeprazole, 20 mg once daily, for an additional 18 days.

Pathologic hypersecretory conditions.

Adults**,** initial: 60 mg/day; then, dose individualized although doses up to 120 mg t.i.d. have been used. Daily doses greater than 80 mg should be divided.

Gastric ulcers.

Adults: 40 mg once daily for 4–8 weeks.

HEALTH CARE CONSIDERATIONS

Administration/Storage

1. Efficacy for more than 8 weeks has not been determined. However, if a client does not respond to 8 weeks of therapy, an additional 4 weeks may help. If there is a recurrence of erosive or symptomatic GERD poorly responsive to usual treatment, an additional 4 to 8 weeks of therapy may be tried.

2. Capsules should be stored in a tight container protected from light and moisture. Store between 15°C and 30°C (59°F and 86°F).

Assessment

1. Record indications for therapy, type, onset, and duration of symptoms.
2. Determine if pregnant.
3. Record abdominal assessments, radiographic/endoscopic findings and *H. pylori* results.
4. Monitor CBC and LFTs; note any hepatic dysfunction.

Client/Family Teaching

1. Antacids can be administered with omeprazole.
2. The capsule should be taken before eating and is to be swallowed whole; it should not be opened, chewed, or crushed.
3. Review drug associated side effects; report if persistent, especially diarrhea.
4. Report any changes in urinary elimination or pain and discomfort.
5. Avoid alcohol and OTC agents.
6. For short-term use only, drug inhibits total gastric acid secretion. Side effects of prolonged therapy and suppression of acid secretion alter bacterial colonization and lead to hypochlorhydria and hypergastrinemia which may cause an increased risk for the development of gastric tumors.

O

Outcome/Evaluate: Promotion of ulcer healing; relief of pain; ↓ gastric acid production

---

Ondansetron hydrochloride

(on-**DAN**-sih-tron)
Pregnancy Category: B
Zofran **(Rx)**
Classification: Antiemetic

Action/Kinetics: Cytotoxic chemotherapy is thought to release serotonin from enterochromoffin cells of the small intestine. The released serotonin may stimulate the vagal afferent nerves through the 5-HT_3 receptors, thus stimulating the vomiting reflex. Ondansetron, a 5-HT_3 antagonist, blocks this effect of serotonin. Whether the drug acts centrally and/or peripherally to antagonize the effect of serotonin is not known. **Time to peak plasma levels, after PO:** 1.7–2.1 hr. **t½, after IV use:** 3.5–4.7 hr; **after PO use:** 3.1–6.2 hr, depending on the age. A decrease in clearance and increase in half-life are observed in clients over 75 years of age, although no dosage adjustment is recommended. Clients less than 15 years of age show a shortened plasma half-life after IV use (2.4 hr). ignificantly metabolized with 5% of a dose excreted unchanged in the urine.

Uses: Parenteral: Prevent N&V resulting from initial and repeated courses of cancer chemotherapy, including high-dose cisplatin. Prophylaxis and treatment of selected cases of postoperative N&V, especially situations where there is multiple retching and long periods of N&V. **Oral:** Prevention of N&V due to initial and repeated courses of cancer chemotherapy. Prevenion of N&V associated with radiotherapy in clients receiving either total body irradiation, single high-dose fraction, or daily fractions to the abdomen. Prevention of postoperative N&V.

Special Concerns: Use with caution during lactation. Safety and effectiveness in children 3 years of age and younger are not known.

Side Effects: *GI:* Diarrhea (most common), constipation, xerostomia, abdominal pain. *CNS:* Headache, dizziness, drowsiness, sedation, malaise, fatigue, anxiety, agitation, extrapyramidal syndrome, ***clonic-tonic seizures.*** *CV:* Tachycardia, chest pain, hypotension, ECG alterations, angina, bradycardia, syncope, vascular occlusive events. *Dermatologic:* Pain, redness, and burning at injection site; cold sensation, pruritus, paresthesia. *Hypersensitivity (rare):* ***Anaphylaxis, bronchospasm, shock,*** SOB, hypotension, angioedema, urticaria. *Miscellaneous:* Rash, ***bronchospasm,*** transient blurred vision, hypokalemia, weakness, fever, musculoskeletal pain, shivers, dysuria, postoperative carbon dioxide-related pain, akathisia, acute dystonic reactions, gynecologic disorder, urinary retention, wound problem.

Laboratory Test Considerations: ↑ AST, ALT.

How Supplied: *Injection:* 2 mg/mL, 32 mg/50 mL; *Oral Solution:* 4 mg/5 mL; *Tablet:* 4 mg, 8 mg

Dosage

- **IM, IV**

Prevention of N&V due to chemotherapy.

Adults and children, 4–18 years: Three doses of 0.15 mg/kg each. The first dose is infused over 15 min starting 30 min before the start of chemotherapy; the second and third doses are given 4 hr and 8 hr, respectively, after the first dose. Alternatively, a single 32-mg dose may be given over 15 min beginning 30 min before the start of chemotherapy.

N&V postoperatively.

Adults: 4 mg over 2–5 min immediately before induction of anesthesia or postoperatively as needed. **Children, 2 to 12 years weighing 40 kg or less:** 0.1 mg/kg over 2–5 min. **Children, 2 to 12 years weighing over 40 kg:** 4 mg over 2–5 min.

• **Tablets**

In clients receiving moderately emetogenic chemotherapy agents.

Adults and children over 12 years of age: 8 mg 30 min before treatment followed by a second 8-mg dose 8 hr after the first dose; **then,** 8 mg b.i.d. for 1–2 days after chemotherapy. **Children, 4–12 years:** 4 mg t.i.d. The first dose is given 30 min before chemotherapy with subsequent doses 4 and 8 hr after the first dose. **Then,** 4 mg q 8 hr for 1–2 days after completion of chemotherapy.

Prevention of N&V due to total body irradiation.

8 mg 1–2 hr before each fraction of radiotherapy administered each day.

Prevention of N&V in single high-dose fraction radiotherapy to the abdomen.

8 mg 1–2 hr before radiotherapy with subsequent doses 8 hr after the first dose for 1–2 days after completion of radiotherapy.

Prevention of N&V due to daily fractionated radiotherapy to the abdomen.

8 mg 1–2 hr before radiotherapy, with subsequent doses 8 hr after the first dose for each day radiotherapy is given.

Prevention of postoperative N&V.

Adults: 16 mg given as a single dose 1 hr before induction of anesthesia.

HEALTH CARE CONSIDERATIONS

See also *Health Care Considerations* for *Antiemetics.*

Administration/Storage

1. With impaired hepatic function, do not exceed 8 mg PO or 8 mg IV daily infused over 15 min; 30 min prior to starting chemotherapy.
2. Tablets may be used to prepare a liquid product with cherry syrup, Syrpalta, Ora Sweet, or Ora Sweet Sugar Free. The concentration is 4 mg/5mL and is stable for 42 days at 4°C (39°F).
3. Suppositories can be made by adding pulverized tablets to a melted fatty acid base, mixing thoroughly, and pouring into suppository molds. They are stable for 30 or more days if stored in light-resistant containers under refrigeration.
4. IV Dilute the 2-mg/mL injection in 50 mL of D5W or 0.9% NaCl injection before administration; infuse over 15 min.
5. The diluted drug is stable at room temperature, with normal lighting, for 48 hr after dilution with 0.9% NaCl; D5W, D5/0.9% NaCl, D5/0.45% NaCl, and 3% NaCl injection.

Assessment

1. Record indications for therapy, onset and duration of symptoms, agents trialed, and outcome.
2. Monitor LFTs; adjust dosage with liver dysfunction.

Client/Family Teaching

1. Take exactly as prescribed in order to ensure desired results.
2. Report any rash, diarrhea, constipation, altered respirations (bronchospasms) or loss of response.

Outcome/Evaluate

• Prevention/control of chemotherapy-induced N&V
• Prophylaxis/relief of postoperative N&V

Oseltamivir phosphate

(oh-sell-**TAM**-ih-vir)

Pregnancy Category: C

Tamiflu **(Rx)**

Classification: Antiviral drug

Action/Kinetics: Hydrolyzed by hepatic esterases to the active oseltamivir carboxylate. May act by inhibiting the flu virus neuraminidase with possible alteration of virus particle aggregation and release. Drug resistance to influenza A virus is possible. Readily absorbed from the GI tract. **t½, oseltamivir carboxylate:** 6–10 hr. Over 99% is eliminated in the urine as oseltamivir carboxylate.

Uses: Treatment of uncomplicated acute influenza A or B infection in adults who have been symptomatic for 2 days or less.

Special Concerns: Use during lactation only if potential benefits outweigh the potential risk to the infant. Efficacy in clients who begin treatment after 40 hr of symptoms, for prophylactic use to prevent influenza, or for repeated treatment courses have not been determined. Safety and efficacy have not been determined in children less than 18 years of age.

Side Effects: *GI:* N&V, diarrhea, abdominal pain. *CNS:* Dizziness, headache, insomnia, vertigo. *Miscellaneous:* Bronchitis, cough, fatigue.

How Supplied: *Capsules:* 75 mg

Dosage

• **Capsules**

Influenza A or B infection.

75 mg b.i.d. for 5 days. Begin treatment within 2 days of onset of flu symptoms.

HEALTH CARE CONSIDERATIONS

Client/Family Teaching

1. Do not double up on doses. Take any missed dose as soon as remembered. If the

missed dose is remembered within 2 hr of the next scheduled dose, take at the usual time and resume usual schedule.
2. Tolerability may be enhanced if taken with food.
3. Initiate treatment as soon as possible at the first appearance of flu S&S.
4. Drug is used to diminish side effects and duration of illness. An annual flu shot is still required.
Outcome/Evaluate: ↓ Intensity/duration of S&S influenza A and B.

Oxacillin sodium

(ox-ah-**SILL**-in)
Pregnancy Category: B
Bactocill **(Rx)**
Classification: Antibiotic, penicillin

See also *Anti-Infectives* and *Penicillins*.
Action/Kinetics: Penicillinase-resistant, acid-stable drug used for resistant staphylococcal infections. **Peak plasma levels: PO,** 1.6–10 mcg after 30–60 min; **IM,** 5–11 mcg/mL after 30 min. **t½:** 30 min.
Uses: Infections caused by penicillinase-producing staphylococci; may be used to initiate therapy when a staphylococcal infection is suspected.
How Supplied: *Capsule:* 250 mg, 500 mg; *Injection:* 1 g/50 mL, 2 g/50 mL; *Powder for injection:* 500 mg, 1 g, 2 g, 10 g; *Powder for reconstitution:* 250 mg/5 mL

Dosage

- **Capsules, Oral Solution**

Mild to moderate infections of the upper respiratory tract, skin, soft tissue.
Adults and children (over 20 kg): 500 mg q 4–6 hr for at least 5 days. **Children less than 20 kg:** 50 mg/kg/day in equally divided doses q 6 hr for at least 5 days.
Septicemia, deep-seated infections.
Parenteral therapy (see below) followed by PO therapy. **Adults:** 1 g q 4–6 hr; **children:** 100 mg/kg/day in equally divided doses q 4–6 hr.

- **IM, IV**

Mild to moderate infections.
Adults and children over 40 kg: 250–500 mg q 4–6 hr. **Children less than 40 kg:** 50 mg/kg/day in equally divided doses q 6 hr.
Severe infections of the lower respiratory tract or disseminated infections.
Adults and children over 40 kg: 1 g q 4–6 hr. **Children less than 40 kg:** 100 mg/kg/day in equally divided doses q 4–6 hr. **Neonates and premature infants, less than 2,000 g:** 50 mg/kg/day divided q 12 hr if less than 7 days of age and 100 mg/kg/day divided q 8 hr if more than 7 days of age. **Neonates and premature infants, more than 2,000 g:** 75 mg/kg/day divided q 8 hr if less than 7 days of age and 150 mg/kg/day divided q 6 hr if more than 7 days of age. Maximum daily dose: **Adults,** 12 g; **children,** 100–300 mg/kg.

HEALTH CARE CONSIDERATIONS

See also *Health Care Considerations* for *Penicillins*.
Administration/Storage
1. Administer IM by deep intragluteal injection, rotate injection sites, and observe for pain and swelling at IM injection site.
IV 2. Reconstitution: Add NaCl or sterile water for injection in amount indicated on vial. Shake until solution is clear. For parenteral use, reconstituted solution may be kept for 3 days at room temperature or 1 week in refrigerator. Discard outdated solutions.
3. IV administration (two methods):
- For rapid, direct administration, add an equal amount of sterile water or isotonic saline to reconstituted dosage (usually 250- to 500-mg vial with 5 mL of solution) and administer over a period of 10 min.
- For IV infusion, add reconstituted solution to either dextrose, saline, or invert sugar solution for a concentration of 0.5–40 mg/mL and administer over a 6-hr period, during which time drug remains potent.
- Observe for pain, redness, and edema at IV injection site and along the course of the vein.

4. Treatment of osteomyelitis may require several months of intensive PO therapy.
5. Do not physically mix other drugs with oxacillin.
Outcome/Evaluate: Improvement in S&S of infection; negative cultures

Oxaprozin

(ox-ah-**PROH**-zin)
Pregnancy Category: C
Daypro **(Rx)**
Classification: Nonsteroidal anti-inflammatory drug

See also *Nonsteroidal Anti-Inflammatory Drugs*.
Uses: Acute and chronic management of rheumatoid arthritis and osteoarthritis.
How Supplied: *Tablet:* 600 mg

Dosage

- **Tablets**

Rheumatoid arthritis.

Adults: 1,200 mg once daily. Lower and higher doses may be required in certain clients.

Osteoarthritis.

Adults: 1,200 mg once daily. For clients with a lower body weight or with a milder disease, 600 mg/day may be appropriate.

Maximum daily dose for either rheumatoid arthritis or osteoarthritis: 1,800 mg (or 26 mg/kg, whichever is lower) given in divided doses.

HEALTH CARE CONSIDERATIONS

See also *Health Care Considerations* for *Nonsteroidal Anti-Inflammatory Drugs.*

Administration/Storage: Regardless of the use, individualize and use the lowest effective dose to minimize side effects.

Assessment:

1. Record type, onset, and symptom characteristics. List other agents used and the outcome.
2. Assess involved joint(s) and determine baseline ROM, the extent of any inflammation and rate pain level.
3. Monitor CBC, liver and renal function studies (q 6–12 months).

Outcome/Evaluate: Relief of joint pain/inflammation with improved mobility

Oxazepam

(ox-**AY**-zeh-pam)

Pregnancy Category: D

Apo-Oxazepam ✱, Novoxapam ✱, Oxpam ✱, PMS-Oxazepam ✱, Serax, Zapex ✱ **(C-IV) (Rx)**

Classification: Antianxiety agent, benzodiazepine

See also *Tranquilizers, Antimanic Drugs, and Hypnotics.*

Action/Kinetics: Absorbed more slowly than most benzodiazepines. **Peak plasma levels:** 2–4 hr. **t½:** 5–20 hr. Broken down in the liver to inactive metabolites, which are excreted through both the urine and feces. Reputed to cause less drowsiness than chlordiazepoxide.

Uses: Anxiety, tension, anxiety with depression. Adjunct in acute alcohol withdrawal.

Special Concerns: Dosage has not been established in children less than 12 years of age; use is not recommended in children less than 6 years of age.

Additional Side Effects: Paradoxical reactions characterized by sleep disorders and hyperexcitability during first weeks of therapy. Hypotension after parenteral administration.

How Supplied: *Capsule:* 10 mg, 15 mg, 30 mg; *Tablet:* 15 mg

Dosage

- **Capsules, Tablets**

Anxiety, mild to moderate.

Adults: 10–30 mg t.i.d.–q.i.d.

Anxiety, tension, irritability, agitation.

Geriatric and debilitated clients: 10 mg t.i.d.; can be increased to 15 mg t.i.d.–q.i.d.

Alcohol withdrawal.

Adults: 15–30 mg t.i.d.–q.i.d.

HEALTH CARE CONSIDERATIONS

See also *Health Care Considerations* for *Tranquilizers, Antimanic Drugs, and Hypnotics.*

Client/Family Teaching

1. Review goals of therapy, dosage, and frequency of administration.
2. Drug may cause dizziness and drowsiness; use caution until drug effects realized.
3. Report any persistant insomnia or hyperactivity.
4. Do not stop abruptly with long-term therapy.

Outcome/Evaluate

- ↓ Symptoms of anxiety and tension
- Control of alcohol withdrawal symptoms

O

Oxcarbazepine

(ox-kar-**BAY**-zeh-peen)

Pregnancy Category: C

Trileptal **(Rx)**

Classification: Anticonvulsant

See also *Anticonvulsants*

Action/Kinetics: Pharmacological activity results from both oxcarbazepine and its monohydroxy metabolite (MHD). Precise mechanism of anticonvulsant effect has not been defined. Oxcarbazepine and MHD block voltage sensitive sodium channels, stabilizing hyperexcited neuronal membranes, inhibiting repetitive firing, and decreasing the propagation of synaptic impulses. These actions are thought to prevent the spread of seizures. Oxcarbazepine and MHD also increase potassium conductance and modulate the activity of high-voltage activated calcium channels. **t½, oxcarbazepine:** 2 hr; **t½, MDH:** 9 hr. **Peak**: 4.5 hr. MHD and inactive metabolites are excreted mainly in the urine.

Uses: Monotherapy or adjunctive therapy in the treatment of partial seizures in adults with epilepsy; adjunctive therapy in the treatment of partial seizures in children 4 to 16 years of age with epilepsy.

Contraindications: Known hypersensitivity to oxcarbazepine or any component. Lactation.

Special Concerns: Oxcarbazepine has been associated with significant hyponatremia (<125 mmol/L). Monitor for signs and symptoms of hyponatremia which usually develops in the first three months of therapy but may occur at any time during therapy. Use with caution in clients with a history of hypersensitivity to carbamazepine due to chemical similarity to oxcarbazepine; cross-sensitivity occurs in 25% to 30% of clients. Stop medication at the first sign of hypersensitivity reaction. May cause drowsiness, dizziness, somnolence, cognitive difficulties, or difficulties with coordination. Clients should be cautioned to avoid operating machinery or driving until they gain experience with their response to this medication. Use with caution in clients receiving other sedative medications or ethanol. Additive sedation may occur. May reduce the effectiveness of oral contraceptives (nonhormonal contraceptive measures are recommended). Do not stop use abruptly; withdraw gradually to reduce risk of increased seizures.

O

Side Effects: Monotherapy, >10%:; *CNS:* Headache, dizziness, somnolence, fatique. *GI:* N&V. *Ophthalmic:* Abnormal vision, diplopia. **<10%:** *CNS:*Anxiety, ataxia, confusion, nervousness, insomnia, tremor, amnesia, exacerbation of seizures, emotional lability, hypoesthesia, fever, vertigo, abnormal coordination, speech disorder.*Dermatologic:*Rash, purpura. *Endocrine/metabolic:* Hyponatremia, hot flashes. *GI:* Diarrhea, dyspepsia, anorexia, abdominal pain, constipation, taste perversion.**Adjunctive Therapy (600 to 2400 mg/day). Frequencies reported in clients receiving other anticonvulsants, >10%:** *CNS:* Headache, dizziness, somnolence, ataxia, fatigue, vertigo. *GI:* N&V, abdominal pain. *Neuromuscular/skeletal:* Abnormal gait. *Ophthalmic:* Diplopia, nystagmus, visual abnormalities.

Additional Side Effects: Rare, severe dermatologic adverse reactions have been reported in postmarketing reports, including Stevens-Johnson syndrome, erythema multiforme, and toxic epidermal necrolysis. A rare, multi-organ hypersensitivity disorder has been described, characterized by rash, fever, lymphadenopathy, abnormal liver function tests, eosinophilia and arthralgia .

OD **Management of Overdose:** *Symptoms:* Include CNS depression (somnolence, ataxia). *Treatment:* Symptomatic and supportive.

Drug Interactions

CYP2C19 inhibitor; CYP3A4/5 enzyme inducer.

Carbamazepine/ ↓ oxcarbazepine serum levels R/T ↑ liver metabolism

Felodipine/ ↓ Plasma felodipine levels; similar effects may occur with other dihydropyridines.

Oral contraceptives/ ↓ Plasma levels of both estrogen and progestin; use alternative contraceptive measures.

Phenobarbital/ ↓ Plasma oxcarbazepine levels R/T ↑ liver metabolism; ↑ plasma levels of phenobarbital

Phenytoin/ ↓ Plasma oxcarbazepine levels R/T ↑ liver metabolism; ↑ plasma levels of phenytoin

Valproic acid/ ↓ Plasma oxcarbazepine levels

Verapamil/ ↓ Plasma oxcarbazepine levels

Laboratory Test Interferences: ↑ Gamma-GT, liver enzymes, serum transaminase. May depress serum T_4without affecting T_3 levels or TSH. Hyponatremia, hyperglycemia, hypocalcemia, hypoglycemia, hypokalemia.

How Supplied: *Tablet:* 150 mg, 300 mg, 600 mg

Dosage

• **Tablets**

Adults, initiation of monotherapy,oral (persons not receiving AEDs): 300 mg twice daily; increase dose by 300 mg/day every third day to a dose of 1200 mg/day. **Adjunctive therapy, initial oral:**300 mg bid; dosage may be increased by 600 mg/day at approximate weekly intervals. Recommended daily dose is 1200 mg/day. Daily doses >1200 mg/day have demonstrated greater efficacy, most patients were unable to tolerate 2400 mg/day due to CNS effects.**Conversion to monotherapy:** (persons receiving antiepileptic drugs at the same time) **Initial:** 300 mg twice daily while simultaneously reducing the dose of AEDs. Withdraw AEDs completely over 3-6 weeks, while increasing the oxcarbazepine dose in increments of 600 mg/day at weekly intervals, reaching maximum oxcarbazipine dose (2400 mg/day) in about 2-4 weeks. Reduce dosages by one-half based on creatinine clearance for renal impairment and elderly.**Children, aged 4-16 years, initial:**8-10 mg/kg twice daily (not to exceed 600 mg/day); given in two equally divided doses. **Maintenance:**Target maintenance dose should be achieved over 2 weeks, and depends on the weight of the child: 20-29 kg: 900 mg/day; 29.1-39 kg: 1200 mg/day; >39 kg: 1800 mg/day.

NOTE: Initiate therapy at 300 mg/day in those with a C_{CR} less than 30 mL/min. May then increase slowly to achieve the desired response.

HEALTH CARE CONSIDERATIONS

See also *Health Care Considerations* for *Anticonvulsants.*

Assessment

1. Record indications for therapy, onset and characteristics of seizures.
2. Monitor seizure frequency, serum sodium (particularly during first 3 months of therapy), and symptoms of CNS depression (dizziness, headache, somnolence).
3. Question the client about and record any carbamazepine allergy.

Client/Family Teaching

1. May be taken with or without food; take with food if the medicine causes stomach upset.
2. Avoid alcohol or other drugs which may cause sedation; do not drive or operate heavy machinery until you know how this medication affects you.
3. Tell the healthcare provider prescribing this medication if you are allergic to carbamazepine, if you have an allergic reaction, or are sleeping excessively.
4. Report symptoms of nausea, general persistent tiredness, headache, lethargy, or confusion to your healthcare provider; blood levels of sodium may need to be checked.
5. Do not rely on oral contraceptives to prevent pregnancy; use barrier contraception.
6. Do not stop this medication without healthcare provider approval; may cause an increase in seizures.

Outcome/Evaluate: Control of seizures.

Oxiconazole nitrate

(ox-ee-**KON**-ah-zohl)
Pregnancy Category: B
Oxistat **(Rx)**
Classification: Antifungal agent, topical

See also *Anti-Infectives.*

Action/Kinetics: Acts by inhibiting ergosterol synthesis, which is required for cytoplasmic membrane integrity of fungi. Active against a broad range of organisms including many strains of *Trichophyton rubrum* and *T. mentagrophytes.* Systemic absorption is low.

Uses: Topical treatment of tinea pedis (athlete's foot), tinea cruris (jock itch), tinea versicolor, and tinea corporis (ringworm) due to *Trichophyton rubrum, T. mentagrophytes,* and *Epidermophyton floccosum.* Cream only to treat tinea versicolor due to *Malassezia furfur* in adults and children.

Contraindications: Ophthalmic or vaginal use.

Special Concerns: Use with caution during lactation.

Side Effects: *Dermatologic:* Pruritus, burning, stinging, irritation, erythema, fissuring, maceration, contact dermatitis, scaling, tingling, pain, dyshidrotic eczema, folliculitis, papules, rash, nodules.

How Supplied: *Cream:* 1%; *Lotion:* 1%

Dosage

- **Cream (1%), Lotion (1%)**

Adults and childen: Apply 1% cream or lotion to cover affected areas and immediately surrounding areas once or twice daily for tinea pedis, tinea corporis, and tinea cruris. Apply cream only to affected areas once daily for tinea versicolor. To prevent recurrence, continue treatment for 2 weeks for tinea corporis, tinea versicolor, and tinea cruris and for 1 month for tinea pedis.

HEALTH CARE CONSIDERATIONS

Assessment

1. Assess and describe area of involvement, note onset, duration, presentation, and symptom characteristics.
2. The diagnosis should be reviewed if no clinical response after the designated treatment period (tinea corporis and tinea cruris require 2 weeks of therapy; tinea pedis requires 1 month of therapy to prevent recurrence).

Client/Family Teaching

1. Wash hands before and after application; use only as directed.
2. Report any itching/burning; discontinue treatment if sensitivity or chemical irritation appear.
3. Follow prescribed therapy; some infections may require 2-4 weeks of daily treatments to ensure no recurrence.
4. For external use only; avoid eye contact.

Outcome/Evaluate: Resolution of fungal infection; symptomatic improvement

Oxybutynin chloride

(ox-ee-**BYOU**-tih-nin)
Pregnancy Category: B

Albert Oxybutynin ✱, Apo-Oxybutynin ✱, Ditropan, Gen-Oxybutynin ✱, Novo-Oxybutynin ✱, Nu-Oxybutyn ✱, Oxybutyn ✱, PMS-Oxybutynin ✱ **(Rx)**
Classification: Antispasmodic

Action/Kinetics: Causes increased vesicle capacity, decreases frequency of uninhibited contractions of the detrusor muscle, and delays initial urgency to void by exerting a direct antispasmodic effect. Has no effect at either the neuromuscular junction or autonomic ganglia. Has 4–10 times the antispasmodic effect of atropine but only one-fifth the anticholinergic activity. **Onset:** 30–60 min; **Time to peak effect:** 3–6 hr; **duration:** 6–10 hr. Eliminated through the urine.
Uses: Neurogenic bladder disease characterized by urinary retention, urinary overflow, incontinence, nocturia, urinary frequency or urgency, reflex neurogenic bladder.
Contraindications: Glaucoma (angle closure), untreated narrow anterior chamber angles, GI obstruction, paralytic ileus, intestinal atony (in elderly or debilitated), megacolon, toxic megacolon complicating ulcerative colitis, severe colitis, myasthenia gravis, obstructive uropathy, unstable CV status in acute hemorrhage.
Special Concerns: *Use with caution when increased cholinergic effect is undesirable and in the elderly.* Safe use in children less than 5 years of age has not been determined. Use with caution in geriatric clients; during lactation; in clients with autonomic neuropathy, renal, or hepatic disease; and in clients with hiatal hernia with reflex esophagitis. Heat stroke and fever (due to decreased sweating) may occur if given at high environmental temperatures.
Side Effects: *GI:* N&V, constipation, bloated feeling, decreased GI motility. *CNS:* Drowsiness, insomnia, weakness, dizziness, restlessness, hallucinations. *EENT:* Dry mouth, decreased lacrimation, mydriasis, amblyopia, cycloplegia. *CV:* Tachycardia, palpitations, vasodilation. *Miscellaneous:* Decreased sweating, urinary hesitancy and retention, impotence, suppression of lactation, ***severe allergic reactions,*** drug idiosyncrasies, urticaria, and other dermal manifestations. *NOTE:* The drug may aggravate symptoms of prostatic hypertrophy, hypertension, coronary heart disease, CHF, hyperthyroidism, cardiac arrhythmias, and tachycardia.
OD **Management of Overdose:** *Symptoms:* Intense CNS disturbances (restlessness, psychoses), circulatory changes (flushing, hypotension) and failure, respiratory failure, paralysis, coma. *Treatment:* Stomach lavage, physostigmine (0.5–2 mg IV; repeat as necessary up to maximum of 5 mg). Supportive therapy, if necessary. Counteract excitement with sodium thiopental (2%) or chloral hydrate (100–200 mL of 2% solution) rectally. Artificial respiration may be necessary if respiratory muscles become paralyzed.
Drug Interactions: See *Cholinergic Blocking Agents.*
How Supplied: *Syrup:* 5 mg/5 mL; *Tablet:* 5 mg

Dosage

- **Syrup, Tablets**

Adults: 5 mg b.i.d.–t.i.d. Maximum dose: 5 mg q.i.d. **Children, over 5 years:** 5 mg b.i.d. Maximum dose: 5 mg t.i.d.

HEALTH CARE CONSIDERATIONS

See also *Health Care Considerations* for *Cholinergic Blocking Agents.*
Administration/Storage: Dispense in tight, light-resistant containers and store at 15°C–30°C (59°F–86°F).
Assessment
1. Record type, onset, frequency, and duration of symptoms.
2. Review conditions that may be aggravated by oxybutynin and note if present (renal, hepatic disease, hiatal hernia, reflux esophagitis).
Client/Family Teaching
1. Take only as directed.
2. Use caution driving a car or in operating dangerous machinery; drug may cause drowsiness and blurred vision.
3. Withhold medication and report if diarrhea occurs (especially with an ileostomy or colostomy); may be symptom of intestinal obstruction.
4. Consume 2–3 L/day of fluids to ensure adequate hydration and to relieve symptoms of dry mouth.
5. Vegetables, fruit, fiber, and fluids should be consumed in adequate quantities to prevent constipation.
6. Wear sunglasses, sunscreen, and protective clothing during exposure; may cause photosensitivity reaction.
7. Avoid overexposure to heat; body needs increased fluids in hot weather because sweating is drug inhibited and heat stroke may occur.
8. Report any loss of effect as dosage may require adjustment.
9. With neurogenic bladder, return as scheduled for cystometry, to evaluate response to therapy, and need for continuation of medication.
Outcome/Evaluate
- Relief of spasms and GU pain
- Normal elimination patterns
- Positive cystometry findings

COMBINATION DRUG

Oxycodone and acetaminophen

(ox-ee-**KOH**-dohn, ah-**SEAT**-ah-**MIN**-oh-fen)

Pregnancy Category: C

Endocet, Oxycocet ✱, Percocet ✱, Percocet-Demi ✱, Roxicet **(C-II) (Rx)**

Classification: Analgesic

See also *Acetaminophen* and *Narcotic Analgesics.*

Content: Endocet and Roxicet Tablets: *Narcotic analgesic:* Oxycodone hydrochloride, 5 mg. *Analgesic:* Acetaminophen, 325 mg. **Roxicet Oral Solution:** *Narcotic analgesic:* Oxycodone hydrochloride, 5 mg/5 mL. *Analgesic:* Acetaminophen, 325 mg/5 mL.

Uses: Relief of moderate to moderately severe pain.

Contraindications: Hypersensitivity to either oxycodone or acetaminophen.

Special Concerns: Can produce drug dependence and has abuse potential. The respiratory depressant effects of oxycodone can be exaggerated in clients with head injury, other intracranial lesions, or a preexisting increase in intracranial pressure. Use with caution in clients who are elderly, are debilitated, have severely impaired hepatic or renal function, are hyperthyroid, have Addison's disease, have prostatic hypertrophy, or have urethral stricture. Use for acute abdominal conditions may obscure the diagnosis or clinical course. Use with caution during lactation. Safety and efficacy in children have not been established.

Side Effects: Commonly, dizziness, lightheadedness, N&V, and sedation; these effects are more common in ambulatory clients than nonambulatory clients. Other side effects include euphoria, dysphoria, constipation, skin rash, and pruritus. See also individual components.

Drug Interactions

Anticholinergic drugs / Production of paralytic ileus

Antidepressants, tricyclic / ↑ Effect of either the tricyclic antidepressant or oxycodone

CNS depressants (including other narcotic analgesics, phenothiazines, antianxiety drugs, sedative-hypnotics, anesthetics, alcohol) / Additive CNS depression

MAO inhibitors / ↑ Effect of either the MAO inhibitor or oxycodone

How Supplied: See Content

Dosage

- **Oral Solution, Tablets**

Analgesic.

Adults: 5 mL of the oral solution q 6 hr or 1 tablet q 6 hr as needed for pain.

HEALTH CARE CONSIDERATIONS

See also *Health Care Considerations* for *Acetaminophen* and *Narcotic Analgesics.*

Assessment

1. Record indications for therapy, type, onset, and duration of symptoms. Use a pain-rating scale to rate pain level.
2. List other agents prescribed and the outcome.
3. Note CNS assessment findings and level of consciousness.

Client/Family Teaching

1. Take only as directed; may take with food to decrease GI upset.
2. Drug may cause dizziness and drowsiness; do not perform activities that require mental or physical alertness and do not change positions abruptly.
3. May cause constipation, N&V, dry mouth, and physical dependence; review interventions to offset side effects.
4. Avoid alcohol and any other CNS depressants without provider approval. (*NOTE:* Oral solution contains small amounts of alcohol.)

Outcome/Evaluate: Pain control

O

COMBINATION DRUG

Oxycodone and Aspirin

(ox-ee-**KOH**-dohn, **ASS**-pih-rin)

Endodan, Oxycodan ✱, Percodan, Percodan-Demi ✱ **(C-II) (Rx)**

Classification: Analgesic

See also *Acetylsalicyic acid* and *Narcotics Analgesics.*

Content: Each tablet contains: *Narcotic analgesics:* oxycodone, 4.5 mg and oxycodone terephthalate, 0.38 mg. *Analgesic:* Aspirin, 325 mg.

Uses: Relief of moderate to moderately severe pain.

Contraindications: Use in children and during pregnancy.

Special Concerns: Oxycodone can produce drug dependence and has abuse potential. The respiratory depressant effects of oxycodone can be exaggerated in clients with head injury, other intracranial lesions, or a preexisting increase in intracranial pressure. Use with caution in clients who are elderly, are debilitated, have severely impaired hepatic or renal function, are hyperthyroid, have Addison's disease, have prostat-

ic hypertrophy, or have urethral stricture. Use for acute abdominal conditions may obscure the diagnosis or clinical course.
Side Effects: Commonly, dizziness, lightheadedness, N&V, and sedation; these effects are more common in ambulatory clients than in nonambulatory clients. Other side effects include euphoria, dysphoria, constipation, skin rash, and pruritus. See also individual components.
Drug Interactions
Aspirin / ↑ Effect of anticoagulants
CNS depressants (including other narcotic analgesics, phenothiazines, antianxiety drugs, sedative-hypnotics, anesthetics, alcohol) / Additive CNS depression

Dosage

- **Tablets**

Analgesic.
Adults: 1 tablet q 6 hr as needed for pain; higher doses may be required in cases of more severe pain or in those who have become tolerant to the analgesic effect of narcotics.

HEALTH CARE CONSIDERATIONS

See also *Health Care Considerations* for *Acetylsalicyic acid* and *Narcotic Analgesics.*
Assessment:
1. Record indications for therapy, type, onset, and duration of symptoms. Use a pain-rating scale to rate pain level. List other agents prescribed and the outcome.
2. Note the presence of PUD or coagulation abnormalities.
Client/Family Teaching
1. Take only as directed; take with food to decrease GI upset.
2. Drug may cause dizziness and drowsiness; avoid activities that require mental or physical alertness.
3. Drug may cause constipation, N&V, dry mouth, and physical dependence; review appropriate interventions to offset side effects.
4. Avoid alcohol and any other CNS depressants without approval.
Outcome/Evaluate: Desired pain control

Oxycodone hydrochloride

(ox-ee-**KOH**-dohn)
Pregnancy Category: C
OxyContin, Percolone CII, Roxicodone, Roxicodone Intensol, Supeudol ✱ **(C-II) (Rx)**
Classification: Narcotic analgesic, morphine type

See also *Narcotic Analgesics.*

Action/Kinetics: Semisynthetic opiate causing mild sedation and little or no antitussive effect. Most effective in relieving acute pain. **Onset:** 15–30 min. **Peak effect:** 60 min. **Duration:** 4–6 hr. t½: 3.2 hr for immediate-release product and 4.5 hr for extended-release. Dependence liability is moderate. Oxycodone terephthalate is available but only in combination with aspirin (e.g., Percodan) or acetaminophen.
Uses: Moderate to severe pain. The extended-release product (OxyContin) is indicated for moderate to severe pain, including that due to cancer, injuries, arthritis, lower back problems, and other musculoskeletal conditions that require treatment for more than a few days.
Additional Contraindications: Use in children.
Special Concerns: OxyContin 80 mg controlled release is indicated only for opiate-tolerant clients.
Additional Drug Interactions: Clients with gastric distress, such as colitis or gastric or duodenal ulcer, and clients who have glaucoma should not receive Percodan, which also contains aspirin.
How Supplied: *Capsule:* 5 mg; *Concentrate:* 20 mg/mL; *Solution:* 5 mg/5 mL; *Tablet:* 5 mg; *Tablet, Extended Release:* 10 mg, 20 mg, 40 mg, 80 mg

Dosage

- **Capsule, Oral Solution, Concentrated Solution, Tablet, Extended Release Tablet**

Analgesia.
Adults: 5 mg q 6 hr.

- **Extended Release Tablet**

Analgesia.
Adults, opioid-naive: 10 mg q 12 hr. **Adults, with prior narcotic therapy:** 10–30 mg b.i.d.

HEALTH CARE CONSIDERATIONS

See also *Health Care Considerations* for *Narcotic Analgesics.*
Assessment: Record onset, location, and duration of pain and characteristics of symptoms. Use a pain-rating scale to rate pain levels. Note other agents trialed and the outcome.
Client/Family Teaching
1. Take medication with food to minimize GI upset.
2. Swallow extended-release tablets whole. Ingesting broken, crushed, or chewed extended-release tablets may lead to rapid release and absorption and the possibility of toxic effects.

3. Use caution; do not perform activities that require mental alertness.
4. Avoid alcohol in any form.

Outcome/Evaluate: Relief of pain

Oxymorphone hydrochloride

(ox-ee-**MOR**-fohn)

Pregnancy Category: C

Numorphan **(C-I) (Rx)**

Classification: Narcotic analgesic, morphine type

See also *Narcotic Analgesics.*

Action/Kinetics: On a weight basis, is 2–10 times more potent as an analgesic than morphine, although potency depends on the route of administration. Produces mild depression of the cough reflex and significant respiratory depression and emesis. **Onset:** 5–10 min. **Peak effect:** 30–60 min. **Duration:** 3–6 hr.

Uses: Moderate to severe pain. **Parenteral:** Preoperative analgesia, to support anesthesia, obstetrics, relief of anxiety in clients with dyspnea associated with acute LV failure and pulmonary edema.

How Supplied: *Injection:* 1 mg/mL, 1.5 mg/mL; *Suppository:* 5 mg

Dosage

- **SC, IM**

  Analgesia.

Adults, initial: 1–1.5 mg q 4–6 hr; dose can be increased carefully until analgesic response obtained.

  Analgesia during labor.

Adults: 0.5–1.0 mg IM.

- **IV**

  Analgesia.

Adults, initial: 0.5 mg.

- **Suppositories**

  Analgesia.

Adults: 5 mg q 4–6 hr. **Not recommended for children under 12 years of age.**

HEALTH CARE CONSIDERATIONS

See also *Health Care Considerations* for *Narcotic Analgesics.*

Administration/Storage

1. Store suppositories in the refrigerator.

IV 2. If the drug is to be administered IV, dilute the dosage in 5 mL of sterile water or NSS and administer over 2–3 min.

Assessment: Record indications for therapy, noting onset, location, duration and characteristics of pain; use scale to rate pain to evaluate effectiveness.

Client/Family Teaching

1. C&DB several times each hour while awake to prevent atelectasis; incentive spirometry may be useful.
2. Drug may aggravate gallbladder conditions; report any abdominal complaints.
3. Use safety precautions; drug causes drowsiness and dizziness.

Outcome/Evaluate: Relief of pain; control of anxiety

P

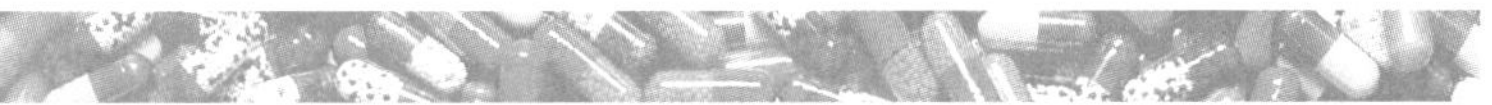

Pancrelipase (Lipancreatin)

(pan-kree-**LY**-payz)

Pregnancy Category: C

Cotazym, Cotazym-S, Creon 5, 10, or 20, Creon 10, or 25 ✱, Digess 8000 ✱, Ilozyme, Ku-Zyme HP, Pancrease, Pancrease MT 4, 10, 16, or 20, Protilase, Ultrase ✱, Ultrase MT12, 20, or 24, Viokase, Viokase ✱, Zymase **(Rx)**

Classification: Digestant

Action/Kinetics: Enzyme concentrate from hog pancreas, which contains lipase, amylase, and protease, enzymes that replace or supplement naturally occurring enzymes. More active at neutral or slightly alkaline pH. Has 12 times the lipolytic activity and 4 times both the proteolytic and amylolytic activity of pancreatin. Certain products have an enteric coating that protects the enzymes from deactivation in the stomach.

Uses: Pancreatic deficiency diseases such as chronic pancreatitis, cystic fibrosis of the pancreas, pancreatectomy, ductal obstructions caused by cancer of the pancreas or common bile duct, steatorrhea of malabsorption syndrome or postgastrectomy or postgastrointestinal surgery. Presumptive test for pancreatic function, especially in insufficiency due to chronic pancreatitis.

Contraindications: Hog protein sensitivity. Acute pancreatitis, acute exacerbation of chronic pancreatic disease.

Special Concerns: Safety for use during lactation and in children less than 6 months of age not established. Methacrylic acid copolymer, which is found in the enteric coating of certain products, may cause fibrosing colonopathy.

Side Effects: *GI:* Nausea, diarrhea, abdominal cramps following high doses. *Other:* Inhalation of the powder is irritating to the skin and mucous membranes and may result in an asthma attack. High doses cause hyperuricemia and hyperuricosuria.

OD **Management of Overdose:** *Symptoms:* Diarrhea, intestinal upset.

Drug Interactions

Calcium carbonate / ↓ Effect of pancreatic enzymes

Iron / Response to oral iron may ↓ if given with pancreatic enzymes

Magnesium hydroxide / ↓ Effect of pancreatic enzymes

How Supplied: *Capsule; Enteric Coated capsule; Enteric Coated tablet; Powder; Tablet*

Dosage

• **Capsules; Enteric-Coated Microspheres, Microtablets, Spheres, Pellets; Powder; Tablets**

Pancreatic insufficiency.

Adults and children over 12 years of age: 4,000–48,000 units of lipase with each meal and with snacks. **Children, 7–12 years:** 4,000–12,000 units of lipase with each meal and snacks; **1–6 years:** 4,000–8,000 units of lipase with each meal and 4,000 units lipase with snacks. **6–12 months:** 2,000 units lipase with each meal. Dosage has not been established in children less than 6 months of age. Severe deficiencies may require up to 64,000–88,000 units of lipase with meals (or the frequency of administration can be increased if side effects are not manifested).

Pancreatectomy or obstruction of pancreatic ducts.

Adults: 8,000–16,000 units of lipase at 2 hr intervals or as directed by a physician.

Cystic fibrosis.

Use 0.7 g of the powder with meals.

HEALTH CARE CONSIDERATIONS

Administration/Storage

1. When administering to young children, may sprinkle capsule contents on food.
2. After several weeks of use, adjust the dosage according to the therapeutic response.
3. Store unopened preparations in tight containers at a temperature not to exceed 25°C (77°F).
4. Do not crush or chew enteric-coated products (i.e., microspheres, microtablets). If unable to swallow, the capsule may be opened and shaken on a small amount of soft, cold food (e.g., applesauce, gelatin) that does not require chewing. Swallow immediately without chewing (the enzymes may irritate the mucosa). Follow with a glass of juice or water to ensure complete swallowing of the product. Enteric-coated products that come in contact with foods with a pH greater than 5.5 will dissolve.
5. Generally, 300 mg of pancrelipase is required to digest every 17 g of dietary fat.
6. Products are not bioequivalent; do not interchange without approval.

Assessment

1. Obtain a thorough health history and record indications for therapy.
2. Determine any sensitivity or allergy to pork, since hog protein is the main constituent of pancrelipase.

Client/Family Teaching

1. Review the appropriate dietary recommendations (usually low fat, high calorie, high protein); utilize a dietitian for dietary counseling and assistance in meal planning. It takes 300 mg of pancrelipase to digest 17 g of dietary fat.
2. Take just before or with meals and snacks and with plenty of liquids to prevent oral mucosal irritation. Omit if dose missed.
3. Report any nausea, cramping, or diarrhea. The dosage needs to be adjusted to control steatorrhea.

Outcome/Evaluate

• Improved digestion/nutritional status with deficiency states
• Control of diarrhea, ↓ steatorrhea

Pantoprazole

(pan-**TOH**-prah-zohl)
Pregnancy Category: B
Protonix **(Rx)**
Classification: Gastric acid secretion inhibitor

Action/Kinetics: Suppresses gastric acid secretion by inhibiting the parietal cell H+/K+ ATP pump. **t½:**1 hr. **Peak:** 2.5 hr after oral ingestion.

Uses: Short-term treatment (8 wk) of erosive esophagitis associated with GERD.

Contraindications: Hypersensitivity to pantoprazole or any component. Lactation.

Special Concerns: Symptomatic response does not eliminate possiblity of gastric malignancy. Not indicated for maintenance therapy. Safety and efficacy for use beyond 16 weeks have not been established. Safety and efficacy in pediatric clients have not been established.

Side Effects: *CNS:* Pain, migraine, anxiety, dizziness. *CV:* Chest pain. *Endocrine/metabolic:* Hyperglycemia, hyperlipidemia. *GI:* Diarrhea, constipation, dyspepsia, gastroenteritis, N&V, rectal disorder. *GU:* Urinary frequency, urinary tract infection. *Hepatic:* Liver function test abnormality, increased SGPT. *Neuromuscular & skeletal:* Weakness, back pain, neck pain, arthralgia, hypertonia. *Respiratory:* Bronchitis, increased cough, dyspnea, pharyngitis, rhinitis, sinusitis, upper respiratory tract infection. *Miscellaneous:* Flu-like syndrome, infection.

Drug Interactions: CYP2C19, CYP3A4 enzyme substrate. The absorption of drugs dependent upon gastric acid pH, (i.e. itraconazole, ketoconazole, and other azole antifungals, ampicillin esters, iron salts) may have decreased absorption when used at the same time. Monitor for a change in effectiveness.

How Supplied: *Tablets, delayed-release:* 40 mg

Dosage

- **Tablets**

Adults: 40 mg daily for up to 8 weeks; an additional 8 weeks may be used in clients who have not healed after an 8-week course.

HEALTH CARE CONSIDERATIONS

Administration/Storage

1. Take with or without food.
2. Do not break, crush, or chew tablets.
3. Do not give through a nasogastric or feeding tube.

Assessment

1. Record reasons for therapy, type, onset and duration symptoms.
2. Record location, extent, and characteristics of abdominal pain.
3. Review UGI findings; note modifications trialed with GERD.
4. Assess other medications the client may be taking where absorption may be altered by a change in gastric pH (itraconazole, ketoconazole, iron salts, ampicillin esters).

Client/Family Teaching

1. Take with or without food.
2. Do not split, chew or crush tablets.
3. Take at the same time each day.
4. Inform prescriber if you are or intend to become pregnant. Discontinue breast-feeding prior to starting this medicine.

Outcome/Evaluate: Healing in clients with erosive esophagitis

Papaverine

(pah-**PAV**-er-een)

Pregnancy Category: C

Pavabid Plateau Caps, Pavagen TD **(Rx)**

Classification: Peripheral vasodilator

Action/Kinetics: Direct spasmolytic effect on smooth muscle, possibly by inhibiting cyclic nucleotide phosphodiesterase, thus increasing levels of cyclic AMP. This effect is seen in the vascular system, bronchial muscle, and in the GI, biliary, and urinary tracts. Large doses produce CNS sedation and sleepiness. May also directly relax cerebral vessels as it increases cerebral blood flow and decreases cerebral vascular resistance. Depresses cardiac conduction and irritability and prolongs the myocardial refractory period. Localized in fat tissues and liver. Steady plasma concentration maintained when drug is given q 6 hr. **Peak plasma levels:** 1–2 hr. **t½:** 30–120 min. Sustained-release products may be poorly and erratically absorbed. Metabolized in the liver and inactive metabolites excreted in the urine.

Uses: Relief of cerebral and peripheral ischemia associated with arterial spasm and myocardial ischemia complicated by arrhythmias.

Contraindications: Complete AV block.

Special Concerns: Safe use during lactation or for children not established. Use with extreme caution in coronary insufficiency and glaucoma.

Side Effects: *CV:* Flushing of face, hypertension, increase in HR and depth of respiration. Large doses can depress AV and intraventricular conduction, causing serious arrhythmias. *GI:* Nausea, anorexia, abdominal distress, constipation or diarrhea, dry mouth and throat. *CNS:* Headache, drowsiness, sedation, vertigo. *Miscellaneous:* Sweating, malaise, pruritus, skin rashes, chronic hepatitis, hepatic hypersensitivity, jaundice, eosinophilia, altered LFTs.

Laboratory Test Considerations: ↑ AST, ALT, and bilirubin.

OD **Management of Overdose:** *NOTE:* Both acute and chronic poisoning may result from use of papaverine. Symptoms are extensions of side effects.

Symptoms (Acute Poisoning): Nystagmus, diplopia, drowsiness, weakness, lassitude, incoordination, coma, cyanosis, ***respiratory depression.*** *Treatment (Acute Poisoning):* Delay absorption by giving tap water, milk, or activated charcoal followed by gastric lavage or induction of vomiting and then a cathartic. Maintin BP and take measures to treat respiratory depression and coma. Hemodialysis is effective.

Symptoms (Chronic Poisoning): Ataxia, blurred vision, drowsiness, anxiety, headache, GI upset, depression, urticaria, erythematous macular eruptions, blood dyscrasias, hypotension. *Treatment (Chronic Poisoning):* Discontinue medication. Monitor and treat blood dyscrasias. Provide symptomatic

P

treatment. Treat hypotension by IV fluids, elevation of legs, and a vasopressor with inotropic effects.

Drug Interactions

Diazoxide IV / Additive hypotensive effect
Levodopa / Papaverine ↓ effect of levodopa by blocking dopamine receptors

How Supplied: *Capsule, Extended Release:* 150 mg; *Injection:* 30 mg/mL

Dosage

- **Capsules, Timed-Release**

Ischemia.

150 mg q 12 hr. May be increased to 150 mg q 8 hr or 300 mg q 12 hr in difficult cases.

HEALTH CARE CONSIDERATIONS

Assessment

1. Record indications for therapy, type, onset, duration, and characteristics of symptoms.
2. Determine any cardiac dysfunction; monitor VS, ECG, and LFTs.
3. Record mental status; assess all extremities for color, warmth, and pulses.

Client/Family Teaching

1. Take with meals or milk to minimize GI upset.
2. Do not perform activities that require mental alertness until drug effects are realized; may cause dizziness or drowsiness.
3. Avoid tobacco products as nicotine may cause vasospasm.

Outcome/Evaluate: ↓ Pain symptoms R/T ischemia

P

Paregoric (Camphorated opium tincture)

(pair-eh-GOR-ick)

Pregnancy Category: C

(C-III) (Rx)

Classification: Antidiarrheal agent, systemic

See also *Narcotic Analgesics.*

Action/Kinetics: The active principle of the mixture is opium (0.04% morphine). The preparation also contains benzoic acid, camphor, and anise oil. Morphine increases the muscular tone of the intestinal tract, decreases digestive secretions, and inhibits normal peristalsis. The slowed passage of the feces through the intestines promotes desiccation, which is a function of the time the feces spend in the intestine. **t½:** 2–3 hr. **Duration:** 4–5 hr.

Uses: Acute diarrhea.

Contraindications: See *Morphine Sulfate.* Use in clients with diarrhea caused by poisoning until toxic substance has been eliminated. Treatment of pseudomembranous colitis due to lincomycin, penicillins, and cephalosporins. Rubbing paregoric on the gums of a teething child. Use to treat neonatal opioid dependence.

Side Effects: See *Narcotic Analgesics.*

Drug Interactions: See *Narcotic Analgesics.*

How Supplied: *Oral Liquid:* 2 mg/5 mL

Dosage

- **Liquid**

Adult: 5–10 mL 1–4 times/day (5 mL contains 2 mg of morphine). **Pediatric:** 0.25–0.5 mL/kg 1–4 times/day.

HEALTH CARE CONSIDERATIONS

See also *Health Care Considerations* for *Narcotic Analgesics.*

Administration/Storage

1. Administer with water to ensure that it reaches the stomach; mixture will have a milky appearance.
2. Store in a light-resistant container.
3. Carefully distinguish between paregoric and tincture of opium. Tincture of opium contains 25 times more morphine than paregoric.
4. Paregoric preparations are subject to the Controlled Substances Act and must be charted accordingly.
5. Have naloxone available to treat any overdosage.

Assessment

1. Record onset, duration, and condition requiring paregoric, level of effectiveness, other agents prescribed and the outcome.
2. Note any hepatic dysfunction or drug dependence.

Client/Family Teaching

1. Adhere to prescribed regimen.
2. Report if the diarrhea persists.
3. Stop medication once diarrhea has abated. Continued use may result in constipation.

Outcome/Evaluate: Relief of diarrhea

Paricalcitol

(pair-ee-KAL-sih-tohl)

Pregnancy Category: C

Zemplar **(Rx)**

Classification: Drug for hyperparathyroidism

Action/Kinetics: Synthetic vitamin D analog that reduces parathyroid hormone levels in chronic renal failure with no significant changes in the incidence of hypercalcemia or hyperphosphatemia. Serum phosphorous, calcium, and calcium x phosphorous product may increase. **Peak levels:** 5 min which decrease quickly within 2 hr. **t½:** About 15 hr. Hepatobiliary excretion is most common.

Uses: Prevention and treatment of secondary hyperparathyroidism associated with chronic renal failure.
Contraindications: Evidence of vitamin D toxicity, hypercalemia, or hypersensitivity to any part of the product. Use of phosphate or vitamin D-related compounds concomitantly with paricalcitol.
Special Concerns: Use with caution during lactation or if given with digitalis compounds. Safety and efficacy have not been determined in children.
Side Effects: *GI:* N&V, GI bleeding, dry mouth. *CV:* Palpitation. *CNS:* Lightheadedness. *Respiratory:* Pneumonia. *Miscellaneous:* Edema, chills, fever, flu, sepsis, not feeling well.
OD **Management of Overdose:** *Symptoms:* Hypercalcemia. Early symptoms include weakness, headache, somnolence, nausea, vomiting, dry mouth, constipation, muscle pain, bone pain, and metallic taste. Late symptoms include anorexia, weight loss, conjunctivitis, pancreatitis, photophobia, rhinorrhea, pruritus, hyperthermia, decreased libido, elevated BUN, hypercholesterolemia, elevated AST and ALT, ectopic calcification, hypertension, cardiac arrhythmias, somnolence, overt psychosis, death (rarely). *Treatment:* Immediately reduce or discontinue therapy. Institute a low calcium diet and withdraw calcium supplements. Mobilize client, give attention to fluid and electrolyte imbalances, assess ECG abnormalities (especially if also taking digitalis), and undertake hemodialysis or peritoneal dialysis against a calcium-free dialysate. Monitor serum calcium levels frequentlly until normal values are obtained.
Drug Interactions: Digitalis toxicity is potentiated by hypercalcemia.
How Supplied: *Injection:* 5 mcg/mL

Dosage

- **Injection**

Treat hyperparathyroidism associated with chronic renal failure.

Initial: 0.04–0.1 mcg/kg (2.8 to 7 mcg) as a bolus dose no more frequently than every other day at any time during dialysis. Doses as high as 0.24 mcg/kg (16.8 mcg) have been used safely. If a satisfactory response is not seen, the dose may be increased by 2 to 4 mcg at 2– 4–week intervals. During any dosage adjustment period, monitor serum calcum and phosphorous levels more frequently. If an elevated calcium level or Ca x P product greater than 75 is noted, immediately reduce or stop the drug until parameters are normal. Then, restart at a lower dose. Doses may need to be decreased as the parathyroid levels decrease in response to therapy.

HEALTH CARE CONSIDERATIONS

Administration/Storage: Store at 25°C (77°F). Discard unused portion.

Assessment

1. Note indications for therapy.
2. Initially and with dose adjustment monitor Ca and P twice weekly and then q mo once dose established. Monitor PTH every 3 mo.

Client/Family Teaching

1. Client must adhere to a dietary regimen of calcium supplementation and phosphorous restriction.
2. Avoid excessive use of aluminum-containing compounds.
3. Drug is used for the prevention and treatment of secondary hyperparathyroidism associated with CRF.
4. May experience nausea, vomiting, and edema; report if persistent or intolerable.

Outcome/Evaluate: ↓ PTH concentrations

Paromomycin sulfate

(pair-oh-moh-**MY**-sin)
Humatin **(Rx)**
Classification: Antibiotic, aminoglycoside

See also *Aminoglycosides.*
Action/Kinetics: Obtained from *Streptomyces rimosus forma paromomycina.* Spectrum of activity resembles that of neomycin and kanamycin. Poorly absorbed from the GI tract and is ineffective against systemic infections when given PO.
Uses: Inhibition of ammonia-forming bacteria in GI tract in hepatic encephalopathy, intestinal amebiasis, preoperative suppression of intestinal flora. Hepatic coma. *Investigational:* Anthelmintic, to treat *Dientamoeba fragilis, Diphyllobothrium latum, Taenia saginata, T. solium, Dipylidium caninum,* and *Hymenolepis nana.*
Contraindications: Intestinal obstruction.
Special Concerns: Use during pregnancy only if benefits outweigh risks. Use with caution in the presence of GI ulceration because of possible systemic absorption.
Additional Side Effects: Diarrhea or loose stools. Heartburn, emesis, and pruritus ani. Superinfections, especially by monilia.
Drug Interactions: Penicillin is inhibited by paromomycin.
How Supplied: *Capsule:* 250 mg

Dosage

- **Capsules**

Hepatic coma.

Adults: 4 g/day in divided doses for 5–6 days.

Intestinal amebiasis.

Adults and children: 25–35 mg/kg/day administered in three doses with meals for 5–10 days.

D. fragilis infections.

25–30 mg/kg/day in three divided doses for 1 week.

H. nana infections.

45 mg/kg/day for 5–7 days.

D. latum, T. saginata, T. solium, D. caninum infections.

Adults: 1 g/ q 15 min for a total of four doses; **pediatric:** 11 mg/kg/15 min for four doses.

HEALTH CARE CONSIDERATIONS

See also *Health Care Considerations* for *Aminoglycosides.*

Administration/Storage: Do not administer parenterally and/or concurrently with penicillin.

Client/Family Teaching

1. Take before or after meals.
2. Report any persistent diarrhea, dehydration, and general weakness.

Outcome/Evaluate: Suppression of intestinal flora

P

Paroxetine hydrochloride

(pah-**ROX**-eh-teen)

Pregnancy Category: B

Paxil **(Rx)**

Classification: Antidepressant

Action/Kinetics: Inhibits neuronal reuptake of serotonin in the CNS resulting in potentiation of serotonergic activity in the CNS. Weak effects on neuronal uptake of norepinephrine and dopamine. Does not cause anticholinergic effects or orthostatic hypotension; slight sedative effects. Completely absorbed from the GI tract. **Time to peak plasma levels:** 5.2 hr. **Peak plasma levels:** 61.7 ng/mL. **t½:** 21–24 hr. **Time to reach steady state:** 7–14 days. Plasma levels are increased in impaired renal and hepatic function as well as in geriatric clients. Extensively metabolized in the liver to inactive metabolites. Approximately two-thirds of the drug is excreted through the urine and one-third is excreted in the feces.

Uses: Treatment of major depressive episodes, panic disorder with or without agoraphobia (as defined in DSM-IV), and obsessive-compulsive disorders (as defined in DSM-III-R). *Investigational:* Headaches, diabetic neuropathy, premature ejaculation.

Contraindications: Use of alcohol and in clients taking MAO inhibitors.

Special Concerns: Use with caution and initially at reduced dosage in elderly clients as well as in those with impaired hepatic or renal function, with a history of mania, with a history of seizures, in clients with diseases or conditions that could affect metabolism or hemodynamic responses, and during lactation. Concurrent administration of paroxetine with lithium or digoxin should be undertaken with caution. Safety and efficacy have not been determined in children.

Side Effects: The side effects listed were observed with a frequency up to 1 in 1,000 clients.

CNS: Headache, somnolence, insomnia, agitation, ***seizures,*** tremor, anxiety, activation of mania or hypomania, dizziness, nervousness, paresthesia, drugged feeling, myoclonus, CNS stimulation, confusion, amnesia, impaired concentration, depression, emotional lability, vertigo, abnormal thinking, akinesia, alcohol abuse, ataxia, ***convulsions, possibility of a suicide attempt*** depersonalization, hallucinations, hyperkinesia, hypertonia, incoordination, lack of emotion, manic reaction, paranoid reaction. *GI:* Nausea, abdominal pain, diarrhea, dry mouth, vomiting, constipation, decreased appetite, flatulence, oropharynx disorder (“lump” in throat, tightness in throat), dyspepsia, increased appetite, bruxism, dysphagia, eructation, gastritis, glossitis, increased salivation, mouth ulceration, ***rectal hemorrhage,*** abnormal LFTs. *Hematologic:* Anemia, leukopenia, lymphadenopathy, purpura. *CV:* Palpitation, vasodilation, postural hypotension, hypertension, syncope, tachycardia, bradycardia, conduction abnormalities, abnormal ECG, hypotension, migraine, peripheral vascular disorder. *Dermatologic:* Sweating, rash, pruritus, acne, alopecia, dry skin, ecchymosis, eczema, furunculosis, urticaria. *Metabolic/Nutritional:* Edema, weight gain, weight loss, hyperglycemia, peripheral edema, thirst. *Respiratory:* Respiratory disorder (cold symptoms or URI), pharyngitis, yawn, increased cough, rhinitis, asthma, bronchitis, dyspnea, epistaxis, hyperventilation, pneumonia, respiratory flu, sinusitis. *GU:* Abnormal ejaculation (usually delay), erectile difficulties, sexual dysfunction, impotence, urinary frequency, urinary difficulty or hesitancy, decreased libido, anorgasmia in women, difficulty in reaching climax/orgasm in women, abortion, amenorrhea, breast pain, cystitis, dysmenorrhea, dysuria, menorrhagia, nocturia, polyuria, urethritis, urinary incontinence, urinary retention, vaginitis. *Musculoskeletal:* Asthenia, back pain, myopathy, myalgia, myasthenia, neck pain, arthralgia, arthritis. *Ophthalmologic:* Blurred vision, abnormality of accommodation, eye pain, mydriasis. *Otic:* Ear pain, otitis media, tinnitus. *Miscellaneous:* Fever, chest pain, trauma, taste perversion or loss, chills, malaise, allergic reaction, ***carcinoma,*** face edema, moniliasis, anorexia.

NOTE: Over 4- to 6-week period, there was evidence of adaptation to side effects such as nausea and dizziness but less adaptation to dry mouth, somnolence, and asthenia.

OD **Management of Overdose:** *Symptoms:* N&V, drowsiness, sinus tachycardia, dilated pupils. *Treatment:*

- Establish and maintain an airway.
- Ensure adequate oxygenation and ventilation.
- Induction of emesis, lavage, or both; following evacuation, 20–30 g activated charcoal may be given q 4–6 hr during the first 24–48 hr after ingestion.
- Take an ECG and monitor cardiac function if there is any evidence of abnormality.
- Provide supportive care with monitoring of VS.

Drug Interactions

Antiarrhythmics, Type IC / Possible ↑ effect due to ↓ liver breakdown
Cimetidine / ↑ Effect of paroxetine due to ↓ breakdown by the liver
Digoxin / Possible ↓ plasma levels
MAO inhibitors / Possibility of serious, and sometimes fatal, reactions including hyperthermia, rigidity, myoclonus, autonomic instability with possible rapid fluctuations in VS, and mental status changes including extreme agitation progressing to delirium and coma
Phenobarbital / Possible ↓ effect of paroxetine due to ↑ breakdown by the liver
Phenytoin / Possible ↓ effect of paroxetine due to ↑ breakdown by the liver; also, paroxetine ↓ levels of phenytoin
Procyclidine / ↓ Dose of procyclidine as significant anticholinergic effects are seen
Theophylline / ↑ Theophylline levels
Tryptophan / Possibility of headache, nausea, sweating, and dizziness when taken together
Warfarin / Possibility of ↑ bleeding tendencies

How Supplied: *Suspension:* 10 mg/5 mL; *Tablet:* 10 mg, 20 mg, 30 mg, 40 mg

Dosage

- **Tablets**

Depression.

Adults: 20 mg/day, usually given as a single dose in the morning. Some clients not responding to the 20-mg dose may benefit from increasing the dose in 10-mg/day increments, up to a maximum of 50 mg/day. Make dose changes at intervals of at least 1 week.

Panic disorders.

Adults, initial: 10 mg/day usually given in the morning; **then,** increase by 10-mg increments each week until a dose of 40 mg/day is reached. Maximum daily dose: 60 mg.

Obsessive-compulsive disorders.

Adults, initial: 20 mg/kg; **then,** increase by 10-mg increments a day in intervals of at least 1 week until a dose of 40 mg/kg is reached. Maximum daily dose: 60 mg.

Headaches.

10–50 mg/day.

Diabetic neuropathy.

10–60 mg/day.

Premature ejaculation in men.

20 mg/day.

NOTE: Geriatric or debilitated clients, those with severe hepatic or renal impairment, **initial:** 10 mg/day, up to a maximum of 40 mg/day for all uses.

HEALTH CARE CONSIDERATIONS

Administration/Storage

1. Even though beneficial effects may be seen in 1–4 weeks, continue therapy as prescribed.
2. Effectiveness is maintained for up to 1 year with daily doses averaging 30 mg.

Assessment

1. Record type, onset, and duration of symptoms, any previous treatment, and the outcome.
2. Note clinical presentation and behavioral manifestations.
3. Record any mania, altered metabolic or hemodynamic states, or seizures.
4. List drugs currently prescribed to ensure no unfavorable interactions. Do not use in combination with a MAO or within 14 days of discontinuing treatment with a MAO.
5. Monitor weight, VS, ECG, electrolytes, CBC, liver and renal function studies; note any dysfunction.
6. During management of overdose, always entertain the possibility of multiple drug involvement.

Client/Family Teaching

1. Take only as directed. Prescriptions will be

P

for small quantities to ensure compliance and to discourage overdose.
2. Do not engage in tasks that require mental alertness until drug effects realized.
3. Avoid alcohol and OTC products.
4. Report excessive weight loss and adjust diet to compensate.
5. Notify provider if pregnancy is suspected or planned.
6. Report any thoughts of suicide or increased suicide ideations. Advise family not to leave severely depressed individuals alone; possibility of a suicide attempt is inherent in depression and may persist until significant remission is observed.
7. Participate in therapy sessions designed to assist with underlying problems.

Outcome/Evaluate
- ↓ Depression
- Improved eating/sleeping patterns; ↑ social involvement/activity
- ↓ Panic attacks; ↓ obsessive repetitive behaviors

COMBINATION DRUG

Pediazole

(PEE-dee-ah-zohl)
Pregnancy Category: C
(Rx)
Classification: Antibacterial

See also *Erythromycins* and *Sulfonamides*.
Content: This product is available as granules that, when reconstituted, provide an oral suspension.

Antibacterial, antibiotic: Erythromycin ethylsuccinate, 200 mg/5 mL erythromycin activity. *Antibacterial, sulfonamide:* Sulfisoxazole, 600 mg/5 mL. See also information on individual components.
Uses: Acute otitis media in children caused by *Haemophilus influenzae*.
Contraindications: Pregnancy at term and in children less than 2 months of age. Use with caution during other times of pregnancy.
How Supplied: See Content

Dosage

- **Oral Suspension**

Usual: Equivalent of 50 mg/kg/day of erythromycin and 150 mg/kg/day of sulfisoxazole, up to a maximum of 6 g/day. **Over 45 kg:** 10 mL q 6 hr; **24 kg:** 7.5 mL q 6 hr; **16 kg:** 5 mL q 6 hr; **8 kg:** 2.5 mL q 6 hr; **less than 8 kg:** Calculate dose according to body weight.

HEALTH CARE CONSIDERATIONS

See also *General Nursing Considerations for All Anti-Infectives* and *Sulfonamides*.

Administration/Storage
1. Refrigerate the reconstituted suspension and use within 14 days.
2. Continue therapy for 10 days.

Client/Family Teaching
1. Review the appropriate method, dosage, and frequency for administration.
2. May take without regard to meals.
3. Keep medication refrigerated; shake well before using.
4. Return as scheduled for F/U to ensure desired response to therapy.

Outcome/Evaluate: Resolution of infection; symptomatic improvement

Pemirolast potassium ophthalmic solution

(peh-MEER-oh-last)
Pregnancy Category: C
Alamast **(Rx)**
Classification: Mast cell stabilizier, ophthalmic drug

Action/Kinetics: Inhibits the antigen-induced release of inflammatory mediators such as histamine and leukotriene C_4, D_4, and E_4, from human mast cells. Also inhibits the chemotaxis of eosinophils into ocular tissue and blocks the release of mediators from human eosinophils. Probably acts by preventing calcium influx into mast cells upon antigen stimulation. A small amount is absorbed systemically.
Uses: Prevent itching of the eye due to allergic conjunctivitis.
Contraindications: Use by injection or PO.
Special Concerns: Use with caution during lactation. Safety and efficacy have not been determined in children less than 3 years of age.
Side Effects: *Ophthalmic:* Burning, dry eye, foreign body sensation, ocular discomfort. *Respiratory:* Rhinitis, cold/flu symptoms, bronchitis, cough, sinusitis, sneezing/nasal congestion. *Miscellaneous:* Headache, allergy, back pain, dysmenorrhea, fever.
How Supplied: *Ophthalmic Solution:* 0.1%

Dosage

- **Ophthalmic Solution**

Allergic conjunctivitis.
1–2 gtt in each affected eye q.i.d. Effect may be evident within a few days but frequently requires up to four weeks.

HEALTH CARE CONSIDERATIONS

Administration/Storage: Store at 15–25°C (59–77°F).

Assessment: Note indications for therapy, onset, duration, and characteristics of symptoms. Identify triggers.

Client/Family Teaching

1. Review administration procedure using 1-2 drops four times per day.
2. To prevent contamination of the dropper tip and solution, do not touch the eyelids or surrounding areas with the dropper tip. Keep bottle tightly closed when not in use.
3. Do not wear contact lenses if eyes are red.
4. Do not use to treat contact lens irritation.
5. Lauralkonium chloride, the preservative used, may be absorbed by soft contact lenses. Wait at least ten minutes after instilling pemirolast before inserting contact lenses.
6. May experience ocular burning, dryness, foreign body sensation, or discomfort as well as URI S&S.

Outcome/Evaluate: Symptomatic relief of allergic conjunctivitis

Pemoline

(PEM-oh-leen)

Pregnancy Category: B

Cylert, Cylert Chewable **(C-IV) (Rx)**

Classification: CNS stimulant

Action/Kinetics: Believed to act by dopaminergic mechanisms. Causes a decrease in hyperactivity and a prolonged attention span in children. **Peak serum levels:** 2–4 hr. **Duration:** Up to 8 hr. **t½:** 12 hr. **Steady state:** 2–3 days; beneficial effects may not be noted for 3–4 weeks. Approximately 50% is bound to plasma protein. Metabolized by the liver, and approximately 50% is excreted unchanged by the kidneys.

Uses: Attention-deficit disorders. Due to possible life-threatening hepatic failure, not usually first-line therapy. *Investigational:* Narcolepsy.

Contraindications: Hypersensitivity to drug. Tourette's syndrome. Children under 6 years of age.

Special Concerns: Safe use during lactation has not been established. Use with caution in impaired renal or kidney function. Chronic use in children may cause growth suppression.

Side Effects: *CNS:* Insomnia (most common). Dyskinesia of the face, tongue, lips, and extremities; precipitation of Tourette's syndrome. Mild depression, headache, nystagmus, dizziness, hallucinations, irritability, ***seizures.*** Exacerbation of behavior disturbances and thought disorders in psychotic children. *GI:* Transient weight loss, gastric upset, nausea. *Miscellaneous:* Skin rash, ***hepatic failure.***

Laboratory Test Considerations: ↑ AST, ALT, serum LDH.

OD **Management of Overdose:** *Symptoms:* Symptoms of CNS stimulation and sympathomimetic effects including agitation, confusion, delirium, euphoria, headache, muscle twitching, mydriasis, vomiting, hallucinations, flushing, sweating, tachycardia, hyperreflexia, tremors, ***hyperpyrexia,*** hypertension, ***seizures (may be followed by coma).*** *Treatment:* Reduce external stimuli. If symptoms are not severe, induce vomiting or undertake gastric lavage. Chlorpromazine can be used to decrease the CNS stimulation and sympathomimetic effects.

How Supplied: *Chew Tablet:* 37.5 mg; *Tablet:* 18.75 mg, 37.5 mg, 75 mg

Dosage

- **Tablets, Chewable Tablets**

  Attention-deficit disorders.

Children, 6 years and older, initial: 37.5 mg/day as a single dose in the morning; increase at 1-week intervals by 18.75 mg until desired response is attained up to maximum of 112.5 mg/day. **Usual maintenance:** 56.25–75 mg/day.

Narcolepsy.

Adults: 50–200 mg/day in two divided doses.

HEALTH CARE CONSIDERATIONS

Administration/Storage: Interrupt treatment once or twice annually to determine whether behavioral symptoms still necessitate drug therapy.

Assessment

1. Record indications for therapy, type, onset, and characteristics of symptoms; describe clinical presentation.
2. List other agents prescribed and the outcome.

Client/Family Teaching

1. Administer early in the morning to minimize insomnia.
2. Do not perform activities that require mental alertness until drug effects are realized.
3. Avoid excessive consumption of caffeine-containing products.
4. Advise school health department of medication regimen.
5. Measure height every month, and weigh child twice/week. Graph all measurements and bring to each visit. Report weight loss or failure to grow.
6. Continue therapy; behavioral changes take 3–4 weeks to occur.

7. Instruct when to interrupt drug administration, and to observe and record behavior without the medication, to determine whether therapy should be resumed.
8. Stress importance of bringing the child in periodically for LFTs to assess for toxicity.
9. Identify signs of overdosage, such as agitation, restlessness, hallucinations, and tachycardia; withhold drug, protect the child, and report immediately.

Outcome/Evaluate: Improved attention span; ↓ hyperactivity with ability to sit quietly and concentrate

Penbutolol sulfate

(pen-**BYOU**-toe-lohl)
Pregnancy Category: C
Levatol **(Rx)**
Classification: Beta-adrenergic blocking agent

See also *Beta-Adrenergic Blocking Agents*.

Action/Kinetics: Has both beta-1- and beta-2-receptor blocking activity. It has no membrane-stabilizing activity but does possess minimal intrinsic sympathomimetic activity. High lipid solubility. **t½:** 5 hr. 80%–98% protein bound. Metabolized in the liver and excreted through the urine.

Uses: Mild to moderate arterial hypertension.

Contraindications: Bronchial asthma or bronchospasms, including severe COPD.

Special Concerns: Dosage has not been established in children. Geriatric clients may manifest increased or decreased sensitivity to the usual adult dose.

How Supplied: *Tablet:* 20 mg

Dosage

- **Tablets**

  Hypertension.

Initial: 20 mg/day either alone or with other antihypertensive agents. **Maintenance:** Same as initial dose. Doses greater than 40 mg/day do not result in a greater antihypertensive effect.

HEALTH CARE CONSIDERATIONS

See also *Health Care Considerations* for *Antihypertensive Agents*.

Administration/Storage: Doses of 10 mg/day are effective but full effects are not evident for 4–6 weeks. The full effect of a 20- to 40-mg dose may not be observed for 2 weeks.

Client/Family Teaching

1. May cause postural hypotension; to avoid, rise slowly from a sitting or lying position.
2. Take only as prescribed; full effects may not be realized for a month or more.
3. May cause an increased sensitivity to cold; dress appropriately.

Outcome/Evaluate: ↓ BP

Penciclovir

(pen-**SIGH**-kloh-veer)
Pregnancy Category: B
Denavir **(Rx)**
Classification: Antiviral drug

See also *Antiviral Drugs*.

Action/Kinetics: Active against herpes simplex viruses (HSVs), including HSV-1 and HSV-2. In infected cells, viral thymidine kinase phosphorylates penciclovir to a monophosphate form which then is converted to penciclovir triphosphate by cellular kinases. Penciclovir triphosphate inhibits HSV polymerase competitively with deoxyguanosine triphosphate which inhibits herpes viral DNA synthesis and replication. Not absorbed through the skin.

Uses: Treatment of recurrent herpes labialis (cold sores) in adults.

Contraindications: Lactation. Application of the drug to mucous membranes.

Special Concerns: Use with caution if applied around the eyes due to the possibility of irritation. The effect of the drug in immunocompromised clients has not been determined. Safety and efficacy have not been determined in children.

Side Effects: *Dermatologic:* Reaction at the site of application, hypesthesia, local anesthesia, erythematous rash, mild erythema. *Miscellaneous:* Headache, taste perversion.

How Supplied: *Cream:* 10 mg/g.

Dosage

- **Cream (10 mg/g)**

  Cold sores.

Apply q 2 hr while awake for 4 days.

HEALTH CARE CONSIDERATIONS

See also *Health Care Considerations* for *Antiviral Drugs*.

Administration/Storage

1. Start treatment as soon as possible during the prodrome or when lesions appear.
2. Use only on the lips and face.

Assessment: Record onset, location, description, and extent of lesions. Note frequency of occurrence and any triggers or prodrome.

Client/Family Teaching

1. Apply q 2 hr while awake for 4 days at first cold sore symptoms.

2. Avoid contact with mucous membranes; apply to lips and face only.
3. Use sunscreens and lip balms with a sunscreen when sun exposed to prevent recurrence and to diminish intersity of outbreaks.
4. Report if lesions do not improve or if a foul odor or purulent drainage appears.

Outcome/Evaluate: ↓ Intensity/pain; clearing of herpes labialis lesions

Penicillamine

(pen-ih-**SILL**-ah-meen)

Pregnancy Category: D

Cuprimine, Depen **(Rx)**

Classification: Antirheumatic, heavy metal antagonist, to treat cystinuria

Action/Kinetics: A chelating agent for mercury, lead, iron, and copper; forms soluble complexes, thus decreasing toxic levels of the metal (e.g., copper in Wilson's disease). Anti-inflammatory activity may be due to its ability to inhibit T-lymphocyte function and therefore decrease cell-mediated immune response. May also protect lymphocytes from hydrogen peroxide generated at the site of inflammation by inhibiting release of lysosomal enzymes and oxygen radicals. Beneficial effects may not be seen for 2 to 3 months when used for rheumatoid arthritis. In cystinuria, is able to reduce excess cystine excretion, probably by disulfide interchange between penicillamine and cystine. This results in penicillamine-cysteine disulfide, which is a complex that is more soluble than cystine and is thus readily excreted. Well absorbed from the GI tract and excreted in urine. Food decreases the absorption of penicillamine over 50%. **Peak plasma levels:** 1–3 hr. About 80% is bound to plasma albumin. **t½:** Approximately 2 hr. Metabolites are excreted through the urine.

Uses: Wilson's disease, cystinuria, and rheumatoid arthritis (severe active disease unresponsive to conventional therapy). Heavy metal antagonist. *Investigational:* Primary biliary cirrhosis. Scleroderma.

Contraindications: Pregnancy, lactation, penicillinase-related aplastic anemia or agranulocytosis, hypersensitivity to drug. Clients allergic to penicillin may cross-react with penicillamine. Renal insufficiency or history thereof.

Special Concerns: Use for juvenile rheumatoid arthritis has not been established. Clients older than 65 years may be at greater risk of developing hematologic side effects.

Side Effects: This drug manifests a large number of potentially serious side effects. Clients should be carefully monitored. *GI:* Altered taste perception (common), N&V, diarrhea, anorexia, GI pain, stomatitis, oral ulcerations, reactivation of peptic ulcer, glossitis, cheilosis, colitis, gingivostomatitis (rare). *CNS:* Tinnitus, myasthenia gravis, peripheral sensory and motor neuropathies (with or without muscle weakness), reversible optic neuritis, polyradiculopathy (rare). *Hematologic:* Thrombocytopenia, leukopenia, ***agranulocytosis, aplastic anemia,*** eosinophilia, monocytosis, red cell aplasia, thrombocytopenia, ***hemolytic anemia,*** leukocytosis, thrombocytosis. *Renal:* Proteinuria, hematuria, nephrotic syndrome, ***Goodpasture's syndrome*** (a severe and ultimately fatal glomerulonephritis). *Allergic:* Rashes (common), lupus-like syndrome, drug fever, pruritus, pemphigoid-type symptoms (e.g., bullous lesions), arthralgia, lymphadenopathy, dermatoses, urticaria, thyroiditis, hypoglycemia, migratory polyarthralgia, polymyositis, allergic alveolitis. *Respiratory:* Obliterative bronchiolitis, pulmonary fibrosis, pneumonitis, bronchial asthma, interstitial pneumonitis. *Dermatologic:* Increased skin friability, excessive skin wrinkling, development of small white papules at venipuncture and surgical sites, alopecia or falling hair, lichen planus, dermatomyositis, nail disorders, ***toxic epidermal necrolysis,*** cutaneous macular atrophy. *Hepatic:* Pancreatitis, hepatic dysfunction, intrahepatic cholestasis, toxic hepatitis (rare). *Other:* Thrombophlebitis, hyperpyrexia, polymyositis, mammary hyperplasia, renal vasculitis (may be fatal), hot flashes, lupus erythematosus–like syndrome.

Laboratory Test Considerations: ↑ Serum alkaline phosphatase, LDH. Positive thymol turbidity test and cephalin flocculation test.

Drug Interactions

Antacids / ↓ Effect of penicillamine due to ↓ absorption from GI tract
Antimalarial drugs / ↑ Risk of blood dyscrasias and adverse renal effects
Cytotoxic drugs / ↑ Risk of blood dyscrasias and adverse renal effects
Digoxin / Penicillamine ↓ effect of digoxin
Gold therapy / ↑ Risk of blood dyscrasias and adverse renal effects
Iron salts / ↓ Effect of penicillamine due to ↓ absorption from GI tract

How Supplied: *Capsule:* 125 mg, 250 mg; *Tablet:* 250 mg

Dosage

• **Capsules, Tablets**

P

Rheumatoid arthritis.
Adults, individualized, initial: 125–250 mg/day. Dosage may be increased at 1- to 3-month intervals by 125- to 250-mg increments until adequate response is attained. **Maximum:** 500–750 mg/day. Up to 500 mg/day can be given as a single dose; higher dosages should be divided. **Maintenance, individualized. Range:** 500–750 mg/day. If the client is in remission for 6 or more months, a gradual stepwise decrease in dose of 125 or 250 mg/day at about 3-month intervals can be attempted.

Wilson's disease.
Dosage is usually calculated on the basis of the urinary excretion of copper. One gram of penicillamine promotes excretion of 2 mg of copper. **Adults and adolescents, usual, initial:** 250 mg q.i.d. Dosage may have to be increased to 2 g/day. A further increase does not produce additional excretion. **Pediatric, 6 months—young children:** 250 mg as a single dose given in fruit juice.

Antidote for heavy metals.
Adults: 0.5–1.5 g/day for 1–2 months; **pediatric:** 30–40 mg/kg/day (600–750 mg/m^2/day) for 1–6 months.

Cystinuria.
Individualized and based on excretion rate of cystine (100–200 mg/day in clients with no history of stones, below 100 mg with clients with history of stones or pain). Initiate at low dosage (250 mg/day) and increase gradually to minimum effective dosage. **Adult, usual:** 2 g/day (range: 1–4 g/day); **pediatric:** 7.5 mg/kg q.i.d. If divided in fewer than four doses, give larger dose at night.

Primary biliary cirrhosis.
Adults: 600–900 mg/day.

P

HEALTH CARE CONSIDERATIONS

Administration/Storage

1. If unable to tolerate dosage for cystinuria, the bedtime dosage should be larger and should be continued.
2. Administer the contents of the capsule in 15–30 mL of chilled juice or pureed fruit if unable to swallow capsules or tablets.
3. When treating rheumatoid arthritis, discontinue if doses up to 1.5 g/day for 2–3 months do not produce improvement.
4. Alternative dosage forms may be prepared if needed. An elixir containing 50 mg/mL may be prepared by dissolving the contents of 48 capsules in 100 mL of water. This is then filtered, and 100 mL of cherry syrup and 30 mL of alcohol stirred in. The volume is then brought up to 240 mL with water. The preparation is shaken well and stored in the refrigerator. Suppositories (750 mg) may be prepared by melting 51 g of cocoa butter and dissolving the contents of 150 capsules in the cocoa butter; the mixture is poured into a prelubricated suppository mold and then frozen and stored in a refrigerator.

Assessment

1. Determine indications, presenting symptoms, other therapies prescribed and outcome.
2. Note if taking any medication with which penicillamine will interact unfavorably; impedes absorption of many drugs.
3. Assess hearing to detect any evidence of hearing loss.
4. Record CNS assessment and neurologic status.
5. With arthritis, assess joints for pain, stiffness, soreness, swelling, and ↓ ROM.
6. Test for pregnancy; drug can cause fetal damage.
7. White papules appearing at the site of venipuncture or at surgical sites may indicate sensitivity to penicillamine or the presence of infection.
8. If to undergo surgery, anticipate dosage reduction to 250 mg/day until wound healing is complete.
9. Monitor CBC, LFTs, and urinalysis. If WBC falls below 3,500/mm^3 or the platelet count falls below 100,000/mm^3, withhold drug and report. If counts are low for three successive lab tests, a temporary interruption of therapy is indicated.
10. A positive ANA test indicates client may develop a lupus-like syndrome in the future. The drug need not be discontinued.

Client/Family Teaching

1. Give on an empty stomach 1 hr before or 2 hr after meals; wait 1 hr after ingestion of any other food, milk, or drug. Report if unable to tolerate dosage for cystinuria as the bedtime dosage should be larger and continued.
2. Take temperature nightly during the first few months of therapy. A fever may indicate a hypersensitivity reaction.
3. Report any evidence of fever, sore throat, chills, bruising, or bleeding; early symptoms of granulocytopenia.
4. If stomatitis occurs, report immediately and stop drug. Practice regular oral hygiene such as brushing teeth with a soft toothbrush, flossing daily, and using alcohol free mouth rinses.
5. Inspect mucosal surfaces at regular intervals. Report if ulcers appear and are severe or

persistent, may need to reduce drug dose as it may interfere with wound healing.
6. Penicillamine increases the body's need for pyridoxine. May be given pyridoxine (25 mg/day po).
7. A loss of taste perception or a metallic taste may develop; relates to zinc chelation and may last for 2 months or more. With N&V or diarrhea, monitor weight and I&O. Report jaundice or other signs of hepatic dysfunction.
8. If to receive an oral iron preparation, at least 2 hr should elapse between ingestion of penicillamine and the dose of therapeutic iron. Iron decreases the cupruretic effects of penicillamine.
9. Skin tends to become friable and susceptible to injury; avoid activities that could injure skin. Elderly should avoid excessive pressure on the shoulders, elbows, knees, toes, and buttocks.
10. Report cloudy urine or urine that is smoky brown (signs of proteinuria and hematuria).
11. Practice reliable birth control; report missed menstrual period or other symptoms of pregnancy.
12. With Wilson's disease:
• Eat a diet low in copper. Exclude foods such as chocolate, nuts, shellfish, mushrooms, liver, molasses, broccoli, and copper-enriched cereals.
• Use distilled or demineralized water if drinking water contains more than 0.1 mg/L copper.
• Unless taking iron supplements, take sulfurated potash or Carbo-Resin with meals to minimize the absorption of copper.
• It may take 1–3 months for neurologic improvements to occur. Therefore, continue the therapy even if no improvements seem evident.
• Check any vitamin preparations being used to ensure that they do not contain copper.
13. If cystinuria occurs, do the following:
• Drink large amounts of fluid to prevent the formation of renal calculi. Drink 500 mL of fluid at bedtime and another pint during the night, when the urine tends to be the most concentrated and most acidic. The greater the fluid intake, the lower the required dose of penicillamine.
• Measure specific gravity and determine pH. The urine specific gravity should be maintained at less than 1.010 and the pH maintained at 7.5–8.0.
• Obtain yearly X-ray of the kidneys to detect presence of renal calculi.
• Eat a diet low in methionine, a major precursor of cystine. Exclude foods high in cystine such as rich meat, soups and broths, milk, eggs, cheeses, and peas.
• If client is pregnant or a child, diets low in methionine are also low in calcium; consider calcium supplementation.
14. With rheumatoid arthritis, continue using other therapies and meds to achieve relief from symptoms; penicillamine may take 4–6 mo to have therapeutic effect. As improvement begins, analgesic drugs and NSAIDs may be slowly discontinued.

Outcome/Evaluate
• ↑ Urinary excretion of copper
• ↓ Cystine excretion and prevention of renal calculi in cystinuria
• ↓ Joint pain, swelling, inflammation, and stiffness with ↑ mobility

COMBINATION DRUG

Penicillin G benzathine and Procaine combined, intramuscular

(pen-ih-**SILL**-in, **BEN**-zah-theen, **PROH**-kain)
Pregnancy Category: B
Bicillin C-R, Bicillin C-R 900/300 **(Rx)**
Classification: Antibiotic, penicillin

See also *Anti-Infectives* and *Penicillins*.
Content: The injection contains the following: *300,000 units/dose:* 150,000 units each of penicillin G benzathine and penicillin G procaine. *600,000 units/dose:* 300,000 units each of penicillin G benzathine and penicillin G procaine. *1,200,000 units/dose:* 600,000 units each of penicillin G benzathine and penicillin G procaine. *2,400,000 units/dose:* 1,200,000 units each of penicillin G benzathine and penicillin G procaine. *Injection, 900/300 per dose.* 900,000 units of penicillin G benzathine and 300,000 units of penicillin G procaine.
Uses: Streptococcal infections (A, C, G, H, L, and M) without bacteremia, of the upper respiratory tract, skin, and soft tissues. Scarlet fever, erysipelas, pneumococcal infections, and otitis media. *Note:* For severe pneumonia, empyema, bacteremia, pericarditis, meningitis, peritonitis, and arthritis of pneumococcal etiology, use aqueous penicillin G during the acute stage.
Contraindications: Use to treat syphilis, gonorrhea, yaws, bejel, and pinta.
Additional Drug Interactions: Aspirin, ethacrynic acid, furosemide, indomethacin, sulfonamides, or thiazide diuretics may

P

compete with penicillin G for renal tubular secretion → prolongation of serum t½ of penicillin

How Supplied: See Content

Dosage

• **IM Only**

Streptococcal infections.

Adults and children over 27 kg: 2,400,000 units, given at a single session using multiple injection sites or, alternatively, in divided doses on days 1 and 3; **children 13.5–27 kg:** 900,000–1,200,000 units; **infants and children under 13.5 kg:** 600,000 units.

Pneumococcal infections, except meningitis.

Adults: 1,200,000 units; **pediatric:** 600,000 units. Give q 2–3 days until temperature is normal for 48 hr.

HEALTH CARE CONSIDERATIONS

See also *Health Care Considerations* for *Penicillins.*

Administration/Storage

1. For adults, administer by deep IM injection in the upper outer quadrant of the buttock. For infants and children, use the midlateral aspect of the thigh.
2. Rotate injection sites for repeated doses.
3. Refrigerate but protect from freezing.

Outcome/Evaluate: Resolution of infection

P

Penicillin G benzathine, intramuscular

(pen-ih-SILL-in, BEN-zah-theen)

Pregnancy Category: B

Bicillin L-A, Megacillin Suspension ✱, Permapen **(Rx)**

Classification: Antibiotic, penicillin

See also *Anti-Infectives* and *Penicillins.*

Action/Kinetics: Penicillin G is neither penicillinase resistant nor acid stable. The product is a long-acting (repository) form of penicillin in an aqueous vehicle; it is administered as a sterile suspension. **Peak plasma levels: IM** 0.03–0.05 unit/mL.

Uses: Infections due to penicillin G sensitive microorganisms susceptible to low and prolonged serum levels. Mild to moderate URTI due to susceptible streptococci. Syphilis, yaws, bejel, and pinta. Prophylaxis of rheumatic fever or chorea. Follow-up prophylactic therapy for rheumatic heart disease and acute glomerulonephritis.

Contraindications: IV use.

Additional Drug Interactions: Aspirin, ethacrynic acid, furosemide, indomethacin, sulfonamides, or thiazide diuretics may compete with penicillin G for renal tubular secretion → prolongation of serum t½ of penicillin

How Supplied: *Injection:* 300,000 U/mL, 600,000 U/mL

Dosage

• **Parenteral Suspension (IM Only)**

URTI due to Group A streptococcus.

Adults: 1,200,000 units as a single dose; **older children:** 900,000 units as a single dose; **children under 27 kg:** 300,000–600,000 units as a single dose; **neonates:** 50,000 units/kg as a single dose.

Early syphilis (primary, secondary, or latent).

Adults: 2,400,000 units as a single dose. **Children:** 50,000 units/kg, up to the adult dose.

Gummas and cardiovascular syphilis.

Adults: 2,400,000 units q 7 days for 3 weeks. **Children:** 50,000 units/kg, up to adult dose.

Neurosyphilis.

Adults: Aqueous penicillin G, 18,000,000–24,000,000 units IV/day for 10–14 days followed by penicillin G benzathine, 2,400,000 units IM q week for 3 weeks.

Yaws, bejel, pinta.

1,200,000 units in a single dose.

Prophylaxis of rheumatic fever and glomerulonephritis.

Following an acute attack, 1,200,000 units once a month or 600,000 units q 2 weeks.

HEALTH CARE CONSIDERATIONS

See also *Health Care Considerations* for *Penicillins.*

Administration/Storage

1. Shake multiple-dose vial vigorously before withdrawing the desired dose because medication tends to clump on standing. Check that all medication is dissolved and that no residue is present at bottom of bottle.
2. Use a 20-gauge needle and do not allow medication to remain in the syringe and needle for long periods of time before administration because the needle may become plugged and the syringe "frozen."
3. Inject slowly and steadily into muscle; *do not massage* injection site.
4. For adults, use the upper outer quadrant of the buttock; for infants and small children, the midlateral aspect of the thigh should be used. Do not administer in the gluteal region in children less than 2 years of age.
5. *Do not administer IV.* Before injection of medication, aspirate to ensure that needle is not in a vein.

6. Rotate and chart site of injections.
7. Divide between two injection sites if dose is large or available muscle mass is small.
8. Refrigerate, but do not freeze.

Client/Family Teaching

1. Must return for repository penicillin injections.
2. Obtain sexual counseling. Sexual partner should also undergo treatment.

Outcome/Evaluate

- Prophylaxis of poststreptococcal rheumatic fever
- Resolution of infection

Penicillin G potassium for injection

(pen-ih-**SILL**-in)
Pregnancy Category: B
Pfizerpen **(Rx)**

Penicillin G (Aqueous) sodium for injection

(pen-ih-**SILL**-in)
Pregnancy Category: B
(Rx)
Classification: Antibiotic, penicillin

See also *Anti-Infectives* and *Penicillins.*

Action/Kinetics: The first choice for treatment of many infections due to low cost. Rapid onset makes it especially suitable for fulminating infections. Is neither penicillinase resistant nor acid stable. **Peak plasma levels: IM or SC,** 6–20 units/mL after 15–30 min **t½:** 30 min.

Uses: Streptococci of groups A, C, G, H, L, and M are sensitive to penicillin G. High serum levels are effective against streptococci of the D group.

Additional Side Effects: Rapid IV administration may cause hyperkalemia and cardiac arrhythmias. Renal damage occurs rarely.

Additional Drug Interactions: Aspirin, ethacrynic acid, furosemide, indomethacin, sulfonamides, or thiazide diuretics may compete with penicillin G for renal tubular secretion → prolongation of serum t½ of penicillin

How Supplied: Penicillin G potassium for injection: *Injection:* 1 million U/50 mL, 2 million U/50 mL, 3 million U/50 mL; *Powder for injection:* 1 million U, 5 million U, 10 million U, 20 million U Penicillin G (Aqueous) sodium for injection: *Powder for injection:* 5 million U

Dosage

- **Penicillin G Potassium and Sodium**

Injections (IM, Continuous IV Infusion)

Serious streptococcal infections (empyema, endocarditis, meningitis, pericarditis, pneumonia).

Adults: 5–24 million units/day in divided doses q 4 to 6 hr. **Pediatric:** 150,000 units/kg/day given in equal doses q 4 to 6 hr. **Infants over 7 days of age:** 75,000 units/kg/day in divided doses q 8 hr. **Infants less than 7 days of age:** 50,000 units/kg/day given in divided doses q 12 hr. For group B streptococcus, give 100,000 units/kg/day.

Meningococcal meningitis/septicemia.

Adults: 1–2 million units IM q 2 hr or 20–30 million units/day continuous IV drip for 14 days or until afebrile for 7 days. Or, 200,000–300,000 units/kg/day q 2–4 hr in divided doses for a total of 24 doses.

Meningitis due to susceptible strains of Pneumococcus or Meningococcus.

Children: 250,000 units/kg/day divided in equal doses q 4 to 6 hr for 7 to 14 days (maximum daily dose: 12–20 million units). **Infants over 7 days of age:** 200,000–300,0000 units/kg/day divided into equal doses given q 6 hr. **Infants less than 7 days of age:** 100,000–150,000 units/kg/day.

Anthrax.

Adults: A minimum of 5 million units/day (up to 12–20 million units have been used).

Clostridial infections.

Adults: 20 million units/day used with an antitoxin.

Actinomycosis.

Adults: *Cervicofacial:* 1–6 million units/day. *Thoracic and abdominal disease:* **initial,** 10–20 million units/day divided into equal doses given q 6 hr IV for 6 weeks followed by penicillin V, PO, 500 mg q.i.d. for 2–3 months.

Rat-bite fever, Haverhill fever.

Adults: 12–20 million units/day q 4 to 6 hr for 3–4 weeks. **Children:** 150,000–250,000 units/kg/day in equal doses q 4 hr for 4 weeks.

Endocarditis due to Listeria.

Adults: 15–20 million units/day q 4 to 6 hr for 4 weeks.

Endocarditis due to Erysipelothrix rhusiopathiae.

Adults: 12–20 million units/day q 4 to 6 hr for 4–6 weeks.

Meningitis due to Listeria.

Adults: 15–20 million units/day q 4 to 6 hr for 2 weeks.

Pasteurella infections causing bacteremia and meningitis.

P

Adults: 4–6 million units/day q 4 to 6 hr for 2 weeks.

Severe fusospirochetal infections of the oropharynx, lower respiratory tract, and genital area.

Adults: 5–10 million units/day q 4 to 6 hr.

Pneumococcal infections causing empyema.

Adults: 5–24 million units/day in divided doses q 4–6 hr.

Pneumococcal infections causing meningitis.

Adults: 20–24 million units/day for 14 days.

Pneumococcal infections causing endocarditis, pericarditis, peritonitis, suppurative arthritis, osteomyelitis, mastoiditis.

Adults: 12–20 million units/day for 2–4 weeks.

Adjunct with antitoxin to prevent diphtheria.

Adults: 2–3 million units/day in divided doses q 4 to 6 hr for 10–12 days. **Children:** 150,000–250,000 units/kg/day in equal doses q 6 hr for 10 days.

Neurosyphilis.

Adults: 18–24 million units/day (3–4 million units q 4 hr) for 10–14 days (can be followed by benzathine penicillin G, 2.4 million units IM weekly for 3 weeks).

Disseminated gonococcal infections.

Adults: 10 million units/day q 4 to 6 hr (for meningococcal meningitis/septicemia, give q 3 hr). **Children, less than 45 kg:** Arthritis, 100,000 units/kg/day in 4 equally divided doses for 7 to 10 days. Endocarditis: 250,000 units/kg/day in equal doses q 4 hr for 4 weeks. Meningitis: 250,000 units/kg/day in equal doses q 4 hr for 10 to 14 days. **Children, over 45 kg:** Arthritis, endocarditis, meningitis: 10 million units/day in 4 equally divided doses (duration depends on type of infection).

Congenital syphilis after the newborn period.

50,000 units/kg IV q 4–6 hr for 10–14 days.

Symptomatic or asymptomatic congenital syphilis in infants.

Infants: 50,000 units/kg IV q 12 hr the first 7 days; then, q 8 hr for a total of 10 days. **Children:** 50,000 units/kg q 4 to 6 hr for 10 days.

HEALTH CARE CONSIDERATIONS

See also *Health Care Considerations* for *Penicillins*.

Administration/Storage

1. IM administration is preferred; discomfort is minimized by using solutions of up to 100,000 units/mL.
2. Use 1%–2% lidocaine solution as diluent for IM (if ordered) to lessen pain at injection site. Do not use procaine as diluent for aqueous penicillin.
3. Electrolyte contents: Penicillin G Sodium (1 mg =1,600 units) contains 2 mEq Na/1 million units; Penicillin G Potassium (1 mg =1,600 units) contains 1.7 mEq K^+ and 0.3 mEq Na/1 million units.
4. **IV** Use sterile water, isotonic saline USP, or D5W and mix with recommended volume for desired strength.
5. For intermittent IV administration (q 6 hr) reconstitute with 100 mL of dextrose or saline solution and infuse over 1 hr.
6. Loosen powder by shaking bottle before adding diluent.
7. Hold vial horizontally and rotate slowly while directing the stream of the diluent against the wall of the vial.
8. Shake vigorously after addition of diluent.
9. Solutions may be stored at room temperature for 24 hr or in refrigerator for 1 week. Discard remaining solution.
10. The following drugs should *not* be mixed with penicillin during IV administration: aminophylline, amphotericin B, ascorbic acid, chlorpheniramine, chlorpromazine, gentamicin, heparin, hydroxyzine, lincomycin, metaraminol, novobiocin, oxytetracycline, phenylephrine, phenytoin, polymyxin B, prochlorperazine, promazine, promethazine, sodium bicarbonate, sodium salts of barbiturates, sulfadiazine, tetracycline, tromethamine, vancomycin, vitamin B complex.

Assessment

1. Record indications for therapy, type, onset, and characteristics of symptoms.
2. Order drug by specifying sodium or potassium salt.
3. Monitor I&O. Dehydration decreases drug excretion and may raise blood level of penicillin G to dangerously high levels causing kidney damage. GI disturbances may lead to dehydration.
4. Very high doses (>20 million units) may cause seizures or platelet dysfunction, especially with impaired renal function.
5. Obtain baseline CBC, liver and renal function studies and cultures.

Outcome/Evaluate

- Symptomatic improvement; negative culture reports
- Resolution of infective process

Penicillin G procaine, intramuscular

(pen-ih-**SILL**-in, **PROH**-caine)

P

Pregnancy Category: B
Ayercillin ✱, Wycillin **(Rx)**
Classification: Antibiotic, penicillin

See also *Anti-Infectives* and *Penicillins*.

Action/Kinetics: Long-acting (repository) form in aqueous or oily vehicle. Destroyed by penicillinase. Because of slow onset, a soluble penicillin is often administered concomitantly for fulminating infections.

Uses: Penicillin-sensitive staphylococci, pneumococci, streptococci, and bacterial endocarditis (for *Streptococcus viridans* and *S. bovis* infections). Gonorrhea, all stages of syphilis. *Prophylaxis:* Rheumatic fever, pre- and postsurgery. Diphtheria, anthrax, fusospirochetosis (Vincent's infection), erysipeloid, rat-bite fever. *Note:* Severe pneumonia, empyema, bacteremia, pericarditis, meningitis, peritonitis, and purulent or septic arthritis due to pneumococcus are better treated with aqueous penicillin G during the acute stage.

Contraindications: Use in newborns due to possible sterile abcesses and procaine toxicity.

Additional Drug Interactions: Aspirin, ethacrynic acid, furosemide, indomethacin, sulfonamides, or thiazide diuretics may compete with penicillin G for renal tubular secretion → prolongation of serum t½ of penicillin

How Supplied: *Injection:* 600,000 U/mL

Dosage

- **IM Only**

Pneumococccal, staphylococcal, streptococcal infections; erysipeloid, rat-bite fever, anthrax, fusospirochetosis.

Adults, usual: 600,000–1 million units/day for 10–14 days. **Children, less than 27.2 kg:** 300,000 units/day.

Bacterial endocarditis (only very sensitive S. viridans or S. bovis infections).

Adults: 600,000–1 million units/day.

Diphtheria carrier state.

300,000 units/day for 10 days.

Diphtheria, adjunct with antitoxin.

300,000–600,000 units/day.

Anthrax (cutaneous), erysipeloid, rate-bite fever.

600,000 to 1 million units/day.

Fusospirochetosis: Vincent's gingivitis, pharyngitis.

600,000 to 1 million units/day. Obtain necessary dental care.

Gonococcal infections.

4.8 million units divided into at least two doses at one visit and given with 1 g PO probenecid (given 30 min before the injections).

Neurosyphilis.

2.4 million units/day for 10 to 14 days (given at two sites) with probenecid 500 mg PO q.i.d.; **then,** benzathine penicillin G, 2.4 million units/week for 3 weeks. *Note:* For yaws, bejel, and pinta, treat the same as syphilis in corresponding stage of disease.

Congenital syphilis in infants, symptomatic and asymptomatic.

50,000 units/kg/day for 10 days.

Syphilis: primary, secondary, latent with negative spinal fluid.

Adults and children over 12 years: 600,000 units/day for 8 days (total of 4.8 million units).

Syphilis: tertiary, neurosyphilis, latent with positive spinal-fluid.

Adults: 600,000 units/day for 10 to 15 days (total of 6 to 9 million units).

HEALTH CARE CONSIDERATIONS

See also *Health Care Considerations* for *Penicillins.*

Administration/Storage

1. Shake multiple-dose vial thoroughly to ensure uniform suspension before injection. If the medication is clumped at the bottom of the vial, shake until clump dissolves.
2. Use a 20-gauge needle and aspirate immediately after withdrawing medication from the vial; otherwise needle may become clogged and syringe may "freeze."
3. Administer into two sites if dose is large or available muscle mass is small.
4. Aspirate to check that the needle is not in a vein.
5. Inject slowly, deep into the muscle.
6. For IM use only. Rotate and chart injection sites. Do not massage after injection.

Assessment: Record indications for therapy, onset of symptoms, any other treatments prescribed, and pretreatment cultures.

Client/Family Teaching

1. Report a wheal or other skin reactions at injection site that may indicate reaction to procaine as well as to penicillin.
2. Obtain sexual counseling; have sexual partner also undergo treatment.
3. With a history of rheumatic fever or congenital heart disease, must use antibiotic prophylaxis prior to any invasive medical/dental procedure.

Outcome/Evaluate: Resolution of infection; infection prophylaxis

P

Penicillin V potassium (Phenoxymethyl-penicillin potassium)

(pen-ih-**SILL**-in)

Pregnancy Category: B

Apo-Pen-VK ✱, Beepen-VK, Nadopen-V ✱, Novo–Pen-VK ✱, Nu-Pen-VK ✱, Penicillin VK, Pen-Vee K, PVF K ✱, Veetids '250' **(Rx)**

Classification: Antibiotic, penicillin

See also *Anti-Infectives* and *Penicillins.*

Action/Kinetics: Related closely to penicillin G. Products are not penicillinase resistant but are acid stable and resist inactivation by gastric secretions. Well absorbed from the GI tract and not affected by foods. **Peak plasma levels:** Penicillin V, **PO:** 2.7 mcg/mL after 30–60 min; penicillin V potassium, **PO:** 1–9 mcg/mL after 30–60 min. **t½:** 30 min. Periodic blood counts and renal function tests are indicated during long-term usage.

Uses: Mild to moderate upper respiratory tract streptococcal infections, including scarlet fever and erysipelas. Mild to moderate upper respiratory tract pneumococcal infections, including otitis media. Mild staphylococcal infections of the skin and soft tissue. Mild to moderate fusospirochetosis (Vincent's infection) of the oropharynx. Prophylaxis of recurrence following rheumatic fever or chorea. *Investigational:* Prophylactially to reduce *S. pneumoniae* septicemia in children with sickle cell anemia, mild to moderate anaerobic infections, Lyme disease.

Contraindications: PO penicillin V to treat severe pneumonia, empyema, bacteremia, pericarditis, meningitis, and arthritis during the acute stage. Prophylactic uses for GU instrumentation or surgery, sigmoidoscopy, or childbirth.

Special Concerns: More and more strains of staphylococci are resistant to penicillin V, necessitating culture and sensitivity studies.

Additional Drug Interactions

Contraceptives, oral / ↓ Effectiveness of oral contraceptives

Neomycin, oral / ↓ Absorption of penicillin V

How Supplied: *Powder for reconstitution:* 125 mg/5 mL, 250 mg/5 mL; *Tablet:* 250 mg, 500 mg

Dosage

- **Oral Solution, Tablets**

Streptococcal infections, including scarlet fever and mild erysipelas.

Adults and children over 12 years: 125–250 mg q 6–8 hr for 10 days. **Children, usual:** 500 mg q 8 hr for pharyngitis.

Staphylococcal infections (including skin and soft tissue), fusospirochetosis of oropharynx.

Adults and children over 12 years: 250 mg q 6–8 hr.

Pneumococcal infections, including otitis media.

Adults and children over 12 years: 250 mg q 6 hr until afebrile for at least 2 days.

Prophylaxis of recurrence of rheumatic fever/chorea.

Adults and children over 12 years: 125–250 mg b.i.d., on a continuing basis.

Prophylaxis of septicemia caused by Staphylococcus pneumoniae *in children with sickle cell anemia.*

125 mg b.i.d.

Anaerobic infections.

250 mg q.i.d. See also *Penicillin G, Procaine, Aqueous, Sterile.*

Lyme disease.

250–500 mg q.i.d. for 10–20 days (for children less than 2 years of age, 50 mg/kg/day in four divided doses for 10–20 days).

NOTE: 250 mg penicillin V is equivalent to 400,000 units.

HEALTH CARE CONSIDERATIONS

See also *Health Care Considerations* for *Penicillins.*

Administration/Storage

1. Administer without regard to meals. Blood levels may be slightly higher when administered on an empty stomach.
2. Do not administer at the same time as neomycin because malabsorption of penicillin V may occur.
3. Store reconstituted solution in the refrigerator; discard unused portion after 14 days.

Client/Family Teaching

1. Clients with a history of rheumatic fever or congenital heart disease need to use and understand the importance of antibiotic prophylaxis prior to any invasive medical or dental procedure.
2. Report if throat and/or ear symptoms do not improve after 48 hr of therapy; may need to reevaluate and alter therapy.
3. With oral administration, if a reaction is going to occur, you usually see it after the second dose. Seek medical intervention immediately if respiratory distress or skin wheals appear.
4. Use an additional nonhormonal form of birth control if taking oral contraceptives because their effectiveness may be diminished.

Outcome/Evaluate

- Symptomatic improvement
- Negative lab C&S reports
- Endocarditis/rheumatic fever prophylaxis

—COMBINATION DRUG—

Pentazocine hydrochloride with Naloxone hydrochloride

(pen-**TAZ**-oh-seen, nah-**LOX**-ohn)
Pregnancy Category: C
Talwin NX **(C-IV) (Rx)**

Pentazocine lactate

(pen-**TAZ**-oh-seen)
Pregnancy Category: C
Talwin **(C-IV) (Rx)**
Classification: Narcotic agonist/antagonist

See also *Narcotic Analgesics.*
Content: Each tablet of pentazocine HCl with naloxone HCl contains: pentazocine HCl, 50 mg, and naloxone HCl, 0.5 mg.
Action/Kinetics: Manifests both narcotic agonist and antagonist properties. Agonist effects are due to combination with kappa and sigma opioid receptors; antagonistic effect is due to an action on mu opioid receptors. Also elevates systemic and pulmonary arterial pressure, systemic vascular resistance, and LV end-diastolic pressure, which results in an increased cardiac workload. One-third as potent as morphine as an analgesic. **Onset: IM,** 15–20 min; **PO,** 15–30 min; **IV,** 2–3 min. **Peak effect: IM,** 15–60 min; **PO,** 60–180 min. **Duration, all routes:** 3 hr. However, onset, duration, and degree of relief depend on both dose and severity of pain. **t½:** 2–3 hr. Extensive first-pass metabolism in the liver.

To reduce the possibility of abuse, the PO dosage form of pentazocine has been combined with naloxone (Talwin NX), which will prevent the effects of IV administered pentazocine but will not affect the efficacy of pentazocine when taken PO. If pentazocine with naloxone is used IV, fatal reactions may occur, which include vascular occlusion, pulmonary emboli, ulceration, and abscesses, and withdrawal in narcotic-dependent individuals.
Uses: PO: Moderate to severe pain. **Parenteral:** Preoperative or preanesthetic medication, obstetrics, supplement to surgical anesthesia. Moderate to severe pain.
Additional Contraindications: Increased ICP or head injury. Use in children under 12 years of age. Use of methadone or other narcotics for pentazocine withdrawal.
Special Concerns: Use with caution in impaired renal or hepatic function, as well as after MI, when N&V are present. Use with caution in women delivering premature infants and in clients with respiratory depression. Safety and efficacy in children less than 12 years of age have not been determined.
Additional Side Effects: *CNS:* Syncope, dysphoria, nightmares, hallucinations, disorientation, paresthesias, confusion, ***seizures.*** *Miscellaneous;* Decreased WBCs, edema of the face, chills. Both psychologic and physical dependence are possible, although the addiction liability is thought to be no greater than for codeine. Multiple parenteral doses may cause severe sclerosis of the skin, SC tissues, and underlying muscle.
How Supplied: Pentazocine hydrochloride with Naloxone hydrochloride: See Content. Pentazocine lactate: *Injection:* 30 mg/mL

Dosage

PENTAZOCINE HYDROCHLORIDE WITH NALOXONE

- **Tablets**

Analgesia.

Adults: 50 mg q 3–4 hr, up to 100 mg. Daily dose should not exceed 600 mg.

PENTAZOCINE LACTATE

- **IM, IV, SC**

Analgesia.

Adults: 30 mg q 3–4 hr; doses exceeding 30 mg IV or 60 mg IM not recommended. Do not exceed a total daily dosage of 360 mg.

Obstetric analgesia.

Adults: 30 mg IM given once; or, 20 mg IV q 2–3 hr for two or three doses.

HEALTH CARE CONSIDERATIONS

See also *Health Care Considerations* for *Narcotic Analgesics.*

Administration/Storage

1. Do not mix soluble barbiturates in the same syringe with pentazocine as a precipitate will form.

IV 2. May be administered undiluted. However, if the drug is to be diluted, place 5 mg of drug into 5 mL of sterile water for injection. Administer each 5 mg or less over a 1-min period.

Assessment

1. Record indications for therapy, characteristics of pain, other agents used and the outcome. Rate pain using a pain-rating scale.
2. Note evidence of head injury or increased ICP; assess mental status. Note history of hepatic, renal, or cardiac dysfunction.

Client/Family Teaching

1. Drug may cause dizziness and drowsiness.
2. Avoid alcohol and any other CNS depressants.

Outcome/Evaluate: Relief of pain

Pentobarbital

(pen-toe-**BAR**-bih-tal)
Pregnancy Category: D
Nembutal **(C-II) (Rx)**

Pentobarbital sodium

(pĕn-toe-**BAR**-bih-tal)
Pregnancy Category: D
Nembutal Sodium, Nova-Rectal ✱, Novo-Pentobarb ✱ **(C-II) (Rx)**
Classification: Sedative-hypnotic, barbiturate type

See also *Barbiturates.*
Action/Kinetics: Short-acting. **t½:** 19–34 hr. Is 60%–70% protein bound.
Uses: PO: Sedative. Short-term treatment of insomnia (no more than 2 weeks). Preanesthetic. **Rectal:** Sedation, short-term treatment of insomnia (no more than 2 weeks). **Parenteral:** Short-term treatment of insomnia (no more than 2 weeks). Preanesthetic. Anticonvulsant in anesthetic doses for emergency treatment of acute convulsive states (e.g., status epilepticus, eclampsia, meningitis, tetanus, and toxic reactions to strychnine or local anesthetics). *Investigational:* Parenterally to induce coma to protect the brain from ischemia and increased ICP following stroke and head trauma.
Special Concerns: Reduce dose in geriatric and debilitated clients and in impaired hepatic or renal function.
How Supplied: Pentobarbital: *Elixir:* 18.2 mg/5 mL. Pentobarbital sodium: *Capsule:* 50 mg, 100 mg; *Injection:* 50 mg/mL; *Suppository:* 30 mg, 60 mg, 120 mg, 200 mg

Dosage
- **Capsules**

Sedation.
Adults: 20 mg t.i.d.–q.i.d. **Pediatric:** 2–6 mg/kg/day, depending on age, weight, and degree of sedation desired.
Preoperative sedation.
Adults: 100 mg. **Pediatric:** 2–6 mg/kg/day (maximum of 100 mg), depending on age, weight, and degree of sedation desired.
Hypnotic.
Adults: 100 mg at bedtime.
- **Suppositories, Rectal**

Hypnotic.
Adults: 120–200 mg at bedtime; **infants, 2–12 months (4.5–9 kg):** 30 mg; **1–4 years (9–18.2 kg):** 30 or 60 mg; **5–12 years (18.2–36.4 kg):** 60 mg; **12–14 years (36.4–50 kg):** 60 or 120 mg.
- **IM**

Hypnotic/preoperative sedation.
Adults: 150–200 mg; **pediatric:** 2–6 mg/kg (not to exceed 100 mg).
Anticonvulsant.
Pediatric, initially: 50 mg; **then,** after 1 min, additional small doses may be given, if needed, until the desired effect is achieved.
- **IV**

Sedative/hypnotic.
Adults: 100 mg followed in 1 min by additional small doses, if required, up to a total of 500 mg.
Anticonvulsant.
Adults, initial: 100 mg; **then,** after 1 min, additional small doses may be given, if needed, up to a total of 500 mg. **Pediatric, initially:** 50 mg; **then,** after 1 min, additional small doses may be given, if needed, until the desired effect is achieved.

HEALTH CARE CONSIDERATIONS

See also *Health Care Considerations* for *Barbiturates.*
Administration/Storage
1. Parental pentobarbital is incompatible with most other drugs; therefore, do not mix other drugs in the same syringe. Do not use if solution is discolored or contains a precipitate.
2. Administer no more than 5 mL IM at one site because of possible tissue irritation (pain, necrosis, gangrene).
3. Parenteral product is not for SC use.
4. Do not divide suppositories.
IV 5. Give IV dose in fractions because pentobarbital is a potent CNS depressant that may cause adverse respiratory and circulatory responses. Adults generally receive 100 mg initially; children and debilitated clients, 50 mg. Subsequent fractions are administered after 1-min observation periods. Overdose or too rapid administration may cause spasms of the larynx and/or pharynx.
6. Do not exceed an IV rate of 50 mg/min.
7. Pentobarbital solutions are highly alkaline.
8. Assess IV site for patency. Interrupt infusion and report any complaint of pain at injection site or in the limb.
Assessment
1. Record indications for therapy, onset and characteristics of symptoms, and other agents prescribed.
2. With insomnia, assist to identify type and any causative factors; review sleep patterns.
3. Obtain baseline liver and renal function studies; anticipate reduced dose with impairment as well as with the debilitated and elderly.
4. Observe for signs of respiratory depression; usually the first sign of drug overdose.
5. During treatment of cerebral edema (bar-

biturate coma), monitor and document ICP readings, and neurologic status.
6. Initiate appropriate safety measures once the medication has been administered. This is particularly important when working with confused or elderly clients.
7. Administer analgesics as needed since sedatives and hypnotics do not control pain.

Client/Family Teaching
1. Drug may cause drowsiness and morning-after "hangover."
2. Avoid alcohol or any other CNS depressants.
3. With insomnia, drug is for short-term use only; with long-term use one can experience rebound insomnia.

Outcome/Evaluate
- Improved sleeping patterns
- Desired level of sedation
- Control of seizures

Pentosan polysulfate sodium

(PEN-toh-san)
Pregnancy Category: B
Elmiron **(Rx)**
Classification: Urinary analgesic

Action/Kinetics: Mechanism for urinary analgesic activity is not known. It appears to adhere to the bladder wall mucosal membrane and may act as a buffer to control cell permeability, thus preventing irritating solutes in the urine from reaching the cells. Also has a weak anticoagulant effect. Less than 3% of an administered dose is absorbed from the GI tract. **t½:** 4.8 hr. Metabolized by the liver and spleen.
Uses: Relief of bladder pain or discomfort associated with interstitial cystitis.
Contraindications: Hypersensitivity to pentosan polysulfate sodium or related compounds.
Special Concerns: Use with caution during lactation, in those with hepatic insufficiency or spleen disorders, and in those who have a history of heparin-induced thrombocytopenia. Safety and efficacy have not been determined in children less than 16 years of age.
Side Effects: *GI:* Diarrhea, N&V, abdominal pain, dyspepsia, anorexia, colitis, constipation, esophagitis, flatulence, gastritis, mouth ulcer. *CNS:* Headache, severe emotional lability or depression, hyperkinesia, dizziness, insomnia. *CV:* Bleeding complications, including ecchymosis, epistaxis, gum hemorrhage. *Hematologic:* Anemia, leukopenia, thrombocytopenia. *Respiratory:* Dyspnea, pharyngitis, rhinitis. *Dermatologic:* Alopecia, rash, pruritus, urticaria, increased sweating. *Ophthalmic:* Amblyopia, conjunctivitis, optic neuritis, retinal hemorrhage. *Miscellaneous:* Hepatic toxicity, liver function abnormalities, allergic reactions, tinnitus, photosensitivity.
Laboratory Test Considerations: ↑ PTT, PT.
How Supplied: *Capsule:* 100 mg

Dosage
- **Capsules**
  Interstitial cystitis.
100 mg t.i.d.

HEALTH CARE CONSIDERATIONS

Administration/Storage: Store at controlled room temperatures of 15°C–30°C (59°F–86°F).

Assessment
1. Record onset, duration, frequency, and characteristics of symptoms. Note other agents trialed and the outcome.
2. Determine any spleen disorder, liver dysfunction, or intolerance to heparin.
3. Obtain baseline CBC and urine for C&S.

Client/Family Teaching
1. Take each capsule as directed with a full glass of water 1 hr before or 2 hr after a meal.
2. Report any unusual bruising or bleeding; drug has a mild anticoagulant effect.
3. Notify provider if pain persists or worsens.

Outcome/Evaluate: Relief of bladder pain/discomfort with interstitial cystitis

P

Pentoxifylline

(pen-tox-EYE-fih-leen)
Pregnancy Category: C
Albert Pentoxifylline ✱, Apo-Pentoxifylline SR ✱, Trental **(Rx)**
Classification: Agent affecting blood viscosity

Action/Kinetics: Drug and active metabolites decrease the viscosity of blood and improve erythrocyte flexibility. Results in increased blood flow to the microcirculation and an increase in tissue oxygen levels. Mechanism may include (1) decreased synthesis of thromboxane A_2, thus decreasing platelet aggregation, (2) increased blood fibrinolytic activity (decreasing fibrinogen levels), and (3) decreased RBC aggregation and local hyperviscosity by increasing cellular ATP. **Peak plasma levels:** 2–4 hr. Significant first-pass effect. **t½:** pentoxifylline, 0.4–0.8 hr; metabolites, 1–1.6 hr. Excreted in the urine.
Uses: Intermittent claudication; not intended to replace surgery. *Investigational:* To im-

prove circulation in clients with cerebrovascular insufficiency, TIAs, sickle cell thalassemia, diabetic angiopathies and neuropathies, high-altitude sickness, strokes, acute and chronic hearing disorders, circulation disorders of the eye, severe recurrent aphthous stomatitis, leg ulcers, asthenozoospermia, and Raynaud's phenomenon.
Contraindications: Intolerance to pentoxifylline, caffeine, theophylline, or theobromine. Recent cerebral or retinal hemorrhage.
Special Concerns: Use with caution in impaired renal function and during lactation. Safety and efficacy in children less than 18 years of age not established. Geriatric clients may be at greater risk for manifesting side effects.
Side Effects: *CV:* Angina, chest pain, hypotension, edema. *GI:* Abdominal pain, flatus/bloating, dyspepsia, salivation, bad taste in mouth, N&V, anorexia, constipation, dry mouth and thirst, cholecystitis. *CNS:* Dizziness, headache, tremor, malaise, anxiety, confusion, depression, ***seizures.*** *Ophthalmologic:* Blurred vision, conjunctivitis, scotomata. *Dermatologic:* Pruritus, rash, urticaria, brittle fingernails, angioedema. *Respiratory:* Dyspnea, laryngitis, nasal congestion, epistaxis. *Miscellaneous:* Flu-like symptoms, leukopenia, sore throat, swollen neck glands, change in weight, earache, malaise.
OD **Management of Overdose:** *Symptoms:* Agitation, fever, flushing, hypotension, nervousness, ***seizures,*** somnolence, tremors, loss of consciousness. *Treatment:* Gastric lavage followed by activated charcoal. Monitor BP and ECG. Support respiration, control seizures, and treat arrhythmias.
Drug Interactions
Antihypertensives / Small ↓ in BP; dose of antihypertensive may need to be ↑
Theophylline / ↑ Theophylline levels → ↑ risk of toxicitiy
Warfarin / Prolonged PT
How Supplied: *Tablet, Extended Release:* 400 mg

Dosage

- **Extended-Release Tablets**

Intermittent claudication.

Adults: 400 mg t.i.d. with meals for at least 8 weeks. If side effects occur, reduce dose to 400 mg b.i.d.

Severe idiopathic recurrent aphthous stomatitis.

400 mg t.i.d. for 1 month.

HEALTH CARE CONSIDERATIONS

Assessment

1. Note any history of sensitivity to caffeine, theophylline, or theobromine.
2. Record indications for therapy and type, onset, and duration of symptoms. List other agents trialed and any studies performed (i.e., Dopplers) to rule out blockage.
3. Determine if pregnant.
4. Monitor CBC and renal function studies.

Client/Family Teaching

1. Take the medication with meals to minimize GI upset.
2. Report any angina and palpitations if evident.
3. Continue the treatment for at least 8 weeks, even though effectiveness may not yet be apparent.
4. Do not perform activities that require mental alertness until drug effects are realized as dizziness and blurred vision may occur.
5. Avoid nicotine-containing products; nicotine constricts blood vessels.
6. Walk every day to the point of pain, rest and then resume walking. Wear cotton socks and comfortable, well-fitting shoes.
7. Report for F/U to evaluate drug effectiveness.

Outcome/Evaluate: ↓ Pain and cramping in lower extremities during activity

COMBINATION DRUG

Percocet

(PER-koh-set)
Pregnancy Category: C
(C-II) (Rx)
Classification: Analgesic

See also *Acetaminophen* and *Narcotic Analgesics.*
Content: Each tablet contains: *Nonnarcotic analgesic:* Acetaminophen, 325 mg. *Narcotic analgesic:* Oxycodone HCl, 5 mg. Also see information on individual components.
Uses: Moderate to moderately severe pain.
Special Concerns: Use with caution during lactation. Safety and effectiveness have not been determined in children. Dependence to oxycodone can occur.
How Supplied: See Content

Dosage

- **Tablets**

Adults, usual: 1 tablet q 6 hr as required for pain.

HEALTH CARE CONSIDERATIONS

See also *Health Care Considerations* for *Narcotic Analgesics* and *Acetaminophen.*
Administration/Storage: Adjust dosage depending on the response of the client, tolerance, and the severity of the pain.
Assessment: Record location, onset, duration, and characteristics of pain. Use a pain-rating

scale to rate pain. List other agents/therapies trialed and the outcome.

Client/Family Teaching

1. May cause dizziness and drowsiness and constipation.
2. Drug is for short-term use; chronic pain conditions require alternative pharmacologic agents.
3. Avoid alcohol and any other CNS depressants.

Outcome/Evaluate: Relief of pain

Pergolide mesylate

(PER-go-lyd)

Pregnancy Category: B

Permax **(Rx)**

Classification: Antiparkinson agent

See also *Antiparkinson Agents*.

Action/Kinetics: Potent dopamine receptor (both D_1 and D_2) agonist. May act by directly stimulating postsynaptic dopamine receptors in the nigrostriatal system, thus relieving symptoms of parkinsonism. Also inhibits prolactin secretion; causes a transient rise in serum levels of growth hormone and a decrease in serum levels of LH. About 90% of the drug is bound to plasma proteins. Metabolized in the liver and excreted through the urine.

Uses: Adjunct with levodopa/carbidopa in Parkinson's disease.

Special Concerns: Use with caution during lactation and in clients prone to cardiac dysrhythmias, preexisting dyskinesia, and preexisting states of confusion or hallucinations. Safety and efficacy have not been determined in children.

Side Effects: The most common side effects are listed. *CV:* Postural hypotension, palpitation, vasodilation, syncope, hypotension, hypertension, ***arrhythmias, MI.*** *GI:* Nausea (common), vomiting, diarrhea, constipation, dyspepsia, anorexia, dry mouth. *CNS:* Dyskinesia (common), dizziness, dystonia, hallucinations, confusion, insomnia, somnolence, anxiety, tremor, depression, abnormal dreams, psychosis, personality disorder, extrapyramidal syndrome, akathisia, paresthesia, incoordination, akinesia, neuralgia, hypertonia, speech disorders. *Musculoskeletal:* Arthralgia, bursitis, twitching, myalgia. *Respiratory:* Rhinitis, dyspnea, hiccup, epistaxis. *Dermatologic:* Sweating, rash. *Ophthalmologic:* Abnormal vision, double vision, eye disorders. *GU:* UTI, urinary frequency, hematuria. *Whole body:* Pain in chest, abdomen, neck, or back; headache, asthenia, flu syndrome, chills, facial edema, infection. *Miscellaneous:* Taste alteration, peripheral edema, anemia, weight gain.

OD **Management of Overdose:** *Symptoms:* Include agitation, hypotension, N&V, hallucinations, involuntary movements, palpitations, tingling of arms and legs. *Treatment:* Activated charcoal (usually recommended instead of or in addition to gastric lavage or induction of vomiting). Maintain BP. An antiarrhythmic drug may be helpful. A phenothiazine or butyrophenone may help any CNS stimulation. Support ventilation.

Drug Interactions

Butyrophenones / ↓ Effect of pergolide due to dopamine antagonist effect
Metoclopramide / ↓ Effect of pergolide due to dopamine antagonist effect
Phenothiazines / ↓ Effect of pergolide due to dopamine antagonist effect
Thioxanthines / ↓ Effect of pergolide due to dopamine antagonist effect

How Supplied: *Tablet:* 0.05 mg, 0.25 mg, 1 mg

Dosage

- **Tablets**

Parkinsonism.

Adults, initial: 0.05 mg/day for the first 2 days; **then,** increase dose gradually by 0.1 or 0.15 mg/day every third day over the next 12 days. The dosage may then be increased by 0.25 mg/day every third day until the therapeutic dosage level is reached. The mean therapeutic daily dosage is 3 mg used concurrently with levodopa/carbidopa (expressed as levodopa) at a dose of 650 mg/day. The effectiveness of doses of pergolide greater than 5 mg/day has not been evaluated.

HEALTH CARE CONSIDERATIONS

See also *Health Care Considerations* for *Antiparkinson Agents*.

Administration/Storage

1. Usually given in divided doses 3 times/day.
2. When determining the therapeutic dose for pergolide, the dosage of concurrent levodopa/carbidopa may be decreased cautiously.

Assessment

1. Note any sensitivity to ergot derivatives.
2. Document/record cardiac arrhythmias.
3. Describe tremor, rigidity, motor fluctuations and movements.

Client/Family Teaching

1. Pergolide is to be taken concurrently with prescribed dose of levodopa/carbidopa. Do not exceed prescribed dosage.
2. Do not perform tasks that require mental alertness until drug effects realized; may cause drowsiness or dizziness.

3. Rise slowly from a sitting or lying position to minimize hypotensive effects. May need to curtail activities until side effects subside.
4. Report for all scheduled lab and medical appointments so that drug therapy may be evaluated and adjusted as needed.

Outcome/Evaluate: Improved levodopa/carbidopa response evidenced by ↓ muscle weakness, ↓ rigidity, ↓ salivation, and improved mobility

Perindopril erbumine

(per-**IN**-doh-pril)

Pregnancy Category: C (first trimester), D (second and third trimesters)

Aceon **(Rx)**

Classification: Antihypertensive, ACE Inhibitor

See also *Angiotensin Converting Enzyme (ACE) Inhibitors.*

Action/Kinetics: Converted in the liver to the active perindoprilat.

Uses: Treatment of essential hypertension, either alone or combined with other antihypertensive classes, especially thiazide diuretics.

Contraindications: Use in those with a history of angioedema related to previous ACE inhibitor therapy.

Special Concerns: Safety and efficacy have not been determined in clients with a C_{CR} less than 30 mL/min. There is a higher incidence of angioedema in blacks compared to nonblacks. Use with caution during lactation. Safety and efficacy have not been determined in children.

P

Side Effects: *GI:* Diarrhea, abdominal pain, N&V, dyspepsia, flatulence, dry mouth, dry mucous membrane, increased appetite, gastroenteritis, ***hepatic necrosis/failure***. *CNS:* Headache, dizziness, sleep disorder, paresthesia, depression, migraine, amnesia, vertigo, anxiety, psychosexual disorder. *CV:* Palpitation, abnormal ECG, ***CVA, MI,*** orthostatic symptoms, hypotension, ventricular extrasystole, vasodilation, syncope, abnormal conduction, heart murmur. *Respiratory:* Cough, sinusitis, URTI, rhinitis, pharyngitis, posterior nasal drip, bronchitis, rhinorrhea, throat disorder, dyspnea, sneezing, epistaxis, hoarseness, pulmonary fibrosis. *Body as a whole:* Asthenia, viral infection, fever, edema, rash, seasonal allergy, malaise, pain, cold/hot sensation, chills, fluid retention, angioedema, ***anaphylaxis***. *Musculoskeletal:* Back pain, upper extremity pain, lower extremity pain, chest pain, neck pain, myalgia, arthralgia, arthritis. *GU:* UTI, male sexual dysfunction, menstrual disorder, vaginitis, kidney stone, flank pain, urinary frequency, urinary retention. *Dermatologic:* Sweating, skin infection, tinea, pruritus, dry skin, erythema, fever blisters, purpura, hematoma. *Miscellaneous:* Hypertonia, ear infection, injury, tinnitus, facial edema, gout, ecchymosis.

Laboratory Test Considerations: ↑ Alkaline phosphatase, uric acid, cholesterol, AST, ALT, creatinine, glucose. ↓ Potassium. Hematuria, proteinuria.

Drug Interactions: Concomitant use of diuretics may cause an excessive ↓ BP.

How Supplied: *Tablets:* 2 mg, 4 mg, 8 mg

Dosage

- **Tablets**

Uncomplicated essential hypertension.

Adults, initial: 4 mg once daily (may also be given in 2 divided doses). May increase dose until BP, when measured just before the next dose, is controlled. **Usual maintenance:** 4–8 mg, up to a maximum of 16 mg/day. For elderly clients, give doses greater than 8 mg/day cautiously.

Use with a diuretic for essential hypertension.

If possible, discontinue the diuretic 2–3 days before beginning perindopril therapy. If BP is not controlled with perindopril, resume the diuretic. When using both drugs, use an initial dose of 2–4 mg of perindopril daily in 1 or 2 divided doses. Carefully supervise until BP has stabilized.

In clients with a C_{CR} greater than 30 mL/min, give an initial dose of 2 mg/day. Daily dose should not exceed 8 mg.

HEALTH CARE CONSIDERATIONS

See also *Health Care Considerations* for *Angiotensin Converting Enzyme (ACE) Inhibitors.*

Assessment

1. Note indications for therapy, other medical conditions, previous agents trialed, and outcome.
2. Monitor electrolytes, urinalysis, renal and LFTs; reduce dose with renal dysfunction.

Client/Family Teaching

1. Take as directed at the same time(s) each day.
2. May experience cough, headaches, palpitations, sinusitis and dizziness; report if persistent.
3. Do not perform activities that require mental alertness until drug effects known.
4. Practice reliable contraception.
5. Continue life style changes useful in controlling BP; i.e.; regular exercise, weight loss, low fat/salt diet, smoking cessation, reduced alcohol intake, and stress reduction.
6. Monitor BP at different times during the day and keep a log for provider review.

Outcome/Evaluate: Control of HTN; ↓ BP

Perphenazine

(per-**FEN**-ah-zeen)

Pregnancy Category: C

Apo-Perphenazine ✱, Phenazine ✱, PMS-Perphenazine ✱, Trilafon **(Rx)**

Classification: Antipsychotic, antiemetic, piperazine-type phenothiazine

See also *Antipsychotic Agents, Phenothiazines.*

Action/Kinetics: Resembles chlorpromazine. High incidence of extrapyramidal effects; strong antiemetic effects; moderate anticholinergic effects; and a low incidence of orthostatic hypotension and sedation. **Onset, IM:** 10 min. **Maximum effect, IM:** 1–2 hr. **Duration, IM:** 6 hr (up to 24 hr).

Uses: Psychotic disorders. IV to treat severe N&V and intractable hiccoughs.

Special Concerns: Use during pregnancy only if benefits clearly outweigh risks. Dosage has not been established in children less than 12 years of age. Geriatric, emaciated, or debilitated clients usually require a lower initial dose.

How Supplied: *Concentrate:* 16 mg/5 mL; *Injection:* 5 mg/mL; *Tablet:* 2 mg, 4 mg, 8 mg, 16 mg

Dosage

- **Concentrate, Tablets**

  Psychoses.

Nonhospitalized clients: 4–8 mg t.i.d. **Hospitalized clients:** 8–16 mg b.i.d.–q.i.d. Avoid doses greater than 64 mg/day.

- **IM**

  Psychotic disorders.

Adults and adolescents, nonhospitalized: 5 mg q 6 hr, not to exceed 15 mg/day. **Hospitalized clients: initial,** 5–10 mg; total daily dose should not exceed 30 mg.

- **IV**

  Severe N&V.

Adults: Up to 5 mg diluted to 0.5 mg/mL with 0.9% sodium chloride injection. Give in divided doses of not more than 1 mg q 1–3 hr. Can also be given as an infusion at a rate not to exceed 1 mg/min. Restrict use to hospitalized recumbent adults. Do not exceed a single dose of 5 mg.

HEALTH CARE CONSIDERATIONS

See also *Health Care Considerations* for *Antipsychotic Agents, Phenothiazines.*

Administration/Storage

1. Dilute each 5.0 mL of oral concentrate with 60 mL of water, homogenized milk, saline, carbonated orange drink, or orange, pineapple, apricot, prune, tomato, and grapefruit juice.
2. Do not mix with caffeinated beverges (e.g., tea, coffee, cola), grape juice, or apple juice as it will precipitate.
3. When rapid action is required, administer IM using 5 mg. Inject deep into the muscle, and repeat at 6-hr intervals as needed. Place client in a recumbent position and retain in that position for at least 1 hr after IM administration.
4. Protect from light and store solutions in an amber-colored container.
5. **IV** For IV use dilute with NSS to a concentration of 0.5 mg/mL and administer 1 mg over at least 1 min.

Assessment

1. Record indications for therapy, describe behavioral manifestations, and note onset of symptoms.
2. List other agents prescribed, duration of therapy, and outcome.
3. Obtain baseline CBC, ECG, and LFTs.
4. Monitor VS closely; may cause hypotension, tachycardia, and/or bradycardia. Supervise activity until drug effects realized.
5. Observe for tardive dyskinesia and other extrapyramidal symptoms; would require a dosage reduction/discontinuation.

Client/Family Teaching

1. May dilute each 5.0 mL of oral concentrate with 60 mL of water, homogenized milk, saline, carbonated orange drink, or orange, pineapple, apricot, prune, tomato, and grapefruit juice.
2. Do not mix with caffeinated beverges (e.g., tea, coffee, cola), grape juice, or apple juice as it will precipitate.
3. May cause drowsiness and dizziness.
4. Report any rash, fever, or urinary retention as well as symptoms of tardive dyskinesia and extrapyramidal symptoms.
5. May discolor urine pinkish brown.
6. Wear protective clothes and sunscreen when sun exposure necessary; may discolor skin a bluish color.
7. Drug impairs body temperature regulation; dress appropriately and avoid temperature extremes.
8. Avoid alcohol and CNS depressants.

Outcome/Evaluate

- ↓ Agitation/excitability or withdrawn behaviors
- Control of severe N&V

P

Phenazopyridine hydrochloride (Phenylazodiamino pyridine HCl)

(fen-**AY**-zoh-**PEER**-ih-deen)
Pregnancy Category: B
Azo-Standard, Baridium, Phenazo ✦, Prodium, Pyridiate, Pyridiate No. 2, Pyridium, Pyronium ✦, Urogesic **(OTC) (Rx)**
Classification: Urinary analgesic

Action/Kinetics: An azo dye with local analgesic and anesthetic effects on the urinary tract. Sixty-five percent excreted unchanged or as metabolites within 24 hr.
Uses: Relief of pain, urgency or frequency, and burning in chronic UTIs or irritation, including cystitis, urethritis and pyelitis, trauma, surgery, or urinary tract instrumentation. As an adjunct to antibacterial therapy. Determine the underlying cause of the irritation.
Contraindications: Renal insufficiency. Use in children less than 12 years of age. Chronic use to treat undiagnosed pain of the urinary tract.
Side Effects: *GI:* Nausea. *Hematologic:* Methemoglobinemia, ***hemolytic anemia*** (especially in clients with G6PD deficiency). *Dermatologic:* Yellowish tinge of the skin or sclerae may indicate accumulation of drug due to renal insufficiency, pruritus, rash. *Miscellaneous:* Renal and hepatic toxicity, headache, anaphylactoid reaction, staining of contact lenses.
Laboratory Test Considerations: Ehrlich's test for urine urobilinogen, phenolsulfonphthalein excretion test for kidney function, urine bilirubin, Clinistix or Tes-Tape, colorimetric laboratory test procedures (e.g., urine ketone tests, urine protein tests, urine steroid determinations).
OD **Management of Overdose:** *Symptoms:* Methemoglobinemia following massive overdoses. Hemolysis due to G6PD deficiency. *Treatment:* Methylene blue, 1–2 mg/kg IV or 100–200 mg PO of ascorbic acid to treat methemoglobinemia.
How Supplied: *Tablet:* 95 mg, 97.2 mg, 100 mg, 200 mg

Dosage

- **Tablets**

Adults: 200 mg t.i.d. with or after meals for not more than 2 days when used together with an antibacterial agent for UTI. **Pediatric, 6–12 years:** 4 mg/kg t.i.d. with food for 2 days.

HEALTH CARE CONSIDERATIONS

Assessment
1. Record indications for therapy, type, onset, and characteristics of symptoms.
2. Assess for any liver/renal dysfunction.

Client/Family Teaching
1. Take with or after meals to prevent GI upset.
2. Use for only 2 days when taken together with an antibacterial agent for UTIs; continue antibiotic for entire prescription.
3. Consume 2–3 L/day of fluids.
4. With diabetes, check finger sticks regularly.
5. May cause staining of contact lenses.
6. Drug turns urine orange-red; may stain fabrics. Wear a sanitary napkin to avoid staining garments. A 0.25% sodium dithionate or sodium hydrosulfite solution, available from a pharmacy, will remove these stains.
7. Report any itching or yellowing of skin.

Outcome/Evaluate: Relief of pain and discomfort with UTI

Phendimetrazine tartrate

(fen-dye-**ME**-trah-zeen)
Pregnancy Category: C
Adipost, Bontrol PDM and Slow-Release, Dital, Dyrexan-OD, Melfiat-105 Unicelles, Plegine, Prelu-2, Rexigen Forte **(C-III) (Rx)**
Classification: Anorexiant

See also *Amphetamines and Derivatives*.
Action/Kinetics: Duration, tablets: 4 hr. **t½:** 5.5 hr (average).
Uses: Short-term (8–12 weeks) treatment of exogenous obesity in conjunction with a weight reduction program including exercise, reduced caloric intake, and behavior modification.
How Supplied: *Capsule:* 35 mg; *Capsule, Extended Release:* 105 mg; *Tablet:* 35 mg

Dosage

- **Capsules, Tablets**

Adults: 35 mg 2–3 times/day 1 hr before meals. **Maximum daily dose:** 70 mg t.i.d.

- **Extended-Release Capsules, Extended-Release Tablets**

Adults: 105 mg/day 30–60 min before the morning meal.

HEALTH CARE CONSIDERATIONS

See *Health Care Considerations* for *Amphetamines* and *Derivatives*.
Assessment: List indications for therapy, noting pretreatment weight, ECG, and labs. Identify other methods trialed and the outcome.

Client/Family Teaching
1. Must combine therapy with exercise and reduced caloric intake in the overall management of obesity.
2. This agent is for short-term therapy only.

Attend formal behavioral modification programs.
Outcome/Evaluate: Control of appetite; weight loss

Phenelzine sulfate

(FEN-ell-zeen)
Pregnancy Category: C
Nardil **(Rx)**
Classification: Antidepressant, monoamine oxidase inhibitor

Action/Kinetics: MAO inhibitor that prevents MAO from metabolizing biogenic amines. Antidepressant effect due to accumulation of biogenic amines in presynaptic granules, increasing the concentration of neurotransmitter released upon nerve stimulation. Slight anticholinergic, sedative, and orthostatic hypotensive effects. **Onset:** Few days to several months. Beneficial effects at doses of 60 mg/day may not be seen for at least 4 weeks. Clinical effects of the drug may be observed for up to 2 weeks after termination of therapy.
Uses: Depression characterized as atypical, nonendogenous, or neurotic; most often used in those clients who have mixed anxiety and depression and phobic or hypochondriacal symptoms. Not usually first-line therapy; reserve for those who have failed to respond to drugs more commonly used. *Investigational:* Alone or as an adjunct to treat bulimia nervosa, agoraphobia with panic attcks, globus hystericus syndrome, and chronic headache. Also for orthostatic hypotension, refractory migraine headaches, narcolepsy, obsessive-compulsive disorder, panic attacks, posttraumatic stress disorder, and social phobia.
Contraindications: Pheochromocytoma, CHF, history of liver disease, abnormal LFTs. Use with other sympathomimetic drugs due to the possibility of hypertensive crisis. Contraindicated with the use of many other drugs (see *Drug Interactions*). Use in children under the age of 16 years.
Special Concerns: Use with caution in combination with antihypertensive drugs, including thiazide diuretics and β-blockers, due to the possibility of severe hypotensive effects. The safe use during pregnancy or lactation has not been determined. Use with caution in geriatric clients.
Side Effects: *CNS:* Dizziness, headache, drowsiness, sleep disturbances (insomnia, hypersomnia), fatigue, weakness, tremors, twitching, myoclonic movements, hyperreflexia, jitteriness, palilalia, euphoria, nystagmus, paresthesias, ataxia, ***shock-like coma,*** toxic delirium, manic reaction, ***convulsions,*** acute anxiety reaction, precipitation of schizophrenia. *GI:* Constipation, dry mouth, GI disturbances, reversible jaundice. Rarely, ***fatal necrotizing hepatocellular damage***. *CV:* Postural hypotension, edema. *GU:* Anorgasmia, ejaculatory disturbances, urinary retention. *Metabolic:* Weight gain, hypernatremia, hypermetabolic syndrome. *Dermatologic:* Skin rash, sweating. *Ophthalmic:* Blurred vision, glaucoma. *Miscellaneous:* Leukopenia, edema of the glottis, fever associated with increased muscle tone.
Laboratory Test Considerations: ↑ Serum transaminases.
OD **Management of Overdose:** *Symptoms:* Drowsiness, dizziness, fainting, irritability, hyperactivity, agitation, severe headache, hallucinations, trismus, opisthotonus, rigidity, convulsions, coma, rapid and irregular pulse, hypertension, hypotension, cardiovascular collapse, precordial pain, respiratory depression, respiratory failure, hyperpyrexia, diaphoresis, cold and clammy skin, death. Symptoms of overdose may be absent or minimal during the initial 12-hr period after ingestion but then slowly increase, reaching a maximum effect within 24 to 48 hr. *Treatment:* If detected early, induction of emesis or gastric lavage followed by a charcoal slurry. Use of IV diazepam for CNS symptoms. For hypotension and CV collapse, IV fluids and, if necessary, BP titration with an IV infusion of a dilute pressor drug. Respirations should be supported by use of supplemental oxygen and mechanical ventilation. Fluid and electrolyte balance must be maintained. Do **not** use phenothiazine derivatives or CNS stimulants.

Drug Interactions
Alcohol / Possibility of excitation, seizures, delirium, hyperpyrexia, circulatory collapse, coma, death
Anesthetics, general / ↑ Hypotensive effect; use together with caution. Discontinue phenelzine at least 10 days before elective surgery
Anticholinergic drugs, atropine / MAO inhibitors ↑ effect of anticholinergic drugs
Antidepressants, tricyclic / Comcomitant use may result in excitation, sweating, tachycardia, tachypnea, hyperpyrexia, disseminated intravascular coagulation, delirium, tremors, convulsions, death. At least 7-10 days should elapse between discontinuing a MAO inhibitor and initiating a new drug. However, such combinations have been used together successfully

P

Antidiabetic drugs / Potentiatioin of hypoglycemic response and delayed recovery from hypoglycemia
Antihypertensive drugs / Exaggerated hypotensive effects
Beta-adrenergic blocking drugs / Exaggerated hypotensive effects; development of bradycardia
Bupropion / Concomitant use contraindicated; allow at least 10 days between discontinuing phenelzine and starting bupropion
Buspirone / Elevated BP
Carbamazepine / Possible hypertensive crisis, severe seizures, coma, or circulatory collapse; do not use together
Dextromethorphan / Possible hyperpyrexia, abnormal muscle movement, psychosis, bizarre behavior, hypotension, coma, and death; do not use together
Fluoxetine / Possibility of hyperthermia, rigidity, myoclonic movements, death. At least 10 days should elapse between discontinuation of phenelzine and initiation of fluoxetine; and, at least 5 weeks should elapse between discontinuing fluoxetine and beginning phenelzine
Guanethidine / Inhibition of the hypotensive effect of guanethidine
Levodopa / Possible hypertensive reactions
Meperidine / Possibility of agitation, excitation, seizures, diaphoresis, delirium, hyperpyrexia, apnea, coma, death; do not use together
Methyldopa / Loss of BP control or signs of central stimulation
Metrizamide / Possible ↓ of seizure threshold
Narcotics / Use with caution with phenelzine
Phenothiazines / ↑ Effect of phenothizines due to ↓ breakdown by the liver; also, ↑ chance of severe extrapyramidal effects and hypertensive crisis
Succinylcholine / ↑ Effect of succinylcholine due to ↓ breakdown in the plasma by pseudocholinesterase
Sulfonamides / Either sulfonamide or phenelzine toxicity
Sumatriptan / ↑ Risk of sumatriptan toxicity
Sympathomimetic drugs—amphetamine, cocaine, dopa, ephedrine, epinephrine, metaraminol, methyldopa, methylphenidate, norepinephrine, phenylephrine, phenylpropanolamine. Many OTC cold products, hay fever medications, and nasal decongestants contain one or more of these drugs / All peripheral, metabolic, cardiac, and central effects are potentiated for up to 2 weeks after termination of MAO inhibitor therapy. Symptoms include acute hypertensive crisis with possible intracranial hemorrhage, hyperthermia, coma, and possibly death
Thiazide diuretics / Exaggerated hypotensive effects
Tryptophan / Possibility of behavioral and neurologic effects, including disorientation, confusion, amnesia, delirium, agitation, hypomania, ataxia, myoclonus, hyperreflexia, shivering, ocular oscillation,and Babinski signs
Tyramine-rich foods—beer, broad beans, certain cheeses (Brie, cheddar, Camembert, Stilton), Chianti wine, chicken livers, caffeine, cola beverages, figs, licorice, liver, pickled or kippered herring, dry sausage (Genoa salami, hard salami, pepperoni, Lebanon bologna), tea, cream, yogurt, yeast extract, and chocolate / Possible precipitation of hypertensive crisis, including severe headache, hyperension, intracranial hemorrhage, death

How Supplied: *Tablets:* 15 mg.

Dosage

- **Tablets**

Treatment of depression.

Adults, initial: 15 mg t.i.d.; **then,** increase the dose to 60 mg/day at a fairly rapid pace (some may require 90 mg/day). **Maintenance:** After the maximum beneficial effect has been observed, the dose should be reduced slowly over several weeks to a range of 15 mg/day or every other day to as high as 45 mg/day or every other day. **Geriatric, initial:** 0.8–1 mg/kg daily in divided doses; **then,** increase s needed to a maximum of 60 mg/day.

HEALTH CARE CONSIDERATIONS

Assessment

1. Record indications for therapy, onset and duration of symptoms, previous agents trialed and the outcome. Note clinical presentation and failure with other classes of antidepressants. Assess for prior use of MAO inhibitors. These drugs have a narrow safety margin and require close supervision and restriction of foods and drugs and use with other medical conditions.
2. List drugs currently prescribed and those used within the past two weeks (especially sympathomimetic drugs) to ensure none interact unfavorably.
3. Obtain pregnancy test; drugs cross placental barrier and may be teratogenic.
4. Monitor VS, ECG, electrolytes, liver and renal function studies; assess for hypertension or arrhythmias.
5. Assess diet for foods that affect MAO inhib-

P

itors (especially tyramine-rich foods). If client has been taking elevated doses of MAO inhibitors over a long period of time, any drug withdrawal should be accomplished by gradually reducing the dosage of drug to a maintenance level before discontinuing the drug entirely.

Client/Family Teaching

1. Take as directed and with meals to decrease GI irritation. Do not administer in the evening because of the risk of insomnia.
2. Avoid taking other drugs while on this therapy and for two week after therapy has been discontinued unless specifically ordered. This includes OTC preparations for coughs, colds, congestion, or allergies.
3. Review list of tyramine-containing foods to avoid (i.e., beer, Chianti wine, chicken livers, caffeine, cola beverages, certain cheeses such as Brie, cheddar, Camembert, and Stilton; figs, licorice, liver, pickled or kippered herring, dried fish, bananas, raisins, tenderizers, game meats, avocados, dry sausage such as Genoa salami, hard salami, pepperoni, and Lebanon bologna; tea, sour cream, yogurt, yeast extract, and chocolate.
4. Several weeks of therapy are required before significant changes may occur . Continue taking if there is improvement since this is necessary to maintain proper blood levels of the drugs as well as the feelings of symptomatic improvement.
5. With diabetes, monitor FS closely and report any major variations; may potentiate the effect of insulin and sulfonylureas.
6. Report any visual changes, stiff neck, photophobia, unusual soreness or sweating, or changes in pupil size immediately as these may signal a hypertensive crisis.
7. Practice reliable birth control during and for several weeks before and after therapy.
8. Frequent mouth rinses, sugarless gum or hard candy, and increased fluid intake may diminish dry mouth side effects.
9. If feeling faint lie down immediately. Rise slowly from a supine position and dangle legs before standing to minimize orthostatic hypotension.
10. Maintain activity in moderation. MAO inhibitors suppress anginal pain which may indicate myocardial ischemia.
11. Report symptoms of CHF, such as rales, SOB, or the presence of peripheral edema.
12. Obtain weight prior to initiating therapy and biweekly therafter. May experience weight loss, nausea, anorexia, and/or diarrhea.
13. Report any increased agitation, anxiety, mania, marked behavioral changes or suicidal ideations. Suicide attempts are more frequent when client emerges from the deepest phases of depression.
14. Note any urinary retention or bladder distension. Retention is more common among the elderly, males and those who are immobilized.
15. Increase fluids to 3 L/day and the intake of fuits, fruit juices, and fiber to avoid constipation.
16. Reports of red-green vision warrant further evaluation as this may indicate eye damage.
17. Therapy requires regular F/U care since the dose will be gradually increased until the desired response is obtained. (Generally if there is no response observed by the third week of therapy, it is not likely client will respond to increased dosages.)

Outcome/Evaluate

- Improvement in mood, energy, and interest levels
- ↓ Somatic complaints; normal sleep patterns
- Improved sense of self and abilty to problem solve

Phenobarbital

(fee-no-**BAR**-bih-tal)
Pregnancy Category: D
Barbilixir ✱, Solfoton **(C-IV) (Rx)**

Phenobarbital sodium

(fee-no-**BAR**-bih-tal)
Pregnancy Category: D
Luminal Sodium **(C-IV) (Rx)**
Classification: Sedative, anticonvulsant, barbiturate type

See also *Barbiturates.*

Action/Kinetics: Long-acting. **t½:** 53–140 hr. **Onset:** 30 to more than 60 min. **Duration:** 10–16 hr. **Anticonvulsant therapeutic serum levels:** 15–40 mcg/mL. **Time for peak effect, after IV:** up to 15 min. Distributed more slowly than other barbiturates due to lower lipid solubility. Is 50%–60% protein bound. Twenty-five percent eliminated unchanged in the urine.

Uses: PO: Sedative, hypnotic (short-term), anticonvulsant (partial and generalized tonic-clonic or cortical focal seizures); emergency control of acute seizure disorders such as status epilepticus, meningitis, tetanus, eclampsia, toxicity of local anesthetics. **Parenteral:** Sedative, hypnotic (short-term), preanesthetic, anticonvulsant, emergency control of acute seizure disorders.

Special Concerns: Reduce the dose in geriatric and debilitated clients,as well as those with impaired hepatic or renal function.

Additional Side Effects: Chronic use may result in headache, fever, and megaloblastic anemia.

How Supplied: Phenobarbital: *Elixir:* 20 mg/5 mL; *Tablet:* 15 mg, 16.2 mg, 30 mg, 60 mg, 100 mg. Phenobarbital sodium: *Injection:* 30 mg/mL, 60 mg/mL, 65 mg/mL, 130 mg/mL

Dosage

PHENOBARBITAL, PHENOBARBITAL SODIUM

- **Capsules, Elixir, Tablets**

Sedation.

Adults: 30–120 mg/day in two to three divided doses. **Pediatric:** 2 mg/kg (60 mg/m^2) t.i.d.

Hypnotic.

Adults: 100–200 mg at bedtime. **Pediatric:** Dose should be determined by provider, based on age and weight.

Anticonvulsant.

Adults: 60–200 mg/day in single or divided doses. **Pediatric:** 3–6 mg/kg/day in single or divided doses.

- **IM, IV**

Sedation.

Adults: 30–120 mg/day in two to three divided doses.

Preoperative sedation.

Adults: 100–200 mg IM only, 60–90 min before surgery. **Pediatric:** 1–3 mg/kg IM or IV 60–90 min prior to surgery.

Hypnotic.

Adults: 100–320 mg IM or IV.

Acute convulsions.

Adults: 200–320 mg IM or IV; may be repeated in 6 hr if needed. **Pediatric:** 4–6 mg/kg/day for 7–10 days to achieve a blood level of 10–15 mcg/mL (or 15 mg/kg/day, IV or IM).

Status epilepticus.

Adults: 15–20 mg/kg IV (given over 10–15 min); may be repeated if needed. **Pediatric:** 15–20 mg/kg given over a 10- to 15-min period.

HEALTH CARE CONSIDERATIONS

See also *Health Care Considerations* for *Barbiturates.*

Administration/Storage

1. When used for seizures, give the major fraction of the dose according to when seizures are likely to occur (i.e., on arising for daytime seizures and at bedtime when seizures occur at night).
2. When used as an anticonvulsant in infants and children, a loading dose of 15–20 mg/kg achieves blood levels of about 20 mcg/mL shortly after administration. To achieve therapeutic blood levels of 10–20 mcg/mL, higher doses per kilogram may be needed compared with adults.
3. When used IM, inject into a large muscle (e.g., gluteus maximus, vastus lateralis). Injection into or near peripheral nerves may cause permanent neurological deficit.
4. In most cases, when used for epilepsy, drug must be taken regularly to avoid seizures, even when no seizures are imminent.
5. When used for seizures, give the lowest dose possible to avoid adding to the depression that may follow seizures.
6. IV Reserve IV use for conditions when other routes are not feasible. There is the possibility of overdose, including respiratory depression, even with slow injection of fractional doses.
7. Freshly prepare the aqueous solution for injection.
8. Some ready-dissolved solutions for injection are available; the vehicle is propylene glycol, water, and alcohol.
9. For IV administration, inject slowly at a rate of 50 mg/min.
10. Avoid extravasation as tissue damage and necrosis may result.

Assessment

1. Record indications for therapy, type, onset, and duration of symptoms.
2. List other agents prescribed and the outcome.
3. Assess liver and renal function studies. Reduce dose with impairment and in debilitated/elderly clients.

Client/Family Teaching

1. Take only as directed and do not stop abruptly.
2. May initially cause drowsiness; assess effects before performing tasks that require mental alertness.
3. Phenobarbital may require an increase in vitamin D consumption; consume foods high in vitamin D.
4. Drug decreases the effect of oral contraceptives; practice other nonhormonal forms of birth control.
5. Avoid alcohol and OTC agents without approval.

Outcome/Evaluate

- Sedation; control of seizures
- Therapeutic anticonvulsant drug levels (10–40 mcg/mL)

Phensuximide

(fen-**SUCKS**-ih-myd)

Milontin **(Rx)**

Classification: Anticonvulsant, succinimide type

See also *Anticonvulsants* and *Succinimides.*

Action/Kinetics: Less effective and less toxic than other succinimides. May color the urine pink, red, or red-brown. **t½:** 5–12 hr. **Peak effect:** 1–4 hr. Excreted through the bile and urine.
Uses: Absence seizures.
Special Concerns: Use with caution in clients with intermittent porphyria.
Additional Side Effects: Kidney damage, hematuria, urinary frequency.
How Supplied: *Capsule:* 0.5 g

Dosage

- **Capsules**

Absence seizures.

Adults and children, initial: 0.5 g b.i.d.; **then,** dose can be increased by 0.5 g/day at 1-week intervals until seizures are controlled or the daily dosage reaches 3 g. May be used with other anticonvulsants in the presence of multiple types of epilepsy.

HEALTH CARE CONSIDERATIONS

See also *Health Care Considerations* for *Anticonvulsants* and *Succinimides.*

Client/Family Teaching

1. May discolor urine a pink-brown. Report changes in elimination such as pain, frequency, or blood.
2. Report loss of seizure control.

Outcome/Evaluate: Control of seizures

Phenylephrine hydrochloride

(fen-ill-**EF**-rin)

Pregnancy Category: C

Nasal: Alconefrin 12, 25, and 50, Children's Nostril, Doktors, Duration, Neo-Synephrine Solution, Nostril, Rhinall, Vicks Sinex. **Ophthalmic:** AK-Dilate, Dionephrine ✱, Mydfrin 2.5%, Neo-Synephrine, Neo-Synephrine Viscous, Phenoptic, Prefrin Liquifilm, Relief. **Parenteral:** Neo-Synephrine. (Rx: Parenteral and Ophthalmic Solutions 2.5% or greater; OTC: Nasal products and ophthalmic solutions 0.12% or less)

Classification: Alpha-adrenergic agent (sympathomimetic)

See also *Sympathomimetic Drugs.*

Action/Kinetics: Stimulates alpha-adrenergic receptors, producing pronounced vasoconstriction and hence an increase in both SBP and DBP; reflex bradycardia results from increased vagal activity. Also acts on alpha receptors producing vasoconstriction in the skin, mucous membranes, and the mucosa as well as mydriasis by contracting the dilator muscle of the pupil. Resembles epinephrine, but it has more prolonged action and few cardiac effects. **IV: Onset,** immediate; **duration,** 15–20 min. **IM, SC: Onset,** 10–15 min; **duration:** 0.5–2 hr for IM and 50–60 min for SC. *Nasal decongestion (topical):* **Onset:** 15–20 min; **duration,** 30 min–4 hr. *Ophthalmic:* **Time to peak effect for mydriasis,** 15–60 min for 2.5% solution and 10–90 min for 10% solution. **Duration:** 0.5–1.5 hr for 0.12%, 3 hr for 2.5%, and 5–7 hr with 10% (when used for mydriasis). Excreted in urine.
Uses: Systemic: Vascular failure in shock, shock-like states, drug-induced hypotension or hypersensitivity. To maintain BP during spinal and inhalation anesthesia; to prolong spinal anesthesia. As a vasoconstrictor in regional analgesia. Paroxysmal SVT. **Nasal:** Nasal congestion due to allergies, sinusitis, common cold, or hay fever. **Ophthalmologic: 0.12%:** Temporary relief of redness of the eye associated with colds, hay fever, wind, dust, sun, smog, smoke, contact lens. **2.5% and 10%:** Decongestant and vasoconstrictor, treatment of uveitis with posterior synechiae, open-angle glaucoma, refraction without cycloplegia, ophthalmoscopic examination, funduscopy, prior to surgery.
Contraindications: Severe hypertension, VT.
Special Concerns: Use with extreme caution in geriatric clients, severe arteriosclerosis, bradycardia, partial heart block, myocardial disease, hyperthyroidism and during pregnancy and lactation. Systemic absorption with nasal or ophthalmic use. Use of the 2.5% or 10% ophthalmic solutions in children may cause hypertension and irregular heart beat. In geriatric clients, chronic use of the 2.5% or 10% ophthalmic solutions may cause rebound miosis and a decreased mydriatic effect.
Side Effects: *CV:* Reflex bradycardia, arrhythmias (rare). *CNS:* Headache, excitability, restlessness. *Ophthalmologic:* Rebound miosis and decreased mydriatic response in geriatric clients, blurred vision.
OD **Management of Overdose:** *Symptoms:* Ventricular extrasystoles, short paroxysms of ventricular tachycardia, sensation of fullness in the head, tingling of extremities. *Treatment:* Administer an alpha-adrenergic blocking agent (e.g., phentolamine).

Additional Drug Interactions

Anesthetics, halogenated hydrocarbon / May sensitize myocardium → serious arrhythmias
Bretylium / ↑ Effect of phenylephrine → possible arrhythmias

How Supplied: *Injection:* 10 mg/mL; *Liquid:* 5 mg/5 mL; *Nasal Solution:* 0.125%,

P

0.25%, 0.5%, 1%; *Ophthalmic Solution:* 0.12%, 2.5%, 10%; *Nasal Spray:* 0.25%, 0.5%, 1%

Dosage

- **IM, IV, SC**

Vasopressor, mild to moderate hypotension.

Adults: 2–5 mg (range: 1–10 mg), not to exceed an initial dose of 5 mg IM or SC repeated no more often than q 10–15 min; or, 0.2 mg (range: 0.1–0.5 mg), not to exceed an initial dose of 0.5 mg IV repeated no more often than q 10–15 min. **Pediatric:** 0.1 mg/kg (3 mg/m^2) IM or SC repeated in 1–2 hr if needed.

Vasopressor, severe hypotension and shock.

Adults: 10 mg by continuous IV infusion using 250–500 mL D5W or 0.9% NaCl injection given at a rate of 0.1–0.18 mg/min initial; **then,** give at a rate of 0.04–0.06 mg/min.

Prophylaxis of hypotension during spinal anesthesia.

Adults: 2–3 mg IM or SC 3–4 min before anesthetic given; subsequent doses should not exceed the previous dose by more than 0.1–0.2 mg. No more than 0.5 mg should be given in a single dose. **Pediatric:** 0.044–0.088 mg/kg IM or SC.

Hypotensive emergencies during spinal anesthesia.

Adults, initial: 0.2 mg IV; dose can be increased by no more than 0.2 mg for each subsequent dose not to exceed 0.5 mg/dose.

Prolongation of spinal anesthesia.

2–5 mg added to the anesthetic solution increases the duration of action up to 50% without increasing side effects or complications.

Vasoconstrictor for regional anesthesia.

Add 1 mg to every 20 mL of local anesthetic solution. If more than 2 mg phenylephrine is used, pressor reactions can be expected.

Paroxysmal SVT.

Initial: 0.5 mg (maximum) given by rapid IV injection (over 20–30 seconds). Subsequent doses are determined by BP and should not exceed the previous dose by more than 0.1–0.2 mg and should never be more than 1 mg.

- **Nasal Solution, Nasal Spray**

Adults and children over 12 years of age: 2–3 gtt of the 0.25% or 0.5% solution into each nostril q 3–4 hr as needed. In resistant cases, the 1% solution can be used but no more often than q 4 hr. **Children, 6–12 years of age:** 2–3 gtt of the 0.25% solution q 3–4 hr as needed. **Infants, greater than 6 months of age:** 1–2 gtt of the 0.16% solution into each nostril q 3–4 hr.

- **Ophthalmic Solution, 0.12%, 2.5%, 10%**

Vasoconstriction, pupillary dilation.

1 gtt of the 2.5% or 10% solution on the upper limbus a few minutes following 1 gtt of topical anesthetic (prevents stinging and dilution of solution by lacrimation). An additional drop may be needed after 1 hr.

Uveitis.

1 gtt of the 2.5% or 10% solution with atropine. To free recently formed posterior synechiae, 1 gtt of the 2.5% or 10% solution to the upper surface of the cornea. Continue treatment the following day, if needed. In the interim, apply hot compresses for 5–10 min t.i.d. using 1 gtt of 1% or 2% atropine sulfate before and after each series of compresses.

Glaucoma.

1 gtt of 10% solution on the upper surface of the cornea as needed. Both the 2.5% and 10% solutions may be used with miotics in clients with open-angle glaucoma.

Surgery.

2.5% or 10% solution 30–60 min before surgery for wide dilation of the pupil.

Refraction.

Adults: 1 gtt of a cycloplegic (homatropine HBr, atropine sulfate, cyclopentolate, tropicamide HCl, or a combination of homatropine and cocaine HCl) in each eye followed in 5 min with 1 gtt of 2.5% phenylephrine solution and in 10 min with another drop of cycloplegic. The eyes are ready for refraction in 50–60 min. **Children:** 1 gtt of atropine sulfate, 1%, in each eye followed in 10–15 min with 1 gtt of phenylephrine solution, 2.5%, and in 5–10 min with a second drop of atropine sulfate, 1%. The eyes are ready for refraction in 1–2 hr.

Ophthalmoscopic examination.

1 gtt of 2.5% solution in each eye. The eyes are ready for examination in 15– 30 min and the effect lasts for 1–3 hr.

Minor eye irritations.

1–2 gtt of the 0.12% solution in the eye(s) up to q.i.d. as needed.

HEALTH CARE CONSIDERATIONS

See also *Health Care Considerations* for *Sympathomimetic Drugs.*

Administration/Storage

1. Store drug in a brown bottle and away from light.
2. Instill a drop of local anesthetic before administering the 10% ophthalmic solution.
3. Instruct clients to blow their noses before administering as a nasal decongestant.
4. IV For IV administration, dilute each 1 mg

with 9 mL of sterile water and administer over 1 min. Further dilution of 10 mg in 500 mL of dextrose, Ringer's, or saline solution may be titrated to client response.
5. When used parenterally, monitor infusion site closely to avoid extravasation. If evident, administer SC phentolamine locally to prevent tissue necrosis.
6. Prolonged exposure to air or strong light may result in oxidation and discoloration. Do not use solution if it changes color, becomes cloudy, or contains a precipitate.

Assessment

1. Record indications for therapy, type, onset, and characteristics of symptoms; note goals of therapy.
2. During IV administration monitor cardiac rhythm and BP continuously until stabilized, noting any evidence of bradycardia or arrhythmias.

Client/Family Teaching

1. Ophthalmic instillations and nasal decongestants may produce systemic sympathomimetic effects; chronic excessive use may cause rebound congestion.
2. Wear sunglasses in bright light. Report if symptoms of photosensitivity and blurred vision persist after 12 hr. Blurred vision should decrease with repeated use.
3. With ophthalmic solution, report if there is no relief of symptoms within 2 days.
4. When using for nasal decongestion, report if no relief of symptoms within 3 days. Rebound nasal congestion may occur with longer therapy.

Outcome/Evaluate

- ↑ BP
- Termination of paroxysmal SVT
- Relief of nasal congestion
- ↓ Conjunctivitis/allergic S&S
- Dilatation of pupils

Phenytoin (Diphenylhydantoin)

(FEN-ih-toyn, dye-fen-ill-hy-DAN-toyn)
Pregnancy Category: C
Dilantin Infatab, Dilantin-125, Novo-Phenytoin ✱, Tremytoine ✱ **(Rx)**

Phenytoin sodium, extended

(FEN-ih-toyn)
Pregnancy Category: C
Dilantin Kapseals **(Rx)**

Phenytoin sodium, parenteral

(FEN-ih-toyn)
Pregnancy Category: C
Dilantin Sodium **(Rx)**

Phenytoin sodium prompt

(FEN-ih-toyn)
Pregnancy Category: C
Diphenylan Sodium **(Rx)**
Classification: Anticonvulsant, hydantoin type; antiarrhythmic (type I)

See also *Anticonvulsants* and *Antiarrhythmic Agents.*

Action/Kinetics: Acts in the motor cortex of the brain to reduce the spread of electrical discharges from the rapidly firing epileptic foci in this area. This is accomplished by stabilizing hyperexcitable cells possibly by affecting sodium efflux. Also, phenytoin decreases activity of centers in the brain stem responsible for the tonic phase of grand mal seizures. Has few sedative effects.

Monitor serum levels because the serum concentrations of phenytoin increase disproportionately as the dosage is increased. Phenytoin extended is designed for once-a-day dosage. It has a slow dissolution rate—no more than 35% in 30 min, 30%–70% in 60 min, and less than 85% in 120 min. Absorption is variable following PO dosage. **Peak serum levels: PO,** 4–8 hr. Since the rate and extent of absorption depend on the particular preparation, the same product should be used for a particular client. **Peak serum levels (following IM):** 24 hr (wide variation). **Therapeutic serum levels:** 5–20 mcg/mL. **t½:** 8–60 hr (average: 20–30 hr). **Steady state:** 7–10 days after initiation. Biotransformed in the liver. Both inactive metabolites and unchanged drug are excreted in the urine.

As an antiarrhythmic, phenytoin increases the electrical stimulation threshold of heart muscle, although it is less effective than quinidine, procainamide, or lidocaine. **Onset:** 30–60 min. **Duration:** 24 hr or more. **t½:** 22–36 hr. **Therapeutic serum level:** 10–20 mcg/mL.

Uses: Chronic epilepsy, especially of the tonic-clonic, psychomotor type. Not effective against absence seizures and may even increase the frequency of seizures in this disorder. Parenteral phenytoin is sometimes used to treat status epilepticus and to control seizures during neurosurgery.

PO for certain PVCs and IV for PVCs and tachycardia. Particularly useful for arrhythmias produced by digitalis overdosage.

Investigational: Paroxysmal choreoathetosis; to treat blistering and erosions in clients with recessive dystrophic epidermolysis bullosa; episodic dyscontrol; trigeminal neuralgia; as a muscle relaxant in neuromyotonia,

P

myotonia congenita, or myotonic muscular dystrophy; to treat cardiac symptoms in overdosage of tricyclic antidepressants. Severe preeclampsia.

Contraindications: Hypersensitivity to hydantoins, exfoliative dermatitis, sinus bradycardia, second- and third-degree AV block, clients with Adams-Stokes syndrome, SA block. Lactation.

Special Concerns: Use with caution in acute, intermittent porphyria. Administer with extreme caution to clients with a history of asthma or other allergies, impaired renal or hepatic function, and heart disease (hypotension, severe myocardial insufficiency). Abrupt withdrawal may cause status epilepticus. Combined drug therapy is required if petit mal seizures are also present.

Side Effects: *CNS:* Most commonly, drowsiness, ataxia, dysarthria, confusion, insomnia, nervousness, irritability, depression, tremor, numbness, headache, psychoses, ***increased seizures.*** Choreoathetosis following IV use. *GI:* Gingival hyperplasia, N&V, either diarrhea or constipation. *Dermatologic:* Various dermatoses including a measles-like rash (common), scarlatiniform, maculopapular, and urticarial rashes. Rarely, drug-induced lupus erythematosus, ***Stevens-Johnson syndrome,*** exfoliative or purpuric dermatitis, and ***toxic epidermal necrolysis.*** Alopecia, hirsutism. Skin reactions may necessitate withdrawal of therapy. *Hematopoietic:* Leukopenia, granulocytopenia, thrombocytopenia, pancytopenia, ***agranulocytosis,*** macrocytosis, megaloblastic anemia, leukocytosis, monocytosis, eosinophilia, simple anemia, ***aplastic anemia, hemolytic anemia.*** *Hepatic:* Liver damage, toxic hepatitis, hypersensitivity reactions involving the liver including hepatocellular degeneration and ***fatal hepatocellular necrosis.*** *Ophthalmic:* Diplopia, nystagmus, conjunctivitis. *Miscellaneous:* Hyperglycemia, chest pain, edema, fever, photophobia, weight gain, ***pulmonary fibrosis,*** lymph node hyperplasia, gynecomastia, periarteritis nodosa, depression of IgA, soft tissue injury at injection site, coarsening of facial features, Peyronie's disease, enlarged lips.

Rapid parenteral administration may cause serious CV effects, including hypotension, arrhythmias, CV collapse, and heart block, as well as CNS depression.

Many clients have a partial deficiency in the ability of the liver to degrade phenytoin, and as a result, toxicity may develop after a small PO dose. Liver and kidney function tests and hematopoietic studies are indicated prior to and periodically during drug therapy.

Laboratory Test Considerations: Alters LFTs, ↑ blood glucose values, and ↓ PBI values. ↑ Gamma globulins. Phenytoin ↓ immunoglobulins A and G. False + Coombs' test.

OD **Management of Overdose:** *Symptoms:* Initially, ataxia, dysarthria, and nystagmus followed by unresponsive pupils, hypotension, and ***coma.*** Plasma levels greater than 40 mcg/mL result in significant decreases in mental capacity. *Treatment:* Treat symptoms. Hemodialysis may be effective. In children, total-exchange transfusion has been used.

Drug Interactions

Acetaminophen / ↓ Effect of acetaminophen due to ↑ breakdown by liver; however, hepatotoxicity may be ↑
Alcohol, ethyl / In alcoholics, ↓ effect of phenytoin due to ↑ breakdown by liver
Allopurinol / ↑ Effect of phenytoin due to ↓ breakdown in liver
Amiodarone / ↑ Effect of phenytoin or amiodarone due to ↓ breakdown by liver
Antacids / ↓ Effect of phenytoin due to ↓ GI absorption
Anticoagulants, oral / ↑ Effect of phenytoin due to ↓ breakdown by liver. Also, possible ↑ anticoagulant effect due to ↓ plasma protein binding
Antidepressants, tricyclic / May ↑ incidence of epileptic seizures or ↑ effect of phenytoin by ↓ plasma protein binding
Barbiturates / Effect of phenytoin may be ↑, ↓, or not changed; possible ↑ effect of barbiturates
Benzodiazepines / ↑ Effect of phenytoin due to ↓ breakdown by liver
Carbamazepine / ↓ Effect of phenytoin or carbamazepine due to ↑ breakdown by liver
Charcoal / ↓ Effect of phenytoin due to ↓ absorption from GI tract
Chloramphenicol / ↑ Effect of phenytoin due to ↓ breakdown by liver
Chlorpheniramine / ↑ Effect of phenytoin
Cimetidine / ↑ Effect of phenytoin due to ↓ breakdown by liver
Clonazepam / ↓ Plasma levels of clonazepam or phenytoin; or, ↑ risk of phenytoin toxicity
Contraceptives, oral / Estrogen-induced fluid retention may precipitate seizures; also, ↓ effect of contraceptives due to ↑ breakdown by liver
Corticosteroids / Effect of corticosteroids ↓ due to ↑ breakdown by liver; also, corticosteroids may mask hypersensitivity reactions due to phenytoin
Cyclosporine / ↓ Effect of cyclosporine due to ↑ breakdown by liver
Diazoxide / ↓ Effect of phenytoin due to ↑ breakdown by liver

Dicumarol / Phenytoin ↓ effect of dicumarol due to ↑ breakdown by liver
Digitalis glycosides / ↓ Effect of digitalis glycosides due to ↑ breakdown by liver
Disopyrimide / ↓ Effect of disopyramide due to ↑ breakdown by liver
Disulfiram / ↑ Effect of phenytoin due to ↓ breakdown by liver
Dopamine / IV phenytoin results in hypotension and bradycardia; also, ↓ effect of dopamine
Doxycycline / ↓ Effect of doxycycline due to ↑ breakdown by liver
Estrogens / See *Contraceptives, oral*
Fluconazole / ↑ Effect of phenytoin due to ↓ breakdown by liver
Folic acid / ↓ Effect of phenytoin
Furosemide / ↓ Effect of furosemide due to ↓ absorption
Haloperidol / ↓ Effect of haloperidol due to ↑ breakdown by liver
Ibuprofen / ↑ Effect of phenytoin
Isoniazid / ↑ Effect of phenytoin due to ↓ breakdown by liver
Levodopa / Phenytoin ↓ effect of levodopa
Levonorgestrel / ↓ Effect of norgestrel
Lithium / ↑ Risk of lithium toxicity
Loxapine / ↓ Effect of phenytoin
Mebendazole / ↓ Effect of mebendazole
Meperidine / ↓ Effect of meperidine due to ↑ breakdown by liver; toxic effects of meperidine may ↑ due to accumulation of active metabolite (normeperidine)
Methadone / ↓ Effect of methadone due to ↑ breakdown by liver
Metronidazole / ↑ Effect of phenytoin due to ↓ breakdown by liver
Metyrapone / ↓ Effect of metyrapone due to ↑ breakdown by liver
Mexiletine / ↓ Effect of mexiletine due to ↑ breakdown by liver
Miconazole / ↑ Effect of phenytoin due to ↓ breakdown by liver
Nitrofurantoin / ↓ Effect of phenytoin
Omeprazole / ↑ Effect of phenytoin due to ↓ breakdown by liver
Phenacemide / ↑ Effect of phenytoin due to ↓ breakdown by liver
Phenothiazines / ↑ Effect of phenytoin due to ↓ breakdown by liver
Phenylbutazone / ↑ Effect of phenytoin due to ↓ breakdown by liver and ↓ plasma protein binding
Primidone / Possible ↑ effect of primidone
Pyridoxine / ↓ Effect of phenytoin
Quinidine / ↓ Effect of quinidine due to ↑ breakdown by liver
Rifampin / ↓ Effect of phenytoin due to ↑ breakdown by liver
Salicylates / ↑ Effect of phenytoin by ↓ plasma protein binding
Sucralfate / ↓ Effect of phenytoin due to ↓ absorption from GI tract
Sulfonamides / ↑ Effect of phenytoin due to ↓ breakdown in liver
Sulfonylureas / ↓ Effect of sulfonylureas
Theophylline / ↓ Effect of both drugs due to ↑ breakdown by liver
Trimethoprim / ↑ Effect of phenytoin due to ↓ breakdown by liver
Valproic acid / ↑ Effect of phenytoin due to ↓ breakdown by liver and ↓ plasma protein binding; phenytoin may also ↓ effect of valproic acid due to ↑ breakdown by liver

How Supplied: Phenytoin: *Chew Tablet:* 50 mg; *Suspension:* 100 mg/4 mL, 125 mg/5 mL; Phenytoin sodium, extended: *Capsule, Extended Release:* 30 mg, 100 mg; Phenytoin sodium, parenteral: *Injection:* 50 mg/mL; Phenytoin sodium prompt: *Capsule:* 100 mg

Dosage

- **Oral Suspension, Chewable Tablets**

Seizures.

Adults, initial: 100 mg (125 mg of the suspension) t.i.d.; adjust dosage at 7- to 10-day intervals until seizures are controlled; **usual, maintenance:** 300–400 mg/day, although 600 mg/day (625 mg of the suspension) may be required in some. **Pediatric, initial:** 5 mg/kg/day in two to three divided doses; **maintenance,** 4–8 mg/kg (up to maximum of 300 mg/day). Children over 6 years may require up to 300 mg/day. **Geriatric:** 3 mg/kg initially in divided doses; **then,** adjust dosage according to serum levels and response. Once dosage level has been established, the extended capsules may be used for once-a-day dosage.

- **Capsules, Extended-Release Capsules**

Seizures.

Adults, initial: 100 mg t.i.d.; adjust dose at 7- to 10-day intervals until control is achieved. An initial loading dose of 12–15 mg/kg divided into two to three doses over 6 hr followed by 100 mg t.i.d. on subsequent days may be preferred if seizures are frequent. **Pediatric:** See dose for Oral Suspension and Chewable Tablets.

Arrhythmias.

Adults: 200–400 mg/day.

- **IV**

Status epilepticus.

Adults, loading dose: 10–15 mg/kg at a rate not to exceed 50 mg/min; **then,** 100 mg PO or IV q 6–8 hr. **Pediatric, loading dose:** 15–20 mg/kg in divided doses of 5–10 mg/kg given at a rate of 1–3 mg/kg/min.

P

Arrhythmias.
Adults: 100 mg q 5 min up to maximum of 1 g.
• **IM**
Dose should be 50% greater than the PO dose.

Neurosurgery.
100–200 mg q 4 hr during and after surgery (during first 24 hr, administer no more than 1,000 mg; after first day, give maintenance dosage).

HEALTH CARE CONSIDERATIONS

See also *Health Care Considerations* for *Anticonvulsants* and *Antiarrhythmic Agents.*

Administration/Storage

1. Full effectiveness of PO administered hydantoins is delayed and may take 6–9 days to be fully established. A similar period of time will elapse before effects disappear completely.
2. When hydantoins are substituted for or added to another anticonvulsant medication, their dosage is gradually increased, while dosage of the other drug is decreased proportionally.
3. Avoid IM, SC, or perivascular injections. Pain, inflammation, and necrosis may be caused by the highly alkaline solutions.
4. If receiving tube feedings of Isocal or Osmolite, the PO absorption of phenytoin may be decreased. Do not administer together.
5. Due to potential differences in bioavailability between PO products, do not interchange brands. Also, when switching from extended to prompt products, dosage adjustments may be required.
6. **IV** Use of IV infusion is not recommended, as the drug is poorly soluble and may form a precipitate. Inject slowly and directly into a large vein through a large-gauge needle or IV catheter.
7. For parenteral preparations:
   • Use only a clear solution.
   • Dilute with special diluent supplied by manufacturer.
   • Shake the vials until the solution is clear. It may take about 10 min for the drug to dissolve.
   • To hasten the process, warm the vial in warm water after adding the diluent.
   • The drug is incompatible with acid solutions.
8. *Do not* add phenytoin to an already running IV solution.
9. If IV infusion is used, a rate of 50 mg/min should not be exceeded in adults or 1–3 mg/kg/min in neonates.
10. Following IV administration, administer NSS through the same needle or IV catheter to avoid local irritation of the vein due to alkalinity of the solution. Do not use dextrose solutions.
11. For treatment of status epilepticus, inject IV slowly at a rate not to exceed 50 mg/min. May repeat the dose 30 min after the initial administration if needed.

Assessment

1. Record indications for therapy, onset and characteristics of symptoms.
2. Note history and nature of seizures, addressing location, frequency, duration, causes, and characteristics.
3. Determine if hypersensitive to hydantoins or has exfoliative dermatitis. Consider fosphenytoin in those unable to tolerate phenytoin.
4. Do not breast-feed following delivery.
5. Monitor ECG hematologic, liver, and renal function studies.

Interventions

1. During IV administration, monitor for hypotension.
2. Monitor serum drug levels:
   • Seven to 10 days may be required to achieve recommended serum levels. Drug is highly protein bound; may order free and bound drug levels to better assess response. The drug is metabolized much more slowly by elderly clients; thus most may be managed with once a day dosing.
   • If receiving drugs that interact with hydantoins or with impaired liver function, obtain level more frequently. Dilantin induces hepatic microsomal enzymes for drug metabolism.
3. Oral form has variable absorption; do not administer with tube feedings. Administer separately, flush, and clamp tube for 20 min to ensure absorption.

Client/Family Teaching

1. May take with food to minimize GI upset. Do not take within 2–3 hr of antacid ingestion.
2. Use care when performing tasks that require mental alertness. Drug may cause drowsiness, dizziness, and blurred vision.
3. Do not substitute products or exchange brands because bioavailability of phenytoin may vary. Seizure control may be lost or toxic blood levels may develop with substitutions.
4. Prompt-release forms cannot be substituted for another unless the dosage is also adjusted.
   • If taking phenytoin extended, do not substitute chewable tablets for capsules. The strengths of the medications are not equal.

• If taking phenytoin extended, check bottle carefully. Chewable tablets are never in the extended form.
• With extended, take only a single dose daily; take only as directed and only in the brand prescribed.
5. If a dose is missed, take as soon as it is remembered. Then resume the usual schedule. Do not double up to make up for the missed dose. If the doses of drug are scheduled throughout the day, and one of the doses is missed, take the drug as soon as it is realized unless it's within 4 hr of the next dose. In that case, omit unless otherwise instructed.
6. Do not take any other agents. Hydantoins interact with many other medications and may require adjustment of the anticonvulsant dose.
7. Avoid alcohol in any form and CNS depressants.
8. With diabetes, monitor FS and report changes; may have to to adjust insulin dosage and/or diet.
9. May cause urine to appear pink, red, or brown; do not be alarmed.
10. To minimize bleeding from the gums and prevent gingival hyperplasia, practice good oral hygiene. Brush teeth with a soft toothbrush, massage the gums, and floss every day. Advise dentist of therapy.
11. Hydantoin has an androgenic effect on the hair follicle. Acne may develop; practice good skin care.
12. Report any excessive hair growth on the face and trunk and any discolorations or skin rash; may require dermatologist referral.
13. Complaints of weakness, ease of fatigue, headaches, or feeling faint may be signs of folic acid deficiency or megaloblastic anemia. Dietitian evaluation as well as hematologic evaluations may be indicated.
14. Report for lab studies as ordered, including CBC, drug levels, and renal and liver function studies.
15. Drug may alter thyroid function results. If thyroid studies are conducted, for ensured accuracy, they should be repeated 10 days after therapy has been discontinued.
16. Do not stop abruptly. Report all bothersome side effects because these may be dose-related.
17. Practice reliable birth control; drug may interfere with oral contraceptives.

Outcome/Evaluate

• Control of seizures
• Termination of ventricular arrhythmias; restoration of stable cardiac rhythm
• Therapeutic drug levels (5–20 mcg/mL)

Phosphorated carbohydrate solution

(FOS-for-ay-ted kar-boh-HIGH-drayt)
Emetrol, Nausea Relief, Nausetrol **(OTC)**
Classification: Antiemetic

See also *Antiemetics.*

Action/Kinetics: A hyperosmolar carbohydrate solution containing fructose, dextrose, and orthophosphoric acid with controlled hydrogen ion concentration. It relieves N&V due to a direct action on the wall of the GI tract that decreases smooth muscle contraction and delays gastric emptying time; the effect is directly related to the amount used.

Uses: Symptomatic relief of nausea due to upset stomach from intestinal flu, stomach flu, and food or drink. *Investigational:* Morning or motion sickness, regurgitation in infants, N&V due to drug therapy or inhaled anesthetics.

Contraindications: Diabetic clients due to the presence of carbohydrates. Individuals with hereditary fructose intolerance.

Special Concerns: Since nausea may be a symptom of a serious condition, a physician should be consulted if symptoms are not relieved or recur often.

Side Effects: *GI:* Abdominal pain and diarrhea due to large doses of fructose.

How Supplied: *Solution:* Liquid

Dosage

• **Oral Solution**

Nausea.

Adults: 15–30 mL at 15-min intervals until vomiting ceases; if the first dose is rejected, the same dosage should be given in 5 min. Should not be taken for more than five doses (1 hr). **Children, 2 to 12 years:** 5–10 mL at 15-min intervals in the same manner as adults.

Regurgitation in infants.

5 or 10 mL, 10–15 min before each feeding; in refractory cases, 10 or 15 mL, 30 min before feeding.

Morning sickness.

15–30 mL on arising; repeat q 3 hr or when nausea threatens.

N&V due to drug therapy or inhalation anesthesia, motion sickness.

Adults and older children: 15 mL; **young children:** 5 mL.

HEALTH CARE CONSIDERATIONS

See also *Health Care Considerations* for *Antiemetics.*

P

Assessment

1. Record indications for therapy, onset and duration of symptoms, other agents utilized and outcome.
2. Note any diabetes or hereditary fructose intolerance.

Client/Family Teaching

1. Do not dilute and do not take PO fluids immediately before a dose or for at least 15 min after a dose.
2. Report if symptoms persist, recur often, or become worse.
3. Increase fluid intake to prevent the development of dehydration.

Outcome/Evaluate: Relief of N&V

Physostigmine salicylate

(fye-zoh-**STIG**-meen)
Pregnancy Category: C
Antilirium **(Rx)**

Physostigmine sulfate

(fye-zoh-**STIG**-meen)
Pregnancy Category: C
Eserine Sulfate **(Rx)**
Classification: Indirectly acting cholinergic-acetylcholinesterase inhibitor

See also *Neostigmine* and *Ophthalmic Cholinergic Agents*.

Action/Kinetics: Reversible acetylcholinesterase inhibitor causing an increased concentration of acetylcholine at nerve endings; antagonizes anticholinergic drugs. Produces miosis, increased accommodation, and a decrease in intraocular pressure with decreased resistance to outflow of aqueous humor. When used for chronic open-angle glaucoma, ciliary muscle contraction may open the intertrabecular spaces, facilitating aqueous humor outflow. **Onset, IV:** 3–5 min. **Duration, IV:** 1–2 hr. **t½:** 1–2 hr. No dosage alteration is necessary in clients with renal impairment. **Onset, miosis:** 20–30 min; **duration, miosis:** 12–36 hr. **Reduction of IOP, peak:** 2–6 hr; **duration:** 12–36 hr.

Uses: Overdosage due to cholinergic blocking drugs (e.g., atropine) and tricyclic antidepressant overdosage. Reduce intraocular pressure in open-angle glaucoma. Friedreich's and other inherited ataxias (FDA has granted orphan status for this use). *Investigational:* Angle-closure glaucoma during or after iridectomy, secondary glaucoma if no inflammation present. Treat delirium tremens (DTs) and Alzheimer's disease. May also antagonize the CNS depressant effect of diazepam.

Contraindications: Active uveal inflammation, any inflammatory disease of the iris or ciliary body, glaucoma associated with iridocyclitis. Asthma, gangrene, diabetes, CV disease, GI or GU tract obstruction, any vagotonic state, in those receiving choline esters or depolarizing neuromuscular blocking drugs.

Special Concerns: Use with caution during lactation, in clients with chronic angle-closure glaucoma, or in clients with narrow angles. Safety and efficacy have not been established for ophthalmic use in children. Reserve systemic use in children for life-threatening situations only. Benzyl alcohol, found in the parenteral product, may cause a fatal "gasping syndrome" in premature infants. The parenteral form also contains sulfites that may cause allergic reactions.

Additional Side Effects: If IV administration is too rapid, bradycardia, hypersalivation, breathing difficulties, and ***seizures*** may occur. Conjunctivitis when used for glaucoma.

OD **Management of Overdose:** *Symptoms:* Cholinergic crisis. *Treatment:* IV atropine sulfate: **Adults:** 0.4–0.6 mg; **infants and children up to 12 years of age:** 0.01 mg/kg q 2 hr as needed (maximum single dose should not exceed 0.4 mg). A short-acting barbiturate may be used for seizures not relieved by atropine.

Drug Interactions

Anticholinesterases, systemic / Additive effects → toxicity
Succinylcholine / ↑ Risk of respiratory and CV collapse

How Supplied: Physostigmine salicylate: *Injection:* 1 mg/mL. Physostigmine sulfate: *Ophthalmic Ointment:* 0.25%

Dosage

- **IM, IV**

Anticholinergic drug overdose.

Adults, IM, IV: 0.5–2 mg at a rate of 1 mg/min; may be repeated if necessary. **Pediatric, IV:** 0.02 mg/kg IM or by slow IV injection (0.5 mg given over a period of at least 1 min). Dose may be repeated at 5–10 min if needed to a maximum of 2 mg if no toxic effects are manifested.

Postanesthesia.

0.5–1 mg given IM or by slow IV (less than 1 mg/min). May be repeated at 10- to 30-min intervals to attain desired response.

- **Ophthalmic Ointment**

Glaucoma.

Adults and children: 1 cm of the 0.25% sulfate ointment applied to the lower fornix up to t.i.d.

HEALTH CARE CONSIDERATIONS

See also *Health Care Considerations* for *Neostigmine,* and *Ophthalmic Cholinergic Agents.*

Administration/Storage

1. The ophthalmic ointment may be used at night for prolonged effect of the medication.
2. Store the ophthalmic ointment tightly closed and protected from heat.

IV 3. May administer IV undiluted: 1 mg/min; 0.5 mg/min for children. Product contains benzyl alcohol.

Assessment: Determine type of overdosage (drug or plant ingestion), amount and time ingested.

Interventions

1. During IV administration, monitor ECG and VS; report any bradycardia, hypersalivation, respiratory difficulty, or seizure activity.
2. Have client void prior to administering. If incontinence occurs, may be caused by too high a dose.

Client/Family Teaching

1. Wash hands before and after administration to prevent contamination and systemic absorption.
2. Some stinging and burning of the eyes may occur. This should disappear with continued use. If painful spasms occur, apply cold compresses. If itching, pain, or tearing persists, do not continue using until medically cleared.
3. During ophthalmic instillation, wipe away any excess medication from around the eyes.
4. Night vision may be impaired.
5. N&V may occur; report if the symptoms persist or are severe.

Outcome/Evaluate

- Reversal of toxic CNS symptoms R/T drug overdosage or plant toxins
- ↓ Intraocular pressures

Phytonadione (Vitamin K_1)

(fye-toe-nah-**DYE**-ohn)

Pregnancy Category: C

Aqua-Mephyton, Mephyton **(Rx)**

Classification: Fat-soluble vitamin

Action/Kinetics: Vitamin K is essential for the hepatic synthesis of factors II, VII, IX, and X, all of which are essential for blood clotting. Vitamin K deficiency causes an increase in bleeding tendency, demonstrated by ecchymoses, epistaxis, hematuria, GI bleeding, and postoperative and intracranial hemorrhage. Phytonadione is similar to natural vitamin K. GI absorption occurs only via intestinal lymphatics and requires the presence of bile salts. Vitamin K is not effective in reversing the anticoagulant effect of heparin. Frequent determinations of PT are indicated during therapy. **IM: Onset,** 1–2 hr. *Control of bleeding:* Parenteral, 3–6 hr. *Normal PT:* 12–14 hr. **PO: Onset,** 6–12 hr.

Uses: Primary and drug-induced hypoprothrombinemia, especially that caused by anticoagulants of the coumarin and phenindione type. Vitamin K cannot reverse the anticoagulant activity of heparin.

Parenteral use for vitamin K malabsorption syndromes. Adjunct during whole blood transfusions. Preoperatively to prevent the danger of hemorrhages in surgical clients who may require anticoagulant therapy.

Certain forms of liver disease. Hemorrhagic states associated with obstructive jaundice, celiac disease, ulcerative colitis, sprue, biliary fistula, cystic fibrosis of the pancreas, regional enteritis, resection of intestine. Prophylaxis of hemorrhagic disease of the newborn.

Contraindications: Severe liver disease.

Special Concerns: Use with caution in clients with sulfite sensitivity and during lactation as phytonadione is excreted in breast milk. Safety and efficacy have not been determined in children. Benzyl alcohol, contained in some preparations, may cause toxicity in newborns.

Side Effects: May be transient flushing of the face, sweating, a sense of constriction of the chest, and weakness. Cramp-like pain, weak and rapid pulse, convulsive movements, chills and fever, hypotension, cyanosis, or hemoglobinuria has been reported occasionally. ***Shock and cardiac and respiratory failure*** may be observed. *Allergic:* Rash, urticaria, ***anaphylaxis.*** *After PO use:* N&V, stomach upset, headache. *After parenteral use:* Flushing, alteration of taste, sweating, hypotension, dizziness, rapid and weak pulse, dyspnea, cyanosis, delayed skin reactions. Pain, swelling, and tenderness at injection site. ***IV administration may cause severe reactions (e.g., shock, cardiac or respiratory arrest, anaphylaxis) leading to death.*** These effects may occur when receiving vitamin K for the first time. *Newborns:* ***Fatal kernicterus,*** hemolysis, jaundice, hyperbilirubinemia (especially in premature infants).

Drug Interactions

Antibiotics / May inhibit the body's production of vitamin K and may lead to bleeding. Vitamin K supplements should be given
Anticoagulants, oral / Vitamin K antagonizes anticoagulant effect
Cholestyramine / ↓ Effect of phytonadione due to ↓ absorption from GI tract
Colestipol / ↓ Effect of phytonadione due to ↓ absorption from GI tract
Hemolytics / ↑ Potential for toxicity

Mineral oil / ↓ Effect of phytonadione due to ↓ absorption from GI tract
Quinidine, Quinine / ↑ Requirement for vitamin K
Salicylates / High doses of salicylates → ↑ requirements for vitamin K
Sulfonamides / ↑ Requirements for vitamin K
Sucralfate / ↓ Effect of phytonadione due to ↓ absorption from GI tract
How Supplied: *Injection:* 1 mg/0.5 mL, 10 mg /mL; *Tablet:* 0.1 mg, 5 mg

Dosage

- **Tablets**

Hypoprothrombinemia, drug-induced.
Adults: 2.5–10 mg (up to 25 mg); dose may be repeated after 12–48 hr if needed.

Vitamin supplement, prothrombogenic, drug-induced hypoprothrombinemia.
Pediatric: 5–10 mg.

- **IM, SC**

Vitamin supplement, prothrombogenic, drug-induced hypoprothrombinemia.
Adults: 2.5–10 mg (up to 25 mg) which may be repeated after 6–8 hr if needed. **Infants:** 1–2 mg; **children:** 5–10 mg.

Prophylaxis of hypoprothrombinemia during prolonged TPN.
Adults, IM: 5–10 mg once weekly; **pediatric:** 2–5 mg IM once weekly.

Infants receiving milk substitutes or who are breastfed.
1 mg/month if vitamin K in diet is less than 0.1 mg/L.

Prevention of hemorrhagic disease in the newborn.
0.5–1 mg IM within 1 hr after delivery. The dose may be repeated in 2–3 weeks if the mother took anticoagulant, anticonvulsant, antituberculosis, or recent antibiotic therapy during pregnancy. Alternatively, 1–5 mg given to the mother 12–24 hr before delivery.

Treatment of hemorrhagic disease in the newborn.
1 mg SC or IM (higher doses may be needed if the mother has been taking oral anticoagulants).

HEALTH CARE CONSIDERATIONS

Administration/Storage

1. Mix suspension (injection) only with water or D5W.
2. Mix colloidal injection with D5W, isotonic NaCl, or D5/NSS.
3. Protect vitamin K from light.
4. Store injectable emulsion or colloidal solutions in cool, 5°C–15°C (41°F–59°F), dark place.
5. Do not freeze.
6. Heparin may be used to reverse effects from overdosage.

Assessment

1. Record sensitivity to sulfites.
2. Note drugs prescribed to ensure none interact.
3. Monitor PT/PTT, liver and hematologic values.
4. Determine history or lab evidence of advanced liver disease. This results in loss of protein synthesis and is not responsive to vitamin K.

Interventions

1. Note any frank bleeding. Test stools, urine, and GI drainage for occult blood.
2. Observe hospitalized clients with poor nutrition (receiving TPN), uremia, recent surgery, and multiple antibiotic therapy for vitamin K deficiency.
3. Administer slowly. Rapid parenteral administration can produce dyspnea, chest and back pain, and even death.
4. With decreased bile secretion, administer bile salts to ensure absorption of PO phytonadione.
5. If receiving bile acid–binding resins such as colestipol or cholestyramine, monitor PT and assess carefully for malabsorption of vitamin K.

Client/Family Teaching

1. Take only as directed.
2. Dietary sources high in vitamin K include dairy products, meats, and green leafy vegetables. The dietary requirement is low since it is also synthesized by colonized bacteria in the intestine.
3. Report any evidence of unusual bruising or bleeding.
4. Use a soft toothbrush, electric razor, and a night light at night; wear shoes and avoid IM shots and flossing to prevent injury with bleeding.
5. Avoid alcohol, aspirin, and ibuprofen compounds (NSAIDs) as well as any other OTC preparations.

Outcome/Evaluate

- Prevention/control of bleeding
- Prophylaxis of hypoprothrombinemia during prolonged TPN
- Prevention of hemorrhagic disease in the newborn

Pilocarpine hydrochloride

(pie-low-**CAR**-peen)
Pregnancy Category: C
Adsorbocarpine, Akarpine, Diocarpine ★, Isopto Carpine, Miocarpine ★, Pilocar, Pilopine HS, Piloptic-½ -1, -2, -3, -4, and -6, Pilopto-Carpine, Pilostat, Salagen, Schein-pharm Pilocarpine ★ **(Rx)**

Pilocarpine ocular therapeutic system

(pie-low-**CAR**-peen)
Pregnancy Category: C
Ocusert Pilo-20 and -40 **(Rx)**
Classification: Direct-acting cholinergic agent (miotic)

See also *Ophthalmic Cholinergic Agents.*
Action/Kinetics: *Hydrochloride Solution:* 4–14 hr. *Hydrochloride Gel:* **Onset:** 60 min; **peak effect:** 3–12 hr; **duration:** 18–24 hr. *Nitrate:* The ocular therapeutic system is placed in the cul-de-sac of the eye for release of pilocarpine. The drug is released from the ocular therapeutic system three times faster during the first few hours and then decreases (within 6 hr) to a rate of 20 or 40 mcg/hr for 1 week. *Ocular system:* **onset:** 60 min. **peak effect:** 1.5–2 hr; **duration:** 7 days. When used to treat dry mouth due to radiotherapy in head and neck cancer clients, pilocarpine stimulates residual functioning salivary gland tissue to increase saliva production.
Uses: HCl: Chronic simple glaucoma (especially open-angle). Chronic angle-closure glaucoma, including after iridectomy. Acute angle-closure glaucoma (alone or with other miotics, epinephrine, beta-adrenergic blocking agents, carbonic anhydrase inhibitors, or hyperosmotic agents). To reverse mydriasis (i.e., after cycloplegic and mydriatic drugs). Pre- and postoperative intraocular tension. The nitrate product is also used for emergency miosis. Salagen (Pilocarpine HCl) has been approved for treatment of radiation-induced dry mouth in head and neck cancer clients, as well as in Sjogren's syndrome. **Ocular Therapeutic System:** Glaucoma alone or with other ophthalmic medications. *Investigational:* Hydrochloride used to treat xerostomia in clients with malfunctioning salivary glands.
Contraindications: Lactation.
Special Concerns: Use with caution during lacation, in those with narrow angles (angle closure may result), in those with known or suspected cholelithiasis or biliary tract disease, and in clients with controlled asthma, chronic bronchitis, or COPD. Safety and efficacy have not been established in children.
Additional Side Effects: The following side effects have been attributed to the pilocarpine ocular system. *Ophthalmic:* Conjunctival irritation, including mild erythema with or without a slight increase in mucous secretion upon initial use.

Oral use (tablets). *Dermatologic:* Sweating, flushing, rash, pruritus. *GI:* N&V, dyspepsia, diarrhea, abdominal pain, taste perversion, anorexia, increased appetite, esophagitis, tongue disorder. *CV:* Hypertension, tachycardia, bradycardia, ECG abnormality, palpitations, syncope. *CNS:* Dizziness, asthenia, headache, tremor, anxiety, confusion, depression, abnormal dreams, hyperkinesia, hypesthesia, nervousness, paresthesias, speech disorder, twitching. *Respiratory:* Sinusitis, rhinitis, pharyngitis, epistaxis, increased sputum, stridor, yawning. *Ophthalmic:* Lacrimation, amblyopia, conjunctivitis, abnormal vision, eye pain, glaucoma. *GU:* Urinary frequency, dysuria, metrorrhagia, urinary impairment. *Body as a whole:* Chills, edema, body odor, hypothermia, mucous membrane abnormality. *Miscellaneous:* Dysphagia, voice alteration, myalgias, seborrhea.
OD **Management of Overdose:** *Treatment:* Titrate with atropine (0.5–1 mg SC or IM) and supportive measures to maintain circulation and respiration. If there is severe cardiovascular depression or bronchoconstriction, epinephrine (0.3–1 mg SC or IV) may be used.
How Supplied: Pilocarpine hydrochloride: *Device:* 20 mcg/hr, 40 mcg/hr; *Ophthalmic gel:* 4%; *Ophthalmic Solution:* 0.25%, 0.5%, 1%, 2%, 3%, 4%, 5%, 6%, 8%; *Tablet:* 5 mg. Pilocarpine ocular therapeutic system: *Device:* 20 mcg/hr, 40 mcg/hr

P

Dosage

PILOCARPINE HYDROCHLORIDE

- **Ophthalmic Gel, 4%**

Glaucoma.

Adults and adolescents: ½-in. ribbon in the lower conjunctival sac of the affected eye(s) once daily at bedtime.

- **Ophthalmic Solution, ¼%, ½%, 1%, 2%, 3%, 4%, 5%, 6%, 8%**

Doses listed are all for adults and adolescents.

Chronic glaucoma.

1 gtt of a 0.5%–4% solution q.i.d.

Acute angle-closure glaucoma.

1 gtt of a 1% or 2% solution q 5–10 min for three to six doses; then, 1 gtt q 1–3 hr until pressure is decreased.

Miotic, to counteract sympathomimetics.

1 gtt of a 1% solution.

Miosis, prior to surgery.

1 gtt of a 2% solution q 4–6 hr for one or two doses before surgery.

Miosis before iridectomy.

1 gtt of a 2% solution for four doses immediately before surgery.

• **Ocular System**

Insert and remove as directed on package insert or by physician. Ocusert Pilo-20 is approximately equal to the 0.5% or 1% drops, while Ocusert Pilo-40 is approximately equal to the 2% or 3% solution.

• **Tablets (Salagen)**

Treat radiation-induced dry mouth in head and neck cancer clients.

Initial: 5 mg t.i.d.; **then,** up to 10 mg t.i.d., if needed.

HEALTH CARE CONSIDERATIONS

See also *Health Care Considerations* for *Ophthalmic Cholinergic Agents.*

Administration/Storage

1. Concentrations greater than 4% of pilocarpine HCl may be more effective in clients with dark pigmented eyes; however, the incidence of side effects increases.
2. Myopia may be observed during the first several hours of therapy with the ocular therapeutic system. Thus, insert the system at bedtime so by morning the myopia is stable.
3. For acute, narrow-angle glaucoma, give pilocarpine in the unaffected eye to prevent angle-closure glaucoma.
4. Store the solution, protected from light, at 8°C–30°C (46°F–86°F). Refrigerate the gel at 2°C–8°C (36°F–46°F) until dispensed. Do not freeze gel; discard any unused portion after 8 weeks. Refrigerate the ocular therapeutic system at 2°C–8°C (36°F–46° F).

P

Assessment: Clients with acute infectious conjunctivitis or keratitis should be carefully evaluated before use of the pilocarpine ocular system.

Client/Family Teaching

1. Review how to insert and how to check the conjunctival sac for presence of the ocular system. Follow these general guidelines for insertion:
• Wash hands.
• Do not permit drug to touch any surface.
• Rinse insert with cool water.
• Pull down lower eyelid.
• Place according to manufacturer's directions.
• System may be moved under closed eyelids to upper eyelid for sleep. Use caution and report any pain as corneal abrasion or irritation may be present.
• Insert at bedtime to diminish side effects; check for presence of ocular system at bedtime and also upon awakening each day. If retention is a problem, the system can be placed in the superior cul-de-sac. The unit can be moved from the lower to upper conjunctival cul-de-sac by gentle digital massage through the eyelid. For best retention, move the unit to the upper conjunctival cul-de-sac before sleep.
• Report if eye irritation, redness, or mucus production persist with the ocular system.
2. If other glaucoma medication (i.e., drops) is used with the gel at bedtime, instill the drops at least 5 min before the gel.
3. Report for periodic tonometric readings to evaluate effectiveness of the drug.
4. Use only as directed. Refrigerate gel and ocular system.

Outcome/Evaluate

• ↓ IOP; pupillary constriction
• ↑ Saliva production; relief of radiation-induced or Sjogren's syndrome dry mouth

Pindolol

(PIN-doh-lohl)

Pregnancy Category: B

Apo-Pindol ✱, Gen-Pindolol ✱, Novo–Pindol ✱, Nu-Pindol ✱, Visken **(Rx)**

Classification: Beta-adrenergic blocking agent

See also *Beta-Adrenergic Blocking Agents.*

Action/Kinetics: Manifests both beta-1 and beta-2 adrenergic blocking activity. Also has significant intrinsic sympathomimetic effects and minimal membrane-stabilizing activity. Moderate lipid solubility. **t½:** 3–4 hr; however, geriatric clients have a variable half-life ranging from 7 to 15 hr, even with normal renal function. Metabolized by the liver, and the metabolites and unchanged (35%–40%) drug are excreted through the kidneys.

Uses: Hypertension (alone or in combination with other antihypertensive agents as thiazide diuretics). *Investigational:* Ventricular arrhythmias and tachycardias, antipsychotic-induced akathisia, situational anxiety.

Contraindications: Bronchial asthma or bronchospasm, including severe COPD.

Special Concerns: Dosage has not been established in children.

Laboratory Test Considerations: ↑ AST and ALT. Rarely, ↑ LDH, uric acid, alkaline phosphatase.

How Supplied: *Tablet:* 5 mg, 10 mg

Dosage

• **Tablets**

Hypertension.

Initial: 5 mg b.i.d. (alone or with other antihypertensive drugs). If no response in 3–4 weeks, increase by 10 mg/day q 3–4 weeks to a maximum of 60 mg/day.

Antipsychotic-induced akathisia.

5 mg/day.

HEALTH CARE CONSIDERATIONS

See also *Health Care Considerations* for *Beta-Adrenergic Blocking Agents* and *Antihypertensive Agents*.

Assessment

1. Record indications for therapy, onset and duration of symptoms, and any other agents trialed.
2. Assess diet, sodium consumption, weight, exercise regimens, and life-style.
3. Record VS and cardiopulmonary assessments.

Outcome/Evaluate: ↓ BP; ↓ restlessness

Pioglitazone hydrochloride

(pie-oh-GLIT-ah-zohn)

Pregnancy Category: C

Actos **(Rx)**

Classification: Oral hypoglycemic agent

See also *Oral Hypoglycemic Agents*.

Action/Kinetics: Depends on the presence of insulin to act. Decreases insulin resistance in the periphery and liver resulting in increased insulin-dependent glucose disposal and decreased hepatic glucose output. It is not an insulin secretagogue. Is an agonist for peroxisome proliferator-activated receptor (PPAR) gamma, which is found in adipose tissue, skeletal muscle, and liver. Activation of these receptors modulates the transcription of a number of insulin responsive genes that control glucose and lipid metabolism. After PO, steady state serum levels are reached within 7 days. **Peak levels:** 2 hr; food slightly delays the time to peak serum levels to 3–4 hr, but does not change the extent of absorption. Extensively protein-bound (over 99%). Metabolized to both active and inactive metabolites. Unchanged drug and metabolites are excreted in the feces. **t½:** 3–7 hr (pioglitazone); 16–24 hr (total pioglitazone).

Uses: Adjunct to diet and exercise in type 2 diabetes. Used either as monotherapy or in combination with a sulfonylurea, metformin, or insulin when diet and exercise plus the single drug does not adequately control blood glucose.

Contraindications: In type I diabetes, diabetic ketoacidosis, active liver disease, with ALT levels that exceed 2.5 times ULN, in clients with NYHA Class II or IV cardiac status, or during lactation.

Special Concerns: Treatment may result in resumption of ovulation in premenopausal anovulatory clients with insulin resistance. Use with caution in clients with edema. Safety and efficacy have not been determined in children.

Side Effects: *Metabolic:* Hypoglycemia, aggravation of diabetes mellitus. *Respiratory:* URTI, sinusitis, pharyngitis. *Miscellaneous:* Headache, myalgia, tooth disorder, anemia, edema.

Laboratory Test Considerations: ↑ ALT, creatine phosphokinase (sporadic and transient); ↓ H&H.

Drug Interactions

Ketoconazole / Significant inhibition of pioglitazone metabolism

Oral contraceptives (containing ethinyl estradiol/norethindrone / ↓ Plasma levels of both hormones; possible loss of contraception

How Supplied: *Tablets:* 15 mg, 30 mg, 45 mg

Dosage

- **Tablets**

Type II diabetes as monotherapy.

Adults: 15 mg or 30 mg once daily in clients not adequately controlled with diet and exercise. Initial dose can be increased up to 45 mg once daily for those who respond inadequately.

Type II diabetes as combination therapy.

If combined with a sulfonylurea, initiate pioglitazone at 15 or 30 mg once daily. The current sulfonylurea dose can be continued unless hypoglycemia occurs; then, reduce the sulfonylurea dose. If combined with metformin, initiate pioglitazone at 15 or 30 mg once daily. The current metformin dose can be continued; it is unlikely the metformin dose will have to be adjusted due to hypoglycemia. If combined with insulin, initiate pioglitazone at 15 or 30 mg once daily. The current insulin dose can be continued unless hypoglycemia occurs or plasma glucose levels decrease to less than 100 mg/dL; then, decrease the insulin dose by 10% to 25%. Individualize further dosage adjustments based on glucose-lowering response.

Daily dose should not exceed 45 mg.

HEALTH CARE CONSIDERATIONS

See also *Health Care Considerations* for *Oral Hypoglycemic Agents*.

Assessment

1. Note indications for therapy, onset and duration of disease, other agents trialed and outcome.
2. List drugs prescribed to ensure none interact.
3. Obtain CBC, HbA1c, renal and LFTs. Ensure clients undergo periodic monitoring of

P

liver enzymes. Evaluate ALT prior to initiation of therapy, every two months for the first year of therapy, and periodically thereafter. Obtain LFTs if symptoms suggest hepatic dysfunction. Discontinue if jaundice is seen.

Client/Family Teaching

1. Take once daily without regard to meals.
2. May cause edema, resumption of ovulation, and hypoglycemia.
3. Report if dark urine, abdominal pain, fatigue or unexplained N&V occur.
4. Practice reliable contraception if pregnancy is not desired.
5. Follow dietary guidelines, perform regular exercise and other life style changes consistent with controlling diabetes.
6. Monitor FS at different times during the day and maintain log for provider review.

Outcome/Evaluate: Control of NIDDM by ↓ insulin resistance; normalization of glucose and HbA1c < 7

Piperazine citrate

(pie-**PER**-ah-zeen)
Pregnancy Category: B
(Rx)
Classification: Anthelmintic

See also *Anthelmintics.*

Action/Kinetics: Acts to paralyze the muscles of parasites; this dislodges the parasites and promotes their elimination by peristalsis. Has little effect on larvae in tissues. Readily absorbed from the GI tract, is partially metabolized by the liver, and the remainder is excreted in urine. Rate of elimination differs among clients although it is excreted nearly unchanged in the urine within 24 hr.

Uses: Pinworm (oxyuriasis) and roundworm (ascariasis) infestations. Particularly recommended for pediatric use.

Contraindications: Impaired liver or kidney function, seizure disorders, hypersensitivity. Lactation.

Special Concerns: Safe use during pregnancy has not been established. Due to neurotoxicity, avoid prolonged, repeated, or excessive use in children.

Side Effects: Piperazine has low toxicity. *GI:* N&V, diarrhea, cramps. *CNS:* Tremors, headache, vertigo, decreased reflexes, paresthesias, ***seizures,*** ataxia, chorea, memory decrement. *Ophthalmologic:* Nystagmus, blurred vision, cataracts, strabismus. *Allergic:* Urticaria, fever, skin reactions, purpura, lacrimation, rhinorrhea, arthralgia, ***bronchospasm,*** cough. *Miscellaneous:* Muscle weakness.

Laboratory Test Considerations: False – or ↓ uric acid values.

Drug Interactions: Concomitant administration of piperazine and phenothiazines may result in an increase in extrapyramidal effects (including violent convulsions) caused by phenothiazines.

How Supplied: *Tablet:* 250 mg

Dosage

- **Syrup, Tablets**

  Pinworms.

Adults and children: 65 mg/kg/day as a single dose for 7 days up to a maximum daily dose of 2.5 g.

Roundworms.

Adults: One dose of 3.5 g/day for 2 consecutive days; **pediatric:** One dose of 75 mg/kg/day for 2 consecutive days, not to exceed 3.5 g/day. For severe infections, repeat therapy after 1 week.

HEALTH CARE CONSIDERATIONS

See also *Health Care Considerations* for *Anthelmintics.*

Assessment

1. Note any evidence of impaired hepatic or renal function.
2. Document/record any seizure disorder or chronic neurologic disease.
3. Determine previous treatments and length of therapy; excessive therapy should be avoided in children due to neurotoxic effects.
4. Use cautiously with severe malnutrition or anemia.

Client/Family Teaching

1. Take on an empty stomach before breakfast or in two divided doses.
2. Report any adverse drug effects immediately.
3. Strict hygiene is required to prevent reinfection.
4. Keep pleasant-tasting medication out of reach of children.
5. Drug causes paralysis of ascariasis parasite and they are expelled live by peristalsis. Flush toilet 2–3 times to ensure that contents are completely removed.

Outcome/Evaluate

- Eradication of infecting parasite
- Negative stool exams and perianal swabs

Pipobroman

(pip-oh-**BROH**-man)
Pregnancy Category: D
Classification: Antineoplastic, alkylating agent.

See also *Antineoplastic Agents* and *Alkylating Agents.*

Action/Kinetics: The mechanism, metabolism, and excretion are not known. Well absorbed from the GI tract.
Uses: Polycythemia vera; chronic granulocytic leukemia in clients refractory to busulfan.
Additional Contraindications: Children under 15 years of age. Lactation. Bone marrow depression due to chemotherapy or X rays.
Special Concerns: Bone marrow depression may not occur for 4 or more weeks after therapy is started.
Side Effects: *Hematologic:* Leukopenia, anemia, thrombocytopenia. *GI:* N&V, diarrhea, abdominal cramps. *Dermatologic:* Skin rashes.
OD **Management of Overdose:** *Symptoms:* Hematologic toxicity, especially with chronic overdosage. *Treatment:* Monitor hematologic status; if necessary, begin vigorous supportive treatment.
How Supplied: *Tablet:* 25 mg

Dosage

- **Tablets**

Polycythemia vera.

1 mg/kg/day. Up to 1.5–3 mg/kg/day may be required in clients refractory to other treatment; do not use such doses until a dose of 1 mg/kg/day has been given for at least 30 days with no improvement. When hematocrit has been reduced to 50%–55%, **maintenance dosage** of 100–200 mcg/kg is instituted.

Chronic granulocytic leukemia.

Initial: 1.5–2.5 mg/kg/day; **maintenance:** 7–175 mg/day, to be instituted when leukocyte count approaches 10,000/mm^3.

HEALTH CARE CONSIDERATIONS

See also *Health Care Considerations* for *Antineoplastic Agents.*

Assessment

1. Record indications for therapy, other agents trialed and the outcome.
2. Obtain baseline hematologic profile and monitor closely for dosing parameters, leukopenia and thrombocytopenia. Bone marrow depression may occur latently in therapy (after 4 weeks) (Nadir: 14–21 days).

Client/Family Teaching

1. Discuss with provider and review literature for benefits/dangers of drug therapy.
2. Report evidence of infection such as fever, shaking chills, SOB, or painful urination; drug may decrease body's ability to fight infections.
3. Nausea, vomiting, or hair loss may occur with this drug.
4. Avoid aspirin-containing products and use alcohol in moderation, if at all.
5. Identify if candidate for sperm/egg harvesting; drug may cause permanent sterility in men and women.
6. Use reliable birth control; may cause birth defects.

Outcome/Evaluate

- ↓ Hematocrit (50%–55%) with polycythemia vera
- Hematologic recovery with leukemia
- Inhibition of malignant cell proliferation

Pirbuterol acetate

(peer-**BYOU**-ter-ohl)
Pregnancy Category: C
Maxair Autohaler **(Rx)**
Classification: Sympathomimetic, bronchodilator

See also *Sympathomimetic Drugs.*
Action/Kinetics: Causes bronchodilation by stimulating beta-2-adrenergic receptors. Has minimal effects on beta-1 receptors. Also inhibits histamine release from mast cells, causes vasodilation, and increases ciliary motility. **Onset, inhalation:** Approximately 5 min. **Time to peak effect:** 30–60 min. **Duration:** 5 hr.
Uses: Alone or with theophylline or steroids for prophylaxis and treatment of bronchospasm in asthma and other conditions with reversible bronchospasms, including bronchitis, emphysema, bronchiectasis, obstructive pulmonary disease.
Contraindications: Cardiac arrhythmias due to tachycardia; tachycardia caused by digitalis toxicity.
Special Concerns: Safety and efficacy have not been determined in children less than 12 years of age.
Additional Side Effects: *CV:* PVCs, hypotension. *CNS:* Hyperactivity, hyperkinesia, anxiety, confusion, depression, fatigue, syncope. *GI:* Diarrhea, dry mouth, anorexia, loss of appetite, bad taste or taste change, abdominal pain, abdominal cramps, stomatitis, glossitis. *Dermatologic:* Rash, edema, pruritus, alopecia. *Miscellaneous:* Flushing, numbness in extremities, weight gain.
How Supplied: *Aerosol Solid w/Adapter:* 0.2 mg/inh

Dosage

- **Inhalation Aerosol**

P

Adults and children over 12 years: 0.2–0.4 mg (1–2 inhalations) q 4–6 hr, not to exceed 12 inhalations (2.4 mg) daily.

HEALTH CARE CONSIDERATIONS

See also *Health Care Considerations* for *Sympathomimetic Drugs*.

Assessment: Record indications for therapy, noting onset, duration, and characteristics of symptoms. Assess lungs and note ECG, CXR, and PFTs.

Client/Family Teaching

1. Review methods, frequency, and indication for administration. Use a chamber (spacer) to enhance dispersion.
2. Report if condition or peak flows deteriorate or if inhaler is ineffective in relieving symptoms at prescribed dosage.

Outcome/Evaluate: Improved airway exchange; ↓ airway resistance

Piroxicam

(peer-**OX**-ih-kam)

Alti-Piroxicam ♣, Apo-Piroxicam ♣, Dom-Piroxicam ♣, Feldene, Gen-Piroxicam ♣, Novo–Pirocam ♣, Nu-Pirox ♣, PMS-Piroxicam ♣, Pro-Piroxicam ♣, Rho-Piroxicam ♣ **(Rx)**

Classification: Nonsteroidal anti-inflammatory drug

See also *Nonsteroidal Anti-Inflammatory Drugs*.

Action/Kinetics: May inhibit prostaglandin synthesis. Effect is comparable to that of aspirin, but with fewer GI side effects and less tinnitus. May be used with gold, corticosteroids, and antacids. **Peak plasma levels:** 1.5–2 mcg/mL after 3–5 hr (single dose). **Steady-state plasma levels** (after 7–12 days): 3–8 mcg/mL. **t½:** 50 hr. **Analgesia, onset:** 1 hr; **duration:** 2–3 days. **Anti-inflammatory activity, onset:** 7–12 days; **duration:** 2–3 weeks. Metabolites and unchanged drug excreted in urine and feces.

Uses: Acute and chronic treatment of rheumatoid arthritis and osteoarthritis. *Investigational:* Juvenile rheumatoid arthritis, primary dysmenorrhea, sunburn.

Contraindications: Safe use during pregnancy has not been determined. Use in children less than 14 years old. Lactation.

Special Concerns: Safety and efficacy have not been established in children. Increased plasma levels and elimination half-life may be observed in geriatric clients (especially women).

Laboratory Test Considerations: Reversible ↑ BUN.

How Supplied: *Capsule:* 10 mg, 20 mg

Dosage

- **Capsules**

  Anti-inflammatory, antirheumatic.

Adults: 20 mg/day in one or more divided doses. Do not assess the effect of therapy for 2 weeks.

HEALTH CARE CONSIDERATIONS

See also *Health Care Considerations* for *Nonsteroidal Anti-Inflammatory Drugs*.

Administration/Storage

1. Steady-state plasma levels may not be reached for 2 weeks.
2. Clients over 70 years of age generally require one-half the usual adult dose of medication.

Assessment

1. Record indications for therapy, symptom characteristics, other agents prescribed, and the outcome.
2. Assess involved joints and note ROM, erythema, swelling, pain, and warmth.

Client/Family Teaching

1. Take with food or milk to decrease GI upset. A stomach protectant (i.e., Cytotec) may be prescribed for those with a history of ulcer disease.
2. Take at anti-inflammatory dose to prevent further joint destruction during acute exacerbations.
3. Therapeutic effects of the medication cannot be evaluated fully for at least 2 weeks after treatment onset.
4. Aspirin decreases the effectiveness of piroxicam and may increase the occurrence of side effects. Avoid aspirin, ethanol, and OTC products.
5. Report any increased abdominal pain, abnormal bruising or bleeding, malaise, or changes in the color of the stool immediately.
6. Drug side effects may not be evident for 7–10 days.
7. Report for scheduled labs.

Outcome/Evaluate: ↓ Joint pain and inflammation with improved mobility

Pneumococcal conjugate vaccine, 7-valent

(**NEW**-moh-**kock**-al)

Pregnancy Category: C

Prevnar **(Rx)**

Classification: Vaccine

Action/Kinetics: Contains saccharides of capsular antigens of serotypes 4, 6B, 9V, 18C, 19F, and 23F, individually conjugated to CRM197 protein.

Uses: Immunization of infants and toddlers against *Streptococcus pneumoniae* infection caused by serotypes included in the vaccine.
Contraindications: Clients with hypersensitivity to the vaccine or any component, including diphtheria toxoid. Current or recent severe or moderate febrile illness. Thrombocytopenia. Any contraindication to IM injection; not for IV use.
Special Concerns: Caution in latex sensitivity. Children with impaired immune response may have a reduced response to active immunization. Use of pneumococcal conjugate vaccine does not replace the use of the 23-valent vaccine in children >24 months of age with sickle cell disease, asplenia, HIV infection, chronic illness, or immunocompromise. Safety and efficacy have not been established in children <6 weeks of age. Not for IV use.
Side Effects: All serious adverse reactions must be reported to the U.S. Department of Health and Human Services (DHHS) Vaccine Adverse Event Reporting System (VAERS) 1-800-822-7967. *CNS:* Fever, irritability, drowsiness, restlessness. *Dermatologic:* Erythema, rash. *GI:* Decreased appetite, vomiting, diarrhea. *Localized:* Induration, tenderness, nodule.

Dosage

- **Injection**

  Immunization

Infants: 0.5 mL at approximately 2-month intervals for 3 consecutive doses, followed by a fourth dose of 0.5 mL at 12-15 months of age. First dose may be given as young as 6 weeks of age, but is usually given at 2 months of age. **Previously unvaccinated older infants and children: 7-11 months:** 0.5 mL for a total of 3 doses; 2 doses at least 4 weeks apart, followed by a third dose after the first birthday, separated from the second dose by at least 2 months. **12-23 months:** 0.5 mL for a total of 2 doses, separated by at least 2 months. **>24 months:** 0.5 mL as a single dose.

HEALTH CARE CONSIDERATIONS

Administration/Storage: Store refrigerated at 2°C to 8°C (36°F to 46°F)
Assessment: Record date, site and route of administration, lot number, and expiration date of vaccine.
Client/Family Teaching: Inform caregiver of child of the correct interval for the next immunization.
Administration: Administer IM in lateral mid-thigh; in older children administer in deltoid muscle.

Podofilox

(poh-**DAHF**-ih-lox)
Pregnancy Category: C
Condyline ✦, Condylox **(Rx)**
Classification: Keratolytic

Action/Kinetics: An antimitotic agent that causes necrosis of visible wart tissue when applied topically. Small amounts are absorbed into the system 1–2 hr after application. **t½:** 1–4.5 hr. The drug does not accumulate following multiple treatments.
Uses: Topical treatment of external genital warts and perianal warts (gel only). *Investigational:* Systemically for treatment of cancer.
Contraindications: Use of solution or gel for mucous membrane warts or solution for perianal warts. Lactation.
Special Concerns: Genital warts must be distinguished from squamous cell carcinoma prior to initiation of treatment. Safety and effectiveness have not been demonstrated in children. Avoid contact with the eyes.
Side Effects: Solution. *Dermatologic:* Commonly, burning, pain, inflammation, erosion, and itching. Also, tenderness, chafing, scarring, vesicle formation, dryness and peeling, tingling, bleeding, ulceration, malodor, crusting edema, foreskin irretraction. *Miscellaneous:* Pain with intercourse, insomnia, dizziness, hematuria, vomiting.

Gel. *Dermatologic:* Commonly, burning, pain, inflammation, erosion, itching, and bleeding. Also, stinging, erythema, desquamation, scabbing, discoloration, tenderness, dryness, crusting, fissures, soreness, ulceration, swelling/edema, tingling, rash, blisters.

Systemic Use. *GI:* N&V, diarrhea, oral ulcers. *Hematologic:* Bone marrow depression, leukocytosis, pancytosis. *CNS:* Altered mental status, lethargy, ***coma, seizures.*** *Miscellaneous:* Peripheral neuropathy, fever, tachypnea, ***respiratory failure,*** hematuria, renal failure.

OD **Management of Overdose:** *Symptoms:* N&V, diarrhea, fever, altered mental status, hematologic toxicity, peripheral neuropathy, lethargy, tachypnea, ***respiratory failure,*** hematuria, leukocytosis, pancytosis, renal failure, ***seizures, coma.*** *Treatment:* Wash the skin free of any remaining drug. General supportive therapy to treat symptoms.
How Supplied: *Solution:* 0.5%, *Gel:* 0.5%

P

Dosage

- **Topical Solution, Topical Gel**

External genital warts, perianal warts (gel only).

Adults, initial: Apply b.i.d. in the morning and evening (i.e., q 12 hr) for 3 consecutive days; **then,** withhold use for 4 consecutive days. The 1-week cycle of treatment may be repeated up to 4 times until there is no visible sign of wart tissue. Consider alternative treatment if the response is incomplete after four treatments.

HEALTH CARE CONSIDERATIONS

Administration/Storage

1. Limit treatment to less than 10 cm^2 of wart tissue and to 0.5 mL or less of the solution or 0.5 g of the gel daily. Higher amounts do not increase efficacy but may increase the incidence of side effects.
2. Do not freeze the solution or gel; avoid exposure to excessive heat.

Assessment

1. Note histologic confirmation of differentiation of lesion from SCC.
2. Record the number and size of condyloma, location, and condition of pretreatment area(s).

Client/Family Teaching

1. Wash hands before and after application. Apply the solution with the cotton-tipped applicator supplied and the gel with either the applicator or a finger. Apply only the minimum amount of solution required to cover the lesion.
2. Allow the solution or gel to dry before allowing the return of opposing skin surfaces to their normal positions.
3. After each treatment, dispose of the used applicator properly.
4. Adhere to the exact dosing instructions (on for 3 days, off for 4 days) to prevent adverse side effects.
5. Avoid contact with the eyes. If contact does occur, immediately flush the eye with large amounts of water and report.

Outcome/Evaluate: Clearing; ↓ number/size of condylomas

Polymyxin B sulfate, parenteral

(pol-ee-**MIX**-in)

Pregnancy Category: C

Aerosporin **(Rx)**

Polymyxin B sulfate, sterile ophthalmic

(pol-ee-**MIX**-in)

Pregnancy Category: C

(Rx)

Classification: Antibiotic, polymyxin

See also *Anti-Infectives.*

Action/Kinetics: Derived from the spore-forming soil bacterium *Bacillus polymyxa.* Bactericidal against most gram-negative organisms; rapidly inactivated by alkali, strong acid, and certain metal ions. Increases the permeability of the plasma cell membrane of the bacterium (i.e., similar to detergents), causing leakage of essential metabolites and ultimately inactivation. **Peak serum levels: IM,** 2 hr. **t½:** 4.3–6 hr. Longer in presence of renal impairment. Sixty percent of drug excreted in urine. Virtually unabsorbed from the GI tract except in newborn infants. Remains in plasma after parenteral administration.

Uses: Systemic: Acute infections of the urinary tract and meninges, septicemia caused by *Pseudomonas aeruginosa.* Meningeal infections caused by *Haemophilus influenzae,* UTIs caused by *Escherichia coli,* bacteremia caused by *Enterobacter aerogenes* or *Klebsiella pneumoniae.* Combined with neomycin for irrigation of the urinary bladder to prevent bacteriuria and bacteremia from indwelling catheters.

Ophthalmic: Conjunctival and corneal infections (e.g., conjunctivitis, keratitis, keratoconjunctivitis, corneal ulcers, blepharitis, blepharoconjunctivitis, acute meibomianitis, dacryocystitis) due to *E. coli, H. influenzae, H. parainfluenzae, K. pneumoniae, E. aerogenes,* and *P. aeruginosa.* Used alone or in combination for ear infections.

Contraindications: Hypersensitivity. A potentially toxic drug to be reserved for the treatment of severe, resistant infections in hospitalized clients. Not indicated for clients with severely impaired renal function or nitrogen retention. Ophthalmic use in dendritic keratitis, vaccinia, varicella, mycobacterial infections of the eye, fungal diseases of the eye, use with steroid combinations after uncomplicated removal of a foreign body from the cornea. Ophthalmic use in deep-seated ophthalmic infections or in those likely to become systemic infections.

Special Concerns: Safe use during pregnancy has not been established.

Side Effects: *Nephrotoxic:* Albuminuria, cylindruria, azotemia, hematuria, proteinuria, leukocyturia, electrolyte loss. *Neurologic:* Dizziness, flushing of face, mental confusion, irritability, nystagmus, muscle weakness, drowsiness, paresthesias, blurred vision, slurred speech, ataxia, ***coma, seizures. Neuromuscular blockade may lead to respirato-***

ry paralysis. *GI:* N&V, diarrhea, abdominal cramps. *Miscellaneous:* Fever, urticaria, skin exanthemata, eosinophilia, ***anaphylaxis.***

Following intrathecal use: Meningeal irritation with fever, stiff neck, headache, increase in leukocytes and protein in the CSF. Nerve-root irritation may result in neuritic pain and urine retention. *Following IM use:* Irritation, severe pain. *Following IV use:* Thrombophlebitis. *Following ophthalmic use:* Burning, stinging, irritation, inflammation, angioneurotic edema, itching, urticaria, vesicular and maculopapular dermatitis.

Laboratory Test Considerations: False + or ↑ levels of urea nitrogen and creatinine. Casts and RBCs in urine.

Drug Interactions

Aminoglycoside antibiotics / Additive nephrotoxic effects

Cephalosporins / ↑ Risk of renal toxicity

Phenothiazines / ↑ Risk of respiratory depression

Skeletal muscle relaxants (surgical) / Additive muscle relaxation

How Supplied: *Powder for injection:* 500,000 U

Dosage

- **IV**

Infections.

Adults and children: 15,000 25,000 units/kg/day (maximum) in divided doses q 12 hr. **Infants,** up to 40,000 units/kg/day.

- **IM**

Not usually recommended due to pain at injection site.

Infections.

Adults and children: 25,000–30,000 units/kg/day in divided doses q 4–6 hr. **Infants,** up to 40,000 units/kg/day.

Both IV and IM doses should be reduced in renal impairment.

- **Intrathecal**

Meningitis.

Adults and children over 2 years: 50,000 units/day for 3–4 days; **then,** 50,000 units every other day until 2 weeks after cultures are negative; **children under 2 years,** 20,000 units/day for 3–4 days or 25,000 units once every other day; dosage of 25,000 units should be continued every other day for 2 weeks after cultures are negative.

- **Ophthalmic Solution**

1–2 gtt 2–6 times/day, depending on the infection. Treatment may be necessary for 1–2 months or longer.

HEALTH CARE CONSIDERATIONS

See also *General Health Care Considerations for All Anti-Infectives.*

Administration/Storage

1. When used in the eye(s), tilt the head back and place the medication in the conjunctival sac. Light finger pressure should be applied on the lacrimal sac for 1 min.
2. To avoid contamination, do not allow the tip of the container to touch any surface.
3. Store and dilute as directed on package insert.
4. Lessen pain on IM injection by reducing drug concentration as much as possible. It is preferable to give drug more frequently in more dilute doses. If ordered, procaine hydrochloride (2 mL of a 0.5%–1.0% solution per 5 units of dry powder) may be used for mixing the drug for IM injection.
5. IV For IV administration, reconstitute 500,000 units with 300–500 mL of D5W and infuse over 60–90 min.
6. *Never use preparations containing procaine hydrochloride for IV or intrathecal use.*

Assessment

1. Note indications: type, onset, and duration of symptoms.
2. Determine kidney function and urinary output; note edema. Assess respiratory function; note any prior problems.
3. Obtain specimens for C&S.
4. Note any muscle weakness and early signs of muscle paralysis related to neuromuscular blockade. Assess for evidence of respiratory paralysis; withhold drug and report.
5. Monitor I&O; reduce dose with impaired renal function; observe for nephrotoxicity, characterized by albuminuria, urinary casts, nitrogen retention, and hematuria.
6. Ambulatory or bedridden clients with neurologic disturbances require supervision.

Client/Family Teaching

1. Avoid hazardous tasks until drug effects realized; may cause dizziness, vertigo, and ataxia.
2. Consume at least 2 L/day of fluids.
3. Report any neurologic disturbances, i.e., dizziness, blurred vision, irritability, circumoral and peripheral numbness and tingling, weakness, and ataxia; usually disappear 24–48 hr after drug discontinued and associated with high drug levels.
4. Anticipate a prolonged regimen of topical application of solution because drug is not toxic when used in wet dressings, and provid-

P

er may wish to prevent emergence of resistant strains.

Outcome/Evaluate: Negative cultures; resolution of infection; symptomatic improvement

Potassium Salts Potassium acetate, parenteral

Pregnancy Category: C

(Rx)

Potassium acetate, Potassium bicarbonate, and Potassium citrate (Trikates)

Oral Solution: Tri-K **(Rx)**

Potassium bicarbonate

K + Care ET **(Rx)**

Potassium bicarbonate and Citric acid

Effervescent Tablets: K+ Care ET

Potassium bicarbonate and Potassium chloride

Effervescent Granules: Neo-K ✱ **(Rx)**. **Effervescent Tablets:** Klorvess, K-Lyte/Cl, K-Lyte/Cl 50, Potassium-Sandoz ✱ **(Rx)**

Potassium bicarbonate and Potassium citrate

Effervescent Tablets: Effer-K, Effervescent Potassium, K-Lyte **(Rx)**

Potassium chloride

Extended-Release Capsules: K-Lease, K-Norm, Micro-K Extencaps, Micro-K 10 Extencaps **(Rx)**. **Injection:** Potassium Chloride for Injection Concentrate **(Rx)**. **Oral Solution:** Cena-K 10% and 20%, K-10 ✱, Kaochlor-10 and -20 ✱, Kaochlor 10%, Kaochlor S-F 10%, Kaon-Cl 20% Liquid, Kay Ciel, KCl 5% ✱, Klorvess 10% Liquid, Potasalan, Rum-K **(Rx)**. **Powder for Oral Solution:** Gen-K, Kay Ciel, K+ Care, K-Lor, Klor-Con Powder, Klor-Con/25 Powder, K-Lyte/Cl Powder, Micro-K LS **(Rx)**. , **Extended-Release Tablets:** Apo-K ✱, K+ 10, Kalium Durules ✱, Kaon-Cl, Kaon-Cl-10, K-Dur 10 and 20, K-Long ✱, Klor-Con 8 and 10, Klotrix, K-Tab, Novolente-K ✱, Slow-K, Slo-Pot 600 ✱, Slow-K ✱, Ten-K **(Rx)**

Potassium chloride, Potassium bicarbonate, and Potassium citrate

Effervescent Granules: Klorvess Effervescent Granules **(Rx)**

Potassium gluconate

Elixir: Kaon, Kaylixir, K-G Elixir, Potassium-Rougier ✱, Royonate ✱ **(Rx)**. **Tablets:** Kaon ✱ **(Rx)**

Potassium gluconate and Potassium chloride

Oral Solution and Powder for Oral Solution: Kolyum **(Rx)**

Potassium gluconate and Potassium citrate

Oral Solution: Twin-K **(Rx)**

Classification: Electrolyte

General Statement: Potassium is the major cation of the body's intracellular fluid. It is essential for the maintenance of important physiologic processes, including cardiac, smooth, and skeletal muscle function, acid-base balance, gastric secretions, renal function, protein and carbohydrate metabolism. Symptoms of hypokalemia include weakness, cardiac arrhythmias, fatigue, ileus, hyporeflexia or areflexia, tetany, polydipsia, and, in severe cases, flaccid paralysis and inability to concentrate urine. Loss of potassium is usually accompanied by a loss of chloride resulting in hypochloremic metabolic alkalosis.

The usual adult daily requirement of potassium is 40–80 mg. In adults, the normal extracellular concentration of potassium ranges from 3.5 to 5 mEq/L with the intracellular levels being 150–160 mEq/L. Extracellular concentrations of up to 5.6 mEq/L are normal in children.

Both hypokalemia and hyperkalemia, if uncorrected, can be fatal; thus, potassium must always be administered cautiously.

Action/Kinetics

Potassium is readily and rapidly absorbed from the GI tract. Though a number of salts can be used to supply the potassium cation, potassium chloride is the agent of choice since hypochloremia frequently accompanies potassium deficiency. Dietary measures can often prevent and even correct potassium deficiencies. Potassium-rich foods include most meats (beef, chicken, ham, turkey, veal), fish, beans, broccoli, brussels sprouts, lentils, spinach, potatoes, milk, bananas, dates, prunes, raisins, avocados, watermelon, cantaloupe, apricots, and molasses.

From 80% to 90% of potassium intake is excreted by the kidney and is partially reabsorbed from the glomerular filtrate.

Uses: PO: Treat hypokalemia due to digitalis intoxication, diabetic acidosis, diarrhea and vomiting, familial periodic paralysis, certain cases of uremia, hyperadrenalism, starvation and debilitation, and corticosteroid or diuretic therapy. Also, hypokalemia with or without metabolic acidosis and following surgical conditions accompanied by nitrogen loss, vomiting and diarrhea, suction drainage, and increased urinary excretion of potassium. Prophylaxis of potassium depletion when dietary intake is not adequate in the following conditions: clients on digitalis and diuretics for CHF, hepatic cirrhosis with ascites, excess aldosterone with normal renal function, significant cardiac arrhythmias, potassium-losing nephropathy, and certain states accompanied by diarrhea. *Investigational:* Mild hypertension.

NOTE: Use potassium chloride when hypokalemia is associated with alkalosis; potassium bicarbonate, citrate, acetate, or gluconate should be used when hypokalemia is associated with acidosis.

IV: Prophylaxis and treatment of moderate to severe potassium loss when PO therapy is not feasible. Potassium acetate is used as an additive for preparing specific IV formulas when client needs cannot be met by usual nutrient or electrolyte preparations. Potassium acetate is also used in the following conditions: marked loss of GI secretions due to vomiting, diarrhea, GI intubation, or fistulas; prolonged parenteral use of potassium-free fluids (e.g., dextrose or NSS); diabetic acidosis, especially during treatment with insulin and dextrose infusions; prolonged diuresis; metabolic alkalosis; hyperadrenocorticism; primary aldosteronism; overdose of adrenocortical steroids, testosterone, or corticotropin; attacks of hereditary or familial periodic paralysis; during the healing phase of burns or scalds; and cardiac arrhythmias, especially due to digitalis glycosides.

Contraindications: Severe renal function impairment with azotemia or oliguria, postoperatively before urine flow has been reestablished. Crush syndrome, Addison's disease, hyperkalemia from any cause, anuria, heat cramps, acute dehydration, severe hemolytic reactions, adynamia episodica hereditaria, clients receiving potassium-sparing diuretics or aldosterone-inhibiting drugs. Solid dosage forms in clients in whom there is a reason for delay or arrest in passage of tablets through the GI tract.

Special Concerns: Safety during lactation and in children has not been established. Geriatric clients are at greater risk of developing hyperkalemia due to age-related changes in renal function. Administer with caution in the presence of cardiac and renal disease. Potassium loss is often accompanied by an obligatory loss of chloride resulting in hypochloremic metabolic alkalosis; thus, the underlying cause of the potassium loss should be treated.

Side Effects: Hypokalemia. *CNS:* Dizziness, mental confusion. *CV:* Arrhythmias; weak, irregular pulse; hypotension, ***heart block,*** ECG abnormalities, ***cardiac arrest.*** *GI:* Abdominal distention, anorexia, N&V, *Neuromuscular:* Weakness, paresthesia of extremities, flaccid paralysis, areflexia, muscle or ***respiratory paralysis,*** weakness and heaviness of legs. *Other:* Malaise.

Hyperkalemia. *CV:* Bradycardia, then tachycardia, ***cardiac arrest.*** *GI:* N&V, diarrhea, abdominal cramps, GI bleeding or obstruction. Ulceration or perforation of the small bowel from enteric-coated potassium chloride tablets. *GU:* Oliguria, anuria. *Neuromuscular:* Weakness, tingling, paralysis. *Other:* Skin rashes, hyperkalemia.

Effects due to solution or IV technique used. Fever, infection at injection site, venous thrombosis, phlebitis extending from injection site, extravasation, venospasm, hypervolemia, hyperkalemia.

OD **Management of Overdose:** *Symptoms:* Mild (5.5–6.5 mEq/L) to moderate (6.5–8 mEq/L) hyperkalemia (may be asymptomatic except for ECG changes). ECG changes include progression in height and peak of T waves, lowering of the R wave, decreased amplitude and eventually disappearance of P waves, prolonged PR interval and QRS complex, shortening of the QT interval, ***ventricular fibrillation, death. Muscle weakness that may progress to flaccid quadriplegia and respiratory failure,*** although dangerous cardiac arrhythmias usually occur before onset of complete paralysis. *Treatment (plasma potassium levels greater than 6.5 mEq/L):* All measures must be monitored by ECG. Measures consist of actions taken to shift potassium ions from plasma into cells by:

- **Sodium bicarbonate:** IV infusion of 50–100 mEq over period of 5 min. May be repeated after 10–15 minutes if ECG abnormalities persist.
- **Glucose and insulin:** IV infusion of 3 g glucose to 1 unit regular insulin to shift potassium into cells.
- **Calcium gluconate—or other calcium salt** (only for clients not on digitalis or other cardiotonic glycosides): IV infusion of 0.5–1 g (5–10 mL of a 10% solution) over period of 2 min. Dosage may be repeated after 1–2 min if ECG remains abnormal. When ECG is approximately normal, the excess potassium should be removed from the body by ad-

P

ministration of polystyrene sulfonate, hemodialysis or peritoneal dialysis (clients with renal insufficiency), or other means.

• **Sodium polystyrene sulfonate, hemodialysis, peritoneal dialysis:** To remove potassium from the body.

Drug Interactions

ACE inhibitors / May cause potassium retention → hyperkalemia
Digitalis glycosides / Cardiac arrhythmias
Potassium-sparing diuretics / Severe hyperkalemia with possibility of cardiac arrhythmias or arrest

How Supplied: Potassium acetate, parenteral: *Injection:* 2 mEq/mL, 4 mEq/mL; Potassium acetate, potassium bicarbonate, and potassium citrate: *Liquid:* 45 mEq/15 mL; Potassium bicarbonate: *Tablet, effervescent:* 25 mEq, 650 mg; Potassium bicarbonate and potassium citrate: *Tablet, effervescent*: 25 mEq; Potassium bicarbonate and potassium chloride: *Granule for reconstitution:* 20 mEq; *Tablet, effervescent*: 25 mEq, 50 mEq; Potassium chloride: *Capsule, extended release:* 8 mEq, 10 mEq; *Injection:* 1.5 mEq/mL, 2 mEq/mL, 10 mEq/50 mL, 10 mEq/100 mL, 20 mEq/50 mL, 20 mEq/100 mL, 30 mEq/100 mL, 40 mEq/100 mL, 100 mEq/L, 200 mEq/L; *Liquid:* 20 mEq/15 mL, 30 mEq/15 mL, 40 mEq/15 mL; *Powder for reconstitution:* 20 mEq, 25 mEq, 200 mEq; *Tablet:* 180 mg; *Tablet, extended release:* 8 mEq, 10 mEq, 20 mEq; Potassium gluconate: *Elixir:* 20 mEq/15 mL; *Tablet:* 486 mg, 500 mg, 550 mg, 595 mg, 610 mg, 620 mg; *Tablet, extended release:* 595 mg; Potassium gluconate and potassium citrate: *Liquid:* 20 mEq/15 mL

Dosage

Highly individualized. Oral administration is preferred because the slow absorption from the GI tract prevents sudden, large increases in plasma potassium levels. Dosage is usually expressed as mEq/L of potassium. The bicarbonate, chloride, citrate, and gluconate salts are usually administered PO. The chloride, acetate, and phosphate may be administered by **slow IV** infusion.

• **IV Infusion**

Serum K less than 2.0 mEq/L.

400 mEq/day at a rate not to exceed 40 mEq/hr. Use a maximum concentration of 80 mEq/L.

Serum K more than 2.5 mEq/L.

200 mEq/day at a rate not to exceed 20 mEq/hr. Use a maximum concentration of 40 mEq/L.

Pediatric: Up to 3 mEq potassium/kg (or 40 mEq/m^2) daily. Adjust the volume administered depending on the body size.

• **Effervescent Granules, Effervescent Tablets, Elixir, Extended-Release Capsules, Extended Release Granules, Extended-Release Tablets, Oral Solution, Powder for Oral Solution, Tablets**

Prophylaxis of hypokalemia.

16–24 mEq/day.

Potassium depletion.

40–100 mEq/day.

NOTE: Usual dietary intake of potassium is 40–250 mEq/day.

For clients with accompanying metabolic acidosis, use an alkalizing potassium salt (potassium bicarbonate, potassium citrate, or potassium acetate).

HEALTH CARE CONSIDERATIONS

Administration/Storage

1. Give PO doses 2–4 times/day. Correct hypokalemia slowly over a period of 3–7 days to minimize risk of hyperkalemia.
2. With esophageal compression, administer dilute liquid solutions of potassium rather than tablets.
3. **IV** Do not administer potassium IV undiluted. Usual method is to administer by slow IV infusion in dextrose solution at a concentration of 40–80 mEq/L and at a rate not to exceed 10–20 mEq/hr.
4. Avoid "layering" of potassium by inverting container during addition of potassium solution and properly agitating the prepared IV solution. Squeezing the plastic container will not prevent KCL from settling to the bottom. Never add potassium to an IV bottle that is hanging.
5. Check site of administration frequently for pain and redness because drug is extremely irritating.
6. In critical clients, KCL may be given slow IV in a solution of saline (unless contraindicated) since dextrose may lower serum potassium levels by producing an intracellular shift.
7. Administer all concentrated potassium infusions and riders with an infusion control device.
8. Have sodium polystyrene sulfonate (Kayexalate) available for oral or rectal administration in the event of hyperkalemia.

Assessment

1. Note indications for therapy; document electrolytes and ECG.
2. Note any impaired renal function. Assess for adequate urinary flow before administering potassium. Impaired function can lead to hyperkalemia.

Interventions

1. Withhold and report if abdominal pain, distention, or GI bleeding develops.
2. Complaints of weakness, fatigue, or the

P

presence of cardiac arrhythmias may be symptoms of hypokalemia indicating a low *intracellular* potassium level, although the level may appear to be within normal limits.
3. Monitor I&O. Withhold drug and report oliguria, anuria, or azoturia.
4. Observe for symptoms of adrenal insufficiency or extensive tissue breakdown.
5. Report complaints of weakness or heaviness of the legs, the presence of a gray pallor, cold skin, listlessness, mental confusion, flaccid paralysis, hypotension, or cardiac arrhythmias (S&S of hyperkalemia).
6. Monitor serum potassium levels during parenteral therapy; normal level is 3.5–5.0 mEq/L.

Client/Family Teaching

1. Dilute or dissolve PO liquids, effervescent tablets, or soluble powders in 3–8 oz of cold water, fruit or vegetable juice, or other suitable liquid and drink slowly. Chill to increase palatability.
2. If GI upset occurs, products can be taken after meals or with food with a full glass of water.
3. Swallow enteric-coated tablets and extended-release capsules and tablets; do not dissolve in the mouth.
4. Salt substitutes should not be used concomitantly with potassium preparations.
5. If receiving potassium-sparing diuretics, such as spironolactone or triamterene, do not take potassium supplements or eat foods high in potassium.
6. Identify high-potassium sources in the diet: spinach, collards, brussel sprouts, beet greens, tomato juice, celery. Once parenteral potassium is discontinued, ingest potassium-rich foods such as citrus juices, bananas, apricots, raisins, and nuts. The daily adult requirement is usually 40–80 mg. A dietitian may assist with meal planning.

Outcome/Evaluate: Correction of potassium deficiency; potassium levels within desired range

Pramipexole

(prah-mih-**PEX**-ohl)
Pregnancy Category: C
Mirapex **(Rx)**
Classification: Antiparkinson drug

Action/Kinetics: Thought to act by stimulating dopamine (especially D_3) receptors in striatum. Rapidly absorbed. **Peak levels:** 2 hr. Food increases time for maximum levels to occur. **t½, terminal:** About 8 hr (12 hr in geriatric clients). Excreted mainly unchanged in urine. Clearance decreases with age.

Uses: Idiopathic Parkinson's disease.
Contraindications: Lactation.
Special Concerns: Safety and efficacy have not been determined in children.
Side Effects: *CNS:* Hallucinations (especially in elderly), dizziness, somnolence, insomnia, confusion, amnesia, hypesthesia, dystonia, akathisia, abnormal thinking, decreased libido, myoclonus. *CV:* Orthostatic hypotension. *Body as a whole:* Asthenia, general edema, malaise, fever. *GI:* Nausea, constipation, anorexia, dysphagia. *Miscellaneous:* Vision abnormalities, impotence, peripheral edema, decreased weight.

Drug Interactions

Butyrophenones / Possible ↓ effect of pramipexole
Cimetidine / ↑ Levodopa levels and half-life
CNS Depressants / Additive CNS depression
Levodopa / ↑ Levodopa levels; also, may cause or worsen pre-existing dyskinesia
Metoclopramide / Possible ↓ effect of pramipexole
Phenothiazines / Possible ↓ effect of pramipexole
Thioxanthines / Possible ↓ effect of pramipexole

How Supplied: *Tablets:* 0.125 mg, 0.25 mg, 0.5 mg, 1 mg, 1.5 mg

Dosage

- **Tablets**

Parkinsonism.

Initial: Start with 0.125 mg t.i.d.; **then,** increase dose by 0.125 mg t.i.d. weekly for seven weeks (i.e., dose at week seven is 1.5 mg t.i.d.). **Maintenance:** 1.5–4.5 mg/day in equally divided doses t.i.d. with or without comcomitant levodopa (about 800 mg/day). Impaired renal function, C_{CR}, over 60 mL/min: Start with 0.125 mg t.i.d., up to maximum of 1.5 mg t.i.d. C_{CR}, 25–59 mL/min: Start with 0.125 mg b.i.d., up to maximum of 1.5 mg b.i.d. C_{CR}, 15–24 mL/min: Start with 0.125 mg once daily, up to maximum of 1.5 mg once daily.

HEALTH CARE CONSIDERATIONS

Administration/Storage

1. Take with food to decrease nausea.
2. Consider decrease in levodopa dose if taken with pramipexole.
3. Discontinue pramipexole over 1 week period.

Assessment

1. Record disease onset, extent of motor function, reflexes, gait, strength of grip, and amount of tremor.

2. With tremor, assess for muscle weakness, muscle rigidity, difficulty walking, or changing directions.
3. Monitor LFTs, VS, ECG, and renal function studies.

Client/Family Teaching

1. Take only as prescribed; may take with food to decrease nausea.
2. Rise slowly from sitting or lying position to prevent postural effects.
3. Do not drive or perform activities that require mental/motor alertness until stabilized on drug. May cause dizziness, fainting, blackouts, hypotension, and sedative effects.
4. Practice reliable contraception.
5. Report any vision problems; obtain regular eye exams.
6. May cause hallucinations; report if evident.
7. Do not stop abruptly; must do so over one week period.

Outcome/Evaluate: Control of Parkinsonian symptoms (e.g., improvement in motor function, reflexes, gait, strength of grip, and amount of tremor)

Pravastatin sodium

(prah-vah-**STAH**-tin)
Pregnancy Category: X
Pravachol **(Rx)**
Classification: Antihyperlipidemic agent

P

Action/Kinetics: Competitively inhibits HMG-CoA reductase, the enzyme catalyzing the conversion of HMG-CoA to mevalonate in the biosynthesis of cholesterol. This results in an increased number of LDL receptors on cell surfaces and enhanced receptor-mediated catabolism and clearance of circulating LDL. Also inhibits LDL production by inhibiting hepatic synthesis of VLDL, the precursor of LDL. Elevated levels of total cholesterol, dLDL cholesterol, and apolipoprotein B (a membrane transport complex for LDL) promote development of atherosclerosis and are lowered by pravastatin. Drug increases survival in heart transplant recipients. Rapidly absorbed from the GI tract. **Peak plasma levels:** 1–1.5 hr. Significant first-pass extraction and metabolism in the liver, which is the site of action of the drug; thus, plasma levels may not correlate well with lipid-lowering effectiveness. **t½, elimination:** 77 hr. Metabolized in the liver; approximately 20% of a PO dose is excreted through the urine and 70% in the feces.

Uses: Adjunct to diet for reducing elevated total and LDL cholesterol levels in clients with primary hypercholesterolemia (type IIa and IIb) and mixed dyslipidemia when the response to a diet with restricted saturated fat and cholesterol has not been effective. Reduce the risk of heart attack with and without established CHD and slow progression of coronary atherosclerosis in those with hypercholesterolemia and heart disease. To reduce the risk of stroke or TIA. *Investigational:* To lower cholesterol levels in those with heterozygous familial hypercholesterolemia, familial combined hyperlipidemia, diabetic dyslipidemia in non-insulin-dependent diabetics, hypercholesterolemia secondary to nephrotic syndrome, homozygous familial hypercholesterolemia in those not completely devoid of LDL receptors but who have a decreased level of LDL receptor activity.

Contraindications: To treat hypercholesterolemia due to hyperalphaproteinemia. Active liver disease; unexplained, persistent elevations in LFTs. Use during pregnancy and lactation and in children less than 18 years of age.

Special Concerns: Use with caution in clients with a history of liver disease, renal insufficiency, or heavy alcohol use.

Side Effects: *Musculoskeletal:* Rhabdomyolysis with renal dysfunction secondary to myoglobinuria, myalgia, myopathy, arthralgias, localized pain, muscle cramps, leg cramps, bursitis, tenosynovitis, myasthenia, tendinous contracture, myositis. *CNS:* CNS vascular lesions characterized by ***perivascular hemorrhage,*** edema, and mononuclear cell infiltration of perivascular spaces; headache, dizziness, psychic disturbances. Dizziness, vertigo, memory loss, anxiety, insomnia, somnolence, abnormal dreams, emotional lability, incoordination, hyperkinesia, torticollis, psychic disturbances. *GI:* N&V, diarrhea, abdominal pain, cramps, constipation, flatulence, heartburn, anorexia, gastroenteritis, dry mouth, rectal hemorrhage, esophagitis, eructation, glossitis, mouth ulceration, increased appetite, stomatitis, cheilitis, duodenal ulcer, dysphagia, enteritis, melena, gum hemorrhage, stomach ulcer, tenesmus, ulcerative stomach. *CV:* Palpitation, vasodilation, syncope, migraine, postural hypotension, phlebitis, arrhythmia. *Hepatic:* Hepatitis (including chronic active hepatitis), fatty change in liver, cirrhosis, ***fulminant hepatic necrosis, hepatoma,*** pancreatitis, cholestatic jaundice, biliary pain. *GU:* Gynecomastia, erectile dysfunction, loss of libido, cystitis, hematuria, impotence, dysuria, kidney calculus, nocturia, epididymitis, fibrocystic breast, albuminuria, breast enlargement, nephritis, urinary frequency, incontinence, retention and urgency, abnormal ejaculation, vaginal or uterine hemorrhage, metrorrhagia, UTI. *Ophthalmic:* Progression of cataracts, lens opacities, ophthalmoplegia. *Hypersensitivity reaction:* Vasculitis, purpura, polymyalgia rheumatica, ***angioedema,*** lupus erythematosus–like syndrome, thrombocytopenia, ***hemolytic anemia,*** leukopenia, positive ANA, arthritis, arthralgia, urticaria, asthenia, ESR increase, fever, chills, photosensitivity, malaise, dyspnea, ***toxic epidermal necrolysis, Stevens-Johnson syndrome.*** *Dermatologic:* Alopecia, pruritus, rash, skin nodules, discoloration of skin, dryness of skin and mucous membranes, changes in hair and nails, contact dermatitis, sweating, acne, urticaria, eczema, seborrhea, skin ulcer. *Neurologic:* Dysfunction of certain cranial nerves resulting in alteration of taste, impairment of extraocular movement, and facial paresis; paresthesia, peripheral neuropathy, tremor, vertigo, memory loss peripheral nerve palsy. *Respiratory:* Common cold, rhinitis, cough. *Hematologic:* Anemia, transient asymptomatic eosinophilia, thrombocytopenia, leukopenia, ecchymosis, lymphadenopathy, petechiae. *Miscellaneous:* Cardiac chest pain, fatigue, influenza.

Laboratory Test Considerations: ↑ CPK, AST, ALT, alkaline phosphatase, bilirubin. Abnormalities in thyroid function tests.

Drug Interactions

Bile acid sequestrants / ↓ Bioavailability of pravastatin
Clofibrate / ↑ Risk of myopathy
Cyclosporine / ↑ Risk of myopathy or rhabdomyolysis
Erythromycin / ↑ Risk of myopathy or rhabdomyolysis
Gemfibrozil / ↑ Risk of myopathy or rhabdomyolysis
Niacin / ↑ Risk of myopathy or rhabdomyolysis
Warfarin / ↑ Anticoagulant effect of warfarin

How Supplied: *Tablet:* 10 mg, 20 mg, 40 mg

Dosage

- **Tablets**

Initial: 10–20 mg once daily at bedtime (geriatric clients should take 10 mg once daily at bedtime). **Maintenance dose:** 10–40 mg once daily at bedtime (maximum dose for geriatric clients is 20 mg/day). Use a starting dose of 10 mg/day at bedtime in renal/hepatic dysfunction and in the elderly.

HEALTH CARE CONSIDERATIONS

See also *Health Care Considerations* for *Antihyperlipidemic Agents.*

Administration/Storage

1. Place on a standard cholesterol-lowering diet for 3–6 months before beginning pravastatin and continue during therapy.
2. Drug may be taken without regard to meals.
3. The maximum effect is seen within 4 weeks during which time periodic lipid determinations should be undertaken.

Assessment

1. Determine that secondary causes for hypercholesterolemia are ruled out. Secondary causes include hypothyroidism, poorly controlled diabetes mellitus, dysproteinemias, obstructive liver disease, nephrotic syndrome, alcoholism, and other drug therapy.
2. Determine if pregnant.
3. Assess for liver disease or alcohol abuse.
4. Document all CAD risk factors.
5. Monitor cholesterol profile, CBC, liver and renal function studies.

Interventions

1. Obtain LFTs prior to pravastatin therapy q 6 weeks during the first 3 months of therapy, q 2–3 months during the remainder of the first year, then at 6-month intervals.
2. Pravastatin should be discontinued if markedly elevated CPK levels occur or myopathy is diagnosed.
3. Pravastatin should be discontinued temporarily in clients experiencing an acute or serious condition (e.g., sepsis, hypotension, major surgery, trauma, uncontrolled epilepsy, or severe metabolic, endocrine, or electrolyte disorders) predisposing to the development of renal failure secondary to rhabdomyolysis.

Client/Family Teaching

1. Review the prescribed dietary recommendations (restricted cholesterol and saturated fats); continue diet during drug therapy.
2. Continue a regular exercise program and strive to attain recommended weight loss.
3. Report any unexplained muscle pain, tenderness, or weakness, especially if accompanied by malaise or fever.
4. Practice reliable birth control; report if pregnancy is suspected as drug therapy hazardous to a developing fetus.

Outcome/Evaluate: ↓ Serum cholesterol and LDL levels; heart attack prophylaxis in those with atherosclerosis and hypercholesterolemia

Praziquantel

(pray-zih-**KWON**-tell)
Pregnancy Category: B
Biltricide **(Rx)**
Classification: Anthelmintic

See also *Anthelmintics.*

P

Action/Kinetics: Causes increased cell permeability in the helminth, resulting in a loss of intracellular calcium with massive contractions, and paralysis of musculature with breakdown of the integrity of the organism. Also causes vacuolization and disintegration of phagocytes to the parasite, resulting in death. **Maximum serum levels:** 1–3 hr. **t½:** 0.8–1.5 hr. Levels in the CSF are approximately 14%–20% of the total amount of the drug in the plasma. Significant first-pass effect. Excreted primarily in the urine.
Uses: Schistosomal infections due to *Schistosoma japonicum, S. mansoni, S. mekongi,* and *S. hematobium*. Liver flukes (*Clonorchis sinensis, Opisthorchis viverrini). Investigational:* Neurocysticercosis, other tissue flukes, and intestinal cestodes. Low doses of oxamniquine and praziquantel as a single-dose treatment of schistosomiasis.
Contraindications: Ocular cysticercosis. Lactation.
Special Concerns: Safety in children less than 4 years of age not established.
Side Effects: *GI:* Nausea, abdominal discomfort. *CNS:* Malaise, headache, dizziness, drowsiness. *Miscellaneous:* Fever, urticaria (rare). *NOTE:* These side effects may also be due to the helminth infection itself.
OD Management of Overdose: *Symptoms:* Extension of side effects. *Treatment:* Administer a fast-acting laxative.
Drug Interactions: Hydantoins may decrease serum praziquantel levels, resulting in ineffective treatment.
How Supplied: *Tablet:* 600 mg

Dosage

- **Tablets**

Schistosomiasis.

Three doses of 20 mg/kg as a 1-day treatment with an interval between doses not less than 4 hr or more than 6 hr.

Chonorchiasis and opisthorchiasis.

Three doses of 25 mg/kg as a 1-day treatment with an interval between doses not less than 4 hr or more than 6 hr.

HEALTH CARE CONSIDERATIONS

See also *Health Care Considerations* for *Anthelmintics.*

Assessment

1. Record indications for therapy, onset, characteristics, duration of symptoms, and source of infestation.
2. Determine if the schistosomiasis or fluke infection is accompanied by cerebral cysticercosis; if so, hospitalize for treatment.
3. Note any liver dysfunction as reduced dosage may be indicated.
4. List drugs currently prescribed to ensure none interact unfavorably or deactivate drug (i.e., hydantoins).

Client/Family Teaching

1. Swallow tablets unchewed with liquid during meals. Keeping the tablets in the mouth may cause gagging or vomiting; do not chew the tablets as their bitter taste can cause retching and vomiting.
2. Use caution while driving or performing tasks requiring alertness; may cause dizziness/drowsiness, .
3. Do not nurse baby on treatment day and for 3 days following.

Outcome/Evaluate: Eradication of parasitic infestation; negative cultures

Prazosin hydrochloride

(PRAY-zoh-sin)
Pregnancy Category: C
Alti-Prazosin ★, Apo-Prazo ★, Minipress, Novo-Prazin ★, Nu-Prazo ★, Rho-Prazosin ★
(Rx)
Classification: Antihypertensive, alpha-1-adrenergic blocking agent

See also *Alpha-1-Adrenergic Blocking Agents* and *Antihypertensive Agents.*
Action/Kinetics: Produces selective blockade of postsynaptic alpha-1-adrenergic receptors. Dilates arterioles and veins, thereby decreasing total peripheral resistance and decreasing DBP more than SBP. CO, HR, and renal blood flow are not affected. Can be used to initiate antihypertensive therapy; most effective when used with other agents (e.g., diuretics, beta-adrenergic blocking agents). **Onset:** 2 hr. Absorption not affected by food. **Maximum effect:** 2–3 hr; **duration:** 6–12 hr. **t½:** 2–3 hr. Full therapeutic effect: 4–6 weeks. Metabolized extensively; excreted primarily in feces.
Uses: Mild to moderate hypertension alone or in combination with other antihypertensive drugs. *Investigational:* CHF refractory to other treatment. Raynaud's disease, BPH.
Special Concerns: Safe use in children has not been established. Use with caution during lactation. Geriatric clients may be more sensitive to the hypotensive and hypothermic effects; may be necessary to decrease the dose in these clients due to age-related decreases in renal function.
Side Effects: First-dose effect: ***Marked hypotension*** and syncope 30–90 min after administration of initial dose (usually 2 or more mg), increase of dosage, or addition of other antihypertensive agent. *CNS:* Dizziness, drowsiness, headache, fatigue, paresthesias, depression, vertigo, nervousness, hallucinations. *CV:* Palpitations, syncope, tachycar-

dia, orthostatic hypotension, aggravation of angina. *GI:* N&V, diarrhea or constipation, dry mouth, abdominal pain, pancreatitis. *GU:* Urinary frequency or incontinence, impotence, priapism. *Respiratory:* Dyspnea, nasal congestion, epistaxis. *Dermatologic:* Pruritus, rash, sweating, alopecia, lichen planus. *Miscellaneous:* Asthenia, edema, symptoms of lupus erythematosus, blurred vision, tinnitus, arthralgia, myalgia, reddening of sclera, eye pain, conjunctivitis, edema, fever.

Laboratory Test Considerations: ↑ Urinary metabolites of norepinephrine, VMA.

OD Management of Overdose: *Symptoms:* Hypotension, ***shock.*** *Treatment:* Keep client supine to restore BP and HR. If shock is manifested, use volume expanders and vasopressors; maintain renal function.

Drug Interactions

Antihypertensives (other) / ↑ Antihypertensive effect

Beta-adrenergic blocking agents / Enhanced acute postural hypotension following the first dose of prazosin

Clonidine / ↓ Antihypertensive effect of clonidine

Diuretics / ↑ Antihypertensive effect

Indomethacin / ↓ Effect of prazosin

Nifedipine / ↑ Hypotensive effect

Propranolol / Especially pronounced additive hypotensive effect

Verapamil / ↑ Hypotensive effect; ↑ sensitivity to prazosin-induced postural hypotension

How Supplied: *Capsule:* 1 mg, 2 mg, 5 mg

Dosage

- **Capsules**

Hypertension.

Individualized: Initial, 1 mg b.i.d.–t.i.d.; **maintenance:** if necessary, increase gradually to 6–15 mg/day in two to three divided doses. Do not exceed 20 mg/day, although some clients have benefitted from doses of 40 mg daily. If used with diuretics or other antihypertensives, reduce dose to 1–2 mg t.i.d. **Pediatric, less than 7 years of age, initial:** 0.25 mg b.i.d.–t.i.d. adjusted according to response. **Pediatric, 7–12 years of age, initial:** 0.5 mg b.i.d.–t.i.d. adjusted according to response.

HEALTH CARE CONSIDERATIONS

See also *Health Care Considerations* for *Antihypertensive Agents* and *Alpha-1-Adrenergic Blocking Agents.*

Administration/Storage: Reduce the dose to 1 or 2 mg t.i.d. if a diuretic or other antihypertensive agent is added to the regimen and then retitrate client.

Client/Family Teaching

1. Take the first dose at bedtime. Also, take the first dose of each increment at bedtime to reduce the incidence of syncope.
2. Do not drive or operate machinery for 24 hr after the first dose; may cause dizziness and drowsiness.
3. Food may delay absorption and minimize side effects of the drug.
4. Avoid rapid postural changes that may precipitate weakness, dizziness, and syncope. Lie down or sit down and put head below knees to avoid fainting if a rapid heartbeat is felt.
5. Avoid dangerous situations that may lead to fainting.
6. Report any bothersome side effects because reduction in dosage may be indicated. Use sips of water and sugarless gum or candies for dry mouth effects.
7. Do not stop medication unless directed.
8. Avoid cold, cough, and allergy medications. The sympathomimetic component of such medications will interfere with the action of prazosin.
9. Comply with prescribed drug regimen; full drug effect may not be evident for 4–6 weeks.

Outcome/Evaluate: ↓ BP; ↓ symptoms of refractory CHF

P

Prednisolone

(pred-**NISS**-oh-lohn)

Pregnancy Category: C

Syrup: Prelone. **Tablets:** Delta-Cortef **(Rx)**

Prednisolone acetate

(pred-**NISS**-oh-lohn)

Pregnancy Category: C

Parenteral: Articulose-50, Key-Pred 25 and 50, Predalone 50, **Ophthalmic Suspension:** Diopred ✱, Econopred, Econopred Plus, Ophtho-Tate ✱, Pred Forte Ophthalmic, Pred Mild Ophthalmic **(Rx)**

Prednisolone acetate and Prednisolone sodium phosphate

(pred-**NISS**-oh-lohn)

Pregnancy Category: C

(Rx)

Prednisolone sodium phosphate

(pred-**NISS**-oh-lohn)

Pregnancy Category: C
Oral Solution: Pediapred **(Rx)**. **Ophthalmic Solution:** AK-Pred Ophthalmic, Inflamase Forte Ophthalmic, Inflamase Mild Ophthalmic **(Rx)**, **Parenteral:** Hydeltrasol, Key-Pred-SP **(Rx)**

Prednisolone tebutate

(pred-**NISS**-oh-lohn)
Pregnancy Category: C
Hydeltra-T.B.A., Prednisol TPA **(Rx)**
Classification: Corticosteroid, synthetic

See also *Corticosteroids*.
Action/Kinetics: Intermediate-acting. Is five times more potent than hydrocortisone and cortisone. Minimal side effects except for GI distress. Moderate mineralocorticoid activity. **Plasma t½:** over 200 min.
Contraindications: Lactation.
Special Concerns: Use with particular caution in diabetes.
How Supplied: Prednisolone: *Syrup:* 5 mg/5 mL, 15 mg/5 mL; *Tablet:* 5 mg. Prednisolone acetate: *Injection:* 25 mg/mL, 50 mg/mL; *Ophthalmic Suspension:* 0.12%, 0.125%, 1%. Prednisolone sodium phosphate: *Liquid:* 5 mg/5 mL; *Ophthalmic Solution:* 0.125%, 1%. Prednisolone tebutate: *Injection:* 20 mg/mL.

Dosage

PREDNISOLONE

- **Tablets, Syrup**

Most uses.
5–60 mg/day, depending on disease being treated.
Multiple sclerosis (exacerbation).
200 mg/day for 1 week; **then,** 80 mg on alternate days for 1 month.
Pleurisy of tuberculosis.
0.75 mg/kg/day (then taper) given concurrently with antituberculosis therapy.

PREDNISOLONE ACETATE

- **IM**

4–60 mg/day. **Not for IV use.**
Multiple sclerosis (exacerbation).
See *Prednisolone.*

- **Intralesional, Intra-articular, Soft Tissue Injection**

4–100 mg (larger doses for large joints).

- **Ophthalmic Suspension (0.12%, 0.125%, 1%)**

Instill 1–2 gtt into the conjunctival sac b.i.d.–q.i.d. During the first 24 to 48 hr, the frequency of dosing may be increased if necessary.

PREDNISOLONE ACETATE AND PREDNISOLONE SODIUM PHOSPHATE

- **IM Only**

20–80 mg acetate and 5–20 mg sodium phosphate every few days for 3–4 weeks.

- **Intra-articular, Intrasynovial**

20–40 mg prednisolone acetate and 5–10 mg prednisolone sodium phosphate.

PREDNISOLONE SODIUM PHOSPHATE

- **PO Solution**

Most uses.
5–60 mg/day in single or divided doses.
Adrenocortical insufficiency.
Pediatric: 0.14 mg/kg (4 mg/m²) daily in three to four divided doses.
Other pediatric uses.
0.5–2 mg/kg (15–60 mg/m²) daily in three to four divided doses.

- **IM, IV**

4–60 mg/day.
Multiple sclerosis (exacerbation).
See *Prednisolone.*

- **Intralesional, Intra-articular, Soft Tissue Injection**

2–30 mg, depending on site and severity of disease.

- **Ophthalmic Solution (0.125%, 1%)**

1–2 gtt into the conjunctival sac q hr during the day and q 2 hr during the night; **then,** after response obtained, decrease dose to 1 gtt/ q 4 hr and then later 1 gtt t.i.d.–q.i.d.

PREDNISOLONE TEBUTATE

- **Intra-articular, Intralesional, Soft Tissue Injection**

4–30 mg, depending on site and severity of disease. Doses higher than 40 mg are not recommended.

HEALTH CARE CONSIDERATIONS

See also *Health Care Considerations* for *Corticosteroids.*

Administration/Storage

1. Before administering, check spelling and dose carefully; is frequently confused with prednisone.
2. Check to see if provider wants PO form administered with an antacid.
3. Prednisolone sodium phosphate oral solution produces a 20% higher peak plasma level than tablets.
4. Shake the suspension well before using.
IV 5. The IV form (sodium phosphate) may be administered at a rate not to exceed 10 mg/min.

Assessment

1. Record indications for therapy, type and onset of symptoms. Note any previous experiences with this drug and the outcome.
2. Monitor VS, CBC, electrolytes, blood sugar, weight, and mental status.

Outcome/Evaluate

- Replacement therapy during adrenocortical hypofunction
- Symptomatic relief of allergic, immune, and inflammatory manifestations

Prednisone

(PRED-nih-sohn)

Pregnancy Category: C

Oral Solution: Prednisone Intensol Concentrate **(Rx)**. **Syrup:** Liquid Pred **(Rx)**. **Tablets:** Alti-Prednisone ✦, Apo-Prednisone ✦, Deltasone, Jaa Prednisone ✦, Meticorten, Novo-Prednisone ✦, Orasone 1, 5, 10, 20, and 50, Panasol-S, Sterapred DS, Winpred ✦ **(Rx)**

Classification: Corticosteroid, synthetic

See also *Corticosteroids*.

Action/Kinetics: Three to five times as potent as cortisone or hydrocortisone. May cause moderate fluid retention. Metabolized in the liver to prednisolone, the active form.

Special Concerns: Dose must be highly individualized.

How Supplied: *Concentrate:* 5 mg/mL; *Solution:* 5 mg/5 mL; *Syrup:* 5 mg/5 mL; *Tablet:* 1 mg, 2.5 mg, 5 mg, 10 mg, 20 mg, 50 mg

Dosage

- **Oral Concentrate, Syrup, Tablets**

Acute, severe conditions.

Initial: 5–60 mg/day in four equally divided doses after meals and at bedtime. Decrease gradually by 5–10 mg q 4–5 days to establish minimum maintenance dosage (5–10 mg) or discontinue altogether until symptoms recur.

Replacement.

Pediatric: 0.1–0.15 mg/kg/day.

COPD.

30–60 mg/day for 1–2 weeks; then taper.

Ophthalmopathy due to Graves' disease.

60 mg/day; **then,** taper to 20 mg/day.

Duchenne's muscular dystrophy.

0.75–1.5 mg/kg/day (used to improve strength).

HEALTH CARE CONSIDERATIONS

See also *Health Care Considerations* for *Corticosteroids*.

Assessment

1. Record indications for therapy, type, onset, and duration of symptoms. List other agents prescribed and the outcome.
2. Monitor CBC, electrolytes, blood sugar, weights, and mental status.

Client/Family Teaching

1. Take with food to decrease GI upset.
2. Do not stop abruptly with long-term therapy.
3. Report any S&S of adrenal insufficiency or loss of effectiveness.
4. Avoid alcohol and OTC agents.

Outcome/Evaluate: Relief of allergic, immune, and inflammatory manifestations

Primaquine phosphate

(PRIM-ah-kwin)

Pregnancy Category: C

(Rx)

Classification: 8-Aminoquinoline, antimalarial

Action/Kinetics: Mechanism of action not known, but the drug binds to and may alter the properties of DNA leading to decreased protein synthesis. Both the gametocyte and exoerythrocyte forms are inhibited. Some gametocytes are destroyed while others cannot undergo maturation division in the gut of the mosquito. Well absorbed from GI tract. **Peak plasma levels:** 1–3 hr. Poorly distributed in body tissues. **t½ elimination:** 4 hr. Rapidly metabolized.

Uses: Only for the radical cure of *Plasmodium vivax* malaria, the prophylaxis of relapse in *P. vivax* malaria, or following the termination of chloroquine phosphate suppressive therapy in areas where *P. vivax* is endemic.

Contraindications: Concomitant use with quinacrine. In clients with rheumatoid arthritis or lupus erythematosus who are acutely ill or who have a tendency to develop granulocytopenia. Concomitant use with other bone marrow depressants or hemolytic drugs.

Special Concerns: Use during pregnancy only when benefits outweigh risks.

Side Effects: *GI:* Abdominal cramps, epigastric distress, N&V. *Hematologic:* Leukopenia. Methemoglobinemia in NADH methemoglobin reductase deficient individuals. Blacks and members of certain Mediterranean ethnic groups (Sardinians, Sephardic Jews, Greeks, Iranians) manifest a high incidence of G6PD deficiency and as a result have a low tolerance for primaquine. These individuals manifest ***marked hemolytic anemia*** following primaquine administration. *Miscellaneous:* Headache, pruritus, interference with visual accommodation, ***cardiac arrhythmias,*** hypertension.

OD **Management of Overdose:** *Symptoms:* Abdominal cramps, vomiting, burning and epigastric distress, cyanosis, methemoglobinemia, anemia, moderate leukocytosis or leukopenia, CNS and CV disturbances. Granulocytopenia and ***acute hemolytic anemia*** in sensitive clients. *Treatment:* Treat symptoms.

Drug Interactions

Bone marrow depressants, hemolytic drugs / Additive side effects

Quinacrine / Quinacrine interferes with metabolic degradation of primaquine and thus enhances its toxic side reactions. **Do**

P

not give primaquine to clients who are receiving or have received quinacrine within the past 3 months.

How Supplied: *Tablet:* 26.3 mg

Dosage

- **Tablets**

Acute attack of vivax malaria, clients with parasitized RBCs.

15 mg (base) daily for 14 days together with chloroquine phosphate (to destroy erythrocytic parasites).

Suppression of malaria.

Adults: 26.3 mg (15 mg base) daily for 14 days or 78.9 mg once a week for 8 weeks; **children:** 0.5 mg/kg/day (0.3 mg/kg base) for 14 days.

HEALTH CARE CONSIDERATIONS

See also *General Health Care Considerations for All Anti-Infectives* and *Antimalarial Drugs, 4-Aminoquinolines.*

Administration/Storage

1. Store in tightly closed containers.
2. For suppression therapy, initiate during the last 2 weeks of or after suppressive therapy with chloroquine or a similar drug.

Assessment

1. Note any history of rheumatoid arthritis or lupus.
2. List other drugs prescribed to ensure no unfavorable interactions.
3. Determine if pregnant. Do not give during first trimester and preferably not until after delivery.
4. Obtain hematologic profile and cultures. Monitor for indications to withdraw drug: dark urine may indicate hemolysis.
5. Assess dark-skinned clients closely. Because of a possible inborn deficiency of G6PD, these clients are particularly susceptible to hemolytic anemia while on primaquine.

Client/Family Teaching

1. Take immediately before or after meals or with antacids to minimize gastric irritation.
2. For suppressive therapy, take drug on same day each week.
3. Monitor color of urine; report darkening or brown discoloration.
4. Must complete a full course of therapy for effective results.
5. Report GI, CNS, and CV disturbances; symptoms of overdose.

Outcome/Evaluate: Termination of acute malarial attacks; suppression of malarial symptoms

Primidone

(PRIH-mih-dohn)

Apo-Primidone ★, Mysoline, Sertan ★ **(Rx)**

Classification: Anticonvulsant, miscellaneous

Action/Kinetics: Closely related to the barbiturates; however, the anticonvulsant mechanism is unknown. Produces a greater sedative effect than barbiturates when used for seizure treatment. Side effects usually subside with use. **Peak plasma levels:** 3 hr. Primidone is converted in the liver to two active metabolites, phenobarbital and phenylethylmalonamide (PEMA). **Peak plasma levels (PEMA):** 7–8 hr. **t½ (primidone):** 5–15 hr; **t½ (PEMA):** 10–18 hr; **t½ (phenobarbital):** 53–140 hr. The appearance of phenobarbital in the plasma may be delayed several days after initiation of therapy. **Therapeutic plasma levels, primadone:** 5–12 mcg/mL; **phenobarbital,** 15–40 mcg/mL. Primidone and metabolites are excreted through the kidneys, although 40% of primidone is excreted unchanged.

Uses: Alone or with other anticonvulsants to treat psychomotor seizures, focal seizures, or tonic-clonic seizures (including those refractory to barbiturate-hydantoin regimens). *Investigational:* Benign familial tremor.

Contraindications: Porphyria. Hypersensitivity to phenobarbital. Lactation.

Special Concerns: Safe use during pregnancy has not been determined. Use during lactation may result in drowsiness in the neonate. Children and geriatric clients may react to primidone with restlessness and excitement. Due to differences in bioavailability, brand interchange is not recommended.

Side Effects: *CNS:* Drowsiness, ataxia, vertigo, fatigue, hyperirritability, emotional disturbances, personality disturbances with mood changes and paranoia. *GI:* N&V, anorexia, painful gums. *Hematologic:* Megaloblastic anemia, thrombocytopenia. *Ophthalmologic:* Diplopia, nystagmus. *Miscellaneous:* Impotence, morbilliform and maculopapular skin rashes. Occasionally has caused hyperexcitability, especially in children. ***Postpartum hemorrhage and hemorrhagic disease of the newborn.*** Symptoms of SLE.

Drug Interactions

See also *Barbiturates.*

Acetazolamide / ↓ Effect of primidone due to ↓ levels

Carbamazepine / ↓ Plasma levels of primidone and phenobarbital and ↑ plasma levels of carbamazepine

Hydantoins / ↑ Plasma levels of primidone, phenobarbital, and PEMA

Isoniazid / ↑ Effect of primidone due to ↓ breakdown by liver
Nicotinamide / ↑ Effect of primidone due to ↓ rate of clearance from body
Succinimides / ↓ Plasma levels of primidone and phenobarbital
How Supplied: *Suspension:* 250 mg/5 mL; *Tablet:* 50 mg, 250 mg

Dosage

- **Oral Suspension, Tablets**

Seizures, in clients on no other anticonvulsant medication.

Adults and children over 8 years, initial: Days 1–3, 100–125 mg at bedtime; days 4–6, 100–125 mg b.i.d.; days 7–9, 100–125 mg t.i.d.; **maintenance:** 250 mg t.i.d.–q.i.d. (may be increased to 250 mg 5–6 times/day; not to exceed 500 mg q.i.d.). **Children under 8 years, initial:** days 1–3, 50 mg at bedtime; days 4–6, 50 mg b.i.d.; days 7–9, 100 mg b.i.d.; **maintenance:** 125 mg b.i.d.–250 mg t.i.d. (10–25 mg/kg in divided doses).

Seizures, in clients receiving other anticonvulsants.

Initial: 100–125 mg at bedtime; **then,** increase to maintenance levels as other drug is slowly withdrawn (transition should take at least 2 weeks).

Benign familial tremor.

750 mg/day.

HEALTH CARE CONSIDERATIONS

See also *Health Care Considerations* for *Anticonvulsants.*

Assessment

1. Record age of seizure onset, frequency of occurrence, characteristics, and cause if known.
2. List other agents prescribed and the outcome.
3. Monitor CBC, liver and renal function studies.

Client/Family Teaching

1. May be taken with food if GI upset occurs.
2. Review the following conditions that should be reported:
   - Hyperexcitability in children
   - Excessive loss of hair
   - Edema of eyelids and legs
   - Visual disturbances
   - Mental status changes
   - Impotence
   - Loss of seizure control
3. Vitamin K may be prescribed during the last month of pregnancy to prevent postpartum hemorrhage in the mother and hemorrhagic disease of the newborn.

Outcome/Evaluate

- Control of refractory seizures
- Therapeutic drug levels (5–12 mcg/mL)

Probenecid

(proh-**BEN**-ih-sid)
Pregnancy Category: B
Benemid, Benuryl ✱ **(Rx)**
Classification: Antigout agent, uricosuric agent

Action/Kinetics: A uricosuric agent that increases the excretion of uric acid by inhibiting the tubular reabsorption of uric acid; this results in a decreased serum level of uric acid. Also inhibits the renal secretion of penicillins and cephalosporins; this effect is often taken advantage of in the treatment of infections because concomitant administration of probenecid will increase plasma levels of antibiotics. **Peak plasma levels:** 2–4 hr. **Time to peak effect, uricosuric:** 0.5 hr; **for suppression of penicillin excretion:** 2 hr. **Therapeutic plasma levels for inhibition of antibiotic secretion:** 40–60 mcg/mL; **therapeutic plasma levels for uricosuric effect:** 100–200 mcg/mL. **t½:** approximately 5–8 hr. **Duration for inhibition of penicillin excretion:** 8 hr. Metabolized in the liver to active metabolites; excreted in urine (5%–10% unchanged). Excretion is increased in alkaline urine.

Uses: Hyperuricemia in chronic gout and gouty arthritis. Adjunct in therapy with penicillins or cephalosporins to elevate and prolong plasma antibiotic levels.

Contraindications: Hypersensitivity to drug, blood dyscrasias, uric acid, and kidney stones. Use for hyperuricemia in neoplastic disease or its treatment. Use in children less than 2 years of age. Concomitant use of salicylates or use with penicillin in renal impairment.

Special Concerns: Use with caution in renal disease, porphyria, G6PD deficiency, history of allergy to sulfa drugs, and peptic ulcer.

Side Effects: *CNS:* Headaches, dizziness. *GI:* Anorexia, N&V, diarrhea, constipation, and abdominal discomfort. *Allergic:* Skin rash, dermatitis, pruritus, drug fever, and rarely ***anaphylaxis.*** *GU:* Nephrotic syndrome, uric acid stones with or without hematuria, urinary frequency, renal colic or costovertebral pain. *Miscellaneous:* Flushing, ***hemolytic anemia (possibly related to G6PD deficiency),*** anemia, sore gums, ***hepatic necrosis, aplastic anemia.***

Initially, the drug may increase frequency of acute gout attacks due to mobilization of uric acid.

Drug Interactions
Acyclovir / Probenecid ↓ renal excretion of acyclovir
Allopurinol / Additive effects to ↓ uric acid serum levels
AZT / ↑ Bioavailability of AZT; possible malaise, myalgia, fever
Benzodiazepines / More rapid onset and longer duration of the effects of benzodiazepines
Cephalosporins / ↑ Effect of cephalosporins due to ↓ excretion by kidney
Ciprofloxacin / 50% ↑ in systemic levels of ciprofloxacin
Clofibrate / ↑ Levels of clofibric acid (active) → ↑ effects
Dapsone / ↑ Effect of dapsone
Dyphylline / ↑ Effect of dyphylline due to ↓ excretion by kidney
Methotrexate / ↑ Effect and toxicity of methotrexate due to ↓ excretion by kidney
NSAIDs / ↑ Effect of NSAIDs due to ↓ excretion by kidney
Pantothenic acid / ↑ Effects of pantothenic acid
Penicillamine / ↓ Effect of penicillamine
Penicillins / ↑ Effect of penicillins due to ↓ excretion by kidney
Pyrazinamide / Probenecid inhibits hyperuricemia produced by pyrazinamide
Rifampin / ↑ Effect of rifampin due to ↓ excretion by kidney
Salicylates / Salicylates inhibit uricosuric activity of probenecid
Sulfinpyrazone / ↑ Effect of sulfinpyrazone due to ↓ excretion by kidney
Sulfonamides / ↑ Effect of sulfonamides due to ↓ plasma protein binding
Sulfonylureas, oral / ↑ Action of sulfonylureas → hypoglycemia
Thiopental / ↑ Effect of thiopental
How Supplied: *Tablet:* 500 mg

Dosage
- **Tablets**

Gout.
Adults, initial: 250 mg b.i.d. for 1 week. **Maintenance:** 500 mg b.i.d. Dosage may have to be increased further (by 500 mg/day q 4 weeks to maximum of 2 g) until urate excretion is less than 700 mg in 24 hr. Colbenemid, a combination tablet containing colchicine (0.5 mg) and probenecid (500 mg), is available.

Adjunct to penicillin or cephalosporin therapy.
Adults: 500 mg q.i.d. Dosage is decreased for elderly clients with renal damage. **Pediatric, 2–14 years, initial:** 25 mg/kg (or 700 mg/m^2); **maintenance,** 10 mg/kg q.i.d. (or 300 mg/m^2 q.i.d.). **For children 50 kg or more:** give adult dosage.

Gonorrhea, uncomplicated.
Adults: 1 g (as a single dose) 30 min before 4.8 million units of penicillin G procaine aqueous; **pediatric, less than 45 kg:** 25 mg/kg (up to a maximum of 1 g) with appropriate antibiotic therapy.

Neurosyphilis.
Adults: 0.5 g q.i.d. with penicillin G procaine aqueous, 2.4 million units/day IM, both for 10–14 days.

Pelvic inflammatory disease.
Adults: 1 g (as a single dose) plus cefoxitin, 2 g IM given concurrently.

HEALTH CARE CONSIDERATIONS

Administration/Storage
1. Do not start therapy until acute gouty attack has subsided. If an acute attack is precipitated during therapy, continue the drug.
2. To prevent kidney stones, take at least 6 to 8 (8-oz) glasses of water.
3. Maintain an alkaline urine by taking sodium bicarbonate, 3–7.5 g/day, or potassium citrate, 7.5 g/day.

Assessment
1. Record indications for therapy, type and onset of symptoms.
2. Determine any PUD, G6PD deficiency, uricemia R/T neoplastic disease, kidney stones, or blood dyscrasia.
3. Assess involved joints, noting pain, inflammation, heat, swelling, deformity, and ROM.
4. Monitor CBC, uric acid, liver and renal function studies. Note urate excretion levels.
5. Hypersensitivity reactions may occur more frequently with intermittent therapy.
6. Assess for toxic plasma antibiotic levels if excretion is inhibited by probenecid; adjust dosage.

Client/Family Teaching
1. Take with food or milk to minimize gastric irritation. Report gastric intolerance so dosage may be corrected without loss of therapeutic effect.
2. Take a liberal amount of fluid (2.5–3 L/day) to prevent the formation of sodium urate stones. Avoid cranberry juice or vitamin C preparations, which acidify urine. Sodium bicarbonate may be used to maintain an alkaline urine to prevent urates from crystallizing and forming kidney stones.
3. Acute gout attacks may initially be more frequent due to mobilization of uric acid. Report any increase in the number of acute attacks at the initiation of therapy since colchicine may need to be added. Continue to take during acute attacks with colchicine unless otherwise specified.
4. Report any unexplained fever, fatigue,

skin rash, persistent GI upset, flushing, increased sweating, headaches, or dizziness.
5. Do not take salicylates or use caffeine or alcohol during uricosuric therapy. Acetaminophen preparations may be used for analgesia.
6. Monitor FS closely; drug may increase hypoglycemic effects of PO antidiabetic agents.

Outcome/Evaluate

- ↓ Uric acid levels; ↓ gout attacks
- ↓ Joint pain and swelling
- Elevated/prolonged antibiotic (penicillin or cephalosporin) levels

Procainamide hydrochloride

(proh-**KAYN**-ah-myd)
Pregnancy Category: C
Apo-Procainamide ✦, Procan SR ✦, Procanbid, Pronestyl, Pronestyl-SR **(Rx)**
Classification: Antiarrhythmic, class IA

See also *Antiarrhythmic Agents.*

Action/Kinetics: Produces a direct cardiac effect to prolong the refractory period of the atria and to a lesser extent the bundle of His-Purkinje system and ventricles. Large doses may cause AV block. Some anticholinergic and local anesthetic effects. **Onset: PO,** 30 min; **IV,** 1–5 min. **Time to peak effect, PO:** 90–120 min; **IM,** 15–60 min; **IV,** immediate. **Duration:** 3 hr. **t½:** 2.5–4.7 hr. **Therapeutic serum level:** 4–8 mcg/mL. **Protein binding:** 15%. From 40% to 70% excreted unchanged. Metabolized in the liver (16%–21% by slow acetylators and 24%–33% by fast acetylators) to the active N-acetylprocainamide (NAPA); has antiarrhythmic properties with a longer half-life than procainamide.

Uses: Documented ventricular arrhythmias (e.g., sustained ventricular tachycardia) that may be life threatening in clients where benefits of treatment clearly outweigh risks. Antiarrhythmic drugs have not been shown to improve survival in clients with ventricular arrhythmias.

Contraindications: Hypersensitivity to drug, complete AV heart block, lupus erythematosus, torsades de pointes, asymptomatic ventricular premature contractions. Lactation.

Special Concerns: There is an increased risk of death in those with non-life-threatening arrhythmias. Although used in children, safety and efficacy have not been established. Use with extreme caution in clients for whom a sudden drop in BP could be detrimental, in CHF, acute ischemic heart disease, or cardiomyopathy. Also, use with caution in clients with liver or kidney dysfunction, preexisting bone marrow failure or cytopenia of any type, development of first-degree heart block while on procainamide, myasthenia gravis, and those with bronchial asthma or other respiratory disorders. May cause more hypotension in geriatric clients; also, in this population, the dose may have to be decreased due to age-related decreases in renal function.

Side Effects: *Body as a whole:* Lupus erythematosus–like syndrome especially in those on maintenance therapy and who are slow acetylators. Symptoms include arthralgia, pleural or abdominal pain, arthritis, pleural effusion, pericarditis, fever, chills, myalgia, skin lesions, hematologic changes. *CV:* Following IV use: Hypotension, ***ventricular asystole or fibrillation, partial or complete heart block.*** Rarely, second-degree heart block after PO use. *GI:* N&V, diarrhea, anorexia, bitter taste, abdominal pain. *Hematologic:* Thrombocytopenia, ***agranulocytosis,*** neutropenia. ***Rarely, hemolytic anemia.*** *Dermatologic:* Urticaria, pruritus, angioneurotic edema, flushing, maculopapular rash. *CNS:* Depression, dizziness, weakness, giddiness, psychoses, hallucinations. *Other:* Granulomatous hepatitis, weakness, fever, chills.

Laboratory Test Considerations: May affect LFTs. False + ↑ in serum alkaline phosphatase. Positive ANA test. High levels of lidocaine and meprobamate may inhibit fluorescence of procainamide and NAPA.

OD Management of Overdose: *Symptoms:* Plasma levels of 10–15 mcg/mL are associated with toxic symptoms. Progressive widening of the QRS complex, prolonged QT or PR intervals, lowering of R and T waves, increased AV block, increased ventricular extrasystoles, ***ventricular tachycardia or fibrillation. IV overdose may result in hypotension, CNS depression, tremor, respiratory depression.*** *Treatment:*

- Induce emesis or perform gastric lavage followed by administration of activated charcoal.
- To treat hypotension, give IV fluids and/or a vasopressor (dopamine, phenylephrine, or norepinephrine).
- Infusion of ⅙ molar sodium lactate IV reduces the cardiotoxic effects.
- Hemodialysis (but not peritoneal dialysis) is effective in reducing serum levels.
- Renal clearance can be enhanced by acidification of the urine and with high flow rates.

P

• A ventricular pacing electrode can be inserted as a precaution in the event AV block develops.

Drug Interactions
Acetazolamide / ↑ Effect of procainamide due to ↓ excretion by kidney
Anticholinergic agents, atropine / Additive anticholinergic effects
Antihypertensive agents / Additive hypotensive effect
Cholinergic agents / Anticholinergic activity of procainamide antagonizes effect of cholinergic drugs
Cimetidine / ↑ Effect of procainamide due to ↑ bioavailability
Disopyramide / ↑ Risk of enhanced prolongation of conduction or depression of contractility and hypotension
Ethanol / Effect of procainamide may be altered, but because the main metabolite is active as an antiarrhythmic, specific outcome not clear
Kanamycin / Procainamide ↑ muscle relaxation produced by kanamycin
Lidocaine / Additive cardiodepressant effects
Magnesium salts / Procainamide ↑ muscle relaxation produced by magnesium salts
Neomycin / Procainamide ↑ muscle relaxation produced by neomycin
Propranolol / ↑ Serum procainamide levels
Quinidine / ↑ Risk of enhanced prolongation of conduction or depression of contractility and hypotension
Ranitidine / ↑ Effect of procainamide due to ↑ bioavailability
Sodium bicarbonate / ↑ Effect of procainamide due to ↓ excretion by the kidney
Succinylcholine / Procainamide ↑ muscle relaxation produced by succinylcholine
Trimethoprim / ↑ Effect of procainamide due to ↑ serum levels

How Supplied: *Capsule:* 250 mg, 375 mg, 500 mg; *Injection:* 100 mg/mL, 500 mg/mL; *Tablet:* 250 mg, 375 mg, 500 mg; *Tablet, extended release:* 250 mg, 500 mg, 750 mg, 1000 mg

Dosage

• **Capsules, Extended-Release Tablets, Tablets**

Adults, initial: 50 mg/kg/day in divided doses q 3 hr. **Usual, 40–50 kg:** 250 mg q 3 hr of standard formulation or 500 mg q 6 hr of sustained-release; **60–70 kg:** 375 mg q 3 hr of standard formulation or 750 mg q 6 hr of sustained-release; **80–90 kg:** 500 mg q 3 hr of standard formulation or 1 g q 6 hr of sustained-release; **over 100 kg:** 625 mg q 3 hr of standard formulation or 1.25 g q 6 hr of sustained-release. **Pediatric:** 15–50 mg/kg/day divided q 3–6 hr (up to a maximum of 4 g/day).

• **Procanbid Extended-Release Tablets**

Life-threatening arrhythmias.

500 or 1,000 mg b.i.d.

• **IM**

Ventricular arrhythmias.

Adults, initial: 50 mg/kg/day divided into fractional doses of 1/8–1/4 given q 3–6 hr until PO therapy is possible. **Pediatric:** 20–30 mg/kg/day divided q 4–6 hr (up to a maximum of 4 g/day).

Arrhythmias associated with surgery or anesthesia.

Adults: 100–500 mg.

• **IV**

Initial loading infusion: 20 mg/min (for up to 25–30 min). **Maintenance infusion:** 2–6 mg/min. **Pediatric, initial loading dose:** 3–5 mg/kg/dose over 5 min (maximum of 100 mg); **maintenance:** 20–80 mcg/kg/min continuous infusion (maximum of 2 g/day).

HEALTH CARE CONSIDERATIONS

See also *Health Care Considerations* for *Antiarrhythmic Agents.*

Administration/Storage

1. Extended-release tablets are not recommended for use in children or for initiating treatment.
2. IM therapy may be used as an alternative to PO in clients with less threatening arrhythmias but who are nauseated or vomiting, who cannot take anything PO (e.g., preoperatively), or who have malabsorptive problems.
3. If more than three IM injections are required, assess the age, renal function, and blood levels of procainamide and NAPA; adjust dosage accordingly.

IV 4. Reserve IV use for emergency situations.

5. For IV initial therapy, dilute the drug with D5W; give a maximum of 1 g slowly to minimize side effects by one of the following methods:

• Direct injection into a vein or into tubing of an established infusion line at a rate not to exceed 50 mg/min. Dilute either the 100- or 500-mg/mL vials prior to injection to facilitate control of the dosage rate. Doses of 100 mg may be given q 5 min until arrhythmia is suppressed or until 500 mg has been given (then wait 10 or more min before resuming administration).

• Loading infusion containing 20 mg/mL (1 g diluted with 50 mL of D5W) given at a constant rate of 1 mL/min for 25–30 min to deliver 500–600 mg.

6. For IV maintenance infusion, the dose is

usually 2–6 mg/min. Administer with an electronic infusion device.
7. Discard solutions that are darker than light amber or otherwise colored. Solutions that have turned slightly yellow on standing may be used. Consult pharmacist if unsure.

Assessment

1. Record indications for therapy, type, onset, and duration of symptoms. List other agents prescribed and the outcome.
2. Assess cardiopulmonary status and note findings.
3. Monitor ECG, CBC, electrolytes, ANA titers, liver and renal function studies.

Interventions

1. Place in a supine position during IV infusion and monitor BP. Discontinue if SBP falls 15 mm Hg or more during administration or if increased SA or AV block is noted.
2. Assess for symptoms of SLE, manifested by polyarthralgia, arthritis, pleuritic pain, fever, myalgia, and skin lesions.

Client/Family Teaching

1. Take with a full glass of water to lessen GI symptoms. Take either 1 hr before or 2 hr after meals.
2. If GI symptoms are severe and persistent may take with meals or with a snack to ensure adherence.
3. Sustained-release preparations should be swallowed whole. They should not be crushed, broken, or chewed. The wax matrix of sustained-release tablets may be evident in the stool and is considered normal.
4. Report any sore throat, fever, rash, chills, bruising, or diarrhea.
5. Do not take any OTC drugs.

Outcome/Evaluate

- Termination of arrhythmias with restoration of stable cardiac rhythm
- Therapeutic drug levels (4–8 mcg/mL)

Procarbazine hydrochloride (MIH, N-Methylhydrazine)

(pro-**KAR**-bah-zeen)

Pregnancy Category: D

Matulane, Natulan ✱ (Abbreviation: PCB)

(Rx)

Classification: Antineoplastic, miscellaneous

See also *Antineoplastic Agents*.

Action/Kinetics: May inhibit synthesis of protein, RNA, and DNA and inhibit transmethylation of methyl groups of methionine into t-RNA. Absences of t-RNA could result in cessation of protein synthesis and subsequently DNA and RNA synthesis. Also, hydrogen peroxide formed during auto-oxidation of the drug may attack protein sulfhydryl groups found in residual protein that is tightly bound to DNA. Rapidly absorbed from GI tract. Drug equilibrates between plasma and CSF (peak CSF levels occur within 30–90 min and peak plasma levels occur within 60 min). **t½, after IV:** 10 min. Metabolized in the liver and kidneys to cytotoxic products. About 70% eliminated in urine, mostly as metabolites, after 24 hr.

Uses: As an adjunct in the treatment of Hodgkin's disease (stage III and stage IV) as part of MOPP (nitrogen mustard, vincristine, procarbazine, prednisone) or ChlVPP (chlorambucil, vinblastine, procarbazine, prednisone) therapies. *Investigational:* Non-Hodgkin's lymphomas, malignant melanoma, primary brain tumors, lung cancer, multiple myeloma, polycythemia vera.

Contraindications: Inadequate bone marrow reserve as shown by bone marrow aspiration (i.e., in clients with leukopenia, thrombocytopenia, or anemia). Lactation. Hypersensitivity to drug.

Special Concerns: Use with caution in impaired kidney or liver function. Due to the possibility of tremors, convulsions, and coma, close monitoring is necessary when used in children.

Side Effects: *GI:* N&V, anorexia, stomatitis, dry mouth, dysphagia, abdominal pain, hematemesis, melena, diarrhea, constipation. *CNS:* Paresthesias, neuropathies, headache, dizziness, depression, apprehension, nervousness, insomnia, nightmares, hallucinations, falling, weakness, fatigue, lethargy, drowsiness, unsteadiness, ataxia, foot drop, decreased reflexes, tremors, confusion, ***coma, convulsions.*** *CV:* Hypotension, tachycardia, syncope. *Respiratory:* Pleural effusion, pneumonitis, cough. *Hematologic:* Leukopenia, anemia, thrombocytopenia, pancytopenia, eosinophilia, ***hemolytic anemia,*** petechiae, purpura, epistaxis, hemoptysis. *GU:* Hematuria, urinary frequency, nocturia. *Dermatologic:* Dermatitis, pruritus, rash, urticaria, herpes, hyperpigmentation, flushing, alopecia. *Ophthalmic:* Retinal hemorrhage, nystagmus, photophobia, diplopia, inability to focus, papilledema. *Hepatic:* Jaundice, hepatic dysfunction. *Miscellaneous:* Gynecomastia in prepubertal and early pubertal boys, pain, myalgia and arthralgia, pyrexia, diaphoresis, chills, intercurrent infections, edema, hoarseness, generalized allergic reactions, hearing loss, slurred speech, second nonlymphoid malignancies (including acute myelocytic leukemia, malignant myelosclerosis) and azoospermia in those treated with

P

procarbazine combined with other chemotherapy or radiation.

OD **Management of Overdose:** *Symptoms:* N&V, diarrhea, enteritis, hypotension, tremors, seizures, coma, hematologic and hepatic toxicity. *Treatment:* Induce vomiting or undertake gastric lavage. IV fluids. Perform frequent blood counts and LFTs.

Drug Interactions

Alcohol / Antabuse-like reaction
Antihistamines / Additive CNS depression
Antihypertensive drugs / Additive CNS depression
Barbiturates / Additive CNS depression
Chemotherapy / Depressed bone marrow activity
Digoxin / ↓ Digoxin plasma levels
Guanethidine / Excitation and hypertension
Hypoglycemic agents, oral / ↑ Hypoglycemic effect
Insulin / ↑ Hypoglycemic effect
Levodopa / Flushing and hypertension within 1 hr of levodopa administration
MAO inhibitors / Possibility of hypertensive crisis
Methyldopa / Excitation and hypertension
Narcotics / Significant CNS depression → possible deep coma and death
Phenothiazines / Additive CNS depression; also, possibility of hypertensive crisis
Reserpine / Excitation and hypertension
Sympathomimetics, indirectly acting / Possibility of hypertensive crisis
Tricyclic antidepressants / Possible toxic and fatal reactions, including excitability, fluctuations in BP, seizures, and coma
Tyramine-containing foods / Possibility of hypertensive crisis

How Supplied: *Capsule:* 50 mg

Dosage

- **Capsules**

When used alone.

Adults: 2–4 mg/kg/day for first week; **then,** 4–6 mg/kg/day until leukocyte count falls below 4,000/mm³ or platelet count falls below 100,000/mm³. If toxic symptoms appear, discontinue drug and resume treatment at rate of 1–2 mg/kg/day; **maintenance:** 1–2 mg/kg/day. **Children, highly individualized:** 50 mg/m²/day for first week; then 100 mg/m² (to nearest 50 mg) until maximum response obtained or until leukopenia or thrombocytopenia occurs. When maximum response is reached, maintain the dose at 50 mg/m²/day.

When used in combination with other antineoplastic drugs (e.g., MOPP or ChIVPP therapies).

100 mg/m² for 14 days.

HEALTH CARE CONSIDERATIONS

See also *Health Care Considerations* for *Antineoplastic Agents.*

Assessment

1. Record indications for therapy and other agents prescribed.
2. Record cardiopulmonary and neurologic assessments.
3. Monitor CBC, uric acid, liver and renal function studies. May cause granulocyte and platelet suppression. Nadir: 14 days; recovery: 21–28 days.

Client/Family Teaching

1. Consult provider before taking any other medication because procarbazine has MAO inhibitory activity. Avoid sympathomimetic drugs and foods with a high tyramine content (yeasts, yogurt, caffeine, chocolate, aged cheese, liver, smoked or pickled fish, fermented sausage, etc.) during and for 2 weeks after completing therapy; may precipitate a hypertensive crisis.
2. Do not drive or perform tasks that require mental alertness until drug effects are realized.
3. Consume adequate fluids (2–3 L/day) to prevent dehydration.
4. Drug increases effect of insulin and oral hypoglycemic agents; report hypoglycemic symptoms because medication adjustment may be necessary.
5. Avoid exposure to sun or to ultraviolet rays because a photosensitive skin reaction may occur. Wear sunscreen, sunglasses, and protective clothing if exposure is necessary.
6. Avoid alcohol; a disulfiram-type reaction may occur.
7. Practice reliable contraception.
8. Report persistent constipation (especially if diet, increased fluids, and bulk are ineffective); laxatives may be needed.

Outcome/Evaluate: Suppression of malignant cell proliferation

Prochlorperazine

(proh-klor-**PAIR**-ah-zeen)
Compazine, Stemetil Suppositories ✦ **(Rx)**

Prochlorperazine edisylate

(proh-klor-**PAIR**-ah-zeen)
Compazine **(Rx)**

Prochlorperazine maleate

(proh-klor-**PAIR**-ah-zeen)
Compazine, Stemetil ✦ **(Rx)**
Classification: Antipsychotic, antiemetic, piperazine-type phenothiazine

See also *Antipsychotic Agents, Phenothiazines.*

Action/Kinetics: Prochlorperazine causes a high incidence of extrapyramidal and antiemetic effects, moderate sedative effects, and a low incidence of anticholinergic effects and orthostatic hypotension. It also possesses significant antiemetic effects.
Uses: Psychotic disorders. Short-term treatment of generalized nonpsychotic anxiety (not drug of choice). Postoperative N&V, radiation sickness, vomiting due to toxins. Severe N&V. *Investigational:* Acute headache.
Contraindications: Use in clients who weigh less than 44 kg or who are under 2 years of age.
Special Concerns: Safe use during pregnancy has not been established. Geriatric, emaciated, and debilitated clients usually require a lower initial dose.
How Supplied: Prochlorperazine: *Suppository:* 2.5 mg, 5 mg, 25 mg; Prochlorperazine Edisylate: *Injection:* 5 mg/mL; *Syrup:* 5 mg/5 mL; Prochlorperazine maleate: *Capsule, extended release:* 10 mg, 15 mg; *Tablet:* 5 mg, 10 mg

Dosage

- **Edisylate Syrup, Maleate Extended-Release Capsules, Tablets**

Psychotic disorders.

Adults and adolescents: 5 or 10 mg t.i.d. or q.i.d. for mild conditions. For severe conditions, for hospitalized, or adequately supervised clients: 10 mg t.i.d. or q.i.d. Dose can be increased gradually q 2–3 days as needed and tolerated. For extended-release capsules, up to 100–150 mg/day can be given. **Pediatric, 2–12 years:** 2.5 mg b.i.d.–t.i.d. Do not give more than 10 mg on the first day.

N&V.

Adults and adolescents: 5–10 mg t.i.d.–q.i.d. (up to 40 mg/day). For extended-release capsules, the dose is 15–30 mg once daily in the morning (or 10 mg q 12 hr, up to 40 mg/day). **Pediatric, 18–39 kg:** 2.5 mg (base) t.i.d. (or 5 mg b.i.d.), not to exceed 15 mg/day; **14–17 kg:** 2.5 mg (base) b.i.d.–t.i.d., not to exceed 10 mg/day; **9–13 kg:** 2.5 mg (base) 1–2 times/day, not to exceed 7.5 mg/day. The total daily dose for children should not exceed 10 mg the first day; on subsequent days, the total daily dose should not exceed 20 mg for children 2–5 years of age or 25 mg for children 6–12 years of age.

Anxiety.

Adults and adolescents: 5 mg t.i.d.–q.i.d. on arising. Or, 15 mg sustained release on arising or 10 mg sustained release q 12 hr. Do not give more than 20 mg/day for more than 12 weeks.

- **IM, Edisylate Injection**

Psychotic disorders, for immediate control of severely disturbed clients.

Adults and adolescents, initial: 10–20 mg; dose can be repeated q 2–4 hr as needed (usually up to three or four doses). If prolonged therapy is needed: 10–20 mg q 4–6 hr. **Children, less than 12 years of age:** 0.03 mg/kg by deep IM injection. After control is achieved (usually after 1 injection), switch to PO at same dosage level or higher.

N&V.

Adults and adolescents: 5–10 mg; repeat the dose q 3–4 hr as needed. **Pediatric, 2–12 years:** 0.132 mg/kg.

N&V during surgery.

Adults and adolescents: 5–10 mg (base) given as a slow injection or infusion 15–30 min before induction of anesthesia; to control symptoms during or after surgery the dose can be repeated once. The rate of infusion should not exceed 5 mg/mL/min.

- **Rectal Suppositories**

Pediatric, 2–12 years: 2.5 mg b.i.d.–t.i.d. with no more than 10 mg given on the first day. No more than 20 mg/day for children 2–5 years of age and 25 mg/day for children 6–12 years of age.

HEALTH CARE CONSIDERATIONS

See also *Health Care Considerations* for *Antipsychotic Agents, Phenothiazines.*

Administration/Storage

1. Store all forms of the drug in tight-closing amber-colored bottles; store suppositories below 37°C (98.6°F).
2. Add desired dosage of concentrate to 60 mL of beverage (e.g., tomato or fruit juice, milk, soup) or semisolid food just before administration to disguise the taste.
3. Due to local irritation, do not give SC.
4. Do not mix with other agents in a syringe.
5. Do not dilute with any material containing the preservative parabens.
6. When given IM to children for N&V, the duration of action may be 12 hr.
7. Parenteral prescribing limits are 20 mg/day for children 2–5 years of age and 25 mg/day for children 6–12 years of age.

Assessment

1. Record indications for therapy, onset and characteristics of symptoms.
2. Assess mental status and note behavioral manifestations.
3. Monitor CBC, LFTs, and ECG.

Interventions

1. Monitor I&O and VS.
2. Auscultate bowel sounds and assess function.
3. Incorporate safety precautions during the treatment of an overdose. If taking spansules, continue treatment until all signs of overdosage are no longer evident. Saline laxatives may be used to hasten the evacuation of pellets that have not yet released their medication.

Client/Family Teaching

1. Do not exceed the prescribed dose of drug.
2. Withhold drug and report if child shows signs of restlessness and excitement.
3. Do not drive or operate machinery until drug effects are realized; drowsiness or dizziness may occur.
4. Report symptoms of extrapyramidal effects and tardive dyskinesia.
5. Use protection when in the sun to prevent photosensitivity reaction.
6. Rise and change positions slowly to prevent orthostatic effects.

Outcome/Evaluate

- Control of N&V
- Reduction in agitation, excitability, or withdrawn behaviors

Progesterone gel

(pro-**JES**-ter-ohn)
Crinone 4%, Crinone 8% **(Rx)**
Classification: Progesterone product

See also Progesterone and Progestins.

Action/Kinetics: t½, absorption: 25–50 hr. **t½, elimination:** 5–20 min. Extensively bound to plasma proteins. Metabolized in liver; excreted through urine and feces.

Uses: Progesterone supplementation or replacement as part of assisted reproductive technology treatment for infertile women with progesterone deficiency. Secondary amenorrhea.

Contraindications: Undiagnosed vaginal bleeding, liver disease or dysfunction, known or suspected malignancy of breast or genital organs, missed abortion, active thrombophlebitis or thromboembolic disease (or history of such). Concurrent use with other local intravaginal therapy.

Special Concerns: Safety and efficacy have not been determined in children.

Side Effects: See Progesterone and Progestins.

How Supplied: *Vaginal applicator:* 90 mg/1.125 g (Crinone 8%), 45 mg 1.125 g (Crinone 4%)

Dosage

- **Vaginal gel: Crinone 8%**

  Assisted reproductive technology.

90 mg once daily for women who require progesterone supplementation. Administer 90 mg b.i.d. in women with partial or complete ovarian failure who require progesterone replacement. If pregnancy occurs, treatment may be continued until placental autonomy has been achieved (up to 10–12 weeks).

- **Vaginal gel: Crinone 4%**

  Secondary amenorrhea.

45 mg every other day up to total of 6 doses. For women who fail to respond, Crinone 8% (90 mg) may be given every other day up to total of 6 doses.

HEALTH CARE CONSIDERATIONS

See also *Health Care Considerations* for *Progesterone and Progestins.*

Administration/Storage

1. Dosage increase from 4% gel can only be accomplished by using 8% gel. Increasing volume of gel does not increase amount absorbed.
2. If other local intravaginal therapy is to be used, wait at least 6-hr before or after Crinone administration.
3. Store at controlled room temperature below 25°C (77°F).

Assessment

1. Record indications for therapy, with physical and GYN findings.
2. Assess for liver disease, breast or genital malignancy, undiagnosed vaginal bleeding, or history of thromboembolic disease; precludes drug therapy.

Client/Family Teaching

1. Review product information sheet on how to use product; use only as directed.
2. Do not use with other intravaginal products; if concurrent therapy prescribed, wait for 6 hr.
3. May experience breast enlargement, constipation, headaches, sleepiness, and perineal pain.
4. Report any overt symptoms or depression.

Outcome/Evaluate: Progesterone replacement/supplementation

Promazine hydrochloride

(**PROH**-mah-zeen)
Pregnancy Category: C
Sparine **(Rx)**
Classification: Antipsychotic, dimethylaminopropyl-type phenothiazine

See also *Antipsychotic Agents, Phenothiazines.*

Action/Kinetics: Significant anticholinergic, sedative, and hypotensive effects; moderate antiemetic effect; and weak extrapyramidal effects. Ineffective in reducing destructive behavior in acutely agitated psychotic clients.

Uses: Psychotic disorders.

Special Concerns: Safe use during pregnancy has not been established. Dosage has not been established in children less than 12 years of age. Geriatric, emaciated, and debilitated clients may require a lower initial dosage.

How Supplied: *Injection:* 25 mg/mL, 50 mg/mL; *Tablet:* 50 mg

Dosage

- **Tablets**

Psychotic disorders.

Adults: 10–200 mg q 4–6 hr; adjust dose as needed and tolerated. Total daily dose should not exceed 1,000 mg. **Pediatric, 12 years and older:** 10–25 mg q 4–6 hr; adjust dose as needed and tolerated.

- **IM**

Psychotic disorders, severe and moderate agitation.

Adults, initial: 50–150 mg; if desired calming effect is not seen after 30 min, give additional doses up to a total of 300 mg. **Maintenance:** 10–200 mg q 4–6 hr as needed and tolerated. Switch to PO therapy as soon as possible. **Pediatric over 12 years:** 10–25 mg q 4–6 hr for chronic psychotic disorders (maximum dose: 1 g/day).

HEALTH CARE CONSIDERATIONS

See also *Health Care Considerations* for *Antipsychotic Agents, Phenothiazines.*

Administration/Storage

1. Dilute concentrate as directed on bottle. Taste can be disguised when given with citrus fruit juice, milk, or flavored drinks.
2. IM administration is preferred. Give in the gluteal region.
3. Reserve parenteral use for bedfast clients. Can be used in ambulatory clients in acute states but take proper precautions.

Assessment: Record indications for therapy, symptom onset, and presenting behaviors. Note other agents trialed and the outcome.

Outcome/Evaluate: Improved behavior patterns with a reduction in agitation, excitability, or withdrawn behaviors

Promethazine hydrochloride

(proh-METH-ah-zeen)

Pregnancy Category: C

Parenteral: Anergan 50, Phenergan, **Suppositories:** Phenergan, **Syrup:** Phenergan Fortis, Phenergan Plain, **Tablets:** Phenergan, PMS Promethazine ✦ **(Rx)**

Classification: Antihistamine, phenothiazine-type

See also *Antihistamines* and *Antiemetics.*

Action/Kinetics: Antiemetic effects are likely due to inhibition of the CTZ. Effective in vertigo by its central anticholinergic effect which inhibits the vestibular apparatus and the integrative vomiting center as well as the CTZ. May cause severe drowsiness. **Onset, PO, IM, PR:** 20 min; **IV:** 3–5 min. **Duration, antihistaminic:** 6–12 hr; **sedative:** 2–8 hr. Slowly eliminated through urine and feces.

Uses: PO and PR for prophylaxis and treatment of motion sickness. Prophylaxis of N&V due to anesthesia or surgery (also postoperatively). Pre- or postoperative sedative, obstetric sedative. Hypersensitivity reactions, including perennial and seasonal allergic rhinitis, vasomotor rhinitis, allergic conjunctivitis, urticaria, angioedema, allergic reactions to blood or plasma, dermographism. Adjunct in the treatment of anaphylaxis or anaphylactoid reactions. Adjunct to analgesics for postoperative pain. IV with meperidine or other narcotics in special surgical procedures as bronchoscopy, ophthalmic surgery, or in poor-risk clients.

Contraindications: Lactation. Comatose clients, CNS depression due to drugs, previous phenothiazine idiosyncrasy, acutely ill or dehydrated children (due to greater susceptibility to dystonias). Children up to 2 years of age. SC or intra-arterial use due to tissue necrosis and gangrene.

Special Concerns: Safe use during pregnancy has not been established. Use in children may cause paradoxical hyperexcitability and nightmares. Geriatric clients are more likely to experience confusion, dizziness, hypotension, and sedation.

Additional Side Effects: Leukopenia and ***agranulocytosis (especially if used with cytotoxic agents)***.

How Supplied: *Injection:* 25 mg/mL, 50 mg/mL; *Suppository:* 12.5 mg, 25 mg, 50 mg; *Syrup:* 6.25 mg/5 mL, 25 mg/5 mL; *Tablet:* 12.5 mg, 25 mg, 50 mg

Dosage

- **Suppositories, Syrup, Tablets**

Hypersensitivity reactions.

P

Adults: 12.5 mg q.i.d. before meals and at bedtime (or 25 mg at bedtime if needed). **Pediatric over 2 years:** 0.125 mg/kg (3.75 mg/m^2) q 4–6 hr; 0.5 mg/kg (15 mg/m^2) at bedtime if needed; or, 6.25–12. mg t.i.d. (or 25 mg at bedtime if needed).

Antiemetic.

Adults: 25 mg (usual); 12.5–25 mg q 4–6 hr as needed. **Pediatric, over 2 years:** 0.25–0.5 mg/kg (7.5–15 mg/m^2) q 4–6 hr as needed (or 12.5–25 mg q 4–6 hr).

Sedation.

Adults: 25–50 mg at bedtime; **pediatric, over 2 years:** 0.5–1 mg/kg (15–30 mg/m^2) or 12.5–25 mg at bedtime.

Motion sickness.

Adults: 25 mg b.i.d. **Pediatric, over 2 years:** 12.5–25 mg b.i.d.

Analgesia adjunct.

Adults: 50 mg with an equal amount of meperidine and an appropriate dose of an atropine-like agent. **Pediatric, over 2 years:** 1.2 mg/kg with an equal amount of meperidine and an atropine-like agent.

• **IM, IV**

Hypersensitivity reactions.

Adults: 25 mg repeated in 2 hr if needed; **pediatric, 2–12 years:** 12.5 mg or less, not to exceed half the adult dose. Resume PO therapy as soon as possible.

Antiemetic.

Adults: 12.5–25 mg q 4 hr if needed. If used postoperatively, reduce doses of concomitant hypnotics, analgesics, or barbiturates. **Pediatric, 2–12 years:** Do not exceed half the adult dose. Do not use when the cause of vomiting is unknown.

Sedation.

Adults: 25–50 mg at bedtime. May be combined with hypnotics for pre- and postoperative sedation. **Pediatric, 2–12 years:** Do not exceed half the adult dose.

Sedation during labor.

Adults: 50 mg during early stages of labor, not to exceed 100 mg/24 hr.

Analgesia adjunct.

Adults: 25–50 mg in combination with reduced doses of analgesics and hypnotics; give atropine-like drugs as needed. **Pediatric, 2–12 years:** 1.2 mg/kg in combination with an equal dose of analgesic or barabiturate and an appropriate dose of an atropine-like drug.

HEALTH CARE CONSIDERATIONS

See also *Health Care Considerations* for *Antihistamines,* and *Antiemetics.*

Administration/Storage: Decrease dosage in dehydrated clients or those with oliguria.

Assessment: Record indications for therapy, type and onset of symptoms. Note age; older clients may manifest more adverse side effects.

Client/Family Teaching

1. Take only as directed and do not exceed dose, as arrhythmias may occur. May take with food or milk to decrease GI upset.
2. When used to prevent motion sickness, take 30–60 min before travel. On successive travel days, take on rising and again before the evening meal.
3. Avoid activities requiring mental alertness until drug effects realized.
4. Do not consume alcohol or any OTC agents.
5. Drug may alter skin testing; stop 72 hr before testing.

Outcome/Evaluate

- Prevention of vertigo
- Control of N&V
- Promotion of sleep
- Control of allergic manifestations

Propafenone hydrochloride

(proh-pah-FEN-ohn)

Pregnancy Category: C

Rythmol **(Rx)**

Classification: Antiarrhythmic, class IC

Action/Kinetics: Manifests local anesthetic effects and a direct stabilizing action on the myocardium. Reduces upstroke velocity (Phase O) of the monophasic action potential, reduces the fast inward current carried by sodium ions in the Purkinje fibers, increases diastolic excitability threshold, and prolongs the effective refractory period. Also, spontaneous activity is decreased. Slows AV conduction and causes first-degree heart block. Has slight beta-adrenergic blocking activity. **Peak plasma levels:** 3.5 hr. **Therapeutic plasma levels:** 0.5–3 mcg/mL. Significant first-pass effect. Most metabolize rapidly (**t^1/$_2$:** 2–10 hr) to two active metabolites: 5-hydroxypropafenone and N-depropylpropafenone. However, approximately 10% (as well as those taking quinidine) metabolize the drug more slowly (**t^1/$_2$:** 10–32 hr). Because the 5-hydroxy metabolite is not formed in slow metabolizers and because steady-state levels are reached after 4–5 days in all clients, the recommended dosing regimen is the same for all clients.

Uses: Documented life-threatening ventricular arrhythmias, such as sustained ventricular tachycardia where the benefits outweigh the risks. Paroxysmal atrial fibrillation or flutter and paroxysmal supraventricular tachycardia associated with disabling symptoms. Do

not use in less severe ventricular arrhythmias even if the client is symptomatic. Antiarrhythmic drugs have not been shown to improve survival in clients with ventricular arrhythmias. *Investigational:* Arrhythmias associated with Wolff-Parkinson-White syndrome.
Contraindications: Uncontrolled CHF, cardiogenic shock, sick sinus node syndrome or AV block in the absence of an artificial pacemaker, bradycardia, marked hypotension, bronchospastic disorders, electrolyte disorders, hypersensitivity to the drug. MI more than 6 days but less than 2 years previously. Lactation.
Special Concerns: There is an increased risk of death in those with non-life-threatening arrhythmias. Use with caution during labor and delivery. Safety and effectiveness have not been determined in children. Use with caution in clients with impaired hepatic or renal function. Geriatric clients may require lower dosage.
Side Effects: *CV:* ***New or worsened arrhythmias.*** First-degree AV block, intraventricular conduction delay, palpitations, PVCs, proarrhythmia, bradycardia, atrial fibrillation, angina, syncope, CHF, ***ventricular tachycardia, second-degree AV block,*** increased QRS duration, chest pain, hypotension, bundle branch block. Less commonly, atrial flutter, AV dissociation, flushing, hot flashes, sick sinus syndrome, sinus pause or arrest, SVT, ***cardiac arrest.*** *CNS:* Dizziness, headache, anxiety, drowsiness, fatigue, loss of balance, ataxia, insomnia. Less commonly, abnormal speech, abnormal dreams, abnormal vision, confusion, depression, memory loss, ***apnea,*** psychosis/mania, vertigo, ***seizures, coma,*** numbness, paresthesias. *GI:* Unusual taste, constipation, nausea and/or vomiting, dry mouth, anorexia, flatulence, abdominal pain, cramps, diarrhea, dyspepsia. Less commonly, gastroenteritis and liver abnormalities (cholestasis, hepatitis, elevated enzymes, hepatitis). *Hematologic:* ***Agranulocytosis,*** increased bleeding time, anemia, granulocytopenia, bruising, leukopenia, purpura, anemia, thrombocytopenia. *Miscellaneous:* Blurred vision, dyspnea, weakness, rash, edema, tremors, diaphoresis, joint pain, possible decrease in spermatogenesis. Less commonly, tinnitus, unusual smell sensation, alopecia, eye irritation, hyponatremia, inappropriate ADH secretion, impotence, increased glucose, kidney failure, lupus erythematosus, muscle cramps or weakness, nephrotic syndrome, pain, pruritus.
Laboratory Test Considerations: ↑ ANA titers.

OD **Management of Overdose:** *Symptoms:* Bradycardia, hypotension, IA and intraventricular conduction disturbances, somnolence. ***Rarely, high-grade ventricular arrhythmias and seizures.*** *Treatment:* To control BP and cardiac rhythm, defibrillation and infusion of dopamine or isoproterenol. If seizures occur, diazepam, IV, can be given. External cardiac massage and mechanical respiratory assistance may be required.
Drug Interactions
Beta-adrenergic blockers / ↑ Plasma levels of beta blockers metabolized by the liver
Cimetidine / ↓ Plasma levels of propafenone
Cyclosporine / ↑ Blood trough levels of cyclosporine; ↓ renal function
Digoxin / ↑ Plasma levels of digoxin necessitating a ↓ in the dose of digoxin
Local anesthetics / May ↑ risk of CNS side effects
Quinidine / ↑ Serum levels of propafenone in rapid metabolizers → possible ↑ effect
Rifampin / ↓ Effect of propafenone due to ↑ clearance
Warfarin / May ↑ plasma levels of warfarin necessitating ↓ dose of warfarin
How Supplied: *Tablet:* 150 mg, 225 mg, 300 mg

Dosage

- **Tablets**

Adults, initial: 150 mg q 8 hr; dose may be increased at a minimum of q 3–4 days to 225 mg q 8 hr and, if necessary, to 300 mg q 8 hr.

P

HEALTH CARE CONSIDERATIONS

See also *Health Care Considerations* for *Antiarrhythmic Agents.*

Administration/Storage

1. Always initiate therapy in a hospital setting.
2. The effectiveness and safety of doses exceeding 900 mg/day have not been determined.
3. There is no evidence that the use of propafenone affects the survival or incidence of sudden death with recent MI or SVT.

Assessment

1. Assess ECG and baseline arrhythmias; note any cardiac problems.
2. Monitor CBC, electrolytes, liver and renal function studies. Determine any renal or hepatic disease.
3. Report any significant widening of the QRS complex or any evidence of second- or third-degree AV block.

4. May induce new or more severe arrhythmias; titrate dose based on client response and tolerance.
5. Increase dose more gradually in elderly clients as well as those with previous myocardial damage.
6. Evaluate hematologic studies for anemia, agranulocytosis, leukopenia, thrombocytopenia, or altered prothrombin and coagulation times.

Client/Family Teaching

1. Drink adequate quantities of fluid (2–3 L/day) and add bulk to the diet to avoid constipation.
2. May experience unusual taste in the mouth; report if interferes with eating and nutritional status.
3. Report any increased or unusual bruising/bleeding or S&S of hepatic dysfunction such as yellow sclera, dark-yellow urine, or yellow tinged skin.
4. Report any urinary tract problems or decreased urinary output.
5. Record BP and pulse readings.

Outcome/Evaluate

- Termination of life-threatening VT; restoration of stable rhythm
- Therapeutic drug levels (0.5–3 mcg/mL)

Propantheline bromide

(proh-**PAN**-thih-leen)
Pregnancy Category: C
Norpanth, Pro-Banthine, Propanthel ✱ **(Rx)**
Classification: Anticholinergic, antispasmodic (quaternary ammonium compound)

P

See also *Cholinergic Blocking Agents.*
Action/Kinetics: Duration: 6 hr. Metabolized in the liver and excreted through the urine.
Uses: Adjunct in peptic ulcer therapy. Spastic and inflammatory disease of GI and urinary tracts. Control of salivation and enuresis. Duodenography. Second-line therapy for urinary incontinence.
Special Concerns: Safety and effectiveness for use in children with peptic ulcer have not been established.
How Supplied: *Tablet:* 7.5 mg, 15 mg

Dosage

- **Tablets**

GI problems.

Adults: 15 mg 30 min before meals and 30 mg at bedtime. Reduce dose to 7.5 mg t.i.d. for mild symptoms, geriatric clients, or clients of small stature. **Pediatric:** 0.375 mg/kg (10 mg/m^2) q.i.d. with dose being adjusted as needed.

Urinary incontinence.

Adults: 7.5–30 mg 3–5 times/day; in some, doses as high as 15–60 mg q.i.d. may be needed.

HEALTH CARE CONSIDERATIONS

See also *Health Care Considerations* for *Cholinergic Blocking Agents.*

Assessment

1. Record indications for therapy, type, onset, and duration of symptoms.
2. With ulcer disease or persistent GI complaints, assess for *H. pylori.*
3. A liquid diet is recommended during initiation of therapy with edematous duodenal ulcer.

Client/Family Teaching

1. May cause drowsiness or dizziness. Do not drive or operate equipment until drug effects realized.
2. May impair visual acuity; dark glasses may be necessary. Report if symptoms are persistent.
3. Increase dietary intake of fluids and fiber to minimize the constipating effects of drug therapy.
4. Report any symptoms of urinary retention and persistent constipation.

Outcome/Evaluate

- Relief of GI pain R/T PUD
- Control of urinary incontinence

Propoxyphene hydrochloride

(proh-**POX**-ih-feen)
Pregnancy Category: C
642 Tablets ✱, Darvon, Dolene, Doloxene, Doraphen, Doxaphene, Novo-Propoxyn ✱, Profene, Progesic, Pro Pox, Propoxycon **(C-IV) (Rx)**

Propoxyphene napsylate

(proh-**POX**-ih-feen)
Pregnancy Category: C
Darvon-N **(C-IV) (Rx)**
Classification: Analgesic, narcotic, miscellaneous

Action/Kinetics: Resembles narcotics with respect to its mechanism and analgesic effect; it is one-half to one-third as potent as codeine. Is devoid of antitussive, anti-inflammatory, or antipyretic activity. When taken in excessive doses for long periods, psychologic dependence and occasionally physical dependence and tolerance will be manifested. **Peak plasma levels:** *hydrochloride:* 2–2.5 hr; *napsylate:* 3–4 hr. **Analgesic onset:** 30–60 min. **Peak analgesic effect:** 2–2.5 hr. **Duration:** 4–6 hr. **Therapeutic serum levels:** 0.05–0.12 mcg/mL. **t½, propoxy-**

phene: 6–12 hr; **norpropoxyphene:** 30–36 hr. Extensive first-pass effect; metabolites are excreted in the urine.
Uses: Relief of mild to moderate pain. Napsylate has been used experimentally to suppress the withdrawal syndrome from narcotics.
Contraindications: Hypersensitivity to drug. Use in children.
Special Concerns: Safe use during pregnancy has not been established. Use with caution during lactation.
Side Effects: *GI:* N&V, constipation, abdominal pain. *CNS:* Sedation, dizziness, lightheadedness, headache, weakness, euphoria, dysphoria. *Other:* Skin rashes, visual disturbances. Propoxyphene can produce psychologic dependence, as well as physical dependence and tolerance.
OD **Management of Overdose:** *Symptoms:* Stupor, respiratory depression, ***apnea,*** hypotension, pulmonary edema, ***circulatory collapse, cardiac arrhythmias,*** conduction abnormalities, ***coma, seizures,*** respiratory-metabolic acidosis. *Treatment:* Maintain an adequate airway, artificial respiration, and naloxone, 0.4–2 mg IV (repeat at 2- to 3-min intervals) to combat respiratory depression. Gastric lavage or administration of activated charcoal may be helpful. Correct acidosis and electrolyte imbalance. Acidosis due to lactic acid may require IV sodium bicarbonate.

Drug Interactions

Alcohol, antianxiety drugs, antipsychotic agents, narcotics, sedative-hypnotics / Concomitant use may lead to drowsiness, lethargy, stupor, respiratory, depression, and coma
Carbamazepine / ↑ Effect of carbamazepine due to ↓ breakdown by liver
CNS depressants / Additive CNS depression
Orphenadrine / Concomitant use may lead to confusion, anxiety, and tremors
Phenobarbital / ↑ Effect of phenobarbital due to ↓ breakdown by liver
Skeletal muscle relaxants / Additive respiratory depression
Warfarin / ↑ Hypoprothrombinemic effects of warfarin

How Supplied: Propoxyphene hydrochloride: *Capsule:* 65 mg; Propoxyphene napsylate: *Tablet:* 100 mg

Dosage

- **Capsules (Hydrochloride)**

Analgesia.

Adults: 65 mg q 4 hr, not to exceed 390 mg/day.

- **Tablets (Napsylate)**

Analgesia.

Adults: 100 mg q 4 hr, not to exceed 600 mg/day. Reduce the dose of propoxyphene in renal or hepatic impairment.

HEALTH CARE CONSIDERATIONS

See also *Health Care Considerations* for *Narcotic Analgesics*.

Assessment

1. Record indications for therapy; note onset, duration, and characteristics of pain. Use a pain-rating scale to assess pain. Note other agents prescribed and outcome.
2. Assess for opiate or alcohol dependency.
3. Monitor liver and renal function studies; reduce dose with dysfunction.
4. Determine if smoker; smoking reduces drug effect by increasing metabolism.
5. Use with caution in the elderly and review drug profile to ensure other prescribed agents do not cause additive CNS effects.

Client/Family Teaching

1. May take with food to decrease GI upset.
2. Avoid activities that require mental alertness; may cause dizziness and drowsiness.
3. Do not smoke or consume alcohol or any OTC agents.

Outcome/Evaluate: Relief of pain

COMBINATION DRUG

Propranolol and Hydrochlorothiazide

(proh-**PRAN**-oh-lohl, hy-droh-**klor**-oh-**THIGH**-ah-zyd)
Pregnancy Category: C
Inderide 40/25, Inderide 80/25, Inderide LA 80/50, Inderide LA 120/50, Inderide LA 160/50 **(Rx)**
Classification: Antihypertensive

See also *Propranolol* and *Hydrochlorothiazide*.
Content: *Antihypertensive/diuretic:* Hydrochlorothiazide, 25 mg (Inderide) or 50 mg (Inderide LA).

Beta-adrenergic blocking agent: Propranolol HCl, 40 or 80 mg (Inderide) or 80, 120, or 160 mg (Inderide LA).

Also see information on individual components.
Uses: Hypertension (not indicated for initial therapy).
Special Concerns: Use with caution during lactation. Safety and effectiveness have not been established in children. The risk of hypothermia is increased in geriatric clients.
How Supplied: See Content

P

Dosage

- **Inderide Tablets**

Individualized: 1–2 tablets b.i.d., up to 320 mg propranolol HCl daily.

- **Inderide LA Capsules**

1 capsule once daily.

HEALTH CARE CONSIDERATIONS

See also *Health Care Considerations* for *Antihypertensive Agents* and individual agents.

Administration/Storage

1. Because of side effects from hydrochlorothiazide, do not use Inderide if propranolol must be given in excess of 320 mg/day.
2. If another antihypertensive agent is required, initial dosage should be one-half the usual dose to prevent an excessive drop in BP.
3. Inderide LA is not a milligram-to-milligram substitute for Inderide because the LA produces lower blood levels.

Client/Family Teaching: Take exactly as prescribed. Continue diet, exercise, and life style changes necessary to ensure BP control.

Outcome/Evaluate: ↓ BP; control of hypertension

Propranolol hydrochloride

(proh-**PRAN**-oh-lohl)

Pregnancy Category: C

Apo-Propranolol ✱, Detensol ✱, Dom-Propranolol ✱, Inderal, Inderal 10, 20, 40, 60, 80, and 90, Inderal LA, Novo-Pranol ✱, Nu-Propranolol ✱, PMS Propranolol ✱, Propranolol Intensol **(Rx)**

Classification: Beta-adrenergic blocking agent; antiarrhythmic (type II)

See also *Beta-Adrenergic Blocking Agents.*

Action/Kinetics: Manifests both beta-1- and beta-2-adrenergic blocking activity. Antiarrhythmic action is due to both beta-adrenergic receptor blockade and a direct membrane-stabilizing action on the cardiac cell. Has no intrinsic sympathomimetic activity and has high lipid solubility. **Onset, PO:** 30 min; **IV:** immediate. **Maximum effect:** 1–1.5 hr. **Duration:** 3–5 hr. **t½:** 2–3 hr (8–11 hr for long-acting). **Therapeutic serum level, antiarrhythmic:** 0.05–0.1 mcg/mL. Completely metabolized by liver and excreted in urine. Although food increases bioavailability, absorption may be decreased.

Uses: Hypertension (alone or in combination with other antihypertensive agents). Angina pectoris, hypertrophic subaortic stenosis, prophylaxis of MI, pheochromocytoma, prophylaxis of migraine, essential tremor. Cardiac arrhythmias including ventricular tachycardias and arrhythmias, tachycardias due to digitalis intoxication, supraventricular arrhythmias, PVCs, resistant tachyarrhythmias due to anesthesia/catecholamines.

Investigational: Schizophrenia, tremors due to parkinsonism, aggressive behavior, antipsychotic-induced akathisia, rebleeding due to esophageal varices, situational anxiety, acute panic attacks, gastric bleeding in portal hypertension, vaginal contraceptive, anxiety, alcohol withdrawal syndrome, winter depression.

Contraindications: Bronchial asthma, bronchospasms including severe COPD.

Special Concerns: It is dangerous to use propranolol for pheochromocytoma unless an alpha-adrenergic blocking agent is already in use.

Laboratory Test Considerations: ↑ Blood urea, serum transaminase, alkaline phosphatase, LDH. Interference with glaucoma screening test.

Additional Side Effects: Psoriasis-like eruptions, skin necrosis, SLE (rare).

Additional Drug Interactions

Haloperidol / Severe hypotension
Hydralazine / ↑ Effect of both agents
Methimazole / May ↑ effects of propranolol
Phenobarbital / ↓ Effect of propranolol due to ↑ breakdown by liver
Propylthiouracil / May ↑ the effects of propranolol
Rifampin / ↓ Effect of propranolol due to ↑ breakdown by liver
Smoking / ↓ Serum levels and ↑ clearance of propranolol

How Supplied: *Capsule, extended release:* 60 mg, 80 mg, 120 mg, 160 mg; *Concentrate:* 80 mg/mL; *Injection:* 1 mg/mL; *Solution:* 20 mg/5 mL, 40 mg/5 mL; *Tablet:* 10 mg, 20 mg, 40 mg, 60 mg, 80 mg

Dosage

- **Tablets, Sustained-Release Capsules, Oral Solution, Concentrate**

Hypertension.

Initial: 40 mg b.i.d. or 80 mg of sustained-release/day; **then,** increase dose to maintenance level of 120–240 mg/day given in two to three divided doses or 120–160 mg of sustained-release medication once daily. Do not exceed 640 mg/day. **Pediatric, initial:** 0.5 mg/kg b.i.d.; dose may be increased at 3- to 5-day intervals to a maximum of 1 mg/kg b.i.d. Calculate the dosage range by weight and not by body surface area.

Angina.

Initial: 80–320 mg b.i.d., t.i.d., or q.i.d.; or, 80 mg of sustained-release once daily; **then,** increase dose gradually to maintenance level of 160 mg/day of sustained-release capsule. Do not exceed 320 mg/day.

Arrhythmias.

10–30 mg t.i.d.–q.i.d. given after meals and at bedtime.

Hypertrophic subaortic stenosis.

20–40 mg t.i.d.–q.i.d. before meals and at bedtime or 80–160 mg of sustained-release medication given once daily.

MI prophylaxis.

180–240 mg/day given in three to four divided doses. Do not exceed 240 mg/day.

Pheochromocytoma, preoperatively.

60 mg/day for 3 days before surgery, given concomitantly with an alpha-adrenergic blocking agent.

Inoperable tumors.

30 mg/day in divided doses.

Migraine.

Initial: 80 mg sustained-release medication given once daily; **then,** increase dose gradually to maintenance of 160–240 mg/day in divided doses. If a satisfactory response has not been observed after 4–6 weeks, discontinue the drug and withdraw gradually.

Essential tremor.

Initial: 40 mg b.i.d.; **then,** 120 mg/day up to a maximum of 320 mg/day.

Aggressive behavior.

80–300 mg/day.

Antipsychotic-induced akathisia.

20–80 mg/day.

Tremors associated with Parkinson's disease.

160 mg/day.

Rebleeding from esophageal varices.

20–180 mg b.i.d.

Schizophrenia.

300–5,000 mg/day.

Acute panic symptoms.

40–320 mg/day.

Anxiety.

80–320 mg/day.

Intermittent explosive disorder.

50–1,600 mg/day.

Nonvariceal gastric bleeding in portal hypertension.

24–480 mg/day.

• **IV**

Life-threatening arrhythmias or those occurring under anesthesia.

1–3 mg not to exceed 1 mg/min; a second dose may be given after 2 min, with subsequent doses q 4 hr. Begin PO therapy as soon as possible. Although use in pediatrics is not recommended, investigational doses of 0.01–0.1 mg/kg/dose, up to a maximum of 1 mg/dose (by slow push), have been used for arrhythmias.

HEALTH CARE CONSIDERATIONS

See also *Health Considerations* for *Beta-Adrenergic Blocking Agents* and *Antihypertensive Agents.*

Administration/Storage

1. Do not administer for a minimum of 2 weeks of MAO inhibitor drug use.

IV 2. If signs of serious myocardial depression occur, slowly infuse isoproterenol (Isuprel) IV.

3. For IV use, dilute 1 mg in 10 mL of D5W and administer IV over at least 1 min. May be further reconstituted in 50 mL of dextrose or saline solution and infused IVPB over 10–15 min.

4. After IV administration, have emergency drugs and equipment available to combat hypotension or circulatory collapse.

Assessment

1. Record indications for therapy, type, onset, duration of symptoms, and other agents prescribed.

2. Note ECG, VS, and cardiopulmonary assessment. Assess for pulmonary disease, bronchospasms, or depression.

3. Report rash, fever, and/or purpura; S&S of hypersensitivity reaction.

4. Monitor VS, I&O. Observe for S&S of CHF (e.g., SOB, rales, edema, and weight gain).

Client/Family Teaching

1. May cause drowsiness; assess drug response before performing activities that require mental alertness.

2. Do not smoke; smoking decreases serum levels and interferes with drug clearance.

3. May mask symptoms of hypoglycemia; monitor FS carefully.

4. Check BP and HR weekly; report any significant changes.

5. Do not stop abruptly; may precipitate hypertension, myocardial ischemia, or cardiac arrhythmias.

6. Dress appropriately; may cause increased sensitivity to cold.

7. Avoid alcohol and any OTC agents containing alpha-adrenergic stimulants or sympathomimetics.

8. Report any persistent side effects, e.g., skin rashes, abnormal bleeding, unusual crying, or feelings of depression.

Outcome/Evaluate

- ↓ BP, ↓ HR
- ↓ Frequency/intensity of angina; prophylaxis of myocardial reinfarction
- Migraine prophylaxis
- Control of tachyarrhythmias
- Desired behavioral changes

P

• Therapeutic drug levels as an antiarrhythmic (0.05–0.1 mcg/mL)

Propylthiouracil

(proh-pill-thigh-oh-**YOUR**-ah-sill)

Pregnancy Category: D

Propyl-Thyracil ✱ **(Rx)**

Classification: Antithyroid preparation

See also *Antithyroid Drugs.*

Action/Kinetics: May be preferred for treatment of thyroid storm, as it inhibits peripheral conversion of thyroxine to triiodothyronine. Rapidly absorbed from the GI tract. **Duration:** 2–3 hr. **t½:** 1–2 hr. **Onset:** 10–20 days. **Time to peak effect:** 2–10 weeks. Eighty percent is protein bound. Metabolized by the liver and excreted through the kidneys.

Special Concerns: Incidence of vasculitis is increased.

Drug Interactions: Propylthiouracil may produce hypoprothrombinemia, adding to the effect of anticoagulants.

How Supplied: *Tablet:* 50 mg

Dosage

• **Tablets**

Hyperthyroidism.

Adults, initial: 300 mg/day (up to 900 mg/day may be required in some clients with severe hyperthyroidism) given as one to four divided doses; **maintenance, usual:** 100–150 mg/day. **Pediatric, 6–10 years, initial:** 50–150 mg/day in one to four divided doses; **over 10 years, initial:** 150–300 mg/day in one to four divided doses. Maintenance for all pediatric use is based on response. **Alternative dose for children, initial:** 5–7 mg/kg/day (150–200 mg/m^2/day) in divided doses q 8 hr; **maintenance:** ⅓–⅔ the initial dose when the client is euthyroid.

Thyrotoxic crisis.

Adults: 200–400 mg q 4 hr during the first day as an adjunct to other treatments.

Neonatal thyrotoxicosis.

10 mg/kg daily in divided doses.

HEALTH CARE CONSIDERATIONS

See also *Health Care Considerations* for *Antithyroid Drugs.*

Client/Family Teaching

1. Take only as directed. May take with meals to decrease GI upset.
2. Avoid dietary sources of iodine (shellfish, kelp, iodized salt).
3. Report any fever, sore throat, enlarged cervical lymph nodes, or rash.
4. Alert provider of unusual bruising/bleeding; report for labs.
5. Report S&S of hypothyroidism (cold intolerance, increased fatigue, mental depression).

Outcome/Evaluate

• Normal metabolism; control of S&S (↑ weight, ↓ sweating, ↓ HR)

• Suppression of thyroid hormones (↓ T_3, T_4) after 3 weeks of therapy

Pseudoephedrine hydrochloride

(soo-doh-eh-**FED**-rin)

Pregnancy Category: B

Allermed, Balminil Decongestant Syrup ✱, Cenafed, Children's Congestion Relief, Children's Sudafed Liquid, Congestion Relief, Contac Cold 12 Hour Relief Non Drowsy ✱, Decofed Syrup, DeFed-60, Dorcol Children's Decongestant Liquid, Efidac/24, Eltor 120 ✱, Genaphed, Halofed, PediaCare Infants' Oral Decongestant Drops, PMS-Pseudoephedrine ✱, Pseudo, Pseudo-Gest, Seudotabs, Sinustop Pro, Sudafed, Sudafed 12 Hour, Triaminic Oral Pediatric Drops ✱ **(OTC)**

Pseudoephedrine sulfate

(soo-doh-eh-**FED**-rin)

Pregnancy Category: B

Afrin Extended-Release Tablets, Drixoral Day ✱, Drixoral N.D. ✱, Drixoral Non-Drowsy Formula **(OTC)**

Classification: Direct- and indirect-acting sympathomimetic, nasal decongestant

See also *Sympathomimetic Drugs.*

Action/Kinetics: Produces direct stimulation of both alpha-(pronounced) and beta-adrenergic receptors, as well as indirect stimulation through release of norepinephrine from storage sites. Results in decongestant effect on the nasal mucosa. Systemic administration eliminates possible damage to the nasal mucosa. **Onset:** 15–30 min. **Time to peak effect:** 30–60 min. **Duration:** 3–4 hr. **Extended-release: duration,** 8–12 hr. Urinary excretion slowed by alkalinization, causing reabsorption of drug.

Uses: Nasal congestion associated with sinus conditions, otitis, allergies. Relief of eustachian tube congestion.

Additional Contraindications: Lactation. Use of sustained-release products in children less than 12 years of age.

Special Concerns: Use with caution in newborn and premature infants due to a higher risk of side effects. Geriatric clients may be more prone to age-related prostatic hypertrophy.

How Supplied: Pseudoephedrine hydrochloride: *Liquid:* 7.5 mg/0.8 mL, 30 mg/5 mL; *Syrup:* 15 mg/5 mL, 30 mg/5 mL; *Tablet:* 30 mg, 60 mg; *Tablet, extended release:* 120 mg, 240 mg. Pseudoephedrine sulfate: *Tablet:* 60 mg

Dosage

HYDROCHLORIDE

- **Oral Solution, Syrup, Tablets**

Decongestant.

Adults: 60 mg q 4–6 hr, not to exceed 240 mg in 24 hr. **Pediatric, 6–12 years:** 30 mg using the oral solution or syrup q 4–6 hr, not to exceed 120 mg in 24 hr; **2–6 years:** 15 mg using the oral solution or syrup q 4–6 hr, not to exceed 60 mg in 24 hr. Individualize the dose for children less than 2 years of age.

- **Extended-Release Capsules, Tablets**

Decongestant.

Adults and children over 12 years: 120 mg q 12 hr or 240 mg q 24 hr. Use is not recommended for children less than 12 years of age.

SULFATE

- **Extended-Release Tablets**

Decongestant.

Adults and children over 12 years: 120 mg q 12 hr. Use is not recommended for children less than 12 years of age.

HEALTH CARE CONSIDERATIONS

See also *Health Care Considerations* for *Sympathomimetic Drugs.*

Client/Family Teaching

1. Avoid taking at bedtime; stimulation may produce insomnia.
2. With hypertension, report headaches, dizziness, or increased BP.
3. Do not crush or chew extended-release products.
4. Report if symptoms do not improve after 3–5 days.

Outcome/Evaluate: Relief of nasal, sinus, or eustachian tube congestion

Psyllium hydrophilic muciloid

(SILL-ee-um hi-droh-FILL-ik)

Effer-syllium, Fiberall Natural Flavor, Fiberall Orange Flavor, Fiberall Wafers, Fibrepur ✱, Hydrocil Instant, Konsyl, Konsyl-D, Metamucil, Metamucil Lemon-Lime Flavor, Metamucil Orange Flavor, Metamucil Sugar Free, Metamucil Sugar Free Orange Flavor, Modane Bulk, Natural Vegetable, Novo-Mucilax ✱, Perdiem Fiber, Prodiem Plain ✱, Reguloid Natural, Reguloid Orange, Reguloid Sugar Free Orange, Reguloid Sugar Free Regular, Serutan, Siblin, Syllact, V-Lax **(OTC)**

Classification: Laxative, bulk-forming

See also *Laxatives.*

Action/Kinetics: Obtained from the fruit of various species of plantago. The powder forms a gelatinous mass with water, which adds bulk to the stools and stimulates peristalsis. Also has a demulcent effect on an inflamed intestinal mucosa. Products may also contain dextrose, sodium bicarbonate, monobasic potassium phosphate, citric acid, and benzyl benzoate. Laxative effects usually occur in 12–24 hr. The full effect may take 2–3 days. Dependence may occur.

Uses: Prophylaxis of constipation in clients who should not strain during defecation. Short-term treatment of constipation; useful in geriatric clients with diminished colonic motor response and during pregnancy and postpartum to reestablish normal bowel function. To soften feces during fecal impaction.

Contraindications: Severe abdominal pain or intestinal obstruction.

Side Effects: Obstruction of the esophagus, stomach, small intestine, and rectum.

Drug Interactions: Do not use concomitantly with salicylates, nitrofurantoin, or cardiac glycosides (e.g., digitalis).

How Supplied: *Capsule*; *Granule*; *Granule for reconstitution*; *Powder for reconstitution:* 3.4 g/15 mL; *Wafer*

P

Dosage

Dose depends on the product. General information on adult dosage follows.

- **Granules/Flakes**

Adults: 1–2 teaspoons 1–3 times/day spread on food or with a glass of water.

- **Powder**

Adults: 1 rounded teaspoon in 8 oz of liquid 1–3 times/day.

- **Effervescent Powder**

Adults: 1 packet in water 1–3 times/day.

- **Chewable Pieces**

Adults: 2 pieces followed by a glass of water 1–3 times/day.

HEALTH CARE CONSIDERATIONS

See Health Care Considerations for *Laxatives.*

Client/Family Teaching

1. Mix powder with plenty of liquid just prior to administering; otherwise, the mixture may become thick and difficult to drink.
2. The powder may be noxious and irritating

when removing from the packets or canister. Open in a well-ventilated area and avoid inhaling particulate matter.
3. Take exactly as directed. Report lack of response or intolerable side effects.
Outcome/Evaluate: Prophylaxis/relief of constipation

Pyrantel pamoate

(pie-**RAN**-tell)
Pregnancy Category: C
Antiminth, Combantrin ✱, Pin-Rid, Pin-X, Reese's Pinworm **(OTC)**
Classification: Anthelmintic

See also *Anthelmintics.*
Action/Kinetics: Has neuromuscular blocking effect which paralyzes the helminth, allowing it to be expelled through the feces. Also inhibits cholinesterases. Poorly absorbed from GI tract. **Peak plasma levels:** 0.05–0.13 mcg/mL after 1–3 hr. Partially metabolized in liver. Fifty percent is excreted unchanged in feces and less than 15% excreted unchanged in urine.
Uses: Pinworm (enterobiasis) and roundworm (ascariasis) infestations. Multiple helminth infections, as it is also effective against roundworm and hookworm.
Contraindications: Pregnancy. Hepatic disease.
Special Concerns: Use with caution in presence of liver dysfunction. Safe use in children less than 2 years of age has not been established.
Side Effects: *GI* (most frequent): Anorexia, N&V, abdominal cramps, diarrhea. *Hepatic:* Transient elevation of AST. *CNS:* Headache, dizziness, drowsiness, insomnia. *Miscellaneous:* Skin rashes.
Drug Interactions: Use with piperazine for ascariasis results in antagonism of the effect of both drugs.
How Supplied: *Suspension:* 144 mg/30 mL, 720 mg/5 mL; *Tablet:* 180 mg

Dosage

- **Liquid Oral Suspension, Tablets**

Adults and children: One dose of 11 mg/kg (maximum). **Maximum total dose:** 1.0 g.

HEALTH CARE CONSIDERATIONS

See also *Health Care Considerations* for *Anthelmintics.*
Client/Family Teaching
1. May be taken without regard to food intake. May take with milk or fruit juices.
2. May cause dizziness or drowsiness; do not engage in activities that require mental alertness.
3. Purging is not required.
4. When treating pinworms, review client/family precautions R/T transmission. (See *Anthelmintics.*)
Outcome/Evaluate: Resolution of infection; negative stool and perianal swabs

Pyridostigmine bromide

(peer-id-oh-**STIG**-meen)
Pregnancy Category: C
Mestinon, Mestinon-SR ✱, Regonol **(Rx)**
Classification: Indirectly acting cholinergic-acetylcholinesterase inhibitor

For all information, see also *Neostigmine.*
Action/Kinetics: Has a slower onset, longer duration of action, and fewer side effects than neostigmine. **Onset, PO:** 30–45 min for syrup and tablets and 30–60 min for extended-release tablets; **IM:** 15 min; **IV:** 2–5 min. **Duration, PO:** 3–6 hr for syrup and tablets and 6–12 hr for extended-release tablets; **IM, IV:** 2–4 hr. Poorly absorbed from the GI tract; excreted in urine up to 72 hr after administration.
Uses: Myasthenia gravis. Antidote for nondepolarizing muscle relaxants (e.g., tubocurarine).
Additional Contraindications: Sensitivity to bromides.
Special Concerns: Safe use during pregnancy and during lactation has not been established. May cause uterine irritability and premature labor if given IV to pregnant women near term. Duration of action may be increased in the elderly.
Additional Side Effects: Skin rash. Thrombophlebitis after IV use.
OD **Management of Overdose:** *Symptoms:* Abdominal cramps, vomiting, diarrhea, epigastric distress, excessive salivation, cold sweating, pallor, blurred vision, urinary urgency, fasciculation and ***paralysis of voluntary muscles*** (including the tongue), miosis, increased BP (may be accompanied by bradycardia), sensation of internal trembling, panic, severe anxiety. *Treatment:* Discontinue medication temporarily. Give atropine, 0.5–1 mg IV (up to 5–10 mg or more may be needed to get HR to 80 beats/min). Supportive treatment including artificial respiration and oxygen.
How Supplied: *Injection:* 5 mg/mL; *Syrup:* 60 mg/5 mL; *Tablet:* 60 mg; *Tablet, extended release:* 180 mg

Dosage

- **Syrup, Tablets**

Myasthenia gravis.
Adults: 60–120 mg q 3–4 hr with dosage adjusted to client response. **Maintenance:** 600 mg/day (range: 60 mg–1.5 g). **Pediatric:** 7 mg/kg (200 mg/m²) daily in five to six divided doses.

- **Sustained-Release Tablets**

Myasthenia gravis.
Adults: 180–540 mg 1–2 times/day with at least 6 hr between doses. Sustained-release tablets not recommended for use in children.

- **IM, IV**

Myasthenia gravis.
Adults, IM, IV: 2 mg (about 1/30 the adult dose) q 2–3 hr.
Neonates of myasthenic mothers.
IM: 0.05–0.15 mg/kg q 4–6 hr.
Antidote for nondepolarizing drugs.
Adults, IV: 10–20 mg with 0.6–1.2 mg atropine sulfate given IV.

HEALTH CARE CONSIDERATIONS

See also *Health Care Considerations* for *Neostigmine.*

Administration/Storage

1. During dosage adjustment, administer in a closely monitored environment.
IV 2. Parenteral dosage is 1/30 of the PO dose. May give undiluted at a rate of 0.5 mg IV over 1 min for myasthenia and at a rate of 5 mg IV over 1 min (with atropine) for reversal of nondepolarizing drug effects.

Assessment

1. Monitor VS and observe for toxic reactions demonstrated by generalized cholinergic stimulation.
2. Assess for muscular weakness; may signal impending myasthenic crisis and cholinergic overdose.
3. Determine the best individualized administration schedule according to client's routines and life-style.

Client/Family Teaching

1. Myasthenia is an autoimmune disease with an unclear etiology. Medications correct acetycholine and cholinesterase imbalance at myoneural junction, which facilitates muscle contraction.
2. Do not crush and do not take extended-release tablets more often than q 6 hr; may be taken with conventional tablets, if prescribed.
3. With rest, muscle weakness and fatigue are temporarily resolved.
4. Rest and report symptoms of toxic reaction and myasthenic crisis.
5. Take medication as prescribed, since too early administration may result in cholinergic crisis whereas too late administration may result in myasthenic crisis.
6. Drug resistance may develop; close medical supervision and prompt reporting of all side effects is paramount.
7. Identify local support groups that may assist client to understand and cope with this disorder.

Outcome/Evaluate

- Improvement in muscle strength/function
- Reversal of nondepolarizing drugs

Pyridoxine hydrochloride (Vitamin B_6)

(peer-ih-**DOX**-een)
Pregnancy Category: A
Nestrex (Rx: Injection; OTC: Tablets)
Classification: Vitamin B complex

Action/Kinetics: A water-soluble, heat-resistant vitamin that is destroyed by light. Acts as a coenzyme in the metabolism of protein, carbohydrates, and fat. As the amount of protein increases in the diet, the pyridoxine requirement increases. However, pyridoxine deficiency alone is rare. **t½:** 2–3 weeks. Metabolized in the liver and excreted through the urine.
Uses: Pyridoxine deficiency including poor diet, drug-induced (e.g., oral contraceptives, isoniazid), and inborn errors of metabolism. *Investigational:* Hydrazine poisoning, PMS, high urine oxalate levels, N&V due to pregnancy.
Special Concerns: Safety and effectiveness have not been established in children.
Side Effects: *CNS:* Unstable gait; decreased sensation to touch, temperature, and vibration; paresthesia, sleepiness; numbness of feet; awkwardness of hands; perioral numbness. *NOTE:* Abuse and dependence have been noted in adults administered 200 mg/day.
OD **Management of Overdose:** *Symptoms:* Ataxia, severe sensory neuropathy. *Treatment:* Discontinue pyridoxine; allow up to 6 months for CNS sensation to return.
Drug Interactions
Chloramphenicol / ↑ Pyridoxine requirements
Contraceptives, oral / ↑ Pyridoxine requirements
Cycloserine / ↑ Pyridoxine requirements
Ethionamide / ↑ Pyridoxine requirements
Hydralazine / ↑ Pyridoxine requirements
Immunosuppressants / ↑ Pyridoxine requirements

P

Isoniazid / ↑ Pyridoxine requirements
Levodopa / Daily doses exceeding 5 mg pyridoxine antagonize the therapeutic effect of levodopa
Penicillamine / ↑ Pyridoxine requirements
Phenobarbital / Pyridoxine ↓ serum levels of phenobarbital
Phenytoin / Pyridoxine ↓ serum levels of phenytoin
How Supplied: *Capsule:* 150 mg, 500 mg; *Enteric coated tablet:* 20 mg; *Injection:* 100 mg/mL; *Tablet:* 10 mg, 25 mg, 32.5 mg, 50 mg, 100 mg, 200 mg, 250 mg, 500 mg; *Tablet, extended release:* 200 mg

Dosage

• **Capsules, Enteric-Coated Tablets, Extended-Release Tablets, Tablets**

Dietary supplement.

Adults: 10–20 mg/day for 2 weeks; **then,** 2–5 mg/day as part of a multivitamin preparation for several weeks. **Pediatric,** 2.5–10 mg/day for 3 weeks; **then,** 2–5 mg/day as part of a multivitamin preparation for several weeks.

Pyridoxine dependency syndrome.

Adults and children, initial: 30–600 mg/day; **maintenance,** 30 mg/day for life. **Infants, maintenance:** 2–10 mg/day for life.

Drug-induced deficiency.

Adults, prophylaxis: 10–50 mg/day for penicillamine or 100–300 mg/day for cycloserine, hydralazine, or isoniazid. **Adults, treatment:** 50–200 mg/day for 3 weeks followed by 25–100 mg/day to prevent relapse. **Adults, alcoholism:** 50 mg/day for 2–4 weeks; if anemia responds, continue pyridoxine indefinitely.

Hereditary sideroblastic anemia.

Adults: 200–600 mg/day for 1–2 months; **then,** 30–50 mg/day for life.

• **IM, IV**

Pyridoxine dependency syndrome.

Adults: 30–600 mg/day. **Pediatric:** 10–100 mg initially.

Drug-induced deficiency.

Adults: 50–200 mg/day for 3 weeks followed by 25–100 mg/day as needed.

Cycloserine poisoning.

Adults: 300 mg/day.

Isoniazid poisoning.

Adults: 1 g for each gram of isoniazid taken.

HEALTH CARE CONSIDERATIONS

Administration/Storage

1. If receiving levodopa, avoid preparations of vitamins containing B_6 as this decreases the availability of levodopa to the brain.

IV 2. May be administered by direct IV or placed in infusion solutions.

Assessment

1. Record indications for therapy.
2. Take a complete drug history. Report cycloserine, isoniazid, or oral contraceptive use as these increase pyridoxine requirements.

Client/Family Teaching

1. Foods high in vitamin B_6 include potatoes, lima beans, broccoli, bananas, chicken breast, liver, whole-grain cereals. Well-balanced diets are the best source of vitamins.
2. If prescribed levodopa, avoid vitamin supplements containing vitamin B_6. More than 5 mg of the vitamin antagonizes levodopa effect. At the same time, concomitant carbidopa administration will prevent effects of vitamin B_6 on levodopa.
3. If taking phenobarbital and/or phenytoin, obtain serum drug levels routinely, as pyridoxine alters serum concentrations.
4. Pyridoxine may inhibit lactation.
5. Identify reasons for drug therapy, e.g., to prevent toxicity (peripheral neuropathy) with long term isoniazid or contraceptive therapy, to replace vitamin B_6 with inborn errors of metabolism or with poor nutrition.

Outcome/Evaluate

• Relief of symptoms of pyridoxine deficiency
• Prophylaxis of drug-induced deficiency; ↓ toxic drug side effects

Q

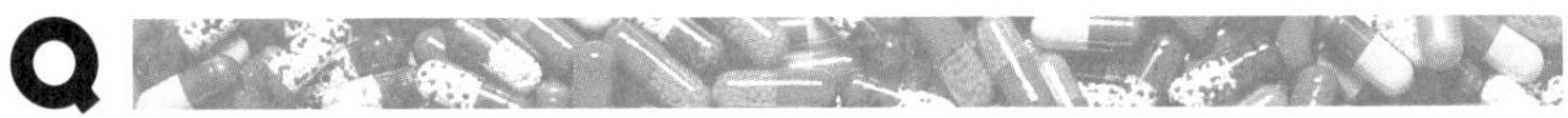

Quetiapine fumarate

(kweh-**TYE**-ah-peen)
Pregnancy Category: C
Seroquel **(Rx)**
Classification: Antipsychotic drug

Action/Kinetics: Mechanism unknown but may act as an antagonist at dopamine D_2 and serotonin $5HT_2$ receptors. Side effects may be due to antagonism of other receptors (e.g., histamine H_1, dopamine D_1, adrenergic alpha-1 and alpha-2, serotonin $5HT_{1A}$). Rapidly absorbed. **Peak plasma levels:** 1.5 hr. Metabolized by liver and excreted through urine and feces. **t½, terminal:** About 6 hr.
Uses: Management of psychoses.
Contraindications: Lactation.

Special Concerns: Use with caution in liver disease, in those at risk for aspiration pneumonia, and in those with history of seizures or conditions that lower seizure threshold (e.g., Alzheimer's). Safety and efficacy have not been determined in children.
Side Effects: Side effects with incidence of 1% or more are listed. *Body as a whole:* Asthenia, rash, fever, weight gain, back pain, flu syndrome. *CNS:* Headache, somnolence, dizziness, hypertonia, dysarthria. *GI:* Constipation, dry mouth, dyspepsia, anorexia, abdominal pain. *CV:* Orthostatic hypotension, syncope, tachycardia, palpitation. *Respiratory:* Pharyngitis, rhinitis, increased cough, dyspnea. *Miscellaneous:* Peripheral edema, sweating, leukopenia, ear pain. *Note:* ***Neuroleptic malignant syndrome*** and ***seizures,*** although rare, may occur.
Laboratory Test Considerations: ↑ ALT during initial therapy, AST, total cholesterol, triglycerides.
OD **Management of Overdose:** *Symptoms:* Drowsiness, sedation, tachycardia, hypotension, dystonic reaction of the head and neck, seizures, obtundation. *Treatment:* Cardiovascular monitoring for arrhythmias. If antiarrhythmic therapy is used, disopyramide, procainamide, and quinidine increase risk of prolongation of QT. Treat hypotension and circulatory shock with IV fluids or sympathomimetic drugs (do not use epinephrine or dopamine as they may worsen hypotension). Use anticholinergic drugs to treat severe extrapyramidal symptoms.
Drug Interactions
Barbiturates / ↓ Effect of quetiapine due to ↑ breakdown by liver
Carbamazepine / ↓ Effect of quetiapine due to ↑ breakdown by liver
Dopamine agonists / Quetiapine antagonizes effect
Glucocorticoids / ↓ Effect of quetiapine due to ↑ breakdown by liver
Levodopa / Quetiapine antagonizes effect
Phenytoin / ↓ Effect of quetiapine due to ↑ breakdown by liver
Rifampin / ↓ Effect of quetiapine due to ↑ breakdown by liver
Thioridazine / ↑ Clearance of quetiapine
How Supplied: *Tablets:* 25 mg, 100 mg, 200 mg

Dosage

- **Tablets**

  Psychoses.

Initial: 25 mg b.i.d., with increases of 25 to 50 mg b.i.d. or t.i.d. on second and third day, as tolerated. Target dose range, by fourth day, is 300 to 400 mg daily. Further dosage adjustments can occur at intervals of two or more days. The antipsychotic dose range is 150 to 750 mg/day.

HEALTH CARE CONSIDERATIONS

Administration/Storage

1. Total daily dose is divided and given two or three times a day.
2. Effectiveness for more than 6 weeks has not been evaluated. Evaluate long-term usefulness periodically. Continue therapy at lowest dose to maintain remission.
3. Slower rate of dose titration and lower target dose is considered for elderly, in hepatic impairment, debilitated clients, and in those predisposed to hypotension.
4. Titration is not required when restarting clients who have had an interval of less than one week off quetiapine. Initial titration schedule is followed if clients have been off drug for more than one week.

Assessment

1. Record clinical presentation and behavioral manifestations.
2. Note any predisposition to hypotensive reactions if debilitated or if hepatic impairment present.
3. Record ophthalmic exam initially, and at 6 mo intervals, to assess for cataract formation.
4. Assess for history of cardiovascular disease; note VS, ECG, and LFTs.

Client/Family Teaching

1. May take with or without food.
2. Do not perform activities that require mental alertness until after titration period and until drug effects realized; may impair judgement and motor skills, and cause sleepiness.
3. Avoid alcohol and any OTC agents without approval.
4. Use reliable contraception; report if pregnancy suspected. Do not breastfeed.
5. Report any evidence of extrapyramidal symptoms; tardive dyskinesia (involuntary movements).
6. Avoid situations where overheating or dehydration may occur.
7. Long-term usefulness must be evaluated periodically while on lowest dose to maintain remission.

Outcome/Evaluate: Control of manifestations of psychotic disorders

Quinapril hydrochloride

(KWIN-ah-prill)

Pregnancy Category: D
Accupril **(Rx)**
Classification: Angiotensin-converting enzyme inhibitor

See also *Angiotensin-Converting Enzyme Inhibitors.*

Action/Kinetics: Onset: 1 hr. **Time to peak serum levels:** 1 hr. **Peak decrease in BP:** 2–6 hr. Metabolized to quinaprilat, the active metabolite. **t½, quinaprilat:** 2–3 hr. **Duration:** 18–24 hr. Significantly bound to plasma proteins. Food reduces absorption. Metabolized with approximately 60% excreted through the urine and 37% excreted in the feces. Also appears to improve endothelial function, an early marker of coronary atherosclerosis.

Uses: Alone or in combination with a thiazide diuretic for the treatment of hypertension. Adjunct with a diuretic or digitalis to treat CHF in those not responding adequately to diuretics or digitalis.

Special Concerns: Use with caution during lactation. Safety and effectiveness have not been determined in children. Geriatric clients may be more sensitive to the effects of quinapril and manifest higher peak quinaprilat blood levels.

Side Effects: *CV:* Vasodilation, tachycardia, ***heart failure,*** palpitations, chest pain, hypotension, ***MI, CVA, hypertensive crisis,*** angina pectoris, orthostatic hypotension, ***cardiac rhythm disturbances, cardiogenic shock***. *GI:* Dry mouth or throat, constipation, diarrhea, N&V, abdominal pain, hepatitis, pancreatitis, ***GI hemorrhage.*** *CNS:* Somnolence, vertigo, insomnia, sleep disturbances, paresthesias, nervousness, depression, headache, dizziness, fatigue. *Hematologic:* ***Agranulocytosis,*** bone marrow depression, thrombocytopenia. *Dermatologic:* ***Angioedema of the lips, tongue, glottis, and larynx;*** sweating, pruritus, exfoliative dermatitis, photosensitivity, dermatopolymyositis, flushing, rash. *Body as a whole:* Malaise, back pain. *GU:* Oliguria and/or progressive azotemia and rarely ***acute renal failure and/or death in severe heart failure.*** Impotence. Worsening renal failure. *Respiratory:* Pharyngitis, cough, asthma, bronchospasm, dyspnea. *Miscellaneous:* Oligohydramnios in fetuses exposed to the drug in utero. Abnormal liver function tests, syncope, hyperkalemia, amblyopia, syncope, malagia, viral infections.

OD **Management of Overdose:** *Symptoms:* Commonly, hypotension. *Treatment:* IV infusion of normal saline to restore blood pressure.

Drug Interactions

Potassium-containing salt substitutes / ↑ Risk of hyperkalemia
Potassium-sparing diuretics / ↑ Risk of hyperkalemia
Potassium supplements / ↑ Risk of hyperkalemia
Tetracyclines / ↓ Absorption of tetracycline due to high magnesium content of quinapril tablets

How Supplied: *Tablet:* 5 mg, 10 mg, 20 mg, 40 mg

Dosage

- **Tablets**

Hypertension.

Initial: 10 or 20 mg once daily; **then,** adjust dosage based on BP response at peak (2–6 hr) and trough (predose) blood levels. The dose should be adjusted at 2-week intervals. **Maintenance:** 20, 40, or 80 mg daily as a single dose or in two equally divided doses. With impaired renal function, the initial dose should be 10 mg if the C_{CR} is greater than 60 mL/min, 5 mg if the C_{CR} is between 30 and 60 mL/min, and 2.5 mg if the C_{CR} is between 10 and 30 mL/min. If the initial dose is well tolerated, the drug may be given the following day as a b.i.d. regimen.

CHF.

Initial: 5 mg b.i.d. If this dose is well tolerated, titrate clients at weekly intervals until an effective dose, usually 20–40 mg daily in two equally divided doses, is attained. Undesirable hypotension, orthostasis, or azotemia may prevent this dosage level from being reached.

HEALTH CARE CONSIDERATIONS

See also *Angiotensin-Converting Enzyme Inhibitors* and *Antihypertensive Agents.*

Administration/Storage

1. If taking a diuretic, discontinue the diuretic 2–3 days prior to beginning quinapril. If the BP is not controlled, reinstitute the diuretic. If the diuretic cannot be discontinued, the initial dose should be 1.25 mg.
2. If the antihypertensive effect decreases at the end of the dosing interval with once-daily therapy, consider either twice-daily administration or increasing the dose.
3. The antihypertensive effect may not be observed for 1–2 weeks.

Assessment

1. Observe infants exposed to quinapril in utero for the development of hypotension, oliguria, and hyperkalemia.
2. If angioedema occurs, stop drug, assess airway, and observe until swelling resolved. Antihistamines may help relieve symptoms.
3. Monitor VS, I&O, weights, electrolytes, CBC, and renal function studies. Agranulocytosis and bone marrow depression seen

Q

more often with renal impairment, especially if collagen vascular disease (e.g., SLE, scleroderma) present.
4. Clients with unilateral or bilateral renal artery stenosis may manifest increased BUN and serum creatinine if given quinapril. Assess renal function closely the first few weeks of therapy.

Client/Family Teaching

1. Take as directed; good reduces absorption.
2. Report any unusual bruising/bleeding or persistent side effects.
3. Any increased SOB, palpitations, swelling, or persistent nonproductive cough should be evaluated.

Outcome/Evaluate: ↓ BP

Quinidine bisulfate

(KWIN-ih-deen)
Pregnancy Category: D
Biquin Durules ✱ **(Rx)**

Quinidine gluconate

(KWIN-ih-deen)
Pregnancy Category: C
Quinaglute Dura-Tabs, Quinalan, Quinate ✱ **(Rx)**

Quinidine polygalacturonate

(KWIN-ih-deen)
Pregnancy Category: C
Cardioquin **(Rx)**

Quinidine sulfate

(KWIN-ih-deen)
Pregnancy Category: C
Apo-Quinidine ✱, Quinidex Extentabs, Quinora **(Rx)**
Classification: Antiarrhythmic, class IA

See also *Antiarrhythmic Agents*.

Action/Kinetics: Reduces the excitability of the heart and depresses conduction velocity and contractility. Prolongs the refractory period and increases conduction time. It also decreases CO and possesses anticholinergic, antimalarial, antipyretic, and oxytocic properties. **PO: Onset:** 0.5–3 hr. **Maximum effects, after IM:** 30–90 min. **t½:** 6–7 hr. **Time to peak levels, PO:** 3–5 hr for gluconate salt, 1–1.5 hr for sulfate salt, and 6 hr for polygalacturonate salt; **IM:** 1 hr. **Therapeutic serum levels:** 2–6 mcg/mL. **Protein binding:** 60%–80%. **Duration:** 6–8 hr for tablets/capsules and 12 hr for extended-release tablets. Metabolized by liver. Urine pH affects rate of urinary excretion (10%–50% excreted unchanged).

Uses: Premature atrial, AV junctional, and ventricular contractions. Treatment and control of atrial flutter, established atrial fibrillation, paroxysmal atrial tachycardia, paroxysmal AV junctional rhythm, paroxysmal and chronic atrial fibrillation, paroxysmal ventricular tachycardia not associated with complete heart block, maintenance therapy after electrical conversion of atrial flutter or fibrillation. The parenteral route is indicated when PO therapy is not feasible or immediate effects are required. *Investigational:* Gluconate salt for life-threatening *Plasmodium falciparum* malaria.

Contraindications: Hypersensitivity to drug or other cinchona drugs. Myasthenia gravis, history of thrombocytopenic purpura associated with quinidine use, digitalis intoxication evidenced by arrhythmias or AV conduction disorders. Also, complete heart block, left bundle branch block, or other intraventricular conduction defects manifested by marked QRS widening or bizarre complexes. Complete AV block with an AV nodal or idioventricular pacemaker, aberrant ectopic impulses and abnormal rhythms due to escape mechanisms. History of drug-induced torsades de pointes or long QT syndrome.

Special Concerns: Safety in children and during lactation has not been established. Use with extreme caution in clients in whom a sudden change in BP might be detrimental or in those suffering from extensive myocardial damage, subacute endocarditis, bradycardia, coronary occlusion, disturbances in impulse conduction, chronic valvular disease, considerable cardiac enlargement, frank CHF, and renal or hepatic disease. Use with caution in acute infections, hyperthyroidism, muscular weakness, respiratory distress, and bronchial asthma. The dose in geriatric clients may have to be reduced due to age-related changes in renal function.

Side Effects: *CV:* Widening of QRS complex, hypotension, ***cardiac asystole,*** ectopic ventricular beats, ***ventricular tachycardia or fibrillation, torsades de pointes,*** paradoxical tachycardia, ***arterial embolism,*** ventricular extrasystoles (one or more every 6 beats), prolonged QT interval, ***complete AV block, ventricular flutter.*** *GI:* N&V, abdominal pain, anorexia, diarrhea, urge to defecate as well as urinate, esophagitis (rare). *CNS:* Syncope, headache, confusion, excitement, vertigo, apprehension, delirium, dementia, ataxia, depression. *Dermatologic:* Rash, urticaria, exfoliative dermatitis, photosensitivity, flushing with intense pruritus, eczema, psoriasis,

Q

pigmentation abnormalities. *Allergic:* Acute asthma, angioneurotic edema, ***respiratory arrest,*** dyspnea, fever, ***vascular collapse,*** purpura, vasculitis, hepatic dysfunction (including granulomatous hepatitis), ***hepatic toxicity.*** *Hematologic:* Hypoprothrombinemia, ***acute hemolytic anemia,*** thrombocytopenic purpura, ***agranulocytosis,*** thrombocytopenia, leukocytosis, neutropenia, shift to left in WBC differential. *Ophthalmologic:* Blurred vision, mydriasis, alterations in color perception, decreased field of vision, double vision, photophobia, optic neuritis, night blindness, scotomata. *Other:* Liver toxicity including hepatitis, lupus nephritis, tinnitus, decreased hearing acuity, arthritis, myalgia, increase in serum skeletal muscle CPK, lupus erythematosus.

Laboratory Test Considerations: False + or ↑ PSP, 17-ketosteroids, PT.

OD Management of Overdose: *Symptoms: CNS:* Lethargy, confusion, ***coma, seizures, respiratory depression or arrest,*** headache, paresthesia, vertigo. CNS symptoms may be seen after onset of CV toxicity. *GI:* Vomiting, diarrhea, abdominal pain, hypokalemia, nausea. *CV:* Sinus tachycardia, ***ventricular tachycardia or fibrillation, torsades de pointes, depressed automaticity and conduction*** (including bundle branch block, sinus bradycardia, SA block, prolongation of QRS and QTc, sinus arrest, AV block, ST depression, T inversion), syncope, ***heart failure.*** Hypotension due to decreased conduction and CO and vasodilation. *Miscellaneous:* Cinchonism, visual and auditory disturbances, hypokalemia, tinnitus, acidosis. *Treatment:*

- Perform gastric lavage, induce vomiting, and administer activated charcoal if ingestion is recent.
- Monitor ECG, blood gases, serum electrolytes, and BP.
- Institute cardiac pacing, if necessary.
- Acidify the urine.
- Use artificial respiration and other supportive measures.
- Infusions of 1/6 molar sodium lactate IV may decrease the cardiotoxic effects.
- Treat hypotension with metaraminol or norepinephrine after fluid volume replacement.
- Use phenytoin or lidocaine to treat tachydysrhythmias.
- Hemodialysis is effective but not often required.

Drug Interactions

Acetazolamide, Antacids / ↑ Effect of quinidine due to ↓ renal excretion
Amiodarone / ↑ Quinidine levels with possible fatal cardiac dysrhythmias
Anticholinergic agents, Atropine / Additive effect on blockade of vagus nerve action
Anticoagulants, oral / Additive hypoprothrombinemia with possible hemorrhage
Barbiturates / ↓ Effect of quinidine due to ↑ breakdown by liver
Cholinergic agents / Quinidine antagonizes effect of cholinergic drugs
Cimetidine / ↑ Effect of quinidine due to ↓ breakdown by liver
Digoxin, Digitoxin / ↑ Symptoms of digoxin or digitoxin toxicity
Disopyramide / Either ↑ disopyramide levels or ↓ quinidine levels
Guanethidine / Additive hypotensive effect
Methyldopa / Additive hypotensive effect
Metoprolol / ↑ Effect of propranolol in fast metabolizers
Neuromuscular blocking agents / ↑ Respiratory depression
Nifedipine / ↓ Effect of quinidine
Phenobarbital, Phenytoin / ↓ Effect of quinidine by ↑ rate of metabolism in liver
Potassium / ↑ Effect of quinidine
Procainamide / ↑ Effects of procainamide with possible toxicity
Propafenone / ↑ Serum propafenone levels in rapid metabolizers
Propranolol / ↑ Effect of propranolol in fast metabolizers
Reserpine / Additive cardiac depressant effects
Rifampin / ↓ Effect of quinidine due to ↑ breakdown by liver
Skeletal muscle relaxants / ↑ Skeletal muscle relaxation
Sodium bicarbonate / ↑ Effect of quinidine due to ↓ renal excretion
Sucralfate / ↓ Serum levels of quinidine → ↓ effect
Thiazide diuretics / ↑ Effect of quinidine due to ↓ renal excretion
Tricyclic antidepressants / ↑ Effect of antidepressant due to ↓ clearance
Verapamil / ↓ Clearance of verapamil → ↑ hypotension, bradycardia, AV block, ventricular tachycardia, and pulmonary edema

How Supplied: Quinidine bisulfate: *Sustained-release tablet:* 250 mg. Quinidine gluconate: *Injection:* 80 mg/mL; *Tablet, extended release:* 324 mg. Quinidine polygalacturonate: *Tablet:* 275 mg. Quinidine sulfate: *Tablet:* 200 mg, 300 mg; *Tablet, extended release:* 300 mg

Dosage

- **Quinidine Bisulfate Sustained-Release Tablets**

Antiarrhythmic.

Initial: Test dose of 200 mg in the morning (to ascertain hypersensitivity). In the evening, administer 500 mg. **Then,** beginning the next day, 500–750 mg/12 hr. **Maintenance:** 0.5–1.25 g morning and evening.

• **Quinidine Polygalacturonate Tablets, Quinidine Sulfate Tablets**

Premature atrial and ventricular contractions.

Adults: 200–300 mg t.i.d.–q.i.d.

Paroxysmal SVTs.

Adults: 400–600 mg q 2–3 hr until the paroxysm is terminated.

Conversion of atrial flutter.

Adults: 200 mg q 2–3 hr for five to eight doses; daily doses can be increased until rhythm is restored or toxic effects occur.

Conversion of atrial flutter, maintenance therapy.

Adults: 200–300 mg t.i.d.–q.i.d. Large doses or more frequent administration may be required in some clients.

• **Quinidine Gluconate Extended-Release Tablets, Quinidine Sulfate Extended-Release Tablets**

All uses.

Adults: 300–600 mg q 8–12 hr.

• **Quinidine Gluconate Injection (IM or IV)**

Acute tachycardia.

Adults, initial: 600 mg IM; **then,** 400 mg IM repeated as often as q 2 hr.

Arrhythmias.

Adults: 330 mg IM or less IV (as much as 500–750 mg may be required).

P. falciparum malaria.

Two regimens may be used. (1) *Loading dose:* 15 mg/kg in 250 mL NSS given over 4 hr; **then,** 24 hr after beginning the loading dose, institute 7.5 mg/kg infused over 4 hr and given q 8 hr for 7 days or until PO therapy can be started. (2) *Loading dose:* 10 mg/kg in 250 mL NSS infused over 1–2 hr followed immediately by 0.02 mg/kg/min for up to 72 hr or until parasitemia decreases to less than 1% or PO therapy can be started.

HEALTH CARE CONSIDERATIONS

See also *Health Care Considerations* for *Antiarrhythmic Agents.*

Administration/Storage

1. A preliminary test dose may be given. **Adults:** 200 mg quinidine sulfate or quinidine gluconate administered PO or IM. **Children:** Test dose of 2 mg/kg of quinidine sulfate.
2. The extended-release forms are not interchangeable.

IV 3. Prepare IV solution by diluting 10 mL of quinidine gluconate injection (800 mg) with 50 mL of D5W; give at a rate of 1 mL/min.

4. Use only colorless clear solution for injection. Light may cause quinidine to crystallize, which turns solution brownish.

Assessment

1. Note any allergic reactions to antiarrhythmic drugs or tartrazine, which is found in some formulations. Perform a test dose; observe for hypersensitivity reactions and check for intolerance.
2. Record indications for therapy, onset, and symptom characteristics.
3. Obtain CXR; monitor electrolytes, CBC, liver and renal function studies.
4. Assess VS and ECG; note heart and lung sounds.

Interventions

1. Report any increased AV block, cardiac irritability, or rhythm suppression during IV administration.
2. Monitor I&O, VS; observe for hypotension. Drug induces urinary alkalization.
3. Report any neurologic deficits/sensory impairment (i.e., numbness, confusion, pyschosis, depression, or involuntary movements).
4. Report any persistent diarrhea. Among the elderly, there is a higher risk of toxicity, reduced CO, and unpredictable effects from drug.
5. Clients with long-standing atrial fibrillation or CHF with atrial fibrillation run a risk of embolization from mural thrombi when converting to sinus rhythm.

Client/Family Teaching

1. Take with food to minimize GI effects.
2. Avoid activities that require mental alertness until drug effects realized; may cause dizziness or blurred vision.
3. Add fruit and grain to diet. A high intake of fruits and vegetables (alkaline-ash foods) may prolong drug half-life.
4. Report any of the following symptoms:
• Severe skin rash, hives or itching
• Severe headache
• Unexplained fever
• Ringing in the ears, buzzing, or hearing loss
• Unusual bruising or bleeding
• Blurred vision
• Irregular heart beat, palpitations, or faintness
• Continued diarrhea
5. Wear dark glasses if photophobic.
6. Report for labs, ECG, PFTs, and eye exams.

Outcome/Evaluate

• Restoration of stable rhythm
• Therapeutic drug levels (2–6 mcg/mL)

Q

Quinine sulfate

(KWYE-nine)
Pregnancy Category: X
Formula Q, Legatrim, M-KYA, Quinamm **(Rx)**
Classification: Antimalarial

Action/Kinetics: Natural alkaloid having antimalarial, antipyretic, analgesic, and oxytocic properties. Use in treating malaria is important due to emergence of resistant forms of vivax and falciparum; no resistant forms of the parasite have been found for quinine. Antimalarial mechanism not known precisely; quinine does affect DNA replication and may raise intracellular pH. Eradicates the erythrocytic stages of plasmodia. Increases the refractory period of skeletal muscle, decreases the excitability of the motor end-plate region, and affects the distribution of calcium within the muscle fiber, thus making it useful for nocturnal leg cramps. Is oxytocic and may cause congenital malformations. Rapidly and completely absorbed from the upper small intestine; widely distributed in body tissues. **Peak plasma levels:** 1–3 hr; **plasma levels following chronic use:** 7 mcg/mL. **t½:** 4–5 hr. Highly bound to protein (70%–85%); about 5% excreted unchanged in urine. Small amounts found in saliva, bile, feces, and gastric juice. Acidifying the urine increases the rate of excretion.

Pharmacokinetics of quinine are affected by malaria, with a decrease in volume of distribution and systemic clearance. Protein binding, which is normally 70% to 85%, increases to more than 90% in clients with cerebral malaria, in pregnancy, and in children.

Uses: Alone or in combination with pyrimethamine and a sulfonamide or a tetracycline for resistant forms of *Plasmodium falciparum*. As alternative therapy for chloroquine, sensitive stains of *P. falciparum, P. malariae, P. ovale,* and *P. vivax*. Mefloquine and clindamycin may also be used with quinine, depending on where the malaria was acquired. *Investigational:* Prevention and treatment of nocturnal recumbency leg cramps.

Contraindications: Use with tinnitus, G6PD deficiency, optic neuritis, history of blackwater fever, and thrombocytopenia purpura associated with previous use of quinine.

Special Concerns: Use with caution in clients with cardiac arrhythmias and during lactation. Hemolysis, with a potential for hemolytic anemia, may occur in clients with G6PD deficiency.

Side Effects: Use of quinine may result in a syndrome referred to as *cinchonism*. Mild cinchonism is characterized by tinnitus, headache, nausea, slight visual disturbances. Larger doses, however, may cause severe CNS, CV, GI, or dermatologic effects.

Allergic: Flushing, cutaneous rashes (papular, scarlatinal, urticarial), fever, facial edema, pruritus, dyspnea, tinnitus, sweating, asthmatic symptoms, visual impairment, gastric upset. *GI:* N&V, epigastric pain, hepatitis. *Ophthalmologic:* Blurred vision with scotomata, photophobia, diplopia, night blindness, decreased visual fields, impaired color vision and perception, amblyopia, mydriasis, optic atrophy. *CNS:* Headache, confusion, restlessness, vertigo, syncope, fever, apprehension, excitement, delirium, hypothermia, dizziness, ***convulsions.*** *Otic:* Tinnitus, deafness. *Hematologic:* Acute hemolysis, hemolytic anemia, thrombocytopenic purpura, agranulocytosis, hypoprothrombinemia. *CV:* Symptoms of angina, ventricular tachycardia, conduction disturbances, vasculitis. *Miscellaneous:* Sweating, hypoglycemia, lichenoid photosensitivity.

OD **Management of Overdose:** *Symptoms:* Dizziness, intestinal cramping, skin rash, tinnitus. With higher doses, symptoms include apprehension, confusion, fever, headache, vomiting, and seizures. *Treatment:*

- Induce vomiting or undertake gastric lavage.
- Maintain BP and renal function.
- If necessary, provide artificial respiration.
- Sedatives, oxygen, and other supportive measures may be required.
- Give IV fluids to maintain fluid and electrolyte balance.
- Treat angioedema or asthma with epinephrine, corticosteroids, and antihistamines.
- Urinary acidification will hasten excretion; however, in the presence of hemoglobinuria, acidification of the urine will increase renal blockade.

Drug Interactions

Acetazolamide / ↑ Blood levels (and therefore potential for toxicity) of quinine due to ↓ rate of elimination
Aluminum-containing antacids / Absorption of quinine ↓ or delayed
Anticoagulants, oral / Additive hypoprothrombinemia due to ↓ synthesis of vitamin K–dependent clotting factors
Cimetidine / ↑ Effect of quinine due to ↓ rate of excretion
Digoxin / ↑ Serum levels of digoxin
Heparin / Effect ↓ by quinine
Mefloquine / ↑ Risk of ECG abnormalities or cardiac arrest; also, ↑ risk of convulsions. Do not use together; delay mefloquine administration at least 12 hr after the last dose of quinine.
Neuromuscular blocking agents (depolarizing and nondepolarizing) / ↑ Respiratory depression and apnea

Rifabutin, Rifampin / ↑ Hepatic clearance of quinine; can persist for several days following discontinuation of the rifampin
Sodium bicarbonate / ↑ Blood levels (and therefore potential for toxicity) of quinine due to ↓ rate of elimination
How Supplied: *Capsule:* 180 mg, 200 mg, 324 mg, 325 mg; *Tablet:* 260 mg

Dosage

- **Capsules, Tablets**

Chloroquine-resistant malaria.
Adults: 650 mg q 8 hr for at least 3 days (7 days in Southeast Asia) along with pyrimethamine, 25 mg b.i.d. for the first 3 days and sulfadiazine, 2 g/day for the first 5 days. There are two alternative regimens: (1) quinine, 650 mg q 8 hr for at least 3 days (7 days in Southeast Asia) along with a tetracycline, 250 mg q 6 hr for 10 days or (2) quinine, 650 mg q 8 hr for 3 days with sulfadoxine, 1.5 g and pyrimethamine, 75 mg as a single dose.
Chloroquine-sensitive malaria.
Adults: 600 mg q 8 hr for 5–7 days. **Pediatric:** 10 mg/kg q 8 hr for 5–7 days.
Nocturnal leg cramps.
Adults: 260–300 mg at bedtime.

HEALTH CARE CONSIDERATIONS

See also *General Health Care Considerations for All Anti-Infectives.*

Administration/Storage

1. Dispense in a light-resistant and child-resistant container; store at controlled room temperatures of 15°C–30°C (59°F–86°F).
IV 2. The parenteral form is available from the Centers for Disease Control if client unable to take PO.

Assessment

1. Record indications for therapy, onset and symptom duration, dates of travel, and other agents trialed.
2. Note any history or evidence of cardiac arrhythmias or disease.
3. Assess leg cramps to determine that they only occur at night when recumbent.
4. Obtain baseline CBC and eye exam and monitor status.

Client/Family Teaching

1. Do not take with antacids. Take with food or after meals to minimize GI irritation.
2. Do not drive a car or operate machinery until drug effects realized; may cause dizziness or blurred vision.
3. Use sunglasses to protect from photophobia.
4. If also taking cimetidine or digoxin, may require dosage adjustment; report side effects.
5. Females should use birth control; drug may harm fetus.
6. Report new ringing in the ears, blurring of vision, and headache, which may be followed by digestive disturbances, impairment of hearing and sight, confusion, and delirium. May indicate intolerance or overdosage and requires immediate medical intervention.

Outcome/Evaluate

- Termination of acute malarial attack/control of malaria symptoms
- Relief of nocturnal leg cramps

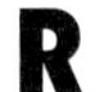
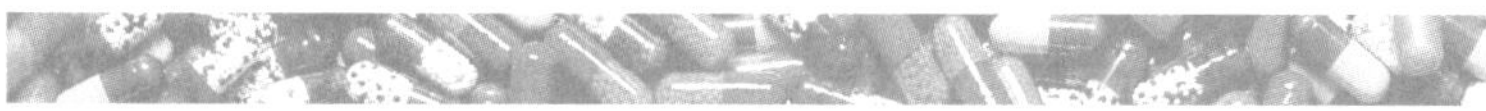

Rabeprazole sodium

(rah-**BEP**-rah-zohl)
Pregnancy Category: B
Aciphex **(Rx)**
Classification: GI drug

Action/Kinetics: Suppresses gastric secretion by inhibiting gastric H^+,K^+ATPase at the secretory surface of parietal cells, i.e., is a gastric proton-pump inhibitor. Blocks the final step of gastric acid secretion. **Peak plasma levels:** 2–5 hr. **t½, plasma:** 1–2 hr. Extensively metabolized in the liver by P450 3A and 2C19. Excreted mainly in the urine.
Uses: Short-term (4–8 weeks) treatment in the healing and symptomatic relief of erosive or ulcerative gastroesophageal reflux disease (GERD). Maintenance of healing and reduction in relapse rates of heartburn symptoms in clients with erosive or ulcerative GERD. Short-term (up to 4 weeks) treatment in healing and symptomatic relief of duodenal ulcers. Long-term treatment of pathological hypersecretory symptoms, including Zollinger-Ellison syndrome.
Contraindications: Known sensitivity to rabeprazole or substituted benzimidazoles. Lactation.
Special Concerns: Safety and efficacy have not been determined in children. Greater sensitivity in some geriatric clients is possible. Symptomatic response to therapy does not preclude presence of gastric malignancy. Use with caution in severe hepatic impairment.

Side Effects: *GI:* Diarrhea, N&V, abdominal pain, dyspepsia, flatulence, constipation, dry mouth, eructation, gastroenteritis, rectal hemorrhage, melena, anorexia, cholelithiasis, mouth ulceration, stomatitis, dysphagia, gingivitis, cholecystitis, increased appetite, abnormal stools, colitis, esophagitis, glossitis, pancreatitis, proctitis. *CNS:* Insomnia, anxiety, dizziness, depression, nervousness, somnolence, hypertonia, neuralgia, vertigo, convulsions, abnormal dreams, decreased libido, neuropathy, paresthesia, tremor, coma, disorientation, delirium. *CV:* Hypertension, ***MI*** , abnormal EEG, migraine, syncope, angina pectoris, bundle branch block, palpitation, sinus bradycardia, tachycardia. *Musculoskeletal:* Myalgia, arthritis, leg cramps, bone pain, arthrosis, bursitis, neck rigidity, rhabdomyolysis. *Respiratory:* Dyspnea, asthma, epistaxis, laryngitis, hiccough, hyperventilation, interstitial pneumonia. *Dermatologic:* Rash, pruritus, sweating, urticaria, alopecia, jaundice, bullous and other skin eruptions. *GU:* Cystitis, urinary frequency, dysmenorrhea, dysuria, kidney calculus, metorrhagia, polyuria. *Endocrine:* Hyperthyroidism, hypothyroidism. *Hematologic:* Anemia, ecchymosis, lymphadenopathy, hypochromic anemia, agranulocytosis, hemolytic anemia, leukopenia, pancytopenia, thrombocytopenia. *Metabolic:* Peripheral edema, edema, weight gain, gout, dehydration, weight loss. *Body as a whole:* Asthenia, fever, allergic reaction, chills, malaise, substernal chest pain, photosensitivity reaction, ***sudden death***. *Ophthalmic:* Cataract, amblyopia, glaucoma, dry eyes, abnormal vision. *Otic:* Tinnitus, otitis media.

Laboratory Test Considerations: ↑ Creatine phosphatase, AST, ALT, TSH, prostatic specific antigen. Abnormal platelets, erythrocytes, LFTs, urine, WBCs. Albuminuria, hypercholesterolemia, hyperglycemia, hyperlipemia, hypokalemia, hyponatremia, leukocytosis, leukorrhea, hyperammonemia.

Drug Interactions

Digoxin / ↑ Plama levels of digoxin R/T changes in gastric pH

Ketoconazole / ↓ Plasma levels of ketoconazole R/T changes in gastric pH

How Supplied: *Tablet, Enteric-Coated:* 20 mg

Dosage

- **Tablet, Enteric-Coated**

Healing of erosive or ulcerative GERD.

Adults: 20 mg once daily for 4–8 weeks. An additional 8 weeks of therapy may be considered for those who have not healed.

Maintenance of healing of erosive or ulcerative GERD.

Adults: 20 mg once daily.

Healing of duodenal ulcers.

Adults: 20 mg once daily after the morning meal for up to 4 weeks. A few clients may require additional time to heal.

Treatment of pathological hypersecretory conditions.

Adults, initial: 60 mg once a day. Adjust dosage to individual client needs (doses up to 100 mg/day and 60 mg b.i.d. have been used). Continue as long as clinically needed.

HEALTH CARE CONSIDERATIONS

Administration/Storage

1. No dosage adjustment is needed in elderly clients, those with renal disease, or in mild to moderate hepatic impairment.
2. Protect tablets from moisture.

Assessment

1. Record indications for therapy, onset, and characteristics of symptoms.
2. List drugs currently prescribed to ensure none interact.

Client/Family Teaching

1. Take as directed. Swallow tablets whole; do not crush, chew, or split tablets.
2. Report any unusual bleeding, acid reflux, abdominal pain or severe lightheadedness.

Outcome/Evaluate

- ↓ Intraesophageal acid exposure
- Healing of duodenal ulcers; symptomatic improvement

Raloxifene hydrochloride

(ral-**OX**-ih-feen)

Pregnancy Category: X

Evista **(Rx)**

Classification: Estrogen receptor modulator

Action/Kinetics: Selective estrogen receptor modulator that reduces bone resorption and decreases overall bone turnover. Considered an estrogen antagonist that acts by combining with estrogen receptors. Has not been associated with endometrial proliferation, breast enlargement, breast pain, or increased risk of breast cancer. Also decreases total and LDL cholesterol levels. Absorbed rapidly after PO; significant first-pass effect. Excreted primarily in feces with small amounts excreted in urine.

Uses: Prevention of osteoporosis in postmenopausal women. Not effective in reducing hot flashes or flushes associated with estrogen deficiency. *Investigational:* Reduce risk of breast cancer in postmenopausal women.

Contraindications: In women who are or who might become pregnant, active or histo-

ry of venous thromboembolic events (e.g., DVT, pulmonary embolism, retinal vein thrombosis). Use in premenopausal women, during lactation, or in pediatric clients. Concurrent use with systemic estrogen or hormone replacement therapy.
Special Concerns: Use with caution with highly protein-bound drugs, including clofibrate, diazepam, diazoxide, ibuprofen, indomethacin, and naproxen. Effect on bone mass density beyond 2 years of treatment is not known.
Side Effects: *CV:* Hot flashes, migraine. *Body as a whole:* Infection, flu syndrome, chest pain, fever, weight gain, peripheral edema. *CNS:* Depression, insomnia. *GI:* Nausea, dyspepsia, vomiting, flatulence, GI disorder, gastroenteritis. *GU:* Vaginitis, UTI, cystitis, leukorrhea, endometrial disorder. *Respiratory:* Sinusitis, pharyngitis, increased cough, pneumonia, laryngitis. *Musculoskeletal:* Arthralgia, myalgia, leg cramps, arthritis. *Dermatologic:* Rash, sweating.
Laboratory Test Considerations: ↑ Apolipoprotein A1, steroid-binding globulin, thyroxine-binding globulin, corticosteroid-binding globulin. ↓ Total cholesterol, LDL cholesterol, fibrinogen, apolipoprotien B, lipoprotein.
Drug Interactions
Cholestryamine / ↓ Absorption of raloxifene
Warfarin / ↓ Prothrombin time
How Supplied: *Tablets:* 60 mg

Dosage
- **Tablets**

Prevention of osteoporosis in postmenopausal women.
Adults: 60 mg once daily.

HEALTH CARE CONSIDERATIONS

Administration/Storage
1. May be taken without regard for meals.
2. Take supplemental calcium and vitamin D if daily dietary intake is inadequate.

Assessment
1. Record indications for therapy; note date of menopause.
2. Assess for history or evidence of CHF, active cancer or blood clots in legs, lungs or eyes.
3. Monitor LFTs; assess for any dysfunction.

Client/Family Teaching
1. Take exactly as directed once daily with or without food; if dietary calcium and vitamin D intake is inadequate, consume supplemental.
2. Drug is used by women after menopause to prevent bones from becoming weak and thin.
3. Avoid prolonged immobilization and restrictions of movement as with travel due to increased risk of venous thromboembolic events. Stop 3 days prior to and during prolonged immobilization such as with surgery or prolonged bedrest.
4. Drug is not effective in reducing hot flashes or flushes associated with low estrogen as it does not stimulate breast or uterus.
5. Regular weight bearing exercises as well as tobacco and alcohol cessation/modification should be practiced.
6. Report any pain in calves or swelling in legs, sudden chest pain, SOB, or coughing up blood, as well as any vision changes.

Outcome/Evaluate: Postmenopausal osteoporosis prophylaxis

Ramipril
(RAM-ih-prill)
Pregnancy Category: D
Altace **(Rx)**
Classification: Angiotensin-converting enzyme inhibitor

See also *Angiotensin-Converting Enzyme Inhibitors.*
Action/Kinetics: Onset: 1–2 hr. **Time to peak serum levels:** 1 hr (1–2 hr for ramiprilat, the active metabolite). **Peak effect:** 3–6 hr. Ramiprilat has approximately six times the ACE inhibitory activity than ramipril. **t½:** 1–2 hr (13–17 hr for ramiprilat); prolonged in impaired renal function. **Duration:** 24 hr. Metabolized in the liver with 60% excreted through the urine and 40% in the feces. Food decreases the rate, but not the extent, of absorption of ramipril.
Uses: Alone or in combination with other antihypertensive agents (especially thiazide diuretics) for the treatment of hypertension. Treatment of CHF following MI to decrease risk of CV death and decrease the risk of failure-related hospitalization and progression to severe or resistant heart failure.
Contraindications: Lactation.
Special Concerns: Geriatric clients may manifest higher peak blood levels of ramiprilat.
Side Effects: *CV:* Hypotension, chest pain, palpitations, angina pectoris, orthostatic hypotension, ***MI, CVA, arrhythmias.*** *GI:* N&V, abdominal pain, diarrhea, dysgeusia, anorexia, constipation, dry mouth, dyspepsia, enzyme changes suggesting pancreatitis, dysphagia,

R

gastroenteritis, increased salivation. *CNS:* Headache, dizziness, fatigue, insomnia, sleep disturbances, somnolence, depression, nervousness, malaise, vertigo, anxiety, amnesia, ***convulsions,*** tremor. *Respiratory:* Cough, dyspnea, URI, asthma, ***bronchospasm***. *Hematologic:* Leukopenia, anemia, eosinophilia. Rarely, decreases in hemoglobin or hematocrit. *Dermatologic:* Diaphoresis, photosensitivity, pruritus, rash, dermatitis, purpura, alopecia, erythema multiforme, urticaria. *Body as a whole:* Paresthesias, angioedema, asthenia, syncope, fever, muscle cramps, myalgia, arthralgia, arthritis, neuralgia, neuropathy, influenza, edema. *Miscellaneous:* Impotence, tinnitus, hearing loss, vision disturbances, epistaxis, weight gain, proteinuria, angioneurotic edema, edema, flu syndrome.
Laboratory Test Considerations: ↓ H&H.
How Supplied: *Capsule:* 1.25 mg, 2.5 mg, 5 mg, 10 mg

Dosage

- **Capsules**

Hypertension.

Initial: 2.5 mg once daily in clients not taking a diuretic; **maintenance:** 2.5–20 mg/day as a single dose or two equally divided doses. *Clients taking diuretics or who have a C_{CR} less than 40 mL/min/1.73 m²:* initially 1.25 mg/day; dose may then be increased to a maximum of 5 mg/day.

CHF following MI.

Initial: 2.5 mg b.i.d. Clients intolerant of this dose may be started on 1.25 mg b.i.d. The target maintenance dose is 5 mg b.i.d.

HEALTH CARE CONSIDERATIONS

See also *Health Care Considerations* for *Angiotensin-Converting Enzyme Inhibitors* and *Antihypertensive Agents.*

Administration/Storage

1. For ease in swallowing, may mix contents of the capsule with water, apple juice, or apple sauce.
2. If the antihypertensive effect decreases at the end of the dosing interval with once-daily dosing, consider either twice-daily administration or an increase in dose.
3. If taking a diuretic, discontinue the diuretic 2–3 days prior to beginning ramipril. If BP is not controlled, reinstitute the diuretic. If the diuretic cannot be discontinued, consider an initial dose of ramipril of 1.25 mg.

Client/Family Teaching

1. Use caution; drug may cause dizziness and postural effects with sudden changes in position.
2. Report any persistent, dry, nonproductive cough, increased SOB, edema, or unusual bruising/bleeding.
3. Do not take any OTC agents without approval.

Outcome/Evaluate

- ↓ BP
- Resolution of S&S of CHF

Ranitidine bismuth citrate

((rah-**NIH**-tih-deen **BIS**-muth))
Pregnancy Category: C, when used with clarithromycin
Pylorid ✱, Tritec **(Rx)**
Classification: Histamine H_2 antagonist/treatment for H. pylori

See also *Histamine H_2 Antagonists*, and *Ranitidine. NOTE:* Since clarithromycin is used with ranitidine bismuth citrate, information on clarithromycin must also be consulted.
Action/Kinetics: A complex of ranitidine and bismuth citrate which is freely soluble in water; solubility decreases as pH is decreased. The complex is more soluble than either ranitidine or bismuth citrate given separately. Is believed the greater solubility of the complex facilitates penetration of the drug into the mucous layer that protects the epithelial cells in the GI mucosa. **Peak levels of ranitidine from complex:** 0.5–5 hr. **t½, elimination, ranitidine from ranitidine bismuth citrate:** 2.8–3.1 hr. Ranitidine is eliminated through the kidneys. **t½, terminal, bismuth:** 11–28 days. Bismuth is excreted primarily in the feces.
Uses: In combination with clarithromycin for treatment of active duodenal ulcers associated with *Helicobacter pylori* infections. *NOTE:* Ranitidine bismuth citrate should not be prescribed alone for the treatment of active duodenal ulcer.
Contraindications: Hypersensitivity to the complex or any of its ingredients. Hangover. Use in those with a history of acute porphyria or in those with a C_{CR} less than 25 mL/min.
Special Concerns: Use with caution during lactation. Safety and efficacy of ranitidine bismuth citrate plus clarithromycin in pediatric clients have not been determined.
Side Effects: See also side effects for *Ranitidine. GI:* N&V, diarrhea, constipation, abdominal discomfort, gastric pain. *CNS:* Headache, dizziness, sleep disorder, tremors (rare). *Hypersensitivity:* Rash, anaphylaxis (rare). *Miscellaneous:* Pruritus, gynecologic problems, taste disturbance, chest symptoms, transient changes in liver enzymes.
Laboratory Test Considerations: False + test for urine protein using Multistix. ↑ ALT, AST.

Drug Interactions
Antacids / Possible ↓ plasma levels of ranitidine and bismuth
Clarithromycin / ↑ Plasma levels of ranitidine and bismuth
How Supplied: *Tablet:* 400 mg

Dosage

- **Tablets**

Eradication of H. pylori *infection.*
Ranitidine bismuth citrate: 400 mg b.i.d. for 4 weeks. *Clarithromycin:* 500 mg t.i.d. for the first 2 weeks of therapy.

HEALTH CARE CONSIDERATIONS

See also *Health Care Considerations* for *Histamine H_2 Antagonists*, and *Ranitidine.*
Administration/Storage
1. Bismuth may cause a temporary and harmless darkening of the tongue or stool; do not confuse with melena.
2. Both ranitidine bismuth citrate and clarithromycin can be taken with or without food.
3. Protect drug from light and store at 2°C–30°C (36°F–86°F).
Assessment
1. Record indications for therapy, onset, duration, and characteristics of symptoms, other agents trialed and the outcome.
2. Check serum *H. pylori* or endoscopic confirmation of disease.
3. Obtain baseline CBC, liver and renal function studies.
4. Determine any experience with these agents. Not for use with acute porphyria, a hangover, or C_{CR} < 25 mL/min.
Client/Family Teaching
1. Take exactly as directed; do not skip doses or try and double up on missed doses. Take missed dose when remembered.
2. The cause for the ulcer is the bacteria *H. pylori;* drug helps kill bacteria. Must be taken with clarithromycin in order to be effective.
3. May experience diarrhea, headache, nausea, vomiting, and itchy skin; report if persistent and use only acetaminophen for headaches.
4. Use sugarless candies or rinse mouth frequently to diminish bad taste.
5. Stools and tongue may appear black in color; do not be alarmed.
6. Do not smoke; smoking slows ulcer healing and may cause a recurrence.
7. Avoid any other medications (prescription or OTC) without approval.
Outcome/Evaluate: Healing of ulcer; ↓ pain and discomfort

Ranitidine hydrochloride

(rah-**NIH**-tih-deen)
Pregnancy Category: B
Alti-Ranitidine HCl ✦, Apo-Ranitidine ✦, Gen-Ranitidine ✦, Novo-Ranidine ✦, Nu-Ranit ✦, Zantac, Zantac-C ✦, Zantac Efferdose, Zantac GELdose Capsules **(Rx)**, Zantac 75 **(OTC)**
Classification: H_2 receptor antagonist

See also *Histamine H_2 Antagonists.*
Action/Kinetics: Competitively inhibits gastric acid secretion by blocking the effect of histamine on histamine H_2 receptors. Both daytime and nocturnal basal gastric acid secretion, as well as food- and pentagastrin-stimulated gastric acid are inhibited. Weak inhibitor of cytochrome P-450 (drug-metabolizing enzymes); thus, drug interactions involving inhibition of hepatic metabolism are not expected to occur. Food increases the bioavailability. **Peak effect: PO,** 1–3 hr; **IM, IV,** 15 min. **t½:** 2.5–3 hr. **Duration, nocturnal:** 13 hr; **basal:** 4 hr. **Serum level to inhibit 50% stimulated gastric acid secretion:** 36–94 ng/mL. From 30% to 35% of a PO dose and from 68% to 79% of an IV dose excreted unchanged in urine.
Uses: Short-term (4–8 weeks) and maintenance treatment of duodenal ulcer. Pathologic hypersecretory conditions such as Zollinger-Ellison syndrome and systemic mastocytosis. Short-term treatment of active, benign gastric ulcers. Maintenance of healing of gastric ulcers. Gastroesophageal reflux disease, including erosive esophagitis. Maintenance of healing of erosive esophagitis. *Investigational:* Prophylaxis of pulmonary aspiration of acid during anesthesia, prevent gastric damage from NSAIDs, prevent stress ulcers, prevent acute upper GI bleeding, as part of multidrug regimen to eradicate Helicobacter pylori.
Contraindications: Cirrhosis of the liver, impaired renal or hepatic function.
Special Concerns: Use with caution during lactation and in clients with decreased hepatic or renal function. Safety and efficacy not established in children.
Side Effects: *GI:* Constipation, N&V, diarrhea, abdominal pain, pancreatitis (rare). *CNS:* Headache, dizziness, malaise, insomnia, vertigo, confusion, anxiety, agitation, depression, fatigue, somnolence, hallucinations. *CV:* Bradycardia or tachycardia, premature ventricular beats following rapid IV use (especially in clients predisposed to cardiac rhythm disturbances), ***cardiac arrest***. *Hematologic:* Thrombocytopenia, granulocytopenia, leukopenia, pancytopenia (sometimes with

R

marrow hypoplasia), ***agranulocytosis, autoimmune hemolytic or aplastic anemia.*** *Hepatic:* Hepatotoxicity, jaundice, hepatitis, increase in ALT. *Dermatologic:* Erythema multiforme, rash, alopecia. *Allergic:* ***Bronchospasm, anaphylaxis,*** angioneurotic edema (rare), rashes, fever, eosinophilia. *Other:* Arthralgia, gynecomastia, impotence, loss of libido, blurred vision, pain at injection site, local burning or itching following IV use.

Laboratory Test Considerations: False + test for urine protein using Multistix.

Drug Interactions

Antacids / Antacids may ↓ the absorption of ranitidine
Diazepam / ↓ Effect of diazepam due to ↓ absorption from GI tract
Glipizide / Ranitidine ↑ effect of glipizide
Procainamide / Ranitidine ↓ excretion of procainamide → possible ↑ effect
Theophylline / Possible ↑ pharmacologic and toxicologic effects of theophylline
Warfarin / Ranitidine may ↑ hypoprothrombinemic effects of warfarin

How Supplied: *Capsule:* 150 mg, 300 mg; *Granule for reconstitution:* 150 mg; *Injection:* 1 mg/mL, 25 mg/mL; *Syrup:* 15 mg/mL; *Tablet:* 75 mg, 150 mg, 300 mg; *Tablet, effervescent:* 150 mg

Dosage

• **Capsules (Soft Gelatin), Effervescent Tablets and Granules, Syrup, Tablets**

Duodenal ulcer, short-term.

Adults: 150 mg b.i.d. or 300 mg at bedtime to heal ulcer, although 100 mg b.i.d. will inhibit acid secretion and may be as effective as the higher dose. **Maintenance:** 150 mg at bedtime.

Pathologic hypersecretory conditions.

Adults: 150 mg b.i.d. (up to 6 g/day has been used in severe cases).

Benign gastric ulcer.

Adults: 150 mg b.i.d. for active ulcer. **Maintenance:** 150 mg at bedtime

Gastroesophageal reflux disease.

Adults: 150 mg b.i.d.

Erosive esophagitis.

Adults: 150 mg q.i.d.

Maintenenace of healing of erosive esophagitis.

Adults: 150 mg b.i.d.

• **IM, IV**

Treatment and maintenance for duodenal ulcer, hypersecretory conditions, gastroesophageal reflux.

Adults, IM: 50 mg q 6–8 hr. **Intermittent IV injection or infusion:** 50 mg q 6–8 hr, not to exceed 400 mg/day. **Continuous IV infusion:** 6.25 mg/hr.

Zollinger-Ellison clients.

Continuous IV infusion: Dilute ranitidine in D5W to a concentration no greater than 2.5 mg/mL with an initial infusion rate of 1 mg/kg/hr. If after 4 hr the client shows a gastric acid output of greater than 10 mEq/hr or if symptoms appear, increase the dose by 0.5-mg/kg/hr increments and measure the acid output. Doses up to 2.5 mg/kg/hr may be necessary.

HEALTH CARE CONSIDERATIONS

See also *Health Care Considerations* for *Histamine H_2 Antagonists.*

Administration/Storage

1. If the C_{CR} is less than 50 mL/min, give 150 mg PO q 24 hr or 50 mg parenterally q 18–24 hr.
2. Give antacids concomitantly for gastric pain although they may interfere with ranitidine absorption.
3. Dissolve Efferdose tablets and granules in 6–8 oz of water before taking.
4. About one-half of clients may heal completely within 2 weeks; thus, endoscopy may show no need for further treatment.
5. No dilution is required for IM use.
6. Store the syrup between 4°C and 25°C (39°F and 77°F).
7. IV For IV injection, dilute 50 mg with 0.9% NaCl injection to a total volume of 20 mL. Give the diluted solution over 5 min or more. For intermittent IV infusion, dilute 50 mg in 100 mL D5W and give over 15–20 min.
8. The premixed injection does not require dilution; give only by slow IV drip over 15–20 min. Do not introduce additives into the solution. If used with a primary IV fluid system, discontinue the primary solution during drug infusion.
9. For continuous IV infusion, add ranitidine injection to D5W
10. The drug is stable for 48 hr at room temperature when mixed with 0.9% NaCl, 5% or 10% dextrose injection, RL injection, or 5% $NaHCO_3$ injection.

Assessment

1. Record indications for therapy, onset and duration of symptoms, other agents used and anticipated treatment period.
2. Assess stomach pain, noting characteristics, frequency of occurrence and things that alter it.
3. Obtain CBC; assess for infections.
4. Note *H. pylori*, UGI, or endoscopy findings.
5. Assess for renal or liver disease.
6. Determine if pregnant.
7. Skin tests using allergens may elicit false negative results; stop drug 24–72 hr prior to testing.

Client/Family Teaching

1. Take with or immediately following meals. Wait 1 hr before taking an antacid.
2. Do not drive or operate machinery until drug effects are realized; dizziness or drowsiness may occur.
3. Avoid alcohol, aspirin-containing products, and beverages that contain caffeine (tea, cola, coffee); these increase stomach acid.
4. Avoid things that may aggravate symptoms, i.e., ETOH, aspirin, NSAIDs, caffeine, and black pepper.
5. Do not smoke; interferes with healing and drug's effectiveness.
6. Report any evidence of diarrhea and maintain adequate hydration.
7. Report any confusion or disorientation.
8. Symptoms of breast tenderness will usually disappear after several weeks; report if persistent and evaluate need to stop drug.
9. Report as scheduled to determine extent of healing and expected length of therapy.

Outcome/Evaluate

- ↓ Gastric acid production
- ↓ Abdominal pain/discomfort
- Endoscopic/radiographic evidence of duodenal ulcer healing

Repaglinide

(re-**PAY**-glin-eyed)

Pregnancy Category: C

Prandin **(Rx)**

Classification: Oral antidiabetic

See also *Antidiabetic Agents, Hypoglycemic Agents*.

Action/Kinetics: Lowers blood glucose by stimulating release of insulin from pancreas. Action depends on functioning beta cells in pancreatic islets. Drug closes ATP-dependent potassium channels in beta-cell membrane due to binding at sites. Blockade of potassium channel depolarizes beta cell which leads to opening of calcium channels. This causes calcium influx which induces insulin secretion. Rapidly and completely absorbed from GI tract. **Peak plasma levels:** 1 hr. Completely metabolized in liver with most excreted in feces.

Uses: Adjunct to diet and exercise in type 2 diabetes mellitus. In combination with metformin to lower blood glucose where hyperglycemia can not be controlled by exercise, diet, or either drug alone.

Contraindications: Lactation. Diabetic ketoacidosis, with or without coma. Type 1 diabetes.

Special Concerns: Use with caution in impaired hepatic function. Safety and efficacy have not been determined in children.

Side Effects: *CV:* Chest pain, angina, ischemia. *GI:* Nausea, diarrhea, constipation, vomiting, dyspepsia. *Respiratory:* URI, sinusitis, rhinitis, bronchitis. *Musculoskeletal:* Arthralgia, back pain. *Miscellaneous:* Hypoglycemia, headache, paresthesia, chest pain, UTI, tooth disorder, allergy.

OD **Management of Overdose:** *Symptoms:* Hypoglycemia. *Treatment:* Oral glucose. Also adjust drug dosage or meal patterns.

Drug Interactions: See *Antidiabetic Agents, Hypoglycemic Agents.*

How Supplied: *Tablets:* 0.5 mg, 1 mg, 2 mg

Dosage

- **Tablets**

Type 2 diabetes mellitus.

Individualize dosage. **Initial:** In those not previously treated or whose HbA1-C is less than 8%, give 0.5 mg. For those previously treated or whose HbA1-C is 8% or more, give 1 or 2 mg before each meal. **Dose range:** 0.5–4 mg taken with meals. **Maximum daily dose:** 16 mg.

HEALTH CARE CONSIDERATIONS

See also *Health Care Considerations* for *Antidiabetic Agents, Hypoglycemic Agents, nref=*.

Administration/Storage

1. May be dosed after meals 2, 3, or 4 times daily, depending on client's meal patterns.
2. Usually taken within 15 min of meal but time may vary from immediately preceding meal to as long as 30 min before meal.
3. When used to replace another oral hypoglycemic, may be started the day after last dose of other drug.
4. If combined with metformin, starting dose and dose adjustments are the same as if repaglinide was used alone.

Assessment

1. Record onset, duration, and characteristics of disease; note other agents/methods trialed and outcome.
2. Monitor VS, HbA1-C, and LFTs.

Client/Family Teaching

1. Take as prescribed.
2. Continue regular exercise, diabetic diet, and lifestyle modifications in order to control BS and prevent organ damage.
3. Record FS for provider review; report any unusual or intolerable side effects.

Outcome/Evaluate: HbA1-C within desired range; control of BS

R

Ribavirin and Interferon alfa-2b recombinant

(rye-bah-VYE-rin/in-ter-FEER-on)
Pregnancy Category: X
Rebetron **(Rx)**
Classification: Drug for chronic hepatitis C

See also *Ribavirin* and *Interferon alfa-2b recombinant. Note:* Rebetron is a combination package containing ribavirin and interferon alfa-2b recombinant. Thus, the information for each drug is to be consulted.

Action/Kinetics: The mechanism of action of the combination in inhibiting the hepatitis C virus is not known.

Uses: Treatment of chronic hepatitis C in clients with compensated liver disease who have relapsed following alpha interferon therapy.

Contraindications: Pregnancy and in those who may become pregnant. Lactation. Hypersensitivity or history thereof to alpha interferons and/or ribavirin. Use in clients with autoimmune hepatitis.

Special Concerns: Use with extreme caution in those with pre-existing psychiatric disorders who report a history of severe depression. Use with caution if C_{CR} is less than 50 mL/min or in pre-existing cardiac disease. Safety and efficacy have not been determined in children less than 18 years of age.

Side Effects: See individual drugs; selected treatment-emergent side effects follow. *Hematologic:* Anemia. *GI:* N&V, anorexia, dyspepsia. *CNS:* Depression, suicidal behavior, dizziness, insomnia, irritability, emotional lability, impaired concentration, nervousness. *Respiratory:* Dyspnea, pulmonary infiltrates, pneumonitis, pneumonia, sinusitis. *Musculoskeletal:* Myalgia, arthralgia, musculoskeletal pain. *Dermatologic:* Alopecia, rash, pruritus. *Body as a whole:* Headache, fatigue, rigors, fever, flu-like symptoms, asthenia, chest pain. *Miscellaneous:* Taste perversion, injection site inflammation or reaction.

Laboratory Test Considerations: ↑ Bilirubin, uric acid. ↓ Hemoglobin, neutrophils.

Drug Interactions: See individual drugs.

How Supplied: Combination packages containing ribavirin (Rebetol) capsules, 200 mg, and interferon alfa-2b recombinant (Introl A) injectable.

Dosage

- **Capsules (Rebetol), SC (Intron A)**
  Chronic hepatitis C.

Adults, 75 kg or less: Rebetol: 2 x 200 mg capsules in the a.m. and 3 x 200 mg capsules in the p.m. Intron A: 3 million I.U. 3 times weekly SC. **Adults, more than 75 kg:** Rebetol: 3 x 200 mg capsules in the a.m. and 3 x 200 mg capsules in the p.m. Intron A: 3 million I.U. three times a week SC. Reduce the dose of Rebetol by 600 mg daily and Intron A by 1.5 million I.U. three times a week if the hemoglobin is less than 10 g/dL.

HEALTH CARE CONSIDERATIONS

See also *Health Care Considerations* for *Ribavirin* and *Interferon alfa-2b recombinant.*

Administration/Storage

1. Continue the drug combination for six months (24 weeks). The safety and efficacy of the combination have not been established beyond 6 months of therapy.
2. Rebetol may be given without regard to food.
3. At provider discretion, the client may self-administer Intron A.
4. Refrigerate Rebetol capsules and Intron A injection between 2°C–8°C (36°F–46°F).

Assessment

1. Detemine disease onset/diagnosis, liver function, previous therapies trialed and when relapsed with alpha interferon therapy.
2. Note any psychiatric history or cardiac disease.
3. Initially obtain a negative pregnancy test and then monthly during therapy and for 6 mo following therapy. Providers should report any pregnancy during or for 6 mo following therapy at 1-800-727-7064.
4. Monitor CBC, renal and LFTs, chemistries and TSH.
5. Obtain eye exam prior to therapy with diabetes and HTN.

Client/Family Teaching

1. Take exactly as directed. The package contains the Rebetol capsules and also the injectable Introl A for SC administration.
2. May experience flu like symptoms which should diminish with continued therapy. Take injections at bedtime to help minimize.
3. Men and women must use reliable birth control during and for 6 mo following therapy; causes severe fetal damage.
4. Report any unusual behaviors, depression, or suicide ideations immediately.
5. Visual problems or decreased acuity should be evaluated by an eye doctor.

Outcome/Evaluate: Treatment of chronic hepatitis C

Rifabutin

(rif-ah-BYOU-tin)
Pregnancy Category: B
Mycobutin **(Rx)**
Classification: Antitubercular drug

Action/Kinetics: Inhibits DNA-dependent RNA polymerase in susceptible strains of *Escherichia coli* and *Bacillus subtilis.* Rapidly absorbed from the GI tract. **Peak plasma levels after a single dose:** 3.3 hr. **Mean terminal t½:** 45 hr. About 85% is bound to plasma proteins. High-fat meals slow the rate, but not the extent, of absorption. About 30% of a dose is excreted in the feces and 53% in the urine, primarily as metabolites. The 25-O-desacetyl metabolite is equal in activity to rifabutin.

Uses: Prevention of disseminated *Mycobacterium avium* complex (MAC) disease in clients with advanced HIV infection.

Contraindications: Hypersensitivity to rifabutin or other rifamycins (e.g., rifampin). Use in active tuberculosis. Lactation.

Special Concerns: Safety and efficacy have not been determined in children, although the drug has been used in HIV-positive children.

Side Effects: *GI:* Anorexia, abdominal pain, diarrhea, dyspepsia, eructation, flatulence, N&V, taste perversion. *Respiratory:* Chest pain, chest pressure or pain with dyspnea. *CNS:* Insomnia, ***seizures,*** paresthesia, aphasia, confusion. *Musculoskeletal:* Asthenia, myalgia, arthralgia, myositis. *Body as a whole:* Fever, headache, generalized pain, flu-like syndrome. *Dermatologic:* Rash, skin discoloration. *Hematologic:* Neutropenia, leukopenia, anemia, eosinophilia, thrombocytopenia. *Miscellaneous:* Discolored urine, nonspecific T wave changes on ECG, hepatitis, hemolysis, uveitis.

Laboratory Test Considerations: ↑ AST, ALT, alkaline phosphatase.

OD **Management of Overdose:** *Symptoms:* Worsening of side effects. *Treatment:* Gastric lavage followed by instillation into the stomach of an activated charcoal slurry.

Drug Interactions: Rifabutin has liver enzyme-inducing properties and may be expected to have similar interactions as does rifampin. However, rifabutin is a less potent enzyme inducer than rifampin.

AZT / ↓ Steady-state plasma levels of AZT after repeated rifabutin dosing

Oral contraceptives / Rifabutin may ↓ the effectiveness of oral contraceptives

How Supplied: *Capsule:* 150 mg

Dosage

- **Capsules**

Prophylaxis of MAC disease in clients with advanced HIV infection.

Adults: 300 mg/day.

HEALTH CARE CONSIDERATIONS

See also *General Health Care Considerations for All Anti-Infectives.*

Assessment

1. Record indications for therapy, noting type, onset, and characteristics of symptoms.
2. Monitor CBC for neutropenia.
3. Ensure that CXR, PPD, and sputum AFB cultures have been performed to rule out active tuberculosis. Clients who develop active tuberculosis during therapy must be covered with appropriate antituberculosis medications.

Client/Family Teaching

1. If N&V or other GI upset occurs, may take doses of 150 mg b.i.d. with food.
2. Urine, feces, saliva, sputum, perspiration, tears, skin, and mucous membranes may be colored brown-orange. Soft contact lenses may be permanently stained.
3. Report any S&S of muscle or eye pain, irritation, or inflammation as well as any persistent vomiting or abnormal bruising/bleeding.
4. Practice nonhormonal form of birth control.

Outcome/Evaluate: Prevention of disseminated *Mycobacterium avium* complex (MAC) with advanced HIV

Rifampin

(rih-**FAM**-pin)

Pregnancy Category: C

Rifadin, Rimactane, Rofact ✱ **(Rx)**

Classification: Primary antitubercular agent

Action/Kinetics: Semisynthetic antibiotic derived from *Streptomyces mediterranei.* Suppresses RNA synthesis by binding to the beta subunit of DNA-dependent RNA polymerase. This prevents attachment of the enzyme to DNA and blockade of RNA transcription. Both bacteriostatic and bactericidal; most active against rapidly replicating organisms. Well absorbed from the GI tract; widely distributed in body tissues. **Peak plasma concentration:** 4–32 mcg/mL after 2–4 hr. **t½:** 1.5–5 hr (higher in clients with hepatic impairment). In normal clients t½ decreases with usage. Metabolized in liver; 60% is excreted in feces.

Uses: All types of tuberculosis. Must be used in conjunction with at least one other tuberculostatic drug (such as isoniazid, ethambutol, pyrazinamide) but is the drug of choice for retreatment. Also for treatment of asymptomatic meningococcal carriers to eliminate *Neisseria meningitidis*. *Investigational:* Used in combination for infections due to *Staphylococcus aureus* and *S. epidermidis* (endocarditis, osteomyelitis, prostatitis); Legionnaire's disease; in combination with dapsone for leprosy; prophylaxis of meningitis due to *Haemophilus influenzae* and gram-negative bacteremia in infants.

Contraindications: Hypersensitivity; not recommended for intermittent therapy.

Special Concerns: Safe use during lactation has not been established. Safety and effectiveness not determined in children less than 5 years of age. Use with extreme caution in clients with hepatic dysfunction.

Side Effects: *GI:* N&V, diarrhea, anorexia, gas, pseudomembranous colitis, pancreatitis, sore mouth and tongue, cramps, heartburn, flatulence. *CNS:* Headache, drowsiness, fatigue, ataxia, dizziness, confusion, generalized numbness, fever, difficulty in concentrating. *Hepatic:* Jaundice, hepatitis. Increases in AST, ALT, bilirubin, alkaline phosphatase. *Hematologic:* Thrombocytopenia, eosinophilia, hemolysis, leukopenia, ***hemolytic anemia.*** *Allergic:* Flu-like symptoms, dyspnea, wheezing, SOB, purpura, pruritus, urticaria, skin rashes, sore mouth and tongue, conjunctivitis. *Renal:* Hematuria, hemoglobinuria, renal insufficiency, acute renal failure. *Miscellaneous:* Visual disturbances, muscle weakness or pain, arthralgia, decreased BP, osteomalacia, menstrual disturbances, edema of face and extremities, adrenocortical insufficiency, increases in BUN and serum uric acid. *NOTE:* Body fluids and feces may be red-orange.

R

Laboratory Test Considerations: ↑ AST, ALT, alkaline phosphatase, BUN, bilirubin, uric acid, BSP retention values. False + Coombs' test.

OD Management of Overdose: *Symptoms:* Shortly after ingestion, N&V, and lethargy will occur. Followed by severe hepatic involvement (liver enlargement with tenderness, increased direct and total bilirubin, change in hepatic enzymes) with unconsciousness. Also, brownish red or orange discoloration of urine, saliva, tears, sweat, skin, and feces. *Treatment:* Gastric lavage followed by activated charcoal slurry introduced into the stomach. Antiemetics to control N&V. Forced diuresis to enhance excretion. If hepatic function is seriously impaired, bile drainage may be required. Extracorporeal hemodialysis may be necessary.

Drug Interactions

Acetaminophen / ↓ Effect of acetaminophen due to ↑ breakdown by liver
Aminophylline / ↓ Effect of aminophylline due to ↑ breakdown by liver
Anticoagulants, oral / ↓ Effect of anticoagulants due to ↑ breakdown by liver
Antidiabetics, oral / ↓ Effect of oral antidiabetic due to ↑ breakdown by liver
Barbiturates / ↓ Effect of barbiturates due to ↑ breakdown by liver
Benzodiazepines / ↓ Effect of benzodiazepines due to ↑ breakdown by liver
Beta-adrenergic blocking agents / ↓ Effect of beta-blocking agents due to ↑ breakdown by liver
Chloramphenicol / ↓ Effect of chloramphenicol due to ↑ breakdown by liver
Clofibrate / ↓ Effect of clofibrate due to ↑ breakdown by liver
Contraceptives, oral / ↓ Effect of oral contraceptives due to ↑ breakdown by liver
Corticosteroids / ↓ Effect of corticosteroids due to ↑ breakdown by liver
Cyclosporine / ↓ Effect of cyclosporine due to ↑ breakdown by liver
Digitoxin / ↓ Effect of digitoxin due to ↑ breakdown by liver
Digoxin / ↓ Serum levels of digoxin
Disopyramide / ↓ Effect of disopyramide due to ↑ breakdown by liver
Estrogens / ↓ Effect of estrogens due to ↑ breakdown by liver
Halothane / ↑ Risk of hepatotoxicity and hepatic encephalopathy
Hydantoins / ↓ Effect of hydantoins due to ↑ breakdown by liver
Isoniazid / ↑ Risk of hepatotoxicity
Ketoconazole / ↓ Effect of either ketoconazole or rifampin
Methadone / ↓ Effect of methadone due to ↑ breakdown by liver
Mexiletine / ↓ Effect of mexiletine due to ↑ breakdown by liver
Quinidine / ↓ Effect of quinidine due to ↑ breakdown by liver
Sulfones / ↓ Effect of sulfones due to ↑ breakdown by liver
Theophylline / ↓ Effect of theophylline due to ↑ breakdown by liver
Tocainide / ↓ Effect of tocainide due to ↑ breakdown by liver
Verapamil / ↓ Effect of verapamil due to ↑ breakdown by liver

How Supplied: *Capsule:* 150 mg, 300 mg; *Powder for injection:* 600 mg

Dosage

- **Capsules, IV**

Pulmonary tuberculosis.

Adults: Single dose of 600 mg/day; **children over 5 years:** 10–20 mg/kg/day, not to exceed 600 mg/day.

Meningococcal carriers.

Adults: 600 mg b.i.d. for 2 days; **children:** 10–20 mg/kg q 12 hr for four doses, not to exceed 600 mg/day.

HEALTH CARE CONSIDERATIONS

See also *General Health Care Considerations for All Anti-Infectives.*

Administration/Storage

1. Administer capsules once daily 1 hr before or 2 hr after meals to ensure maximum absorption.
2. A PO suspension (10 mg/mL) may be prepared as follows: The contents of either four 300-mg rifampin capsules or eight 150-mg capsules are emptied into a 4-oz amber glass bottle. Add 20 mL of simple syrup; shake vigorously; then add 100 mL of simple syrup and shake again. The suspension is stable for 4 weeks when stored at room temperature or in the refrigerator.
3. Check to be sure that there is a desiccant in the bottle containing capsules of rifampin because these are relatively moisture sensitive.
4. If administered concomitantly with PAS, give drugs 8–12 hr apart because the acid interferes with the absorption of rifampin.
5. When used for tuberculosis, continue therapy for 6–9 months.
6. IV Reconstitute 600-mg vial using 10 mL of sterile water for injection. Gently swirl vial to dissolve. The resultant solution contains 60 mg/mL rifampin; it is stable at room temperature for 24 hr.
7. Add the volume of reconstituted solution needed to 500 mL of D5W and infuse over 3 hr, or it may be added to 100 mL D5W and infused over 30 min. Sterile saline may be used when dextrose is contraindicated; however, the stability of rifampin is slightly less.
8. The diluted solution must be used within 4 hr or drug may precipitate from solution.
9. Injectable solution appears dark reddish brown.

Assessment

1. Record indications for therapy, type, onset, and duration of symptoms.
2. List any previous therapy.
3. Monitor CBC, cultures, liver and renal function studies; note any dysfunction.
4. Document any GI disturbances or auditory nerve impairment.
5. Obtain baseline CXR; auscultate and describe/record lung sounds and characteristics of sputum. Note PPD skin test results.

Client/Family Teaching

1. Take drug on an empty stomach 1 hr before or 2 hr after meals; report if GI upset occurs.
2. Must take daily for months to effectively treat tuberculosis. Do not stop or skip doses of medication.
3. Avoid alcohol; increases risk of liver toxicity.
4. Headache, drowsiness, confusion, fever, and muscle and joint aches may occur during the first few weeks of therapy; report if symptoms persist or increase in intensity.
5. Rifampin may impart a red-orange color to urine, feces, saliva, sputum, and tears; may *permanently* discolor contact lenses.
6. Practice alternative birth control since oral contraceptives not effective; drug has teratogenic properties.

Outcome/Evaluate

- Adjunct in treating tuberculosis
- Prophylaxis of meningitis due to *H. influenzae* and gram-negative bacteremia in infants

COMBINATION DRUG

Rifampin and Isoniazid

(rih-**FAM**-pin/**eye**-s**NYE**-ah-zid)

Pregnancy Category: C

Rifamate, Rimactane/INH Dual Pack **(Rx)**

Classification: Antitubercular drug combination

See also *Rifampin* and *Isoniazid.*

Content: Each capsule contains the following antituberculosis drugs: rifampin, 300 mg, and isoniazid, 150 mg.

Uses: Pulmonary tuberculosis following completion of initial therapy. Concomitant treatment with pyridoxine is recommended in malnourished clients, in those predisposed to neuropathy (e.g., alcoholics, diabetics), and in adolescents.

Contraindications: To treat meningococcal infections or asymptomatic carriers of *Neisseria meningitidis* to eliminate meningococci from the nasopharynx. In those who have previous isoniazid-induced hepatic injury or who have had severe side effects to isoniazid.

Special Concerns: Use with caution in impaired liver function, as rifampin and isoniazid can cause liver dysfunction and fatal hepatitis, respectively. Use with caution, if at all, during lactation.

Side Effects: See individual entries for *Rifampin* and *Isoniazid.*

How Supplied: See Content

Dosage

- **Capsules**

  Pulmonary tuberculosis.

Adults: Two capsules once daily.

R

HEALTH CARE CONSIDERATIONS

See also *Health Care Considerations* for *Rifampin* and *Isoniazid.*

Assessment

1. Record symptom onset, source of contact, other agents prescribed.
2. Note previous experience with this drug. Renal hypersensitivity has been reported when therapy was resumed after interruption.
3. Note any alcohol abuse.
4. Monitor CBC, CXR, liver and renal function studies; note dysfunction.

Client/Family Teaching

1. Take exactly as prescribed (should be taken either 1 hr before or 2 hr after a meal); do not skip doses or share medications.
2. Body secretions (urine, feces, tears, sputum, sweat) and skin may become discolored orange-red. Soft contact lenses may become permanently stained.
3. Report any numbness or tingling in hands and feet (S&S of peripheral neuropathy or toxicity). Coadministration of pyridoxine may help prevent CNS toxic effects.
4. Report symptoms of fatigue, weakness, malaise, N&V, and anorexia (symptoms of hepatitis).
5. Practice alternative birth control since oral contraceptives not effective; drug has teratogenic properties.
6. Therapy will be continued until bacterial conversion and maximal improvement is noted.

Outcome/Evaluate: Successful treatment and resolution of tubercle bacilli

R

COMBINATION DRUG

Rifampin, Isoniazid, and Pyrazinamide

(rih-**FAM**-pin/**eye**-soh-**NYE**-ah-zid/pie-rah-**ZIN**-ah-myd)

Pregnancy Category: C

Rifater **(Rx)**

Classification: Antitubercular drug combination

See also *Rifampin* and *Isoniazid.*

Content: Each tablet contains the following antituberculosis drugs: rifampin, 120 mg; isoniazid, 50 mg; and pyrazinamide, 300 mg.
Uses: Initial phase of the short-course (2-month) treatment of pulmonary tuberculosis. Either streptomycin or ethambutol may be added unless the likelihood of resistance to isoniazid or rifampin is low. Concomitant treatment with pyridoxine is recommended in malnourished client's, in those predisposed to neuropathy (e.g., alcoholics, diabetics), and in adolescents. The 2-month treatment with Rifater is followed by a 4-month course of therapy with rifampin and isoniazid (Rifamate).
Contraindications: Hypersensitivity to any of the components. Severe hepatic damage, acute gout. Lactation.
Special Concerns: Use with caution in impaired liver function, as rifampin and isoniazid can cause liver dysfunction and fatal hepatitis, respectively. Use with caution in diabetes mellitus. Safety and efficacy have not been determined in children less than 15 years of age.
Side Effects: For side effects caused by isoniazid or rifampin, consult those drug entries. The side effects due to pyrazinamide follow. *Hepatic:* Hepatotoxicity, porphyria. *GI:* N&V, anorexia. *Hematologic:* Thrombocytopenia, sideroblastic anemia with erythroid hyperplasia, vacuolation of erythrocytes, and increased serum concentration. *Hypersensitivity:* Rashes, urticaria, pruritus. *Miscellaneous:* Hyperuricemia, gout, mild arthralgia and myalgia, fever, acne, photosensitivity, dysuria, interstitial nephritis.
How Supplied: See Content.

Dosage

- **Tablets**

Short-course treatment of pulmonary tuberculosis.

Clients weighing less than 44 kg: 4 tablets/day given at the same time. **Clients weighing 45–54 kg:** 5 tablets/day given at the same time. **Clients weighing more than 55 kg:** 6 tablets/day given at the same time.

HEALTH CARE CONSIDERATIONS

See also *Health Care Considerations* for *Rifampin* and *Isoniazid.*

Administration/Storage

1. Intended for use during the first 2 months of therapy.
2. Protect tablets from excessive humidity; store at room temperature.

Assessment

1. Record symptom onset, characteristics, source of contact, other agents prescribed, and outcome.
2. Monitor CBC, CXR, serum uric acid, and LFTs; note dysfunction.
3. Note/record any alcohol abuse.
4. Assess those with preexisting liver disease or those at risk for drug-related hepatitis (e.g., alcoholics) closely. The drug should be withdrawn if signs of hepatocellular damage or hyperuricemia accompanied by an acute gouty arthritis occur. However, if hyperuricemia accompanied by an acute gouty ar-

thritis occurs without liver dysfunction, can transfer to a regimen that does not contain pyrazinamide.

Client/Family Teaching

1. Take tablets either 1 hr before or 2 hr after a meal with a full glass of water and 1 hr before antacids.
2. Therapy is short-term (2 months) and will be followed by a 4-month course of rifamate.
3. Avoid tyramine- (cheese, red wine) and histamine- (skipjack, tuna, other tropical fish) containing foods.
4. Drug contains rifampin, which may cause a red-orange discoloration to body secretions (sweat, sputum, urine, feces, tears) and skin. Soft contact lenses may become permanently stained.
5. Report any numbness or tingling in hands and feet; S&S of peripheral neuropathy or toxicity. Coadministration of pyridoxine may help prevent CNS toxic effects.
6. Report symptoms of fatigue, weakness, malaise, N&V, and anorexia (symptoms of hepatitis).
7. Avoid alcohol or any alcohol-containing products.

Outcome/Evaluate: Treatment of pulmonary tuberculosis/resolution of tubercle bacilli infection.

Rifapentine

(rih-fah-**PEN**-teen)
Pregnancy Category: C
Priftin **(Rx)**
Classification: Antituberculosis drug

Action/Kinetics: Similar activity to rifampin. Inhibits DNA–dependent RNA polymerase in susceptible strains of *Mycobacterium tuberculosis*, but not in mammalian cells. Is bactericidal against both intracellular and extracellular organisms. Food increases amount absorbed. **Maximum levels:** 5–6 hr. **Steady state conditions:** 10 days after 600 mg/day. Metabolized to the active 25–desacetyl rifapentine. Both the parent drug and active metabolite are significantly bound to plasma proteins. **t½:** 13.2 hr for parent drug, 13.4 hr for active metabolite. Excreted in the feces (70%) and the urine (17%).

Uses: Treatment of pulmonary tuberculosis. Must be used with at least one other antituberculosis drug.

Contraindications: Hypersensitivity to other rifamycins (e.g., rifampin or rifabutin). Lactation.

Special Concerns: Experience is limited in HIV-infected clients. Organisms resistant to other rifamycins are likely to be resistant to rifapentine. Use with caution in clients with abnormal liver tests or liver disease. Safety and efficacy have not been determined in children less than 12 years of age.

Side Effects: Side effects listed occurred in 1% or more of clients and were seen when rifapentine was used in combination with other antituberculosis drugs (e.g., isoniazid, pyrazinamide, ethambutol). *GI:* N&V, dyspepsia, diarrhea, hemoptysis. *CNS:* Anorexia, headache, dizziness. *GU:* Pyuria, proteinuria, hematuria, urinary casts. *Dermatologic:* Rash, acne, maculopapular rash. *Hematologic:* Neutropenia, lymphopenia, anemia, leukopenia, thrombocytosis. *Miscellaneous:* Hyperuricemia (probably due to pyrizinamide), hypertension, pruritus, arthralgia, pain, red coloration of body tissues and fluids.

Laboratory Test Considerations: ↑ ALT, AST. Inhibition of standard microbiological assays for serum folate and vitamin B_{12}.

Drug Interactions

Cytochrome P450 / Rifapentine is an inducer of certain cytochromes P450 → reduced activity of a number of drugs (See *Rifampin*). Dosage adjustment may be required
Indinavir / Three-fold ↑ in clearance of indinavir.

How Supplied: *Tablets:* 150 mg

Dosage

- **Tablets**

Tuberculosis, intensive phase.
600 mg (four 150 mg tablets) twice weekly with an interval of 72 hr or more between doses continued for 2 months.

Tuberculosis, continuation phase
Continue rifapentine therapy once weekly for 4 months in combination with isoniazid or another antituberculosis drug. If the client is still sputum-smear- or culture-positive, if resistant organisms are present, or if the client is HIV-positive, follow ATS/CDC treatment guidelines.

R

HEALTH CARE CONSIDERATIONS

Administration/Storage

1. Give concomitant pyridoxine in the malnourished, those predisposed to neuropathy (e.g., alcoholics, diabetics), and in adolescents.
2. Give rifapentine in combination as part of a regimen that includes other antituberculosis drugs, especially on days when rifapentine is not given.
3. May be given with food if stomach upset, nausea, or vomiting occurs.

Assessment

1. Determine onset, duration, and characteristics of disease.
2. Obtain chemistries, CBC, and LFTs; assess sputum culture. Monitor LFTs every two to four weeks during therapy.
3. List other drugs prescribed to ensure none interact.

Client/Family Teaching

1. Take exactly as directed. May take with food if stomach upset, nausea, or vomiting occurs.
2. Vitamin B_6 is prescribed for clients who are malnourished or predisposed to neuropathy, and in adolescents.
3. May stain body fluids/tissues (tears, urine, saliva, sweat, skin, teeth, feces, tongue) a red-orange color.
4. Drug is administered less frequently and in conjunction with other antitubercular agents. During the two-month intensive phase, drug is taken every three days. Following this phase, rifapentine is given once a week for four months in combinations with isoniazid or other agent for susceptible organisms called the continuation phase for TB. A more frequent dosing pattern is used in HIV infected clients. Adherence to prescribed regimen is of utmost importance.
5. Report any N&V, fever, darkened urine, pain or swelling of the joints, or yellow discolorations of the skin and eyes.

Outcome/Evaluate

- Treatment of pulmonary TB
- Prevention of disseminated *Mycobacterium avium* complex disease with HIV infection

R

Riluzole

(RIL-you-zohl)
Pregnancy Category: C
Rilutek **(Rx)**
Classification: Drug for amyotrophic lateral sclerosis

Action/Kinetics: Mechanism not known. Possible effects include (a) inhibition of glutamate release, (b) inactivation of voltage-dependent sodium channels, and (c) interference with intracellular events that follow transmitter binding at excitatory amino acid receptors. Well absorbed following PO use; high-fat meals decrease absorption. **t½, elimination, after repeated doses:** 12 hr. About 96% is bound to plasma proteins. Extensively metabolized, mainly in the liver, and excreted in the urine.

Uses: Treatment of clients with ALS; the drug extends both survival and time to tracheostomy.

Contraindications: Lactation.

Special Concerns: Use with caution in hepatic and renal impairment due to decreased excretion and higher plasma levels. Use with caution in the elderly, as age-related changes in renal and hepatic function may cause a decreased clearance. Clearance of riluzole in Japanese clients is 50% lower compared with Caucasians; clearance may also be lower in women. Safety and efficacy have not been determined in children.

Side Effects: Side effects listed occurred at a frequency of 0.1% or more. *GI:* N&V, diarrhea, anorexia, abdominal pain, dyspepsia, flatulence, dry mouth, stomatitis, tooth disorder, oral moniliasis, dysphagia, constipation, increased appetite, intestinal obstruction, fecal impaction, ***GI hemorrhage,*** GI ulceration, gastritis, fecal incontinence, jaundice, hepatitis, glossitis, gum hemorrhage, pancreatitis, tenesmus, esophageal stenosis. *Body as a whole:* Asthenia, malaise, weight loss or gain, peripheral edema, flu syndrome, hostility, abscess, ***sepsis,*** photosensitivity reaction, cellulitis, facial edema, hernia, peritonitis, reaction at injection site, chills, ***attempted suicide,*** enlarged abdomen, neoplasm. *CNS:* Dizziness (more common in women), vertigo, somnolence, circumoral paresthesia, headache, aggravation reaction, hypertonia, depression, insomnia, agitation, tremor, hallucination, personality disorders, abnormal thinking, coma, paranoid reaction, manic reaction, ataxia, extrapyramidal syndrome, hypokinesis, emotional lability, delusions, apathy, hypesthesia, incoordination, confusion, ***convulsion,*** amnesia, increased libido, stupor subdural hematoma, abnormal gait, delirium, depersonalization, facial paralysis, hemiplegia, decreased libido. *CV:* Hypertension, tachycardia, phlebitis, palpitation, postural hypotension, ***heart arrest, heart failure,*** syncope, hypotension, migraine, peripheral vascular disease, angina pectoris, ***MI,*** ventricular extrasystoles, ***cerebral hemorrhage,*** atrial fibrillation, bundle branch block, CHF, pericarditis, lower extremity embolus, ***myocardial ischemia, shock.*** *Hematologic:* Neutropenia, anemia, leukocytosis, leukopenia, ecchymosis. *Respiratory:* Decreased lung function, pneumonia, rhinitis, increased cough, sinusitis, apnea, bronchitis, dyspnea, respiratory disorder, increased sputum, hiccup, pleural disorder, asthma, epistaxis, hemoptysis, yawn, hyperventilation, lung edema, hypoventilation, ***lung carcinoma,*** hypoxia, laryngitis, pleural effusion, pneumothorax, respiratory moniliasis, stridor. *Musculoskeletal:* Arthralgia, back pain, leg cramps, dysarthria, myoclonus, arthrosis, myasthenia, ***bone neoplasm.*** *GU:* Urinary retention, urinary urgency, urine abnormality, urinary incontinence, kidney calculus, hematuria, impotence, ***prostate carcinoma,*** kidney pain, metrorrhagia, priapism. *Dermatologic:* Pruritus, eczema, alopecia, exfoliative dermatitis, skin ulceration, urticaria, psoriasis, seborrhea, skin disorder, fungal dermatitis. *Metabolic:* Gout, respiratory acidosis, edema, thirst, hypokalemia, hyponatremia. *Miscellaneous:* Accidental or intentional injury, ***death,*** diabetes mellitus, thyroid neoplasia, amblyopia, ophthalmitis.

Laboratory Test Considerations: ↑ Gamma glutamyl transferase, alkaline phosphatase, gamma globulins. Abnormal liver function tests, + direct Coombs' test.

Drug Interactions

Amitriptyline / ↓ Elimination of riluzole → higher plasma levels

Caffeine / ↓ Elimination of riluzole → higher plasma levels

Charcoal-broiled foods / ↑ Elimination of riluzole → lower plasma levels

Omeprazole / ↑ Elimination of riluzole → lower plasma levels

Quinolones / ↓ Elimination of riluzole → higher plasma levels

Rifampin / ↑ Elimination of riluzole → lower plasma levels

Smoking (cigarettes) / ↑ Elimination of riluzole → lower plasma levels

Theophyllines / ↓ Elimination of riluzole → higher plasma levels

How Supplied: *Tablets*: 50 mg.

Dosage

- **Tablets**

Treatment of ALS.

50 mg q 12 hr. Higher daily doses will not increase the beneficial effect but will increase the incidence of side effects.

HEALTH CARE CONSIDERATIONS

Administration/Storage

1. Take 1 hr before or 2 hr after a meal to avoid decreased bioavailability. Take at the same time each day. If a dose is missed, take the next tablet as originally planned.
2. Protect from bright light.

Assessment

1. Record symptom onset, characteristics, presentation, ethnic background, and familial associations.
2. Assess renal and LFTs. Elevations of several liver functions, especially bilirubin, should preclude drug use.
3. Monitor LFTs. SGPT levels should be measured q month during the first 3 months of therapy, q 3 months for the remainder of the first year, and then periodically.

Client/Family Teaching

1. Take 1 hr before or 2 hr after meals to maintain drug bioavailability.
2. Take as prescribed at the same time each day. Do not double up if dose is missed or forgotten.
3. Report any febrile illnesses.
4. Drug may cause dizziness, drowsiness, or vertigo. Do not perform activities that require mental alertness until drug effects realized.
5. Severe dry mouth symptoms may require use of salagen.
6. Do not smoke. Avoid alcohol, as alcohol may potentiate liver toxicity.

Outcome/Evaluate: Extension of survival or time to tracheostomy with ALS

Rimantadine hydrochloride

(rih-**MAN**-tih-deen)

Pregnancy Category: C

Flumadine **(Rx)**

Classification: Antiviral agent

See also *Antiviral Drugs* and *Amantadine.*

Action/Kinetics: May act early in the viral replication cycle, possibly by inhibiting the uncoating of the virus. A virus protein specified by the virion M_2 gene may play an important role in the inhibition of the influenza A virus by rimantadine. Has little or no activity against influenza B virus. Plasma trough levels following 100 mg b.i.d. for 10 days range from 118 to 468 ng/mL; however, levels are higher in clients over the age of 70 years. Metabolized in the liver, and both unchanged drug (25%) and metabolites excreted through the urine.

Uses: In adults for prophylaxis and treatment of illness caused by strains of influenza A virus. In children for prophylaxis against influenza A virus.

Contraindications: Hypersensitivity to amantadine, rimantadine, or other drugs in the adamantine class. Lactation.

Special Concerns: Use with caution in clients with renal or hepatic insufficiency. An increased incidence of seizures is possible in clients with a history of epilepsy who have received amantadine. Influenza A virus strains resistant to rimantadine can emerge during treatment and be transmitted, causing symptoms of influenza. Safety and efficacy of rimantadine in the treatment of symptomatic influenza infections in children have not been established. Safety and efficacy for prophylax-

R

is of infections have not been determined in children less than 1 year of age. The incidence of side effects in geriatric clients is higher than in other clients.

Side Effects: GI and CNS side effects are the most common. *GI:* N&V, anorexia, dry mouth, abdominal pain, diarrhea, dyspepsia, constipation, dysphagia, stomatitis. *CNS:* Insomnia, dizziness, headache, nervousness, fatigue, asthenia, impairment of concentration, ataxia, somnolence, agitation, depression, gait abnormality, euphoria, hyperkinesia, tremor, hallucinations, confusion, ***convulsions,*** agitation, diaphoresis, hypesthesia. *Respiratory:* Dyspnea, ***bronchospasm,*** cough. *CV:* Pallor, palpitation, hypertension, ***cerebrovascular disorder, cardiac failure,*** pedal edema, heart block, tachycardia, syncope. *Miscellaneous:* Tinnitus, taste loss or change, parosmia, eye pain, rash, nonpuerperal lactation, increased lacrimation, increased frequency of micturition, fever, rigors.

OD **Management of Overdose:** *Symptoms:* Extensions of side effects including the possibility of agitation, hallucinations, ***cardiac arrhythmias, and death.*** *Treatment:* Supportive therapy. IV physostigmine at doses of 1–2 mg IV in adults and 0.5 mg in children, not to exceed 2 mg/hr, has been reported to be beneficial in treating overdose for amantadine (a related drug).

Drug Interactions

Acetaminophen / ↓ Peak concentration and area under the curve for rimantadine

Aspirin / ↓ Peak plasma levels and area under the curve for rimantadine

Cimetidine / ↓ Clearance of rimantadine

How Supplied: *Syrup:* 50 mg/5 mL; *Tablet:* 100 mg

Dosage

- **Syrup, Tablets**

Prophylaxis.

Adults and children over 10 years of age: 100 mg b.i.d. In clients with severe hepatic dysfunction (C_{CR} < 10 mL/min) and in elderly nursing home clients, reduce the dose to 100 mg/day. **Children, less than 10 years of age:** 5 mg/kg once daily, not to exceed a total dose of 150 mg/day.

Treatment.

Adults: 100 mg b.i.d. In clients with severe hepatic dysfunction and in elderly nursing home clients, reduce the dose to 100 mg/day.

HEALTH CARE CONSIDERATIONS

See also *Health Care Considerations* for *Amantadine.*

Administration/Storage: For treatment of influenza A virus infections, initiate therapy as soon as possible, preferably within 48 hr after onset of S&S. Continue treatment for approximately 7 days from the initial onset of symptoms.

Assessment

1. Record indications for therapy, noting onset and duration of symptoms or exposure.
2. Determine when immunized.
3. List other drugs prescribed to ensure none interact unfavorably.
4. Assess liver and renal function studies to determine any dysfunction; reduce dosage with severe hepatic dysfunction and with elderly nursing home clients.
5. Note/record any history of epilepsy; assess for loss of seizure control.

Client/Family Teaching

1. Take only as directed; do not share meds.
2. Initiate as soon as symptoms appear and continue for 7 days.
3. Drug may cause dizziness.
4. Early annual vaccination is the method of choice for influenza prophylaxis. The 2- to 4-week time frame required to develop an antibody response can be managed with rimantadine.

Outcome/Evaluate: Prevention/ ↓ severity of influenza A virus

Rimexolone

(rih-**MEX**-ah-lohn)

Pregnancy Category: C

Vexol **(Rx)**

Classification: Corticosteroid, ophthalmic

See also *Corticosteroids.*

Action/Kinetics: Very low plasma levels seen after ophthalmic use.

Uses: Treatment of postoperative inflammation following ocular surgery. Treatment of anterior uveitis.

Contraindications: Use in epithelial herpes simplex keratitis; vaccinia, varicella, and most other viral infections of the cornea or conjunctiva; mycobacterial infections of the eye; fungal infections of the eye; any acute, untreated eye infection.

Special Concerns: Acute purulent ocular infections may be masked if used in bacterial, fungal, or viral eye infections. Safety and efficacy have not been determined in children.

Side Effects: *Ophthalmic:* Elevated IOP, blurred vision, discharge, discomfort, ocular pain, foreign body sensation, hyperemia, pruritus, sticky sensation, increased fibrin, dry eye, conjunctival edema, corneal staining, keratitis, tearing, photophobia, edema, irrita-

tion, corneal ulcer, browache, lid margin crusting, corneal edema, infiltrate, corneal erosion. *Respiratory;* Pharyngitis, rhinitis. *Miscellaneous:* Headache, taste perversion. *Prolonged use:* Ocular hypertension, glaucoma, optic nerve damage, defects in visual acuity and visual fields, posterior subcapsular formation, secondary ocular infections, perforation of the globe where there is thinning of the cornea or sclera.
How Supplied: *Ophthalmic Suspension:* 1%

Dosage

• **Ophthalmic Suspension**

Postoperative inflammation following ocular surgery.

Adults: 1–2 gtt in the conjunctival sac(s) q.i.d. beginning 24 hr after surgery and continuing for 2 weeks.

Anterior uveitis.

Adults: 1–2 gtt in the conjunctival sac(s) q hr during waking hours during the first week and 1 gtt q 2 hr during the second week; then, taper the dose until uveitis is resolved.

HEALTH CARE CONSIDERATIONS

See also *Health Care Considerations* for *Corticosteroids.*

Administration/Storage: Store upright between 4°C–30°C (40°F–86°F). Shake well before use.

Client/Family Teaching

1. Use ATC exactly as directed.
2. Wash hands before instillation and avoid contact with the container and surrounding eye structure.
3. Report any adverse reactions, increased pain, or vision changes.

Outcome/Evaluate: ↓ Ocular inflammation; control of uveitis

Risedronate sodium

(rih-**SEH**-droh-nayt)

Pregnancy Category: C

Actonel **(Rx)**

Classification: Biphosphonate for Paget's disease

Action/Kinetics: Inhibits osteoclasts, thus leading to decreased bone resorption. Rapidly absorbed; food decreases absorption. **t½, initial:** 1.5 hr; **terminal:** 220 hr. Excreted unchanged in the urine.
Uses: Treatment of Paget's disease in those who (1) have a serum alkaline phosphatase level at least two times the upper limit of normal, (2) are symptomatic, or (3) are at risk for future complications from the disease.
Contraindications: Use in those with C_{CR} less than 30 mL/min. Hypocalcemia. Lactation.
Special Concerns: May cause upper GI disorders, including dysphagia, esophagitis, esophageal ulcer, or gastric ulcer. Use with caution in those with a history of UGI disorders. Safety and efficacy have not been determined in children.
Side Effects: *GI:* Diarrhea, abdominal pain, nausea, constipation, belching, colitis. *CNS:* Headache, dizziness. *Body as a whole:* Flu syndrome, chest pain, asthenia, neoplasm. *Musculoskeletal:* Arthralgia, bone pain, leg cramps, myasthenia. *Respiratory:* Sinusitis, bronchitis. Ophthalmic: Amblyopia, dry eye. *Miscellaneous:* Peripheral edema, skin rash, tinnitus.
OD **Management of Overdose:** *Symptoms:* Hypocalemia. *Treatment:* Gastric lavage to remove unabsorbed drug. Milk or antacids to bind risedronate. IV calcium.

Drug Interactions

Antacids, calcium-containing / ↓ Absorption of risedronate
Bone imaging agents / Risedronate interferes with these agents
Calcium / ↓ Absorption of risedronate
NSAIDs / Possible additive GI side effects

How Supplied: *Tablets:* 30 mg

Dosage

• **Tablets**

Treat Paget's disease.

Adults: 30 mg once daily for 2 months.

HEALTH CARE CONSIDERATIONS

Administration/Storage

1. Before starting therapy, treat hypocalcemia and other disturbances of bone and mineral metabolism.
2. Following post-treatment observation for 2 months, retreatment may be considered if serum alkaline phosphatase is not normal. For retreatment, the dose and duration of therapy is the same as for initial treatment.

Assessment

1. Record onset and characteristics of disease; list other agents trialed.
2. Obtain chemistries, alkaline phosphatase, Ca, liver and renal function studies; avoid if $C_{CR} < 30$ mL/min.

Client/Family Teaching

1. Take sitting or standing with a full glass of water at least 30 min before the first food or drink of the day.
2. To facilitate delivery to the stomach and minimize GI side effects, take in an upright position with 6 to 8 oz of water. Avoid lying down for 30 min after taking the drug.

R

3. Therapy is once a day for two months.
4. If dietary intake is not adequate, consume supplemental calcium and vitamin D.
5. Antacids and calcium may interfere with drug; take at different times during the day with food.
6. Report any swallowing difficulty, throat or abdominal pain.

Outcome/Evaluate: Remission of Paget's disease with ↓ bone resorption, ↓ pain and ↓ alkaline phosphatase levels

Risperidone

(ris-**PAIR**-ih-dohn)

Pregnancy Category: C

Risperdal **(Rx)**

Classification: Antipsychotic

Action/Kinetics: Mechanism may be due to a combination of antagonism of dopamine (D_2) and serotonin ($5\text{-}HT_2$) receptors. Also has high affinity for the alpha-1, alpha-2, and histamine-1 receptors. Metabolized significantly in the liver to the active metabolite 9-hydroxyrisperidone, which has equal receptor-binding activity as risperidone. Thus, the effect is likely due to both the parent compound and the metabolite. Food does not affect either the rate or extent of absorption. The ability to convert risperidone to 9-hydroxyrisperidone is subject to genetic variation. A low percentage of Asians have the ability to metabolize the drug. **Peak plasma levels, risperidone:** 1 hr; **peak plasma levels, 9-hydroxyrisperidone:** 3 hr for extensive metabolizers and 17 hr for poor metabolizers. **t½, risperidone and 9-methylrisperidone:** 3 and 21 hr, respectively, for extensive metabolizers and 20 and 30 hr, respectively, for poor metabolizers. Clearance is decreased in geriatric clients and in clients with hepatic and renal impairment.

Uses: Treatment of psychotic disorders.

Contraindications: Lactation.

Special Concerns: Use with caution in clients with known CV disease (including history of MI or ischemia, heart failure, conduction abnormalities), cerebrovascular disease, and conditions that predispose the client to hypotension (e.g., dehydration, hypovolemia, use of antihypertensive drugs). Use with caution in clients who will be exposed to extreme heat or when taken with other CNS drugs or alcohol. The effectiveness of risperidone for more than 6–8 weeks has not been studied. Safety and effectiveness have not been established for children.

Side Effects: ***Neuroleptic malignant syndrome:*** Hyperpyrexia, muscle rigidity, altered mental status, autonomic instability (i.e., irregular pulse or BP, tachycardia, diaphoresis, cardiac dysrhythmia), elevated CPK, rhabdomyolysis, ***acute renal failure, death.*** *CNS:* Tardive dyskinesia (especially in geriatric clients), somnolence, insomnia, agitation, anxiety, aggressive reaction, extrapyramidal symptoms, headache, dizziness, increased dream activity, decreased sexual desire, nervousness, impaired concentration, depression, apathy, catatonia, euphoria, increased libido, amnesia, increased duration of sleep, dysarthria, vertigo, stupor, paresthesia, confusion. *GI:* Constipation, nausea, dyspepsia, vomiting, abdominal pain, increased or decreased salivation, toothache, anorexia, flatulence, diarrhea, increased appetite, stomatitis, melena, dysphagia, hemorrhoids, gastritis. *CV:* Prolongation of the QT interval that might lead to ***torsades de pointes,***. Orthostatic hypotension, tachycardia, palpitation, hypertension or hypotension, ***AV block, MI.*** *Respiratory:* Rhinitis, coughing, URI, sinusitis, pharyngitis, dyspnea. *Body as a whole:* Arthralgia, back pain, chest pain, fever, fatigue, rigors, malaise, edema, flu-like symptoms, increase or decrease in weight. *Hematologic:* Purpura, anemia, hypochromic anemia. *GU:* Polyuria, polydipsia, urinary incontinence, hematuria, dysuria, menorrhagia, orgastic dysfunction, dry vagina, erectile dysfunction, nonpuerperal lactation, amenorrhea, female breast pain, leukorrhea, mastitis, dysmenorrhea, female perineal pain, intermenstrual bleeding, ***vaginal hemorrhage,*** failure to ejaculate. *Dermatologic:* Rash, dry skin, seborrhea, increased pigmentation, increased or decreased sweating, acne, alopecia, hyperkeratosis, pruritus, skin exfoliation. *Ophthalmic:* Abnormal vision, abnormal accommodation, xerophthalmia. *Miscellaneous:* Increased prolactin, photosensitivity, diabetes mellitus, thirst, myalgia, epistaxis.

Laboratory Test Considerations: ↑ CPK, serum prolactin, AST, ALT. Hyponatremia.

OD **Management of Overdose:** *Symptoms:* Exaggeration of known effects, especially drowsiness, sedation, tachycardia, hypotension, and extrapyramidal symptoms. *Treatment:* Establish and secure airway, and ensure adequate oxygenation and ventilation. Follow gastric lavage with activated charcoal and a laxative. Monitor CV system, including continuous ECG readings. Provide general supportive measures. Treat hypotension and circulatory collapse with IV fluids or sympathomimetic drugs; however, do not use epinephrine and dopamine, as beta stimulation may worsen hypotension due to risperidone-induced alpha blockade. Anticholinergic drugs can be given for severe extrapyramidal symptoms.

Drug Interactions
Carbamazepine / ↑ Clearance of risperidone following chronic use of carbamazepine
Clozapine / ↓ Clearance of risperidone following chronic use of clozapine
Levodopa / Risperidone antagonizes the effects of levodopa and dopamine agonists
How Supplied: *Solution:* 1 mg/mL; *Tablet:* 1 mg, 2 mg, 3 mg, 4 mg

Dosage

- **Oral Solution, Tablets**

Antipsychotic.

Adults, initial: 1 mg b.i.d. Once daily dosing can also be used. Can be increased by 1 mg b.i.d. on the second and third days, as tolerated, to reach a dose of 3 mg b.i.d. by the third day. Further increases in dose should occur at intervals of about 1 week. **Maximal effect:** 4–6 mg/day. Doses greater than 6 mg/day were not shown to be more effective and were associated with greater incidence of side effects. Safety of doses greater than 16 mg/day have not been studied. **Maintenance:** Use lowest dose that will maintain remission. The initial dose is 0.5 mg b.i.d. for clients who are elderly or debilitated, those with severe renal or hepatic impairment, and those predisposed to hypotension or in whom hypotension would pose a risk. Dosage increases in these clients should be in increments of 0.5 mg b.i.d. Dosage increases above 1.5 mg b.i.d. should occur at intervals of about 1 week.

HEALTH CARE CONSIDERATIONS

See also *Health Care Considerations* for *Antipsychotic Drugs.*

Administration/Storage

1. Use a lower starting dose in geriatric clients and those with impaired renal or hepatic function. The PO solution may ease administration to geriatric clients and those in an acute-care setting.
2. When restarting clients who have had an interval of risperidone, follow the initial 3-day dose titration schedule.
3. If switching from other antipsychotic drugs to risperidone, immediate discontinuation of the previous antipsychotic drug is recommended when starting risperidone therapy. When switching from a depot antipsychotic injection, initiate risperidone in place of the next scheduled shot.

Assessment

1. Record indications for therapy; note onset and duration as well as presenting behavioral manifestations and mental status.
2. Perform appropriate baseline assessments. Electrolyte imbalance, bradycardia, and concomitant administration with drugs that prolong the QT interval may increase the risk of torsades de pointes.
3. Reduce dose with severe liver, cardiac, or renal dysfunction.
4. Note any history of drug dependency.
5. Observe for altered mental status, muscle rigidity, dyskinetic movements, or overt changes in VS.
6. The antiemetic effect of risperidone may mask the S&S of overdose with certain drugs or conditions such as intestinal obstruction, Reye's syndrome, and brain tumor.

Client/Family Teaching

1. Take only as directed; do not share meds or stop abruptly.
2. Drug may impair judgment, motor skills, and thinking and cause blurred vision; determine drug effects before engaging in activities that require mental alertness.
3. Rise slowly from a lying to a sitting position, dangle legs before standing; may cause orthostatic hypotension.
4. May alter temperature regulation; avoid exposure to extreme heat.
5. Wear protective clothing, sunscreen, hat, and sunglasses when sun exposure is necessary; may cause a photosensitivity reaction.
6. Report abnormal bruising/bleeding or yellow skin discoloration.
7. Practice birth control. Report if pregnancy is suspected or desired.
8. Avoid alcohol and any other OTC agents or CNS depressants.
9. Risperidone elevates serum prolactin levels. Explore the potential relationship of prolactin and human breast cancer development; report evidence/history of breast cancer.
10. Any suicide ideations or bizarre behavior should be reported immediately. Due to the possibility of suicide attempts with schizophrenia, advise that close supervision of high-risk clients is necessary and that prescriptions will be written for the smallest quantity of tablets. Stress importance of close F/U.

Outcome/Evaluate: Improved behavior patterns with ↓ agitation, ↓ hyperactivity, and reality orientation

Ritonavir

(rih-**TOH**-nah-veer)
Pregnancy Category: B
Norvir **(Rx)**
Classification: Antiviral drug, protease inhibitor

See also *Anitiviral Drugs.*

Action/Kinetics: A peptidomimetic inhibitor of both the HIV-1 and HIV-2 proteases. Inhibition of HIV protease results in the enzyme incapable of processing the "gag-pool" polyprotein precursor that leads to production of noninfectious immature HIV particles. **Peak concentrations after 600 mg of the solution:** 2 hr after fasting and 4 hr after nonfasting. **t½:** 3–5 hr. Metabolized by the cytochrome P450 system. Metabolites and unchanged drug are excreted through both the feces and urine.

Uses: Alone or in combination with nucleoside analogues (ddC or AZT) for the treatment of HIV infection. Use of ritonavir may result in a reduction in both mortality and AIDS-defining clinical events. Clinical benefit has not been determined for periods longer than 6 months.

Special Concerns: Not considered a cure for HIV infection; clients may continue to manifest illnesses associated with advanced HIV infection, including opportunistic infections. Also, therapy with ritonavir has not been shown to decrease the risk of transmitting HIV to others through sexual contact or blood contamination. Use with caution in those with impaired hepatic function and during lactation. Hemophiliacs treated with protease inhibitors may manifest spontaneous bleeding episodes. Safety and efficacy have not been determined in children less than 12 years of age.

Side Effects: Side effects listed are those with a frequency of 2% or greater. *GI:* N&V, diarrhea, taste perversion, anorexia, flatulence, constipation, abdominal pain, dyspepsia, local throat irritation. *Nervous:* Circumoral paresthesia, peripheral paresthesia, dizziness, insomnia, paresthesia, somnolence, abnormal thinking. *Body as a whole:* Asthenia, headache, malaise, fever. *Dermatologic:* Sweating, rash. *Miscellaneous:* Vasodilation, hyperlipidemia, myalgia, pharyngitis.

Laboratory Test Considerations: ↑ Triglycerides, AST, ALT, GGT, CPK, uric acid.

OD Management of Overdose: *Symptoms:* Extension of side effects. *Treatment:* General supportive measures, including monitoring of VS and observing the clinical status. Elimination of unabsorbed drug may be assisted by emesis or gastric lavage, with attention given to maintaining a patent airway. Activated charcoal may also help in removing any unabsorbed drug. Dialysis is not likely to be of benefit in removing the drug from the body.

Drug Interactions: Ritonavir is expected to produce large increases in the plasma levels of a number of drugs, including amiodarone, astemizole, bepridil, bupropion, cisapride, clozapine, encainide, erythromycin, flecainide, meperidine, methylphenidate, pentoxifylline, phenothiazines, piroxicam, propafenone, propoxyphene, quinidine, rifabutin, tefenadine, and warfarin. This may lead to an increased risk of arrhythmias, hematologic complications, seizures, or other serious adverse effects.

Ritonavir may produce a decrease in the plasma levels of the following drugs: atovaquone, clofibrate, daunorubicin, diphenoxylate, metoclopramide, and sedative/hypnotics.

Coadministration of ritonavir with the following drugs may cause extreme sedation and respiratory depression and thus should not be combined: alprazolam, clorazepate, diazepam, estazolam, flurazepam, midazolam, triazolam, and zolpidem.

Clarithromycin / ↑ Clarithromycin levels; reduce clarithromycin dose
Desipramine / Significant ↑ despiramine levels; reduce desipramine dose
Ethinyl estradiol / ↓ Ethyinyl estradiol levels; use alternative contraceptive
Propulsid / ↑ Risk of serious cardiac arrhythmias
Saquinavir / Significant ↑ in saquinavir blood levels
Theophylline / ↓ Theophylline levels

How Supplied: *Capsules:* 100 mg; *Oral Solution:* 600 mg/7.5 mL.

Dosage

- **Capsules, Oral Solution**

  Treatment of HIV infection.

600 mg b.i.d. If nausea is experienced upon initiation of therapy, dose escalation may be tried as follows: 300 mg b.i.d. for 1 day, 400 mg b.i.d. for 2 days, 500 mg b.i.d. for 1 day, and then 600 mg b.i.d. thereafter.

HEALTH CARE CONSIDERATIONS

See also *Health Care Considerations* for *Antiviral Drugs.*

Administration/Storage

1. Clients prescribed combination regimens with nucleoside analogues may improve GI tolerance by starting therapy with ritonavir alone and then adding the nucleoside before completing 2 weeks of ritonavir monotherapy.
2. Store capsules in the refrigerator at 2°C–8°C (36°F–46°F) and protect from light. Keep PO solution under the same conditions until dispensed. Refrigeration of the solution is recommended after dispensing; however, this is not necessary if the solution is stored in the original container, used within 30 days, and kept below 25°C (77°F).

Assessment
1. Record symptom onset, serum confirmation of diagnosis, and other agents trialed with the outcome.
2. Monitor CBC, T-lymphocytes (CD_4), viral load, and LFTs. Document/record impaired liver function; drug hepatically metabolized via P450 system.
3. List other agents prescribed to ensure none interact unfavorably.

Client/Family Teaching
1. Take with food, if possible. Taste may be improved by mixing with chocolate milk, Ensure, or Advera within 1 hr of dosing.
2. Take each day as prescribed. Do not alter dosage or discontinue without approval. If a dose is missed, the next dose should be taken as soon as possible; if a dose is skipped, do not double the next dose.
3. Use reliable birth control and barrier protection; drug does not reduce the risk of transmitting disease through sexual contact or blood contamination.
4. Drug is not a cure for HIV; illnesses associated with advanced HIV infection may still occur, including opportunistic infections.

Outcome/Evaluate: Inhibition of disease progression and death with HIV infection

Rivastigmine tartrate

(rih-vah-**STIG**-meen)
Pregnancy Category: B
Exelon **(Rx)**
Classification: Acetylcholinesterase inhibitor; cholinergic agent

Action/Kinetics: It is thought that a deficiency of cortical acetylcholine may account for some of the symptoms of Alzheimer's disease. Rivastigmine increases acetylcholine in the central nervous system through reversible inhibition of its hydrolysis by cholinesterase. **t½:**1.5 hr. **Peak:** 1 hr.
Uses: Mild to moderate dementia from Alzheimer's disease.
Contraindications: Hypersensitivity to rivastigmine, other carbamate derivatives, or other components of the formulation.
Special Concerns: Significant nausea, vomiting, anorexia, and weight loss are associated with use; occurs more frequently in women and during the titration phase. Use with caution in clients with a history of peptic ulcer disease or concurrent NSAID use. Use with caution in clients undergoing anesthesia who will receive succinylcholine-type muscle relaxation, clients with sick sinus syndrome, bradycardia or supraventricular conduction conditions, urinary obstruction, seizure disorders, or pulmonary conditions such as asthma or COPD.
Side Effects: >10%: *CNS:* Dizziness, headache. *GI:* Nausea, vomiting, diarrhea, anorexia, abdominal pain.**<10%:** *CNS:* Fatigue, insomnia, confusion, depression, anxiety, malaise, somnolence, hallucinations, aggressiveness. *CV:* Syncope, hypertension. *GI:* Dyspepsia, constipation, flatulence, weight loss, eructation. *GU:* UTI.*Neuromuscular/skeletal:* Weakness, tremor. *Respiratory:* Rhinitis. *Miscellaneous:* ↑ Sweating, flu-like syndrome
OD **Management of Overdose:** In cases of asymptomatic overdoses, rivastigmine should be held for 24 hrs. *Symptoms:* Cholinergic crisis, caused by significant acetylcholinesterase inhibition, is characterized by severe nausea, vomiting, salivation, sweating, bradycardia, hypotension, respiratory depression, collapse, and convulsions. *Treatment:* Supportive and symptomatic. Dialysis would not be helpful.
Drug Interactions
Anticholinergic agents/ Rivastigmine may ↓ effects
Beta-blockers without ISA activity/ ↑ risk of bradycardia
Calcium channel blockers (diltiazem or verapamil)/ ↑ risk of bradycardia. Cholinergic agonist effects may be ↑ with rivastigmine.
Digoxin/ ↑ risk of bradycardia
Depolarizing neuromuscular blocking agents/Rivastigmine may ↑ effects
How Supplied: *Capsule:* 1.5 mg, 3 mg, 4.5 mg, 6 mg. *Oral solution:* 2 mg /mL (120 mL).

Dosage
• **Oral**
Adults,initial: 1.5 mg b.i.d. to start; **then,** if tolerated for at least 2 weeks, increase to 3 mg b.i.d. Increases to 4.5 mg b.i.d. and 6 mg b.i.d. should only be attempted after at least 2 weeks at the previous dose. Maximum dose is 6 mg b.i.d. If adverse events occur such as nausea, vomiting, abdominal pain, or loss of appetite, the client (or caregiver) should be instructed to discontinue treatment for several doses; then, restart at the same or next lower dosage level. Antiemetics have been used to control GI symptoms. In renal or hepatic impairment, titrate the dose to the individual client response. Use lowest possible dose. May consider waiting >2 weeks between dosage adjustments.

HEALTH CARE CONSIDERATIONS

Administration/Storage: Give with food.

R

Assessment

1. Record/describe clinical presentation; other agents trialed.
2. Note any history of asthma, COPD, NSAID use, or PUD.
3. Note ECG reading.
4. Assess which oral preparation is best for the individual client.

Client/Family Teaching

1. Take with meals at breakfast and dinner. Swallow whole, do not chew, break or crush capsule. A liquid is available for clients who cannot swallow capsules.
2. Watch for nausea, vomiting, loss of appetitie or weight loss. Notify healthcare provider if any of these occur.
3. May swallow solution directly from syringe or mix with water, juice or soda. Stir well. Drink all of mixture within 4 hours of mixing. Do not mix with other liquids.
4. Avoid use of ethanol while taking this medication.

Outcome/Evaluate: Assess cognitive function at periodic intervals. Monitor weight.

Rizatriptan benzoate

(rise-ah-**TRIP**-tan)

Pregnancy Category: C

Maxalt, Maxalt-MLT **(Rx)**

Classification: Antimigraine drug

Action/Kinetics: Binds to $5\text{-HT}_{IB/ID}$ receptors, resulting in cranial vessel vasocontriction, inhibition of neuropeptide release, and reduced transmission in trigeminal pain pathways. Completely absorbed after PO use; rate of absorption of Maxalt-MLT is somewhat slower. **Peak plasma levels, Maxalt:** 1–1.5 hr; **Maxalt-MLT:** 1.6–2.5 hr. Food has no effect on bioavailability, but will delay time to reach peak levels by an hr. **t½:** 2–3 hr. Metabolized by MAO-A; most is excreted through the urine. Is a significant first-pass effect.

Uses: Acute treatment of migraine attacks in adults with or without aura.

Contraindications: Use in children less than 18 years of age, as prophylactic therapy of migraine, or use in the management of hemiplegic or basilar migraine. Use in those with ischemic heart disease or vasospastic coronary artery disease, uncontrolled hypertension, within 24 hr of treatment with another 5-HT_1 agonist or an ergotamine-containing or ergot-type medication (e.g., dihydroergotamine, methysergide). Use concurrently with MAO inhibitors or use of rizatriptan within 2 weeks of discontinuing a MAO inhibitor. Strongly recommended the drug not be given in unrecognized coronary artery disease (CAD) predicted by the presence of risk factors, including hypertension, hypercholesterolemia, smoking, obesity, diabetes, strong family history of CAD, female with surgical or physiological menopause, or males over 40, unless a CV evaluation reveals the client is free from CAD or ischemic myocardial disease.

Special Concerns: Safety and efficacy have not been determined for use in cluster headache or in children. Use with caution during lactation, with diseases that may alter the absorption, metabolism, or excretion of drugs; in dialysis clients, and in moderate hepatic insufficiency. Maxalt-MLT tablets contain phenylalanine; may be of concern to phenylketonurics.

Side Effects: *CV:* ***Acute MI, coronary artery vasospasm, life-threatening disturbances in cardiac rhythm (VT, ventricular fibrillation), death, cerebral hemorrhage, subarachnoid hemorrhage, stroke, hypertensive crisis.*** Also, transient myocardial ischemia, peripheral vascular ischemia, colonic ischemia with abdominal pain and bloody diarrhea, palpitation, tachycardia, cold extremities, hypertension, arrhythmia, bradycardia. *GI:* Nausea, dry mouth, abdominal distention, vomiting, dyspepsia, thirst, acid regurgitation, dysphagia, constipation, flatulence, tongue edema. *CNS:* Somnolence, headache, dizziness, paresthesias, hypesthesia, decreased mental acuity, euphoria, tremor, nervousness, vertigo, insomnia, anxiety, depression, disorientation, ataxia, dysarthria, confusion, dream abnormality, abnormal gait, irritability, impaired memory, agitation, hyperesthesia. *Pain and pressure sensations:* Chest tightness/pressure and/or heaviness; pain/tightness/pressure in the precordium, neck, throat, jaw; regional pain, tightness, pressure, or heaviness; or unspecified pain. *Musculoskeletal:* Muscle weakness, stiffness, myalgia, muscle cramps, musculoskeletal pain, arthralgia, muscle spasm. *Respiratory:* Dyspnea, pharyngitis, nasal irritation, nasal congestion, dry throat, URI, yawning, dry nose, epistaxis, sinus disorder. *GU:* Urinary frequency, polyuria, menstrual disorder. *Dermatologic:* Flushing, sweating, pruritus, rash, urticaria. *Body as a whole:* Asthenia, fatigue, chills, heat sensitivity, hangover effect, warm/cold sensations, dehydration, hot flashes. *Ophthalmic:* Blurred vision, dry eyes, burning eye, eye pain, eye irritation, tearing. *Miscellaneous:* Facial edema, tinnitus, ear pain.

Drug Interactions

Dihydroergotamine / Additive vasospastic reactions; do not use within 24 hr of each other

MAO Inhibitors / ↑ Plasma levels of rizatriptan; do not use together

Methysergide / Additive vasospastic reactions; do not use within 24 hr of each other
Propranolol / ↑ Plasma levels of rizatriptan
How Supplied: *Orally Disintegrating Tablets:* 5 mg, 10 mg; *Tablets:* 5 mg, 10 mg.

Dosage

- **Oral Disintegrating Tablets, Tablets**

Acute treatment of migraine.

Adults: Single dose of 5 mg or 10 mg of Maxalt or Maxalt-MLT. Doses should be separated by at least 2 hr, with no more than 30 mg taken in any 24-hr period.

HEALTH CARE CONSIDERATIONS

Administration/Storage

1. In clients receiving propranolol, use the 5-mg dose of Maxalt, up to a maximum of 3 doses in any 24-hr period.
2. Store Maxalt and Maxalt-MLT tablets at room temperature.

Assessment

1. Note/record characteristics of migraines, when diagnosed, other agents trialed and the outcome.
2. Determine any evidence of heart disease, uncontrolled HTN, DM, or allergies. Assess risk factors for CAD. Clients over age 40 should be carefully screened for CAD.
3. List all meds consumed to ensure none interact. Reduce dose if prescribed propranolol.

Client/Family Teaching

1. For Maxalt-MLT, do not remove the blister from the outer pouch until just before dosing. Peel open the blister (do not push through the blister) with dry hands and place the orally-disintegrating tablet on the tongue. It will dissolve and be swallowed in the saliva; fluids are not needed which facilitates ease of administration.
2. May cause dizziness, drowsiness, or pressure sensation in the upper chest; do not operate equipment or drive until effects realized.
3. Do not take within 24 hr of any other prescription drug used to treat headaches or depression.
4. Review patient information sheet provided for side effects; report if persistent or intolerable.
5. If headache returns or only a partial response is attained, may repeat dose after waiting at least 2 hr. Do not exceed 30 mg in a 24-hr period.

Outcome/Evaluate: Treatment of migraine headache

Rofecoxib

(roh-feh-KOX-ib)
Pregnancy Category: C
Vioxx **(Rx)**
Classification: NSAID, COX-2 inhibitor

See also *Nonsteroidal Anti-Inflammatory Drugs.*
Action/Kinetics: NSAID that acts by inhibiting prostaglandin synthesis via inhibition of cyclooxygenase-2 (COX-2). **Peak levels:** 2–3 hr. The tablets and oral suspension are bioequivalent. Bound to plasma protein (87%). Metabolized in the liver and excreted in the urine (72%) and feces (14%, including unchanged drug). **t½:** 17 hr.
Uses: Relieve signs and symptoms of osteoarthritis, acute pain in adults, and treatment of dysmenorrhea.
Contraindications: Advanced renal disease. Use in clients who manifested asthma, urticaria, or allergic-type reactions after taking aspirin or other NSAIDs. Use in late pregnancy due to premature closure of the ductus arteriosus. Lactation.
Special Concerns: Use with extreme caution in those with a prior history of ulcer disease or GI bleeding. Use with caution in fluid retention, hypertension, or heart failure. Most fatal GI events are in elderly or debilitated clients. Safety and efficacy have not been determined in children less than 18 years of age.
Side Effects: Side effects listed occurred in at least 2% of clients. *GI:* Diarrhea, nausea, constipation, heartburn, epigastric discomfort, dyspepsia, abdominal pain. *CNS:* Headache. *Respiratory:* Bronchitis, upper respiratory tract infection. *CV:* Hypertension. *GU:* UTI. *Body as a whole:* Lower extremity edema, asthenia, fatigue, dizziness, flu-like disease, fever. *Miscellaneous:* Back pain, sinusitis, post-dental extraction alveolitis.
Laboratory Test Considerations: ↑ ALT, AST.

Drug Interactions

ACE inhibitors / ↓ ACE inhibitor effect
Antacids (Mg-Al containing, Calcium carbonate) / ↓ Absorption of rofecoxib
Aspirin / ↑ Risk of GI ulceration and other complications
Furosemide / ↓ Natriuertic effect of furosemide
Lithium / ↑ Risk of lithium toxicity
Methotrexate / ↑ Risk of methotrexate toxicity
Rifampin / ↓ Plasma levels of rifampin R/T ↑ liver metabolism
Thiazide diurtetics / ↓ Natriuretic effect of thiazides

R

Warfarin / ↑ PT

How Supplied: *Oral Suspension:* 12.5 mg/5 mL, 25 mg/mL; *Tablets:* 12.5 mg, 25 mg

Dosage

- **Oral Suspension, Tablets**

  Osteoarthritis.

Adults, initial: 12.5 mg once daily, up to a maximum of 25 mg once daily.

Acute pain, primary dysmenorrhea.

Adults, initial: 50 mg once daily; **then,** 50 mg once daily as needed.

HEALTH CARE CONSIDERATIONS

See also *Health Care Considerations* for *Nonsteroidal Anti-Inflammatory Drugs.*

Administration/Storage

1. Can be given without regard to meals.
2. Seek the lowest dose for each client.
3. Use for more than 5 days for pain has not been studied.
4. Store the tablets and oral suspension between 15–30°C (59–86°F).

Assessment

1. Record indications for therapy, onset and characteristics of disease, ROM, deformity/loss of function, instability, pain level, other agents trialed and the outcome.
2. Determine any GI bleed or ulcer history, sulfonamide allergy or aspirin or other NSAID-induced asthma/sensitivity, urticaria, or allergic-type reactions.
3. Assess for liver/renal dysfunction; monitor lytes, renal and LFTs.

Client/Family Teaching

1. Take as directed at the same time each day.
2. Report any GI discomfort as drug may cause GI bleeding, ulcerations or perforation.
3. Report weight gain, swelling of ankles, chest pain, or SOB.

Outcome/Evaluate: Relief of joint pain/inflammation with improved mobility

Ropinirole hydrochloride

(roh-**PIN**-ih-roll)

Pregnancy Category: C

Requip **(Rx)**

Classification: Antiparkinson agent

See also *Antiparkinson Agents.*

Action/Kinetics: Mechanism is not known but believed to involve stimulation of postsynaptic D_2 dopamine receptors in caudate-putamen in brain. Causes decreases in both systolic and diastolic BP at doses above 0.25 mg. Rapidly absorbed. **Peak plasma levels:** 1–2 hr. Food reduces maximum concentration. **t½, elimination:** 6 hr. First pass effect; extensively metabolized in liver.

Uses: Treat signs and symptoms of idiopathic Parkinson's disease.

Contraindications: Lactation.

Special Concerns: Safety and efficacy have not been determined in children.

Side Effects: *CNS:* Hallucinations, cause and/or exacerbate pre-existing dyskinesia. *CV:* Syncope (sometimes with bradycardia), postural hypotension.

OD **Management of Overdose:** *Symptoms:* Agitation, increased dyskinesia, grogginess, sedation, orthostatic hypotension, chest pain, confusion, N&V. *Treatment:* General suppportive measures. Maintain vital signs. Gastric lavage.

Drug Interactions

Ciprofloxacin / Significant ↑ in ropinirole plasma levels

Estrogens / ↓ Oral clearance of ropinirole

How Supplied: *Tablets:* 0.25 mg, 0.5 mg, 1 mg, 2 mg, 5 mg.

Dosage

- **Tablets**

  Parkinson's disease.

Week 1: 0.25 mg t.i.d. **Week 2:** 0.5 mg t.i.d. **Week 3:** 0.75 mg t.i.d. **Week 4:** 1 mg t.i.d. After week 4, daily dose, if necessary, may be increased by 1.5 mg/day on weekly basis up to dose of 9 mg/day. This may be followed by increase of up to 3 mg/day weekly to total dose of 24 mg/day.

HEALTH CARE CONSIDERATIONS

See also *Health Care Considerations* for *Antiparkinson Agents,* .

Administration/Storage

1. If taken with l-dopa, decrease dose of l-dopa gradually, as tolerated.
2. When discontinued, do so gradually over 7-day period. Reduce frequency of administration to twice daily for 4 days. For remaining 3 days, reduce frequency to once daily prior to complete withdrawal.

Assessment

1. Record disease onset, extent of motor function, reflexes, gait, strength of grip, and amount of tremor.
2. With tremor, note extent, muscle weakness, muscle rigidity, difficulty walking or changing direction.
3. Monitor VS, ECG.

Client/Family Teaching

1. May be taken with or without food.
2. May cause dizziness and syncope, use caution; report if persists.
3. Report any loss of effect or evidence of dyskinesia.

4. Do not stop abruptly. Drug must be gradually withdrawn over seven day period.
Outcome/Evaluate: Control of tremor

Rosiglitazone maleate

(roh-sih-**GLIH**-tah-zohn)
Pregnancy Category: C
Avelox **(Rx)**
Classification: Oral hypoglycemic agent.

See also *Antidiabetic Agents: Hypoglycemic Agents.*

Action/Kinetics: Improves blood glucose levels by improving insulin sensitivity in type II diabetes insulin resistance. Active only in the presence of insulin. A highly selective and potent agonist for the peroxisome proliferator-activated receptor (PPAR)-gamma which is found in adipose tissue, skeletal muscle, and liver. Activation of these receptors regulates the transcription of insulin-responsive genes involved in the control of glucose production, transport, and use. The genes also participate in regulation of fatty acid metabolism. **Peak plasma levels:** 1 hr (over 99% bioavailable). Food decreases the rate of absorption but not the total amount absorbed. Approximately 99.8% bound to plasma proteins. **t½, distribution:** 3–4 hr. Extensively metabolized in the liver and excreted in the urine and feces.

Additional Uses: As an adjunct to diet and exercise to improve glycemic control in type II diabetes. Used either as monotherapy or in combination witih metformin when diet, exercise, and rosiglitazone alone do not control blood glucose.

Contraindications: Type I diabetes, diabetic ketoacidosis, active liver disease, if serum ALT levels are 2.5 times ULN, in clients with NYHA Class III and IV cardiac status (unless the expected benefit outweighs the potential risk), and during lactation.

Special Concerns: Treatment may result in resumption of ovulation in premenopausal anovulatory clients with insulin resistance. Use with caution in clients with edema. Safety and efficacy have not been determined in clients less than 18 years of age.

Side Effects: *Respiratory:* URTI, sinusitis. *Metabolic:* Hyperglycemia, hypoglycemia. *Miscellaneous:* Injury, headache, back ache, fatigue, diarrhea, anemia, edema.

Laboratory Test Considerations: ↑ ALT. ↓ H&H. Changes in serum lipids. Hyperbilirubinemia.

How Supplied: *Tablets:* 2 mg, 4 mg, 8 mg

Dosage

- **Tablets**

Type II diabetes, monotherapy.

Adults, initial: 4 mg once daily or in divided doses b.i.d. If the response is inadequate after 12 weeks, the dose can be increased to 8 mg as a single dose once daily or in divided doses b.i.d. A dose of 4 mg b.i.d. resulted in the greatest decrease in fasting blood glucose and HbA1c.

Type II diabetes, combination therapy with metformin.

Adults, initial: 4 mg once daily or in divided doses b.i.d. If the response is inadequate after 12 weeks, the dose can be increased to 8 mg as a single dose once daily or in divided doses b.i.d.

HEALTH CARE CONSIDERATIONS

See also *Health Care Considerations* for *Antidiabetic Agents: Hypoglycemic Agents.*

Assessment

1. Record disease onset, other agents trialed, dietary/exercise adherance.
2. Record any history of CAD and NYHA class.
3. List agents prescribed to ensure none interact.
4. Monitor liver enzymes following initiation of therapy, every 2 months during the first year of use, and periodically thereafter. If ALT levels increase to 3X ULN at any time, recheck liver enzymes as soon as possible. If ALT levels remain greater than 3X ULN, discontinue therapy.
5. Monitor fasting blood glucose and HbA1c levels.

Client/Family Teaching

1. Take once daily without regard to meals.
2. May cause edema, resumption of ovulation, and hypoglycemia.
3. Report if dark urine, abdominal pain fatigue or unexplained N&V occur.
4. Practice reliable contraception if pregnancy is not desired.
5. Follow dietary guidelines, perform regular exercise and other life style changes consistent with controlling diabetes.
6. Monitor FS at different times during the day and maintain log for provider review.

Outcome/Evaluate: Control of NIDDM by ↓ insulin resistance; HbA1c < 7

R

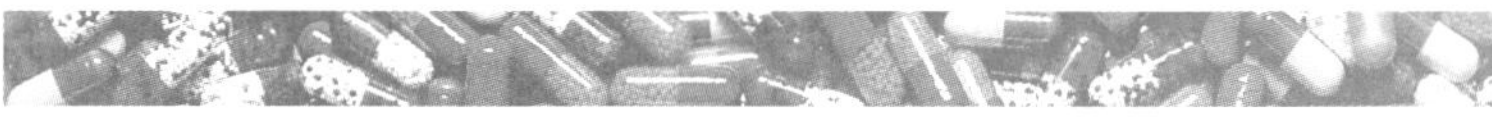

Sacrosidase

(sac-roh-SIGH-dace)
Pregnancy Category: C
Sucraid **(Rx)**
Classification: Enzyme

Action/Kinetics: Enzyme replacement for those with genetic sucrase deficiency. In the absence of sucrase, sucrose is not metabolized and is thus not absorbed from the intestine. This results in osmotic water retention, loose stools, excessive gas, bloating, abdominal cramps, nausea, and vomiting. Chronic malabsorption of disaccharides may result in malnutrition.
Uses: Oral replacement therapy for sucrase deficiency, which is part of congenital sucrase-isomaltase deficiency. Safe and effective for use in children.
Contraindications: Hypersensitivity to yeast, yeast products, or glycerin.
Side Effects: *GI:* Abdominal pain, N&V, diarrhea, constipation. *CNS:* Insomnia, headache, nervousness. *Miscellaneous:* Hypersensitivity reactions, dehydration.
How Supplied: *Solution:* 8500 IU/mL

Dosage

- **Solution**

Treat sucrase deficiency.

Clients 15 kg or less: 1 mL (8500 IU)—1 full measuring scoop or 22 drops per meal or snack. **Clients over 15 kg:** 2 mL (17,000 IU)—2 full measuring scoops or 44 drops per meal or snack. Dosage may be measured with the 1 mL measuring scoop provided or by drop count method using the guide of 1 mL equals 22 drops from the sacrosidase container tip.

S

HEALTH CARE CONSIDERATIONS

Administration/Storage: Store in the refrigerator at 2°C–8°C (36°F–46°F). Protect from heat and light.
Assessment
1. Record frequency and characteristics of symptoms of CSID (congenital sucrase-isomaltase deficiency) i.e., watery diarrhea, abdominal cramps, bloating, gas, and chronic malabsorption symptoms.
2. Record any sensitivity to yeast or yeast products as drug is derived from baker's yeast.
3. Assess height and weight and monitor.
Client/Family Teaching
1. Drug is used to replace sucrase enzyme deficiency states. It catalyzes the hydrolysis of sucrose to glucose and fructose in the small intestine.
2. Restriction of starch in the diet may still be necessary (drug does not provide replacement for the deficiency of isomaltase or catalyze the hydrolysis of starch) and will be evaluated for each patient.
3. Sacrosidase is fully soluble with water, milk, and infant formula but the product is heat sensitive. Serve cold or at room temperature.
4. Do not reconstitute or take with fruit juice, as the acidity may decrease enzyme activity.
5. About one-half of the dose is taken at the beginning of each meal or snack and the remainder at the end of each meal or snack.
6. Store in the refrigerator. Discard bottles of sacrosidase 4 weeks after first opening due to the potential for bacterial growth.
Outcome/Evaluate: Enzyme replacement therapy with sucrase deficiency/ CSID

Salmeterol xinafoate

(sal-MET-er-ole)
Pregnancy Category: C
Serevent **(Rx)**
Classification: Beta-2 adrenergic agonist

See also *Sympathomimetic Drugs.*
Action/Kinetics: Selective for beta-2 adrenergic receptors, located in the bronchi and heart. Acts by stimulating intracellular adenyl cyclase, the enzyme that converts ATP to cyclic AMP. Increased AMP levels cause relaxation of bronchial smooth muscle and inhibition of release of mediators of immediate hypersensitivity, especially from mast cells. Significantly bound to plasma proteins. Cleared by hepatic metabolism.
Uses: Long-term maintenance treatment of asthma or bronchospasm associated with COPD. Prevention of bronchospasms in clients over 12 years of age with reversible obstructive airway disease, including nocturnal asthma. Prevention of exercise-induced bronchospasms. Inhalation powder for long-term maintenance treatment of asthma in clients aged 12 years or older.
Contraindications: Use in clients who can be controlled by short-acting, inhaled beta-2 agonists. Use to treat acute symptoms of asthma or in those who have worsening or deteriorating asthma. Lactation.

Special Concerns: Not a substitute for PO or inhaled corticosteroids. The safety and efficacy of using salmeterol with a spacer or other devices has not been studied adequately. Use with caution in impaired hepatic function; with cardiovascular disorders, including coronary insufficiency, cardiac arrhythmias, and hypertension; with convulsive disorders or thyrotoxicosis; and in clients who respond unusually to sympathomimetic amines. Because of the potential of the drug interfering with uterine contractility, use of salmeterol during labor should be restricted to those in whom benefits clearly outweigh risks. Safety and efficacy have not been determined in children less than 12 years of age.
Side Effects: *Respiratory:* Paradoxical bronchospasms, upper or lower respiratory tract infection, nasopharyngitis, disease of nasal cavity/sinus, cough, pharyngitis, allergic rhinitis, laryngitis, tracheitis, bronchitis. *Allergic:* ***Immediate hypersensitivity reactions,*** including urticaria, rash, and ***bronchospasm.*** *CV:* Palpitations, chest pain, increased BP, tachycardia. *CNS:* Headache, sinus headache, tremors, nervousness, malaise, fatigue, dizziness, giddiness. *GI:* Stomachache. *Musculoskeletal:* Joint pain, back pain, muscle cramps, muscle contractions, myalgia, myositis, muscle soreness. *Miscellaneous:* Flu, dental pain, rash, skin eruption, dysmenorrhea.
Laboratory Test Considerations: ↓ Serum potassium.
OD **Management of Overdose:** *Symptoms:* Tachycardia, arrhythmia, tremors, headache, muscle cramps, hypokalemia, hyperglycemia. *Treatment:* Supportive therapy. Consider judicious use of a beta-adrenergic blocking agent, although these drugs can cause bronchospasms. Cardiac monitoring is necessary. Dialysis is not an appropriate treatment of overdosage.
Drug Interactions
MAO Inhibitors / Potentiation of the effect of salmeterol
Tricyclic antidepressants / Potentiation of the effect of salmeterol
How Supplied: *Metered dose inhaler:* 21 mcg/inh; *Powder for Inhalation:* 46 mcg/inh

Dosage
- **Metered Dose Inhaler**

Maintenance of bronchodilation, prevention of symptoms of asthma, including nocturnal asthma.
Adults and children over 12 years of age: Two inhalations (42 mcg) b.i.d. (morning and evening, approximately 12 hr apart).

Prevention of exercise-induced bronchospasms.
Adults and children over 12 years of age: Two inhalations (42 mcg) at least 30–60 min before exercise. Additional doses should not be used for 12 hr.
- **Inhalation Powder (Diskus)**

Maintenance treatment of asthma or bronchospasm associated with COPD.
Adults and children over 12 years of age: 50 mcg (one inhalation) b.i.d. in the morning and evening.
NOTE: Even though the metered dose inhaler and the inhalation powder are used for the same conditions, they are not interchangeable.

HEALTH CARE CONSIDERATIONS

See also *Health Care Considerations* for *Sympathomimetic Drugs.*
Administration/Storage
1. Ensure that doses are spaced q 12 hr.
2. The safety of more than 8 inhalations per day of short-acting beta-2 agonists with salmeterol has not been established.
3. If a previously effective dose fails to provide the usual response, contact provider immediately.
4. If using salmeterol twice daily, do not use additional doses to prevent exercise-induced bronchospasms.
5. Use only with the actuator provided. Do not use the actuator with other aerosol medications.
6. Store between 2°C and 30°C (36°F and 86°F). Store the canister nozzle end down and protect from freezing temperatures and direct sunlight.
7. Do not spray in the eyes.
8. Shake canister well before using at room temperature; therapeutic effect may diminish if cold.
9. For the inhalation of powder (Diskus), a built-in dose counter shows the number of doses remaining.

Assessment
1. Record onset, duration, and characteristics of symptoms; note agents trialed and outcome.
2. Determine any cardiac or liver dysfunction, thyrotoxicosis, hypertension, or seizure disorders.
3. Record pulmonary function status and lung sounds.
4. Monitor VS, liver enzymes, PFTs (ABGs, PEFR, and FEV).

Client/Family Teaching
1. Review proper use (with actuator) and

S

obtain instruction. Record peak flows and identify critical zones.
2. Use only as prescribed and do not exceed prescribed dosage and administration frequency (drug effects last 12 hr).
3. Do not use this drug during an acute asthma attack.
4. Review procedure for use of the short-acting beta-2 agonist prescribed to treat symptoms of asthma that occur between the salmeterol dosing schedule. Increased utilization warrants medical evaluation (e.g., when used more than 4 times/day or more than one canister of 200 inhalations/8 weeks).
5. May experience palpitations, chest pain, headaches, tremors, and nervousness as side effects.
6. Report immediately if chest pain, fast pounding irregular heart beat, hives, increased wheezing, or difficulty breathing occurs.
7. Take 30–60 min before activity to prevent acute bronchospasms.
8. Salmeterol does not replace inhaled or systemic steroids; do not stop prescribed steroid therapy abruptly without approval.
9. Identify appropriate support groups that may assist client to cope and live a normal life with asthma.
10. Stop smoking; avoid smokey environments and any other triggers that may aggravate breathing condition.

Outcome/Evaluate

- Prevention and control of asthmatic symptoms (e.g., decreased wheezing, dyspnea, orthopnea, and cough)
- Control of bronchospasms with COPD
- Prevention of exercise-induced bronchospasms

Saquinavir mesylate

((sah-**KWIN**-ah-veer))
Pregnancy Category: B
Fortovase, Invirase **(Rx)**
Classification: Antiviral drug, protease inhibitor

See also *Antiviral Drugs*.

Action/Kinetics: HIV protease cleaves viral polyprotein precursors to form functional proteins in HIV-infected cells. Cleavage of viral polyprotein precursors is required for maturation of the infectious virus. Saquinavir inhibits the activity of HIV protease and prevents the cleavage of viral polyproteins. Has a low bioavailability after PO use, probably due to incomplete absorption and first-pass metabolism. A high-fat meal or high-calorie meal increases the amount of drug absorbed. Over 98% bound to plasma protein. About 87% metabolized in the liver by the cytochrome P450 system. Both metabolites and unchanged drug are excreted mainly through the feces. It is believed the bioavailability of Fortovase is greater than Invirase.

Uses: Combined with AZT or zalcitabine (ddC) for treatment of advanced HIV infection in selected clients. No data are available regarding the benefit of combination therapy of saquinavir with AZT or ddC on HIV disease progression or survival.

Contraindications: Lactation. Use with astemizole, cisapride, ergot derivatives, midazolam, terfenadine, triazolam.

Special Concerns: Photoallergy or phototoxicity may occur; take protective measures against exposure to ultraviolet or sunlight until tolerance is assessed. Use with caution in those with hepatic insufficiency. Hemophiliacs treated with protease inhibitors for HIV infections may manifest spontaneous bleeding episodes. Safety and efficacy have not been determined in HIV-infected children or adolescents less than 16 years of age.

Side Effects: Side effects listed are for saquinavir combined with either AZT or ddC. *GI:* Diarrhea, abdominal discomfort, nausea, dyspepsia, abdominal pain, ulceration of buccal mucosa, cheilitis, constipation, dysphagia, eructation, blood-stained or discolored feces, gastralgia, gastritis, GI inflammation, gingivitis, glossitis, ***rectal hemorrhage,*** hemorrhoids, hepatomegaly, hepatosplenomegaly, melena, pain, painful defecation, pancreatitis, parotid disorder, pelvic salivary glands disorder, stomatitis, tooth disorder, vomiting, frequent bowel movements, dry mouth, alteration in taste. *CNS:* Headache, paresthesia, numbness of extremity, dizziness, peripheral neuropathy, ataxia, confusion, ***convulsions,*** dysarthria, dysesthesia, hyperesthesia, hyperreflexia, hyporeflexia, face numbness, facial pain, paresis, poliomyelitis, progressive multifocal leukoencephalopathy, spasms, tremor, agitation, amnesia, anxiety, depression, excessive dreaming, euphoria, hallucinations, insomnia, reduced intellectual ability, irritability, lethargy, libido disorder, overdose effect, psychic disorder, somnolence, speech disorder. *Musculoskeletal:* Musculoskeletal pain, myalgia, arthralgia, arthritis, back pain, muscle cramps, musculoskeletal disorder, stiffness, tissue changes, trauma. *Body as a whole:* Allergic reaction, chest pain, edema, fever, intoxication, external parasites, retrosternal pain, shivering, wasting syndrome, weight decrease, abscess, angina tonsillaris, candidiasis, hepatitis, herpes simplex, herpes zoster, infections (bacterial, mycotic, staphylococcal), influenza, lymphadenopathy, tumor. *CV:* Cyanosis, heart murmur, heart valve disorder, hypertension, hypotension, syncope, distended vein, HR disorder. *Metabolic:* Dehydration, hyperglycemia, weight decrease, worsening of existing diabetes mellitus. *Hematologic:* Anemia, microhemorrhages, pancytopenia, splenomegaly, thrombocytopenia. *Respiratory:* Bronchitis, cough, dyspnea, epistaxis, hemoptysis, laryngitis, pharyngitis, pneumonia, respiratory disorder rhinitis, sinusitis, URTI. *GU:* Enlarged prostate, vaginal discharge, micturition disorder, UTI. *Dermatologic:* Acne, dermatitis, seborrheic dermatitis, eczema, erythema, folliculitis, furunculosis, hair changes, hot flushes, photosensitivity reaction, changes in skin pigment, maculopapular rash, skin disorder, skin nodules, skin ulceration, increased sweating, urticaria, verruca, xeroderma. *Ophthalmic:* Dry eye syndrome, xerophthalmia, blepharitis, eye irritation, visual disturbance. *Otic:* Earache, ear pressure, decreased hearing, otitis, tinnitus.

Laboratory Test Considerations: ↑ CPK, serum amylase, AST, ALT, total bilirubin. ↓ Neutrophils. Abnormal phosphorus.

Drug Interactions

Astemizole / Possibility of serious or life-threatening cardiac arrhythmias or prolonged sedation

Carbamazepine / ↓ Blood levels of saquinavir

Cisapride / Possibility of serious or life-threatening cardiac arrhythmias or prolonged sedation

Clarithromycin / ↑ Blood levels of both drugs

Dexamethasone / ↓ Blood levels of saquinavir

Ergot derivatives / Possibility of serious or life-threatening cardiac arrhythmias or prolonged sedation

Ketcconazole / ↑ Blood levels of saquinavir

Midazolam / Possibility of serious or life-threatening cardiac arrhythmias or prolonged sedation

Phenobarbital / ↓ Blood levels of saquinavir

Phenytoin / ↓ Blood levels of saquinavir

Rifampin / ↓ Blood levels of saquinavir

Ritonavir / ↑ Blood levels of saquinavir

Terfenadine / Possibility of serious or life-threatening cardiac arrhythmias or prolonged sedation

Triazolam / Possibility of serious or life-threatening cardiac arrhythmias or prolonged sedation

How Supplied: *Capsules:* 200 mg.

Dosage

- **Fortovase Capsules**

HIV infections in combination with AZT or ddC.

Six 200-mg capsules (i.e., 1,200 mg) taken t.i.d. with meals or up to 2 hr after meals.

- **Invirase Capsules**

HIV infections in combination with AZT or ddC.

Three 200-mg capsules of saquinavir t.i.d. taken within 2 hr of a full meal. The recommended doses of AZT or ddC as part of combination therapy are: AZT, 200 mg t.i.d., or ddC, 0.75 mg t.i.d. However, base dosage adjustments of AZT or ddC on the known toxicity profile of the individual drug. This form of the drug will be phased out.

HEALTH CARE CONSIDERATIONS

See also *Health Care Considerations* for *Antiviral Drugs*.

Administration/Storage

1. Take within 2 hr of a full meal. If taken without food, blood levels may not be sufficiently high to exert an antiviral effect.
2. Doses less than 200 mg t.i.d. of Invirase are not recommended; lower doses have not shown antiviral activity.
3. Fortovase Capsules must be refrigerated in tightly closed bottles.

Assessment

1. Record onset, duration, and type of symptoms manifested.
2. Monitor CBC, T-lymphocytes/viral load, renal and LFTs.
3. List drugs currently prescribed; drug is metabolized hepatically via cytochrome P450 system.
4. If serious or severe toxicity occurs, interrupt therapy until cause is determined or toxicity resolves.

Client/Family Teaching

1. Take only as prescribed and within 2 hr of a full meal, as blood levels markedly reduced when taken without food.
2. Drug is not a cure for HIV infections. It does not prevent the occurrence or decrease the frequency of opportunistic infections associated with HIV.
3. Avoid sun exposure; take protective measures against UV or sunlight until tolerance assessed.
4. Continue to use barrier contraception and safe sex; drug does not inhibit disease transmission.
5. Long-term drug effects are still unknown; report any unusual side effects.

Outcome/Evaluate: Control of progression of HIV infections

S

Scopolamine hydrobromide

(scoh-**POLL**-ah-meen)
Pregnancy Category: C
Hyoscine Hydrobromide, Isopto Hyoscine Ophthalmic, Scopace **(Rx)**

Scopolamine transdermal therapeutic system

(scoh-**POLL**-ah-meen)
Pregnancy Category: C
Transderm-Scop, Transderm-V ✱ **(Rx)**
Classification: Anticholinergic, antiemetic

See also *Cholinergic Blocking Agents*.
Action/Kinetics: Anticholinergic with CNS depressant effects; produces amnesia when given with morphine or meperidine. In the presence of pain, delirium may be produced. Causes pupillary dilation and paralyzes the muscle required to accommodate for close vision (cycloplegia). This enables the physician to examine the inner structure of the eye, including the retina, as well as to examine refractive errors of the lens without automatic accommodation by the client. Tolerance may develop if scopolamine is used alone. When used for refraction: **peak for mydriasis,** 20–30 min; **peak for cycloplegia,** 30–60 min; **duration:** 24 hr (residual cycloplegia and mydriasis may last for 3–7 days). Recovery time can be reduced by using 1–2 gtt pilocarpine (1% or 2%). To reduce absorption, apply pressure over the nasolacrimal sac for 2–3 min.

The transdermal therapeutic system contains 1.5 mg scopolamine, which is slowly released from a mineral oil–polyisobutylene matrix. Approximately 0.5 mg is released from the system per day.

S

Uses: Ophthalmic: For cycloplegia and mydriasis in diagnostic procedures. Preoperatively and postoperatively in the treatment of iridocyclitis. Dilate the pupil in treatment of uveitis or posterior synechiae. *Investigational:* Prophylaxis of synechiae, treatment of iridocyclitis. **Parenteral:** Antiemetic, antivertigo. Preanesthetic sedation and obstetric amnesia. Antiarrhythmic during anesthesia and surgery. **Oral:** Prevention of motion sickness. **Transdermal:** Antiemetic, antivertigo. Prevention of motion sickness.
Additional Contraindications: Use of the transdermal system in children or lactating women. Ophthalmic use in glaucoma or infants less than 3 months of age. Use for prophylaxis of excess secretions in children less than 4 months of age.
Special Concerns: Use with caution in children, infants, geriatric clients, diabetes, hypo- or hyperthyroidism, narrow anterior chamber angle.
Additional Side Effects: Disorientation, delirium, increased HR, decreased respiratory rate. *Ophthalmologic:* Blurred vision, stinging, increased intraocular pressure. Long-term use may cause irritation, photophobia, conjunctivitis, hyperemia, or edema.
How Supplied: Scopolamine hydrobromide: *Injection:* 0.4 mg/mL, 1 mg/mL; *Ophthalmic Solution:* 0.25%; *Tablet:* 0.4 mg. Scopolamine transdermal therapeutic system: *Film, extended release:* 0.33 mg/24 hr, 0.5 mg/24 hr

Dosage

- **Ophthalmic Solution**

Cycloplegia/mydriasis.

Adults: 1–2 gtt of the 0.25% solution in the conjunctiva 1 hr prior to refraction; **children:** 1 gtt of the 0.25% solution b.i.d. for 2 days prior to refraction.

Uveitis.

Adults and children: 1 gtt of the 0.25% solution in the conjunctiva 1–4 times/day, depending on the severity of the condition.

Treatment of posterior synechiae.

Adults and children: 1 gtt of the 0.25% solution q min for 5 min. (1 gtt of either a 2.5% or 10% solution of phenylephrine instilled q min for 3 min will enhance the effect of scopolamine.)

Postoperative mydriasis.

Adults: 1 gtt of the 0.25% solution once daily. For dark brown irides, administration 2 or 3 times/day may be required.

Pre- or Postoperative iridocyclitis.

Adults and children: 1 gtt of the 0.25% solution 1–4 times/day as required. Individualize the pediatric dose based on age, weight, and severity of the inflammation.

- **Injection (IM, IV, SC)**

Anticholinergic, antiemetic.

Adults: 0.3–0.6 mg (single dose). **Pediatric:** 0.006 mg/kg (0.2 mg/m^2) as a single dose.

Prophylaxis of excessive salivation and respiratory tract secretions in anesthesia.

Adults: 0.2–0.6 mg 30–60 min before induction of anesthesia. **Pediatric (given IM): 8–12 years:** 0.3 mg; **3–8 years:** 0.2 mg; **7 months–3 years:** 0.15 mg; **4–7 months:** 0.1 mg. Not recommended for children less than 4 months of age.

Adjunct to anesthesia, sedative-hypnotic.

Adults: 0.6 mg t.i.d–q.i.d.

Adjunct to anesthesia, amnesia.

Adults: 0.32–0.65 mg.

- **Tablets**

Prevent motion sickness.

0.4–0.8 mg taken 1 hr before travel.

- **Transdermal System**

Antiemetic, antivertigo.

Adults: 1 transdermal system placed on the postauricular skin to deliver either 1 mg or

0.33 mg over 3 days (apply at least 4 hr before antiemetic effect is required). The Canadian product should be applied about 12 hr before the antiemetic effect is desired.

HEALTH CARE CONSIDERATIONS

See also *Health Care Considerations* for *Cholinergic Blocking Agents.*

Administration/Storage

1. Give drops into the conjunctival sac followed by digital pressure for 2–3 min after instillation.
2. Do not give alone for pain because it may cause delirium; use an analgesic or sedative as needed.
3. Protect solution from light.

Assessment

1. Record indications for therapy, type and onset of symptoms.
2. With eyedrops, check for angle-closure glaucoma; may precipitate an acute glaucoma crisis.
3. Some clients may experience toxic delirium with therapeutic doses. Observe closely and have physostigmine available to reverse effects.

Client/Family Teaching

1. Do not drive a car or operate dangerous machinery until drug effects realized; may cause drowsiness, confusion, disorientation, and, when used ophthalmologically, blurred vision and dilated pupils.
2. Wear dark glasses if photosensitivity occurs and report if eye pain occurs. May temporarily impair vision.
3. Wait 5 min before instilling other eye drops.
4. With the transdermal system:
   • Wash hands before and after application
   • Apply at least 4 hr before desired effect
   • Apply to a clean, nonhairy site, behind the ear
   • Use pressure to apply the patch to ensure contact with the skin
   • Replace with a new system if patch becomes dislodged
   • System is water-proof so bathing and swimming are permitted
   • System effects last for 3 days
   • NOT for use in children
5. Report any extrapyramidal symptoms, urinary retention, and constipation. Increase fluids and bulk to prevent constipation.
6. Use gum, sugarless candies, and frequent mouth rinses to alleviate symptoms of dry mouth.
7. Avoid alcohol and any other CNS depressants.

Outcome/Evaluate

• Control of vomiting
• Preoperative sedation; postoperative amnesia
• Desired mydriasis
• Prevention of motion sickness

Secobarbital sodium

(see-koh-**BAR**-bih-tal)

Pregnancy Category: D

Novo-Secobarb ✦, Seconal Sodium **(C-II)** **(Rx)**

Classification: Barbiturate sedative-hypnotic

See also *Barbiturates.*

Action/Kinetics: Short-acting. Distributed quickly due to high lipid solubility. **Onset:** 10–15 min. **t½:** 15–40 hr. **Duration:** 3–4 hr. Is 46%–70% protein bound.

Uses: Short-term treatment of insomnia (2 weeks or less).

Special Concerns: Elderly or debilitated clients may be more sensitive to the drug and require reduced dosage.

How Supplied: *Capsule:* 100 mg

Dosage

• **Capsule**

Hypnotic.

Adults: 100 mg at bedtime.

HEALTH CARE CONSIDERATIONS

See also *Health Care Considerations* for *Barbiturates.*

Administration/Storage

1. Reduce dosage in impaired hepatic or renal function.
2. Following prolonged use, taper dosage and withdraw drug slowly to prevent withdrawal symptoms.

Client/Family Teaching

1. Do not perform activities that require mental alertness until drug effects realized.
2. Avoid alcohol and any other CNS depressants.
3. Take analgesics as prescribed; does not control pain.
4. Drug may cause dependency. Review alternative methods that assist with sleeping, such as relaxation techniques, daily exercise, no napping, stress reduction, no caffeine, and/or white noise simulator.

Outcome/Evaluate: Improved sleeping patterns with less frequent awakenings

Sertraline hydrochloride

(**SIR**-trah-leen)

Pregnancy Category: B
Zoloft **(Rx)**
Classification: Antidepressant

Action/Kinetics: Believed to act by inhibiting CNS neuronal uptake of serotonin. No significant affinity for adrenergic, cholinergic, dopaminergic, histaminergic, serotonergic, GABA, or benzodiazepine receptors. Steady-state plasma levels are usually reached after 1 week of once daily dosing but is increased to 2–3 weeks in older clients. **Time to peak plasma levels:** 4.5–8.4 hr. **Peak plasma levels:** 20–55 ng/mL. **Time to reach steady state:** 7 days. **Terminal elimination t½:** 1–4 days (including active metabolite). Washout period is 7 days. Food decreases the time to reach peak plasma levels. Undergoes significant first-pass metabolism, significant (98%) binding to serum proteins. Excreted through the urine (40%–45%) and feces (40%–45%). Metabolized to N-desmethylsertraline, which has minimal antidepressant activity.

Uses: Treatment of depression with reduced psychomotor agitation, anxiety, and insomnia. Obsessive-compulsive disorders in adults and children as defined in DSM-III-R. Treatment of panic disorder, with or without agoraphobia.

Contraindications: Use in combination with a MAO inhibitor or within 14 days of discontinuing treatment with a MAO inhibitor.

Special Concerns: Use with caution in hepatic or renal dysfunction, with seizure disorders, during lactation, and in diseases or conditions that may affect hemodynamic responses or metabolism. Safety and efficacy have not been determined in children. The plasma clearance may be lower in elderly clients. The possibility of a suicide attempt is possible in depression and may persist until significant remission occurs.

Side Effects: A large number of side effects is possible; listed are those side effects with a frequency of 0.1% or greater. *GI:* Nausea and diarrhea (common), dry mouth, constipation, dyspepsia, vomiting, flatulence, anorexia, abdominal pain, thirst, increased salivation, increased appetite, gastroenteritis, teeth-grinding, dysphagia, eructation, taste perversion or change. *CV:* Palpitations, hot flushes, edema, hypertension, hypotension, peripheral ischemia, postural hypotension or dizziness, syncope, tachycardia. *CNS:* Headache (common), insomnia (common), somnolence, agitation, nervousness, anxiety, dizziness, tremor, fatigue, impaired concentration, yawning, paresthesia, hypoesthesia, twitching, hypertonia, confusion, ataxia or abnormal coordination, abnormal gait, hyperesthesia, hyperkinesia, abnormal dreams, aggressive reaction, amnesia, apathy, delusion, depersonalization, depression, aggravated depression, emotional lability, euphoria, hallucinations, neurosis, paranoid reaction, ***suicide ideation or attempt,*** abnormal thinking, hypokinesia, migraine, nystagmus, vertigo. *Dermatologic:* Rash, acne, excessive sweating, alopecia, pruritus, cold and clammy skin, facial edema, erythematous rash, maculopapular rash, dry skin. *Musculoskeletal:* Myalgia, arthralgia, arthrosis, dystonia, muscle cramps or weakness. *GU:* Urinary frequency, micturition disorders, menstrual disorders, dysmenorrhea, dysuria, painful menstruation, intermenstrual bleeding, sexual dysfunction and decreased libido, nocturia, polyuria, dysuria, urinary incontinence. *Respiratory:* Rhinitis, pharyngitis, yawning, bronchospasm, coughing, dyspnea, epistaxis. *Ophthalmologic:* Blurred vision, abnormal vision, abnormal accommodation, conjunctivitis, diplopia, eye pain, xerophthalmia. *Otic:* Tinnitus, earache. *Body as a whole:* Asthenia, fever, chest pain, chills, back pain, weight loss or weight gain, generalized edema, malaise, flushing, hot flashes, rigors, lymphadenopathy, purpura.

Laboratory Test Considerations: ↑ AST or ALT, total cholesterol, triglycerides. ↓ Serum uric acid.

OD **Management of Overdose:** *Symptoms:* Intensification of side effects. *Treatment:*

- Establish and maintain an airway, ensuring adequate oxygenation and ventilation.
- Activated charcoal, with or without sorbitol, may be as or more effective than emesis or lavage.
- Cardiac and VS should be monitored.
- Provide general supportive measures and symptomatic treatment.
- Since sertraline has a large volume of distribution, it is unlikely that dialysis, forced diuresis, hemoperfusion, or exchange transfusion will be beneficial.

Drug Interactions: Because sertraline is highly bound to plasma proteins, its use with other drugs that are also highly protein bound may lead to displacement, resulting in higher plasma levels of the drug and possibly increased side effects.

Alcohol / Concurrent use is not recommended in depressed clients
Benzodiazepines / ↓ Clearance of benzodiazepines metabolized by hepatic oxidation
Cimetidine / ↑ Half-life and blood levels of sertraline
Diazepam / ↑ Plasma levels of desmethyldiazepam (significance not known)
MAO inhibitors / Serious and possibly fatal reactions including hyperthermia, rigidity, autonomic instability with possible rapid

fluctuation of VS, myoclonus, changes in mental status (e.g., extreme agitation, delirium, coma)
Warfarin / ↑ PT and delayed normalization of PT
How Supplied: *Tablet:* 25 mg, 50 mg, 100 mg

Dosage

- **Tablets**

Depression.

Adults, initial: 50 mg once daily either in the morning or evening. Clients not responding to a 50-mg dose may benefit from doses up to a maximum of 200 mg/day.

Obsessive-compulsive disorder.

Adults: 50–200 mg/day. **Children, 6 to 12 years:** 25 mg once a day; **adolescents, 13 to 17 years:** 50 mg once a day.

Panic attacks.

Adults, initial: 25 mg/day for the first week; **then,** dosage ranges from 50–200 mg/day, based on response and tolerance.

HEALTH CARE CONSIDERATIONS

Administration/Storage

1. Clients responding during an initial 8-week treatment period will likely benefit during an additional 8-week treatment period. The effectiveness of sertraline has not been evaluated for more than 16 weeks, although it is generally recognized that acute periods of depression require several months or longer of sustained drug therapy. Shown to be effective up to 52 weeks for depression.
2. Do not increase dosage at intervals of less than 1 week.
3. Beneficial effects may not be observed for 2–4 weeks after treatment is started.
4. Use for more than 12 weeks for panic attacks has not been studied.

Assessment

1. Record indications for therapy, type, onset, and symptom characteristics.
2. List other drugs trialed and the outcome.
3. Note any seizure disorder.
4. Assess life-style, i.e., recent loss (death of loved one), stress, job change/loss, alcohol/drug use, or other factors that may contribute to depression.
5. Monitor ECG, liver and renal function studies.

Client/Family Teaching

1. Take only as directed and remain under close medical supervision.
2. Do not perform activities that require mental and physical alertness until drug effects are realized.
3. Review side effects, noting those that require immediate medical attention.
4. Loss of appetite, persistent nausea, and diarrhea with excessive weight loss should be reported.
5. Report any suicidal thoughts or aggression. Attend counseling and maintain contact with provider so drug utilization can be assessed, as the risk of suicide is tantamount in a depressive phase.
6. Avoid OTC agents, alcohol, and any other CNS depressants.
7. Use reliable contraception; report if pregnancy suspected.

Outcome/Evaluate

- Improved eating/sleeping pattern
- ↓ Levels of agitation and anxiety
- Relief of symptoms of depression

Sevelamer hydrochloride

(seh-**VEL**-ah-mer)
Pregnancy Category: C
Renagel **(Rx)**
Classification: Urinary tract product for end-stage renal disease (ESRD)

Action/Kinetics: A polymeric phosphate binder that decreases intestinal phosphate absorption. A decrease in serum phosphate decreases ectopic calcification and osteitis fibrosa. Also lowers LDL and total serum cholesterol. Is not absorbed into the systemic circulation.
Uses: To reduce serum phosphorous in ESRD in clients on hemodialysis.
Contraindications: Hypophosphatemia, bowel obstruction.
Special Concerns: No well controlled studies in lactating mothers. Use with caution in dysphagia, swallowing disorders, severe GI motility disorders, or major GI tract surgery. Safety and efficacy have not been determined in children.
Side Effects: *GI:* Diarrhea, dyspepsia, vomiting. *CV:* Hypotension or hypertension, thrombosis. *Body as a whole:* Infection, pain, headache. *Respiratory:* Increased cough.
Drug Interactions: Sevelamer may bind antiarrhythmic or anticonvulsant drugs → ↓ absorption.
How Supplied: *Capsules:* 340 mg

Dosage

- **Capsules**

Hyperphosphatemia in ESRD

Adults, initial: 2–4 capsules with each meal, based on the following serum phosphorus levels: **Greater than 6 but less**

S

than 7.5 mg/dL: 2 capsules t.i.d.; **7.5 mg/dL or more but less than 9 mg/dL:** 3 capsules t.i.d.; **9 mg/dL or more:** 4 capsules t.i.d. Adjust dosage to lower serum phosphorus to 6 mg/dL or less. Increase or decrease the dose by 1 capsule/meal as needed.

HEALTH CARE CONSIDERATIONS

Assessment

1. Note disease onset, dietary compliance, other agents trialed, and time on hemodialysis.
2. Assess for low P levels and bowel obstruction; determine any dysphagia, swallowing or severe GI motility disorders, or major GI surgery.
3. Monitor serum P, Ca, Cl, and bicarbonate levels.

Client/Family Teaching

1. Take with meals and adhere to prescribed diet for ESRD.
2. Space doses of concomitant drugs by 1 or more hr before or 3 hr after sevelamer.
3. Swallow whole. Do not chew capsules or take apart because the capsule contents expand in water.
4. Dosage is prescribed/adjusted according to serum phosphorus levels.
5. May experience diarrhea, vomiting, GI upset, headaches, and pain; report if persistent.

Outcome/Evaluate: ↓ Serum phosphorus to 6 mg/dL or less

Sibutramine hydrochloride monohydrate

(sih-**BYOU**-trah-meen)
Pregnancy Category: C
Meridia **(Rx) (C-IV)**
Classification: Anti-obesity drug

Action/Kinetics: Main effect is likely due to primary and secondary amine metabolites of sibutramine. Inhibits reuptake of norepinephrine (NE) and serotonin (5HT), resulting in enhanced NE and 5HT activity and reduced food intake. Significant improvement in serum uric acid. Rapidly absorbed from GI tract. Extensive first-pass metabolism in liver. **Peak plasma levels of active metabolites:** 3–4 hr. **t½, sibutramine:** 1.1 hr; **t½, active metabolites:** 14–16 hr. Excreted in urine and feces.

Uses: Management of obesity, including weight loss and maintenance of weight loss. Recommended for obese clients with initial body mass index of 30 kg/m^2 or more or 27 kg/m^2 in presence of hypertension, diabetes, or dyslipidemia. Use in conjunction with reduced calorie diet. Safety and efficacy have not been determined for more than 1 year.

Contraindications: Lactation. Use in clients receiving MAO inhibitors, who have anorexia nervosa, those taking centrally-acting appetite suppressant drugs, those with history of coronary artery disease, CHF, arrhythmias, or stroke. Use in severe renal impairment or hepatic dysfunction. Use with serotonergic drugs, such as fluoxetine, fluvoxamine, paroxetine, sertraline, venlafaxine, sumatriptan, and dihydroergotamine; also, use with dextromethorphan, meperidine, pentazocine, fentanyl, lithium, or tryptophan.

Special Concerns: Use with caution in geriatric clients. Safety and efficacy have not been determined in children less than 16 years of age. Use with caution in narrow angle glaucoma, history of seizures, or with drugs that may raise BP (e.g., phenylpropanolamine, ephedrine, pseudoephedrine). Exclude organic causes (e.g., untreated hypothyroidism) before use.

Side Effects: *Body as a whole:* Headache, back pain, flu syndrome, injury/accident, asthenia, chest pain, neck pain, allergic reaction. *GI:* Dry mouth, anorexia, abdominal pain, constipation, N&V, rectal disorder, increased appetite, dyspepsia, gastritis. *CNS:* Insomnia, dizziness, paresthesia, nervousness, anxiety, depression, somnolence, CNS stimulation, emotional lability. *CV:* Increased blood pressure, tachycardia, vasodilation, migraine, palpitation. *Dermatologic:* Sweating, rash, herpes simplex, acne. *Musculoskeletal:* Arthralgia, myalgia, tenosynovitis, joint disorder. *Respiratory:* Rhinitis, pharyngitis, sinusitis, increase cough, laryngitis. *GU:* Dysmenorrhea, UTI, vaginal monilia, metrorrhagia. *Otic:* Ear disorder, ear pain. *Miscellaneous:* Thirst, generalized edema, taste perversion.

How Supplied: *Capsules:* 5 mg, 10 mg, 15 mg

Dosage

- **Capsules**

  Obesity.

Adults, initial: 10 mg once daily (usually in morning) with or without food. If there is inadequate weight loss, dose may be titrated after 4 weeks to total of 15 mg once daily. Do not exceed 15 mg daily.

HEALTH CARE CONSIDERATIONS

Administration/Storage

1. May be taken with or without food.
2. Re-evaluate therapy if client has not lost at least 4 pounds in first 4 weeks of treatment.
3. Allow at least 2 weeks to elapse between discontinuation of MAO inhibitor and initia-

tion of sibutramine and between discontinuation of sibutramine and initiation of MAO inhibitor.
4. Store at controlled room temperature. Protect from heat and moisture and dispense in tight, light-resistant container.

Assessment

1. Record indications for therapy, length of weight problem, other agents/therapies trialed and outcome.
2. Assess for anorexia nervosa and MAO use.
3. Obtain weight and calculate BMI.
4. Monitor ECG, VS and labs; assess for increased BP or increased HR.

Client/Family Teaching

1. Take only as directed with or without food. Do not exceed prescribed dosage.
2. Continue regular exercise, weight counselling, and low calorie diet during therapy.
3. Review package insert before starting therapy and review with each refill.
4. Report any signs of allergic reaction including rash or hives.
5. Avoid all OTC agents and report all prescribed meds to prevent interactions.
6. Report regularly for F/U visits and lab work; record BP and pulse for provider review.

Outcome/Evaluate: Desired weight loss

Sildenafil citrate

(sill-**DEN**-ah-fill)
Pregnancy Category: B
Viagra **(Rx)**
Classification: Drug for erectile dysfunction

Action/Kinetics: Nitric oxide activates the enzyme guanylate cyclase, which causes increased levels of guanosine monophosphate (cGMP) and subsequently smooth muscle relaxation in the corpus cavernosum and allowing inflow of blood. Sildenafil enhances effect of nitric oxide by inhibiting phosphodiesterase type 5 which is responsible for degradation of cGMP in the corpus cavernosum. When sexual stimulation causes local release of nitric oxide, inhibition of phosphodiesterse type 5 by sildenafil causes increased levels of cGMP in the corpus cavernosum and thus smooth muscle relaxation and inflow of blood resulting in an erection. Drug has no effect in absence of sexual stimulation. Rapidly absorbed after PO use. Absorption is decreased when taken with high fat meal. Metabolized in liver where it is converted to active metabolite (N-desmethyl sildenafil). **t½, sildenafil and metabolite:** 4 hr. Excreted mainly in feces (80%) with about 13% excreted in urine. Reduced clearance is seen in geriatric clients.

Uses: Treatment of erectile dysfunction.

Contraindications: Concomitant use with organic nitrates in any form or with other treatments for erectile dysfunction. Use in newborns, children, or women.

Special Concerns: Use with caution in clients with anatomical deformation of penis, in those with predisposition to priapism (e.g., sickle cell anemia, multiple myeloma, leukemia), in bleeding disorders or active peptic ulceration, and in those with genetic disorders of retinal phosphodiesterases.

Side Effects: Listed are side effects with incidence of 2% or greater. *CNS:* Headache, dizziness. *GI:* Dyspepsia, diarrhea. *Dermatologic:* Flushing, rash. *Ophthalmic:* Mild and transient predominantly color tinge to vision, increased sensitivity to light, blurred vision. *Respiratory:* Nasal congestion, respiratory tract infection. *Miscellaneous:* UTI, back pain, flu syndrome, arthralgia. *Note:* Death has occurred in some clients following use of the drug.

OD Management of Overdose: *Symptoms:* Extension of side effects. *Treatment:* Standard supportive measures.

Drug Interactions

Cimetadine / ↑ Plasma levels of sildenafil
Erythromycin / ↑ Plasma levels of sildenafil
Itraconazole / ↑ Plasma levels of sildenafil
Ketoconazole / ↑ Plasma levels of sildenafil
Mibefradil / ↑ Plasma levels of sildenafil
Rifampin / ↓ Plasma levels of sildenafil

How Supplied: *Tablets:* 25 mg, 50 mg, 100 mg

Dosage

- **Tablets**

Treat erectile dysfunction.

For most clients, 50 mg no more than once daily, as needed, about 1 hr before sexual activity. Take anywhere from 0.5 hr to 4 hr before sexual activity. Depending on tolerance and effectiveness, dose may be increased to maximum of 100 mg or decreased to 25 mg. Consider a starting dose of 25 mg in those with hepatic or renal impairment or if taken with erythromycin, itraconzole, or ketoconazole.

HEALTH CARE CONSIDERATIONS

Assessment

1. Note onset and cause of erectile dysfunction, i.e., organic, psychogenic, or combined.
2. Assess cardiovascular status and obtain

S

ECG. Clients using nitrates should not use this drug or should be nitrate free for 24 hr prior to use.
3. List drugs prescribed as some may potentiate drug effects.
4. Assess for any retinal or bleeding disorders or active ulcers.
5. Note any conditions that may predispose client to priapism, i.e., multiple myelomas, sickle cell anemia, or leukemia.
6. Assess for any anatomical deformation of penis (Peyronie's disease, angulation, or cavernosal fibrosis).

Client/Family Teaching
1. Take only as directed; high fat meal may slow absorption.
2. May experience headache, flushing, upset stomach, stuffy nose, or abnormal vision; report any unusual, persistant or bothersome effects.
3. Do not use any other agent for erections with this therapy. Effects may be evident the day after therapy; assess before taking additional drug.
4. Report all meds currently prescribed to ensure none alter effects.
5. Practice safe sex; drug does not prevent disease transmission.
6. Plan some form of stimulation after ingestion to ensure desired erection obtained.
7. Do not share meds or prescriptions due to potential for adverse interactions and effects.

Outcome/Evaluate: Acquisition and maintenance of penile erection

Simvastatin

(sim-vah-**STAH**-tin)
Pregnancy Category: X
Zocor **(Rx)**
Classification: Antihyperlipidemic

S

See also *Antihyperlipidemic Agents HMG–CoA Reductase Inhibitors*.

Action/Kinetics: Inhibits HMG-CoA reductase, an enzyme that is necessary to convert HMG-CoA to mevalonate (an early step in the biosynthesis of cholesterol). Levels of VLDL and LDL cholesterol and plasma triglycerides are reduced while the plasma concentration of HDL cholesterol is increased. Does not reduce basal plasma cortisol or testosterone levels or impair renal reserve. **Peak therapeutic response:** 4–6 weeks. Approximately 85% absorbed; significant first-pass effect with less than 5% of a PO dose reaching the general circulation. Significantly bound to plasma proteins. **t½:** 3 hr. Metabolites excreted in the feces (60%) and urine (13%).

Uses: Adjunct to diet for the reduction of elevated total and LDL cholesterol levels in types IIa and IIb hypercholesterolemia when the response to diet and other approaches has been inadequate. In coronary heart disease and hypercholesterolemia to reduce risk of total mortality by reducing coronary death; to reduce the risk of non-fatal MI; to reduce the risk for undergoing myocardial revascularization procedures; to reduce the risk of stroke or TIAs. *Investigational:* Heterozygous familial hypercholesterolemia, familial combined hyperlipidemia, diabetic dyslipidemia in non-insulin-dependent diabetes, hyperlipidemia secondary to the nephrotic syndrome, and homozygous familial hypercholesterolemia in clients with defective LDL receptors.

Contraindications: Active liver disease or unexplained persistent increases in LFTs. Use in pregnancy, during lactation, or in children.

Special Concerns: Use with caution in clients who have a history of liver disease/consume large quantities of alcohol or with drugs that affect steroid levels or activity. Higher plasma levels may be observed in clients with hepatic and severe renal insufficiency. Safety and efficacy have not been determined in children less than 18 years of age.

Side Effects: *Musculoskeletal:* Rhabdomyolysis with renal dysfunction secondary to myoglobinuria, myopathy, arthralgias. *GI:* N&V, diarrhea, abdominal pain, constipation, flatulence, dyspepsia, pancreatitis, anorexia, stomatitis. *Hepatic:* Hepatitis (including chronic active hepatitis), cholestatic jaundice, cirrhosis, fatty change in liver, ***fulminant hepatic necrosis, hepatoma.*** *Neurologic:* Dysfunction of certain cranial nerves resulting in alteration of taste, impairment of extraocular movement, and facial paresis. Paresthesia, peripheral neuropathy, peripheral nerve palsy. *CNS:* Headache, tremor, vertigo, memory loss, anxiety, insomnia, depression. *Hypersensitivity Reactions:* Although rare, the following symptoms have been noted. ***Angioedema, anaphylaxis,*** lupus erythematous–like syndrome, vasculitis, purpura, thrombocytopenia, leukopenia, ***hemolytic anemia,*** polymyalgia rheumatica, positive ANA, ESR increase, arthritis, arthralgia, asthenia, urticaria, photosensitivity, chills, fever, flushing, malaise, dyspnea, ***toxic epidermal necrolysis, erythema multiforme (including Stevens-Johnson syndrome).*** *GU:* Gynecomastia, loss of libido, erectile dysfunction. *Ophthalmologic:* Lens opacities, ophthalmoplegia. *Hematologic:* Transient asymptomatic eosinophilia, anemia, thrombocytopenia, leukopenia. *Miscellaneous:* URI, asthenia, alopecia, edema.

Laboratory Test Considerations: ↑ CPK, AST, ALT.

Additional Drug Interactions

Gemfibrozil / Possible severe myopathy or rhabdomyolysis

Warfarin / ↑ Anticoagulant effect of warfarin

How Supplied: *Tablet:* 5 mg, 10 mg, 20 mg, 40 mg, 80 mg

Dosage

- **Tablets**

Adults, initially: 20 mg once daily in the evening; **maintenance:** 5–80 mg/day as a single dose in the evening. Consider a starting dose of 5 mg/day for clients on immunosuppressives or those with LDL less than 190 mg/dL and 10 mg/day for clients with LDL greater than 190 mg/dL. For geriatric clients, the starting dose should be 5 mg/day with maximum LDL reductions seen with 20 mg or less daily.

HEALTH CARE CONSIDERATIONS

See also *Health Care Considerations* for *Antihyperlipidemic Agents HMG–CoA Reductase Inhibitors*.

Administration/Storage

1. Place client on a standard cholesterol-lowering diet for 3–6 months before starting simvastatin. Continue the diet during drug therapy.
2. May be given without regard to meals.
3. Dosage may be adjusted at intervals of at least 4 weeks.

Assessment

1. Monitor CBC, cholesterol profile, liver and renal function studies. Schedule LFTs at the beginning of therapy and semiannually for the first year of therapy. Special attention should be paid to elevated serum transaminase levels.
2. List all medications prescribed to ensure none interact unfavorably.
3. Assess level of adherence to weight reduction, exercise, and cholesterol-lowering diet.
4. Note any alcohol abuse.

Client/Family Teaching

1. A low-cholesterol diet must continue to be followed during drug therapy. Consult dietitian for assistance in meal planning and food preparation.
2. Report any S&S of infections, unexplained muscle pain, tenderness/weakness (especially if accompanied by fever or malaise), surgery, trauma, or metabolic disorders.
3. Review importance of following a low-cholesterol diet, regular exercise, low alcohol consumption, and not smoking in the overall plan to reduce serum cholesterol levels.

Outcome/Evaluate: ↓ Serum triglycerides and LDL cholesterol levels

Sodium bicarbonate

(**SO**-dee-um bye-**KAR**-bon-ayt)

Pregnancy Category: C

Arm and Hammer Pure Baking Soda, Bell/ans, Citrocarbonate, Neut, Soda Mint (Rx and OTC)

Classification: Alkalinizing agent, antacid, electrolyte

Action/Kinetics: The antacid action is due to neutralization of hydrochloric acid by forming sodium chloride and carbon dioxide (1 g of sodium bicarbonate neutralizes 12 mEq of acid). Provides temporary relief of peptic ulcer pain and of discomfort associated with indigestion. Although widely used by the public, sodium bicarbonate is rarely prescribed as an antacid because of its high sodium content, short duration of action, and ability to cause alkalosis (sometimes desired). Is also a systemic and urinary alkalinizer by increasing plasma and urinary bicarbonate, respectively.

Uses: Treatment of hyperacidity, severe diarrhea (where there is loss of bicarbonate). Alkalization of the urine to treat drug toxicity (e.g., due to barbiturates, salicylates, methanol). Treatment of acute mild to moderate metabolic acidosis due to shock, severe dehydration, anoxia, uncontrolled diabetes, renal disease, cardiac arrest, extracorporeal circulation of blood, severe primary lactic acidosis. Prophylaxis of renal calculi in gout. During sulfonamide therapy to prevent renal calculi and nephrotoxicity. Neutralizing additive solution to decrease chemical phlebitis and client discomfort due to vein irritation at or near the site of infusion of IV acid solutions. *Investigational:* Sickle cell anemia.

Contraindications: Chloride loss due to vomiting or from continuous GI suction. With diuretics known to produce a hypochloremic alkalosis. Metabolic and respiratory alkalosis. Hypocalcemia in which alkalosis may cause tetany. Hypertension, convulsions, CHF, and other situations where administration of sodium can be dangerous. As a systemic alkalinizer when used as a neutralizing additive solution. As an antidote for strong mineral acids because carbon dioxide is formed, which may cause discomfort and even perforation.

S

Special Concerns: Use with caution in impaired renal function, toxemia of pregnancy, with oliguria or anuria, during lactation, in edema, CHF, liver cirrhosis, with low-salt diets, and in geriatric or postoperative clients with renal or CV insufficiency with or without CHF.

Side Effects: *GI:* Acid rebound, gastric distention. *Milk-alkali syndrome:* Hypercalcemia, metabolic alkalosis (dizziness, cramps, thirst, anorexia, N&V, hyperexcitability, tetany, diminished breathing, ***seizures***), renal dysfunction. *Miscellaneous:* Systemic alkalosis after prolonged use. *Following rapid infusion:* Hypernatremia, alkalosis, hyperirritability, tetany, fluid or solute overload. Extravasation following IV use may manifest ulceration, sloughing, cellulitis, or tissue necrosis at the site of injection.

OD **Management of Overdose:** *Symptoms:* Severe alkalosis that may be accompanied by tetany or hyperirritability. *Treatment:* Discontinue sodium bicarbonate. Reverse symptoms of alkalosis by rebreathing expired air from a paper bag or using a rebreathing mask. Use an IV infusion of ammonium chloride solution, 2.14%, to control severe cases. Treat hypokalemia by IV sodium chloride or potassium chloride. Calcium gluconate will control tetany.

Drug Interactions

Amphetamines / ↑ Effect of amphetamines by ↑ renal tubular reabsorption
Antidepressants, tricyclic / ↑ Effect of tricyclics by ↑ renal tubular reabsorption
Benzodiazepines / ↓ Effect due to ↑ alkalinity of urine
Chlorpropamide / ↑ Rate of excretion due to alkalinization of the urine
Ephedrine / ↑ Effect of ephedrine by ↑ renal tubular reabsorption
Erythromycin / ↑ Effect of erythromycin in urine due to ↑ alkalinity of urine
Flecainide / ↑ Effect due to ↑ alkalinity of urine
Iron products / ↓ Effect due to ↑ alkalinity of urine
Ketoconazole / ↓ Effect due to ↑ alkalinity of urine
Lithium carbonate / Excretion of lithium is proportional to amount of sodium ingested. If client on sodium-free diet, may develop lithium toxicity because less lithium is excreted
Mecamylamine / ↓ Excretion due to alkalinization of the urine
Methenamine compounds / ↓ Effect of methenamine due to ↑ alkalinity of urine
Methotrexate / ↑ Renal excretion due to alkalinization of the urine
Nitrofurantoin / ↓ Effect of nitrofurantoin due to ↑ alkalinity of urine
Procainamide / ↑ Effect of procainamide due to ↓ excretion by kidney
Pseudoephedrine / ↑ Effect of pseudoephedrine due to ↑ tubular reabsorption
Quinidine / ↑ Effect of quinidine by ↑ renal tubular reabsorption
Salicylates / ↑ Rate of excretion due to alkalinization of the urine
Sulfonylureas / ↓ Effect due to ↑ alkalinity of urine
Sympathomimetics / ↓ Renal excretion due to alkalinization of the urine
Tetracyclines / ↓ Effect of tetracyclines due to ↑ excretion by kidney

How Supplied: *Granule, effervescent*; *Injection:* 4%, 4.2%, 5%, 7.5%, 8.4%; *Powder*; *Tablet:* 325 mg, 520 mg, 648 mg, 650 mg

Dosage

- **Effervescent Powder**

Antacid.

Adults: 3.9–10 g in a glass of cold water after meals. **Geriatric and pediatric, 6–12 years:** 1.9–3.9 g after meals.

- **Oral Powder**

Antacid.

Adults: ½ teaspoon in a glass of water q 2 hr; adjust dosage as required.

Urinary alkalinizer.

Adults: 1 teaspoon in a glass of water q 4 hr; adjust dosage as required. Dosage not established for this form for children.

- **Tablets**

Antacid.

Adults: 0.325–2 g 1–4 times/day; pediatric, 6–12 years: 520 mg; may be repeated once after 30 min.

Urinary alkalinizer.

Adults, initial: 4 g; **then,** 1–2 g q 4 hr. **Pediatric:** 23–230 mg/kg/day; adjust dosage as needed.

- **IV**

Cardiac arrest.

Adults: 200–300 mEq given rapidly as a 7.5% or 8.4% solution. In emergencies, 300–500 mL of a 5% solution given as rapidly as possible without overalkalinizing the client. **Infants, less than 2 years of age, initial:** 1–2 mEq/kg/min given over 1–2 min; **then,** 1 mEq/kg q 10 min of arrest. Do not exceed 8 mEq/kg/day.

Severe metabolic acidosis.

90–180 mEq/L (about 7.5–15 g) at a rate of 1–1.5 L during the first hour. Adjust to needs of client.

Less severe metabolic acidosis.

Add to other IV fluids. **Adults and older children:** 2–5 mEq/kg given over a 4- to 8-hr period.

Neutralizing additive solution.
One vial of neutralizing additive solution added to 1 L of commonly used parenteral solutions, including dextrose, NaCl, and Ringer's.

HEALTH CARE CONSIDERATIONS

Administration/Storage

IV 1. Hypertonic solutions must be administered by trained personnel. Avoid extravasation as tissue irritation or cellulitis may result.
2. Determine IV dose by arterial blood pH, pCO_2, and base deficit; may be given IV push in an arrest situation or may be diluted in dextrose or saline solution and administered over 4–8 hr.
3. Administer isotonic solutions slowly; too-rapid administration may result in death due to cellular acidity. Check rate of flow frequently.
4. If only the 7.5% or 8.4% solution is available, dilute 1:1 with D5W when used in infants for cardiac arrest.
5. Do not exceed a rate of administration of 8 mEq/kg/day in infants with cardiac arrest to guard against hypernatremia, induction of intracranial hemorrhage, and decreasing CSF pressure.
6. In the event of severe alkalosis or tetany, have available a parenteral solution of calcium gluconate and 2.14% ammonium chloride .
7. Do not add to calcium-containing solutions, except where compatibility has been established.
8. Norepinephrine and dobutamine are incompatible with $NaHCO_3$.

Assessment

1. Note any history of renal impairment or CHF.
2. Assess for edema, which may indicate inability to utilize $NaHCO_3$. May try potassium bicarbonate (sodium content is 27%).
3. If on low continuous or intermittent NG suctioning or vomiting, assess for evidence of excessive chloride loss.
4. Record I&O. Observe for dry skin and mucous membranes, polydipsia, polyuria, and air hunger; may indicate a reversal of metabolic acidosis.
5. With acidosis, assess for the relief of dyspnea and hyperpnea.
6. If prescribed to counteract metabolic acidosis, monitor electrolytes and ABGs (pH, pCO_2, and HCO_3). Test urine periodically with nitrazine paper to determine if becoming alkaline.

Client/Family Teaching

1. If routinely taking excessive PO preparations of sodium bicarbonate to relieve gastric distress, a rebound reaction may occur, resulting either in an increased acid secretion or systemic alkalosis. Persistent symptoms of gastric distress require medical intervention.
2. Continuous, routine ingestion of sodium bicarbonate may cause formation of phosphate crystals in the kidney and fluid retention.
3. Consuming sodium bicarbonate with milk or calcium may result in a milk-alkali syndrome. Report immediately if anorexia, N&V, or mental confusion occurs.
4. Avoid OTC preparations that contain sodium bicarbonate, such as Alka-Seltzer or Fizrin.

Outcome/Evaluate

- Reversal of metabolic acidosis
- ↑ Urinary and serum pH
- ↓ Gastric discomfort

Sodium chloride

(**SO**-dee-um **KLOR**-eyed)

Pregnancy Category: C

Topical: Ayr Saline, HuMIST Saline Nasal, Na-Sal Saline Nasal, Ocean Mist, Saline From Otrivin ✦, Salinex Nasal Mist., Thalaris ✦, **Ophthalmic:** Adsorbonac Ophthalmic, AK-NaCl, Cordema ✦, Hypersal 5%, Muro-128 Ophthalmic, Muroptic-5, **Parenteral:** Sodium Chloride IV Infusions (0.45%, 0.9%, 3%, 5%), Sodium Chloride Injection for Admixtures (50, 100, 625 mEq/vial), Sodium Chloride Diluent (0.9%), Concentrated Sodium Chloride Injection (14.6%, 23.4%) (parenteral is Rx; topical and ophthalmic are OTC)

Classification: Electrolyte

Action/Kinetics: Sodium is the major cation of the body's extracellular fluid. It plays a crucial role in maintaining the fluid and electrolyte balance. Excess retention of sodium results in overhydration (edema, hypervolemia), which is often treated with diuretics. Abnormally low levels of sodium result in dehydration. Normally, the plasma contains 136–145 mEq sodium/L and 98–106 mEq chloride/L. The average daily requirement of salt is approximately 5 g.

Uses: PO: Prophylaxis of heat prostration or muscle cramps, chloride deficiency due to diuresis or salt restriction, prevention or treatment of extracellular volume depletion.

Parenteral:

0.9% (Isotonic) NaCl. To restore sodium and chloride losses; to dilute or dissolve drugs for IV, IM, or SC use; flushing of IV catheters; extracellular fluid replacement; priming solu-

S

tion for hemodialysis; initiate and terminate blood transfusions so RBCs will not hemolyze; metabolic alkalosis when there is fluid loss and mild sodium depletion.

0.45% (Hypotonic) NaCl. Fluid replacement when fluid loss exceeds depletion of electrolytes; hyperosmolar diabetes when dextrose should not be used (need for large volume of fluid but without excess sodium ions).

3% or 5% (Hypertonic) NaCl. Hyponatremia and hypochloremia due to electrolyte losses; to dilute body water significantly following excessive fluid intake; emergency treatment of severe salt depletion.

Concentrated NaCl. Additive in parenteral therapy for clients with special needs for sodium intake.

Bacteriostatic NaCl. Used only to dilute or dissolve drugs for IM, IV, or SC injection.

Topical: Relief of inflamed, dry, or crusted nasal membranes; irrigating solution. **Ophthalmic:** Use hypertonic solutions to decrease corneal edema due to bullous keratitis; as an aid to facilitate ophthalmoscopic examination in gonioscopy, biomicroscopy, and funduscopy.

Contraindications: Congestive heart failure, severely impaired renal function, hypernatremia, fluid retention. Use of the 3% or 5% solutions in elevated, normal, or only slightly depressed levels of plasma sodium and chloride. Use of bacteriostatic NaCl injection in newborns.

Special Concerns: Use with caution in CV, cirrhotic, or renal disease; in presence of hyperproteinemia, hypervolemia, urinary tract obstruction, and CHF; in those with concurrent edema and sodium retention and in clients receiving corticosteroids or corticotropin; and during lactation. Use with caution in geriatric or postoperative clients with renal or CV insufficiency with or without CHF.

Side Effects: Hypernatremia. Excessive NaCl may lead to hypopotassemia and acidosis. Fluid and solute overload leading to dilution of serum electrolyte levels, CHF, overhydration, ***acute pulmonary edema*** (especially in clients with CV disease or in those receiving corticosteroids or other drugs that cause sodium retention). Too rapid administration may cause local pain and venous irritation.

Postoperative intolerance of NaCl: Cellular dehydration, weakness, asthenia, disorientation, anorexia, nausea, oliguria, increased BUN levels, distention, deep respiration.

Symptoms due to solution or administration technique: Fever, abscess, tissue necrosis, infection at injection site, venous thrombosis or phlebitis extending from injection site, local tenderness, extravasation, hypervolemia.

Inadvertent administration of concentrated NaCl (i.e., without dilution) will cause sudden hypernatremia with the possibility of CV shock, extensive hemolysis, CNS problems, necrosis of the cortex of the kidneys, local tissue necrosis (if given extravascularly).

OD **Management of Overdose:** *Symptoms:* Irritation of GI mucosa, N&V, abdominal cramps, diarrhea, edema. Hypernatremia symptoms include: irritability, restlessness, ***weakness, seizures,*** coma, tachycardia, hypertension, fluid accumulation, ***pulmonary edema, respiratory arrest.*** *Treatment:* Supportive measures, including gastric lavage, induction of vomiting, provide adequate airway and ventilation, maintain vascular volume and tissue perfusion. Magnesium sulfate given as a cathartic.

How Supplied: *Dressing*; *Injection:* 0.45%, 0.9%, 2.5%, 3%, 5%, 14.6%, 23.4%; *Inhalation solution:* 0.45%, 0.9%, 3%, 10%; *Irrigation solution:* 0.45%, 0.9%; *Nasal solution:* 0.4%, 0.75%; *Ophthalmic ointment:* 5%; *Ophthalmic solution:* 0.44%, 2%, 5%; *Powder for reconstitution*; *Tablet:* 250 mg, 1 g

Dosage

- **Tablets (Including Extended-Release and Enteric-Coated)**

Heat cramps/dehydration.

0.5–1 g with 8 oz water up to 10 times/day; total daily dose should not exceed 4.8 g.

- **IV**

Individualized. Daily requirements of sodium and chloride can be met by administering 1 L of 0.9% NaCl.

To calculate sodium deficit. Amount of sodium to be given to raise serum sodium to the desired level:

Total body water (TBW): sodium deficit (mEq) = TBW × (desired plasma Na – observed plasma Na).

- **Ophthalmic Solution 2% or 5%**

1–2 gtt in eye q 3–4 hr.

- **Ophthalmic Ointment 5%**

A small amount (approximately 1/4 in.) to the inside of the affected eye(s) (i.e., by pulling down the lower eyelid) q 3–4 hr.

HEALTH CARE CONSIDERATIONS

Administration/Storage

IV 1. Give hypertonic injections of NaCl slowly through a small-bore needle placed well within the lumen of a large vein (to minimize irritation). Avoid infiltration.

2. Concentrated NaCl injection must be diluted before use.

3. Flush IV catheters before and after the

medications are given using 0.9% NaCl for injection.
4. Incompatibilities may occur when mixing NaCl injection with other additives; inspect the final product for cloudiness or a precipitate immediately after mixing, before administration, and periodically during administration. Do not store these mixtures.

Assessment

1. Record indications for therapy; monitor electrolytes, ECG, liver and renal function studies.
2. Observe for S&S of hypernatremia: flushed skin, elevated temperature, rough dry tongue, and edema. Symptoms of hyponatremia may include N&V, muscle cramps, dry mucous membranes, increased HR, and headaches.
3. Monitor VS and I&O. Assess urine specific gravity and serum sodium levels. Report if urine specific gravity is above 1.020 and serum sodium level is above 146 mEq/L.
4. Note level of consciousness and periodically assess heart and lung sounds.
5. When administering IV the 0.45% NaCl is hypotonic, the 0.9% NaCl is isotonic, and the 3% and 5% NaCl solutions are hypertonic.

Outcome/Evaluate

- Prophylaxis of heat prostration during exposure to high temperatures or during increased activity
- Prevention of chloride deficiency R/T excessive diuresis or salt restriction or excessive sweating

Sodium hyaluronate/ Hylan G-F 20

(SO-dee-um **high**-ah-**LUR**-ah-nayt)
Hyalgan, Synvisc **(Rx)**
Classification: Hyaluronic acid derivative

Action/Kinetics: Hyaluronic acid occurs naturally in body tissues and fluids. It is secreted by cells in synovial membranes and, in healthy synovial joints, maintains viscosity of synovial fluid and supports lubricating and shock-absorbing properties of the cartilage. In osteoarthritis, synovial fluid is decreased in viscosity and elasticity. Sodium hyaluronate and hylan G-F 20 replace diseased synovial fluid. Following intra-articular use, hylan G-F 20 permeates cartilage and slowly moves through joint tissues; it then passes through the lymph system into systemic circulation. Hyaluronic acid is metabolized by hyaluronidase in synovium.
Uses: Treatment of pain in osteoarthritis of knee in those who have not responded adequately to conservative non-drug therapy and to acetaminophen.
Contraindications: Hypersensivity to hyaluronan. Use in infections or skin diseases in area of injection site or with skin disinfectants containing quaternary ammonium salts (drug may precipitate). Concomitant use with other intra-articular injectables.
Special Concerns: Safety and efficacy on intra-articular use in areas other than knee or use for conditions other than osteoarthritis have not been determined. Use with caution in severely inflamed knee joints, when lymphatic or venous stasis exists in treatment leg, during lactation, and in those allergic to avian proteins, feathers and egg products. Safety and efficacy may be altered by dilutional effects. Safety and efficacy have not been determined during pregnancy or in children.
Side Effects: *Sodium hyaluronate (Hyalgan):* Injection site pain, skin reaction (ecchymosis, rash), pruritus.

Hylan G-F 20 (Synvisc): Knee pain, swelling, thorax and back rash, pruritus, calf cramps, hemorrhoid problems, ankle edema, muscle pain, tonsillitis with nausea, tachyarrhythmia, phlebitis with varicosities, low back sprain.
How Supplied: Sodium Gyaluronate: *Injection:* 8 mg/mL, 10 mg/mL; Hylan G-F 20: *Injection:* 8 mg/mL

Dosage

- **Intra-articular injection**

Osteoarthritis of knee.

Hyalgan: 2 mL once weekly for total of 5 injections using 20 gauge needle. *Synvisc:* 2 mL once weekly for total of 3 injections using 18-20 gauge needle. For both drugs, inject local anesthetic (e.g., lidocaine) SC prior to administration. Pain relief may not be noted until after last injection.

HEALTH CARE CONSIDERATIONS

Administration/Storage

1. If treatment is bilateral,use separate 2 mL vial/syringe for each knee.
2. Do not prepare injection site with skin disinfectants containing quaternary ammonium salts.
3. Remove joint effusion before giving drug. Do not use same syringe for removing fluid and injecting hyaluronic acid derivatives. However, use the same needle for injecting hylan G-F 20.
4. Drug products are intended for single use. Use immediately once opened and discard unused portion.

S

5. Safety and efficacy of repeat cycles have not been determined.
6. Store in original package at 25°C–30°C (77°F–86°F). Protect from light; do not freeze.

Assessment

1. Document other therapy utilized (nonpharmacologic and analgesic) and outcome.
2. Assess for effusion and remove prior to administering therapy.
3. Drug is derived from chicken/rooster coombs; assess for allergy to egg products, feathers, or avian proteins.

Client/Family Teaching

1. Review drug information sheet.
2. Drug is administered by provider into knee joint once weekly for 3-5 weeks, depending on agent used.
3. May experience swelling and pain in treated joints.
4. Do not perform strenuous or prolonged (>1 hr) weight bearing activities such as tennis or jogging within 48 hr of injection.
5. Pain relief usually lasts for up to 6 mo and may not be evident until after last injection.

Outcome/Evaluate: Control of osteoarthritis knee pain; ↑ mobility

Somatrem

(SO-mah-trem)
Pregnancy Category: C
Protropin **(Rx)**

Somatropin

(so-mah-TROH-pin)
Pregnancy Category: C, Serostim is B
Genotropin, Humatrope, Norditropin, Nutropin, Nutropin AQ, Saizen, Serostim **(Rx)**
Classification: Growth hormone

S

Action/Kinetics: Both somatrem and somatropin are derived from recombinant DNA technology. Somatrem contains the same sequence of amino acids (191) as human growth hormone derived from the pituitary gland plus one additional amino acid (methionine). Somatropin has the identical sequence of amino acids as does human growth hormone of pituitary origin. These agents stimulate linear growth by increasing somatomedin-C serum levels, which, in turn, increases the incorporation of sulfate into proteoglycans, thereby stimulating skeletal growth. They also increase the number and size of muscle cells, increase synthesis of collagen, increase protein synthesis, and increase internal organ size. Serum insulin levels increase (indicative of insulin resistance), and there is acute mobilization of lipid. **Peak plasma levels, somatotropin:** 7.5 hr after SC. **t½, somatotropin:** 3.8 hr after SC and 4.9 hr after IM.

Uses: Treat growth failure associated with chronic renal insufficiency up to the time of renal transplantation. Except for Serostim to stimulate linear growth of children who suffer from lack of adequate levels of endogenous growth hormone. Humatrope and Genotropin have been approved for the treatment of somatropin deficiency syndrome in adults. In adults, Humatrope produces increased lean muscle mass and exercise capacity, decreased body fat, and normalized high-density lipoprotein cholesterol levels. Humatrope, Nutropin, and Nutropin AQ for long-term treatment of short stature associated with Turner's syndrome. Serostim is approved for the treatment of AIDS wasting (i.e., cachexia). *Investigational:* Short children due to intrauterine growth retardation.

Contraindications: In clients in whom epiphyses have closed. Active intracranial lesions, sensitivity to benzyl alcohol (somatrem); sensitivity to m-cresol or glycerin (diluent in Humatrope). Use of Genotropin to treat acute catabolism in critically ill clients. *NOTE:* Hypothyroidism (which may be induced by the drug) decreases the response to somatrem.

Special Concerns: Use with caution during lactation. Concomitant use of glucocorticoids may decrease the response to growth hormone.

Side Effects: Development of persistent antibodies to growth hormone (30%–40% taking somatrem and 2% taking somatropin). Development of insulin resistance; hypothyroidism. Sodium retention and mild edema (especially in adults). Slipped capital femoral epiphysis or avascular necrosis of the femoral head in children with advanced renal osteodystrophy. Intracranial hypertension manifested by papilledema, visual changes, headache, N&V. *In adults:* Hyperglycemia, glucosuria; mild, transient edema; headache, weakness, muscle pain. *In children:* Injection site pain, leukemia.

Nutropin AQ: CTS, increased growth of preexisting nevi, gynecomastia, peripheral edema (rare), pancreatitis (rare). *Somatropin:* In adults, headache, localized muscle pain, weakness, mild hyperglycemia, glucosuria, mild transient edema during early treatment.

OD Management of Overdose: *Symptoms:* In acute overdose, hypoglycemia followed by hyperglycemia. Long-term overdose can result in S&S of acromegaly or gigantism.

Drug Interactions: Glucocorticoids inhibit the effect of somatrem on growth.

How Supplied: Somatrem:*Powder for injection:* 5 mg, 10 mg;Somatropin: *Injection:* 5 mg/mL; *Powder for injection:* 1.5 mg, 5 mg, 5.8 mg, 6 mg, 10 mg

Dosage

SOMATREM (PROTROPIN)

• **IM, SC**

Individualized. Usual: Up to 0.1 mg/kg (0.26 IU/kg) 3 times/week, not to exceed a weekly dosage of 0.30 mg/kg (about 0.90 IU/kg). The incidence of side effects increases if the dose is greater than 0.1 mg/kg.

SOMATROPIN (GENOTROPIN)

• **SC**

0.16–0.24 mg/kg/week divided into 6 or 7 SC injections.

SOMATROPIN (HUMATROPE)

• **IM, SC**

Adults: Individualized. Initial: 0.006 mg/kg/day (0.018 IU/kg/day) or less SC. May be increased, depending on need, to a maximum of 0.0125 mg/kg/day (0.0375 IU/kg/day). **Pediatric:** 0.18 mg/kg/week (0.54 IU/kg/week) SC or IM divided into equal doses given either on 3 alternate days or 6 times a week. Maximum weekly dose is 0.3 mg/kg (0.9 IU/kg) divided into equal doses and given on 3 alternate days.

SOMATRIPIN (NORDITROPIN)

• **SC**

0.024–0.034 mg/kg 6 to 7 times a week.

SOMATROPIN (NUTROPIN, NUTROPIN AQ)

• **SC**

Growth hormone deficiency.

Individualized. Usual: Give a weekly dose of 0.3 mg/kg (about 0.9 IU/kg).

Chronic renal insufficiency.

Individualized. Usual: Give a weekly dose of 0.35 mg/kg (about 1.05 IU/kg). This dose can be given up to the time of renal transplantation.

Turner Syndrome.

Give a weekly dose of 0.375 (or less) mg/kg (about 1.125 IU/kg) divided into equal doses 3 to 7 times/week.

SOMATROPIN (SAIZEN)

• **IM, SC**

0.06 mg/kg (about 0.18 IU/kg) 3 times weekly. Discontinue when epiphyses fuse.

SOMATROPIN (SEROSTIM)

• **SC**

Weight > 55 kg: 6 mg daily; **45–55 kg:** 5 mg daily; **35–45 kg:** 4 mg daily; **less than 35 kg:** 0.1 mg/kg. Give daily dose at bedtime.

HEALTH CARE CONSIDERATIONS

Administration/Storage

1. Somatrem should be prescribed only by a physician experienced in the diagnosis and treatment of pituitary disorders.
2. Due to the development of insulin resistance, evaluate for possible glucose intolerance.
3. Reconstitue the powder for injection for somatrem *only* with bacteriostatic water for injection (benzyl alcohol preserved).
4. If used in newborns, reconstitute with water for injection because benzyl alcohol can be toxic to newborns.
5. Inject only reconstituted somatrem solution that is clear and without particulate matter.
6. Be sure needle used for injection is at least 1 in. or longer so that the injection reaches muscle layer.
7. Use reconstituted somatrem within 7 days; do not freeze.
8. Genotropin is supplied in a two-chamber cartridge with the drug in the front chamber and the diluent in the rear chamber. Use a reconstitution device to co-mix the drug and diluent following the directions on the package. Gently tip the cartridge upside down a few times until complete dissolution occurs. Do not shake.
9. For Genotropin, the 1.5-mg cartridge may be refrigerated for 24 hr or less because it contains no preservative. Use once and discard any remaining solution. The 5.8- and 13.8-mg cartridges contain a preservative and may be stored under refrigeration for up to 14 days.
10. Give Genotropin in the thigh, buttocks, or abdomen; rotate the site daily to help prevent liopatrophy.
11. Humatrope is reconstituted by adding 1.5–5 mL of the diluent supplied for each 5-mg vial. Do not shake the vial. Do not give the reconstituted solution if it is cloudy or contains particulate material. Use a small enough syringe to ensure accuracy when the solution is withdrawn from the vial.
12. If sensitivity to the diluent for Humatrope occurs, reconstitute with sterile water for injection. The following guidelines must be followed.
   - Use only one dose per reconstituted vial.
   - Refrigerate solutions if not used immediately after reconstitution.
   - Use the reconstituted dose within 24 hr.
   - After the dose is administered, discard any unused portion.
13. Reconstitute either the 4- or 8-mg vial of Norditropin with 2 mL diluent. Avoid direct sunlight. Refrigerate and use reconstituted vials within 14 days after dissolution.
14. Give Norditropin in the thighs; rotate and vary injection sites.

15. Reconstitute Nutropin by adding bacteriostatic water for injection, 1–5 mL for each 5-mg vial and 1–10 mL for each 10-mg vial. For use in newborns, use water for injection as the benzyl alcohol (preservative) used in the bacteriostatic water may cause toxicity.
16. Use the following guidelines when giving Nutropin for clients who require dialysis:
• Give hemodialysis clients Nutropin at night just prior to going to sleep or at least 3–4 hr after dialysis in order to prevent hematoma formation due to heparin.
• Give chronic cycling peritoneal dialysis clients Nutropin in the morning after dialysis completed .
• Give chronic ambulatory peritoneal dialysis clients Nutropin in the evening at the time of the overnight exchange.
17. Reconstitute Saizen with 1 to 3 mL bacteriostatic water for injection. Reconstituted solutions are stable, under refrigeration, for 14 days. Avoid freezing.
18. Reconstitute Serostim with 1 mL sterile water for injection. Use within 24 hr of reconstitution and refrigerate reconstituted solution.
19. Except for Genotropin, when reconstituting somatrem or somatropin, do not shake the vial. Rather, swirl with a gentle rotary motion. The solution should be clear immediately after reconstitution.
20. Before reconstitution, store vials at 2°C–8°C (36°F–46°F).

Assessment

1. Record indications for therapy, age of client, and any other therapy trialed.
2. Determine that X-ray evidence of bone growth (wrists, hands) has been conducted. Record height and weight monthly. Generally a growth increase of 2 cm/year should be attained in order for treatment to be continued.
3. If growth is slow in the absence of rising antibody titers, hypopituitarism should be ruled out; untreated hypothyroidism or excessive glucocorticoid replacement can impair growth.
4. Monitor blood sugar and thyroid function studies; assess for diabetes or hypothyroidism. With diabetes, assess for hyperglycemia and acidosis.
5. Note any limps or knee/hip pain because a slipped capital epiphysis may occur.

Client/Family Teaching

1. Keep and review drug literature with guidelines for administration, drug preparation, and storage, after instructed by provider.
2. Report as scheduled for F/U.
3. Report any adverse effects or any limps or knee or hip pain.
4. The cost per year is based on client's weight and typically runs $10,000–$30,000.

Outcome/Evaluate: Desired skeletal growth; (growth hormone replacement with deficiency)

Sotalol hydrochloride

(SOH-tah-lol)
Pregnancy Category: B
Alti-Sotalol ✱, Apo-Sotalol ✱, Betapace, Gen-Sotalol ✱, Linsotalol ✱, Novo-Sotalol ✱, Nu-Sotalol ✱, Rylosol ✱, Sotacor ✱ **(Rx)**
Classification: Beta-adrenergic blocking agent

See also *Beta-Adrenergic Blocking Agents*.
Action/Kinetics: Blocks both beta-1- and beta-2-adrenergic receptors; has no membrane-stabilizing activity or intrinsic sympathomimetic activity. Has both Group II and Group III antiarrhythmic properties (dose dependent). Significantly increases the refractory period of the atria, His-Purkinje fibers, and ventricles. Also prolongs the QTc and JT intervals. **t½:** 12 hr. Not metabolized; excreted unchanged in the urine.
Uses: Treatment of documented ventricular arrhythmias such as life-threatening sustained VT.
Contraindications: Use in asymptomatic PVCs or supraventricular arrhythmias due to the proarrhythmic effects of sotalol. Congenital or acquired long QT syndromes. Use in clients with hypokalemia or hypomagnesemia until the imbalance is corrected, as these conditions aggravate the degree of QT prolongation and increase the risk for torsades de pointes.
Special Concerns: Clients with sustained ventricular tachycardia and a history of CHF appear to be at the highest risk for serious proarrhythmia. Dose, presence of sustained ventricular tachycardia, females, excessive prolongation of the QTc interval, and history of cardiomegaly or CHF are risk factors for torsades de pointes. Use with caution in clients with chronic bronchitis or emphysema and in asthma if an IV agent is required. Use with extreme caution in clients with sick sinus syndrome associated with symptomatic arrhythmias due to the increased risk of sinus bradycardia, sinus pauses, or sinus arrest. Reduce dosage in impaired renal function. Safety and efficacy in children have not been established.
Additional Side Effects: *CV:* ***New or worsened ventricular arrhythmias, including sustained VT or ventricular fibrillation that might be fatal. Torsades de pointes.***
How Supplied: *Tablet:* 80 mg, 120 mg, 160 mg, 240 mg

Dosage

- **Tablets**

Ventricular arrhythmias.

Adults, initial: 80 mg b.i.d. The dose may be increased to 240 or 320 mg/day after appropriate evaluation. **Usual:** 160–320 mg/day given in two or three divided doses. Clients with life-threatening refractory ventricular arrhythmias may require doses ranging from 480 to 640 mg/day (due to potential proarrhythmias, use these doses only if the potential benefit outweighs the increased risk of side effects).

HEALTH CARE CONSIDERATIONS

See also *Health Care Considerations* for *Beta-Adrenergic Blocking Agents.*

Administration/Storage

1. Adjust dosage gradually, allowing 2–3 days between increments in dosage. This allows steady-state plasma levels to be reached and QT intervals to be monitored.
2. Undertake initiation of and increases in dosage in a hospital with facilities for cardiac rhythm monitoring. Dosage must be individualized only after appropriate clinical assessment.
3. Proarrhythmias can occur during initiation of therapy and with each dosage increment.
4. In clients with impaired renal function, alter the dosing interval as follows: if C_{CR} is 30–60 mL/min, the dosing interval is 24 hr; if C_{CR} is 10–30 mL/min, the dosing interval should be 36–48 hr. If C_{CR} is less than 10 mL/min, dose must be individualized. Undertake dosage adjustments in clients with impaired renal function only after five to six doses at the intervals described.
5. Before initiating sotalol, withdraw previous antiarrhythmic therapy with careful monitoring for a minimum of 2–3 plasma half-lives if condition permits.
6. Do not initiate sotalol after amiodarone is discontinued until the QT interval is normalized.

Assessment

1. Perform a thorough health history; note any cardiomegaly or CHF.
2. Obtain ECG and note/document QT interval; note symptoms associated with arrhythmia.
3. Client should be in a closely monitored environment with VS and ECG monitored during initiation and adjustment of sotalol.
4. Monitor VS, I&O, electrolytes, magnesium level, liver and renal function studies.

Client/Family Teaching

1. Take on an empty stomach as food decreases absorption.
2. Take exactly as directed and do not stop abruptly; drug controls symptoms but does not cure condition.
3. Avoid activites that require mental alertness until drug effects realized; may cause dizziness/drowsiness.
4. Report increased chest pain/SOB, night cough, swelling of feet and ankles, increased fatigue, low heart rate, or unsteady gait.
5. Avoid alcohol and OTC agents.
6. Continue dietary and exercise guidelines as prescribed and healthy life-style changes.

Outcome/Evaluate: Control/conversion of life-threatening arrhythmias to stable cardiac rhythm

Sparfloxacin

(spar-**FLOX**-ah-sin)

Pregnancy Category: C

Zagam **(Rx)**

Classification: Fluoroquinolone antibiotic

See also *Fluoroquinolones.*

Action/Kinetics: Well absorbed. **Peak serum levels:** 4–5 hr. 50% excreted in the urine.

Uses: Community acquired pneumonia due to *Chlamydia pneumoniae, Haemophilus influenzae, Haemophilus parainfluenzae, Moraxella catarrhalis, Mycoplasma pneumoniae,* or *Streptococcus pneumoniae.* Acute bacterial exacerbations of chronic bronchitis caused by *C. pneumoniae, Enterobacter cloacae, H. influenzae, H. parainfluenzae, Klebsiella pneumoniae, M. catarrhalis, Staphylococcus aureus,* or *S. pneumoniae.*

Special Concerns: Safety and efficacy have not been determined in children less than 18 years of age.

How Supplied: *Tablets:* 200 mg.

Dosage

- **Tablets**

Community-acquired pneumonia, acute bacterial exacerbations of chronic bronchitis.

Adults over 18 years of age: Two - 200 mg tablets taken on the first day as a loading dose. Then, one - 200 mg tablet q 24 hr for a total of 10 days of therapy (i.e., a total of 11 tablets). For clients with a C_{CR} less than 50 mL/min, the loading dose is two - 200 mg tablets taken on the first day. Then, one - 200 mg

S

tablet q 48 hr for a total of 9 days (i.e., a total of 6 tablets).

HEALTH CARE CONSIDERATIONS

See also *Health Care Considerations* for *Antiviral Drugs*, .

Assessment

1. Record onset, location, duration, and characteristics of symptoms.
2. Monitor CBC, cultures, and renal function studies; reduce dose with impaired renal function.

Client/Family Teaching

1. Take exactly as directed; may be taken with or without food.
2. Complete entire prescription and do not skip or double up on doses unless directed.
3. Report any unusual side effects or lack of response after 72 hr.

Outcome/Evaluate

- Symptomatic improvement
- Resolution of infection

Spectinomycin hydrochloride

(speck-tin-oh-**MY**-sin)

Pregnancy Category: B

Trobicin **(Rx)**

Classification: Antibiotic, miscellaneous

See also *Anti-Infectives*.

Action/Kinetics: Produced by *Streptomyces spectabilis*. It inhibits bacterial protein synthesis by binding to ribosomes (30S subunit), thereby interfering with transmission of genetic information crucial to life of microorganism. Mainly bacteriostatic. Only given IM. **Peak plasma concentration:** 100 mcg/mL (2-g dose) after 1 hr and 160 mcg/mL (4-g dose) after 2 hr. **t½:** 1.2–2.8 hr. Not significantly bound to protein. Excreted in urine.

S

Uses: Acute gonorrheal proctitis and urethritis in males and acute gonorrheal cervicitis and proctitis in females due to susceptible strains of *Neisseria gonorrhoeae*. For pharyngeal infections, use only in those intolerant to cephalosporins or quinolones. It is ineffective against pharyngeal infections and against syphilis; is a poor drug to choose when mixed infections are present.

Contraindications: Sensitivity to drug.

Special Concerns: Safe use during pregnancy, in infants, and in children has not been established. Benzyl alcohol in the product may cause a fatal gasping syndrome in infants.

Side Effects: A single dose of spectinomycin has caused soreness at the site of injection, urticaria, dizziness, nausea, chills, fever, and insomnia. Multiple doses have caused a decrease in H&H and C_{CR} and an increase in alkaline phosphatase, BUN, and ALT. In single or multiple doses, decrease in urine output.

How Supplied: *Powder for injection:* 2 g

Dosage

- **IM Only**

Gonorrheal urethritis in males, proctitis, and cervicitis.

2 g. In geographic areas where antibiotic resistance is known to be prevalent, give 4 g divided between two gluteal injection sites.

Alternative regimen for urethral, endocervical, or rectal gonococcal infections in clients who cannot take ceftriaxone.

Adults and children weighing more than 45 kg: Spectinomycin, 2 g, as a single dose followed by doxycycline. **Children weighing less than 45 kg:** 40 mg/kg given IM once.

Gonococcal infections in pregnancy where client is allergic to beta-lactams.

2 g followed by erythromycin.

Disseminated gonococcal infection where client is allergic to beta-lactams.

2 g q 12 hr.

HEALTH CARE CONSIDERATIONS

See also *General Health Care Considerations for All Anti-Infectives.*

Administration/Storage

1. Powder is stable for 3 years.
2. Benzyl alcohol in the product may cause a fatal gasping syndrome in infants.
3. Use reconstituted solution within 24 hr.
4. Inject deeply into the upper, outer quadrant of the gluteus muscle.
5. Injections may be divided between two sites for clients requiring 4 g. Rotate and document injection sites.

Client/Family Teaching

1. Return for serologic tests monthly for at least 3 months if syphilis suspected; with gonorrhea, report for a repeat serologic test 3 months after treatment.
2. Obtain counseling and encourage treatment of sexual partners.
3. Abstain from intercourse until infection is resolved; follow safe sex practices to prevent reinfections.

Outcome/Evaluate

- Negative serology/cultures for gonorrhea
- Symptomatic improvement with gonorrheal urethritis, cervicitis, and/or proctitis

Spironolactone

(speer-oh-no-**LAK**-tohn)

Pregnancy Category: D

Aldactone, Novo-Spiroton ✦ **(Rx)**
Classification: Diuretic, potassium-sparing

See also *Diuretics, Thiazides*.

Action/Kinetics: Mild diuretic that acts on the distal tubule to inhibit sodium exchange for potassium, resulting in increased secretion of sodium and water and conservation of potassium. An aldosterone antagonist. Manifests a slight antihypertensive effect. Interferes with synthesis of testosterone and may increase formation of estradiol from testosterone, thus leading to endocrine abnormalities. **Onset:** Urine output increases over 1–2 days. **Peak:** 2–3 days. **Duration:** 2–3 days, and declines thereafter. Metabolized to an active metabolite (canrenone). **t½:** 13–24 hr for canrenone. Canrenone is excreted through the urine (primary) and the bile. Almost completely bound to plasma protein.

Uses: Primary hyperaldosteronism, including diagnosis, short-term preoperative treatment, long-term maintenance therapy for those who are poor surgical risks and those with bilateral micronodular or macronodular adrenal hyperplasia. To treat edema when other approaches are inadequate or ineffective (e.g., CHF, cirrhosis of the liver, nephrotic syndrome). Essential hypertension (usually in combination with other drugs). Prophylaxis of hypokalemia in clients taking digitalis. *Investigational:* Hirsutism, treat symptoms of PMS, with testolactone to treat familial male precocious puberty (short-term treatment), acne vulgaris.

Contraindications: Acute renal insufficiency, progressive renal failure, hyperkalemia, and anuria. Clients receiving potassium supplements, amiloride, or triamterene.

Special Concerns: Use during pregnancy only if benefits clearly outweigh risks. Use with caution in impaired renal function. Geriatric clients may be more sensitive to the usual adult dose.

Side Effects: *Electrolyte:* Hyperkalemia, hyponatremia (characterized by lethargy, dry mouth, thirst, tiredness). *GI:* Diarrhea, cramps, ulcers, gastritis, gastric bleeding, vomiting. *CNS:* Drowsiness, ataxia, lethargy, mental confusion, headache. *Endocrine:* Gynecomastia, menstrual irregularities, impotence, bleeding in postmenopausal women, deepening of voice, hirsutism. *Dermatologic:* Maculopapular or erythematous cutaneous eruptions, urticaria. *Miscellaneous:* Drug fever, breast carcinoma, gynecomastia, hyperchloremic metabolic acidosis in hepatic cirrhosis (decompensated), ***agranulocytosis***. *NOTE:* Spironolactone has been shown to be tumorigenic in chronic rodent studies.

Laboratory Test Considerations: Interference with radioimmunoassay for digoxin. False + plasma cortisol (as determined by fluorometric assay of Mattingly).

Drug Interactions

Anesthetics, general / Additive hypotension
ACE inhibitors / Significant hyperkalemia
Anticoagulants, oral / Inhibited by spironolactone
Antihypertensives / Potentiation of hypotensive effect of both agents. Reduce dosage, especially of ganglionic blockers, by one-half
Captopril / ↑ Risk of significant hyperkalemia
Digitalis / ↑ Half-life of digoxin → ↓ clearance. Spironolactone may ↓ inotropic effect of digoxin. Spironolactone both ↑ and ↓ elimination t½ of digitoxin
Diuretics, others / Often administered concurrently because of potassium-sparing effect of spironolactone. Severe hyponatremia may occur. Monitor closely
Lithium / ↑ Chance of lithium toxicity due to ↓ renal clearance
Norepinephrine / ↓ Responsiveness to norepinephrine
Potassium salts / Since spironolactone conserves potassium excessively, hyperkalemia may result. Rarely used together
Salicylates / Large doses may ↓ effects of spironolactone
Triamterene / Hazardous hyperkalemia may result from combination

How Supplied: *Tablet:* 25 mg, 50 mg, 100 mg

Dosage

- **Tablets**

Edema.

Adults, initial: 100 mg/day (range: 25–200 mg/day) in two to four divided doses for at least 5 days; **maintenance:** 75–400 mg/day in two to four divided doses. **Pediatric:** 3.3 mg/kg/day as a single dose or as two to four divided doses.

Antihypertensive.

Adults, initial: 50–100 mg/day as a single dose or as two to four divided doses—give for at least 2 weeks; **maintenance:** adjust to individual response. **Pediatric:** 1–2 mg/kg in a single dose or in two to four divided doses.

Hypokalemia.

Adults: 25–100 mg/day as a single dose or two to four divided doses.

Diagnosis of primary hyperaldosteronism.

Adults: 400 mg/day for either 4 days (short-test) or 3–4 weeks (long-test).

Hyperaldosteronism, prior to surgery.

Adults: 100–400 mg/day in two to four doses prior to surgery.

S

Hyperaldosteronism, chronic-therapy.
Use lowest possible dose.
Hirsutim.
50–200 mg/day.
Symptoms of PMS.
25 mg q.i.d. beginning on day 14 of the menstrual cycle.
Familial male precocious puberty, short-term.
Spironolactone, 2 mg/kg/day, and testolactone, 20–40 mg/kg/day, for at least 6 months.
Acne vulgaris.
100 mg/day.

HEALTH CARE CONSIDERATIONS

See also *Health Care Considerations* for *Diuretics, Thiazides.*

Administration/Storage

1. When used as the sole drug to treat edema, maintain the initial dose for at least 5 days. After that, adjustments may be made. If the dosage is not effective, a second diuretic may be added, especially one that acts in the proximal tubules.
2. When administered to small children, tablets may be crushed and given as suspension in cherry syrup.
3. Food may increase the absorption of spironolactone.
4. Protect the drug from light.

Assessment

1. Record indications for therapy, other agents prescribed, and the outcome.
2. If history of cardiac disease, be alert for cardiac irregularities R/T hypokalemia.
3. Monitor ABGs, ECG, CBC, blood sugar, uric acid, serum electrolytes, and liver and renal function studies. Record VS, I&O, and weights.
4. If client develops dysuria, urinary frequency, or renal spasm, obtain a urinalysis and urine culture.
5. Assess for drug tolerance characterized by edema and reduced urine output.

Client/Family Teaching

1. Take with a snack or meals to minimize GI upset. Report if nausea, bloating, anorexia, vomiting, or diarrhea persist.
2. Record BP for provider review.
3. Avoid foods or salt substitutes high in potassium; drug is potassium-sparing.
4. Record weight twice a week. Report any evidence of edema or weight gain/loss of more than 5 lb (2.2 kg) weekly.
5. Do not drive/operate dangerous machinery until drug effects realized; may cause drowsiness or ataxia.
6. Drug may cause gynecomastia and diminished libido by reducing testosterone levels.
7. Report if deep, rapid respirations, headaches, or mental slowing occurs; may indicate hyperchloremic metabolic acidosis.
8. Drug is metabolized in the liver. Report jaundice, tremors, or mental confusion; may develop hepatic encephalopathy with liver disease.

Outcome/Evaluate

- Enhanced diuresis with ↓ edema
- ↓ BP
- Antagonism of high levels of aldosterone
- Prevention of hypokalemia in those taking digitalis and/or other diuretics

COMBINATION DRUG

Spironolactone and Hydrochlorothiazide

(speer-oh-no-**LAK**-tohn)
(hy-droh-**klor**-oh-**THIGH**-ah-zyd)
Pregnancy Category: D
Aldactazide, Aldactazide 25 and 50 ✱, Novo-Spirozine ✱ **(Rx)**
Classification: Antihypertensive, diuretic

See also *Spironolactone* and *Hydrochlorothiazide.*
Content: Spironolactone - Hydrochlorothiazide: *Tablets:* 25 mg - 25 mg, 50 mg - 50 mg
Action/Kinetics: This drug is a combination of a thiazide and potassium-sparing diuretic.
Uses: Congestive heart failure, essential hypertension, nephrotic syndrome. Edema and/or ascites in cirrhosis of the liver.
Contraindications: Use in pregnancy only if benefits outweigh risks.
How Supplied: See Content

Dosage

- **Tablets**

Edema.
Adults, usual: 100 mg of each drug daily (range: 25–200 mg), given as single or divided doses. **Pediatric, usual:** equivalent to 1.65–3.3 mg/kg spironolactone.
Essential hypertension.
Adults, usual: 50–100 mg of each drug daily in single or divided doses.

HEALTH CARE CONSIDERATIONS

See Health Care Considerations for *Hydrochlorothiazide* and *Spironolactone.*

Outcome/Evaluate

- Enhanced diuresis; ↓ edema
- ↓ BP

Stavudine

(STAH-vyou-deen)
Pregnancy Category: C
Zerit
Classification: Antiviral agent

See also *Antiviral Agents.*
Action/Kinetics: Inhibits replication of HIV due to phosphorylation by cellular kinases to stavudine triphosphate, which has antiviral activity. The mechanism for the antiviral activity includes inhibition of HIV reverse transcriptase by competing with the natural substrate deoxythymidine triphosphate and by causing DNA chain termination, thereby inhibiting viral DNA synthesis. Rapidly absorbed. **Peak plasma levels:** 1 hr or less. **t½, terminal:** Approximately 1.2 hr. About 40% of the drug is eliminated through the kidney.
Uses: Treatment of adults with advanced HIV infection who cannot tolerate approved therapies or who have experienced significant clinical or immunologic deterioration while receiving such therapies (or for whom such therapies are contraindicated).
Contraindications: Lactation.
Special Concerns: The effect of stavudine on the clinical progression of HIV infection, such as incidence of opportunistic infections or survival, has not been determined.
Side Effects: *Neurologic:* Peripheral neuropathy (common), including numbness, tingling, or pain in feet or hands. *CNS:* Insomnia, anxiety, depression, nervousness, dizziness, confusion, migraine, somnolence, tremor, neuralgia, dementia. *GI:* Diarrhea, N&V, anorexia, dyspepsia, constipation, ulcerative stomatitis, aphthous stomatitis, pancreatitis. *Body as a whole:* Headache, chills, fever, asthenia, abdominal pain, back pain, malaise, weight loss, allergic reactions, flu syndrome, lymphadenopathy, pelvic pain, neoplasms, death. *CV:* Chest pain, vasodilation, hypertension, peripheral vascular disorder, syncope. *GU:* Dysuria, genital pain, dysmenorrhea, vaginitis, urinary frequency, hematuria, impotence, urogenital neoplasm. *Respiratory:* Dyspnea, pneumonia, asthma. *Dermatologic:* Rash, sweating, pruritus, maculopapular rash, benign skin neoplasm, urticaria, exfoliative dermatitis. *Ophthalmic:* Conjunctivitis, abnormal vision.
Laboratory Test Considerations: ↑ AST, ALT.
How Supplied: *Capsule:* 15 mg, 20 mg, 30 mg, 40 mg; *Powder for Injection:* 1 mg/mL

Dosage

- **Capsules**

Advanced HIV infections.
Adults, initial: 40 mg b.i.d. for clients weighing 60 or more kg and 30 mg b.i.d. for clients weighing less than 60 kg. In clients developing peripheral neuropathy, the following dosage schedule may be used if symptoms of neuropathy resolve completely: 20 mg b.i.d. for clients weighing 60 or more kg and 15 mg b.i.d. for clients weighing less than 60 kg.

The following dosage schedule is recommended for clients with impaired renal function: (a) C_{CR} greater than 50 mL/min: 40 mg q 12 hr for clients weighing 60 or more kg and 30 mg q 12 hr for clients weighing less than 60 kg; (b) C_{CR} 26–50 mL/min: 20 mg q 12 hr for clients weighing 60 or more kg and 15 mg q 12 hr for clients weighing less than 60 kg; (c) C_{CR} 10–25 mL/min: 20 mg q 24 hr for clients weighing 60 or more kg and 15 mg q 24 hr for clients weighing less than 60 kg. Insufficient data are available to recommend doses for a C_{CR} less than 10 mL/min or for clients undergoing dialysis.

HEALTH CARE CONSIDERATIONS

See *Health Care Considerations* for *Antiviral Agents.*
Administration/Storage: The interval between PO doses is 12 hr.
Assessment
1. Record onset of symptoms, other agents prescribed, and date confirmed; note date of intolerance.
2. Obtain baseline CBC, CD_4 counts/viral load, PT/PTT, liver and renal function studies. Reduce dose with impaired renal function.

Client/Family Teaching
1. May be taken without regard to meals.
2. Take exactly as prescribed, do not exceed prescribed dose, and do not share medications.
3. Drug is not a cure, but alleviates/manages the symptoms of HIV infections. May continue to acquire illnesses associated with AIDS or ARC, including opportunistic infections; must remain under close medical supervision.
4. The risk of transmission of HIV to others through blood or sexual contact is not reduced with drug therapy. Review the criteria and precautions for safe sex and do not share needles.
5. Insomnia and GI upset usually resolve after 3–4 weeks of therapy.
6. Report any S&S of infection (i.e., sore throat, swollen glands, fever).

7. Report symptoms of peripheral neuropathy characterized by numbness and tingling or pain in the hands and/or feet and discontinue drug if evident. Symptoms may temporarily worsen following cessation of drug therapy but, once resolved, drug may be reintroduced at a lower dose.
8. Report for all scheduled lab studies and follow-up visits to assess response to therapy and to identify any adverse drug effects.
9. Identify local support groups that may assist client/family to understand and cope with this disease.

Outcome/Evaluate: Clinical/immunologic improvement with AIDS and ARC

Sucralfate

(sue-**KRAL**-fayt)

Pregnancy Category: B

Apo-Sucralfate ✦, Carafate, Novo-Sucralate ✦, Nu-Sucralfate ✦, Sulcrate ✦, Sulcrate Suspension Plus ✦ **(Rx)**

Classification: Antiulcer drug

Action/Kinetics: Thought to form an ulcer-adherent complex with albumin and fibrinogen at the site of the ulcer, protecting it from further damage by gastric acid. May also form a viscous, adhesive barrier on the surface of the gastric mucosa and duodenum. It adsorbs pepsin, thus inhibiting its activity. May be used in conjunction with antacids. Approximately 90% excreted in the feces. **Duration:** 5 hr.

Uses: Short-term treatment (up to 8 weeks) of active duodenal ulcers. Maintenance for duodenal ulcer at decreased dosage after healing of acute ulcers. *Investigational:* Hasten healing of gastric ulcers, chronic treatment of gastric ulcers. Treatment of reflux and peptic esophagitis. Treatment of aspirin- and NSAID-induced GI symptoms; prevention of stress ulcers and GI bleeding in critically ill clients. The suspension has been used to treat oral and esophageal ulcers due to chemotherapy, radiation, or sclerotherapy.

Note: Even though healing of ulcers may result, the frequency or severity of subsequent attacks is not altered.

Special Concerns: Safety for use in children and during lactation has not been fully established. A successful course resulting in healing of ulcers will not alter posthealing frequency or severity of duodenal ulceration.

Side Effects: *GI:* Constipation (most common); also, N&V, diarrhea, indigestion, flatulence, dry mouth, gastric discomfort. *Hypersensitivity:* Urticaria, ***angioedema, respiratory difficulty,*** rhinitis. *Miscellaneous:* Back pain, dizziness, sleepiness, vertigo, rash, pruritus, facial swelling, ***laryngospasm.***

Drug Interactions
Antacids containing aluminum / ↑ Total body burden of aluminum
Anticoagulants / ↓ Hypoprothrombinemic effect of warfarin
Cimetidine / ↓ Absorption of cimetidine due to binding to sucralfate
Ciprofloxacin / ↓ Absorption of ciprofloxacin due to binding to sucralfate
Digoxin / ↓ Absorption of digoxin due to binding to sucralfate
Ketoconazole / ↓ Bioavailability of ketoconazole
Norfloxacin / ↓ Absorption of norfloxacin due to binding to sucralfate
Phenytoin / ↓ Absorption of phenytoin due to binding to sucralfate
Quinidine / ↓ Quinidine levels → ↓ effect
Ranitidine / ↓ Absorption of ranitidine due to binding to sucralfate
Tetracycline / ↓ Absorption of tetracycline due to binding to sucralfate
Theophylline / ↓ Absorption of theophylline due to binding to sucralfate

How Supplied: *Suspension:* 1 g/10 mL; *Tablet:* 1 g

Dosage

• **Suspension, Tablets**

Adults: usual: 1 g q.i.d. (10 mL of the suspension) 1 hr before meals and at bedtime (it may also be taken 2 hr after meals). Take for 4–8 weeks unless X-ray films or endoscopy have indicated significant healing. **Maintenance (tablets only):** 1 g b.i.d.

HEALTH CARE CONSIDERATIONS

Assessment

1. Record indications for therapy, noting onset and characteristics of symptoms.
2. List other agents prescribed and the outcome.
3. Ensure that tablets are reconstituted prior to administering through the NGT. Generally when placed in a medicine cup with a small amount of water and left for 10–15 min, the tablets will dissolve completely.
4. Assess and monitor gastric pH; maintain pH above 5.
5. Monitor CBC and serum phosphate levels. Drug binds phosphate and may lead to hypophosphatemia.

Client/Family Teaching

1. Take on an empty stomach 1 hr before or 2 hr after meals. If antacids are used, take 30 min before or after sucralfate.
2. Do not crush or chew tablets.
3. Take exactly as prescribed. It binds to proteins at the site of the lesions to create a

protective barrier that prevents diffusion of hydrogen ions at a normal gastric pH.
4. May cause constipation; increase fluids and bulk and regular exercise.
5. Avoid smoking, alcohol, and caffeine to prevent a recurrence of duodenal ulcers. Even though healing of ulcers may result, the frequency or severity of subsequent attacks is not altered.
6. Report as scheduled for follow-up, upper GI, endoscopy, and labs.

Outcome/Evaluate

- ↓ Abdominal pain/discomfort
- Prophylaxis of GI bleeding
- Healing of duodenal ulcers

Sulconazole nitrate

(sul-**KON**-ah-zohl)
Pregnancy Category: C
Exelderm **(Rx)**
Classification: Antifungal, topical

Action/Kinetics: This broad-spectrum antifungal and antiyeast agent inhibits growth of *Trichophyton mentagrophytes, Epidermophyton floccosum, Microsporum canis,* and *Malassezia furfur* as well as certain gram-positive bacteria.
Uses: Treatment of tinea cruris (jock itch), tinea corporis (ringworm), and tinea versicolor. Efficacy has not been demonstrated for tinea pedis (athlete's foot).
Contraindications: Ophthalmic use.
Special Concerns: Use with caution during lactation. Safety and efficacy have not been demonstrated in children.
Side Effects: *Dermatologic:* Burning, itching, stinging, redness.
How Supplied: *Cream:* 1%; *Solution:* 1%

Dosage

- **Cream, Solution (1% each)**

A small amount of the cream or solution is gently massaged into the affected area and surrounding skin once or twice daily.

HEALTH CARE CONSIDERATIONS

Client/Family Teaching

1. Review how to apply medication; use only as directed.
2. Drug is for external use only. Avoid contact with the eyes.
3. Relief of symptoms usually occurs within a few days, with clinical improvement occurring within 1 week. Report if symptoms do not improve after 4–6 weeks as an alternate diagnosis should be considered.
4. To reduce the chance of recurrent tinea cruris, tinea corporis, and tinea versicolor, treat for 3 weeks. Tinea pedis should be treated for 4 weeks.

Outcome/Evaluate:

- ↓ Skin irritation
- Symptomatic improvement; restoration of normal skin integrity

Sulfacetamide sodium

(sul-fah-**SEAT**-ah-myd)
AK-Sulf, Balsulph ✱, Bleph-10, Bleph-10 Liquifilm ✱, Cetamide, Diosulf ✱, Isopto-Cetamide, I-Sulfacet, Ocu-Sul-10, Ocu-Sul-15, Ocu-Sul-30, Ocusulf-10, Ophthacet, PMS-Sulfacetamide Sodium ✱, Sebizon, Sodium Sulamyd, Spectro-Sulf, Steri-Units Sulfacetamide, Sulf-10, Sulfair, Sulfair 10, Sulfair 15, Sulfair Forte, Sulfamide, Sulfex 10% ✱, Sulten-10 **(Rx)**
Classification: Sulfonamide, topical

See also *Sulfonamides.*
Uses: Topically for conjunctivitis, corneal ulcer, and other superficial ocular infections. As an adjunct to systemic sulfonamides to treat trachoma.
Contraindications: In infants less than 2 months of age. Use in the presence of epithelial herpes simplex keratitis, vaccinia, varicella, and other viral diseases of the cornea and conjunctiva. Mycobacterial or fungal infections of the ocular structures. After uncomplicated removal of a corneal foreign body.
Special Concerns: Safe use during pregnancy and lactation or in children less than 12 years of age has not been established. Use with caution in clients with dry eye syndrome. Ophthalmic ointments may retard corneal wound healing.
Side Effects: *When used topically:* Itching, local irritation, periorbital edema, burning and transient stinging, headache, bacterial or fungal corneal ulcers. *NOTE:* Sulfonamides may cause serious systemic side effects, including severe hypersensitivity reactions. Symptoms include fever, skin rash, GI disturbances, bone marrow depression, ***Stevens-Johnson syndrome, toxic epidermal necrolysis,*** exfoliative dermatitis, photosensitivity. Fatalities have occurred.
Drug Interactions: Preparations containing silver are incompatible with sulfacetamide sodium.
How Supplied: *Lotion:* 10%; *Ophthalmic Ointment:* 10%; *Ophthalmic Solution:* 10%, 15%, 30%

Dosage

- **Ophthalmic Solution, 10%, 15%, 20%**

S

Conjunctivitis or other superficial ocular infections.
1–2 gtt in the conjunctival sac q 1–4 hr. Doses may be tapered by increasing the time interval between doses as the condition improves.

Trachoma.
2 gtt q 2 hr with concomitant systemic sulfonamide therapy.

• **Ophthalmic Ointment (10%)**
Apply approximately 1/4 in. into the lower conjunctival sac 3–4 times/day and at bedtime. Alternatively, 0.5–1 in. is placed in the conjunctival sac at bedtime along with use of drops during the day.

For cutaneous infections.
Apply locally (10%) to affected area b.i.d.–q.i.d.

• **Lotion**

Seborrheic dermatitis.
Apply 1–2 times/day (for mild cases, apply overnight).

Cutaneous bacterial infections.
Apply b.i.d.–q.i.d. until infection clears.

HEALTH CARE CONSIDERATIONS

See also *General Health Care Considerations for All Anti-Infectives* and for *Sulfonamides.*

Administration/Storage: Solutions will darken in color if left standing for long periods; discard these products.

Assessment
1. Record indications for therapy, onset, duration, and characteristics of symptoms.
2. List other agents prescribed and the outcome.
3. Note any allergy to sulfa drugs.

Client/Family Teaching
1. Medication is for topical use only.
2. When used for seborrheic dermatitis of the scalp, apply at bedtime and allow to remain overnight. The hair and scalp may be washed the following morning or at least once a week. Apply lotion for 8–10 consecutive nights.
3. If hair and scalp are oily or if there is debris, shampoo scalp before application.
4. Ophthalmic products may cause sensitivity to bright light; wear sunglasses to minimize.
5. Report any purulent eye drainage as this inactivates sulfacetamide.
6. If prescribed additional eye drops, wait 5 min after sulfacetamide instillation.
7. Do not wear contact lenses until infection is resolved.

Outcome/Evaluate: Resolution of inflammation/infection

Sulfadiazine

(sul-fah-**DYE**-ah-zeen)
Pregnancy Category: C
Microsulfon **(Rx)**

Sulfadiazine sodium

(sul-fah-**DYE**-ah-zeen)
Pregnancy Category: C
(Rx)
Classification: Sulfonamide

See also *Sulfonamides.*

Action/Kinetics: Short-acting; often combined with other anti-infectives.

Uses: UTIs caused by *Escherichia coli, Klebsiella, Enterobacter, Staphylococcus aureus, Proteus mirabilis, and Proteus vulgaris.* Chancroid, inclusion conjunctivitis, adjunct in treating chloroquine-resistant strains of *Plasmodium falciparum,* meningitis caused by *Haemophilus influenzae,* meningococcal meningitis for sulfonamide-sensitive group A strains, nocardiosis, with penicillin to treat acute otitis media caused by *H. influenzae,* rheumatic fever prophylaxis, adjunct with pyrimethamine for toxoplasmosis in selected immunocompromised clients (e.g., those with AIDS, neoplastic disease, or congenital immune compromise), trachoma.

Contraindications: Use in infants less than 2 months of age unless combined with pyrimethamine to treat congenital toxoplasmosis.

Special Concerns: Safe use during pregnancy has not been established.

How Supplied: *Tablet:* 500 mg

Dosage

• **Tablets**

General use.
Adults, loading dose: 2–4 g; **maintenance:** 2–4 g/day in 3 to 6 divided doses; **infants over 2 months, loading dose:** 75 mg/kg/day (2 g/m²); **maintenance:** 150 mg/kg/day (4 g/m²/day) in 4 to 6 divided doses, not to exceed 6 g/day.

Rheumatic fever prophylaxis.
Under 30 kg: 0.5 g/day; **over 30 kg:** 1 g/day.

As adjunct with pyrimethamine in congenital toxoplasmosis.
Infants less than 2 months: 25 mg/kg q.i.d. for 3 to 4 weeks. **Children greater than 2 months:** 25–50 mg/kg q.i.d. for 3 to 4 weeks.

HEALTH CARE CONSIDERATIONS

See also *General Health Care Considerations for All Anti-Infectives* and for *Sulfonamides.*

Assessment: Record indications for therapy, onset, duration, and characteristics of symptoms. Obtain appropriate labs/cultures.
Outcome/Evaluate
- Negative culture reports
- Rheumatic fever prophylaxis during invasive procedures

Sulfamethoxazole

(sul-fah-meth-**OX**-ah-zohl)
Pregnancy Category: C
Apo-Sulfamethoxazole ✤, Gantanol **(Rx)**
Classification: Sulfonamide, intermediate-acting

See also *Sulfonamides.*
Action/Kinetics: t½: 8.6 hr.
Uses: UTIs caused by *Escherichia coli, Klebsiella, Enterobacter, Staphylococcus aureus, Proteus mirabilis, and Proteus vulgaris.* Chancroid, inclusion conjunctivitis, adjunct in treating chloroquine-resistant strains of *Plasmodium falciparum,* meningococcal meningitis for sulfonamide-sensitive group A strains, nocardiosis, with penicillin to treat acute otitis media caused by *H. influenzae,* adjunct with pyrimethamine for toxoplasmosis in selected immunocompromised clients (e.g., those with AIDS, neoplastic disease, or congenital immune compromise), trachoma.
Special Concerns: May be an increased risk of severe side effects in elderly clients.
How Supplied: *Tablet:* 500 mg

Dosage
- **Tablets**

Mild to moderate infections.
Adults, initially: 2 g; **then,** 1 g in morning and evening.
Severe infections.
Adults, initially: 2 g; **then,** 1 g t.i.d. **Infants over 2 months, initial:** 50–60 mg/kg; **then,** 25–30 mg/kg in morning and evening, not to exceed 75 mg/kg/day. Alternative dosing: 50–60 mg/kg/day divided q 12 hr, not to exceed 3 g/24 hr.

HEALTH CARE CONSIDERATIONS

See also *General Health Care Considerations for All Anti-Infectives* and for *Sulfonamides.*
Client/Family Teaching
1. Take only as directed and complete entire prescription.
2. May cause dizziness; assess response prior to any activity requiring mental alertness.
3. Use sunglasses, sunscreens, and protective clothing during sun exposure as a photosensitivity reaction may occur.

Outcome/Evaluate: Resolution of infection; symptomatic improvement

Sulfasalazine

(sul-fah-**SAL**-ah-zeen)
Pregnancy Category: B
Alti-Sulfasalazine ✤, Azulfidine, Azulfidine EN-Tabs, PMS Sulfasalazine ✤, Salazopyrin ✤, Salazopyrin-EN Tabs ✤, SAS-500 ✤ **(Rx)**
Classification: Sulfonamide

See also *Sulfonamides.*
Action/Kinetics: About one-third of the dose of sulfasalazine is absorbed from the small intestine while two-thirds passes to the colon, where it is split to 5-aminosalicylic acid and sulfapyridine. The drug does not affect the microflora.
Uses: Ulcerative colitis. Azulfidine EN-tabs are also used to treat rheumatoid arthritis in clients who do not respond well to NSAIDs. *Investigational:* Ankylosing spondylitis, collagenous colitis, Crohn's disease, psoriasis, juvenile chronic arthritis, psoriatic arthritis.
Additional Contraindications: Children below 2 years. In persons with marked sulfonamide, salicylate, or related drug hypersensitivity. Intestinal or urinary obstruction.
Special Concerns: Use with caution during lactation.
Side Effects: Most common include anorexia, headache, N&V, gastric distress, reversible oligospermia. Less frequently, pruritus, urticaria, fever, Heinz body anemia, hemolytic anemia, cyanosis.
Drug Interactions
Digoxin / ↓ Absorption of digoxin
Folic acid / ↓ Absorption of folic acid
How Supplied: *Enteric Coated Tablet:* 500 mg; *Tablet:* 500 mg

Dosage
- **Enteric-Coated Tablets, Tablets**

Ulcerative colitis.
Adults, initial: 3–4 g/day in divided doses (1–2 g/day may decrease side effects); **maintenance:** 500 mg q.i.d. **Pediatric, over 2 years of age, initial:** 40–60 mg/kg/day in 3 to 6 equally divided doses; **maintenance:** 30 mg/kg/day in 4 divided doses.
For desensitization to sulfasalazine.
Reinstitute at level of 50–250 mg/day; **then,** give double dose q 4–7 days until desired therapeutic level reached. Do not attempt in those with a history of agranulocytosis or who have experienced anaphylaxis previously with sulfasalazine.

S

Collagenous colitis.
2–3 g/day.
Psoriasis.
3–4 g/day.
Juvenile chronic arthritis.
50 mg/kg.
Psoriatic arthritis.
2 g/day.

HEALTH CARE CONSIDERATIONS

See also *General Health Care Considerations for All Anti-Infectives* and for *Sulfonamides.*

Assessment

1. Record indications for therapy, including onset, location, duration, and characteristics of symptoms.
2. Record frequency, quantity, and consistency of stool production as well as characteristics of abdominal pain.
3. Note joint deformity, pain, ROM, inflammation, and swelling with rheumatoid arthritis.
4. Monitor CBC, renal function studies, and urinalysis; with colitis, send stool for analysis.

Client/Family Teaching

1. Take with food to reduce GI upset.
2. Take exactly as ordered; intermittent therapy (2 weeks on, 2 weeks off) is generally recommended.
3. Drug may discolor urine or skin a yellow-orange color.
4. Take at least 2–3 L/day of water to decrease incidence of crystalluria and stone formation.
5. Avoid prolonged exposure to sunlight; may increase sensitivity. Wear protective clothing, sunglasses, and sunscreen.

Outcome/Evaluate

- ↓ Frequency of loose stools; ↓ abdominal pain; ↓ colon inflammation
- Relief of pain from joint deformity, swelling, and inflammation

S

Sulfinpyrazone

(sul-fin-**PEER**-ah-zohn)

Antazone ✦, Anturane, Apo-Sulfinpyrazone ✦, Novo–Pyrazone ✦, Nu-Sulfinpyrazone ✦
(Rx)

Classification: Antigout agent, uricosuric

Action/Kinetics: Inhibits tubular reabsorption of uric acid, thereby increasing its excretion. Also exhibits antithrombotic and platelet inhibitory actions. **Peak plasma levels:** 1–2 hr. **Therapeutic plasma levels:** Up to 160 mcg/mL following 800 mg/day for uricosuria. **Duration:** 4–6 hr (up to 10 hr in some). **t½:** 3–8 hr. Metabolized by the liver. Approximately 45% of the drug is excreted unchanged by the kidney, and a small amount is excreted in the feces.

Uses: Chronic and intermittent gouty arthritis. Not effective during acute attacks of gout and may even increase the frequency of acute episodes during the initiation of therapy. However, do not discontinue during acute attacks. Concomitant administration of colchicine during initiation of therapy is recommended. *Investigational:* To decrease sudden death during first year after MI.

Contraindications: Active peptic ulcer or symptoms of GI inflammation or ulceration. Blood dyscrasias. Sensitivity to phenylbutazone or other pyrazoles. Use to control hyperuricemia secondary to treatment of malignancies.

Special Concerns: Use with caution in pregnant women. Dosage has not been established in children. Use with extreme caution in clients with impaired renal function and in those with a history of peptic ulcers.

Side Effects: *GI:* N&V, abdominal discomfort. May reactivate peptic ulcer. *Hematologic:* Leukopenia, ***agranulocytosis,*** anemia, thrombocytopenia, ***aplastic anemia.*** *Miscellaneous:* Skin rash (which usually disappears with usage), ***bronchoconstriction in aspirin-induced asthma.*** Acute attacks of gout may become more frequent during initial therapy. Give concomitantly with colchicine at this time.

OD Management of Overdose: *Symptoms:* N&V, diarrhea, epigastric pain, labored respiration, ataxia, seizures, coma. *Treatment:* Supportive measures.

Drug Interactions

Acetaminophen / ↑ Risk of acetaminophen hepatotoxicity; ↓ effect of acetaminophen
Anticoagulants / ↑ Effect of anticoagulants due to ↓ plasma protein binding
Niacin / ↓ Uricosuric effect of sulfinpyrazone
Salicylates / Inhibit uricosuric effect of sulfinpyrazone
Theophylline / ↓ Effect of theophylline due to ↑ plasma clearance
Tolbutamide / ↑ Risk of hypoglycemia
Verapamil / ↓ Effect of verapamil due to ↑ plasma clearance

How Supplied: *Capsule:* 200 mg; *Tablet:* 100 mg

Dosage

- **Capsules, Tablets**

Gout.

Adults, initial: 200–400 mg/day in two divided doses with meals or milk. Clients who are transferred from other uricosuric agents can receive full dose at once. **Maintenance:** 100–400 mg b.i.d. Maintain full dosage without interruption even during acute attacks of gout.

Following MI.
Adults: 300 mg q.i.d. or 400 mg b.i.d.

HEALTH CARE CONSIDERATIONS

Assessment

1. Assess joint(s) for pain, deformity, ROM, and inflammation.
2. Monitor CBC and uric acid levels.

Client/Family Teaching

1. If GI upset occurs, take with food, milk, or antacids. May still reactivate peptic ulcer.
2. Consume at least ten to twelve 8-oz glasses of fluid daily to prevent the formation of uric acid stones. Avoid cranberry juice or vitamin C preparations, as these acidify urine; acidification may cause formation of uric acid stones.
3. Sodium bicarbonate may be ordered to alkalinize the urine to prevent urates from crystallizing in acid urine and forming kidney stones.
4. Avoid alcohol and aspirin; may interfere with drug effectiveness.
5. During *acute* attacks of gout, concomitant administration of colchicine is indicated.

Outcome/Evaluate

- ↓ Frequency and intensity of gout attacks
- ↓ Serum uric acid levels

Sulfisoxazole

(sul-fih-**SOX**-ah-zohl)
Pregnancy Category: C
Apo-Sulfisoxazole ✦, Novo-Soxazole ✦, Sulfizole ✦ **(Rx)**

Sulfisoxazole diolamine

(sul-fih-**SOX**-ah-zohl)
Pregnancy Category: C
(Rx)
Classification: Sulfonamide, short-acting

See also *Sulfonamides.*
Action/Kinetics: t½: 5.9 hr.
Uses: UTIs caused by *Escherichia coli, Klebsiella, Enterobacter, Staphylococcus aureus, Proteus mirabilis, and Proteus vulgaris.* Chancroid, inclusion conjunctivitis, adjunct in treating chloroquine-resistant strains of *Plasmodium falciparum,* meningitis caused by *Haemophilus influenzae,* meningococcal meningitis for sulfonamide-sensitive group A strains, nocardiosis, with penicillin to treat acute otitis media caused by *H. influenzae,* adjunct with pyrimethamine for toxoplasmosis in selected immunocompromised clients (e.g., those with AIDS, neoplastic disease, or congenital immune compromise). Ophthalmically as an adjunct with systemic sulfonamides to treat trachoma.
Additional Contraindications: Use in infants less than 2 months of age except as adjunct with pyrimethamine to treat congenital toxoplasmosis. Use in the presence of epithelial herpes simplex keratitis, vaccinia, varicella, and other viral diseases of the cornea and conjunctiva. Mycobacterial or fungal infections of the ocular structures. After uncomplicated removal of a corneal foreign body.
Special Concerns: Safety and efficacy of the ophthalmic products have not been established in children. Use with caution in clients with severe dry eye.
Additional Side Effects: *Following ophthalmic use:* Blurred vision, itching, local irritation, epithelial keratitis, reactive hyperemia, conjunctival edema, burning, headache or browache, transient stinging.
Additional Drug Interactions: Sulfisoxazole may ↑ effects of thiopental due to ↓ plasma protein binding.
How Supplied: Sulfisoxazole: *Tablet:* 500 mg. Sulfisoxazole acetyl: *Suspension:* 500 mg/5 mL Sulfisoxazole diolamine: *Ophthalmic Solution:* 4%

Dosage

- **Tablets**

Adults, loading dose: 2–4 g; **maintenance:** 4–8 g/day in 4 to 6 divided doses, depending on severity of the infection. **Infants over 2 months, initial:** 75 mg/kg/day; **maintenance:** 150 mg/kg/day (4 g/m²/day) in 4 to 6 divided doses, not to exceed 6 g/day.

- **Ophthalmic Solution (4%)**

Conjunctivitis or corneal ulcer.
1–2 gtt into conjunctival sac q 1–4 hr, depending on the severity of the infection. Dose may be tapered by increasing the time interval between doses as the condition improves.
Trachoma.
2 gtt q 2 hr with concomitant systemic therapy.

HEALTH CARE CONSIDERATIONS

See also *General Health Care Considerations for All Anti-Infectives* and *Sulfonamides.*
Administration/Storage: Solutions will darken in color if left standing for long periods; discard these products.

Assessment

1. Record type, onset, and characteristics of

symptoms. List other agents trialed and the outcome.
2. Monitor CBC and cultures.

Client/Family Teaching
1. Ophthalmic use may cause sensitivity to bright light; wear sunglasses to minimize.
2. With ophthalmic use, report if no improvement after 7–8 days, if the condition worsens, or if pain, increased redness, itching, or swelling of the eye occurs.

Outcome/Evaluate: Negative cultures; symptomatic improvement

Sulindac

(sul-IN-dak)
Apo-Sulin ✦, Clinoril, Novo-Sundac ✦, Nu-Sulindac ✦ **(Rx)**
Classification: Nonsteroidal anti-inflammatory drug

See also *Nonsteroidal Anti-Inflammatory Drugs.*

Action/Kinetics: Biotransformed in the liver to a sulfide, the active metabolite. **Peak plasma levels of sulfide:** after fasting, 2 hr; after food, 3–4 hr. **Onset, anti-inflammatory effect:** within 1 week; **duration, anti-inflammatory effect:** 1–2 weeks. **t½,** of sulindac: 7.8 hr; of metabolite: 16.4 hr. Excreted in both urine and feces.

Uses: Acute and chronic treatment of rheumatoid arthritis, osteoarthritis, ankylosing spondylitis, acute gouty arthritis; acute, painful shoulder; tendinitis, bursitis. *Investigational:* Juvenile rheumatoid arthritis, sunburn.

Contraindications: Use with active GI lesions or a history of recurrent GI lesions.

Special Concerns: Safety and efficacy have not been established for children. Safe use during pregnancy has not been established. Use with caution during lactation.

Additional Side Effects: Hypersensitivity, pancreatitis, GI pain (common), maculopapular rash. Stupor, ***coma,*** hypotension, and diminished urine output.

Additional Drug Interactions: Sulindac ↑ effect of warfarin due to ↓ plasma protein binding.

How Supplied: *Tablet:* 150 mg, 200 mg

Dosage

- **Tablets**

Osteoarthritis, rheumatoid arthritis, ankylosing spondylitis.
Adults: 150 mg b.i.d.

Acute painful shoulder, acute gouty arthritis.
Adults: 200 mg b.i.d. for 7–14 days.

Antigout.
Adults: 200 mg b.i.d. for 7 days.

HEALTH CARE CONSIDERATIONS

See also *Health Care Considerations* for *Nonsteroidal Anti-Inflammatory Drugs.*

Administration/Storage: For acute conditions, reduce dosage when satisfactory response is attained.

Assessment
1. Record type, onset, and characteristics of symptoms.
2. Determine baseline ROM; describe location of pain, inflammation, and swelling; note functional class of arthritis.
3. Monitor CBC, liver and renal function studies; reduce dosage with renal dysfunction.

Client/Family Teaching
1. Take with food to decrease GI upset and consume plenty of water. A stomach protectant (i.e., misoprostol) may be prescribed with a history of ulcer disease.
2. Do not take aspirin because plasma levels of sulindac will be reduced. Avoid alcohol.
3. Report any incidence of unexplained bleeding such as oozing of blood from the gums, nosebleeds, or excessive bruising.
4. Drug may cause dizziness; assess response prior to any activity requiring mental alertness.
5. When used for arthritis, a favorable response usually occurs within 1 week.

Outcome/Evaluate: ↓ Joint pain and inflammation with ↑ mobility

Sumatriptan succinate

(soo-mah-TRIP-tan)
Pregnancy Category: C
Imitrex
Classification: Antimigraine drug

Action/Kinetics: Selective agonist for a vascular 5-HT_1 receptor subtype (probably 5-HT_{1D}) located on cranial arteries, on the basilar artery, and the vasculature of the dura mater. Activates the 5-HT_1 receptor, causing vasoconstriction and therefore relief of migraine. Transient increases in BP may be observed. No significant activity at 5-HT_2 or 5-HT_3 receptor subtypes; alpha-1-, alpha-2-, or beta-adrenergic receptors; dopamine-1 or dopamine-2 receptors; muscarinic receptors; or benzodiazepine receptors. **Time to peak effect after SC:** 12 min after a 6-mg SC dose. **t½ distribution, after SC:** 15 min; **terminal t½:** 115 min. Approximately 22% of a SC dose is excreted in the urine as unchanged drug and 38% as metabolites. Rapidly absorbed after PO administration, although bioavailability is low due to incomplete absorption and a first-pass effect (bioavailability may be significantly increased in those with impaired liver function). **PO, elimination t½:** About 2.5 hr. About 60% of a PO dose is excreted through the urine and 40% in the feces.

Uses: Treatment of acute migraine attacks with or without aura. Photophobia, phonophobia, N&V associated with migraine attacks are also relieved. Intended to relieve migraine, but not to prevent or reduce the number of attacks experienced. Acute treatment of cluster headaches (injection only).

Contraindications: Hypersensitivity to sumatriptan. IV use due to the possibility of coronary vasospasm. SC use in clients with ischemic heart disease, history of MI, documented silent ischemia, Prinzmetal's angina, or uncontrolled hypertension. Concomitant use with ergotamine-containing products or MAO inhibitor therapy (or within 2 weeks of discontinuing an MAO inhibitor). Use in clients with hemiplegic or basilar migraine. Use in women who are pregnant, think they may be pregnant, or are trying to get pregnant.

Special Concerns: Use with caution during lactation, in clients with impaired hepatic or renal function, and in clients with heart conditions. Clients with risk factors for CAD (e.g., men over 40, smokers, postmenopausal women, hypertension, obesity, diabetes, hypercholesterolemia, family history of heart disease) should be screened before initiating treatment. Safety and efficacy have not been determined for use in children.

Side Effects: Side effects listed are for either SC or PO use of the drug. *CV:* Coronary vasospasm in clients with a history of CAD. ***Serious and/or life-threatening arrhythmias, including atrial fibrillation, ventricular fibrillation, ventricular tachycardia, MI, marked ischemic ST elevations,*** chest and arm discomfort representing angina pectoris. Flushing, hypertension, hypotension, bradycardia, tachycardia, palpitations, pulsating sensations, ECG changes (including nonspecific ST- or T-wave changes, prolongation of PR or QTc intervals, sinus arrhythmia, nonsustained ventricular premature beats, isolated junctional ectopic beats, atrial ectopic beats, and delayed activation of the right ventricle), syncope, pallor, abnormal pulse, vasodilatation, atherosclerosis, bradycardia, cerebral ischemia, CV lesion, heart block, peripheral cyanosis, thrombosis, transient myocardial ischemia, vasodilation, Raynaud's syndrome. *At injection site:* Pain, redness. *Atypical sensations:* Sensation of warmth, cold, tingling, or paresthesia. Localized or generalized feeling of pressure, burning, numbness, and tightness. Feeling of heaviness, feeling strange, tight feeling in head. *CNS:* Fatigue, dizziness, drowsiness, vertigo, sedation, headache, anxiety, malaise, confusion, euphoria, agitation, relaxation, chills, tremor, shivering, prickling or stinging sensations, phonophobia, depression, euphoria, facial pain, heat sensitivity, incoordination, monoplegia, sleep disturbances, shivering. *EENT:* Throat discomfort, discomfort in nasal cavity or sinuses. Vision alterations, eye irritation, photophobia, lacrimation, otalgia, feeling of fullness in ear, disorders of sclera, mydriasis. *GI:* Abdominal discomfort, dysphagia, discomfort of mouth and tongue, gastroesophageal reflux, diarrhea, peptic ulcer, retching, flatulence, eructation, gallstones, taste disturbances, GI bleeding, hematemesis, melena. *Respiratory:* Dyspnea, diseases of the lower respiratory tract, hiccoughs, influenza, asthma. *Dermatologic:* Erythema, pruritus, skin rashes, skin eruptions, skin tenderness, dry or scaly skin, tightness or wrinkling of skin. *GU:* Dysuria, dysmenorrhea, urinary frequency, renal calculus, breast tenderness, increased urination, intermenstrual bleeding, nipple discharge, abortion, hematuria. *Musculoskeletal:* Weakness, neck pain or stiffness, myalgia, muscle cramps, joint disturbances (pain, stiffness, swelling, ache), muscle stiffness, need to flex calf muscles, backache, muscle tiredness, swelling of the extremities, tetany. *Endocrine:* Elevated TSH levels, galactorrhea, hyperglycemia, hypoglycemia, hypothyroidism, weight gain or loss. *Miscellaneous:* Chest, jaw, or neck tightness. Sweating, thirst, polydipsia, chills, fever, dehydration.

Laboratory Test Considerations: Disturbance of LFTs.

OD **Management of Overdose:** *Symptoms*: Tremor, ***convulsions,*** inactivity erythema of extremities, reduced respiratory rate, cyanosis, ataxia, mydriasis, injection site reactions (desquamation, hair loss, scab formation), paralysis. *Treatment:* Continuous monitoring of client for at least 10 hr and especially when signs and symptoms persist.

Drug Interactions

Ergot drugs / Prolonged vasospastic reactions

Monoamine oxidase A inhibitors / ↑ t½ of sumatriptan

Selective Serotonin Reuptake Inhibitors (SSRIs) / Rarely, weakness, hyperreflexia, and incoordination

How Supplied: *Injection:* 6 mg/0.5 mL; *Kit:* 6 mg/0.5 mL; *Nasal spray*: 5 mg, 20 mg; *Tablet:* 25 mg, 50 mg

S

Dosage

- **SC**

Migraine headaches.

Adults: 6 mg. A second injection may be given if symptoms of migraine come back but no more than two injections (6 mg each) should be taken in a 24-hr period and at least 1 hr should elapse between doses.

- **Tablets**

Adults: 25 mg with fluids as soon as symptoms of migraine appear. A second dose may be taken if symptoms return but not sooner than 2 hr following the first dose. **Maximum recommended dose:** 100 mg, with no more than 300 mg taken in a 24-hr period.

- **Nasal Spray**

A single dose of 5, 10, or 20 mg given in one nostril. The 20 mg dose increases the risk of side effects. The 10-mg dose may be given as a single 5-mg dose in each nostril. If the headache returns, repeat the dose once after 2 hr; not to exceed a total daily dose of 40 mg. The safety of treating an average of more than 4 headaches in a 30-day period has not been studied.

HEALTH CARE CONSIDERATIONS

Administration/Storage

1. No increased beneficial effect has been found with the administration of a second 6-mg dose in clients not responding to the first injection.
2. If side effects are dose limiting, a dose lower than 6 mg may be given; in such cases, only the single-dose vial dosage form should be used, as the autoinjection form delivers 6 mg.
3. Consideration should be given to administering the first dose of sumatriptan in the provider's office due to the possibility (although rare) of coronary events.
4. Is equally effective at whatever stage of the attack given; advisable to take as soon as possible after the onset of a migraine attack.
5. Store away from heat (no higher than 30°C; 86°F) and light.

Assessment

1. Record headache characteristics, including onset, frequency, type, and duration of symptoms.
2. Determine any cardiac problems or ischemic CV disease.
3. Review neurologic exam and CT/MRI results. A clear diagnosis of migraine should be made; the drug should not be given for headaches due to other neurologic events.
4. Assess ECG, liver, and renal function studies. Monitor VS; expect transient increases in BP.
5. Parenteral form is for SC use only. IV use may cause coronary vasospasm.

Client/Family Teaching

1. Review the appropriate method for administration. With SC form, administer (or have client self-administer) first dose in office to assess response.
2. Printed instructions concerning how to load the autoinjector, administer the medication, and remove the syringe, are enclosed and provided by the manufacturer.
3. The injection is given just below the skin as soon as migraine symptoms appear or any time during the attack. A second injection may be administered 1 hr later if migraine symptoms return; do *not* exceed two injections in 24 hr.
4. Practice safe handling, storage, and disposal of syringes.
5. Pain and tenderness may be evident at injection site for up to an hour after administration.
6. For tablets, take a single dose with fluids as soon as symptoms appear; a second dose may be taken if symptoms return, but no sooner than 2 hr after the first dose. If there is no response to the first tablet, do not take a second tablet without consulting the provider.
7. Check expiration date before use and discard all outdated drugs.
8. Report if chest, jaw, throat, and neck pain occur after injection; this should be medically evaluated before using more Imitrex.
9. Severe chest pain or tightness, wheezing, palpitations, facial swelling, or rashes/hives should be immediately reported.
10. Symptoms of flushing, tingling, heat and heaviness, as well as dizziness or drowsiness may occur and should be reported before taking more sumatriptan.
11. Practice barrier contraception and do not use Imitrex if pregnancy is suspected.

Outcome/Evaluate: Reversal of acute migraine attack; relief of symptoms

Suprofen

(sue-**PROH**-fen)

Pregnancy Category: C

Profenal **(Rx)**

Classification: Nonsteroidal anti-inflammatory drug, ophthalmic use

See also *Nonsteroidal Anti-Inflammatory Drugs.*

Action/Kinetics: By inhibiting prostaglandin synthesis, suprofen reverses prostaglandin-induced vasodilation, leukocytosis, increased vascular permeability, and increased intraocular pressure. Also inhibits

miosis, which occurs during cataract surgery.
Uses: Inhibition of intraoperative miosis.
Contraindications: Dendritic keratitis.
Special Concerns: Use with caution during lactation, in clients sensitive to aspirin and other NSAIDs, and in surgical clients with a history of bleeding tendencies or who are on drugs that prolong bleeding time. Safety and efficacy have not been established in children.
Side Effects: *Ophthalmic:* Ocular irritation, transient burning, and stinging on installation. Redness, itching, discomfort, pain, iritis, allergy, chemosis, photophobia, punctate epithelial staining.
Drug Interactions: Acetylcholine and carbachol may be ineffective if used in combination with suprofen.

How Supplied: *Solution:* 1%

Dosage

- **Ophthalmic Solution**

Day before surgery.

2 gtt into the conjunctival sac q 4 hr during waking hours.

Day of surgery.

2 gtt into the conjunctival sac 3, 2, and 1 hr prior to surgery.

HEALTH CARE CONSIDERATIONS

See also *Health Care Considerations* for *Nonsteroidal Anti-Inflammatory Drugs.*
Outcome/Evaluate: Control of inflammation; inhibition of abnormal pupillary contractions

Tacrine hydrochloride (THA, Tetrahydro-aminoacridine)

(TAH-krin)
Pregnancy Category: C
Cognex **(Rx)**
Classification: Psychotherapeutic drug for Alzheimer's disease

Action/Kinetics: During early stages of Alzheimer's disease, cholinergic neuronal pathways that project from the basal forebrain to the cerebral cortex and hippocampus may be affected. Symptoms of dementia may be due to a deficiency of acetylcholine. As a reversible CNS cholinesterase inhibitor, tacrine elevates acetylcholine levels in the cerebral cortex. There is no evidence tacrine alters progression of dementia. Rapidly absorbed after PO administration. **Maximal plasma levels:** 1–2 hr. Food will affect the bioavailability of tacrine. Extensively metabolized in the liver. Undergoes first-pass metabolism; can be overcome by increasing the dose. **Elimination t½:** 2–4 hr. The average plasma levels are about 50% higher in females. Also, the mean tacrine levels in smokers are about one-third the levels of nonsmokers.
Uses: Treatment of mild to moderate dementia of the Alzheimer's type.
Contraindications: Hypersensitivity to tacrine or acridine derivatives. Use in clients previously treated with tacrine who developed jaundice (elevated total bilirubin > 3 mg/dL).
Special Concerns: May cause bradycardia—important in sick sinus syndrome. Use with caution in clients at risk for developing ulcers as the drug increases gastric acid secretion. Use with caution in clients with a history of abnormal liver function as indicated by abnormalities in serum ALT, AST, bilirubin, and GGT levels. Use with caution in clients with a history of asthma. There may be worsening of cognitive function following abrupt discontinuation of the drug. Safety and efficacy have not been determined in children with dementing illness.
Side Effects: *Hepatic:* Increased transaminase levels (most common reason for stopping the drug during treatment). *GI:* N&V, diarrhea, dyspepsia, anorexia, abdominal pain, flatulence, constipation, glossitis, gingivitis, dry mouth or throat, stomatitis, increased salivation, dysphagia, esophagitis, gastritis, gastroenteritis, ***GI hemorrhage,*** stomach ulcer, hiatal hernia, hemorrhoids, bloody stools, diverticulitis, fecal impaction, fecal incontinence, ***rectal hemorrhage,*** cholelithiasis, cholecystitis, increased appetite. *Musculoskeletal:* Myalgia, fracture, arthralgia, arthritis, hypertonia, osteoporosis, tendinitis, bursitis, gout, myopathy. *CNS:* ***Precipitation of seizures*** (may also be due to Alzheimer's), dizziness, confusion, ataxia, insomnia, somnolence, tremor, agitation, depression, abnormal thinking, anxiety, hallucinations, hostility, migraine, ***convulsions,*** vertigo, syncope, hyperkinesia, paresthesia, abnormal dreams, dysarthria, aphasia, amnesia, twitching, hypesthesia, delirium, paralysis, bradykinesia, move-

T

ment disorders, cogwheel rigidity, paresis, neuritis, hemiplegia, Parkinson's disease, neuropathy, extrapyramidal syndrome, decreased or absent reflexes, tardive dyskinesia, dysesthesia, dystonia, encephalitis, ***coma,*** apraxia, oculogyric crisis, akathisia, oral facial dyskinesia, Bell's palsy, nervousness, apathy, increased libido, paranoia, neurosis, ***suicidal episodes,*** psychosis, hysteria. *Respiratory:* Rhinitis, URI, coughing, pharyngitis, sinusitis, bronchitis, pneumonia, dyspnea, epistaxis, chest congestion, asthma, hyperventilation, lower respiratory infection, hemoptysis, lung edema, ***lung cancer, acute epiglottitis.*** *CV:* Hypotension, hypertension, ***heart failure, MI, CVA,*** angina pectoris, TIA, phlebitis, venous insufficiency, abdominal aortic aneurysm, atrial fibrillation or flutter, palpitation, tachycardia, bradycardia, ***pulmonary embolus, heart arrest,*** premature atrial contractions, ***AV block,*** bundle branch block. *Dermatologic:* Rash, facial and skin flushing, increased sweating, acne, alopecia, dermatitis, eczema, dry skin, herpes zoster, psoriasis, cellulitis, cyst, furunculosis, herpes simplex, hyperkeratosis, basal cell carcinoma, skin cancer, desquamation, seborrhea, squamous cell carcinoma, skin ulcer, skin necrosis, ***melanoma.*** *GU:* Bladder outflow obstruction, urinary frequency, urinary incontinence, UTI, hematuria, renal stone, kidney infection, glycosuria, dysuria, polyuria, nocturia, pyuria, cystitis, urinary retention, urinary urgency, ***vaginal hemorrhage,*** genital pruritus, breast pain, urinary obstruction, impotence, ***prostate cancer, bladder tumor, renal tumor, renal failure, breast cancer, ovarian carcinoma,*** epididymitis. *Body as a whole:* Headache, fatigue, chest pain, weight decrease, back pain, asthenia, chill, fever, malaise, peripheral edema, facial edema, dehydration, weight increase, cachexia, lipoma, heat exhaustion, sepsis, ***cholinergic crisis, death.*** *Hematologic:* Anemia, lymphadenopathy, leukopenia, thrombocytopenia, hemolysis, pancytopenia. *Ophthalmologic:* Conjunctivitis, cataract, dry eyes, eye pain, visual field defect, diplopia, amblyopia, glaucoma, hordeolum, vision loss, ptosis, blepharitis. *Otic:* Deafness, earache, tinnitus, inner ear infection, otitis media, labyrinthitis, inner ear disturbance. *Miscellaneous:* Purpura, hypercholesterolemia, diabetes mellitus, hypothyroid, hyperthyroid, unusual taste.

OD **Management of Overdose:** *Symptoms:* Cholinergic crisis characterized by severe N&V, sweating, bradycardia, salivation, hypotension, ***collapse, seizures, and increased muscle weakness (may paralyze respiratory muscles leading to death).*** *Treatment:* General supportive measures. IV atropine sulfate, titrated to effect, may be given in an initial dose of 1–2 mg IV with subsequent doses based on the response.

Drug Interactions

Anticholinergic drugs / Tacrine interferes with the action of these drugs
Bethanechol / Tacrine → synergistic effect with bethanechol
Cholinesterase inhibitors / Tacrine → synergistic effect with cholinesterase inhibitors
Cimetidine / Cimetidine ↑ maximum levels of tacrine
Succinylcholine / Tacrine ↑ muscle relaxation due to succinylcholine
Theophylline / Tacrine ↑ plasma levels of theophylline; ↓ theophylline dose recommended.

How Supplied: *Capsule:* 10 mg, 20 mg, 30 mg, 40 mg

Dosage

- **Capsules**

Alzheimer's disease.

Initial: 10 mg q.i.d. for at least 6 weeks; **then,** after 6 weeks, increase the dose to 20 mg q.i.d., providing there are no significant transaminase elevations and the client tolerates the treatment. Based on the degree of tolerance, the dose may be titrated, at 6-week intervals, to 30 or 40 mg q.i.d.

If transaminase elevations occur, modify the dose as follows:

- If transaminase levels are less than or equal to 2 × ULN, continue treatment according to recommended titration and monitoring schedule.
- If transaminse levels are greater than 2 but equal to or less than 3 × ULN, treatment is continued according to recommended titraiton but levels are monitored weekly until they return to normal levels.
- If transaminase levels are more than 3 but equal to or less than 5 × ULN, the daily dose is reduced by 40 mg/day. Monitor ALT/SGPT levels weekly. Dose titration is resumed and every other week monitoring is undertaken when levels return to within normal limits.
- If transaminase levels are greater than 5 × ULN, stop treatment. Monitor closely for signs and symptoms associated with hepatitis; monitor levels until they are within normal limits.

Clients who are required to stop treatment due to elevated transaminase levels may be rechallenged once levels return to within normal range. Weekly monitoring of serum ALT/SGPT levels should be undertaken after rechallenging occurs. If rechallenged, the initial dose is 10 mg t.i.d. with levels monitored

T

weekly. After 6 weeks on this dose, the client may begin dose titration if transaminase levels are acceptable.

HEALTH CARE CONSIDERATIONS

Administration/Storage

1. Take drug between meals, if possible. If GI upset occurs, may take with meals; however, the plasma level will be decreased by 30%–40%.
2. Do not increase the initial dose for 6 weeks as there is the potential for delayed onset of transaminase elevations.

Assessment

1. Assess mental status. Record onset and duration of symptoms and if this is a first drug trial or a rechallenge. If a rechallenge, document serum bilirubin and SGPT from previous treatment.
2. Note any ECG evidence of sick sinus syndrome or any ulcer disease, asthma, or liver disease.
3. List drugs currently prescribed to ensure none interact unfavorably. Drug is a cholinesterase inhibitor; notify anesthesia before procedures.
4. Monitor ECG, hematologic, liver, and renal profiles. Serum transaminase levels (ALT/SGPT) should be monitored weekly for the first 18 weeks and then every 3 months unless dose is increased or the transaminase levels are mildly elevated; follow guidelines under *Dosage*.
5. Monitor VS; may cause bradycardia.
6. Observe and record response carefully; drug is titrated according to client tolerance.

Client/Family Teaching

1. Take between meals unless GI upset is experienced. With meals, the plasma drug level will be decreased by 30%–40%
2. Take at regularly spaced intervals. Do not increase dose for the first 6 weeks until response and tolerance assessed.
3. Clinical manifestations of mild to moderate dementia in Alzheimer's disease are thought to be related to a deficiency of acetylcholine. Tacrine is thought to act to elevate acetylcholine concentrations in the cerebral cortex. As the disease progresses, tacrine's effect may lessen.
4. Report any new symptoms or any increase in existing symptoms.
5. Smoking may interfere with serum drug levels.
6. During initiation of therapy, N&V and diarrhea may be evident; report if persistent or bothersome. Delayed-onset side effects that should be reported include rashes and yellow skin/stool discolorations.
7. Do not stop abruptly. Abrupt withdrawal may cause a decline in cognitive function and also contribute to behavioral disturbances.
8. Identify appropriate resources and support groups that may assist the family and caregivers in understanding and coping with this disorder.

Outcome/Evaluate: Improved level of cognitive functioning with Alzheimer's disease

---

Tamoxifen

(tah-**MOX**-ih-fen)

Pregnancy Category: D

Apo-Tamox ✤, Gen-Tamoxifen ✤, Nolvadex, Nolvadex-D ✤, Novo-Tamoxifen ✤, Tamofen ✤, Tamone ✤ **(Rx)**

Classification: Antiestrogen

See also *Antineoplastic Agents*.

Action/Kinetics: Antiestrogen believed to compete with estrogen for estrogen-binding sites in target tissue (breast); also blocks uptake of estradiol. **Steady-state plasma levels (after 10 mg b.i.d. for 3 months):** 120 ng/mL for tamoxifen and 336 ng/mL for N-desmethyl tamoxifen. **Steady-state levels, tamoxifen:** About 4 weeks; **for N-desmethyltamoxifen:** About 8 weeks (**t½ for metabolite:** about 14 days). Metabolized to the equally active N-desmethyltamoxifen. Tamoxifen and metabolites are excreted mainly through the feces. Objective response may be delayed 4–10 weeks with bone metastases.

Uses: Adjuvant treatment of axillary node-negative or node-positive breast cancer in women following total or segmental mastectomy, axillary dissection, and breast irradiation. Metastatic breast cancer in premenopausal women as an alternative to oophorectomy or ovarian irradiation (especially in women with estrogen-positive tumors). Advanced metastatic breast cancer in men. Prophylaxis of breast cancer in high-risk women. *Investigational:* Mastalgia, gynecomastia (to treat pain and size), pancreatic carcinoma, advanced or recurrent endometrial and hepatocellular carcinoma.

Contraindications: Lactation.

Special Concerns: Use with caution in clients with leukopenia or thrombocytopenia. Women should not become pregnant while taking tamoxifen. Although the risk of breast cancer is significantly lowered, this benefit must be weighed against an increased risk of

T

endometrial cancer, pulmonary embolism, and DVT.

Side Effects: *GI:* N&V, distaste for food, anorexia, diarrhea, abdominal cramps. *CV:* Peripheral edema, superficial phlebitis, DVT, ***pulmonary embolism, thromboembolic disorders (especially when tamoxifen is combined with other cytotoxic agents).*** *CNS:* Depression, dizziness, lightheadedness, headache, fatigue. *Hepatic:* Rarely, fatty liver, cholestasis, hepatitis, ***hepatic necrosis.*** *GU:* Hot flashes, vaginal bleeding and discharge, menstrual irregularities, pruritus vulvae, ovarian cysts, hyperplasia of the uterus, polyps, uterine carcinoma. *Other:* Skin rash, skin changes, hypercalcemia, musculoskeletal pain, hyperlipidemias, weight gain or loss, increased bone and tumor pain, mild to moderate thrombocytopenia and leukopenia, retinopathy, hair thinning or partial loss, fluid retention, coughing. In men, may be loss of libido and impotency. Impotence and loss of libido in males after discontinuing therapy.

Laboratory Test Considerations: ↑ Serum calcium (transient), thyroid-binding globulin in postmenopausal women, BUN, AST, alkaline phosphatase, bilirubin, creatinine.

Drug Interactions

Anticoagulants / ↑ Hypoprothrombinemic effect

Bromocriptine / ↑ Serum levels of tamoxifen and N-desmethyl tamoxifen

How Supplied: *Tablet:* 10 mg, 20 mg

Dosage

- **Tablets**

Breast cancer.

10–20 mg b.i.d. (morning and evening) or 20 mg daily. Doses of 10 mg b.i.d.–t.i.d. for 2 years and 10 mg b.i.d. for 5 years have been used. There is no evidence that doses greater than 20 mg daily are more effective.

Mastalgia.

10 mg/day for 4 months.

HEALTH CARE CONSIDERATIONS

See also *Health Care Considerations* for *Antineoplastic Agents.*

Assessment

1. Record onset, duration, and characteristics of symptoms.
2. Assess hematologic profile and monitor. Drug may cause granulocyte suppression. Nadir: 14 days; recovery: 21 days.
3. The effect of the steroid and osteolytic metastases may result in hypercalcemia. Report symptoms of hypercalcemia (insomnia, lethargy, anorexia, N&V, coma, and vascular collapse).
4. With increased pain, administer adequate analgesics.

Client/Family Teaching

1. Review side effects that should be reported; a reduction in dosage or discontinuation may be indicated.
2. Increased bone and lumbar pain or local disease flares should subside and may be associated with a good (tumor) response to medication. Take analgesics as needed.
3. Consume 2–3 L/day of fluids to minimize hypercalcemia.
4. Exercise to reduce calcium levels, improve circulation, and prevent thrombophlebitis. (Perform ROM exercises if bedridden.)
5. Record weights weekly; report excessive weight gain or evidence of peripheral edema.
6. May cause "hot flashes" dress accordingly.
7. Wear protective clothing, sunscreens, and sunglasses to prevent photosensitivity reactions.
8. Practice safe, nonhormonal methods of contraception during and for 1 mo following therapy.
9. Report decreased visual acuity. Have regular eye exams, especially if higher than usual dosage.
10. Obtain regular GYN exams; report menstrual irregularities, abnormal vaginal bleeding, change in discharge, or pelvic pain/pressure.
11. Although the risk of breast cancer is significantly lowered, there is also an increased risk of endometrial cancer, pulmonary embolism, and DVT.

Outcome/Evaluate

- Suppression of tumor growth and malignant cell proliferation
- Relief of breast pain
- Prophylaxis of breast cancer in high-risk women

Tamsulosin hydrochloride

(tam-**SOO**-loh-sin)

Pregnancy Category: B

Flomax **(Rx)**

Classification: Alpha-1 adrenergic blocking agent

Action/Kinetics: Blockade of alpha-1 receptors (probably $alpha_{1A)}$ in prostate results in relaxation of smooth muscles in bladder neck and prostate; thus, urine flow rate is improved and there is a decrease in symptoms of BPH. Food interferes with the rate of absorption. **t½, elimination:** 5–7 hr. Significantly bound to plasma proteins. Extensively metabolized in liver; excreted through urine and feces.

Uses: Treatment of signs and symptoms of BPH. Rule out prostatic carcinoma before using tamsulosin.

Contraindications: Use to treat hypertension, with other alpha-adrenergic blocking agents, or in women or children.

Special Concerns: Use with caution with concurrent administration of warfarin.

Side Effects: *Body as a whole:* Headache, infection, asthenia, back pain, chest pain. *CV:* Postural hypotension, syncope. *GI:* Diarrhea, nausea, tooth disorder. *CNS:* Dizziness, vertigo, somnolence, insomnia, decreased libido. *Respiratory:* Rhinitis, pharyngitis, increased cough, sinusitis. *GU:* Abnormal ejaculation. *Miscellaneous:* Amblyopia.

OD **Management of Overdose:** *Symptoms:* Hypotension. *Treatment:* Keep client in supine position to restore BP and normalize HR. If this is inadequate, consider IV fluids. Vasopressors may also be used; monitor renal function.

Drug Interactions: Cimetidine causes significant ↓ in clearance of tamsulosin.

How Supplied: *Capsules:* 0.4 mg

Dosage

- **Capsules**

Benign prostatic hypertrophy.

Adult males: 0.4 mg daily given about 30 min after same meal each day. If, after 2 to 4 weeks, clients have not responded, dose can be increased to 0.8 mg daily.

HEALTH CARE CONSIDERATIONS

Administration/Storage

1. If dose is discontinued or interrupted for several days after either 0.4 mg or 0.8 mg dose, start therapy again with 0.4 mg dose.
2. Store at 20°C–25°C (68°F–77°F).

Assessment

1. Record indications for therapy, onset, and characteristics of symptoms. Note BPH score.
2. List drugs prescribed to ensure none interact; especially cimetidine and coumadin.
3. Note PSA levels and digital rectal exam.

Client/Family Teaching

1. Take as directed, do not chew, crush, or open capsule.
2. Do not perform activities that require mental/physical alertness until drug effects realized; may cause dizziness and syncope.

Outcome/Evaluate: Improvement in BPH symptoms; decreased nocturia

Tazarotene

(taz-**AR**-oh-teen)

Pregnancy Category: X

Tazorac **(Rx)**

Classification: Antipsoriasis topical drug

Action/Kinetics: A retinoid prodrug converted by deesterification to active cognate carboxylic acid of tazarotene. Mechanism not known. Little systemic absorption. **t½, after topical use:** About 18 hr. Parent drug and metabolite are further metabolized and excreted through urine and feces.

Uses: Stable plaque psoriasis. Mild to moderate facial acne vulgaris.

Contraindications: Pregnancy. Use on eczematous skin. Use of cosmetics or skin medications that have strong drying effect.

Special Concerns: Use with caution during lactation. Safety and efficacy have not been determined in children less than 12 years of age. Psoriasis may worsen from month 4 to 12 compared with first 3 months of therapy. Use with caution with drugs that cause photosensitivity.

Side Effects: *Dermatologic:* Pruritus, photosensitivity, burning/stinging, erythema, worsening of psoriasis, skin pain, irritation, rash, desquamation, contact dermatitis, skin inflammation, fissuring, bleeding, dry skin, localized edema, skin discoloration.

OD **Management of Overdose:** *Symptoms:* Marked redness, peeling, discomfort. *Treatment:* Decrease or discontinue dose.

Drug Interactions: ↑ Risk of photosensitivity when used with fluoroquinolones, phenothiazines, sulfonamides, tetracyclines, thiazides.

How Supplied: *Gel:* 0.05%, 0.1%

Dosage

- **Gel**

Acne vulgaris, Psoriasis.

After skin is dry following cleaning, apply thin film (2 mg/cm^2) on lesions once daily in evening. Cover entire affected area. For psoriasis, do not apply to more than 20% of body surface area.

HEALTH CARE CONSIDERATIONS

Administration/Storage: Avoid application to unaffected skin due to increased susceptibility to irritation.

Assessment

1. Record condition requiring treatment; may photograph to assess response.
2. Determine if pregnant and begin therapy during menstrual cycle.

Client/Family Teaching
1. Cleanse face gently, pat dry, apply a thin film in evening only where lesions are present.
2. Apply once daily as directed. Avoid contact with eyes and mouth; rinse thoroughly if contact occurs.
3. Report excessive itching, redness, burning, or peeling of skin. Stop therapy until skin integrity restored.
4. Avoid weather extremes such as wind or cold; may increase irritation.
5. Practice reliable contraception; drug causes fetal damage.
6. May experience photosensitivity reaction; use sunscreens and protective clothing if exposed.

Outcome/Evaluate: Clearing of psoriasis placques/acne lesions

Telmisartan

(tell-mih-SAR-tan)

Pregnancy Category: C (first trimester), D (second and third trimesters)

Micardis **(Rx)**

Classification: Antihypertensive, angiotensin II receptor antagonist

Action/Kinetics: Angiotensin II receptor (AT_1) antagonist that blocks the vasoconstrictor and aldosterone-secreting effects of angiotensin II by blocking binding of angiotensin II to the AT_1 receptors. Over 99.5% bound to plasma protein. **t½, terminal:** About 24 hr. Excreted mainly in the feces by way of the bile.

Uses: Alone or in combination to treat hypertension.

Contraindications: Lactation.

Special Concerns: Control of BP in Black clients is less than in White clients. Use with caution in impaired hepatic function or in biliary obstructive disorders. Safety and efficacy have not been determined in children less than 18 years of age.

T

Side Effects: *GI:* Diarrhea, dyspepsia, heartburn, N&V, abdominal pain. *CNS:* Dizziness, headache, fatigue, anxiety, nervousness. *Musculoskeletal:* Pain, including back and neck pain; myalgia. *Respiratory:* URI, sinusitis, cough, pharyngitis, influenza. *Miscellaneous:* Chest pain, UTI, peripheral edema, hypertension.

Laboratory Test Considerations: ↑ Creatinine (in small number of clients).

OD **Management of Overdose:** *Symptoms:* Hypotension, dizziness, tachycardia or bradycardia. *Treatment:* Supportive for hypotension.

Drug Interactions: ↑ Digoxin peak plasma and trough levels.

How Supplied: *Tablets:* 40 mg, 80 mg

Dosage

- **Tablets**

Antihypertensive.

Adults, initial: 40 mg/day. **Maintenance:** 20–80 mg/day. If additional BP reduction is desired beyond that achieved with 80 mg/day, add a diuretic.

HEALTH CARE CONSIDERATIONS

Administration/Storage: May be taken with or without food.

Assessment
1. Record onset and duration of disease, other agents trialed and the outcome.
2. Symptomatic hypotension may occur in clients who are volume- or salt-depleted. Correct prior to using telmisartan, use a lower starting dose and monitor closely.
3. With renal dialysis may develop orthostatic hypotension; monitor BP closely.
4. Monitor ECG, labs, and VS. With hepatic dysfunction, use cautiously.

Client/Family Teaching
1. Take as directed at the same time daily with or without food.
2. Regular exercise, low-salt diet, and life-style changes (i.e., no smoking, low alcohol, low-fat diet, low stress, adequate rest) contribute to enhanced BP control.
3. Use effective contraception; report pregnancy as drug during second and third trimesters associated with fetal injury and morbidity.

Outcome/Evaluate: BP control

Temazepam

(teh-MAZ-eh-pam)

Pregnancy Category: X

Apo-Temazepam ✦, Dom-Temazepam ✦, Gen-Temazepam ✦, Novo-Temazepam ✦, Nu-Temazepam ✦, PMS-Temazepam ✦, Restoril **(C-IV) (Rx)**

Classification: Benzodiazepine hypnotic

See also *Tranquilizers, Antimanic Drugs, and Hypnotics.*

Action/Kinetics: Benzodiazepine derivative. Disturbed nocturnal sleep may occur the first one or two nights following discontinuance of the drug. Prolonged administration is not recommended because physical dependence and tolerance may develop. See also *Flurazepam.* **Peak blood levels:** 2–4 hr. **t½, initial:** 0.4–0.6 hr; **final:** 10 hr. **Steady-state plasma levels:** 382 ng/mL (2.5 hr after 30-mg dose). Accumulation of the drug is minimal following multiple dosage.

Significantly bound (98%) to plasma protein. Metabolized in the liver to inactive metabolites.

Uses: Insomnia in clients unable to fall asleep, with frequent awakenings during the night and/or early morning awakenings.

Contraindications: Pregnancy.

Special Concerns: Use with caution in severely depressed clients. Use during lactation may cause sedation and feeding problems in the infant. Geriatric clients may be more sensitive to the effects of temazepam.

Side Effects: *CNS:* Drowsiness (after daytime use) and dizziness are common. Lethargy, confusion, euphoria, weakness, ataxia, lack of concentration, hallucinations. In some clients, paradoxical excitement (less than 0.5%), including stimulation and hyperactivity, occurs. *GI:* Anorexia, diarrhea. *Other:* Tremors, horizontal nystagmus, falling, palpitations. Rarely, blood dyscrasias.

How Supplied: *Capsule:* 7.5 mg, 15 mg, 30 mg

Dosage

- **Capsules**

Adults, usual: 15–30 mg at bedtime. **In elderly or debilitated clients, initial:** 15 mg; **then,** adjust dosage to response.

HEALTH CARE CONSIDERATIONS

See also *Health Care Considerations* for *Tranquilizers, Antimanic Drugs, and Hypnotics.*

Assessment

1. Note indications for therapy, onset and duration of symptoms.
2. Assess sleep patterns; identify factors contributing to insomnia.

Client/Family Teaching

1. Take only as directed and do not increase dose.
2. May cause daytime drowsiness. Avoid activities that require mental alertness until drug effects realized.
3. Avoid alcohol and CNS depressants; may increase CNS depression.
4. Avoid tobacco; decreases drug's effect.
5. Review nonpharmacologic methods of sleep induction.
6. For short-term use only. Long-term use can cause dependence and withdrawal symptoms. After more than 3 weeks of continuous use may experience rebound insomnia.

Outcome/Evaluate: Improved sleeping patterns; ↓ awakenings

Terazosin

(ter-**AY**-zoh-sin)

Pregnancy Category: C

Hytrin **(Rx)**

Classification: Antihypertensive, alpha-1-adrenergic receptor blocking agent

Action/Kinetics: Blocks postsynaptic alpha-1-adrenergic receptors, leading to a dilation of both arterioles and veins, and ultimately, a reduction in BP. Both standing and supine BPs are lowered with no reflex tachycardia. Also relaxes smooth muscle of the prostate and bladder neck. Usefulness in BPH is due to alpha-1 receptor blockade, which relaxes the smooth muscle of the prostate and bladder neck and relieves pressure on the urethra. Bioavailability is not affected by food. **Onset:** 15 min. **Peak plasma levels:** 1–2 hr. **t½:** 9–12 hr. **Duration:** 24 hr. Excreted unchanged and as inactive metabolites in both the urine and feces.

Uses: Alone or in combination with diuretics or beta-adrenergic blocking agents to treat hypertension. Treat symptoms of benign prostatic hyperplasia.

Special Concerns: Use with caution during lactation. Safety and efficacy have not been determined in children. Geriatric clients may be more sensitive to the hypotensive and hypothermic effects of terazosin.

Side Effects: *First-dose effect:* Marked postural hypotension and syncope. *CV:* Palpitations, tachycardia, postural hypotension, syncope, ***arrhythmias,*** chest pain, vasodilation. *CNS:* Dizziness, headache, somnolence, drowsiness, nervousness, paresthesia, depression, anxiety, insomnia, vertigo. *Respiratory:* Nasal congestion, dyspnea, sinusitis, epistaxis, bronchitis, ***bronchospasm,*** cold or flu symptoms, increased cough, pharyngitis, rhinitis. *GI:* Nausea, constipation, diarrhea, dyspepsia, dry mouth, vomiting, flatulence, abdominal discomfort or pain. *Musculoskeletal:* Asthenia, arthritis, arthralgia, myalgia, joint disorders, back pain, pain in extremities, neck and shoulder pain, muscle cramps. *Miscellaneous:* Peripheral edema, weight gain, blurred vision, impotence, chest pain, fever, gout, pruritus, rash, sweating, urinary frequency, UTI, tinnitus, conjunctivitis, abnormal vision, edema, facial edema.

Laboratory Test Considerations: ↓ H&H, WBCs, albumin.

OD **Management of Overdose:** *Symptoms:* Hypotension, drowsiness, shock. *Treatment:* Restore BP and HR. Client should be kept supine; vasopressors may be

T

indicated. Volume expanders can be used to treat shock.

How Supplied: *Capsule:* 1 mg, 2 mg, 5 mg, 10 mg

Dosage

- **Capsules**

Hypertension.

Individualized, initial: 1 mg at bedtime (this dose is not to be exceeded); **then,** increase dose slowly to obtain desired response. **Range:** 1–5 mg/day; doses as high as 20 mg may be required in some clients. Doses greater than 20 mg daily do not provide further BP control.

Benign prostatic hyperplasia.

Initial: 1 mg/day; dose should be increased to 2 mg, 5 mg, and then 10 mg once daily to improve symptoms and/or urinary flow rates. Doses greater than 20 mg daily have not been studied.

HEALTH CARE CONSIDERATIONS

See also *Health Considerations* for *Antihypertensive Agents.*

Administration/Storage

1. The initial dosing regimen must be carefully observed to minimize severe hypotension.
2. Monitor BP 2–3 hr after dosing and at the end of the dosing interval to ensure BP control has been maintained.
3. Consider an increase in dose or b.i.d. dosing if BP control is not maintained at 24-hr interval.
4. To prevent dizziness or fainting due to a drop in BP, take the initial dose at bedtime; the daily dose can be given in the morning.
5. If terazosin must be discontinued for more than a few days, reinstitute the initial dosing regimen if restarted.
6. Due to additive effects, use caution when combined with other antihypertensive agents.
7. When treating BPH, a minimum of 4–6 weeks of 10 mg/day may be needed to determine if a beneficial effect has occurred.

Assessment

1. Record onset, duration, and characteristics of symptoms.
2. Assess prostate gland, PSA level, and BPH score.
3. A gradual increase in dose, i.e., 1 mg/day for 7 days, then 2 mg/day for 7 days, then 3 mg/day for 7 days, then 4 mg/day for 7 days, and then 5 mg /day, may assist to diminish adverse effects and enhance compliance, especially in the elderly.

Client/Family Teaching

1. Take initial dose at bedtime to minimize side effects. Do not stop abruptly. Use caution when performing activities that require mental alertness until drug effects realized.
2. Do not drive or undertake hazardous tasks for 12 hr after the first dose and after increasing dose or reinstituting therapy.
3. Avoid symptoms of orthostatic hypotension by rising slowly from a sitting or lying position and waiting until symptoms subside.
4. Record weight 2 times/week; report persistent side effects or excessive weight gain or ankle edema.
5. Report if nocturia persists or increases.

Outcome/Evaluate

- Control of BP
- Improvement in BPH symptoms

Terbinafine hydrochloride

(ter-**BIN**-ah-feen)

Pregnancy Category: B

Lamisil **(Rx)**

Classification: Antifungal agent

Action/Kinetics: Inhibits squalene epoxidase, a key enzyme in the sterol biosynthesis in fungi. Results in ergosterol deficiency and a corresponding accumulation of squalene leading to fungal cell death. Approximately 75% of cutaneously absorbed drug is excreted in the urine, mostly as metabolites. Well absorbed following PO administration, with first-pass metabolism being about 40%. **Peak plasma levels:** 1 mcg/mL within 2 hr. Food enhances absorption. Over 99% bound to plasma proteins. Slowly excreted from adipose tissue and skin. Extensively metabolized, with about 70% of the dose eliminated in the urine. Renal or hepatic disease decreases clearance from the body.

Uses: Topical use: Interdigital tinea pedis (athletes' foot), tinea cruris (jock itch), or tinea corporis (ringworm) due to *Epidermophyton floccosum, Trichophyton mentagrophytes,* or *T. rubrum.* Plantar tinea pedis. Tinea versicolor due to *Malassezia furfur. Investigational:* Cutaneous candidiasis and tinea versicolor. **Oral use:** Onychomycosis of the toenail or fingernail due to dermatophytes.

Contraindications: Ophthalmic or intravaginal use. PO use in preexisting liver disease or renal impairment (C_{CR} less than 50 mL/min). Lactation.

Special Concerns: Safety and efficacy have not been determined in children less than 12 years of age.

Side Effects: *Following topical use. Dermatologic:* Irritation, burning, itching, dryness.

Following oral use. GI: Diarrhea, dyspepsia, abdominal pain, nausea, flatulence. *Dermatologic:* Rash, pruritus, urticaria. *Other:* Headache, taste or visual disturbances. Rarely, symptomatic idiosyncratic hepatobiliary dysfunction (including cholestatic hepatitis), serious skin reactions, severe neutropenia, allergic reactions (including ***anaphylaxis***).

Laboratory Test Considerations: Liver enzyme abnormalities that are two or more times the upper limit of the normal range. ↓ Absolute neutrophil counts.

Drug Interactions

Cimetidine / Terbinafine clearance is ↓ by one-third

Cyclosporine / ↑ Clearance of cyclosporine

Rifampin / ↑ Clearance (100%) of terbinafine

Terfenadine / ↓ Clearance of terbinafine

How Supplied: *Cream:* 1%; *Spray:* 1%; *Tablet:* 250 mg

Dosage

- **Cream**

Interdigital tinea pedis.

Apply to cover the affected and immediately surrounding areas b.i.d. until symptoms are significantly improved. Maintain therapy for a minimum of 1 week and not more than 4 weeks.

Tinea cruris or tinea corporis.

Apply to cover the affected and immediately surrounding areas 1–2 times/day until symptoms are significantly improved. Maintain therapy for a minimum of 1 week and not more than 4 weeks.

- **Spray**

Tinea pedis, Tinea versicolor.

Spray b.i.d. for one week.

Tinea corporis, Tinea cruris.

Spray once daily for one week.

- **Tablets**

Onychomycosis.

250 mg/day for 6 weeks if fingernails are affected and 250 mg/day for 12 weeks if toenails are affected. Alternatively, intermittent dosing may be used: 500 mg daily for 1 week each month (use 2 months for fingernails and 4 months for toenails). The optimal clinical effect is observed several months after mycologic cure and cessation of treatment due to slow period for outgrowth of healthy nails.

HEALTH CARE CONSIDERATIONS

Administration/Storage

1. Avoid contact of the cream with eyes, nose, mouth, or other mucous membranes.
2. Avoid occlusive dressings.
3. For topical use, many clients treated for 1–2 weeks continue to improve during the 2–4 weeks after drug therapy has been completed. Do not consider clients therapeutic failures until they have been observed for a period of 2–4 weeks off therapy.
4. Store the cream between 5°C and 30°C (41°F and 86°F). Protect tablets from light and store below 25°C (77°F).

Assessment

1. Describe clinical presentation and note location, onset, duration, and characteristics of symptoms.
2. If presentation unclear, document infected tissue scrapings to confirm diagnosis.
3. Note any liver or renal dysfunction.

Client/Family Teaching

1. Cream is for topical dermatologic use only; review method for application.
2. Wash hands before and after topical application. Use a clean towel and washcloth; avoid sharing.
3. Avoid contact of cream with mouth, nose, eyes, and other mucous membranes; do not cover treated areas with occlusive dressing.
4. Take tablets with food to ensure maximal absorption.
5. Report symptoms of increased irritation or possible sensitization such as redness, itching, burning, blistering, swelling, or oozing.
6. Use for prescribed time; do not skip or double up on doses.
7. Continued improvement in skin condition and/or mycotic nails may be noted for 2–4 weeks after therapy.

Outcome/Evaluate

- Improvement in dermatologic condition
- Clearing/healing of mycotic nail beds

T

Terbutaline sulfate

(ter-**BYOU**-tah-leen)

Pregnancy Category: B

Brethaire, Brethine, Bricanyl **(Rx)**

Classification: Sympathomimetic, direct-acting; bronchodilator

See also *Sympathomimetic Drugs.*

Action/Kinetics: Specific beta-2 receptor stimulant, resulting in bronchodilation and relaxation of peripheral vasculature. Minimum beta-1 activity. Action resembles that of isoproterenol. **PO: Onset:** 30 min; **maximum effect:** 2–3 hr; **duration:** 4–8 hr. **SC: Onset,** 5–15 min; **maximum effect:** 30 min–1 hr; **duration:** 1.5–4 hr. **Inhalation: Onset,** 5–30 min; **time to peak effect:** 1–2 hr; **duration:** 3–6 hr.

Uses: Bronchodilator in asthma, bronchitis, emphysema, bronchiectasis, pulmonary obstructive disease, and other conditions associated with reversible bronchospasms. Relief of reversible bronchospasms in clients age six and up who suffer from obstructive airway diseases. *Investigational:* Inhibit premature labor.
Contraindications: Lactation.
Special Concerns: Safe use in children less than 12 years of age not established.
Laboratory Test Considerations: ↑ Liver enzymes.
Additional Side Effects: *CV:* PVCs, ECG changes (e.g., atrial premature beats, AV block, sinus pause, ST-T wave depression, T-wave inversion, sinus bradycardia, atrial escape beat with aberrant conduction), tachycardia. *Respiratory:* Wheezing. *Miscellaneous:* Hypersensitivity reactions (including vasculitis), flushing, sweating, bad taste or taste change, muscle cramps, CNS stimulation, pain at injection site.
How Supplied: *Metered dose inhaler:* 0.2 mg/inh; *Injection:* 1 mg/mL; *Tablet:* 2.5 mg, 5 mg

Dosage

- **Tablets**

Bronchodilation.

Adults and children over 15 years: 5 mg t.i.d. q 6 hr during waking hours, not to exceed 15 mg q 24 hr. If disturbing side effects are observed, dose can be reduced to 2.5 mg t.i.d. without loss of beneficial effects. Anticipate use of other therapeutic measures if client fails to respond after second dose. **Children 12–15 years:** 2.5 mg t.i.d., not to exceed 7.5 mg q 24 hr.

Premature labor.

2.5 mg q 4–6 hr until term.

- **SC**

Bronchodilation.

Adults: 0.25 mg. May be repeated 1 time after 15–30 min if no significant clinical improvement is noted. If client does not respond to the second dose, undertake other measures. Do not exceed a dose of 0.5 mg over 4 hr.

- **IV Infusion**

Premature labor.

10 mcg/min initially; **then,** increase rate by 0.005 mg/min q 10 min until contractions cease or a maximum dose of 80 mcg/min is reached. Continue the minimum effective dose for 4–8 hr after contractions cease. Terbutaline may also be given SC for preterm labor.

- **Metered Dose Inhaler**

Bronchodilation.

Adults and children over 12 years: 0.2–0.5 mg (1–2 inhalations) q 4–6 hr. Inhalations should be separated by 60-sec intervals. Dosage may be repeated q 4–6 hr.

HEALTH CARE CONSIDERATIONS

See also *Health Care Considerations* for *Sympathomimetic Drugs.*

Assessment

1. Record type, onset, duration, and characteristics of symptoms.
2. Auscultate and record lung assessments and PFTs. Observe respiratory client for evidence of drug tolerance and rebound bronchospasm.
3. Determine onset, frequency, and duration of contractions and fetal HR with preterm labor.
4. Observe mother for headache, tremor, anxiety, palpitations, symptoms of pulmonary edema, and tachycardia. Assess fetus for distress; report increased contractions. Monitor both for symptoms of hypoglycemia and mother for hypokalemia.

Client/Family Teaching

1. Take oral medication with meals to minimize GI upset.
2. Report any persistent or bothersome side effects. Do not increase dose or frequency if symptoms are not relieved. Report so dose can be reevaluated.
3. Increase fluid intake to help liquefy secretions.
4. With preterm labor, notify provider immediately if labor resumes or unusual side effects are noted.

Outcome/Evaluate

- Improved airway exchange
- Inhibition of premature labor

Terconazole nitrate

(ter-**KON**-ah-zohl)
Pregnancy Category: C
Terazol ★, Terazol 3, Terazol 7 **(Rx)**
Classification: Antifungal, vaginal

Action/Kinetics: May exert its antifungal activity by disrupting cell membrane permeability leading to loss of essential intracellular materials. Also inhibits synthesis of triglycerides and phospholipids as well as inhibiting oxidative and peroxidative enzyme activity. When used for *Candida,* terconazole inhibits transformation of blastospores into the invasive mycelial form.
Uses: Vulvovaginitis caused by *Candida.* Ineffective in infections due to *Trichomonas* or *Haemophilus vaginalis.*

Special Concerns: During lactation, consider discontinuing nursing or the drug. Safety and efficacy have not been established in children.
Side Effects: *GU:* Vulvovaginal burning, irritation, or itching; dysmenorrhea, pain of the female genitalia. *Miscellaneous:* Headache (most common), body pain, photosensitivity, abdominal pain, chills, fever.
How Supplied: *Vaginal cream:* 0.4%, 0.8%; *Vaginal suppository:* 80 mg

Dosage

- **Vaginal Cream (0.4%, 0.8%)**

One applicator full (5 g) intravaginally, once daily at bedtime for 7 consecutive days for the 0.4% cream and for 3 consecutive days for the 0.8% cream.

- **Vaginal Suppository**

One 80-mg suppository once daily at bedtime for 3 consecutive days.

HEALTH CARE CONSIDERATIONS

Assessment

1. Obtain a thorough health history because recurrent candidiasis may be caused by oral contraceptives, antibiotics, or diabetes whereas intractable candidiasis may be the result of undetected diabetes mellitus or reinfection.
2. Prior to a second course of therapy, the diagnosis should be confirmed to rule out other pathogens associated with vulvovaginitis.

Client/Family Teaching

1. Review the appropriate method for administration and cleansing (the cream should be inserted high into the vagina). Sitz baths and vaginal douches may also be used.
2. Discontinue use and report if any burning, irritation, or pain occurs.
3. May stain clothes; use sanitary napkins during therapy and change frequently because damp sanitary napkins may harbor infecting organisms.
4. To avoid reinfection, refrain from sexual intercourse. Advise partner to use a condom as med may also irritate partner.
5. Use for prescribed time frame even if symptoms subside.
6. Continue to use during menses to ensure a full course of therapy.

Outcome/Evaluate: Resolution of fungal infections; symptomatic improvement

Testolactone

(tes-toe-**LACK**-tohn)

Pregnancy Category: C
Teslac **(C-III) (Rx)**
Classification: Antineoplastic, androgen

See also *Antineoplastic Agents.*
Action/Kinetics: Synthetic steroid related to testosterone. May act to reduce synthesis of estrone from adrenal androstenedione by inhibiting steroid aromatase activity. Well absorbed from the GI tract. Metabolized in the liver and unchanged drug and metabolites are excreted through the urine. Does not cause virilization.
Uses: Palliative treatment of advanced disseminated mammary cancer in postmenopausal women or in premenopausal ovariectomized clients. Is effective in only 15% of clients.
Contraindications: Breast cancer in men. Lactation. Premenopausal women with intact ovaries.
Special Concerns: Safety and efficacy have not been determined in children.
Laboratory Test Considerations: ↑ Plasma calcium, urinary excretion of creatine (24 hr) and 17-ketosteroids. ↓ Estradiol levels using radioimmunoassays.
Additional Side Effects: *GI:* N&V, glossitis, anorexia. *CNS:* Numbness or tingling of fingers, toes, face. *Miscellaneous:* Inflammation and irritation at injection site; increased BP. Hypercalcemia. Maculopapular erythema, alopecia, aches and edema of the extremities, nail growth disturbances. See also *Testosterone.*
Drug Interactions: Testolactone may ↑ effect of oral anticoagulants.
How Supplied: *Tablet:* 50 mg

Dosage

- **Tablets**

250 mg q.i.d. Continue therapy for 3 months unless there is active progression of the disease.

HEALTH CARE CONSIDERATIONS

See also *Health Care Considerations* for *Antineoplastic Agents* and *Testosterone.*
Assessment: Record indications for therapy, noting onset, location, and duration of symptoms and other agents or therapies trialed.

Interventions

1. Reduce dose of anticoagulants with concomitant therapy and monitor INR.
2. The effect of the steroid and osteolytic metastases may result in hypercalcemia. Assess for symptoms of hypercalcemia (insom-

T

nia, lethargy, anorexia, N&V). Encourage high fluid intake (2–3 L/day) to minimize hypercalcemia.
3. Monitor BP and report any significant increases >20 mm Hg DBP.
4. Perform ROM exercises on bedridden clients and encourage others to exercise to reduce calcium levels, improve circulation, and prevent thrombophlebitis.

Outcome/Evaluate: ↓ Tumor size and spread

Testosterone aqueous suspension

(tess-**TOSS**-ter-ohn)

Pregnancy Category: X

Histerone 100, Malogen Aqueous ✦, Tesamone 100, Testandro **(Rx) (C-III)**

Testosterone cypionate (in oil)

(tess-**TOSS**-ter-ohn)

Pregnancy Category: X

depAndro 100 and 200, Depotest 100 and 200, Depo-Testosterone, Depo-Testosterone Cypionate ✦, Duratest-100 and -200, Scheinpharm Testone-Cyp ✦ **(Rx) (C-III)**

Testosterone enanthate (in oil)

(tess-**TOSS**-ter-ohn)

Pregnancy Category: X

Andro L.A. 200, Andropository-200, Delatestryl, Durathate-200, Everone 200, Malogex LA ✦, PMS-Testosterone Enanthate ✦ **(Rx) (C-III)**

Testosterone propionate (in oil)

(tess-**TOSS**-ter-ohn)

Pregnancy Category: X

Malogen in Oil ✦ **(Rx) (C-III)**

Testosterone transdermal system

(tess-**TOSS**-ter-ohn)

Pregnancy Category: X

Androderm, Testoderm, Testoderm TTS, Testoderm with Adhesive **(Rx) (C-III)**

Classification: Androgen, natural hormone and salts of natural hormone

Action/Kinetics: Treatment with testosterone and its congeners is complicated by the fact that the exogenous supply of the hormone may depress secretion of the natural hormone through inhibitory effects on the pituitary. Too large a dose may cause permanent damage. Treatment is usually associated with a feeling of well-being. Following PO use, 44% of testosterone is cleared by the liver in the first pass. Thus, the parenteral forms are used. **t½, testosterone cypionate after IM:** 8 days. Ninety percent is excreted through the urine as metabolites and 6% is excreted through the feces. Testosterone and testosterone propionate are considered short-acting; testosterone enanthate and testosterone cypionate are long-acting.

Following use of Testoderm on the scrotal skin: **Maximum serum levels:** 2–4 hr with return to baseline in about 2 hr after system is removed. Serum levels reach a plateau in 3–4 weeks. Will not produce sufficient serum levels if applied to nongenital skin. Following use of Androderm to nonscrotal skin, there is continual absorption over 24 hr. Application of two systems at 10:00 p.m. results in serum testosterone levels similar to normal circadian variation with maximum levels occurring in the early morning hours and minimum levels in the evening.

Uses: Parenteral products: Replacement therapy in males for congenital or acquired primary hypogonadism or for congenital or acquired hypogonadotropic hypogonadism. Delayed puberty. In postmenopausal women to treat inoperable metastatic breast carcinoma or in premenopausal women following oophorectomy. Postpartum breast engorgement (evidence for effectiveness is lacking). *Investigational:* Male contraceptive (testosterone enanthate).

Transdermal products: Replacement therapy for acquired or congenital primary hypogonadism or for acquired or congenital secondary hypogonadotropic hypogonadism.

Contraindications: Serious renal, hepatic, or cardiac disease due to edema formation. Prostatic or breast (males) carcinoma. Use in pregnancy (masculinization of female fetus) and lactation. Discontinue if hypercalcemia occurs.

Special Concerns: Use with caution in young males who have not completed their growth (because of premature epiphyseal closure). Androgens may also cause virilization in females or precocious sexual development in males. Geriatric clients may manifest an increased risk of prostatic hypertrophy or prostatic carcinoma. Androgen therapy occasionally seems to accelerate metastatic breast carcinoma in women.

Side Effects: *Hepatic:* Liver toxicity is the most serious side effect. Jaundice, cholestasis, alterations in BSP retention, AST, and ALT. Rarely, ***hepatic necrosis, hepatocellular neoplasms,*** peliosis hepatis, acute intermittent porphyria in clients with this disease. *GI:* N&V, diarrhea, anorexia, symptoms of peptic ulcer. *CNS:* Headache, anxiety, increased or decreased libido, insomnia, excitation, paresthesias, sleep apnea syndrome, ***CNS hemorrhage,*** chills, choreiform movements, habituation, confusion (toxic doses). *GU:* Testicular atrophy with inhibition of testicular function (e.g., oligospermia), impotence, epididymitis, irritable bladder, prepubertal phallic enlargement, gynecomastia. *Electrolyte:* Retention of sodium, chloride, calcium, potassium, phosphates. Edema. *Miscellaneous:* Acne, flushing, suppression of clotting factors (II, V, VII, X), polycythemia, leukopenia, rashes, dermatitis, ***anaphylaxis (rare),*** muscle cramps, hypercholesterolemia, male-pattern baldness, acne, seborrhea, hirsutism. Hypercalcemia, especially in immobilized clients or those with metastatic breast carcinoma. Virilization in women.

In females, menstrual irregularities (including amenorrhea), virilization, clitoral enlargement, hirsutism, increased libido, baldness (male pattern), virilization of external genitalia of female fetus.

In males, decreased ejaculatory volume, oligospermia (high doses), gynecomastia, increased frequency and duration of penile erections.

In children, disturbances of growth, premature closure of epiphyses, precocious sexual development.

Inflammation and pain at site of IM or SC injection.

NOTE: Side effects of the cypionate and enanthate products are not readily reversible due to the long duration of action of these dosage forms.

The patch may cause itching, irritation, erythema, or discomfort of the scrotum (Testoderm) or on skin areas where applied (Androderm). Potentially, small amounts of testosterone may be transferred to a sex partner.

Laboratory Test Considerations: Altered thyroid function tests. False + or ↑ BSP, alkaline phosphatase, bilirubin, cholesterol, and acid phosphatase (in women). Alteration of glucose tolerance tests.

Drug Interactions

Anticoagulants, oral / Anabolic steroids ↑ effect of anticoagulants

Antidiabetic agents / Additive hypoglycemia

Barbiturates / ↓ Effect of androgens due to ↑ breakdown by liver

Corticosteroids / ↑ Chance of edema

Phenylbutazone / Certain androgens ↑ effect of phenylbutazone

How Supplied: Testosterone aqueous suspension: *Injection:* 50 mg/mL, 100 mg/mL. Testosterone cypionate: *Injection:* 200 mg/mL. Testosterone enanthate: *Injection:* 100 mg/mL, 200 mg/mL. Testosterone propionate: *Injection:* 100 mg/mL. Testosterone transdermal system: *Film, extended release:* 2.5 mg/24 hr, 4 mg/24 hr, 5 mg/24 hr, 6 mg/24 hr

Dosage

Testosterone aqueous suspension and Testosterone propionate in oil

- **IM Only**

Replacement therapy.

25–50 mg 2–3 times/week.

Breast cancer.

50–100 mg 3 times/week.

Growth stimulation in Turner's syndrome or constitutional delay of puberty.

40–50 mg/m²/dose given monthly for 6 months.

Male hypogonadism, initiation of pubertal growth.

40–50 mg/m²/month until growth rate falls to prepubertal levels (about 5 cm/year).

Male hypogonadism, during terminal growth phase.

100 mg/m²/month until growth ceases.

Male hypogonadism, maintain virilization.

100 mg/m² twice monthly or 50–400 mg/dose q 2–4 weeks.

Postpartum breast engorgement.

25–50 mg of testostrone propionate for 3–4 days.

Testosterone enanthate and cypionate

- **IM Only**

Hypogonadism, replacement therapy.

50–400 mg q 2–4 weeks.

Delayed puberty.

50–200 mg q 2–4 weeks for no more than 4–6 months.

Palliation of inoperable breast cancer in women.

200–400 mg q 2–4 weeks.

- **Transdermal System**

Replacement therapy (congenital or acquired primary hypogonadism, congenital or acquired hypogonadotropic hypogonadism).

Testoderm: One 6-mg patch applied daily on clean, dry scrotal skin that has been dry-shaved to remove hair. Clients with a smaller scrotum can use a 4-mg patch. The patch should be worn for 22–24 hr/day for 6–8 weeks. *Testoderm TTS:* One 5-mg patch applied to the arm, back, or upper buttocks each day. The patch can be removed and reapplied if the client wants to swim, bathe, or vigorously exercise.

T

Androderm: Initial dose, usual: Two systems applied nightly for 24 hr providing a total dose of 5 mg/day. The systems are applied to a clean, dry area of the skin on the back, abdomen, upper arms, or thighs.

HEALTH CARE CONSIDERATIONS

Administration/Storage

1. Redissolve crystals of testosterone enanthate or cypionate by warming and shaking the vial.
2. If needle or syringe is wet, the product may become cloudy; this does not affect potency.
3. For IM oil-based suspensions, warm the unopened vial in warm water to decrease the viscosity of the oil. Vigorously rotate the vial to resuspend the medication in the oil. A film may appear on the sides of the vial. When no more suspended particles are observed on the bottom or sides of the vial, the drug has been suspended appropriately. Administer the needle deep into the muscle; give slowly.
4. When parenteral injection is to be used, testosterone propionate is more effective than testosterone because it is released more slowly.
5. Continue therapy for at least 2 months for a satisfactory response and for 5 months for an objective response.
6. When used for delayed puberty, consider the chronological and skeletal ages when determining initial and subsequent doses. Use is for a limited time (e.g., 4–6 mo).
7. The patch is made of a cloth and copolymer that sticks to the skin without a sticky adhesive. Warm the patch in the hands before application. Wear loose clothing to keep the patch in place.
8. Prior to sexual activity, remove the Testoderm patch from the scrotum and wash the scrotal area to remove residue.
9. Do not apply the Androderm patch to bony areas such as the shoulders or hips; it is *not* to be applied to the scrotum. Sites of application should be rotated, with an interval of 7 days between applications to the same site. Areas should not be oily, damaged, or irritated.
10. Apply Androderm immediately after opening the pouch and removing the protective liner. Press the system firmly in place, making sure there is good contact with the skin, especially around the edges of the patch. Excessive heat or pressure can cause the drug reservoir to burst.
11. Do not use damaged patches. Discard systems safely to prevent accidental application or ingestion by children, pets, or others.

T

Assessment

1. Record indications for therapy, type, onset, and characteristics of symptoms.
2. Assess for any cardiac, renal, or hepatic dysfunction. Document neurologic status, BP, respirations, heart sounds, and GU function.
3. Note hair distribution and skin texture.
4. Check prescribed medications for any drugs that may interact unfavorably (i.e., anticoagulants, hypoglycemic agents, and mineralocorticoids).
5. Determine if pregnant.
6. Monitor CBC, serum glucose, calcium, electrolytes, cholesterol, liver and renal function studies. Treatment with aplastic anemia has resulted in several cases of hepatocellular carcinoma.

Interventions

1. Monitor for signs of mental depression such as insomnia, lack of interest in personal appearance, and withdrawal from social contacts.
2. Monitor weight, BP, pulse, and serum electrolytes. Auscultate lung sounds and note any JVD. Report edema, as sodium retention and edema can be easily treated with diuretics.
3. Assess for relaxation of the skeletal muscles and pain deep in the bones. The discomfort in the bones is caused by a honeycombing; often caused by increased calcium levels.
4. Flank pain may be caused by kidney stones from excessively high serum calcium levels. Administer large amounts of fluids to prevent renal calculi. If hypercalcemia is the result of metastases, initiate other appropriate therapy.
5. Observe for jaundice, malaise, complaints of RUQ pain, pruritus, or a change in the color/consistency of stools. Document LFTs.
6. Observe for easy bruising, bleeding, complaints of sore throat or the development of a fever. Obtain CBC to rule out polycythemia and leukopenia.
7. With a child, monitor closely for growth retardation and development of precocious puberty. Use with caution as the effect on the CNS in developing children is still being explored.
   - Review therapy with parents; often intermittent to allow for periods of normal bone growth.
   - Regular X rays to monitor bone maturation and effects on epiphyseal centers; obtain q 6 mo.
   - Record height and weight regularly.
8. If female, report the signs of virilization, such as deepening of the voice, hirsuitism,

acne, menstrual irregularity, and clitoral enlargement. Usually only evident with doses exceeding 200–300 mg/month.
9. Increased libido in females may be early sign of drug toxicity.
10. Report if acne is severe; may be necessary to change dose.
11. May alter serum lipid levels enhancing susceptibility to arteriosclerotic heart disease in women; monitor cholesterol panel periodically.

Client/Family Teaching

1. Review method for administration/application, dosage, frequency of administration, site preparation, and time of application for the transdermal patch.
2. Report any unusual incidents of bleeding/bruising. Androgens suppress clotting factors (II, V, VII, and X); polycythemia and leukopenia may occur.
3. If drug received via pellets, sloughing can occur; report.
4. In older males, urinary obstruction may occur as a result of BPH.
5. Parents of children receiving testosterone should record weight twice a week and height every 2–3 mo. X rays will be performed periodically on prepubertal children to assess effect on bone growth.
6. Women with metastatic breast cancer need lab tests of serum and urine calcium levels, alkaline phosphatase, and serum cholesterol. If the serum cholesterol level is high, the dosage of drug may need to be changed. Follow a low-cholesterol diet and see dietitian for further assistance with diet.
7. Facial hair and acne in females are reversible once drug withdrawn.
8. Drug may cause irregularities in the menstrual cycle; in postmenopausal women may cause withdrawal bleeding.
9. Use reliable birth control during and for several weeks after therapy withdrawn. Report if pregnancy suspected; increased risk of fetal abnormalities with this drug.
10. Males should report gynecomastia or priapism; may necessitate drug withdrawal (at least temporarily).
11. Report any tingling of the fingers and toes or loss of appetite.
12. Follow a diet high in calories, proteins, vitamins, minerals, and other nutrients. Restrict sodium to reduce edema.
13. With diabetes, hypoglycemia may occur. Report extreme variations as diet and/or dose of antidiabetic agents may require modification.
14. Review potential for drug abuse. High doses of androgens for enhancement of athletic performance can result in serious irreversible side effects and permanent physical damage.

Outcome/Evaluate

- Replacement therapy with control of S&S of androgen deficiency
- Male contraceptive agent
- Suppression of breast tumor size and spread

Tetracycline hydrochloride

(teh-trah-**SYE**-kleen)

Pregnancy Category: D

Achromycin Ophthalmic Ointment, Achromycin Ophthalmic Suspension, Actisite Periodontal Fiber, Apo-Tetra ✱, Jaa Tetra ✱, Nor-Tet, Novo-Tetra ✱, Nu-Tetra ✱, Panmycin, Robicaps, Sumycin 250 and 500, Sumycin Syrup, Tetracap, Tetracyn ✱, Topicycline Topical Solution **(Rx)**

Classification: Antibiotic, tetracycline

See also *General Information* on *Tetracyclines*.

Action/Kinetics: t½: 7–11 hr. From 40% to 70% excreted unchanged in urine; 65% bound to serum proteins. Always express dose as the hydrochloride salt.

Additional Uses: Ophthalmic: Superficial ophthalmic infections due to *Staphylococcus aureus, Streptococcus, Streptococcus pneumoniae, Escherichia coli, Neisseria,* and *Bacteroides*. Prophylaxis of *Neisseria gonorrhoeae* in newborns. With oral therapy for treatment of *Chlamydia trachomatis*. **Topical:** Acne vulgaris, prophylaxis or treatment of infection following skin abrasions, minor cuts, wounds, or burns. **Tetracycline fiber:** Adult periodontitis. *Investigational:* Pleural sclerosing agent in malignant pleural effusions (administered by chest tube); in combination with gentamicin for *Vibrio vulnificus* infections due to wound infection after trauma or by eating contaminated seafood. Mouthwash (use suspension) to treat nonspecific mouth ulcerations, canker sores, aphthous ulcers. Possible drug of choice for stage I Lyme disease.

Contraindications: Use of the topical ointment in or around the eyes. Ophthalmic products to treat fungal diseases of the eye, dendritic keratitis, vaccinia, varicella, mycobacterial eye infections, or following removal of a corneal foreign body.

Special Concerns: Use tetracycline fiber with caution in clients with a history of oral candidiasis. Use of the fiber in chronic abscesses has not been evaluated. Safety and ef-

T

ficacy of the fiber have not been determined in children.

Additional Side Effects: Temporary blurring of vision or stinging following administration. Dermatitis and photosensitivity following ophthalmic use. *Use of the tetracycline fiber:* Oral candidiasis, glossitis, staining of the tongue, severe gingival hyperplasia, minor throat irritation, pain following placement in an abscessed area, throbbing pain, hypersensitivity reactions.

How Supplied: Tetracycline: *Syrup:* 125 mg/5 mL; Tetracycline hydrochloride: *Capsule:* 100 mg, 250 mg, 500 mg; *Ointment:* 3%; *Tablet:* 250 mg, 500 mg

Dosage

- **Capsules, Syrup, Tablets**

Mild to moderate infections.

Adults, usual: 500 mg b.i.d. or 250 mg q.i.d.

Severe infections.

Adult: 500 mg q.i.d. **Children over 8 years:** 25–50 mg/kg/day in four equal doses.

Brucellosis.

500 mg q.i.d. for 3 weeks with 1 g streptomycin IM b.i.d. for first week and once daily the second week.

Syphilis.

Total of 30–40 g over 10–15 days.

Gonorrhea.

Initially, 1.5 g; **then,** 500 mg q 6 hr until 9 g has been given.

Gonorrhea sensitive to penicillin.

Initially, 1.5 g; **then,** 500 mg q 6 hr for 4 days (total: 9 g).

GU or rectal Chlamydia trachomatis infections.

500 mg q.i.d. for minimum of 7 days.

Severe acne.

Initially, 1 g/day; **then,** 125–500 mg/day (long-term).

NOTE: The CDC have established treatment schedules for STDs.

Initially, 1 g/day; **then,** 125–500 mg/day (long-term).

- **Topical**

Acne.

Apply topical solution to affected areas in the morning and at night, making sure that skin is completely wet after each application.

Infections.

Apply OTC ointment (3%) to affected areas 1–4 times/day. A sterile bandage may be used.

- **Tetracycline Fiber**

Adult periodontitis.

Place the fiber into the periodontal pocket until the pocket is filled (amount of fiber will vary with pocket depth and contour) ensuring that the fiber is in contact with the base of the pocket. Retain the fiber in place for 10 days, after which it is to be removed. The effectiveness of subsequent therapy with the fiber has not been assessed.

HEALTH CARE CONSIDERATIONS

See also *Health Care Considerations* for *Tetracyclines* and *General Health Care Considerations for All Anti-Infectives.*

Administration/Storage

1. The tetracycline fiber product consists of a monofilament of ethylene/vinyl acetate copolymer evenly dispersed with tetracycline. The fiber provides for continuous release of tetracycline for 10 days; releases about 2 mcg/cm/hr of tetracycline.
2. Avoid actions that may dislodge the fiber; i.e., chewing hard, crusty, or sticky foods; brushing or flossing near any treated areas; engaging in hygienic practices that might dislodge the fiber; probing the treated area with tongue or fingers.
3. Contact the dentist if the fiber is dislodged or falls out before the next scheduled visit or if pain or swelling occurs.

Assessment

1. Record indications for therapy, type, onset, duration, and characteristics of symptoms.
2. Monitor cultures, CBC, liver and renal function studies.

Client/Family Teaching

1. Take PO form 1 hr before or 2 hr after meals with a full glass of water. Avoid dairy products, antacids, or iron preparations for 2 hr of ingestion.
2. May cause photosensitivity reaction; avoid exposure to sunlight and wear protective clothing and sunscreen when exposed.
3. Transient blurring of vision or stinging may occur when instilled into the eye.
4. Ointment may stain clothing.
5. Drug may cause increased yellow-brown discoloration and softening of teeth and bones. *Not* advised for children under 8 years of age.
6. With oral application for gum disease, review proper care of site(s), foods to avoid, and proper cleaning while avoiding floss or pics for the entire length of therapy. Symptoms that require immediate reporting include pain, abnormal discharge, fever, swelling, expulsion of fiber; return as scheduled for removal and follow-up.

Outcome/Evaluate

- Resolution of infection; symptomatic improvement
- ↓ Acne lesions

Thalidomide

(thah-**LID**-ah-myd)

Pregnancy Category: X

Thalomid **(Rx)**

Classification: Dermatologic drug

Action/Kinetics: Immunomodulatory drug; mechanism of action not known. Drug may suppress excessive tumor necrosis factor–alpha (TNF–α) production and down–modulation of selected cell surface adhesion molecules involved in leukocyte migration. **Peak plasma levels:** 2.9–5.7 hr. High fat meals increase the time to peak plasma levels to about 6 hr. **t½:** 5–7 hr. Metabolized in the plasma and excreted in the urine.

Uses: Acute treatment of moderate to severe erythema nodosum leprosum (ENL). Maintenance therapy for prevention and suppression of the cutaneous symptoms of erythema nodosum leprosum recurrence.

Contraindications: Never to be used in pregnancy or in those who could become pregnant while taking the drug (even a single 50 mg dose can cause severe birth defects). Use in males unless the client meets several conditions (see package insert). Use as monotherapy for ENL in the presence of moderate to severe neuritis. Lactation.

Special Concerns: Due to possible birth defects, thalidomide is marketed only under a special restricted distribution program called the "System for Thalidomide Education and Prescribing Safety (STEPS). Under this program only prescribers and pharmacists registered with the program are allowed to prescribe and dispense the drug. Safety and efficacy have not been determined in children less than 12 years of age.

Side Effects: *Note:* Only the most common side effects are listed. **Human teratogenicity.** *GI:* Constipation, diarrhea, nausea, oral moniliasis, tooth pain, abdominal pain. *CNS:* Drowsiness, somnolence, dizziness, tremor, vertigo, headache. *Neurologic:* Peripheral neuropathy. *CV:* Orthostatic hypotension, bradycardia. *Respiratory:* Pharyngitis, rhinitis, sinusitis. *Hematologic:* Neutropenia. *Hypersensitivity:* Erythematous macular rash, fever, tachycardia, hypotension. *Dermatologic:* Photosensitivity, rash, dermatitis, fungal nail disorder, pruritus. *Musculoskeletal:* Back pain, neck pain, neck rigidity. *Miscellaneous:* HIV viral load increase, impotence, peripheral edema, accidental injury, asthenia, chills, facial edema, malaise, pain.

Drug Interactions

Alcohol / Enhanced sedative effects

Barbiturates / Enhanced sedative effects

Chlorpromazine / Enhanced sedative effects

Reserpine / Enhanced sedative effects

How Supplied: *Capsules:* 50 mg

Dosage

- **Capsules**

Cutaneous ENL, initial therapy.

Adults, initial: 100–300 mg once daily with water, preferably at bedtime and at least 1 hr after the evening meal. Clients weighing less then 50 kg should be started at the low end of the dose range. In those with severe cutaneous ENL or who have required higher doses previously, dosing may be started at doses up to 400 mg once daily at bedtime or in divided doses with water 1 hr after meals. Continue initial dosing until signs and symptoms of active reaction have been eliminated (usually at least 2 weeks). Following this, taper clients off medication in 50 mg decrements q 2 to 4 weeks.

Maintenance therapy for prevention and suppression of ENL recurrence.

Maintain on the minimum dose (see initial therapy) necessary to control the reaction. Attempt tapering of medication q 3 to 6 months, in decrements of 50 mg q 2 to 4 weeks.

HEALTH CARE CONSIDERATIONS

Administration/Storage

1. The product is supplied only to pharmacists registered with the STEPS program. The drug is dispensed in no more than a 1–month supply and only on presentation of a new prescription written within the previous 14 days.
2. Specific informed consent and compliance with the mandatory client registry and survey are required of all male and female clients prior to dispensing the drug. The drug must not be repackaged.

Assessment

1. Record characteristics of leprosy, noting number of painful skin nodules and any systemic manifestations (fever, neuritis, malaise). List other agents trialed and outcome.
2. Obtain negative pregnancy test. Drug is teratogenic; only one dose taken during pregnancy can cause severe birth defects. Pregnancy tests will be performed weekly during the first month of therapy and then monthly thereafter with regular menses and every two weeks with irregular menses.
3. Drug will only be dispensed under a restricted distribution program (STEPS) requiring written consent.

4. If HIV-seropositive, monitor viral load the first and third month of treatment and then every 3 mo.

Client/Family Teaching

1. Take as prescribed at least one hr after evening meal or at bedtime unless otherwise directed.
2. May cause dizziness/drowsiness; avoid activities that require mental acuity.
3. Avoid alcohol and CNS depressants.
4. Women of child bearing age must practice two methods of reliable birth control or abstain continously from heterosexual sexual intercourse. Males must always wear a latex condom when engaging in sexual intercourse with women of childbearing age, despite successful vasectomy.
5. Report any numbness, tingling, pain, or burning in the hands or feet. Peripheral neuropathy may occur and may be irreversible.
6. During therapy do not donate blood or sperm.
7. Drug is continued until S&S of active reaction subsides (approx. 2 weeks). The dosage may then be tapered by provider every 2-4 weeks.
8. Drug will be dispensed in a one month supply only and upon presentation of a valid prescription written within past 14 days.
9. Drug therapy requires informed consent and compliance with the mandatory patient registry and survey prior to dispensing.

Outcome/Evaluate: Suppression of cutaneous manifestations with ENL

Theophylline

(thee-OFF-ih-lin)

Pregnancy Category: C

Immediate-release Capsules, Tablets, Liquid Products: Accurbron, Aquaphyllin, Asmalix, Bronkodyl, Elixomin, Elixophyllin, Lanophyllin, Lixolin, Pulmophylline ✦, Quibron-T/SR ✦, Quibron-T Dividose, Slo-Phyllin, Solu-Phyllin, Somnophyllin-T, Theo, Theoclear-80, Theolair, Theolixir ✦, Theomar, Theostat-80, Truxophyllin. **Timed-release Capsules and Tablets:** Aerolate III, Aerolate Jr., Aerolate Sr., Apo-Theo LA ✦, Novo-Theophyl SR ✦, Quibron-T/SR Dividose, Respid, Slo-Bid Gyrocaps, Slo-Phyllin Gyrocaps, Somophyllin-CRT, Sustaire, Theo-24, Theo 250, Theobid Duracaps, Theoclear L.A.-130 Cenules, Theoclear L.A.-260 Cenules, Theocot, Theochron, Theochron-SR ✦, Theo-Dur, Theo-SR ✦, Theolair ✦, Theolair-SR, Theospan-SR, Theo-SR ✦, Theo-Time, Theophylline SR, Theovent Long-Acting, Uni-Dur, Uniphyl **(Rx)**

Classification: Antiasthmatic, bronchodilator

See also *Theophylline Derivatives*.

Action/Kinetics: Time to peak serum levels, oral solution: 1 hr; **uncoated tablets:** 2 hr; **chewable tablets:** 1–1.5 hr; **enteric-coated tablets:** 5 hr; **extended-release capsules and tablets:** 4–7 hr. In healthy adults, about 60% is bound to plasma protein whereas in neonates 36% is bound to plasma protein.

Additional Uses: Oral liquid: Neonatal apnea as a respiratory stimulant. Theophylline and dextrose injection: Respiratory stimulant in neonatal apnea and Cheyne-Stokes respiration.

How Supplied: *Capsule, extended release:* 50 mg, 65 mg, 75 mg, 100 mg, 125 mg, 130 mg, 200 mg, 260 mg, 300 mg, 400 mg; *Elixir:* 80 mg/15 mL; *Solution:* 80 mg/15 mL; *Syrup:* 80 mg/15 mL; *Tablet:* 100 mg, 125 mg, 200 mg, 250 mg, 300 mg; *Tablet, extended release:* 100 mg, 200 mg, 250 mg, 300 mg, 400 mg, 450 mg, 500 mg, 600 mg

Dosage

- **Capsules, Tablets, Elixir, Oral Solution, Syrup**

See *Dosage* for *Oral Solution, Tablets*, under *Aminophylline*.

- **Extended-Release Capsules, Extended-Release Tablets**

See *Dosage* for *Extended-Release Tablets*, under *Aminophylline*.

- **Elixir, Oral Solution, Oral Suspension, Syrup**

Bronchodilator, chronic therapy.

9–12 years: 20 mg/kg/day; **6–9 years:** 24 mg/kg/day.

Neonatal apnea.

Loading dose: Using the equivalent of anhydrous theophylline administered by NGT, 5 mg/kg; **maintenance:** 2 mg/kg/day in two to three divided doses given by NGT.

HEALTH CARE CONSIDERATIONS

See also *Health Care Considerations* for *Theophylline Derivatives*.

Administration/Storage

1. Dosage is individualized to maintain serum levels of 10–20 mcg/mL.
2. Calculate dosage based on lean body weight (theophylline does not distribute to body fat).
3. Monitor serum theophylline levels in chronic therapy, especially if the maximum maintenance doses are used or exceeded.
4. The extended-release tablets or capsules are not recommended for children less than 6 years of age. Dosage for once-a-day products has not been established in children less than 12 years of age.

Assessment

1. Record onset, duration, and characteristics

of symptoms, other agents prescribed, and the outcome.
2. Describe pulmonary assessment findings and note PFTs and ABGs.
3. If switching from IV therapy, wait 4 hr before administering intermediate-release forms; may administer extended-release when IV d/c.

Client/Family Teaching

1. Take with food or milk to minimize GI upset.
2. Take only as prescribed; more is not better.
3. Do not crush or break slow-release forms of the drug.
4. Avoid cigarette smoking; decreases drug's effectiveness.
5. Caffeine- and xanthine-containing beverages and foods (chocolate, coffee, colas) and daily intake of charbroiled foods should be avoided; tend to increase drug side effects.
6. Consume at least 2 L/day of fluids to decrease secretion viscosity.
7. Do not take any OTC cough, cold, or breathing preparations without provider approval.
8. Report if symptoms do not improve or worsen with therapy.
9. Report any adverse side effects; report for serum drug levels.

Outcome/Evaluate

• Improved airway exchange; ease in secretion removal and breathing
• Stimulation of respirations in the neonate
• Therapeutic serum drug levels (10–20 mcg/mL)

Thiabendazole

(thigh-ah-**BEN**-dah-zohl)
Pregnancy Category: C
Mintezol **(Rx)**
Classification: Anthelmintic

See also *Anthelmintics*.

Action/Kinetics: Interferes with the enzyme fumarate reductase, which is specific to several helminths. Readily absorbed from the GI tract. **Peak plasma levels:** 1–2 hr. **t½:** 0.9–2 hr. Most excreted within 24 hr, mainly through the urine.

Uses: Primarily for threadworm infections, cutaneous larva migrans, visceral larva migrans when these infections occur alone or if pinworm is also present. Use in the following infections only if specific therapy is not available or cannot be used or if a second drug is desirable: hookworm, whipworm, large roundworm. To reduce symptoms of trichinosis during the invasive phase.

Contraindications: Lactation. Use in mixed infections with ascaris as it may cause worms to migrate.

Special Concerns: Safety and efficacy not established in children less than 13.6 kg. Use with caution in clients with hepatic disease or impaired hepatic function.

Side Effects: *GI:* N&V, anorexia, diarrhea, epigastric distress. *CNS:* Dizziness, drowsiness, headache, irritability, weariness, giddiness, numbness, psychic disturbances, collapse, ***seizures.*** *Allergic:* Pruritus, ***angioedema,*** flushing of face, chills, fever, skin rashes, ***Stevens-Johnson syndrome, anaphylaxis,*** lymphadenopathy, conjunctival injection, erythema multiforme. *Hepatic:* Jaundice, cholestasis, parenchymal liver damage. *GU:* Crystalluria, hematuria, enuresis, foul odor of urine. *Ophthalmic:* Blurred vision, abnormal sensation in the eyes, yellow appearance of objects, drying of mucous membranes. *Miscellaneous:* Tinnitus, hypotension, hyperglycemia, transient leukopenia, perianal rash, appearance of live *Ascaris* in nose and mouth.

Laboratory Test Considerations: Rarely, ↑ AST and cephalin flocculation.

OD **Management of Overdose:** *Symptoms:* Psychic changes, transient vision changes. *Treatment:* Induce vomiting or perform gastric lavage. Treat symptoms.

Drug Interactions: ↑ Serum levels of xanthines to potentially toxic levels due to ↓ breakdown by liver.

How Supplied: *Chew Tablet:* 500 mg; *Suspension:* 500 mg/5 mL

Dosage

• **Oral Suspension, Chewable Tablets**

Over 68 kg: 1.5 g/dose; **less than 68 kg:** 22 mg/kg/dose.

HEALTH CARE CONSIDERATIONS

See also *Health Care Considerations* for *Anthelmintics.*

Administration/Storage

1. Take with food to reduce stomach upset.
2. Chew chewable tablets before swallowing.
3. Cleansing enemas are not required after drug therapy.
4. For strongyloidiasis, cutaneous larva migrans, hookworm, whipworm, or roundworm; two doses daily are given for 2 days. For trichinelliasis, give two doses daily for 2–4 days. For visceral larva migrans, give two doses/day for 7 successive days.

Assessment

1. Record indications for therapy, onset and

T

duration of symptoms, and how and when acquired.
2. List agents currently prescribed to ensure none interact.

Client/Family Teaching

1. Administer with food or after meals to decrease stomach upset; chew tablets thoroughly.
2. Report any CNS disturbances, including muscular weakness and loss of mental alertness.
3. Do not operate hazardous machinery; drug may cause dizziness and drowsiness.
4. May notice a urine odor 24 hr following ingestion; this is normal.
5. Report any evidence of rash, fever, or itching immediately.

Outcome/Evaluate

- Negative consecutive stool cultures
- Eradication of infestation

Thiamine hydrochloride (Vitamin B$_1$)

(THIGH-ah-min)

Pregnancy Category: A (parenteral use)
Thiamilate (Rx: Injection; OTC: Tablets)

Action/Kinetics: Water-soluble vitamin, stable in acid solution. Decomposed in neutral or acid solutions. Required for the synthesis of thiamine pyrophosphate, a coenzyme required in carbohydrate metabolism. The maximum amount absorbed PO is 8–15 mg/day although absorption may be increased by giving in divided doses with food.

Uses: Prophylaxis and treatment of thiamine deficiency states and associated neurologic and CV symptoms. Prophylaxis and treatment of beriberi. Alcoholic neuritis, neuritis of pellagra, and neuritis of pregnancy. To correct anorexia due to thiamine insufficiency. *Investigational:* Treatment of subacute necrotizing encephalomyelopathy, maple syrup urine disease, pyruvate carboxylase deficiency, hyperalaninemia.

Special Concerns: Use with caution during lactation.

Side Effects: ***Serious hypersensitivity reactions;*** thus, intradermal testing is recommended if sensitivity is suspected. *Dermatologic:* Pruritus, urticaria, sweating, feeling of warmth. *CNS:* Weakness, restlessness. *Other:* Nausea, tightness in throat, ***angioneurotic edema,*** cyanosis, ***hemorrhage into the GI tract, pulmonary edema, CV collapse. Death has been reported.*** *Following IM use:* Induration, tenderness.

Drug Interactions: Because vitamin B$_1$ is unstable in neutral or alkaline solutions, the vitamin should not be used with substances that yield alkaline solutions, such as citrates, barbiturates, carbonates, or erythromycin lactobionate IV.

How Supplied: *Enteric Coated Tablet:* 20 mg; *Injection:* 100 mg/mL; *Tablet:* 25 mg, 50 mg, 100 mg, 250 mg, 500 mg

Dosage

- **Tablets, Enteric-Coated Tablets**

Mild beriberi or maintenance following severe beriberi.

Adults: 5–10 mg/day (as part of a multivitamin product); **infants:** 10 mg/day.

Treatment of deficiency.

Adults: 5–10 mg/day; **pediatric:** 10–50 mg/day.

Alcohol-induced deficiency.

Adults: 40 mg/day.

Dietary supplement.

Adults: 1–2 mg/day; **pediatric:** 0.3–0.5 mg/day for infants and 0.5 mg/day for children.

Genetic enzyme deficiency disease.

10–20 mg/day (up to 4 g/day has been used in some clients).

- **Slow IV**

Wet beriberi with myocardial failure.

Adults: 10–30 mg t.i.d.

- **IM**

Beriberi.

10–20 mg t.i.d. for 2 weeks. Give a PO multivitamin product containing 5–10 mg/day thiamine for 1 month to cause body saturation.

Recommended dietary allowance.

Adult males: 1.2–1.5 mg; **adult females:** 1.1 mg.

HEALTH CARE CONSIDERATIONS

Administration/Storage

IV 1. May administer direct IV undiluted over at least 5 min or may be reconstituted in dextrose or saline solution and administered with daily solution therapy.
2. Drug may enhance the effects of neuromuscular blocking agents. Have epinephrine available to treat for anaphylactic shock if large dose of thiamine ordered.

Assessment

1. Record type, onset, and characteristics of symptoms.
2. List other agents prescribed to ensure none interact.
3. Note neurologic assessment and clinical presentation.

Client/Family Teaching: Review dietary sources high in thiamine (enriched and whole grain cereals, meats, especially pork, and fresh vegetables); consult dietitian for assistance in meal plan/preparation.

Outcome/Evaluate

- Prophylaxis of deficiency
- Prevention/reduction of neuritis symptoms

Thioguanine

(thigh-oh-**GWON**-een)

Pregnancy Category: D

Lanvis ✱, TG, 6-Thioguanine (Abbreviation: 6-TG) **(Rx)**

Classification: Antimetabolite, purine analog

See also *Antineoplastic Agents.*

Action/Kinetics: Purine antagonist that is cell-cycle specific for the S phase of cell division. Converted to 6-thioguanylic acid, which in turn interferes with the synthesis of guanine nucleotides by competing with hypoxanthine and xanthine for the enzyme phosphoribosyltransferase (HGPRTase). Ultimately the synthesis of RNA and DNA is inhibited. Resistance to the drug may result from increased breakdown of 6-thioguanylic acid or loss of HGPRTase activity. Partially absorbed (30%) from GI tract. **t½:** 80 min. Detoxified by liver and excreted in the urine. More effective in children than in adults. Cross-resistance with mercaptopurine. Perform platelet counts weekly; discontinue drug if abnormally large fall in blood count is noted, indicating severe bone marrow depression.

Uses: Acute and nonlymphocytic leukemias (usually in combination with other drugs such as cyclophosphamide, cytarabine, prednisone, vincristine). Chronic myelogenous leukemia (not first-line therapy).

Contraindications: Resistance to mercaptopurine or thioguanine. Lactation.

Laboratory Test Considerations: ↑ Uric acid in blood and urine.

Additional Side Effects: Loss of vibration sense, unsteadiness of gait. ***Hepatotoxicity,*** myelosuppression (common), hyperuricemia. Adults tend to show a more rapid fall in WBC count than children.

OD Management of Overdose: *Symptoms:* N&V, hypertension, malaise, and diaphoresis may be seen immediately, which may be followed by myelosuppression and azotemia. ***Severe hematologic toxicity.*** *Treatment:* Induce vomiting if client is seen immediately after an acute overdosage. Treat symptoms. Hematologic toxicity may be treated by platelet transfusions (for bleeding) and granulocyte transfusions. Antibiotics are indicated for sepsis.

How Supplied: *Tablet:* 40 mg

Dosage

- **Tablets**

Individualized and determined by hematopoietic response.

Adults and pediatric, initial: 2 mg/kg/day (or 75–100 mg/m²) given at one time. From 2 to 4 weeks may elapse before beneficial results become apparent. Compute dose to nearest multiple of 20 mg. If no response, dosage may be increased to 3 mg/kg/day. **Usual maintenance dose (even during remissions):** 2–3 mg/kg/day (or 100 mg/m²). Dosage of thioguanine does not have to be decreased during administration of allopurinol (to inhibit uric acid production).

HEALTH CARE CONSIDERATIONS

See also *Health Care Considerations* for *Antineoplastic Agents.*

Assessment

1. Record indications for therapy, onset, duration, and characteristics of symptoms; list other agents trialed and the outcome.
2. Monitor CBC, uric acid, liver and renal function studies. Obtain CBC weekly and LFTs monthly during course of therapy; may cause granulocyte and platelet suppression. Nadir: 10 days; recovery: 21 days.

Interventions

1. Provide assistance to those who may experience loss of vibration sense and have unsteady gait (may be unable to rely on canes).
2. Expect hyperuricemia after tumor lysis, which may be reduced with administration of allopurinol, by preventing purine breakdown and excessive uric acid formation.

Client/Family Teaching

1. Take on an empty stomach for best results.
2. Increase fluid intake (2–3 L/day) to minimize hyperuricemia and hyperuricosuria.
3. Withhold drug and report if jaundice, decreased urine output, diarrhea, S&S of anemia (fatigue, dyspnea), or extremity swelling occurs.
4. Any sore throat, fever, or flu-like symptoms as well as increased bruising and bleeding tendencies require immediate reporting.
5. Avoid crowds, vaccinia, and persons with infectious diseases.
6. Practice reliable contraception.

Outcome/Evaluate

- Suppression of malignant cell proliferation
- Hematologic evidence of leukemia remission

T

Thioridazine hydrochloride

(thigh-oh-**RID**-ah-zeen)

Pregnancy Category: C

Apo-Thioridazine ✦, Mellaril, Mellaril-S, Novo-Ridazine ✦, PMS-Thioridazine ✦, Thioridazine HCl Intensol Oral **(Rx)**

Classification: Antipsychotic, piperidine-type phenothiazine

See also *Antipsychotic Agents, Phenothiazines.*

Action/Kinetics: High incidence of hypotension; moderate incidence of sedative and anticholinergic effects and weak antiemetic and extrapyramidal effects. May be used in clients intolerant of other phenothiazines. **Peak plasma levels** (after PO administration): 1–4 hr. May impair its own absorption at higher doses due to the strong anticholinergic effects. **t½:** 10 hr. Metabolized in the liver to both active and inactive metabolites.

Uses: Management of psychotic disorders. Short-term treatment of moderate to marked depression with variable levels of anxiety in adults. Treat psychoneurotic symptoms in geriatric clients, including agitation, anxiety, depressed mood, tension, sleep disturbances, and fears. **In children:** Treat severe behavioral problems marked by combativeness or explosive hyperexcitable behavior. Short-term treatment of hyperactive children showing excessive motor activity with accompanying impulsivity, short attention span, aggressivity, mood lability, and poor frustration tolerance.

Special Concerns: Safe use during pregnancy has not been established. Dosage has not been established in children less than 2 years of age. Geriatric, emaciated, or debilitated clients usually require a lower initial dose.

T

Additional Side Effects: More likely to cause pigmentary retinopathy than other phenothiazines.

How Supplied: *Oral Concentrate:* 30 mg/mL, 100 mg/mL; *Tablet:* 10 mg, 15 mg, 25 mg, 50 mg, 100 mg, 150 mg, 200 mg

Dosage

- **Oral Suspension, Oral Solution, Tablets**

Psychotic disorders.

Adults, initial: 50–100 mg t.i.d. Increase gradually to a maximum of 800 mg/day, if needed to control symptoms. Then, reduce gradually to the minimum maintainence dose. Dose range: 200–800 mg/day divided into two to four doses.

Psychoneurotic symptoms.

Initial: 25 mg t.i.d. Dose range: 10 mg b.i.d.–q.i.d. in milder cases to 50 mg t.i.d. or q.i.d. Dose range: 20–200 mg/day.

Behavioral disorders in children.

Ages 2 to 12: 0.5 mg/kg/day to a maximum of 3 mg/kg/day. For moderate disorders, initially use 10 mg b.i.d.–t.i.d. For hospitalized, severely disturbed or psychotic children: 25 mg b.i.d.–t.i.d.

HEALTH CARE CONSIDERATIONS

See also *Health Care Considerations* for *Antineoplastic Agents.*

Administration/Storage: Dilute each dose of concentrate just before administration with distilled water, acidified tap water, or suitable juices. Preparation and storage of bulk dilutions are not recommended.

Assessment

1. Record mental status; assess behavioral manifestations. Note behaviors requiring treatment and presence/type of hallucinations if evident.
2. Monitor ECG, CBC, liver and renal function studies.

Client/Family Teaching

1. Take only as directed; do not stop abruptly, as withdrawal may activate N&V, gastritis, dizziness, tachycardia, headache, and insomnia.
2. Drug may cause drowsiness.
3. Wear protective clothing and sunscreens to prevent a photosensitivity reaction.
4. May cause retinal deposits viewed as a "browning of vision."
5. May impair temperature regulation; avoid temperature extremes and dress appropriately.
6. Doses exceeding 300 mg/day may cause reversible T-wave abnormalities on ECG. Doses above 800 mg/day have been associated with retinal deposits and cardiac toxicity.

Outcome/Evaluate

- ↓ Agitation, combativeness or explosive hyperexcitable behaviors and improved coping mechanisms
- ↓ Anxiety levels; ↓ depression; ↓ sleep disturbances

Thiothixene

(thigh-oh-**THICKS**-een)

Pregnancy Category: C

Navane, Thiothixene HCl Intensol **(Rx)**

Classification: Antipsychotic, miscellaneous

Action/Kinetics: Mechanism of action may be due to blockade of postsynaptic dopamine receptors in the brain, especially at subcortical levels in the reticular formation, hypothalamus, and limbic system. Also causes cholinergic and alpha-adrenergic blocking effects, adrenergic potentiating effects, antiserotonin effects, and prevention of uptake of biogenic amines. This results in significant extrapyramidal symptoms and antiemetic effects and minimal sedation, orthostatic hypotension, and anticholinergic symptoms. The margin between a therapeutically effective dose and one that causes extrapyramidal symptoms is narrow. Well absorbed from the GI tract. **Peak plasma levels, PO:** 1–3 hr. **t½:** 34 hr. A therapeutic response may occur within 1 to 6 hr following IM use and within a few days to several weeks following PO use. Metabolized in the liver and excreted in the feces as both unchanged drug and metabolites.

Uses: Symptomatic treatment of psychotic disorders, including withdrawn, apathetic schizophrenia, delusions, and hallucinations.

Contraindications: Use in clients with circulatory collapse, comatose states, CNS depression due to any cause, and blood dyscrasias. Hypersensitivity to thiothixene and possibly phenothiazine derivatives. Use in children less than 12 years of age.

Special Concerns: Use with caution in CV disease, glaucoma, and prostatic hypertrophy, and in those exposed to extreme heat. Use with extreme caution in those with a history of seizure disorders, alcohol withdrawal, and in clients who develop akathisia and restlessness. Use during pregnancy only when potential benefits outweigh possible risks to the mother and/or fetus.

Side Effects: Since thiothixene has pharmacologic properties similar to phenothiazines, the side effects associated with phenothiazines should also be consulted. *CNS:* Drowsiness, extrapyramidal symptoms (especially akathisia and dystonia), persistent tardive dyskinesia (especially in female geriatric clients), lethargy, dizziness, restlessness, lightheadedness, agitation, insomnia, hyperpyrexia, weakness, fatigue. Rarely, seizures and paradoxical exacerbation of psychoses. *GI:* Dry mouth, constipation, increased salivation, adynamic ileus, anorexia, N&V, diarrhea, increase in appetite and weight, cholestatic jaundice. *CV:* Orthostatic hypotension, tachycardia, syncope, ECG changes. *Ophthlamic:* Blurred vision, miosis, mydriasis. *Hypersensitivity:* Rash, pruritus, urticaria, photosensitivity, ***anaphylaxis (rare)***. *GU:* Impotence, lactation, moderate breast enlargement in women, amenorrhea. *Hematologic:* Leukopenia, leukocytosis. *Miscellaneous:* ***Neuroleptic malignant syndrome.*** Increased sweating, nasal congestion, impotence, leg cramps, polydypsia, peripheral edema, fine lenticular pigmentation.

Laboratory Test Considerations: ↑ Serum transaminase, alkaline phosphatase, uric acid excretion. ↓ Prothrombin time.

OD **Management of Overdose:** *Symptoms:* Muscle twitching, drowsiness, dizziness. In severe cases, symptoms include rigidity, weakness, torticollis, tremor, salivation, dysphagia, disturbance of gait, CNS depression, coma. *Treatment:* General supportive measures, including maintaining an adequate airway and oxygenation. Gastric lavage, if overdose found early. Hypotension and circulatory collapse may be treated with IV fluids and/or vasopressor agents (epinephrine is not to be used). Antiparkinson drugs may be used to treat extrapyramidal symptoms. Do *not* use analeptic drugs.

Drug Interactions

Anticholinergic drugs / Additive or potentiation of anticholinergic effect

CNS depressants / Additive or potentiation of depressant effect

Hypotensive drugs / Additive or potentiation of hypotensive effect

How Supplied: *Capsules:* 1 mg, 2 mg, 5 mg, 10 mg, 20 mg; *Concentrate:* 5 mg/mL

Dosage

- **Capsules, Concentrate**

Mild to moderate psychoses.

Adults, initial: 2 mg t.i.d., increased to 15 mg/day if necessary.

Severe psychoses.

Adults, initial: 5 mg b.i.d., increased to 60 mg/day if necessary. The usual optimum dose is 20–30 mg/day. Doses greater than 60 mg/day rarely increase the therapeutic effect.

HEALTH CARE CONSIDERATIONS

See also *Health Care Considerations* for *Antipsychotics*.

Administration/Storage: For maintenance therapy, a single daily dose may be adequate.

Assessment

1. Record onset, duration, and characteristics of symptoms. List other agents trialed and the outcome.
2. Assess baseline mental status, noting mood, behavior, and any evidence of depression.
3. List drugs currently prescribed to ensure none interact.
4. Avoid drug with CNS depression, circulatory collapse, coma, blood dyscrasias, or uncontrolled seizure disorder.
5. Monitor CBC, LFTs, and ECG.

T

Client/Family Teaching
1. Take exactly as prescribed; do not stop abruptly.
2. Drug may cause sedation, orthostatic hypotension, and visual disturbances. Do not engage in activities that require mental alertness.
3. Drug may cause tardive dyskinesias (slow, automatic movements) and extrapyramidal symptoms (tremor, twisting repetitive jerks); report so dosage can be adjusted or other meds prescribed to combat symptoms.
4. Consume plenty of fluids to prevent dehydration and constipation.
5. Report any elevation in body temperature, feeling of weakness, or sore throat; S&S of blood dyscrasias.
6. May cause a photosensitivity reaction; use suncsreen and protective clothing when exposed.
7. Avoid alcohol, OTC agents or CNS depressants.
8. Drug may cause menstrual irregularity, false positive pregnancy test, breast enlargement, decreased libido, and a pink brown discoloration of urine.
9. Report any evidence of yellow skin discoloration or RUQ abdominal pain as drug may cause cholestatic jaundice.
10. Report as scheduled for F/U ECG, lab work, psychotherapy, prescription renewal, and evaluation of mental status.

Outcome/Evaluate: ↓ Excitable, withdrawn, agitated, or paranoid behaviors.

Tiagabine hydrochloride

(tye-**AG**-ah-been)
Pregnancy Category: C
Gabatril **(Rx)**
Classification: Anticonvulsant, miscellaneous

T

See also *Anticonvulsants.*

Action/Kinetics: Mechanism not known but activity of GABA, an inhibitory neurotransmitter, may be enhanced. Drug may block uptake of GABA into presynaptic neurons allowing more GABA to bind to post-synaptic cells. This prevents propagation of neural impulses that contribute to seizures due to GABA-ergic action. **Peak plasma levels:** About 45 min when fasting. High fat meals decrease rate but not extent of absorption. Metabolized in liver; excreted in urine and feces. **t½, elimination:** 7–9 hr. Diurnal effect occurs with levels being lower in evening compared with morning.

Uses: Adjunctive therapy for partial seizures.

Contraindications: Lactation.

Special Concerns: Safety and efficacy have not been determined in children less than 12 years old.

Side Effects: *CNS:* Dizziness, asthenia, somnolence, nervousness, tremor, insomnia, difficulty with concentration or attention, ataxia, confusion, speech disorder, difficulty with memory, paresthesia, depression, emotional lability, abnormal gait, hostility, nystagmus, problems with language, agitation. *GI:* N&V, diarrhea, increased appetite, mouth ulceration. *Respiratory:* Pharyngitis, increased cough. *Dermatologic:* Rash, pruritus. *Miscellaneous:* Abdominal pain, unspecified pain, vasodilation, myasthenia.

OD **Management of Overdose:** *Symptoms:* Somnolence, impaired consciousness, agitation, confusion, speech difficulties, depression, weakness, myoclonus. *Treatment:* Emesis or gastric lavage, maintain an airway. General supportive treatment.

Drug Interactions
Carbamazepine / ↑ Clearance due to ↑ metabolism
Phenobarbital / ↑ Clearance due to ↑ metabolism
Phenytoin / ↑ Clearance due to ↑ metabolism
Valproate / ↑ Clearance due to ↑ metabolism

How Supplied: *Tablets:* 4 mg, 12 mg, 16 mg, 20 mg

Dosage
- **Tablets**

Partial seizures.

Adults and children over 18 years, initial: 4 mg once daily. Total daily dose may be increased by 4 to 8 mg at weekly intervals until clinical effect is observed or daily dose is 56 mg/day. **Children, 12 to 18 years, initial:** 4 mg once daily. Total daily dose may be increased by 4 mg at beginning of week 2. Thereafter, dose may be increased by 4 to 8 mg at weekly intervals until clinical effect is seen or dose is 32 mg/day. For all ages, give total daily dose in 2 to 4 divided doses.

HEALTH CARE CONSIDERATIONS

See also *Health Care Considerations* for *Anticonvulsants.*

Administration/Storage
1. It is not necessary to modify dose of concomitant anticonvulsant drugs, unless clinically indicated.
2. Dose must be titrated in those taking enzyme-inducing anticonvulsant drugs; consult package insert.

Assessment
1. Record indications for therapy, characteristics of seizures, other agents trialed and outcome.

2. Monitor LFTs; decrease dosage or dosing intervals with dysfunction.

Client/Family Teaching

1. Take with food as directed.
2. Do not perform activities requiring mental alertness until drug effects realized; may cause dizziness, sleepiness, or confusion.
3. Report any increased frequency or loss of seizure control, rash, weakness, or visual disturbances.
4. Do not stop abruptly; may trigger seizures.
5. Practice reliable contraception; do not breast feed.

Outcome/Evaluate: Control of seizures

Ticlopidine hydrochloride

(tie-**KLOH**-pih-deen)

Pregnancy Category: B

Ticlid **(Rx)**

Classification: Platelet aggregation inhibitor

Action/Kinetics: Irreversibly inhibits ADP-induced platelet-fibrinogen binding and subsequent platelet-platelet interactions. This results in inhibition of both platelet aggregation and release of platelet granule constituents as well as prolongation of bleeding time. **Peak plasma levels:** 2 hr. **Maximum platelet inhibition:** 8–11 days after 250 mg b.i.d. **Steady-state plasma levels:** 14–21 days. **t½, elimination:** 4–5 days. After discontinuing therapy, bleeding time and other platelet function tests return to normal within 14 days. Rapidly absorbed; bioavailability is increased by food. Highly bound (98%) to plasma proteins. Extensively metabolized by the liver with approximately 60% excreted through the kidneys; 23% is excreted in the feces (with one-third excreted unchanged). Clearance of the drug decreases with age.

Uses: To reduce the risk of fatal or nonfatal thrombotic stroke in clients who have manifested precursors of stroke or who have had a completed thrombotic stroke. Due to the risk of neutropenia or agranulocytosis, use should be reserved for clients who are intolerant to aspirin therapy. *Investigational:* Chronic arterial occlusion, coronary artery bypass grafts, intermittent claudication, open heart surgery, primary glomerulonephritis, subarachnoid hemorrhage, sickle cell disease, uremic clients with AV shunts or fistulas.

Contraindications: Use in the presence of neutropenia and thrombocytopenia, hemostatic disorder, or active pathologic bleeding such as bleeding peptic ulcer or intracranial bleeding. Severe liver impairment. Lactation.

Special Concerns: Use with caution in clients with ulcers (i.e., where there is a propensity for bleeding). Consider reduced dosage in impaired renal function. Geriatric clients may be more sensitive to the effects of the drug. Severe hematological side effects (including thrombotic thrombocytopenic purpura) may occur within a few days of the start of ticlopidine therapy. Safety and effectiveness have not been established in children less than 18 years of age.

Side Effects: *Hematologic:* Neutropenia, ***agranulocytosis,*** thrombocytopenia, pancytopenia, thrombotic thrombocytopenia purpura, immune thrombocytopenia, ***hemolytic anemia with reticulocytosis.*** *GI:* Diarrhea, N&V, GI pain, dyspepsia, flatulence, anorexia, GI fullness. *Bleeding complications:* Ecchymosis, hematuria, epistaxis, conjunctival hemorrhage, ***GI bleeding,*** perioperative bleeding, ***intracerebral bleeding (rare).*** *Dermatologic:* Maculopapular or urticarial rash, pruritus, urticaria. *CNS:* Dizziness, headache. *Neuromuscular:* Asthenia, SLE, peripheral neuropathy, arthropathy, myositis. *Miscellaneous:* Tinnitus, pain, allergic pneumonitis, vasculitis, hepatitis, cholestatic jaundice, nephrotic syndrome, hyponatremia, serum sickness.

Laboratory Test Considerations: ↑ Alkaline phosphatase, ALT, AST, serum cholesterol, and triglycerides.

Drug Interactions

Antacids / ↓ Plasma levels of ticlopidine
Aspirin / Ticlopidine ↑ effect of aspirin on collagen-induced platelet aggregation
Carbamazepine / ↑ Plasma levels of carbamazepine → toxicity
Cimetidine / ↓ Clearance of ticlopidine probably due to ↓ breakdown by liver
Digoxin / Slight ↓ in digoxin plasma levels
Theophylline / ↑ Plasma levels of theophylline due to ↓ clearance

How Supplied: *Tablet:* 250 mg

Dosage

- **Tablets**

Reduce risk of thrombotic stroke.
250 mg b.i.d.

HEALTH CARE CONSIDERATIONS

Administration/Storage

1. To increase bioavailability and decrease GI discomfort, take with food or just after eating.
2. If switched from an anticoagulant or fibrinolytic drug to ticlopidine, discontinue the former drug before initiation of ticlopidine therapy.
3. IV methylprednisolone (20 mg) may nor-

T

malize prolonged bleeding times, usually within 2 hr.

Assessment

1. Note any liver disease, bleeding disorders, or ulcer disease.
2. Ascertain aspirin intolerance.
3. Determine baseline hematologic profile (e.g., CBC, PT, PTT, INR), liver and renal function studies.
4. Monitor blood biweekly to screen for possibly fatal thrombotic thrombocytopenic purpura.

Client/Family Teaching

1. Take with food or after meals to minimize GI upset.
2. It may take longer than usual to stop bleeding; report unusual bleeding as severe hematological side effects may occur.
3. Brush teeth with a soft-bristle tooth brush, use an electric razor for shaving, wear shoes when ambulating, use caution and avoid injury, as bleeding times may be prolonged.
4. During the first 3 months of therapy, neutropenia can occur, resulting in an increased risk of infection. Come for scheduled blood tests and report any symptoms of infection (e.g., fever, chills, sore throat).
5. Any severe or persistent diarrhea, SC bleeding, skin rashes, or evidence of cholestasis (e.g., yellow skin or sclera, dark urine, light-colored stools) should be reported.

Outcome/Evaluate: Prevention of a complete or recurrent cerebral thrombotic event

Tiludronate disodium

(tye-**LOO**-droh-nayt)

Pregnancy Category: C

Skelid **(Rx)**

Classification: Bone growth regulator

Action/Kinetics: Inhibits activity of osteoclasts and decreases bone turnover. Does not interfere with bone mineralization. Poorly absorbed from GI tract when fasting and in presence of food. **Peak serum levels:** 2 hr. Not metabolized; excreted in urine. **t½:** About 150 hr.

Uses: Treatment of Paget's disease where level of serum alkaline phosphatase is at least twice upper limit of normal, in those who are symptomatic, or who are at risk for future complications of disease.

Contraindications: Not recommended for those with C_{CR} less than 30 mL/min.

Special Concerns: Use with caution during lactation and in those with dysphagia, symptomatic esophageal disease, gastritis, duodenitis, or ulcers. Safety and efficacy have not been determined in children.

Side Effects: *GI:* Diarrhea, N&V, dyspepsia, flatulence, tooth disorder, abdominal pain, constipation, dry mouth, gastritis. *Body as whole:* Pain, back pain, accidental injury, flu-like symptoms, chest pain, asthenia, syncope, fatigue, flushing. *CNS:* Headache, dizziness, paresthesia, vertigo, anorexia, somnolence, anxiety, nervousness, insomnia. *CV:* Dependent edema, peripheral edema, hypertension, syncope. *Musculoskeletal:* Arthralgia, arthrosis, pathological fracture, involuntary muscle contractions. *Respiratory:* Rhinitis, sinusitis, URTI, coughing, pharyngitis, bronchitis. *Dermatologic:* Rash, skin disorder, pruritus, increased sweating, Stevens-Johnson type syndrome (rare). *Ophthalmic:* Cataract, conjunctivitis, glaucoma. *Miscellaneous:* Hyperparathyroidism, vitamin D deficiency, UTI, infection.

OD **Management of Overdose:** *Symptoms:* Hypocalcemia. *Treatment:* Supportive.

Drug Interactions

Antacids, aluminum- or magnesium-containing / ↓ Bioavailability of tiludronate when taken 1 hr before tiludronate
Aspirin / ↓ Bioavailability of tiludronate by 50% when taken 2 hr after tiludronate
Calcium / ↓ Bioavailability of tiludronate when taken at same time
Indomethacin / ↑ Bioavailability of tiludronate by two- to four-fold

How Supplied: *Tablets:* 200 mg

Dosage

- **Tablets**

Paget's disease.

Adults: Single 400 mg dose/day taken with 6 to 8 oz of plain water for period of only 3 months.

HEALTH CARE CONSIDERATIONS

Administration/Storage

1. Take calcium or mineral supplements at least 2 hr before or after tiludronate. Take aluminum- or magnesium-containing antacids at least 2 hr after tiludronate.
2. Allow an interval of 3 months to assess response.
3. Do not remove tablets from the foil strips until just before use.

Client/Family Teaching

1. Take with 6 to 8 oz of plain water. Do not take within 2 hr of food. Beverages other than water, food, and some medications reduce absorption of tiludronate.
2. Do not take aspirin, indomethacin, or calcium or mineral supplements within 2 hr of taking drug.
3. Do not remove tablets from foil strips until they are to be used.

4. May experience nausea, diarrhea, and GI upset; report if severe.
5. Report any rashes, itching, hives, severe stomach pains, bloody or black tarry stools.
6. Consume diet high in calcium and vitamin D.

Outcome/Evaluate: Inhibition of Paget's disease progression

Timolol maleate

(TIE-moh-lohl)

Pregnancy Category: C

Apo-Timol ✱, Apo-Timop ✱, Beta-Tim ✱, Blocadren, Gen-Timolol ✱, Med-Timolol ✱, Novo-Timol ✱, Nu-Timolol ✱, Tim-Ak ✱, Timoptic, Timoptic in Acudose, Timoptic-XE **(Rx)**

Classification: Ophthalmic agent, beta-adrenergic blocking agent

See also *Beta-Adrenergic Blocking Agents.*

Action/Kinetics: Exerts both beta-1- and beta-2-adrenergic blocking activity. Has minimal sympathomimetic effects, direct myocardial depressant effects, or local anesthetic action. Does not cause pupillary constriction or night blindness. The mechanism of the protective effect in MI is not known. **Peak plasma levels:** 1–2 hr. **t½:** 4 hr. Metabolized in the liver. Metabolites and unchanged drug excreted through the kidney.Also reduces both elevated and normal IOP, whether or not glaucoma is present; thought to act by reducing aqueous humor formation and/or by slightly increasing outflow of aqueous humor. Does not affect pupil size or visual acuity. For use in eye: **Onset:** 30 min. **Maximum effect:** 1–2 hr. **Duration:** 24 hr.

Uses: Tablets: Hypertension (alone or in combination with other antihypertensives such as thiazide diuretics). Within 1–4 weeks of MI to reduce risk of reinfarction. Prophylaxis of migraine. *Investigational:* Ventricular arrhythmias and tachycardias, essential tremors.

Ophthalmic solution (Timoptic): Lower IOP in chronic open-angle glaucoma, selected cases of secondary glaucoma, ocular hypertension, aphakic (no lens) clients with glaucoma. *Ophthalmic gel forming solution (Timoptic-XE):* Reduce elevated IOP in glaucoma.

Contraindications: Hypersensitivity to drug. Bronchial asthma or bronchospasm including severe COPD.

Special Concerns: Use ophthalmic preparation with caution in clients for whom systemic beta-adrenergic blocking agents are contraindicated. Safe use in children not established.

Side Effects: *Systemic following use of tablets:* See *Beta-Adrenergic Blocking Agents.*

Following use of ophthalmic product: Few. Occasionally, ocular irritation, local hypersensitivity reactions, slight decrease in resting HR.

Laboratory Test Considerations: ↑ BUN, serum potassium, and uric acid. ↓ H&H.

Drug Interactions: When used ophthalmically, possible potentiation with systemically administered beta-adrenergic blocking agents.

How Supplied: *Gel forming solution:* 0.25%, 0.5%; *Ophthalmic solution:* 0.25%, 0.5%; *Tablet:* 5 mg, 10 mg, 20 mg

Dosage

- **Tablets**

Hypertension.

Initial: 10 mg b.i.d. alone or with a diuretic; **maintenance:** 20–40 mg/day (up to 80 mg/day in two doses may be required), depending on BP and HR. If dosage increase is necessary, wait 7 days.

MI prophylaxis in clients who have survived the acute phase.

10 mg b.i.d.

Migraine prophylaxis.

Initially: 10 mg b.i.d. **Maintenance:** 20 mg/day given as a single dose; total daily dose may be increased to 30 mg in divided doses or decreased to 10 mg, depending on the response and client tolerance. If a satisfactory response for migraine prophylaxis is not obtained within 6–8 weeks using the maximum daily dose, discontinue the drug.

Essential tremor.

10 mg/day.

- **Ophthalmic Solution (Timoptic 0.25% or 0.5%)**

Glaucoma.

1 gtt of 0.25%–0.50% solution in each eye b.i.d. If the decrease in intraocular pressure is maintained, reduce dose to 1 gtt once a day.

- **Ophthalmic Gel-Forming Solution (Timoptic-XE 0.25% or 0.5%)**

Glaucoma.

1 gtt once daily.

HEALTH CARE CONSIDERATIONS

See also *Health Care Considerations* for *Beta-Adrenergic Blocking Agents* and *Antihypertensive Agents.*

Administration/Storage

Ophthalmic Solution

1. When transferred from another antiglauco-

T

ma agent, continue old medication on day 1 of timolol therapy (1 gtt of 0.25% solution). Then, discontinue former therapy. Initiate with 0.25% solution. Increase to 0.50% solution if response is insufficient. Further dosage increases are ineffective.
2. When transferred from several antiglaucoma agents, individualize the dose. If one of the agents is a beta-adrenergic blocking agent, discontinue it before starting timolol. Dosage adjustments should involve one drug at a time at 1-week intervals. Continue the antiglaucoma drugs with the addition of timolol, 1 gtt of 0.25% solution b.i.d. (if response is inadequate, 1 gtt of 0.5% solution may be used b.i.d.). The following day, discontinue one of the other antiglaucoma agents while continuing the remaining agents or discontinue based on client response.
3. Before using the gel, invert the closed container and shake once before each use.
4. Administer other ophthalmics at least 10 min before the gel.
5. The ocular hypotensive effect has been maintained when switching clients from timolol solution given b.i.d. to the gel once daily.

Assessment

1. Record indications for therapy, onset, duration, and characteristics of symptoms.
2. Monitor liver and renal function studies.

Client/Family Teaching

1. Review procedure for ophthalmic administration.
• Apply finger lightly to lacrimal sac for 1 min following administration.
• Regular intraocular measurements by an ophthalmologist are required because ocular hypertension may recur without any overt signs or symptoms.
2. When tablets used for long-term prophylaxis against MI, do not interrupt therapy; abrupt withdrawal may precipitate reinfarction.
3. Report any evidence of rash, dizziness, heart palpitations, SOB, edema, or depression.
4. Do not perform tasks such as driving or operating machinery until drug effects are realized; may cause dizziness.
5. May cause increased sensitivity to cold; dress appropriately.
6. With diabetes, monitor FS as drug may mask S&S of hypoglycemia.
7. Continue life-style modifications (i.e., weight reduction, regular exercise, reduced intake of sodium and alcohol, and no smoking) in the overall goal of BP control.

Outcome/Evaluate

- ↓ BP
- Myocardial reinfarction prophylaxis
- Migraine prophylaxis
- ↓ Intraocular pressures

Tioconazole

(tie-oh-**KON**-ah-zohl)
Pregnancy Category: C
Gynecure ✱, Monistat 1, Trosyd AF ✱, Trosyd J ✱, Vagistat-1 **(Rx) (OTC)**
Classification: Antifungal, vaginal

Action/Kinetics: Antifungal activity thought to be due to alteration of the permeability of the cell membrane of the fungus, causing leakage of essential intracellular compounds. The systemic absorption of the drug in nonpregnant clients is negligible.
Uses: *Candida albicans* infections of the vulva and vagina. Also effective against *Torulopsis glabrata*. OTC for recurrent vaginal yeast infections in those who have previously been diagnosed and have the same symptoms again.
Contraindications: Use of a vaginal applicator during pregnancy may be contraindicated.
Special Concerns: Safety and effectiveness have not been determined during lactation or in children.
Side Effects: *GU:* Burning, itching, irritation, vulvar edema and swelling, discharge, vaginal pain, dysuria, dyspareunia, nocturia, desquamation, dryness of vaginal secretions.
How Supplied: *Ointment:* 6.5%

Dosage

• **Vaginal Ointment, 6.5%**

One applicator full (about 4.6 g) should be inserted intravaginally at bedtime for 3 days. If needed, the treatment period can be extended to 6 days. Monistat 1 is intended as a one-dose product.

HEALTH CARE CONSIDERATIONS

Administration/Storage

1. The ointment base may interact with rubber and latex; thus, avoid use of condoms or diaphragms for 3 days following treatment.
2. After use of Monistat 1, symptomatic improvement is usually seen within 3 days and complete relief within 7 days.

Assessment: Obtain a thorough health history and carefully evaluate symptoms and sources of infection.

Client/Family Teaching

1. Review appropriate method for administration (the cream should be inserted high into the vagina). Administer just prior to bedtime.

2. Continue to take for prescribed time frame even if symptoms subside. Report if burning, irritation, or pain occurs.
3. May stain clothes; use sanitary napkins during therapy and change frequently because damp napkins may harbor infecting organisms.
4. To avoid reinfection, refrain from sexual intercourse. The ointment base may interact with rubber and latex; avoid condoms or diaphragms for 3 days after treatment.
5. Use during menses to ensure a full course of therapy. Effectiveness is not altered by menstruation.
6. With Monistat 1, a one-dose product, symptomatic improvement is usually seen within 3 days and complete relief within 7 days.

Outcome/Evaluate: Resolution of fungal infection; symptomatic improvement

Tizanidine hydrochloride

(tye-**ZAN**-ih-deen)
Pregnancy Category: C
Zanaflex **(Rx)**
Classification: Skeletal muscle relaxant, centrally-acting

See also Skeletal Muscle Relaxants, Centrally Acting.

Action/Kinetics: Acts on central α-2 adrenergic receptors; reduces spasticity by increasing presynaptic inhibition of motor neurons possibly by reducing release of excitatory amino acids. Greatest effects are on polysynaptic pathways. Also may reduce postsynaptic excitatory transmitter activity, decrease the firing rate of noradrenergic locus ceruleas neurons, and inhibit synaptic transmission of nociceptive stimuli in the spinal pathways. **Peak effect:** 1–2 hr. **Duration:** 3–6 hr. Extensive first pass metabolism. **t½:** About 2.5 hr. Excreted in urine and feces. Elderly clear drug more slowly.

Uses: Acute and intermittent management of muscle spasticity.

Contraindications: Use with α-2-adrenergic agonists.

Special Concerns: Use with caution in renal impairment, in elderly and during laction. Use with extreme caution in hepatic insufficiency. Safety and efficacy have not been determined in children.

Side Effects: *Note:* Side effects listed are those with a frequency of 0.1% or greater. *CV:* Hypotension, vasodilation, postural hypotension, syncope, migraine, arrhythmia. *GI:* Hepatotoxicity, dry mouth, constipation, pharyngitis, vomiting, abdominal pain, diarrhea, dyspepsia, dysphagia, cholelithiasis, fecal impaction, flatulence, ***GI hemorrhage*** hepatitis, melena. *CNS:* Dizziness, dyskinesia, nervousness, somnolence, sedation, hallucinations, psychotic-like symptoms, depression, anxiety, paresthesia, tremor, emotional lability, seizures, paralysis, abnormal thinking, vertigo, abnormal dreams, agitation, depersonalization, euphoria, stupor, dysautonomia, neuralgia. *GU:* Urinary frequency, UTI, urinary urgency, cystitis, menorrhagia, pyelonephritis, urinary retention, kidney calculus, enlarged uterine fibroids, vaginal moniliasis, vaginitis. *Hematologic:* Ecchymosis, anemia, leukopenia, leukocytosis. *Musculoskeletal:* Myasthenia, back pain, pathological fracture, arthralgia, arthritis, bursitis. *Respiratory:* Sinusitis, pneumonia, bronchitis, rhinitis. *Dermatologic:* Rash, sweating, skin ulcer, pruritus, dry skin, acne, alopecia, urticaria. *Body as a whole:* Flu syndrome, weight loss, infection, ***sepsis, cellulitis, death,*** allergic reaction, moniliasis, malaise, asthenia, fever, abscess, edema. *Ophthalmic:* Glaucoma, amblyopia, conjunctivitis, eye pain, optic neuritis, retinal hemorrhage, visual field defect. *Otic:* Ear pain, tinnitus, deafness, otitis media. *Miscellaneous:* Speech disorder.

Laboratory Test Considerations: ↑ ALT. Abnormal LFTs. Hypercholesterolemia, hyperlipemia, hypothyroidism, adrenal cortical insufficiency, hyperglycemia, hypokalemia, hyponatremia, hypoproteinemia.

Drug Interactions

Alcohol / ↑ Side effects of tizanidine; additive CNS depressant effects
Alpha-2-Adrenergic agonists / Additive hypotensive effects
Oral contraceptives / ↓ Clearance of tizanidine

How Supplied: *Tablets:* 4 mg

Dosage

- **Tablets**

Muscle spasticity.

Initial: 4 mg; **then,** increase dose gradually in 2 to 4 mg steps to optimum effect. Dose can be repeated at 6–8-hr intervals, to maximum of 3 doses/24 hr, not to exceed 36 mg/day. There is no experience with repeated, single, daytime doses greater than 12 mg or total daily doses of 36 mg or more.

HEALTH CARE CONSIDERATIONS

See also *Health Care Considerations* for *Skeletal Muscle Relaxants, Centrally Acting.*

T

Assessment: Monitor VS, liver, and renal function studies.

Client/Family Teaching

1. Do not perform activities that require mental alertness; drug causes sedation.
2. Report if hallucinations or delusions experienced.
3. May cause orthostatic hypotension; avoid sudden changes in position.
4. Avoid alcohol and any other CNS depressants.
5. Report loss of effect, ↓ ROM, or worsening of symptoms.

Outcome/Evaluate: ↓ Spasticity; ↑ muscle relaxation

Tobramycin sulfate

(toe-brah-**MY**-sin)

Pregnancy Category: D (B for ophthalmic use)

Inhalation: TOBI, **Parenteral:** Nebcin, Nebcin Pediatric, **Ophthalmic:** AKTob Ophthalmic Solution, Tobrex Ophthalmic Ointment, Tobrex Ophthalmic Solution **(Rx)**

Classification: Antibiotic, aminoglycoside

See also *Aminoglycosides.*

Action/Kinetics: Similar to gentamicin and can be used concurrently with carbenicillin. **Therapeutic serum levels: IM,** 4–8 mcg/mL. **t½:** 2–2.5 hr. **Toxic serum levels:** > 12 mcg/mL (peak) and > 2 mcg/mL (trough).

Uses: Systemic: (1) Complicated and recurrent UTIs due to *Pseudomonas aeruginosa, Proteus, Escherichia coli, Klebsiella, Enterobacter, Serratia, Staphylococcus aureus, Citrobacter,* and *Providencia.* (2) Lower respiratory tract infections due to *P. aeruginosa, Klebsiella, Enterobacter, E. coli, Serratia,* and *S. aureus* (penicillinase– and non–penicillinase producing). (3) Intra-abdominal infections (including peritonitis) due to *E. coli, Klebsiella,* and *Enterobacter.* (4) Septicemia in neonates, children, and adults due to *P. aeruginosa, E. coli,* and *Klebsiella.* (5) Skin, bone, and skin structure infections due to *P. aeruginosa, Proteus, E. coli, Klebsiella, Enterobacter,* and *S. aureus.* (6) Serious CNS infections, including meningitis. Can be used with penicillins or cephalosporins in serious infections when results of susceptibility testing are not yet known.

Ophthalmic: Treat superficial ocular infections due to *Staphylococcus, S. aureus, Streptococcus, S. pneumoniae,* beta-hemolytic streptococci, *Corynebacterium, E. coli, Haemophilus aegyptius, H. ducreyi, H. influenzae, H. parainfluenzae, Klebsiella pneumoniae, Neisseria, N. gonorrhoeae, Proteus, Acinetobacter calcoaceticus, Enterobacter, Enterobacter aerogenes, Serratia marcescens, Moraxella, Pseudomonas aeruginosa,* and *Vibrio.*

Inhalation: Management of lung infections (*P. aeruginosa*) in cystic fibrosis clients.

Contraindications: Ophthalmically to treat dendritic keratitis, vaccinia, varicella, fungal or mycobacterial eye infections, after removal of a corneal foreign body. Lactation.

Special Concerns: Use with caution in premature infants and neonates. Ophthalmic ointment may retard corneal epithelial healing.

Additional Side Effects: *Ophthalmic use:* Transient irritation, burning, stinging, itching, inflammation, angioneurotic edema, urticaria, vesicular and maculopapular dermatitis.

OD Management of Overdose: *Symptoms (Ophthalmic Use):* Edema, lid itching, punctate keratitis, erythema, lacrimation.

Additional Drug Interactions: With carbenicillin or ticarcillin, tobramycin may have an increased effect when used for *Pseudomonas* infections.

How Supplied: *Inhalation Solution:* 60 mg/mL; *Injection:* 10 mg/mL, 40 mg/mL; *Powder for injection:* 60 mg, 80 mg, 1.2 g; *Ophthalmic Ointment:* 0.3%; *Ophthalmic Solution:* 0.3%

Dosage

- **IM, IV**

Non-life-threatening serious infections.

Adults: 3 mg/kg/day in three equally divided doses q 8 hr.

Life-threatening infections.

Up to 5 mg/kg/day in three or four equal doses. **Pediatric:** Either 2–2.5 mg/kg q 8 hr or 1.5–1.9 mg/kg q 6 hr; **neonates 1 week of age or less:** up to 4 mg/kg/day in two equal doses q 12 hr.

Impaired renal function.

Initially: 1 mg/kg; **then,** maintenance dose calculated according to information supplied by manufacturer.

- **Ophthalmic Ointment (0.3%)**

Acute infections.

0.5-in. ribbon q 3–4 hr until improvement is noted.

Mild to moderate infections.

0.5-in. ribbon b.i.d.–t.i.d.

- **Ophthalmic Solution (0.3%)**

Acute infections.

Initial: 1–2 gtt q 15–30 min until improvement noted; **then,** reduce dosage gradually.

Moderate infections.

1–2 gtt 2–6 times/day.

- **Inhalation Solution**

T

Pseudomonas aeruginosa in cystic fibrosis. Dose using a nebulizer b.i.d. for 10–15 min in cycles of 28 days on and then 28 days off. See package insert for detailed instructions for administration.

HEALTH CARE CONSIDERATIONS

See also *Health Care Considerations* for *Aminoglycosides.*

Administration/Storage

1. Use the inhalation solution as close as possible to q 12 hr, but not less than q 6 hr.
2. Do not mix TOBI with dornase alfa in the nebulizer.
IV 3. Prepare IV solution by diluting drug with 50–100 mL of dextrose or saline solution; infuse over 30–60 min.
4. Use proportionately less diluent for children than for adults.
5. Do not mix with other drugs for parenteral administration.
6. Discard solution of drug containing up to 1 mg/mL after 24 hr at room temperature.
7. Store drug at room temperature no longer than 2 years.

Client/Family Teaching

1. Drink plenty of fluids (2–3 L/day) during parenteral drug therapy.
2. With eye infections, avoid wearing contact lenses until infection is cleared and provider approves.
3. Report if symptoms do not improve or if they worsen after 3 days of therapy.

Outcome/Evaluate

- Negative cultures; resolution of infection
- Therapeutic drug levels (peak: 4–10 mcg/mL; trough: 1–2 mcg/mL)

Tocainide hydrochloride

(toe-**KAY**-nyd)
Pregnancy Category: C
Tonocard **(Rx)**
Classification: Antiarrhythmic, class IB

See also *Antiarrhythmic Agents.*

Action/Kinetics: Similar to lidocaine. Decreases the excitability of cells in the myocardium by decreasing sodium and potassium conductance. Increases pulmonary and aortic arterial pressure and slightly increases peripheral resistance. Effective in both digitalized and nondigitalized clients. **Peak plasma levels:** 0.5–2 hr. **t½:** 11–15 hr. **Therapeutic serum levels:** 4–10 mcg/mL. **Duration:** 8 hr. Approximately 10% is bound to plasma protein. From 28% to 55% is excreted unchanged in the urine. Alkalinization decreases the excretion of the drug although acidification does not produce any changes in excretion.

Uses: Life-threatening ventricular arrhythmias, including ventricular tachycardia. Has not been shown to improve survival in clients with ventricular arrhythmias. *Investigational:* Myotonic dystrophy, trigeminal neuralgia.

Contraindications: Allergy to amide-type local anesthetics, second- or third-degree AV block in the absence of artificial ventricular pacemaker. Lactation.

Special Concerns: Increased risk of death when used in those with non-life-threatening cardiac arrhythmias. Safety and efficacy have not been established in children. Use with caution in clients with impaired renal or hepatic function (dose may have to be decreased). Geriatric clients may have an increased risk of dizziness and hypotension; the dose may have to be reduced in these clients due to age-related impaired renal function.

Side Effects: *CV:* ***Increased arrhythmias,*** increased ventricular rate (when given for atrial flutter or fibrillation), CHF, tachycardia, hypotension, ***conduction disturbances,*** bradycardia, chest pain, LV failure, palpitations. *CNS:* Dizziness, vertigo, headache, tremors, confusion, disorientation, hallucinations, ataxia, paresthesias, numbness, nervousness, altered mood, anxiety, incoordination, walking disturbances. *GI:* N&V, anorexia, diarrhea. *Respiratory:* ***Pulmonary fibrosis, fibrosing alveolitis,*** interstitial pneumonitis, ***pulmonary edema,*** pneumonia. *Hematologic:* Leukopenia, ***agranulocytosis,*** hypoplastic anemia, ***aplastic anemia,*** bone marrow depression, neutropenia, ***thrombocytopenia and sequelae as septicemia and septic shock.*** *Musculoskeletal:* Arthritis, arthralgia, myalgia. *Dermatologic:* Rash, skin lesion, diaphoresis. *Other:* Blurred vision, visual disturbances, nystagmus, tinnitus, hearing loss, lupus-like syndrome.

Laboratory Test Considerations: Abnormal LFTs (esp. in early therapy). ↑ ANA.

OD **Management of Overdose:** *Symptoms:* Initially are CNS symptoms including tremor (see above). GI symptoms may follow (see above). *Treatment:* Gastric lavage and activated charcoal may be useful. In the event of respiratory depression or arrest or seizures, maintain airway and provide artificial ventilation. An IV anticonvulsant (e.g., diazepam, thiopental, thiamylal, pentobarbital, secobarbital) may be required if seizures are persistent.

T

Drug Interactions
Cimetidine / ↓ Bioavailability of tocainide
Metoprolol / Additive effects on wedge pressure and cardiac index
Rifampin / ↓ Bioavailability of tocainide
How Supplied: *Tablet:* 400 mg, 600 mg

Dosage

- **Tablets**

Antiarrhythmic.

Adults, individualized, initial: 400 mg q 8 hr, up to a maximum of 2,400 mg/day; **maintenance:** 1,200–1,800 mg/day in divided doses. Total daily dose of 1,200 mg may be adequate in clients with liver or kidney disease.

Myotonic dystrophy.

800–1,200 mg/day.

Trigeminal neuralgia.

20 mg/kg/day in three divided doses.

HEALTH CARE CONSIDERATIONS

See also *Health Care Considerations* for *Antiarrhythmic Agents.*

Assessment

1. Record indications for therapy, type, onset, and characteristics of symptoms.
2. Monitor ECG, CBC, electrolytes, liver and renal function studies; correct potassium deficits.
3. Record/document cardiac and pulmonary assessment findings.

Client/Family Teaching

1. Take with food to minimize GI upset.
2. Do not drive or operate machinery until drug effects are realized; may cause drowsiness or dizziness.
3. Report any abnormal bruising, bleeding, fever, sore throat, or chills (S&S of blood dyscrasia).
4. Pulmonary symptoms such as wheezing, coughing, or dyspnea should be reported immediately; may indicate pulmonary fibrosis.

Outcome/Evaluate

- Control of lethal ventricular arrhythmias
- ↓ Muscle spasm and pain
- Therapeutic drug levels (4–10 mcg/mL)

Tolazamide

(toll-**AZ**-ah-myd)
Pregnancy Category: C
Tolinase **(Rx)**
Classification: Sulfonylurea, first-generation

See also *Antidiabetic Agents, Hypoglycemic Agents.*

Action/Kinetics: Effective in some with a history of coma or ketoacidosis; may be effective in clients who do not respond well to other oral antidiabetics. Use with insulin is not recommended for maintenance. **Onset:** 4–6 hr. **t½:** 7 hr. **Time to peak levels:** 3–4 hr. **Duration:** 12–24 hr. Metabolized in liver to metabolites with minor hypoglycemic activity. Excreted through the kidneys (85%) and feces (7%).

Additional Contraindications: Renal glycosuria.

Additional Drug Interactions: Concomitant use of alcohol and tolazamide may → photosensitivity.

How Supplied: *Tablet:* 100 mg, 250 mg, 500 mg

Dosage

- **Tablets**

Diabetes.

Adults, initial: 100 mg/day if fasting blood sugar is less than 200 mg/100 mL, or 250 mg/day if fasting blood sugar is greater than 200 mg/100 mL. Adjust dose to response, not to exceed 1 g/day. If more than 500 mg/day is required, give in two divided doses, usually before the morning and evening meals. **Elderly, malnourished, underweight clients or those not eating properly:** 100 mg once daily with breakfast, adjusting dose by increments of 50 mg/day each week. Doses greater than 1 g/day will probably not improve control.

HEALTH CARE CONSIDERATIONS

See also *Health Care Considerations* for *Antidiabetic Agents, Hypoglycemic Agents.*

Client/Family Teaching

1. Take 30 min before meals for best results; do not take if vomiting or unable to eat.
2. Monitor fingersticks and maintain a record (different times on different days) for provider review.
3. Avoid alcohol as a disulfiram-like reaction may occur.
4. Use caution; may cause dizziness.
5. Use nonhormonal contraception.
6. Wear protective clothing and a sunscreen to prevent a photosensitivity reaction.

Outcome/Evaluate: Serum glucose/HbA1-C levels within desired range

Tolbutamide

(toll-**BYOU**-tah-myd)
Pregnancy Category: C
APO-Tolbutamide ✱, Novo-Butamide ✱, Orinase **(Rx)**

Tolbutamide sodium

(toll-**BYOU**-tah-myd)

Pregnancy Category: C
🍁Orinase Diagnostic **(Rx)**
Classification: Sulfonylurea, first-generation

See also *Antidiabetic Agents, Hypoglycemic Agents.*
Action/Kinetics: Onset: 1 hr. **t½:** 4.5–6.5 hr. **Time to peak levels:** 3–4 hr. **Duration:** 6–12 hr. Changed in liver to inactive metabolites. Excreted through the kidney (75%) and feces (9%).
Additional Uses: Most useful for clients with poor general physical status who should receive a short-acting compound.

Tolbutamide sodium is used to diagnose pancreatic islet cell tumors. It causes blood glucose, in the presence of a tumor, to drop quickly after IV administration and remain low for 3 hr.
Additional Side Effects: Melena (dark, bloody stools) in some clients with a history of peptic ulcer. Relapse or secondary failure may occur a few months after therapy has been started. May cause hyponatremia and a mild goiter.
Additional Drug Interactions
Alcohol / Photosensitivity reactions
Sulfinpyrazone / ↑ Effect of tolbutamide due to ↓ breakdown by liver
How Supplied: Tolbutamide: *Tablet:* 500 mg; Tolbutamide sodium: *Powder for injection:* 1 g

Dosage
- **Tablets**

Diabetes mellitus.
Adults, initial: 1–2 g/day. Adjust dosage depending on response, up to 3 g/day. **Usual maintenance:** 0.25–3 g/day). A daily dose greater than 2 g is seldom required.

HEALTH CARE CONSIDERATIONS

See also *Health Care Considerations* for *Antidiabetic Agents, Oral.*
Client/Family Teaching
1. Take 30 min before meals for best results. May take as a single dose before breakfast or as divided doses before the morning and evening meals. Divided doses may improve GI tolerance.
2. Maintain log of fingersticks for provider review.
3. Drug may cause dizziness.
4. Avoid alcohol and any OTC meds without approval.
5. May cause a photosensitivity reaction; wear protective clothing and sunscreen when exposed.
6. Use a nonhormonal form of birth control.

Outcome/Evaluate
- Serum glucose/HbA1-C levels within desired range
- Pancreatic islet cell tumor presence

Tolcapone
(TOHL-kah-pohn)
Pregnancy Category: C
Tasmar **(Rx)**
Classification: Antiparkinson drug

Action/Kinetics: Reversible inhibitor of catechol-O-methyltransferase (COMT), resulting in an increase in plasma levodopa. When given with levodopa/carbidopa, plasma levels of levodopa are more sustained, allowing for more constant dopaminergic stimulation of the brain. May also increase side effects of levodopa. Rapidly absorbed from the GI tract; **peak levels:** 2 hr. Food given within 1 hr before or 2 hr after PO use decreases bioavailability by 10%–20%. Over 99.9% bound to plasma protein. **t½, elimination:** 2–3 hr. Almost completely metabolized in the liver; excreted in the urine (60%) and feces (40%).
Uses: Adjunct to levodopa and carbidopa for the treatment of idiopathic Parkinson's disease.
Contraindications: Use with a nonselective MAO inhibitor.
Special Concerns: Use with caution in severe renal or hepatic impairment and during lactation.
Side Effects: *GI:* N&V, anorexia, diarrhea, constipation, xerostomia, abdominal pain, dyspepsia, flatulence. *CNS:* Hallucinations, dyskinesias, sleep disorder, dystonia, excessive dreaming, somnolence, confusion, dizziness, headache, syncope, loss of balance, hyperkinesia, paresthesia, hypokinesia, agitation, irritability, mental deficiency, hyperactivity, panic reaction, euphoria, hypertonia. *CV:* Orthostatic hypotension, chest pain, hypotension, chest discomfort. *Respiratory:* URTI, dyspnea, sinus congestion. *Musculoskeletal:* Muscle cramps, stiffness, arthritis, neck pain. *GU:* Hematuria, UTIs, urine discoloration, micturition disorder, uterine tumor. *Dermatologic:* Increased sweating, dermal bleeding, skin tumor, alopecia. *Ophthalmic:* Cataract, eye inflammation. *Body as a whole:* Falling, fatigue, influenza, burning, malaise, fever.

Note: Clients over 75 years of age may develop more hallucinations but less dystonia. Females may develop somnolence more frequently than males.

T

Laboratory Test Considerations: ↑ AST, ALT.

OD **Management of Overdose:** *Symptoms:* Nausea, vomiting, dizziness, possibility of respiratory difficulties. *Treatment:* Hospitalization is advised. Give supportive care.

How Supplied: *Tablets:* 100 mg, 200 mg

Dosage

- **Tablets**

Adjunct for Parkinsonism.

Initial: 100 or 200 mg t.i.d. with or without food, up to a maximum of 600 mg/day. Do not increase the dose to 200 mg t.i.d. in those with moderate to severe liver cirrhosis.

HEALTH CARE CONSIDERATIONS

Administration/Storage

1. Even though 200 mg t.i.d. is reasonably well tolerated, the prescriber may start with 100 mg t.i.d. due to the potential for increased dopaminergic side effects and the possibility of adjustment of the concomitant levodopa/carbidopa dose.
2. A suggested dosing regimen is to give the first dose of tolcapone of the day with the first dose of levodopa/carbidopa; subsequent doses of tolcapone can be given 6 to 12 hr later.
3. Reductions in the daily dose of levodopa may be required.
4. Tolcapone can be used with either the immediate or sustained–release formulations of levodopa/carbidopa.

Assessment

1. Record indications for therapy, characteristics/duration of symptoms, and other agents trialed.
2. List drugs currently prescribed to ensure none interact unfavorably.
3. May cause severe hepatotoxicity. Do not use with clinical evidence of liver disease or if ALT or AST 2x ULN. When used, monitor LFTs q 2 weeks for the first year of therapy, then q 4 weeks for the next six months and then q 8 weeks for the remainer of use. Stop drug with any evidence of liver dysfunction.

Client/Family Teaching

1. Take as directed. Drug increases the action of levodopa by decreasing its metabolism in the peripheral tissues. If taken without levodopa there is no treatment benefit.
2. Do not drive or perform activities requiring mental alertness until drug effects realized; may cause sedation.
3. Stop drug and report any evidence of liver dysfunction: fatigue, loss of appetite, yellow skin discoloration, or clay colored stools.
4. Rise slowly from a sitting or lying position to prevent orthostatic effects.
5. May experience nausea initially and an increase in involuntary repetitive movements; these should subside. Six weeks into therapy may experience diarrhea; report if persistent or severe.
6. May discolor urine bright yellow.
7. Practice reliable birth control; do not nurse.
8. Report any unusual symptoms or side effects; labs will be required every 2 weeks during the first year of therapy to protect from liver toxicity.

Outcome/Evaluate: Control of S&S Parkinson's disease

Tolmetin sodium

(TOLL-met-in)

Pregnancy Category: C

Novo-Tolmetin ✦, Tolectin ✦, Tolectin 200, Tolectin 600, Tolectin DS **(Rx)**

Classification: Nonsteroidal, anti-inflammatory, analgesic

See also *Nonsteroidal Anti-Inflammatory Drugs.*

Action/Kinetics: Peak plasma levels: 30–60 min. **t½:** 1 hr. **Therapeutic plasma levels:** 40 mcg/mL. **Onset, anti-inflammatory effect:** within 1 week; **duration, anti-inflammatory effect:** 1–2 weeks. Inactivated in liver and excreted in urine.

Uses: Acute and chronic treatment of rheumatoid arthritis and osteoarthritis. Juvenile rheumatoid arthritis. *Investigational:* Sunburn.

Special Concerns: Use with caution during lactation. Dosage has not been determined in children less than 2 years of age.

Laboratory Test Considerations: Tolmetin metabolites give a false + test for proteinuria using sulfosalicylic acid.

How Supplied: *Capsule:* 400 mg; *Tablet:* 200 mg, 600 mg

Dosage

- **Capsules, Tablets**

Rheumatoid arthritis, osteoarthritis.

Adults: 400 mg t.i.d. (one dose on arising and one at bedtime); adjust dosage according to client response. **Maintenance:** *rheumatoid arthritis,* 600–1,800 mg/day in three to four divided doses; *osteoarthritis,* 600–1,600 mg/day in three to four divided doses. Doses larger than 1,800 mg/day for rheumatoid arthritis and osteoarthritis are not recommended.

Juvenile rheumatoid arthritis.

2 years and older, initial: 20 mg/kg/day in three to four divided doses to start; **then,** 15–30 mg/kg/day. Doses higher than 30 mg/kg/day are not recommended. Benefi-

T

cial effects may not be observed for several days to a week.

HEALTH CARE CONSIDERATIONS

See also *Health Care Considerations* for *Nonsteroidal Anti-Inflammatory Drugs.*

Assessment

1. Record indications for therapy; note joint pain, deformity, swelling, inflammation, and ROM.
2. Monitor CBC and renal function studies.

Client/Family Teaching

1. Doses should be spaced so that one dose is taken in the morning on arising, one during the day, and one at bedtime.
2. May administer with meals, milk, a full glass of water, or antacids if gastric irritation occurs. Never administer with sodium bicarbonate. The elderly are particularly susceptible to gastric irritation and should take with milk, meals, or an antacid.
3. Assess response; drug may cause drowsiness or dizziness.
4. Report any unusual bruising or bleeding or evidence of edema.
5. It may take several weeks before effects are evident.
6. Avoid alcohol and any OTC meds without approval.
7. Report for labs to evaluate renal function and hematologic parameters.

Outcome/Evaluate: ↓ Joint pain and inflammation; ↑ mobility

Tolnaftate

(toll-**NAF**-tayt)

Absorbine Footcare, Aftate for Athlete's Foot, Aftate for Jock Itch, Genaspor, NP-27, Pitrex ✸, Quinsana Plus, Tinactin, Tinactin for Jock Itch, Tinactin Plus ✸, Ting, Zeasorb-AF **(OTC)**

Classification: Topical antifungal

See also *Anti-Infectives.*

Action/Kinetics: Exact mechanism not known; is thought to stunt mycelial growth causing a fungicidal effect.

Uses: Tinea pedis, tinea cruris, tinea corporis, and tinea versicolor. Fungal infections of moist skin areas.

Contraindications: Scalp and nail infections. Avoid getting into eyes. Use in children less than 2 years of age.

Side Effects: Mild skin irritation.

How Supplied: *Cream:* 1%; *Ointment:* 1%; *Powder:* 1%; *Solution:* 1%; *Spray:* 1%

Dosage

- **Topical: Aerosol Powder, Aerosol Solution, Cream, Ointment, Powder, Solution, Spray Solution**

Apply b.i.d. for 2–3 weeks although treatment for 4–6 weeks may be necessary in some instances.

HEALTH CARE CONSIDERATIONS

See also *General Health Care Considerations for All Anti-Infectives.*

Assessment

1. Inspect source of infection; record presentation because the choice of vehicle is important for effective therapy.
   - Powders are used in mild conditions as adjunctive therapy.
   - For primary therapy and prophylaxis, creams, liquids, or ointments are used, especially if the area is moist.
   - Liquids and solutions are used if the area is hairy.
2. Assess cultures; use concomitant therapy if bacterial or *Candida* infections are also present.

Client/Family Teaching

1. Skin should be thoroughly cleaned and dried before applying.
2. Use care; do not rub medication into or near the eye.
3. Report any bothersome side effects; local relief of symptoms should be evident within the first 24–48 hr. Report if no improvement noted within 10 days.
4. Continue to use as directed, despite improvement of symptoms. Takes 2–6 weeks to clear infection.

Outcome/Evaluate

- Symptomatic relief; skin healing
- Eradication of fungal infection

T

Tolterodine tartrate

(tohl-**TER**-oh-deen)

Pregnancy Category: C

Detrol **(Rx)**

Classification: Urinary tract drug

Action/Kinetics: Acts as a competitive muscarinic receptor antagonist in the bladder to cause increased bladder control. Metabolized by first pass effect in the liver to the active 5–hydroxymethyl derivative, which has similar activity as tolterodine. Rapidly absorbed with peak serum levels within 1–2 hr. Food increases bioavialability. Highly bound to plasma proteins. Excreted in the urine.

Uses: Treat overactive bladder with symptoms of urinary frequency, urgency, or urge incontinence.

Contraindications: Urinary retention, gastric retention, uncontrolled narrow–angle glaucoma, lactation.

Special Concerns: Use with caution in renal impairment, in bladder outflow obstruction, in GI obstructive disorders (e.g., pyloric stenosis), and in those being treated for narrow–angle glaucoma. Doses greater than 1 mg b.i.d. not to be given to those with significantly decreased hepatic function. Safety and efficacy have not been determined in children.

Side Effects: *GI:* Dry mouth (common), dyspepsia, constipation, abdominal pain, N&V, diarrhea, flatulence. *CNS:* Headache, vertigo, dizziness, somnolence, paresthesia, nervousness. *Respiratory:* URI, bronchitis, coughing, pharyngitis, rhinitis, sinusitis. *Dermatologic:* Rash, erythema, dry skin, pruritus. *GU:* UTI, dysuria, micturition frequency, urinary retention. *Ophthalmic:* Abnormalities with vision, including accommodation. *Musculoskeletal:* Arthralgia, back pain, chest pain. *Miscellaneous:* Fatigue, flu–like symptoms, infection, hypertension, weight gain, fall, fungal infection.

OD **Management of Overdose:** *Symptoms:* Significant anticholinergic symptoms. *Treatment:* Symptomatic. Monitor ECG.

Drug Interactions

Clarithromycin / ↑ Plasma levels of tolterodine due to ↓ break down by liver; do not give doses of tolterodine >1 mg b.i.d.

Erythromycin / ↑ Plasma levels of tolterodine due to ↓ break down by liver; do not give doses of tolterodine >1 mg b.i.d.

Itraconazole / ↑ Plasma levels of tolterodine due to ↓ break down by liver; do not give doses of tolterodine >1 mg b.i.d.

Ketoconazole / ↑ Plasma levels of tolterodine due to ↓ break down by liver; do not give doses of tolterodine >1 mg b.i.d.

Miconazole / ↑ Plasma levels of tolterodine due to ↓ break down by liver; do not give doses of tolterodine >1 mg b.i.d.

How Supplied: *Tablets:* 1 mg, 2 mg

Dosage

- **Tablets**

Treat overactive bladder.

Initial: 2 mg b.i.d. Dose may be lowered to 1 mg b.i.d. based on individual response and side effects. Adjust dose to 1 mg b.i.d. in those with significantly reduced hepatic function or who are currently taking drugs that are inhibitors of cytochrome P450 3A4 (see *Drug Interactions*).

HEALTH CARE CONSIDERATIONS

Assessment

1. Note indications for therapy, onset, duration, and characteristics of incontinence and symptoms.
2. List drugs currently prescribed to ensure none interact or alter dosage.
3. Determine any evidence of urinary retention or gastric retention; GI obstructive disorders or glaucoma.
4. Monitor renal and LFTs; decrease dose with hepatic dysfunction.

Client/Family Teaching

1. Take as directed with or without food.
2. Drug is used to help reduce the frequency and urgency associated with urination. It is not for stress incontinence or UTI but is for treatment of an overactive bladder.
3. May experience dizziness and headache; report if persistent.
4. There is a user support number. Call 1-800-896-8596 to enroll and to receive free information/updates and a 24-hr hotline access.

Outcome/Evaluate: ↑ Bladder control with ↓ urinary frequency, urgency, or urge incontinence

Topiramate

(toh-**PYRE**-ah-mayt)

Pregnancy Category: C

Topamax **(Rx)**

Classification: Anticonvulsant, miscellaneous

See also *Anticonvulsants.*

Action/Kinetics: Precise mechanism not known. The following effects may contribute to the anticonvulsant activity. (1) Action potentials seen repetitively by sustained depolarization of neurons are blocked in a time-dependent manner, suggesting an effect to block sodium channels. (2) Increases the frequency at which GABA activates $GABA_A$ receptors, thus enhancing the ability of GABA to cause a flux of chloride ions into neurons (i.e., enhanced effect of the inhibitory transmitter, $GABA_A$). (3) Antagonizes the ability of kainate to activate the kainate/AMPA subtype of excitatory amino acid aspartate, thus reducing the excitatory effect. Rapidly absorbed; **peak plasma levels:** About 2 hr. **t½, elimination:** 21 hr. Steady state is reached in about 4 days in those with normal renal function. Excreted mostly unchanged in the urine.

Uses: Adjunct to treat partial onset seizures in adults.

Contraindications: Lactation.

Special Concerns: Use with caution in impaired hepatic and renal function. Safety and efficacy have not been determined in children.

Side Effects: *Note:* Side effects with an incidence of 0.1% or greater are listed. *CNS:* Psychomotor slowing, including difficulty with concentration and speech or language problems. Somnolence, fatigue, dizziness, ataxia, nystagmus, paresthesia, nervousness, difficulty with memory, tremor, confusion, depression, abnormal coordination, agitation, mood problems, aggressive reaction, hypoesthesia, apathy, emotional lability, depersonalization, hypokinesia, vertIgo, stupor, ***clonic/tonic seizures,*** hyperkinesia, hypertonia, insomnia, personality disorder, impotence, hallucinations, euphoria, psychosis, decreased libido, ***suicide attempt,*** hyporeflexia, neuropathy, migraine, apraxia, hyperesthesia, dyskinesia, hyperreflexia, dysphonia, scotoma, dystonia, coma, encephalopathy, upper motor neuron lesion, paranoid reaction, delusion, paranoia, delirium, abnormal dreaming, neuroses. *GI:* Nausea, dyspepsia, anorexia, abdominal pain, constipation, dry mouth, gingivitis, halitosis, diarrhea, vomiting, fecal incontinence, flatulence, gastroenteritis, gum hyperplasia, hemorrhoids, increased appetite, tooth caries, stomatitis, dysphagia, melena, gastritis, increased saliva, hiccough, gastroesophageal reflux, tongue edema, esophagitis, gall bladder disorder, gingival bleeding. *CV:* Palpitation, hypertension, hypotension, postural hypotension, AV block, bradycardia, bundle branch block, angina pectoris, vasodilation. *Body as a whole:* Asthenia, back pain, chest pain, flu-like symptoms, leg pain, hot flashes, body odor, edema, rigors, fever, malaise, syncope, enlarged abdomen. *Respiratory:* URI, pharyngitis, sinusitis, dyspnea, coughing, bronchitis, asthma, ***bronchospasm, pulmonary embolism.*** *Dermatologic:* Acne, alopecia, dermatitis, nail disorder, folliculitis, dry skin, urticaria, skin discoloration, eczema, photosensitivity reaction, erythematous rash, seborrhea, decreased sweating, abnormal hair texture, facial edema. *GU:* Breast pain, renal stone formation, dysmenorrhea, menstrual disorder, hematuria, intermenstrual bleeding, leukorrhea, menorrhagia, vaginitis, amenorrhea, UTI, micturition frequency, urinary incontinence, dysuria, renal calculus, ejaculation disorder, breast discharge, urinary retention, renal pain, nocturia, albuminuria, polyuria, oliguria. *Musculoskeletal:* Arthralgia, muscle weakness, arthrosis, osteoporosis, myalgia, leg cramps. *Metabolic:* Increased weight, decreased weight, dehydration, xeropthalmia. *Hematologic:* Anemia, leukopenia, lymphadenopathy, eosinophilia, lymphopenia, granulocytopenia, lymphocytosis, thrombocytothemia, purpura, thrombocytopenia. *Dermatologic:* Rash, pruritus, increased sweating, flushing. *Ophthalmic:* Diplopia, abnormal vision, eye pain, conjunctivitis, abnormal accommodation, photophobia, abnormal lacrimation, strabismus, color blindness, myopia, mydriasis, ptosis, visual field defect. *Miscellaneous:* Decreased hearing, epistaxis, taste perversion, tinnitus, taste loss, parosmia, goiter, basal cell carcinoma.

Laboratory Test Considerations: ↑ AST, ALT, alkaline phosphatase, creatinine. Hypokalemia, hypocalcemia, hyperlipemia, acidosis, hyperglycemia, hyperchloremia.

OD **Management of Overdose:** *Symptoms:* See side effects. *Treatment:* Gastric lavage or induction of emesis if ingestion is recent. Supportive treatment. Hemodialysis.

Drug Interactions

Alcohol / CNS depression and cognitive and neuropsychiatric side effects

Carbamazepine / ↓ Plasma levels of topiramate

Carbonic anhydrase inhibitors / ↑ Risk of renal stone formation

CNS depressants / CNS depression and cognitive and neuropsychiatric side effects

Oral contraceptives / ↓ Effect of oral contraceptives

Phenytoin / ↓ Plasma levels of topiramate and ↑ plasma levels of phenytoin

Valproic acid / ↓ Plasma levels of both topiramate and valproic acid

How Supplied: *Tablets:* 25 mg, 100 mg, 200 mg.

Dosage

- **Tablets**

Adjunctive therapy for treatment of partial onset seizures.

Initial: 50 mg/day; **then,** titrate to an effective dose of 400 mg/day in 2 divided doses. Titrate by adding 50 mg each week for eight weeks, until the dose is 400 mg/day. Doses greater than 400 mg/day have not been shown to improve the response. If C_{CR} < 70 mL/1.73 m^2, use one half of the usual adult dose.

HEALTH CARE CONSIDERATIONS

See also *Health Care Considerations* for *Anticonvulsant Drugs.*

Assessment

1. Record age at onset, type, and characteristics of seizures.

T

2. Monitor CBC, liver and renal function studies; reduce dose with renal dysfunction.
3. List drugs currently prescribed to ensure none interact or lose effectiveness; MAO inhibitors may promote kidney stones.
4. Record baseline psychomotor and mental status; assess for psychomotor slowing, speech or expression problems, difficulty concentrating, fatigue, or sleepiness.

Client/Family Teaching

1. Take exactly as prescribed. Due to the bitter taste of the drug, do not break tablets. Can be taken without regard for meals.
2. Distinguish if drug affects motor or mental capacity before driving or performing activities that require mental alertness; may cause dizziness, confusion, drowsiness, and altered concentration.
3. Increase fluid intake to decrease substance concentration as drug may precipitate renal stone formation by increasing urinary pH and reducing urinary citrate excretion.
4. Use reliable, nonhormonal form of birth control; drug may compromise efficacy of PO contraceptives.
5. Do not stop drug abruptly due to risk of increased seizure frequency.
6. Review list of side effects, noting those that require attention.

Outcome/Evaluate: Adjunctive therapy in the control of partial onset seizures.

Toremifene citrate

(TOR-em-ih-feen)
Pregnancy Category: D
Fareston **(Rx)**
Classification: Antineoplastic, hormone

See also *Antineoplastic Agents.*

Action/Kinetics: Antiestrogen that binds to estrogen receptors and may cause estrogenic, antiestrogenic, or both effects, depending on duration of treatment, genders, and endpoint/target organ selected. Antitumor effect is likely due to antiestrogenic effect, i.e., competes for estrogen at receptor and blocks growth-stimulating effects of estrogen in tumor. Well absorbed from GI tract. **Peak plasma levels:** 3 hr. **t½, distribution:** About 4 hr. **t½, elimination:** About 5 days. Extensively metabolized in liver and mainly excreted in feces.

Uses: Metastatic breast cancer in postmenopausal women with positive estrogen-receptor (ER) or ER unknown tumors.

Contraindications: Use with history of thromboembolic disease or in pediatric clients.

Special Concerns: Hypercalcemia and tumor flare in some breast cancer clients with bone metastases during first weeks of treatment. Use with caution during lactation.

Side Effects: *CV:* ***Cardiac failure, MI, pulmonary embolism, CVA,*** TIA. *GI:* Constipation, nausea. *Hematologic:* Leukopenia, thrombocytopenia. *Dermatologic:* Skin discoloration, dermatitis, alopecia, pruritus. *Ophthalmic:* Cataracts, dry eyes, abnormal visual fields, corneal keratopathy, glaucoma, reversible corneal opacity. *CNS:* Tremor, vertigo, depression. *Miscellaneous:* Dyspnea, paresis, anorexia, asthenia, jaundice, rigors, vaginal bleeding.

Laboratory Test Considerations: ↑ AST, alkaline phosphatase, bilirubin. Hypercalcemia.

Drug Interactions

Carbamazepine / ↓ Blood levels of toremifene due to ↑ breakdown in liver
Clonazepam / ↓ Blood levels of toremifene due to ↑ breakdown in liver
Erythromycin / Inhibition of breakdown of toremifene
Ketoconazole / Inhibition of breakdown of toremifene
Macrolide antibiotics / Inhibition of breakdown of toremifene
Phenobarbital / ↓ Blood levels of toremifene due to ↑ breakdown in liver
Phenytoin / ↓ Blood levels of toremifene due to ↑ breakdown in liver
Warfarin / ↑ PT

How Supplied: *Tablets:* 60 mg

Dosage

- **Tablets**

Metastatic breast cancer.

Adults: 60 mg once daily. Continue until disease progression is observed.

HEALTH CARE CONSIDERATIONS

See also *Health Care Considerations* for *Antineoplastic Agents.*

Assessment

1. Record indications for therapy, characteristics of symptoms, other agents trialed and outcome.
2. Note any history or evidence of thromboembolic disorders.
3. Monitor CBC, calcium, and LFTs.

Client/Family Teaching

1. Take once daily as directed.
2. Report any unusual vaginal bleeding.
3. May experience "tumor flare," syndrome of diffuse musculoskeletal pain and erythema with increased size of tumor lesions that regress later; if accompanied by hypercalcemia must stop drug.

Outcome/Evaluate: Control of malignant cell proliferation

T

Torsemide

(TOR-seh-myd)
Pregnancy Category: B
Demadex **(Rx)**
Classification: Loop diuretic

See also *Diuretics, Loop.*
Action/Kinetics: Onset, IV: Within 10 min; **PO:** within 60 min. **Peak effect, IV:** Within 60 min; **PO:** 60–120 min. **Duration:** 6–8 hr. **t½:** 210 min. Metabolized by the liver and excreted through the urine. Food delays the time to peak effect by about 30 min, but the overall bioavailability and the diuretic activity are not affected.
Uses: Congestive heart failure, acute or chronic renal failure, hepatic cirrhosis, hypertension.
Contraindications: Lactation.
Special Concerns: Clients sensitive to sulfonamides may show allergic reactions to torsemide. Safety and efficacy in children have not been determined.
Side Effects: *CNS:* Headache, dizziness, asthenia, insomnia, nervousness, syncope. *GI:* Diarrhea, constipation, nausea, dyspepsia, edema, ***GI hemorrhage,*** rectal bleeding. *CV:* ECG abnormality, chest pain, atrial fibrillation, hypotension, ***ventricular tachycardia,*** shunt thrombosis. *Respiratory:* Rhinitis, increase in cough. *Musculoskeletal:* Arthralgia, myalgia. *Miscellaneous:* Sore throat, excessive urination, rash.
Laboratory Test Considerations: Hyperglycemia, hyperuricemia, hypokalemia, hypovolemia.
How Supplied: *Injection:* 10 mg /mL; *Tablet:* 5 mg, 10 mg, 20 mg, 100 mg

Dosage

- **Tablets, IV**

  Congestive heart failure.

Adults, initial: 10 or 20 mg once daily.
Chronic renal failure.
Adults, initial: 20 mg once daily.
Hepatic cirrhosis.
Adults, initial: 5 or 10 mg once daily given with an aldosterone antagonist or a potassium-sparing diuretic.
Hypertension.
Adults, initial: 5 mg once daily. If this dose does not lead to an adequate decrease in BP within 4–6 weeks, the dose may be increased to 10 mg once daily. If the 10-mg dose is not adequate, an additional antihypertensive agent is added to the treatment regimen.

HEALTH CARE CONSIDERATIONS

See also *Health Care Considerations* for *Diuretics, Loop.*

Administration/Storage

1. If the response is inadequate for the initial dose used for CHF, chronic renal failure, or hepatic cirrhosis, the dose can be doubled until the desired diuretic response is obtained. Doses greater than 200 mg for CHF or chronic renal failure and greater than 40 mg for hepatic cirrhosis have not been adequately studied.
2. May be given without regard for meals.
3. It is not necessary to adjust the dose for geriatric clients.
4. IV Give the IV dose slowly over a period of 2 min or as a continuous infusion.
5. Oral and IV doses are therapeutically equivalent; may switch to and from the IV form with no change in dose.

Assessment

1. Record indications for therapy, type and onset of symptoms. List agents trialed and the outcome.
2. Note any sensitivity to sulfonamides.
3. Monitor VS, weight, I&O, blood sugar, uric acid, and potassium; drug may increase blood sugar and uric acid levels.
4. Record pulmonary, renal, and CV assessments.

Client/Family Teaching

1. Take only as directed. May take with food to decrease GI upset.
2. With hypertension, keep a BP log for provider review.
3. Report immediately any chest pain, increased SOB, or sudden weight gain with edema.
4. Drug may cause dizziness, lightheadedness, and fatigue.
5. Rise slowly from a sitting or lying position to minimize orthostatic drug effects.
6. May experience blurred vision, yellowing of vision, or sensitivity to sunlight. Report any unusual or persistent symptoms.

Outcome/Evaluate

- ↓ Edema; ↑ diuresis; ↓ BP
- Reduction of interdialysis weight gain and promotion of Na, Cl, and water excretion

Tramadol hydrochloride

(TRAM-ah-dol)
Pregnancy Category: C
Ultram **(Rx)**
Classification: Analgesic, centrally acting

T

Action/Kinetics: A centrally acting analgesic not related chemically to opiates. Precise mechanism is not known. It may bind to mu-opioid receptors and inhibit reuptake of norepinephrine and serotonin. The analgesic effect is only partially antagonized by the antagonist naloxone. Causes significantly less respiratory depression than morphine. In contrast to morphine, tramadol does not cause release of histamine. Produces dependence of the mu-opioid type (i.e., like codeine or dextropropoxyphene); however, there is little evidence of abuse. Tolerance occurs but is relatively mild; the withdrawal syndrome is not as severe with other opiates. Rapidly absorbed after PO administration. Food does not affect the rate or extent of absorption. **Onset:** 1 hr. **Peak effect:** 2–3 hr. **Peak plasma levels:** 2 hr. **t½, plasma:** Approximately 7 hr after multiple doses. Extensively metabolized by one of the P-450 isoenzymes. Excreted in the urine, with about 30% excreted unchanged and 60% as metabolites. The M-metabolite is active.

Uses: Management of moderate to moderately severe pain.

Contraindications: Hypersensitivity to tramadol. In acute intoxication with alcohol, hypnotics, centrally acting analgesics, opiates, or psychotropic drugs. Use in clients with past or present addiction or opiate dependence or in those with a prior history of allergy to codeine or opiates. Use for obstetric preoperative medication or for postdelivery analgesia in nursing mothers. Use in children less than 16 years of age, as safety and efficacy have not been determined.

Special Concerns: Use with great caution in those taking MAO inhibitors, as tramadol inhibits norepinephrine and serotonin uptake. Dosage reduction is recommended with impaired hepatic or renal function and in clients over 75 years of age. Use with caution in increased intracranial pressure or head injury, in epilepsy, or in clients with an increased risk for seizures, including head trauma, metabolic disorders, alcohol or drug withdrawal, and CNS infections. Tramadol may complicate the assessment of acute abdominal conditions.

Side Effects: *CNS:* Dizziness, vertigo, headache, somnolence, CNS stimulation, anxiety, confusion, incoordination, euphoria, nervousness, sleep disorders, ***seizures,*** paresthesia, cognitive dysfunction, hallucinations, tremor, amnesia, concentration difficulty, abnormal gait, migraine, development of drug dependence. *GI:* Nausea, constipation, vomiting, dyspepsia, dry mouth, diarrhea, abdominal pain, anorexia, flatulence, GI bleeding, hepatitis, stomatitis, dysgeusia. *CV:* Vasodilation, syncope, orthostatic hypotension, tachycardia, abnormal ECG, hypertension, myocardial ischemia, palpitations. *Dermatologic:* Pruritus, sweating, rash, urticaria, vesicles. *Body as a whole:* Asthenia, malaise, allergic reaction, accidental injury, weight loss, ***suicidal tendency.*** *GU:* Urinary retention, urinary frequency, menopausal symptoms, dysuria, menstrual disorder. *Miscellaneous:* ***Anaphylaxis,*** visual disturbances, cataracts, deafness, tinnitus, hypertonia, dyspnea.

Laboratory Test Considerations: ↑ Creatinine, liver enzymes. ↓ Hemoglobin. Proteinuria.

OD **Management of Overdose:** *Symptoms:* Extension of side effects, especially ***respiratory depression and seizures.*** *Treatment:* Naloxone will reverse some, but not all, of the symptoms of overdose. General supportive treatment, with special attention to maintenance of adequate respiration. Diazepam or barbiturates may help if seizures occur. Hemodialysis is not helpful.

Drug Interactions

Alcohol / Enhanced respiratory depression
Anesthetics, general / Enhanced respiratory depression
Carbamazepine / ↓ Effect of tramadol due to ↑ metabolism induced by carbamazepine
CNS depressants / Additive CNS depression
MAO Inhibitors / Tramadol may ↑ the risk of seizures in those taking MAO inhibitors
Naloxone / Use of naloxone for tramadol overdose may ↑ risk of seizures.
Quinidine / Quinidine inhibits the isoenzyme that metabolizes tramadol → ↑ levels of tramadol and ↓ levels of M1

How Supplied: *Tablet:* 50 mg

Dosage

- **Tablets**

Management of pain.

Adults: 50–100 mg q 4–6 hr, as needed, but not to exceed 400 mg/day. For moderate pain, 50 mg, initially, may be adequate, and for severe pain, 100 mg, initially, is often more effective. For clients over 75 years of age, the recommended dose is no more than 300 mg/day in divided doses. In impaired renal function with a C_{CR} less than 30 mL/min, the dosing interval should be increased to 12 hr, with a maximum daily dose of 200 mg. The recommended dose for clients with cirrhosis is 50 mg q 12 hr.

HEALTH CARE CONSIDERATIONS

See also *Health Care Considerations* for *Narcotic Analgesics*.

T

Assessment
1. Record indications for therapy, location, onset, and characteristics of symptoms. Use a pain-rating scale to rate pain.
2. Assess for history of drug addiction, allergy to opiates or codeine, or seizures; drug may increase the risk of convulsions.
3. Monitor liver and renal function studies; reduce dose with dysfunction and if over 75 years old.

Client/Family Teaching
1. Take only as directed. May be taken without regard to meals. Do not exceed single or daily doses of tramadol to enhance pain relief.
2. Do not perform activities that require mental alertness; drug may impair mental or physical performance.
3. Review list of side effects (nausea, dizziness, constipation, somnolence, pruritus, and constipation) that one may experience; report if persistent or intolerable.
4. May mask abdominal pathology and obscure intracranial pathology due to miosis. Alert provider and carry ID of drugs currently prescribed.

Outcome/Evaluate: Pain control

Trandolapril

(tran-**DOHL**-ah-pril)

Pregnancy Category: C (first trimester); D (second and third trimesters)

Mavik **(Rx)**

Classification: Antihypertensive

See also *Angiotensin Converting Enzyme (ACE) Inhibitors.*

Action/Kinetics: Rapidly absorbed; food slows rate, but not amount absorbed. **Onset:** 2–4 hr. **Peak plasma levels, trandolapril:** 30–60 min; **trandolaprilat:** 4–10 hr. **t½, trandolapril:** About 5 hr; **t½, trandoprilat:** About 10 hr. **Peak effect:** 4–10 hr. Metabolized in liver to active trandolaprilat. **Duration:** 24 hr. About ⅓ trandolaprilat is excreted in urine and ⅔ in feces.

Uses: Hypertension, alone or in combination with other antihypertensives such as hydrochlorothiazide. To treat heart failure after MI or ventricular dysfunction after MI.

Contraindications: In those with history of angioedema with ACE inhibitors.

Special Concerns: Safety and efficacy have not been determined in children.

Side Effects: See also *ACE Inhibitors. Hypersensitivity:* ***Angioedema.*** *CNS:* Dizziness, headache, fatigue, insomnia, paresthesias, drowsiness, vertigo, anxiety. *GI:* Diarrhea, dyspepsia, gastritis, abdominal pain, vomiting, constipation, pancreatitis. *CV:* Hypotension, bradycardia, chest pain, ***cardiogenic shock*** , intermittent claudication, stroke. *Respiratory:* Cough, dyspnea, URTI, epistaxis, throat inflammation. *Hepatic:* ***Hepatic failure,*** including cholestatic jaundice, ***fulminant hepatic necrosis, death.*** *Dermatologic:* Photosensitivity, pruritus, rash. *GU:* UTI, impotence, decreased libido. *Miscellaneous:* Neutropenia, syncope, myalgia, asthenia, muscle cramps, hypocalemia, intermittent claudication, edema, extremity pain, gout.

Laboratory Test Considerations: Hyperkalemia, hypocalcemia. ↑ Serum uric acid, BUN, creatinine.

Drug Interactions
Diuretics / Excessive hypotensive effects
Diuretics, potassium-sparing: ↑ Risk of hyperkalemia
Lithium / ↑ Risk of lithium toxicity

How Supplied: *Tablet:* 1 mg, 2 mg, 4 mg.

Dosage

- **Tablets**

Hypertension.

Initial: 1 mg once daily in nonblack clients and 2 mg once daily in black clients. Adjust dosage according to response; usually, adjustments are made at intervals of 1 week. **Maintenance, usual:** 2–4 mg once daily. Those inadequately treated with once-daily dosing can be treated with twice-daily dosing. If BP is still not adequately controlled, diuretic may be added. If C_{CR} is less than 30 mL/min or if there is hepatic cirrhosis, initial dose is 0.5 mg daily.

Heart failure post–MI/Left ventricular dysfunction post–MI.

Initial: 1 mg/day. Then, increase the dose, as tolerated, to a target dose of 4 mg/day. If 4 mg is not tolerated, continue with the highest tolerated dose.

HEALTH CARE CONSIDERATIONS

See also *Health Care Considerations* for Angiotensin Converting Enzyme (ACE) Inhibitors.

Administration/Storage: If client is on diuretic, discontinue 2 to 3 days prior to beginning therapy with trandolapril to reduce likelihood of hypotension. If diuretic can not be discontinued, use initial dose of trandolapril of 0.5 mg. Titrate subsequent dosage.

Assessment
1. Record indications for therapy, disease onset, other agents trialed and outcome.
2. Monitor liver and renal function studies; reduce dosage with impairment.

Client/Family Teaching
1. Take only as directed.
2. May experience cough, dizziness, and diarrhea; report if persistent.
3. Practice reliable contraception, stop drug and report if pregnancy suspected.
4. Continue lifestyle changes i.e., regular exercise, smoking/alcohol cessation, low fat, low salt diet in overall goal of BP control.

Outcome/Evaluate
- ↓ BP
- Control of heart failure/ventricular dysfunction after MI

Tranylcypromine sulfate

(tran-ill-SIP-roh-meen)
Pregnancy Category: C
Parnate **(Rx)**
Classification: Antidepressant, monoamine oxidase inhibitor

Action/Kinetics: A MAO inhibitor with a rapid onset of activity. Due to inhibition of MAO, the concentration of epinephrine, norepinephrine, and serotonin increases in storage sites throughout the nervous system. This increase has been alleged to be the basis for the antidepressant effects. MAO activity recovers in 3–5 days after drug withdrawal. No orthostatic hypotensive effect; slight anticholinergic and sedative effects. **t½:** 2.4–2.8 hr.

Uses: Treatment of major depressive episode without melancholia. Not a first line of therapy; is used when clients have failed to respond to other drug therapy. *Investigational:* Alone or as an adjunct to treat bulimia, obsessive compulsive disorder, and manifestations of psychotic disorders. Also, treatment of social phobia, seasonal affective disorders, adjunct to treat multiple sclerosis, and to treat idiopathic orthostatic hypotension (e.g., Shy-Drager syndrome) refractory to conventional therapy.

Contraindications: Use in those with a confirmed or suspected CV defect or in anyone with CV disease, hypertension, or history of headache. In the presence of pheochromocytoma. History of liver disease or in those with abnormal liver function. Use in combination with a large number of other drugs, especially other MAO inhibitors, tricyclic antidepressants, serotonin-reuptake inhibitors, buspirone, sympathomimetics, meperidine, CNS depressants (e.g., alcohol and narcotics), hypotensive drugs, excessive caffeine, and dextromethorphan (see *Drug Interactions*). Use with tyramine-containing foods (see *Drug Interactions*).

Special Concerns: Assess benefits versus risks before using during pregnancy and lactation. Use with caution in clients taking antiparkinson drugs, in impaired renal function, in those with seizure disorders, in diabetics, in hyperthyroid clients, and in those taking disulfiram. Geriatric clients may be more sensitive to the drug.

Side Effects: *CNS:* Anxiety, agitation, headaches (without elevation of BP), manic symptoms, restlessness, insomnia, weakness, drowsiness, dizziness, significant anorexia. *GI:* Dry mouth, nausea, diarrhea, abdominal pain, constipation. *CV:* Tachycardia, edema, palpitation. *GU:* Impotence, urinary retention, impaired ejaculation. *Musculoskeletal:* Muscle spasm, tremors, myoclonic jerks, numbness, paresthesia. *Hematologic:* Anemia, leukopenia, agranulocytosis, thrombocytopenia. *Miscellaneous:* Blurred vision, chills, impotence, hepatitis, skin rash, impaired water excretion, tinnitus.

OD **Management of Overdose:** *Symptoms:* Insomnia, restlessness, anxiety, agitation, mental confusion, incoherence, hypotension, dizziness, weakness, drowsiness, shock, hypertension with severe headache. Rarely, hypertension accompanied by twitching or myoclonic fibrillation of skeletal muscles with ***hyperprexia, generalized rigidity, and coma.*** The toxic effects may be delayed or prolonged following the last dose of the drug; thus, observe closely for at least a week. *Treatment:* Gastric lavage, if performed early. General supportive measures. Treat hypertensive crisis using phentolamine 5 mg IV. External cooling to treat hyperprexia. Standard measures to treat circulatory shock. Myoclonic effects may be relieved by using barbiturates; however, tranylcypromine may prolong the effects of barbiturates.

Drug Interactions
Alcohol / Possibility of excitation, seizures, delirium, hyperpyrexia, circulatory collapse, coma, death
Anesthetics, general / Hypotensive effect; use together with caution. Phenelzine should be discontinued at least 10 days before elective surgery
Anticholinergic drugs, atropine / MAO inhibitors effect of anticholinergic drugs
Antidepressants, tricyclic / Comcomitant use may result in excitation, sweating, tachycardia, tachypnea, hyperpyrexia, disseminated intravascular coagulation, delirium, tremors, convulsions, death. At least 7-10 days should elapse between discontinuing a MAO inhibitor and initiating a new drug. However, such combinations have been used together successfully

Antihypertensive drugs / Exaggerated hypotensive effects
Beta-adrenergic blocking drugs / Exaggerated hypotensive effects
Buspirone / Elevated BP
Dextromethorphan / Brief episodes of psychosis or bizarre behavior
Fluoxetine / Possibility of hyperthermia, rigidity, myoclonic movements, death. At least 10 days should elapse between discontinuation of phenelzine and initiation of fluoxetine; and, at least 5 weeks should elapse between discontinuing fluoxetine and beginning phenelzine
MAO Inhibitors / Concomitant use of tranylcypromine with other MAO inhibitors may cause a hypertensive crisis or severe seizures
Meperidine / See *Narcotics*
Narcotics / Possibility of excitation, seizures, delirium, hyperpyrexia, circulatory collapse, coma, death
Selective serotonin reuptake inhibitors /See *Fluoxetine*
Sympathomimetic drugs—amphetamine, cocaine, dopa, ephedrine, epinephrine, metaraminol, methyldopa, methylphenidate, norepinephrine, phenylephrine, phenylpropanolamine. Many OTC cold products, hay fever medications, and nasal decongestants contan one or more of these drugs / All peripheral, metabolic, cardiac, and central effects are potentiated for up to 2 weeks after termination of MAO inhibitor therapy. Symptoms include acute hypertensive crisis with possible intracranial hemorrhage, hyperthermia, coma, and possibly death
Thiazide diuretics / Exaggerated hypotensive effects
Tryptophan / Possibility of behavioral and neurologic effects, including disorientation, confusion, amnesia, delirium, agitation, hypomania, ataxia, myoclonus, hyperreflexia, shivering, ocular oscillation,and Babinski signs
Tyramine-rich foods—beer, broad beans, certain cheeses (Brie, cheddar, Camembert, Stilton), Chianti wine, chicken livers, caffeine, cola beverages, figs, licorice, liver, pickled or kippered herring, dry sausage (Genoa salami, hard salami, pepperoni, Lebanon bologna), tea, cream, yogurt, yeast extract, and chocolate / Possible precipitation of hypertensive crisis, including severe headache, hyperension, intracranial hemorrhage, death

How Supplied: *Tablets:* 10 mg.

Dosage

- **Tablets**

Major depressive syndrome without melancholia.

Individualize the dose. **Usual effective dose:** 30 mg/day given in divided doses. If there are no signs of improvement in 2 weeks, the dose can be increased by 10 mg/day at intervals of 1 to 3 weeks, up to a maximum of 60 mg/day.

HEALTH CARE CONSIDERATIONS

Administration/Storage

1. Improvement should be observed within 2 days to three weeks after beginning treatment.
2. Gradually withdraw when discontinuing therapy.

Assessment

1. Record indications for therapy, onset and duration of symptoms, previous agents trialed and the outcome. Note clinical presentation and failure with other classes of antidepressants. These drugs have a narrow safety margin and require close supervision and restriction of foods and drugs and use with other medical conditions.
2. List all drugs currently prescribed and those used within the past two weeks (especially sympathomimetic drugs) to ensure none interact.
3. Determine if pregnant; drugs cross placenal barrier and may be teratogenic.
4. Monitor VS, ECG, electrolytes, liver and renal function studies.
5. Determine if on any special diet and if foods on the diet affect MAO inhibitors (e.g.; tyramine-rich foods).

Interventions

1. Monitor VS q 4 to 8 hr when initiating therapy and at regular intervals thereafter to detect any hypertension or arrhythmias.
2. Observe for symptoms of CHF, e.g.; rales, SOB, or peripheral edema.
3. Monitor closely for indications of suicidal ideations. Suicide attempts are more frequent when the client emerges from the deepest phases of depression.

Client/Family Teaching

1. Take as directed and with meals to decrease GI irritation. Do not take in the evening; may cause insomnia.
2. Avoid taking other drugs while on this therapy and for two week after therapy has been discontinued. This includes OTC preparations for coughs, colds, congestion, or allergic reactions.
3. Review list of tyramine-containing foods to avoid (i.e. beer, Chianti wine, chicken livers, caffeine, cola beverages, certain cheeses

T

such as Brie, cheddar, Camembert, and Stilton; figs, licorice, liver, pickled or kippered herring, dried fish, bananas, raisins, tenderizers, game meats, avocados, dry sausage such as Genoa salami, hard salami, pepperoni, and Lebanon bologna; tea, sour cream, yogurt, yeast extract, and chocolate.
4. Several weeks of therapy are required before significant changes in condition may be evident. Report increased agitation, anxiety, mania, suicidal ideations, or any marked changes in behavior. Must continue taking even if there appears to be improvement; continued therapy is necessary to maintain proper blood levels of the drug.
5. Report any visual changes, stiff neck, photophobia, unusual soreness or sweating, or changes in pupil size immediately; may signal a hypertensive crisis.
6. Practice reliable birth control during and for several weeks before and after therapy.
7. Use frequent mouth rinses, sugarless gum or hard candy, and increased fluids for dry mouth effects.
8. If feeling faint lie down immediately. Rise slowly from a supine position and dangle legs before standing to minimize orthostatic hypotension.
9. Maintain activity in moderation. MAO inhibitors suppress anginal pain which may indicate myocardial ischemia.
10. May experience weight loss, nausea, anorexia, and/or diarrhea. If weight gain becomes significant, i.e., more than 5 lb/week for more than 2 weeks, may need reducing diet or a change in drug or dosage.
11. Report any urinary retention or bladder distension. Retention is more common among elderly, males and those immobilized.
12. Increase fluids to 3 L/day and the intake of fuits, fruit juices, and fiber to avoid constipation.
13. Report any red-green vision as this may indicate eye damage.
14. If taking elevated doses of MAO inhibitors over a long period of time, any drug withdrawal should be accomplished by gradually reducing the dosage to a maintenance level before discontinuing entirely.
15. Need regular F/U care since the dose will be gradually increased until the desired response is obtained. (Generally if there is no response observed by the third week of therapy, it is unlikely client will respond to increased dosages.)

Outcome/Evaluate

- Improvement in mood, energy, and interest levels; ↓ somatic complaints
- Normal sleep patterns
- Improved sense of self and abilty to problem solve

T

Trazodone hydrochloride

(TRAYZ-oh-dohn)

Pregnancy Category: C

Alti-Trazodone ✦, Alti-Trazodone Dividose ✦, Apo-Trazodone ✦, Apo-Trazodone D ✦, Desyrel, Desyrel Dividose, Dom-Trazodone ✦, Gen-Trazodone ✦, Novo-Trazodone ✦, Nu-Trazodone ✦, Nu-Trazodone-D ✦, PMS-Trazodone ✦, Trazon, Trazorel ✦, Trialodine **(Rx)**

Classification: Antidepressant, miscellaneous

Action/Kinetics: A novel antidepressant that does not inhibit MAO and is also devoid of amphetamine-like effects. Response usually occurs after 2 weeks (75% of clients), with the remainder responding after 2–4 weeks. May inhibit serotonin uptake by brain cells, therefore increasing serotonin concentrations in the synapse. May also cause changes in binding of serotonin to receptors. Causes moderate sedative and orthostatic hypotensive effects and slight anticholinergic effects. **Peak plasma levels:** 1 hr (empty stomach) or 2 hr (when taken with food). **t½, initial:** 3–6 hr; **final:** 5–9 hr. **Effective plasma levels:** 800–1,600 ng/mL. **Time to reach steady state:** 3–7 days. Three-fourths of those with a therapeutic effect respond by the end of the second week of therapy. Metabolized in liver and excreted through both the urine and feces.

Uses: Depression with or without accompanying anxiety. *Investigational:* In combination with tryptophan for treating aggressive behavior. Panic disorder or agoraphobia with panic attacks. Treatment of cocaine withdrawal. Chronic pain including diabetic neuropathy.

Contraindications: During the initial recovery period following MI. Concurrently with electroshock therapy.

Special Concerns: Use with caution during lactation. Safety and efficacy in children less than 18 years of age have not been established. Geriatric clients are more prone to the sedative and hypotensive effects.

Side Effects: *General:* Dermatitis, edema, blurred vision, constipation, dry mouth, nasal congestion, skeletal muscle aches and pains. *CV:* Hypertension or hypotension, syncope, palpitations, tachycardia, SOB, chest pain. *GI:* Diarrhea, N&V, bad taste in mouth, flatulence. *GU:* Delayed urine flow, priapism, hematuria, increased urinary frequency. *CNS:* Nightmares, confusion, anger, excitement, decreased ability to concentrate, dizziness, disorientation, drowsiness, lightheadedness, fatigue, insomnia, nervousness, impaired memory. Rarely, hallucinations, impaired speech, hypomania. *Other:* Incoordination, tremors, paresthesias, decreased libido, appetite disturbances, red eyes, sweating or clamminess, tinnitus, weight gain or loss, anemia, hypersalivation. Rarely, akathisia, muscle twitching, increased libido, impotence, retrograde ejaculation, early menses, missed periods.

OD **Management of Overdose:** *Symptoms: **Respiratory arrest, seizures,*** ECG changes, hypotension, priapism as well as an increase in the incidence and severity of side effects noted above (vomiting and drowsiness are the most common). *Treatment:* Treat symptoms (especially hypotension and sedation). Gastric lavage and forced diuresis to remove the drug from the body.

Drug Interactions

Alcohol / ↑ Depressant effects of alcohol
Antihypertensives / Additive hypotension
Barbiturates / ↑ Depressant effects of barbiturates
Clonidine / Trazodone ↓ effect of clonidine
CNS depressants / ↑ CNS depression
Digoxin / Trazodone may ↑ serum digoxin levels
MAO inhibitors / Initiate therapy cautiously if trazodone is to be used together with MAO inhibitors
Phenytoin / Trazodone may ↑ serum phenytoin levels

How Supplied: *Tablet:* 50 mg, 100 mg, 150 mg, 300 mg

Dosage

- **Tablets**

Antidepressant.

Adults and adolescents, initial: 150 mg/day; **then,** increase by 50 mg/day every 3–4 days to maximum of 400 mg/day in divided doses (outpatients). Inpatients may require up to, but not exceeding, 600 mg/day in divided doses. **Maintenance:** Use lowest effective dose. **Geriatric clients:** 75 mg/day in divided doses; dose can then be increased, as needed and tolerated, at 3- to 4-day intervals.

Treat aggressive behavior.

Trazodone, 50 mg b.i.d., with tryptophan, 500 mg b.i.d. Dosage adjustments may be required to reach a therapeutic response or if side effects develop.

Panic disorder or agoraphobia with panic attacks.

300 mg/day.

HEALTH CARE CONSIDERATIONS

Administration/Storage

1. Initiate dose at the lowest possible level; increase gradually.
2. Beneficial effects may be observed within 1 week with optimal effects seen within 2 weeks.

Assessment

1. Record indications for therapy, onset of symptoms, and any associated causative factors.
2. Note any history of recent MI.
3. Monitor ECG, CBC, liver and renal function studies.

Client/Family Teaching

1. Take with food to enhance absorption and minimize dizziness and/or lightheadedness. Take major portion of dose at bedtime to reduce daytime side effects.
2. Use caution when driving or when performing other hazardous tasks; may cause drowsiness or dizziness.
3. Avoid alcohol and CNS depressants.
4. Report any persistent/bothersome side effects.
5. Use sugarless gum or candies and frequent mouth rinses to diminish dry mouth effects.
6. Inform surgeon if elective surgery is planned to minimize interaction with anesthetic agent.
7. Encourage family to share responsibility for drug therapy to optimize treatment, prevent overdosage, and observe for any suicidal cues. Clients taking antidepressants and emerging from the deepest phases of depression are more prone to suicide.
8. May take 2–4 weeks for full drug effects to be realized.

Outcome/Evaluate:

- ↓ Depression (e.g., improved sleeping/eating patterns, ↓ fatigue, and ↑ social interactions)
- Control of overwhelming anxiety/panic symptoms

Tretinoin (Retinoic acid, Vitamin A acid)

(TRET-ih-noyn)

Pregnancy Category: C (Topical products), D (Oral products)

Avita, Renova, Retin-A, Retin-A Micro, Retisol-A ✱, StieVA-A ✱, StieVA-A Forte ✱, Vesanoid, Vitinoin ✱ **(Rx)**

Classification: Antiacne drug

T

Action/Kinetics: Topical tretinoin is believed to decrease microcomedone formation by decreasing the cohesiveness of follicular epithelial cells. Also believed to increase mitotic activity and increase turnover of follicular epithelial cells as well as decrease keratin synthesis. Some systemic absorption occurs (approximately 5% is recovered in the urine).

The mechanism of action for PO use in acute promyelocytic leukemia (APL) is not known. Absorption is enhanced when the drug is taken with food. **Time to peak levels:** 1–2 hr. Is over 95% bound to plasma proteins (mainly to albumin). **Terminal elimination t½:** 0.5–2 hr in APL clients. Metabolized by the liver, with about two-thirds excreted in the urine and one-third in the feces.

Uses: Dermatologic: *Avita, Retin-A:* Acne vulgaris. *Retin-A* and *Renova:* As an adjunct to comprehensive skin care and sun avoidance to treat fine wrinkles, mottled hyperpigmentation, and roughness of facial skin caused by age and the sun. For those individuals who do not achieve palliation using comprehensive skin care and sun avoidance programs alone. *Investigational (Retin-A):* Treat various forms of skin cancer. Dermatologic conditions including lamellar ichthyosis, mollusca contagiosa, verrucae plantaris, verrucae planae juveniles, ichthyosis vulgaris, bullous congenital ichthyosiform, and pityriasis rubra pilaris. To enhance the percutaneous absorption of topical minoxidil.

Oral: To induce remission in APL. After induction therapy with tretinoin, clients should be given a standard consolidation or maintenance chemotherapy regimen for APL, unless contraindicated.

Contraindications: Eczema, sunburn. Use if inherently sensitive to sunlight or if taking other drugs that increase sensitivity to sunlight. Use of Renova if client is also taking drugs known to be photosensitizers (e.g., fluoroquinolones, phenothiazines, sulfonamides, tetracyclines, thiazides). Those allergic to parabens (preservative in the gelatin capsules). Use of PO form during lactation. Use around the eyes, mouth, angles of the nose, and mucous membranes.

Special Concerns: Use with caution during lactation. Safety and effectiveness have not been determined in children. Excessive sunlight and weather extremes (e.g., wind and cold) may be irritating. Use Avita and Renova with caution with concomitant topical medications, medicated or abrasive soaps, shampoos, cleansers, cosmetics with a strong drying effect, permanent wave solutions, electrolysis, hair depilatories or waxes, and products with high concentrations of alcohol, astringents, spices, or lime. Safety and efficacy of Renova have not been determined in children less than 18 years of age, in individuals over the age of 50 years, or in individuals with moderately or heavily pigmented skin. Use of the PO form has resulted in retonic acid-APL syndrome, especially during the first month of treatment. The safety and efficacy of oral tretinoin at doses less than 45 mg/m²/day have not been evaluated in children.

Side Effects: Following topical use. *Dermatologic:* Red, edematous, crusted, or blistered skin; hyperpigmentation or hypopigmentation, increased susceptibility to sunlight, erythema, pruritus, burning, dryness. Excessive application will cause redness, peeling, or discomfort with no increase in results.

Following oral use. *Retinoic acid-APL syndrome:* Fever, dyspnea, weight gain, radiographic pulmonary infiltrate, pleural or pericardial effusions. Occasional impaired myocardial contractility and episodic hypotension; possibility of concomitant leukocytosis. ***Progressive hypoxemia with possible fatal outcome.*** Respiratory symptoms, including upper respiratory tract disorders, respiratory insufficiency, pneumonia, rales, expiratory wheezing, lower respiratory tract disorders, bronchial asthma, ***pulmonary or larynx edema,*** unspecified pulmonary disease. *Pseudotumor cerebri (especially in children):* Papilledema, headache, N&V, visual disturbances. *Typical retinoid toxicity (similar to ingestion of high doses of vitamin A):* Headache, fever, dryness of skin and mucous membranes, bone pain, N&V, rash, mucositis, pruritus, increased sweating, visual disturbances, ocular disorders, alopecia, skin changes, changed visual acuity, bone inflammation, visual field defects. *Body as a whole:* Malaise, shivering, ***hemorrhage, DIC,*** infections, peripheral edema, pain, chest discomfort, edema, weight increase, anorexia, weight decrease, myalgia, flank pain, cellulitis, facial edema, fluid imbalance, pallor, lymph disorders, acidosis, hypothermia, ascites. *GI:* ***GI hemorrhage,*** abdominal pain, various GI disorders, diarrhea, constipation, dyspepsia, abdominal distension, hepatosplenomegaly, hepatitis, ulcer, unspecified liver disorders. *CV:* Arrhythmias, flushing, hypotension, hypertension, phlebitis, ***cardiac failure, cardiac arrest, stroke,*** MI, enlarged heart, heart murmur, ischemia, myocarditis, pericarditis, pulmonary hypertension, secondary cardiomyopathy. *CNS:* Dizziness, paresthesias, anxiety, insomnia, depression, confusion, ***cerebral hemorrhage,***

intracranial hypertension, agitation, hallucinations, abnormal gait, agnosia, aphasia, asterixis, cerebellar edema, cerebellar disorders, ***convulsions, coma,*** CNS depression, dysarthria, encephalopathy, facial paralysis, hemiplegia, hyporeflexia, hypotaxia, no light reflex, neurologic reaction, spinal cord disorder, tremor, leg weakness, unconsciousness, dementia, forgetfulness, somnolence, slow speech. *GU:* Renal insufficiency, dysuria, acute renal failure, micturition frequency, renal tubular necrosis, enlarged prostate. *Otic:* Earache, feeling of fullness in the ears, hearing loss, unspecified auricular disorders, irreversible hearing loss. *Other:* Erythema nodosum, basophilia, hyperhistaminemia, Sweet's syndrome, organomegaly, hypercalcemia, pancreatitis, myositis.

Laboratory Test Considerations: Elevated LFTs following use of PO product.

Drug Interactions: Concomitant use with sulfur, resorcinol, benzoyl peroxide, or salicylic acid may cause significant skin irritation.

How Supplied: *Cream:* 0.025%, 0.05%, 0.1%; *Gel:* 0.01%, 0.025%, 0.1%; *Liquid:* 0.05%; *Capsules:* 10 mg

Dosage

- **Cream, Gel, or Liquid**

  Acne vulgaris.

Apply lightly over the affected areas once daily at bedtime. Beneficial effects many not be seen for 2–6 weeks.

- **Cream, 0.025%, 0.05%, 0.1%**

  Palliation for skin conditions.

Apply a pea-sized amount once daily at bedtime, using only enough to lightly cover the entire affected area. Up to 6 months of therapy may be needed before effects are seen.

- **Capsules**

  APL.

Adults: 45 mg/m²/day given as two evenly divided doses. Given until complete remission is obtained. Discontinue 30 days after achieving complete remission or after 90 days of treatment, whichever comes first.

HEALTH CARE CONSIDERATIONS

Administration/Storage

1. Apply the liquid carefully with the fingertip, cotton swab, or gauze pad only to affected areas.
2. Excessive amounts of the gel will cause a "pilling" effect which minimizes the likelihood of overapplication.
3. Wash hands thoroughly immediately after applying tretinoin.
4. Before applying Renova, wash the face gently with a mild soap and pat the skin dry, waiting 20–30 min before applying. When applied, take care to avoid contact with eyes, ears, nostrils, and mouth.
5. Do not freeze Renova cream.
6. Treatment with Renova for more than 24 weeks does not appear to increase improvement. The results of continued irritation of the skin for more than 48 weeks are not known.

Assessment

1. Record indications for therapy, type, onset, and characteristics of symptoms.
2. With acne, thoroughly describe pretreatment skin condition; obtain photographs to compare with results of therapy.
3. Determine if pregnant.
4. Monitor hematologic, liver, and renal function studies.

Client/Family Teaching

Topical:

1. Keep away from normal skin, mucous membranes, eyes, ears, mouth, nostrils, and the angles of the nose.
2. Wash with mild soap and warm water and pat skin dry. Wait 20–30 min before applying tretinoin.
3. On application there will be a transitory feeling of warmth and stinging.
4. Wash hands thoroughly before and immediately after applying tretinoin.
5. Expect dryness and peeling of skin from the affected areas.
6. May be more sensitive to wind and cold. Do not apply to wind or sunburned skin or to open wounds.
7. Avoid alcohol-containing preparations such as shaving lotions and creams, perfumes, cosmetics with drying effects, skin cleansers, and medicated soaps.
8. Initially, the lesions may worsen. This is caused by the effect of the drug on deep lesions that had been previously undetected. Report if lesions become severe; drug should be discontinued until skin integrity restored.
9. Improvement should be evident in 6 weeks but therapy should be continued for at least 3 months.
10. Practice reliable birth control.
11. Avoid excessive exposure to sunlamps and to the sun. If exposed, use a sunscreen and protective clothing over affected areas.

Oral:

1. Drug will be administered until complete remission is obtained. It will be stopped 30 days after remission or after 90 days of therapy, whichever comes first. This does not replace standard maintenance chemotherapy for APL.

2. Take with food to enhance absorption.
3. Take exactly as prescribed; do not exceed or skip doses.
4. Review list of potential drug side effects, noting those that require immediate reporting. Avoid pregnancy.

Outcome/Evaluate

- ↓ Size/number of acne eruptions
- Clearing of skin condition; symptomatic improvement
- Remission with APL

Triamcinolone

(try-am-SIN-oh-lohn)

Pregnancy Category: C

Dental Paste: Kenalog in Orabase, Oracort, Oralone **(Rx)**. **Tablets:** Aristocort, Atolone, Kenacort **(Rx)**

Triamcinolone acetonide

(try-am-SIN-oh-lohn)

Pregnancy Category: C

Dental Paste: Oracort ✱. **Inhalation Aerosol:** Azmacort, Nasacort, Nasacort AQ **(Rx)**. **Parenteral:** Kenaject-40, Kenalog-10 and -40, Scheinpharm Triamcine-A ✱, Tac-3 and -40, Triam-A, Triamonide 40, Tri-Kort, Trilog **(Rx)**. **Topical Aerosol:** Kenalog **(Rx)**. **Topical Cream:** Aristocort, Aristocort A, Delta-Tritex, Flutex, Kenac, Kenalog, Kenalog-H, Kenonel, Triacet, Triaderm ✱, Trianide Mild, Trianide Regular, Triderm, Trymex **(Rx)**. **Topical Lotion:** Kenalog, Kenonel **(Rx)**. **Topical Ointment:** Aristocort, Aristocort A, Kenac, Kenalog, Kenonel, Triaderm ✱, Trymex, **Topical Spray:** Nasacort AQ **(Rx)**

Triamcinolone diacetate

(try-am-SIN-oh-lohn)

Pregnancy Category: C

Parenteral: Amcort, Aristocort Forte, Aristocort Intralesional, Aristocort Parenteral ✱, Articulose L.A., Kenacort Diacetate, Triam-Forte, Triamolone 40, Trilone, Tristoject. **Syrup:** Aristocort Syrup ✱ **(Rx)**

Triamcinolone hexacetonide

(try-am-SIN-oh-lohn)

Pregnancy Category: C

Aristospan Intra-Articular, Aristospan Intralesional **(Rx)**

Classification: Corticosteroid, synthetic

See also *Corticosteroids*.

Action/Kinetics: More potent than prednisone. Intermediate-acting. Has no mineralocorticoid activity. **Onset:** Several hours. **Duration:** One or more weeks. **t½:** Over 200 min.

Additional Uses: Pulmonary emphysema accompanied by bronchospasm or bronchial edema. Diffuse interstitial pulmonary fibrosis. With diuretics to treat refractory CHF or cirrhosis of the liver with ascites. Multiple sclerosis. Inflammation following dental procedures. Triamcinolone acetonide for PO inhalation is used for maintenance treatment of asthma. Triamcinolone hexacetonide is restricted to intra-articular or intralesional treatment of rheumatoid arthritis and osteoarthritis.

Special Concerns: Use during pregnancy only if benefits clearly outweigh risks. Use with special caution with decreased renal function or renal disease. Dose must be highly individualized.

Additional Side Effects: Intra-articular, intrasynovial, or intrabursal administration may cause transient flushing, dizziness, local depigmentation, and rarely, local irritation. Exacerbation of symptoms has also been reported. A marked increase in swelling and pain and further restricted joint movement may indicate septic arthritis. Intradermal injection may cause local vesicular ulceration and persistent scarring. ***Syncope and anaphylactoid reactions*** have been reported with triamcinolone regardless of route of administration.

How Supplied: Triamcinolone: *Tablet:* 1 mg, 2 mg, 4 mg, 8 mg. Triamcinolone acetonide: *Metered dose inhaler (nasal):* 55 mcg/inh; *Metered dose inhaler (oral)* 100 mcg/inh; *Cream:* 0.025%, 0.1%, 0.5%; *Nasal Spray: Injection:* 3 mg/mL, 10 mg/mL, 40 mg/mL; *Lotion:* 0.025%, 0.1%; *Ointment:* 0.025%, 0.05%, 0.1%, 0.5%; *Paste:* 0.1%, 55 mcg/inh; *Topical Spray:* 0.147 mg/g. Triamcinolone diacetate: *Injection:* 25 mg/mL, 40 mg/mL. Triamcinolone hexacetonide: *Injection:* 5 mg/mL, 20 mg/mL.

Dosage

TRIAMCINOLONE

- **Tablets**

Adrenocortical insufficiency (with mineralocorticoid therapy).

4–12 mg/day.

Acute leukemias (children).

1–2 mg/kg.

Acute leukemia or lymphoma (adults).

16–40 mg/day (up to 100 mg/day may be necessary for leukemia).

Edema.

16–20 mg (up to 48 mg may be required until diuresis occurs).

Tuberculosis meningitis.

32–48 mg/day.

Rheumatic disease, dermatologic disorders, bronchial asthma.

8–16 mg/day.

SLE.

20–32 mg/day.

Allergies.
8–12 mg/day.
Hematologic disorders.
16–60 mg/day.
Ophthalmologic diseases.
12–40 mg daily.
Respiratory diseases.
16–48 mg/day.
TRIAMCINOLONE ACETONIDE
• **IM Only (Not for IV Use)**
2.5–60 mg/day, depending on the disease and its severity.
• **Intra-articular, Intrabursal, Tendon Sheaths**
2.5–5 mg for smaller joints and 5–15 mg for larger joints, although up to 40 mg has been used.
• **Intradermal**
1 mg/injection site (use 3 mg/mL or 10 mg/mL suspension only).
• **Topical: 0.025%, 0.1%, 0.5% Ointment or Cream; 0.025%, 0.1% Lotion; Paste: 0.1%; Aerosol—to deliver 0.2 mg)**
Apply sparingly to affected area b.i.d.–q.i.d. and rub in lightly.
• **Metered Dose Inhaler (Azmacort)**
Adults, usual: 2 inhalations (200 mcg) t.i.d.–q.i.d. or 4 inhalations (400 mcg) b.i.d., not to exceed 1,600 mcg/day. High initial doses (1,200–1,600 mcg/day) may be needed in some clients with severe asthma. **Pediatric, 6–12 years:** 1–2 inhalations (100–200 mcg) t.i.d.–q.i.d. or 2–4 inhalations b.i.d., not to exceed 1,200 mcg/day. Use in children less than 6 years of age has not been determined.
• **Intranasal Spray (Nasacort)**
Seasonal and perennial allergic rhinitis.
Adults and children over 12 years of age: 2 sprays (110 mcg) into each nostril once a day (i.e., for a total dose of 220 mcg/day). The dose may be increased to 440 mcg/day given either once daily or q.i.d. (1 spray/nostril).
TRIAMCINOLONE DIACETATE
• **IM Only**
40 mg/week.
• **Intra-articular, Intrasynovial**
5–40 mg.
• **Intralesional, Sublesional**
5–48 mg (no more than 12.5 mg/injection site and 25 mg/lesion).
TRIAMCINOLONE HEXACETONIDE
Not for IV use.
• **Intra-articular**
2–6 mg for small joints and 10–20 mg for large joints.
• **Intralesional/Sublesional**
Up to 0.5 mg/sq. in. of affected area.

HEALTH CARE CONSIDERATIONS

See also *Health Care Considerations* for *Corticosteroids.*

Administration/Storage

1. Initially, use the aerosol concomitantly with a systemic steroid. After 1 week, initiate a gradual withdrawal of systemic steroid. Make the next reduction after 1–2 weeks, depending on the response. If symptoms of insufficiency occur, the dose of systemic steroid can be increased temporarily. Also, the dose of systemic steroid may need to be increased in times of stress or a severe asthmatic attack.
2. Do not use the acetonide products if they clump due to exposure to freezing temperatures.
3. A single IM dose of the diacetate provides control from 4–7 days up to 3–4 weeks.
4. Triamcinolone acetonide nasal spray for allergic rhinitis may be effective as soon as 12 hr after initiation of therapy. Reevaluate if improvement is not seen within 2–3 weeks.
5. For best results, store the canister at room temperature and shake well before use.
6. Nasacort AQ is viscous at rest but a liquid when shaken. This allows the drug to stay in the nasal airways at the site of inflammation for up to 2 hr.

Assessment

1. Record indications for therapy; note type, onset, and characteristics of symptoms.
2. Assess area/condition requiring treatment and describe findings.
3. Monitor blood sugar, CBC, electrolytes, and renal function.

Client/Family Teaching

1. Take at the same time each day.
2. Ingest a liberal amount of protein; with regular use may experience gradual weight loss, associated with anorexia, muscle wasting, and weakness. See dietitian for assistance in meal plans/preparation.
3. Lie down if feeling faint; report if syncopal episodes persist and interfere with daily activities.
4. Report any evidence of abnormal bruising, bleeding, weight gain, edema, or dyspnea.
5. Drug may suppress reactions to skin allergy testing.
6. With topical therapy, apply to clean, slightly moist skin. Report if area does not improve with therapy or if symptoms worsen.
7. With nasal spray or inhaler, review appropriate method of administration and

proper care and storage of equipment. Always rinse mouth and equipment after use.
8. Report immediately any new onset of depression as well as aggravation of existing depressive symptoms.

Outcome/Evaluate

- ↓ Immune and inflammatory responses in autoimmune disorders and allergic reactions
- Improved airway exchange
- Restoration of skin integrity
- Relief of pain/inflammation; improved joint mobility

Triamterene

(try-**AM**-ter-een)
Pregnancy Category: B
Dyrenium **(Rx)**
Classification: Diuretic, potassium-sparing

See also *Diuretics*.
Action/Kinetics: Acts directly on the distal tubule to promote the excretion of sodium—which is exchanged for potassium or hydrogen ions—bicarbonate, chloride, and fluid. It increases urinary pH and is a weak folic acid antagonist. **Onset:** 2–4 hr. **Peak effect:** 6–8 hr. **Duration:** 7–9 hr. **t½:** 3 hr. From one-half to two-thirds of the drug is bound to plasma protein. Metabolized to hydroxytriamterene sulfate, which is also active. About 20% is excreted unchanged through the urine.
Uses: Edema due to CHF, hepatic cirrhosis, nephrotic syndrome, steroid therapy, secondary hyperaldosteronism, and idiopathic edema. May be used alone or with other diuretics. *Investigational:* Prophylaxis and treatment of hypokalemia, adjunct in the treatment of hypertension.
Contraindications: Hypersensitivity to drug, severe or progressive renal insufficiency, severe hepatic disease, anuria, hyperkalemia, hyperuricemia, gout, history of nephrolithiasis. Lactation.
Special Concerns: Safety and efficacy have not been determined in children.
Side Effects: *Electrolyte:* Hyperkalemia, electrolyte imbalance. *GI:* Nausea, vomiting (may also be indicative of electrolyte imbalance), diarrhea, dry mouth. *CNS:* Dizziness, drowsiness, fatigue, weakness, headache. *Hematologic:* Megaloblastic anemia, thrombocytopenia. *Renal:* Azotemia, interstitial nephritis. *Miscellaneous:* ***Anaphylaxis,*** photosensitivity, hypokalemia, jaundice, muscle cramps, rash.
Laboratory Test Considerations: Triamterene may impart blue fluorescence to urine, interfering with fluorometric assays (e.g., lactic dehydrogenase, quinidine). ↑ BUN, creatinine. ↑ Serum uric acid in clients predisposed to gouty arthritis.
OD **Management of Overdose:** *Symptoms:* Electrolyte imbalance, especially hyperkalemia. Also, nausea, vomiting, other GI disturbances, weakness, hypotension, reversible acute renal failure. *Treatment:* Immediately induce vomiting or perform gastric lavage. Evaluate electrolyte levels and fluid balance and treat if necessary. Dialysis may be beneficial.
Drug Interactions
Amantadine / ↑ Toxic effects of amantadine due to ↓ renal excretion
Angiotensin-converting enzyme inhibitors / Significant hyperkalemia
Antihypertensives / Potentiated by triamterene
Captopril / ↑ Risk of significant hyperkalemia
Cimetidine / ↑ Bioavailability and ↓ clearance of triamterene
Digitalis / Inhibited by triamterene
Indomethacin / ↑ Risk of nephrotoxicity and acute renal failure
Lithium / ↑ Chance of lithium toxicity due to ↓ renal clearance
Potassium salts / Additive hyperkalemia
Spironolactone / Additive hyperkalemia
How Supplied: *Capsule:* 50 mg, 100 mg

Dosage

- Capsules.

Diuretic.
Adults, initial: 100 mg b.i.d. after meals; **maximum daily dose:** 300 mg.

HEALTH CARE CONSIDERATIONS

See also *Health Care Considerations* for *Diuretics*.

Administration/Storage

1. Minimize nausea by giving the drug after meals.
2. Dosage is usually reduced by one-half when another diuretic is added to the regimen.

Assessment

1. Record indications for therapy; list agents prescribed to ensure none interact.
2. Assess for alcoholism, megaloblastic anemia may occur because triamterene is a weak antagonist of folic acid.
3. Monitor ECG, CBC, uric acid, electrolytes, and renal function.

Client/Family Teaching

1. Take with food to minimize GI upset/nausea.
2. Report any sore throat, rash, or fever (S&S of blood dyscrasia).

3. Persistent headaches, drowsiness, vomiting, restlessness, mental wandering, lethargy, and foul breath may be signs of uremia; report.
4. Drug may cause dizziness.
5. Avoid alcohol and OTC agents. Also avoid potassium supplements, salt substitutes that contain potassium, and foods high in potassium; drug is potassium-sparing.
6. Urine may appear pale fluorescent blue.
7. Avoid direct sunlight for prolonged periods; may cause a photosensitivity reaction. Use sunscreens, sunglasses, hat, and long sleeves and pants when exposed.

Outcome/Evaluate: ↓ Edema; ↑ diuresis; ↓ BP

COMBINATION DRUG

Triamterene and Hydrochlorothiazide Capsules

(try-**AM**-ter-een, hy-droh-**klor**-oh-**THIGH**-ah-zyd)

Pregnancy Category: C

Dyazide **(Rx)**

Triamterene and Hydrochlorothiazide Tablets

(try-**AM**-teh-reen, hy-droh-**kloh**-roh-**THIGH**-ah-zyd)

Pregnancy Category: C

Apo-Triazide ✱, Dyazide, Maxzide, Maxide-25 MG, Novo-Triamzide ✱, Nu-Triazide ✱, Pro-Triazide ✱ **(Rx)**

Classification: Diuretic, antihypertensive

See also *Hydrochlorothiazide* and *Triamterene*.

Content: Capsules. *Diuretic:* Hydrochlorothiazide, 25 or 50 mg. *Diuretic:* Triamterene, 50 or 100 mg. **Tablets.** *Diuretic:* Hydrochlorothiazide, 25 or 50 mg. *Diuretic:* Triamterene, 37.5 or 75 mg. (In Canada the tablets contain 25 mg of hydrochlorothiazide and 50 mg triamterene.)

Uses: To treat hypertension or edema in clients who manifest hypokalemia on hydrochlorothiazide alone. In clients requiring a diuretic and in whom hypokalemia cannot be risked (i.e., clients with cardiac arrhythmias or those taking digitalis). Usually not the first line of therapy, except for clients in whom hypokalemia should be avoided.

Contraindications: Clients receiving other potassium-sparing drugs such as amiloride and spironolactone. Use in anuria, acute or chronic renal insufficiency, significant renal impairment, preexisting elevated serum potassium.

Special Concerns: Use with caution during lactation. Geriatric clients may be more sensitive to the hypotensive and electrolyte effects of this combination; also, age-related decreases in renal function may require a decrease in dosage.

How Supplied: See Content

Dosage

- **Capsules**

  Hypertension or edema.

Adults: Triamterene/hydrochlorothiazide: 37.5 mg/25 mg—1–2 capsules given once daily with monitoring of serum potassium and clinical effect. Triamterene/hydrochlorothiazide: 50 mg/25 mg—1–2 capsules b.i.d. after meals. Some clients may be controlled using 1 capsule every day or every other day. No more than 4 capsules should be taken daily.

- **Tablets**

  Hypertension or edema.

Adults: Triamterene/hydrochlorothiazide: 37.5 mg/25 mg—1–2 tablets/day (determined by individual titration with the components). Or, triamterene/hydrochlorothiazide: 75 mg/50 mg—1 tablet daily.

HEALTH CARE CONSIDERATIONS

See also *Health Care Considerations* for *Antihypertensive Agents, Triamterene,* and *Hydrochlorothiazide.*

Administration/Storage: Monitor clients who are transferred from less bioavailable formulations of triamterene and hydrochlorothiazide for serum potassium levels following the transfer.

Outcome/Evaluate

- Control of hypertension
- Resolution of edema

T

Triazolam

(try-**AYZ**-oh-lam)

Pregnancy Category: X

Alti-Triazolam ✱, Apo-Triazo ✱, Gen-Triazolam ✱, Halcion, Novo-Triolam ✱ **(C-IV) (Rx)**

Classification: Benzodiazepine sedative-hypnotic

See also *Tranquilizers, Antimanic Drugs, and Hypnotics.*

Action/Kinetics: Decreases sleep latency, increases the duration of sleep, and decreases the number of awakenings. **Time to peak plasma levels:** 0.5–2 hr. **t½:** 1.5–5.5 hr. Metabolized in liver; inactive metabolites excreted in the urine.

Uses: Insomnia (short-term management, not to exceed 1 month). May be beneficial in preventing or treating transient insomnia from a sudden change in sleep schedule.
Contraindications: Use concomitantly with itraconazole, ketoconazole, nefazodone. Lactation (may cause sedation and feeding problems in infants).
Special Concerns: Safety and efficacy in children under 18 years of age not established. Geriatric clients may be more sensitive to the effects of triazolam.
Side Effects: *CNS:* Rebound insomnia, anterograde amnesia, headache, ataxia, decreased coordination, "traveler's" amnesia. Psychologic and physical dependence. *GI:* N&V.
How Supplied: *Tablet:* 0.125 mg, 0.25 mg

Dosage

- **Tablets**

Adults, initial: 0.25–0.5 mg before bedtime. **Geriatric or debilitated clients, initial:** 0.125 mg; **then,** depending on response, 0.125–0.25 mg before bedtime.

HEALTH CARE CONSIDERATIONS

See also *Health Care Considerations* for *Tranquilizers, Antimanic Drugs, and Hypnotics.*

Assessment

1. Record indications for therapy, onset, duration, and characteristics of symptoms.
2. Assess mental status and note behavioral manifestations.
3. Monitor CBC and LFTs.
4. Evaluate sleep patterns; determine underlying cause of insomnia so that source may be removed. With simple insomnia, try nonpharmacologic interventions to induce sleep, such as soft music, guided imagery, or progressive muscle relaxation.
5. Initiate safety precautions (i.e., side rails, supervised ambulation, frequent observations), especially with elderly and confused clients.
6. Assess for tolerance and for psychologic and physical dependence. Monitor closely for CNS toxic effects especially during prolonged therapy (longer than 2 weeks).

Client/Family Teaching

1. Take only as directed. Store away from bedside.
2. Avoid alcohol and CNS depressants.
3. Use caution when driving or operating machinery until daytime sedative effects evaluated.
4. Drug is for short-term use only; may cause physical and psychologic dependence. Try warm baths/milk, and other methods to induce sleep, such as white noise simulator, soft music, guided imagery, or progressive muscle relaxation, rather than become dependent on drugs for insomnia.
5. Report unusual side effects including hallucinations, nightmares, depression, or periods of confusion.

Outcome/Evaluate: Improved sleeping patterns; insomnia relief

Trientine hydrochloride

(TRY-en-teen)
Pregnancy Category: C
Syprine **(Rx)**
Classification: Chelating agent

Action/Kinetics: A chelating agent that binds copper, thus facilitating its excretion from the body.
Uses: Wilson's disease (a metabolic defect resulting in excess copper accumulation) who are intolerant of penicillamine.
Contraindications: Use in cystinuria, rheumatoid arthritis, biliary cirrhosis.
Special Concerns: Use with caution during lactation. Safety and effectiveness in children have not been determined although the drug has been used in children as young as 6 years of age.
Side Effects: Iron deficiency anemia, SLE.
How Supplied: *Capsule:* 250 mg

Dosage

- **Capsules**

Wilson's disease.
Adults, initial: 750 mg/day–1.25 g/day in divided doses b.i.d., t.i.d., or q.i.d.; **then,** may increase to a maximum of 2 g/day. **Children less than 12 years of age, initial:** 500–750 mg/day in divided doses b.i.d., t.i.d., or q.i.d.; **then,** may increase to a maximum of 1.5 g/day.

HEALTH CARE CONSIDERATIONS

Administration/Storage

1. Increase the daily dose only if the response is not adequate or the serum copper level is consistently greater than 20 mcg/dL.
2. At 6- to 12-month intervals, determine the optimal long-term maintenance dosage.
3. If the contents of the capsule come in contact with any site on the body, promptly wash with water to avoid contact dermatitis.
4. Store capsules at 2°C–8°C (36°F–46°F).

Assessment: Monitor CBC and serum copper levels. Note previous treatment regimens and results.

Client/Family Teaching

1. Take on an empty stomach at least 1 hr be-

fore or 2 hr after meals and at least 1 hr apart from any other drug, food, or milk.
2. Swallow capsules whole with water; do not chew or open capsules.
3. Iron deficiency anemia may develop in children, in menstruating or pregnant women, or as a result of the low-copper diet necessary to treat Wilson's disease. Iron may given but allow 2 hr between administration of iron and trientine.
4. Record temperature nightly for the first month of treatment; report any fever or skin eruptions.
5. Report for labs; serum copper levels will be followed, and periodically a 24-hr urine for copper. Free serum copper is the most reliable way to monitor the effectiveness of therapy. Clients responsive to therapy will have less than 10 mcg/dL of free copper in the serum.

Outcome/Evaluate: ↓ Serum copper levels; relief of S&S of toxicity

Trifluoperazine

(try-**flew**-oh-**PER**-ah-zeen)
Pregnancy Category: C
Apo-Trifluoperazine ✦, Novo-Trifluzine ✦, PMS-Trifluoperazine ✦, Stelazine, Terfluzine ✦ **(Rx)**
Classification: Antipsychotic, antiemetic, piperazine-type phenothiazine

See also *Antipsychotic Agents, Phenothiazines.*

Action/Kinetics: Causes a high incidence of extrapyramidal symptoms and antiemetic effects and a low incidence of sedation, orthostatic hypotension, and anticholinergic side effects. **Maximum therapeutic effect:** Usually 2–3 weeks after initiation of therapy.

Uses: To manage psychotic disorders. Suitable for clients with apathy or withdrawal. Short-term treatment of nonpsychotic anxiety (not the drug of choice).

Special Concerns: Use during pregnancy only when benefits clearly outweigh risks. Dosage has not been established in children less than 6 years of age. Geriatric, emaciated, or debilitated clients usually require a lower initial dose.

How Supplied: *Injection:* 2 mg/mL; *Tablet:* 1 mg, 2 mg, 5 mg, 10 mg

Dosage

- **Oral Solution, Tablets**

Psychotic disorders.

Adults and adolescents, initial: 2–5 mg (base) b.i.d.; **maintenance:** 15–20 mg/day in two or three divided doses. **Pediatric, 6–12 years:** 1 mg (base) 1–2 times/day; adjust dose as required and tolerated.

Anxiety.

Adults and adolescents: 1–2 mg b.i.d, not to exceed 6 mg/day. Not to be given for this purpose longer than 12 weeks.

- **IM**

Pyschoses.

Adults: 1–2 mg q 4–6 hr, not to exceed 10 mg/day. Switch to PO therapy as soon as possible. **Pediatric:** *Severe symptoms only:* 1 mg 1–2 times/day.

HEALTH CARE CONSIDERATIONS

See also *Health Care Considerations* for *Antipsychotic Agents, Phenothiazines.*

Administration/Storage

1. Dilute concentrate just before administration with 60 mL of juice (tomato or fruit), carbonated drinks, water, milk, orange or simple syrup, coffee, tea, or semisolid foods (e.g., applesauce, pudding, soup).
2. Protect liquid forms from light.
3. Discard strongly colored solutions.
4. Avoid skin contact with liquid form to prevent contact dermatitis.
5. To prevent cumulative effects, allow at least 4 hr between injections.

Assessment

1. Record indications for therapy, onset of symptoms, and behavioral manifestations.
2. Note other agents prescribed and the outcome.
3. Assess mental status and note findings.
4. Monitor CBC, ECG, and LFTs.

Outcome/Evaluate

- Reduction in paranoid, excitable, or withdrawn behaviors
- ↓ Levels of anxiety, agitation, and tension

T

Trihexyphenidyl hydrochloride

(try-hex-ee-**FEN**-ih-dill)
Pregnancy Category: C
Aparkane ✦, Apo-Trihex ✦, Artane, Artane Sequels, Novo-Hexidyl ✦, PMS-Trihexyphenidyl ✦, Trihexy-2 and -5, Trihexyphen ✦ **(Rx)**
Classification: Antiparkinson agent, anticholinergic

See also *Cholinergic Blocking Agents* and *Antiparkinson Drugs.*

Action/Kinetics: Synthetic anticholinergic, which relieves rigidity but has little effect on tremors. Causes a direct antispasmodic effect on smooth muscle. High incidence of side effects. Small doses cause CNS depres-

sion, whereas larger doses may result in CNS excitation. **Onset, PO:** 60 min. **Duration, PO:** 6–12 hr.
Uses: Adjunct in the treatment of all types of parkinsonism (often used as adjunct with levodopa). Drug-induced extrapyramidal symptoms. Sustained-release medication is for maintenance dosage only.
Additional Contraindications: Arteriosclerosis and hypersensitivity to drug.
Additional Side Effects: Serious CNS stimulation (restlessness, insomnia, delirium, agitation) and psychotic manifestations.
Additional Drug Interactions: ↑ Effectiveness of levodopa if used together; such combined use not recommended in clients with psychoses.
How Supplied: *Elixir:* 2 mg/5 mL; *Tablet:* 2 mg, 5 mg

Dosage

- **Elixir, Tablets**

  Parkinsonism.

Initial (day 1): 1–2 mg; **then,** increase by 2 mg q 3–5 days until daily dose is 6–10 mg given in divided doses. Some clients may require 12–15 mg/day (especially those with postencephalitic parkinsonism).

Adjunct with levodopa.

Adults: 3–6 mg/day in divided doses.

Drug-induced extrapyramidal reactions.

Initial: 1 mg/day; **then,** increase as needed to total daily dose of 5–15 mg.

HEALTH CARE CONSIDERATIONS

See also *Health Care Considerations* for *Cholinergic Blocking Agents* and *Antiparkinson Drugs.*

Assessment: Assess for and note extent of involuntary movements, drooling, pill rolling, and muscle spasms/rigidity. Note mental status.

Client/Family Teaching

1. Take with or after meals to minimize GI upset.
2. May cause dizziness or drowsiness and othostatic effects.
3. Increase fluids and bulk in diet to prevent constipation.
4. May impair perspiration; avoid overheating and hot weather exposures. Report urinary retention.
5. This drug has a high incidence of side effects; report as early detection and intervention are imperative.
6. Report any evidence of extrapyramidal symptoms or increase in restlessness, insomnia, agitation, or psychotic manifestations; dosage may need adjusting.

Outcome/Evaluate

- Control of S&S of Parkinsonism
- Prevention of drug-induced extrapyramidal symptoms

Trimethobenzamide hydrochloride

(try-meth-oh-**BENZ**-ah-myd)
Pregnancy Category: C
Arrestin, Hymetic, Tebamide, T-Gen, Ticon, Tigan **(Rx)**
Classification: Antiemetic

See also *Antiemetics.*
Action/Kinetics: Related to the antihistamines but with weak antihistaminic properties. Less effective than the phenothiazines but has fewer side effects. Not suitable as sole agent for severe emesis. Can be used PR. Appears to control vomiting by depressing the CTZ in the medulla. **Onset: PO and IM,** 10–40 min. **Duration:** 3–4 hr after PO and 2–3 hr after IM. 30%–50% of drug excreted unchanged in urine in 48–72 hr.
Uses: Nausea and vomiting.
Contraindications: Hypersensitivity to drug, benzocaine, or similar local anesthetics. Use of suppositories for neonates; IM use in children.
Special Concerns: Use during pregnancy only if benefits outweigh risks. Use with caution during lactation.
Side Effects: *CNS:* Depression of mood, disorientation, headache, drowsiness, dizziness, ***seizures, coma,*** Parkinson-like symptoms. *Other:* Hypersensitivity reactions, hypotension, blood dyscrasias, jaundice, muscle cramps, opisthotonos, blurred vision, diarrhea, allergic skin reactions. *After IM injection:* Pain, burning, stinging, redness at injection site.
Drug Interactions: Concomitant use with atropine-like drugs and CNS depressants including alcohol should be avoided.
How Supplied: *Capsule:* 100 mg, 250 mg; *Injection:* 100 mg/mL; *Suppository:* 100 mg, 200 mg

Dosage

- **Capsules**

Adults: 250 mg t.i.d.–q.i.d.; **pediatric, 13.6–40.9 kg:** 100–200 mg t.i.d.–q.i.d.

- **Suppositories**

Adults: 200 mg t.i.d.–q.i.d.; **pediatric, under 13.6 kg:** 100 mg t.i.d.–q.i.d.; **13.6–40.9 kg:** 100–200 mg t.i.d.–q.i.d.

- **IM**

Adults only: 200 mg t.i.d.–q.i.d. *IM route not to be used in children.*

HEALTH CARE CONSIDERATIONS

See also *Health Considerations* for *Antiemetics.*

Administration/Storage

1. Inject drug IM deeply into the upper, outer quadrant of the gluteus muscle. To minimize local reaction, use care to avoid escape of fluid from the needle.
2. Do not administer suppositories to clients allergic to benzocaine or similar anesthetics.

Assessment

1. Identify cause for N&V.
2. Record any sensitivity to benzocaine. Assess for any skin reaction (first sign of hypersensitivity to the drug).
3. Note any local reaction to the suppositories.

Client/Family Teaching

1. Use only as directed; report any adverse drug effects.
2. Do not drive or operate machinery until drug effects are realized; may cause drowsiness and dizziness.
3. Avoid alcohol and any other CNS depressants.

Outcome/Evaluate: Prevention/control of N&V

—COMBINATION DRUG—

Trimethoprim and Sulfamethoxazole

(try-**METH**-oh-prim, sul-fah-meh-**THOX**-ah-zohl)

Pregnancy Category: C

Apo-Sulfatrim ✦, Bactrim, Bactrim DS, Bactrim IV, Bactrim Pediatric, Bactrim Roche ✦, Cotrim, Cotrim D.S., Cotrim Pediatric, Novo-Trimel ✦, Novo-Trimel D.S. ✦, Nu-Cotrimix ✦, Pro-Trin ✦, Roubac ✦, Septra, Septra DS, Septra Injection ✦, Septra IV, Sulfatrim, Trisulfa ✦, Trisulfa DS ✦ **(Rx)**

Classification: Antibacterial

See also *Sulfonamides.*

Content: These products contain the antibacterial agents sulfamethoxazole and trimethoprim. See also *Sulfamethoxazole.*

Oral Suspension: Sulfamethoxazole, 200 mg and trimethoprim, 40 mg/5 mL.

Tablets: Sulfamethoxazole, 400 mg and trimethoprim, 80 mg/tablet.

Double Strength (DS) Tablets: Sulfamethoxazole, 800 mg and trimethoprim, 160 mg/tablet.

Concentrate for injection: Sulfamethoxazole, 80 mg and trimethoprim, 16 mg/mL.

Uses: PO, Parenteral: UTIs due to *Escherichia coli, Klebsiella, Enterobacter, Pseudomonas mirabilis* and *vulgaris,* and *Morganella morganii.* Enteritis due to *Shigella flexneri* or *S. sonnei. Pneumocystis carinii* pneumonitis in children and adults. **PO:** Acute otitis media in children due to *Haemophilus influenzae* or *Streptococcus pneumoniae.* Traveler's diarrhea in adults due to *E. coli.* Prophylaxis of *P. carinii* pneumonia in immunocompromised clients (including those with AIDS). Acute exacerbations of chronic bronchitis in adults due to *H. influenzae* or *S. pneumoniae. Investigational:* Cholera, salmonella, nocardiosis, prophylaxis of recurrent UTIs in women, prophylaxis of neutropenic clients with *P. carinii* infections or leukemia clients to decrease incidence of gram-negative rod bacteremia. Treatment of acute and chronic prostatitis. Decrease chance of urinary and blood bacterial infections in renal transplant clients.

Additional Contraindications: Infants under 2 months of age. During pregnancy at term. Megaloblastic anemia due to folate deficiency. Lactation.

Special Concerns: Use with caution in impaired liver or kidney function and in clients with possible folate deficiency. AIDS clients may not tolerate or respond to this product.

Laboratory Test Considerations: Jaffe alkaline picrate reaction overestimation of creatinine by 10%.

Additional Drug Interactions

Cyclosporine / ↓ Effect of cyclosporine; ↑ risk of nephrotoxicity
Dapsone / ↑ Effect of both dapsone and trimethoprim
Methotrexate / ↑ Risk of methotrexate toxicity due to displacement from plasma protein binding sites
Phenytoin / ↑ Effect of phenytoin due to ↓ hepatic clearance
Sulfonylureas / ↑ Hypoglycemic effect of sulfonylureas
Thiazide diuretics / ↑ Risk of thrombocytopenia with purpura in geriatric clients
Warfarin / ↑ PT
Zidovudine / ↑ Serum levels of AZT due to ↓ renal clearance

How Supplied: See Content

Dosage

• **Oral Suspension, Double-Strength Tablets, Tablets**

UTIs, shigellosis, bronchitis, acute otitis media.

Adults: 1 DS tablet, 2 tablets, or 4 teaspoonfuls of suspension q 12 hr for 10–14 days. **Pediatric:** Total daily dose of 8 mg/kg trimethoprim and 40 mg/kg sulfamethoxazole di-

T

vided equally and given q 12 hr for 10–14 days. (*NOTE:* For shigellosis, give adult or pediatric dose for 5 days.) For clients with impaired renal function the following dosage is recommended: C_{CR} of 15–30 mL/min: one-half the usual regimen and for C_{CR} less than 15 mL/min: use is not recommended.

Chancroid.

1 DS tablet b.i.d. for at least 7 days (alternate therapy: 4 DS tablets in a single dose).

Pharyngeal gonococcal infection due to penicillinase-producing Neisseria gonorrhoeae.

720 mg trimethoprim and 3,600 mg sulfamethoxazole once daily for 5 days.

Prophylaxis of P. carinii pneumonia.

Adults: 160 mg trimethoprim and 800 mg sulfamethoxazole q 24 hr. **Children:** 150 mg/m^2 of trimethoprim and 750 mg/m^2 sulfamethoxazole daily in equally divided doses b.i.d. on three consecutive days per week. Do not exceed a total daily dose of 320 mg trimethoprim and 1,600 mg sulamethoxazole.

Treatment of P. carinii pneumonia.

Adults and children: Total daily dose of 15–20 mg/kg trimethoprim and 100 mg/kg sulfamethoxazole divided equally and given q 6 hr for 14–21 days.

Prophylaxis of P. carinii pneumonia in immunocompromised clients.

1 DS tablet daily.

Traveler's diarrhea.

Adults, 1 DS tablet q 12 hr for 5 days.

Prostatitis, acute bacterial.

1 DS tablet b.i.d. until client is afebrile for 48 hr; treatment may be required for up to 30 days.

Prostatitis, chronic bacterial.

1 DS tablet b.i.d. for 4–6 weeks.

- **IV**

UTIs, shigellosis, acute otitis media.

Adults and children: 8–10 mg/kg/day (based on trimethoprim) in two to four divided doses q 6, 8, or 12 hr for up to 14 days for severe UTIs or 5 days for shigellosis.

Treatment of P. carinii pneumonia

Adults and children: 15–20 mg/kg/day (based on trimethoprim) in 3–4 divided doses q 6–8 hr for up to 14 days.

HEALTH CARE CONSIDERATIONS

See also *General Health Care Considerations for All Anti-Infectives* and for *Sulfonamides.*

Administration/Storage

IV 1. Administer IV infusion over a 60–90 min period.
2. Each 5-mL vial must be diluted to 125 mL with D5W and used within 6 hr. If the amount of fluid should be restricted, each 5 mL can be diluted up to 75 mL with D5W and used within 2 hr. Do not refrigerate the diluted solution.
3. Do not mix the IV infusion with any other drugs or solutions.
4. If the diluted IV infusion is cloudy or precipitates after mixing, discard and prepare a new solution.

Assessment

1. Record indications for therapy, onset, duration, and characteristics of symptoms.
2. Monitor cultures, CBC, liver and renal function studies; reduce dose with renal dysfunction.
3. Assess for megaloblastic anemia; drug inhibits ability to produce folinic acid. Simultaneous administration of folinic acid (6–8 mg/day) may prevent antifolate drug effects.
4. Record if clients infected with AIDS virus; may be intolerant to this product.

Client/Family Teaching

1. Take only as directed. Complete entire prescription and do not share.
2. Report any symptoms of drug fever, vasculitis, N&V, rash, joint pain/swelling or CNS disturbances.
3. Consume 2.5–3 L of fluids/day.

Outcome/Evaluate

- Resolution of infection; negative cultures
- *P. carinii* pneumonia prophylaxis

Trimipramine maleate

(try-**MIP**-rah-meen)

Pregnancy Category: C

Apo-Trimip ✱, Novo-Tripramine ✱, Nu-Trimipramine ✱, Rhotrimine ✱, Surmontil **(Rx)**

Classification: Antidepressant, tricyclic

See also *Antidepressants, Tricyclic.*

Action/Kinetics: Causes moderate anticholinergic and orthostatic hypotensive effects and significant sedative effects. **Effective plasma levels:** 180 ng/mL. **Time to reach steady state:** 2–6 days. **t½:** 7–30 hr.

Uses: Treatment of symptoms of depression. PUD. Seems more effective in endogenous depression than in other types of depression.

Contraindications: Use in children less than 12 years of age.

How Supplied: *Capsule:* 25 mg, 50 mg, 100 mg

Dosage

- **Capsules**

Antidepressant.

Adults, outpatients, initial: 75 mg/day in divided doses up to 150 mg/day, but not to exceed 200 mg/day; **maintenance:** 50–150 mg/day. Total dose can be given at bedtime. **Adults, hospitalized, initial:** 100 mg/day in divided doses up to 200 mg/day. If no improvement in 2–3 weeks, increase to 250–300 mg/day. **Adolescent/geriatric clients, initial:** 50 mg/day up to 100 mg/day. Not recommended for children.

HEALTH CARE CONSIDERATIONS

See also *Health Care Considerations* for *Antidepressants, Tricyclic.*
Administration/Storage: To minimize relapse, continue maintenance therapy for about 3 months.
Assessment: Record indications for therapy, onset, duration, and characteristics of symptoms. Note any predisposing factors/events.
Outcome/Evaluate
- ↓ Depressive symptoms
- Control of symptoms of PUD

Tripelennamine hydrochloride

(try-pell-**EN**-ah-meen)
PBZ, PBZ-SR, Pyribenzamine ✱ **(Rx)**
Classification: Antihistamine, ethylenediamine derivative

See also *Antihistamines.*
Action/Kinetics: GI effects more pronounced than other antihistamines. Moderate sedative effects and low to no anticholinergic activity. **Duration:** 4–6 hr.
Contraindications: Use in neonates.
Special Concerns: Safe use during pregnancy has not been established. Geriatric clients may be more sensitive to the usual adult dose.
Side Effects: Low incidence. Moderate sedation, mild GI distress, paradoxical excitation, hyperirritability.
How Supplied: *Tablet:* 25 mg, 50 mg; *Tablet, Extended Release:* 100 mg

Dosage
- **Tablets**

Adults, usual: 25–50 mg q 4–6 hr; as little as 25 mg or as high as 600 mg may be given to control symptoms. **Pediatric:** 5 mg/kg/day or 150 mg/m²/day divided into 4–6 doses, not to exceed 300 mg/day.
- **Extended-Release Tablets**

Adults: 100 mg q 8–12 hr as needed, up to a maximum of 600 mg/day. Do not use sustained-release form in children.

HEALTH CARE CONSIDERATIONS

See also *Health Care Considerations* for *Antihistamines.*
Administration/Storage: Swallow extended-release tablets whole; never crush or chew.
Outcome/Evaluate: ↓ Allergic manifestations

COMBINATION DRUG

Tylenol with Codeine Elixir or Tablets

(**TIE**-leh-noll, **KOH**-deen)
Pregnancy Category: C
(Tablets are C-III and Elixir is C-V) **(Rx)**
Classification: Analgesic

See also *Acetaminophen* and *Narcotic Analgesics.*
Content: *Nonnarcotic analgesic:* Acetaminophen, 300 mg in each tablet, and 120 mg/5 mL elixir. *Narcotic analgesic:* Codeine phosphate, 15 mg (No. 2 Tablets), 30 mg (No. 3 Tablets), 60 mg (No. 4 Tablets), and 12 mg/5 mL (Elixir).
Uses: Tablets: Mild to moderately severe pain. **Elixir:** Mild to moderate pain.
Special Concerns: Use with caution during lactation. Safety has not been determined in children less than 3 years of age. May be habit-forming due to the codeine component.
How Supplied: See Content

Dosage
- **Tablets, Capsules**

Analgesia.
Adults, individualized, usual: 1–2 No. 2 or No. 3 Tablets or No. 3 Capsules q 2–4 hr as needed for pain. Or, 1 No. 4 Tablet or Capsule q 4 hr as required. Maximum 24-hr dose is 360 mg codeine phosphate and 4,000 mg acetaminophen. **Pediatric:** Dosage equivalent to 0.5 mg/kg codeine.
- **Elixir**

Analgesia.
Adults, individualized, usual: 15 mL q 4 hr as needed; **pediatric, 7–12 years:** 10 mL t.i.d.–q.i.d.; **3–6 years:** 5 mL t.i.d.–q.i.d.

HEALTH CARE CONSIDERATIONS

See also *Health Care Considerations* for *Narcotic Analgesics* and *Acetaminophen.*
Administration/Storage
1. Adjust dosage depending on client response and severity of pain.
2. Doses of codeine greater than 60 mg do

T

not provide additional analgesia but may lead to an increased incidence of side effects.

Assessment: Record location, onset, duration, and characteristics of symptoms. Use a pain-rating scale to rate/evaluate pain.

Client/Family Teaching

1. Take only as directed.
2. Report any loss of pain control because drug and/or dosage may require adjustment.
3. Increase fluids and bulk in diet to prevent constipation.

Outcome/Evaluate: Relief of pain

COMBINATION DRUG

Tylox

(TIE-lox)

Pregnancy Category: C

(C-II) (Rx)

Classification: Analgesic

See also *Acetaminophen* and *Narcotic Analgesics*.

Content: Each capsule contains: *Nonnarcotic analgesic:* Acetaminophen, 500 mg. *Narcotic analgesic:* Oxycodone HCl, 5 mg.

Uses: Relief of moderate to moderately severe pain.

Special Concerns: Use with caution during lactation. Safety and effectiveness have not been determined in children. Drug dependence can develop due to the oxycodone component.

How Supplied: See Content

Dosage

- **Capsules**

  Analgesia.

Adults, individualized, usual: 1 capsule q 6 hr as required for pain.

HEALTH CARE CONSIDERATIONS

See also *Health Care Considerations* for *Narcotic Analgesics* and *Acetaminophen*.

Administration/Storage

1. Adjust the dose depending on the response of the client and the severity of the pain.
2. As the dose of oxycodone is increased, the incidence of side effects increases. Do not use high doses for severe or intractable pain.

Assessment: Record location, onset, duration, and characteristics of symptoms. Use a pain-rating scale to rate pain.

Client/Family Teaching

1. Take only as directed.
2. Report any loss of pain control; drug and/or dosage may require adjustment.

Outcome/Evaluate: Control of pain

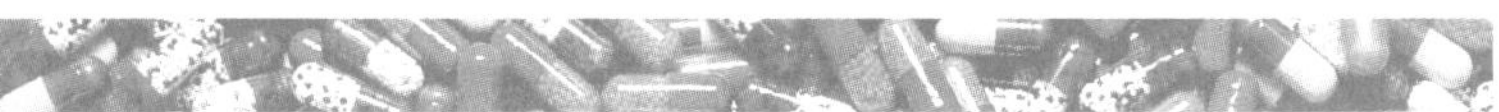

Urofollitropin for injection

(YOUR-oh-foll-ee-troh-pin)

Pregnancy Category: X

Metrodin **(Rx)**

Urofollitropin for injection, purified

(YOUR-oh-foll-ee-troh-pin)

Pregnancy Category: X

Fertinex, Fertinorm HP ✱ **(Rx)**

Classification: Ovarian stimulant

Action/Kinetics: Prepared from the urine of postmenopausal women. Is a gonadotropin that stimulates follicular growth in the ovaries of women without primary ovarian failure. Because treatment with urofollitropin only causes growth and maturation of a follicle, HCG must also be given to effect ovulation.

Time to peak effect: 32–36 hr after HCG.

Uses: To cause ovulation in women with polycystic ovarian disease; such clients should have an elevated LH/FSH ratio and should have failed to respond to therapy with clomiphene. In conjunction with HCG to stimulate development and maturation of ovarian follicles and subsequent ovulation in clients with polycystic ovary syndrome and infertility. Use of the purified urofollitropin is said to cause less discomfort than use of the less purified urofollitropin product.

Contraindications: Primary ovarian failure (as indicated by high levels of both LH and FSH), adrenal dysfunction, thyroid dysfunction, pituitary tumor, abnormal uterine bleeding of unknown cause, ovarian cysts, enlarged ovaries (not as a result of polycystic disease), infertility due to causes other than failure to ovulate. Pregnancy.

Special Concerns: Use with caution in lactation. There is the potential for multiple births.

Side Effects: *Ovarian hyperstimulation syndrome:* Severe ovarian enlargement, abdominal pain or distention, N&V, diarrhea, dyspnea, oliguria, ascites, pleural effusion, hypovolemia, electrolyte imbalance, ***hemoperitoneum, thromboembolic events.*** *Ovarian:* Hyperstimulation resulting in ovarian enlargement with abdominal distention or pain. *GI:* N&V, diarrhea, bloating, abdominal cramps. *CV:* Thromboembolic events resulting in venous thrombophlebitis, arterial occlusion, ***pulmonary embolism, pulmonary infarction, CVA.*** *Respiratory:* Atelectasis, ***acute respiratory distress syndrome.*** *Pyrogenic or allergic reaction:* Chills, fever, muscle aches or pains, joint pain, headache, fatigue, malaise. *Dermatologic:* Hives, dry skin, loss of hair, rash. *Other:* Headache, ***ectopic pregnancy,*** breast tenderness.

OD Management of Overdose: *Symptoms:* Hyperstimulation of the ovary, multiple gestations.

How Supplied: *Powder for injection:* 75 IU, 150 IU

Dosage

- **IM (Metrodin)**

Polycystic ovary syndrome.

Adults, initial: 75 IU urofollitropin daily for 7–12 days followed by 5,000–10,000 IU HCG 24 hr after the last dose of urofollitropin. If ovulation has occurred but pregnancy has not resulted, this dosage regimen may be repeated for two more courses of therapy. If pregnancy still has not resulted, the dose of urofollitropin may be increased to 150 IU/day for 7–12 days followed by 5,000–10,000 IU HCG 24 hr after the last dose of urofollitropin. This regimen may be repeated for two additional courses if pregnancy has not occurred.

In vitro fertilization.

Adults: 150 IU/day beginning on day 2 or 3 of the cycle followed by 5,000–10,000 IU of HCG 1 day after the last dose of urofollitropin. Treatment is usually limited to 10 days.

- **SC (Fertinex)**

Induction of ovulation in polycystic ovary syndrome and infertility.

Adults: 75–300 IU urofollitropin daily with HCG, as above.

HEALTH CARE CONSIDERATIONS

Administration/Storage

1. Reconstitute the powder for injection by dissolving in 1–2 mL of sterile saline immediately before use.
2. Discard any unused drug.
3. Protect from light and store at 3°C–25°C (37°F–77°F).

Assessment

1. A thorough gynecologic and endocrinologic evaluation and examination should be completed before initiating urofollitropin therapy.
2. Note any renal or thyroid dysfunction or abnormal uterine bleeding from an unknown cause.
3. Monitor CBC, electrolytes, liver and renal function studies.

Client/Family Teaching

1. Treatment usually consists of daily injections for 7–12 days.
2. Engage in daily intercourse, beginning 1 day prior to the administration of HCG until ovulation occurs.
3. During the treatment and for 2 weeks thereafter, client should be examined at least every other day for hyperstimulation of the ovaries; if evident, the drug will be stopped immediately.
4. Avoid having intercourse if symptoms of hyperstimulation occur (sudden abdominal pain or tenderness). A ruptured ovarian cyst could occur resulting in hemoperitoneum.
5. This drug enhances the risk of multiple births.
6. Report all side effects to the provider and report for all scheduled exams.

Outcome/Evaluate: Stimulation of ovulation to enhance fertility

Ursodiol

(ur-so-**DYE**-ohl)

Pregnancy Category: B

Actigall, Urso, Ursofalk ✱ **(Rx)**

Classification: Gall stone solubilizer

Action/Kinetics: Naturally occurring bile acid that inhibits the hepatic synthesis and secretion of cholesterol; it also inhibits intestinal absorption of cholesterol. Acts to solubilize cholesterol in micelles and to cause dispersion of cholesterol as liquid crystals in aqueous media. Undergoes a significant first-pass effect where it is conjugated with either glycine or taurine and then secreted into hepatic bile ducts.

Uses: Dissolution of gallstones in clients with radiolucent, noncalcified gallstones (<20 mm) in whom elective surgery would be risky (i.e., systemic disease, advanced age, idiosyncratic reactions to general anesthesia) or in those who refuse surgery. Prevent gallstones in obese clients undergoing rapid weight loss. Primary biliary cirrhosis (Urso).

Contraindications: Clients with calcified cholesterol stones, radiopaque stones, or radiolucent bile pigment stones. Acute cholecystitis, cholangitis, biliary obstruction, gallstone pancreatitis, biliary-gastrointestinal fistula, allergy to bile acids, chronic liver disease. Provide appropriate specifc treatment in those with variceal bleeding, hepatic encephalopathy, ascites, or in need of an urgent liver transplant.

Special Concerns: Use with caution during lactation. Safety and efficacy have not been determined in children. Safety for use beyond 24 months is not known.

Side Effects: *GI:* N&V, dyspepsia, metallic taste, abdominal pain, biliary pain, cholecystitis, constipation, stomatitis, flatulence, diarrhea. *Skin:* Pruritus, rash, dry skin, urticaria. *CNS:* Headache, fatigue, anxiety, depression, sleep disorders. *Other:* Sweating, thinning of hair, back pain, arthralgia, myalgia, rhinitis, cough.

OD **Management of Overdose:** *Symptoms:* Diarrhea. *Treatment:* Treat with supportive measures.

Drug Interactions

Antacids, aluminum-containing / ↓ Effect of ursodiol due to ↓ absorption from GI tract
Cholestyramine / ↓ Effect of ursodiol due to ↓ absorption from GI tract
Clofibrate / ↓ Effect of ursodiol by ↑ hepatic cholesterol secretion
Colestipol / ↓ Effect of ursodiol due to ↓ absorption from GI tract
Contraceptives, oral / ↓ Effect of ursodiol by ↑ hepatic cholesterol secretion
Estrogens / ↓ Effect of ursodiol by ↑ hepatic cholesterol secretion

How Supplied: *Capsule:* 300 mg; *Tablet:* 250 mg

Dosage

- **Capsules**

Gallstones.

Adults: 8–10 mg/kg/day in two or three divided doses, usually with meals.

Prevent gallstones in rapid weight loss in obesity.

Adults: 300 mg b.i.d. during period of weight loss.

- **Tablets**

Primary biliary cirrhosis.

Adults: 13–15 mg/kg/day given in 4 divided doses with food.

U

HEALTH CARE CONSIDERATIONS

Administration/Storage

1. If partial stone dissolution is not observed within 12 months, the drug will probably not be effective.
2. For the first year of therapy, perform gallbladder ultrasound every 6 mo to determine response.

Assessment

1. Record indications for therapy, expected duration, and any conditions that may preclude therapy.
2. Drug is not indicated for calcified cholesterol, radiopaque, or radiolucent bile pigment stones.
3. Obtain ultrasound of gallbladder and LFTs; monitor q 6 mo.
4. Determine if pregnant.

Client/Family Teaching

1. Avoid taking antacids unless prescribed. Many antacids have an aluminum base, which adsorbs the drug.
2. Ursodiol therapy may take up to 24 months; drug will need to be taken 2–3 times/day for stones.
3. Stones may recur after the dissolution of the current stones.
4. With primary biliary cirrhosis, take tablets in 4 divided doses with food.
5. Report any persistent N&V, abdominal pain, diarrhea, presence of a metallic taste in the mouth, headaches, itching, rash, or altered bowel function.
6. Any new-onset headache, anxiety, depression, and sleep disorders should be reported.
7. Practice reliable birth control to avoid pregnancy. The use of estrogens and oral contraceptives may decrease effectiveness of the drug; use alternative birth control.
8. Report for follow-up medical visits, lab studies, and ultrasonography to evaluate the effectiveness of therapy.
9. Ursodiol therapy will be continued for 1–3 months following stone dissolution and then reconfirm status of stones with ultrasound.

Outcome/Evaluate

- Radiographic evidence of a reduction or complete dissolution of radiolucent, noncalcified gallstones.
- Reversal of intracellular accumulation of toxic bile acids

V

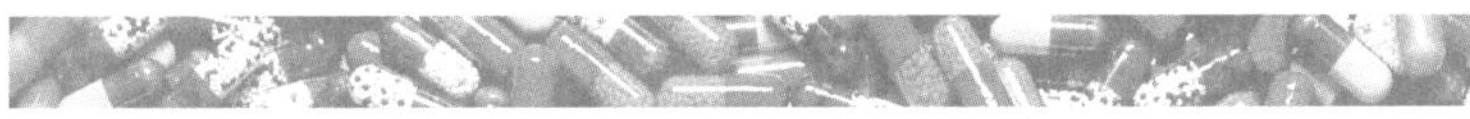

Valacyclovir hydrochloride

(val-ah-SIGH-kloh-veer)
Pregnancy Category: B
Valtrex **(Rx)**
Classification: Antiviral drug

See also *Antiviral Drugs.*

Action/Kinetics: Rapidly converted to acyclovir, which has inhibitory activity against herpes simplex virus types 1 (HSV-1) and 2 (HSV-2) and varicella-zoster virus. Acts by inhibiting replication of viral DNA by competitive inhibition of viral DNA polymerase, incorporation and termination of the growing viral DNA chain, and inactivation of the viral DNA polymerase. Rapidly absorbed after PO administration and is rapidly and nearly completely converted to acyclovir and l-valine by first-pass intestinal or hepatic metabolism. **Time to peak levels:** Approximately 1.5 hr. **Peak plasma levels:** Less than 0.5 mcg/mL of valacyclovir at all doses. **t½, acyclovir:** 2.5–3.3 hr. Approximately 50% is excreted through the urine.

Uses: Treatment of recurrent episodes of genital herpes in immunocompetent adults. Treatment of herpes zoster in immunocompetent adults. Suppression of genital herpes in adults who have experienced previous outbreaks.

Contraindications: Hypersensitivity or intolerance to acyclovir or valacyclovir. Use in immunocompromised individuals. Lactation.

Special Concerns: Use with caution in renal impairment or in those taking potentially nephrotoxic drugs. Dosage reduction may be necessary in geriatric clients depending on the renal status. Safety and efficacy have not been determined in children.

Side Effects: *GI:* N&V, diarrhea, constipation, abdominal pain, anorexia. *CNS:* Headache, dizziness. *Miscellaneous:* Asthenia, precipitation of acyclovir in renal tubules resulting in acute renal failure and anuria.

OD **Management of Overdose:** *Symptoms:* Precipitation of acyclovir in renal tubules if the solubility (2.5 mg/mL) is exceeded in the intratubular fluid. *Treatment:* Hemodialysis until renal function is restored. About 33% of acyclovir in the body is removed during a 4-hr hemodialysis session.

Drug Interactions: Administration of cimetidine and/or probenecid decreased the rate, but not the extent, of conversion of valacyclovir to acyclovir. Also, the renal clearance of acyclovir was decreased.

How Supplied: *Tablet:* 500 mg, 1 g

Dosage

- **Tablets**

Herpes zoster (shingles).

Adults: 1 g t.i.d. for 7 days. *Dosage with renal impairment:* C_{CR}, 30–49 mL/min: 1 g q 12 hr; C_{CR}, 10–29 mL/min: 1 g q 24 hr; and, C_{CR}, less than 10 mL/min: 500 mg q 24 hr.

Recurrent genital herpes.

Adults: 500 mg b.i.d. for 5 days. *Dosage with renal impairment:* C_{CR}, 30–49 mL/min: 500 mg q 12 hr; C_{CR}, 10–29 mL/min: 500 mg q 24 hr; and, C_{CR}, less than 10 mL/min: 500 mg q 24 hr.

Suppression of genital herpes.

Adults: 1 g once daily (500 mg once daily for those who have 9 or fewer recurrences per year).

HEALTH CARE CONSIDERATIONS

See also *Health Care Considerations* for *Antiviral Drugs.*

Administration/Storage: Begin therapy as soon as possible after herpes zoster has been diagnosed. The drug is most effective when started within 48 hr after the onset of rash. For recurrent genital herpes, initiate at the first S&S of a flare.

Assessment

1. Record indications for therapy and onset. With herpes zoster, note dermatone(s) location and characteristics of lesions. Drug is most effective if initiated within 48 hr of rash or within 72 hr of symptoms.
2. With recurrent genital herpes, note extent of lesions; initiate at first S&S of outbreak.
3. Monitor CBC and renal function studies; reduce dose if C_{CR} below 50 mL/min.

Client/Family Teaching

1. Take exactly as prescribed; do not share meds or skip or double up on doses.
2. May take without regard to meals.
3. Vesicles usually become red or pustular after 4 or 5 days and by the 7th to 10th day dry up and crust over. The acute phase is completed by approximately 3 weeks, when the scabs slough from the skin.
4. Immunocompromised clients usually experience a more severe case and the disease course usually doubles.
5. During the acute stage, cover the area and avoid contact with immunocomprom-

ised individuals, pregnant women, or anyone else that has not had the chicken pox virus.

6. Report any persistent pain once lesions have healed (postherpetic neuralgia) or if there is ocular involvement or any other unusual symptoms or behaviors.

7. Report any recurrence since these tend to be rare and may signal an underlying malignancy or immune system dysfunction.

8. With genital herpes, abstain from sexual contact during acute outbreaks to prevent infecting partner; use condoms during all other times.

Outcome/Evaluate

- ↓ Duration/progression of herpes zoster outbreak with reduced healing time; symptomatic relief
- ↓ Pain, ↓ duration, and ↓ intensity with genital herpes outbreak

Valproic acid

(val-**PROH**-ick)

Pregnancy Category: D

Alti-Valproic ✦, Depakene, Deproic ✦, Gen-Valproic ✦, Novo-Valproic ✦, PMS-Valproic Acid ✦ **(Rx)**

Divalproex sodium

(die-val-**PROH**-ex)

Pregnancy Category: D

Depakote, Epival ✦ **(Rx)**

Classification: Anticonvulsant, miscellaneous

See also *Anticonvulsants*.

Action/Kinetics: The following information also applies to divalproex sodium (Depakote, Epival ✦). The precise anticonvulsant action is unknown; may increase brain levels of the neurotransmitter GABA. Other possibilities include acting on postsynaptic receptor sites to mimic or enhance the inhibitory effect of GABA, inhibiting an enzyme that catabolizes GABA, affecting the potassium channel, or directly affecting membrane stability. Absorption is more rapid with the syrup (sodium salt) than capsules. **Peak levels, with syrup:** 15 min–2 hr. Equivalent PO doses of divalproex sodium and valproic acid deliver equivalent amounts of valproate ion to the system. **Peak serum levels, capsules and syrup:** 1–4 hr (delayed if the drug is taken with food); **peak serum levels, enteric-coated tablet (divalproex sodium):** 3–4 hr. **t½:** 9–16 hr, with the lower time usually seen in clients taking other anticonvulsant drugs (e.g., primidone, phenytoin, phenobarbital, carbamazepine). **t½, children less than 10 days:** 10–67 hr; **t½, children over 2 months:** 7–13 hr. **t½, cirrhosis or acute hepatitis:** Up to 18 hr. **Therapeutic serum levels:** 50–100 mcg/mL. Approximately 90% bound to plasma protein. Metabolized in the liver and inactive metabolites are excreted in the urine; small amounts of valproic acid are excreted in the feces.

Uses: Alone or in combination with other anticonvulsants for treatment of simple and complex absence seizures (petit mal). As an adjunct in multiple seizure patterns that include absence seizures. Alone or as adjunct to treat complex partial seizures that occur either in isolation or in association with other types of seizures. Divalproex sodium delayed release used for the acute treatment of manic episodes in bipolar disorder and for prophylaxis of migraine headaches. *Investigational:* Alone or in combination to treat atypical absence, myoclonic, and grand mal seizures; also, atonic, complex partial, elementary partial, and infantile spasm seizures. Prophylaxis of febrile seizures in children, to treat anxiety disorders/panic attacks, and subchronically to treat minor incontinence after ileoanal anastomosis. Management of anxiety disorders or panic attacks.

Contraindications: Liver disease or dysfunction.

Special Concerns: Use with caution during lactation. Use with caution in children 2 years of age or less as they are at greater risk for developing fatal hepatotoxicity. Use lower doses in geriatric clients because they may have increased free, unbound valproic acid levels in the serum. Safety and efficacy of divalproex sodium have not been determined for treating acute mania in children less than 18 years of age or for treating migraine in children less than 16 years of age.

Side Effects: *GI:* (most frequent): N&V, indigestion. Also, abdominal cramps, abdominal pain, dyspepsia, diarrhea, constipation, anorexia with weight loss or increased appetite with weight gain. *CNS:* Sedation, psychosis, depression, emotional upset, aggression, hyperactivity, deterioration of behavior, tremor, headache, dizziness, somnolence, dysarthria, incoordination, coma (rare). *Ophthalmologic:* Nystagmus, diplopia, "spots before eyes." *Hematologic:* Thrombocytopenia, leukopenia, eosinophilia, anemia, bone marrow suppression, relative lymphocytosis, hypofibrinogenemia, myelodysplastic-type syndrome. *Dermatologic:* Transient alopecia, petechiae, erythema multiforme, skin rashes. photosensitivity, pruritus, ***Stevens-Johnson syndrome***. *Hepatic:* Hepatotoxicity. Also, minor increases in AST, ALT, LDH, serum bilirubin, and serum alkaline phosphatase values. *Endocrine:* Menstrual irregularities, secondary amenorrhea, breast enlargement, galactorrhea, swelling of parotid gland, abnormal thyroid function tests. *Miscellaneous:* Also asterixis, weakness, asthenia, bruising, hematoma formation, frank hemorrhage, acute pancreatitis, hyperammonemia, hyperglycinemia, hypocarnitinemia, edema of arms and legs, weakness, inappropriate ADH secretion, Fanconi's syndrome (rare and seen mostly in children), lupus erythematosus, fever, enuresis, hearing loss.

Laboratory Test Considerations: False + for ketonuria. Altered thyroid function tests.

OD **Management of Overdose:** *Symptoms:* Motor restlessness, asterixis, visual hallucinations, somnolence, heart block, ***deep coma.*** *Treatment:* Perform gastric lavage if client is seen early enough (valproic acid is absorbed rapidly). Undertake general supportive measures making sure urinary output is maintained. Naloxone has been used to reverse the CNS depression (however, it could also reverse the anticonvulsant effect). Hemodialysis and hemoperfusion have been used with success.

Drug Interactions

Alcohol / ↑ Incidence of CNS depression
Carbamazepine / Variable changes in levels of carbamazepine with possible loss of seizure control
Charcoal / ↓ Absorption of valproic acid from the GI tract
Chlorpromazine / ↓ Clearance and ↑ t½ of valproic acid → ↑ pharmacologic effects
Cimetidine / ↓ Clearance and ↑ t½ of valproic acid → ↑ pharmacologic effects
Clonazepam / ↑ Chance of absence seizures (petit mal) and ↑ toxicity due to clonazepam
CNS depressants / ↑ Incidence of CNS depression
Diazepam / ↑ Effect of diazepam due to ↓ plasma binding and ↓ metabolism
Erythromycin / ↑ Serum valproic acid levels → valproic acid toxicitiy
Ethosuximide / ↑ Effect of ethosuximide due to ↓ metabolism
Felbamate / ↑ Mean peak valproic acid levels
Lamotrigine / ↓ Valproic acid serum levels and ↑ lamotrigine serum levels (reduce dose of lamotrigine)
Phenobarbital / ↑ Effect of phenobarbital due to ↓ breakdown by liver
Phenytoin / ↑ Effect of phenytoin due to ↓ breakdown by liver or ↓ effect of valproic acid due to ↑ metabolism
Salicylates (aspirin) / ↑ Effect of valproic acid due to ↓ plasma protein binding and ↓ metabolism
Warfarin sodium / ↑ Effect of valproic acid due to ↓ plasma protein binding. Also, additive anticoagulant effect
AZT / ↓ Clearance of AZT in HIV-seropositive clients

How Supplied: Valproic acid: *Capsule:* 250 mg; *Syrup:* 250 mg/5 mL; Divalproex sodium: *Enteric Coated Capsule:* 125 mg; *Enteric Coated Tablet:* 125 mg, 250 mg, 500 mg

Dosage

- **Capsules, Syrup, Enteric-Coated Capsules and Tablets (Divalproex)**

Complex partial seizures.

Adults and children 10 years and older: 10–15 mg/kg/day. Increase by 5–10 mg/kg/week until seizures are controlled or side effects occur, up to a maximum of 60 mg/kg/day. If the total daily dose exceeds 250 mg, divide the dose. Dosage of concomitant anticonvulsant drugs can usually be reduced by about 25% every 2 weeks. Divalproex sodium may be added to the regimen at a dose of 10–15 mg/kg/day; the dose may be increased by 5–10 mg/kg/week to achieve the optimal response (usually less than 60 mg/kg/day).

Simple and complex absence seizures.

Initial: 15 mg/kg/day, increasing at 1-week intervals by 5–10 mg/kg/day until seizures are controlled or side effects occur.

Acute manic episodes in bipolar disorder (use divalproex).

Initial: 250 mg t.i.d.; **then,** increase dose q 2–3 days until a trough serum level of 50 mcg/mL is reached. The maximum dose is 60 mg/kg/day.

Prophylaxis of migraine (divalproex sodium).

250 mg/day b.i.d., although some may require up to 1,000 mg daily.

- **Rectal**

Intractable status epilepticus that has not responded to other treatment.

Adults: 200–1,200 mg q 6 hr rectally with phenytoin and phenobarbital. **Children:** 15–20 mg/kg.

V

HEALTH CARE CONSIDERATIONS

See also *Health Considerations* for *Anticonvulsants.*

Administration/Storage

1. Divide daily dosage if it exceeds 250 mg/day.

2. To minimize GI irritation, initiate at a lower dose, give with food, or use the delayed-release form (Depakote).
3. To minimize CNS depression, give at bedtime.
4. To avoid local irritation, swallow valproic acid capsules whole. However, capsules can either be swallowed whole or the contents sprinkled on teaspoonful of a soft food (e.g., applesauce, pudding) and swallowed immediately without chewing.
5. Do not administer valproic acid syrup to clients whose *sodium* intake must be restricted. Consult provider if a sodium-restricted client is unable to swallow capsules.
6. In clients taking valproic acid, conversion to divalproex sodium can be undertaken at the same total daily dose and dosing schedule.
7. Reduce the starting dose in geriatric clients, depending on the response. Younger children will require larger maintenance doses, especially if they are receiving enzyme-inducing drugs.

Assessment

1. Note indications for therapy, type, onset, and duration of symptoms.
2. Record characteristics of seizure activity, including onset and prodrome if evident.
3. Identify type, frequency, and duration of behaviors that warrant therapy; list other agents prescribed and the outcome.
4. Monitor LFTs due to increased potential for hepatoxicity.

Client/Family Teaching

1. Take with or after meals to minimize GI upset and at bedtime to minimize sedative effects.
2. Take only as directed and do not stop suddenly; seizures may occur with seizure disorder.
3. Do not drive or perform activities that require mental alertness until drug effects realized and seizure control verified.
4. Report any unexplained fever, sore throat, skin rash, yellow skin discoloration, or unusual bruising/bleeding.
5. With diabetes, drug may cause a false positive urine test for ketones. Report symptoms of ketoacidosis (dry mouth, thirst, and dry flushed skin).
6. Report any loss of seizure control.
7. Avoid alcohol and any other CNS depressants or OTC products without approval.
8. Report for periodic CBC, serum glucose/acetone, and LFTs.

Outcome/Evaluate

- Control of seizures
- Migraine headache prophylaxis
- Control of manic episodes
- Therapeutic drug levels (50–100 mcg/mL)

V

Valsartan

(val-**SAR**-tan)
Pregnancy Category: C (1st trimester), D (2nd and 3rd trimesters)
Diovan **(Rx)**
Classification: Antihypertensive, angiotensin II receptor blocker

Action/Kinetics: Angiotensin II receptor blocker specific for AT_1 receptors, which are responsible for cardiovascular effects of angiotensin II. Drug blocks vasoconstrictor and aldosterone-secreting effects of angiotensin II. **Peak plasma levels:** 2–4 hr. Highly bound to plasma proteins. **t½, terminal:** 11–15 hr. Eliminated mostly unchanged in feces (80%) and urine (about 20%).
Uses: Treat hypertension alone or in combination with other antihypertensive drugs.
Contraindications: Lactation.
Special Concerns: Use with caution in impaired hepatic and renal function. Safety and efficacy have not been determined in children.
Side Effects: *CNS:* Headache, dizziness, fatigue, anxiety, insomnia, paresthesia, somnolence. *GI:* Abdominal pain, diarrhea, nausea, constipation, dry mouth, dyspepsia, flatulence. *Respiratory:* URI, cough, rhinitis, sinusitis, pharyngitis, dyspnea. *Body as a whole:* Viral infection, edema, asthenia, allergic reaction. *Musculoskeletal:* Arthralgia, back pain, muscle cramps, myalgia. *Dermatologic:* Pruritus, rash. *Miscellaneous:* Palpitations, vertigo, neutropenia, impotence.
Laboratory Test Considerations: ↓ Hemoglobin and hematocrit. ↑ Serum potassium, liver chemistries.
How Supplied: *Capsules:* 80 mg, 160 mg

Dosage

- **Capsules**

Hypertension.

Adults, initial: 80 mg once daily as monotherapy. **Dose range:** 80–320 mg once daily. If additional antihypertensive effect is needed, dose may be increased to 160 mg or 320 mg once daily or diuretic may be added.

HEALTH CARE CONSIDERATIONS

Administration/Storage

1. May be given with or without food.
2. Antihypertensive effect is usually seen within 2 weeks with maximum reduction after 4 weeks.

Assessment

1. Record disease onset, characteristics of symptoms, other agents trialed and the outcome.
2. Obtain liver and renal function studies; note dysfunction.

Client/Family Teaching
1. May take with or without food and with other prescribed antihypertensive agents.
2. Change positions slowly and avoid dehydration to prevent postural effects and dizziness.
3. Practice reliable contraception; report if pregnancy suspected as drug may cause fetal death.
4. Continue low fat, low sodium diet, regular exercise, weight loss, smoking and alcohol cessation, and stress reduction in overall goal of BP control.
5. May experience headaches, coughing, diarrhea, nausea, and joint aches; report if persistent.

Outcome/Evaluate: ↓ BP

Vancomycin hydrochloride

(van-koh-**MY**-sin)
Pregnancy Category: C, (B for capsules only)
Vancocin, Vancoled **(Rx)**
Classification: Antibiotic, miscellaneous

See also *Anti-Infectives.*

Action/Kinetics: Appears to bind to bacterial cell wall, arresting its synthesis and lysing the cytoplasmic membrane by a mechanism that is different from that of penicillins and cephalosporins. May also change the permeability of the cytoplasmic membranes of bacteria, thus inhibiting RNA synthesis. Bactericidal for most organisms and bacteriostatic for enterococci. Poorly absorbed from the GI tract. Diffuses in pleural, pericardial, ascitic, and synovial fluids after parenteral administration. **Peak plasma levels, IV:** 33 mcg/mL 5 min after 0.5-g dosage. **t½, after PO:** 4–8 hr for adults and 2–3 hr for children; **t½, after IV:** 4–11 hr for adults and ranging from 2–3 hr in children to 6–10 hr for newborns. The half-life is increased markedly in the presence of renal impairment (240 hr has been noted). Primarily excreted in urine unchanged. Auditory and renal function tests are indicated before and during therapy.

Uses: PO: Antibiotic-induced pseudomembranous colitis due to *Clostridium difficile.* Staphylococcal enterocolitis. Severe or progressive antibiotic-induced diarrhea caused by *C. difficile* that is not responsive to the causative antibiotic being discontinued; also for debilitated clients.

IV: Severe staphylococcal infections in clients who have not responded to penicillins or cephalosporins, who cannot receive these drugs, or who have resistant infections. Infections include lower respiratory tract infections, bone infections, endocarditis, septicemia, and skin and skin structure infections. Alone or in combination with aminoglycosides to treat endocarditis caused by *Streptococcus viridans* or *S. bovis.* Must combine with an aminoglycoside to treat endocarditis due to *Streptococcus faecalis.* Used with rifampin, an aminoglycoside (or both) to treat early onset prosthetic valve endocarditis caused by *Staphylococcus epidermidis* or other diphtheroids. Prophylaxis of bacterial endocarditis in pencillin-allergic clients who have congenital heart disease or rheumatic or other acquired or valvular heart disease if such clients are undergoing dental or surgical procedures of the upper respiratory tract. The parenteral dosage form may be given PO to treat pseudomembranous colitis or staphylococcal enterocolitis due to *C. difficile.*

Contraindications: Hypersensitivity. Minor infections. Lactation.

Special Concerns: Use with extreme caution in the presence of impaired renal function or previous hearing loss. Geriatric clients are at a greater risk of developing ototoxicity.

Side Effects: Ototoxicity (may lead to deafness; deafness may progress after drug is discontinued), nephrotoxicity (may lead to uremia). *Red-neck syndrome:* Sudden and profound drop in BP with or without a maculopapular rash over the face, neck, upper chest, and extremities. *CV:* Exaggerated hypotension (due to rapid bolus administration), including ***shock and possibly cardiac arrest.*** *GU:* Renal failure (rare), interstitial nephritis (rare). *Respiratory:* Wheezing, dyspnea. *Dermatologic:* Urticaria, pruritus, macular rashes, exfoliative dermatitis, ***Stevens-Johnson syndrome, toxic epidermal necrolysis,*** vasculitis. *Allergic:* Drug fever, hypersensitivity, ***anaphylaxis.*** *At injection site:* Tissue irritation, including pain, tenderness, necrosis, thrombophlebitis. *Miscellaneous:* Nausea, chills, tinnitus, eosinophilia, neutropenia (reversible), pseudomembranous colitis.

Drug Interactions
Aminoglycosides / ↑ Risk of nephrotoxicity
Anesthetics / Risk of erythema and histamine-like flushing in children
Muscle relaxants, nondepolarizing / ↑ Neuromuscular blockade

How Supplied: *Capsule:* 125 mg, 250 mg; *Powder for injection:* 500 mg, 1 g, 5 g, 10 g; *Powder for reconstitution:* 250 mg/5 mL, 500 mg/6 mL

Dosage

- **Capsules, Oral Solution**

Adults: 0.5–2 g/day in three to four divided doses for 7–10 days. Alternatively, 125 mg t.i.d.–q.i.d. for *C. difficile* may be as effective as the 500-mg dosage. **Children:** 40 mg/kg/day in three to four divided doses for 7–10 days, not to exceed 2 g/day. **Neonates:** 10 mg/kg/day in divided doses.

• **IV**

Severe staphylococcal infections.

Adults: 500 mg q 6 hr or 1 g q 12 hr. **Children:** 10 mg/kg/6 hr. **Infants and neonates, initial:** 15 mg/kg for one dose; **then,** 10 mg/kg q 12 hr for neonates in the first week of life and q 8 hr thereafter up to 1 month of age.

Prophylaxis of bacterial endocarditis in dental, oral, or upper respiratory tract procedures in penicillin-allergic clients.

Adults: 1 g vancomycin over 1 hr plus 1.5 mg/kg gentamicin (IV or IM), not to exceed 80 mg, 1 hr before the procedure. May repeat once, 8 hr after the initial dose. **Children:** 20 mg/kg vancomycin plus 2 mg/kg gentamicin (IV or IM), not to exceed 80 mg, 1 hr before the procedure. May repeat once, 8 hr after the initial dose.

HEALTH CARE CONSIDERATIONS

See also *General Health Care Considerations for All Anti-Infectives.*

Administration/Storage

1. Reduce dosage in renal disease; see package insert for procedure.
2. The PO solution is prepared by adding 115 mL distilled water to the 10-g container. The appropriate dose of PO solution may be mixed with 1 oz of water or flavored syrup to improve the taste. The diluted drug may also be given by NGT.
3. The parenteral form may be administered PO by diluting the 1-g vial with 20 mL distilled or deionized water (each 5 mL contains about 250 mg vancomycin).
IV 4. For IV use, dilute each 500-mg vial with 10 mL of sterile water. This may be further diluted in 200 mL of dextrose or saline solution and infused over 60 min.
5. Intermittent infusion is the preferred route, but continuous IV drip may be used.
6. Avoid rapid IV administration because this may result in hypotension, nausea, warmth, and generalized tingling. Administer over 1 hr in at least 200 mL of NSS or D5W.
7. Avoid extravasation during injections; may cause tissue necrosis.
8. Reduce risk of thrombophlebitis by rotating injection sites or adding additional diluent.
9. Aqueous solution is stable for 2 weeks.
10. Once rubber stopper is punctured, ampule should be refrigerated to maintain stability.

Assessment

1. Record indications for therapy, type, onset, and characteristics of symptoms.
2. Assess renal and auditory functions (including 8th CN function).
3. Monitor CBC, cultures, and renal function studies; reduce dose with renal dysfunction.

Interventions

1. Record weight, VS, and I&O; ensure adequate hydration.
2. Report any adverse drug effects, such as:
• Ototoxicity, demonstrated by tinnitus, progressive hearing loss, dizziness, and/or nystagmus; may occur latently
• Nephrotoxicity, demonstrated by albuminuria, hematuria, anuria, casts, edema, and uremia
3. During IV administration ensure that peak and trough drug levels are performed at the prescribed dosing interval, usually 30 min prior to scheduled IV dose (trough) and 1 hr following IV dose (peak) to accurately assess serum levels.

Outcome/Evaluate

• Negative cultures
• Relief of S&S R/T infection
• Serum levels within therapeutic range (trough 1–5 mcg/mL; peak 20–50 mcg/mL)

Venlafaxine hydrochloride

(ven-lah-**FAX**-een)
Pregnancy Category: C
Effexor, Effexor XR **(Rx)**
Classification: Antidepressant, miscellaneous

Action/Kinetics: Not related chemically to any of the currently available antidepressants. A potent inhibitor of the uptake of neuronal serotonin and norepinephrine in the CNS and a weak inhibitor of the uptake of dopamine. Has no anticholinergic, sedative, or orthostatic hypotensive effects. The major metabolite—O-desmethylvenlafaxine (ODV)—is active. The drug and metabolite are eliminated through the kidneys. **t½, venlafaxine:** 5 hr; **t½, ODV:** 11 hr. **Time to reach steady state:** 3–4 days. The half-life of the drug and metabolite are increased in clients with impaired liver or renal function. Food has no effect on the absorption of venlafaxine.

Uses: Treatment of depression.

Contraindications: Use with a MAO inhibitor or within 14 days of discontinuation of a MAO inhibitor. Use of alcohol.

Special Concerns: Use with caution with impaired hepatic or renal function, during lactation, in clients with a history of mania, and in those with diseases or conditions that could affect the hemodynamic responses or metabolism. Although it is possible for a geriatric client to be more sensitive, dosage adjustment is not necessary. Use for more than 4–6 weeks has not been evaluated.

Side Effects: Side effects with an incidence of 0.1% or greater are listed. *CNS:* Anxiety, nervousness, insomnia, mania, hypomania, ***seizures, suicide attempts,*** dizziness, somnolence, tremors, abnormal dreams, hypertonia, paresthesia, decreased libido, agitation, confusion, abnormal thinking, depersonalization, depression, twitching, migraine, emotional lability, trismus, vertigo, apathy, ataxia, circumoral paresthesia, CNS stimulation, euphoria, hallucinations, hostility, hyperesthesia, hyperkinesia, hypertonia, hypotonia, incoordination, increased libido, myoclonus, neuralgia, neuropathy, paranoid reaction, psychosis, psychotic depression, sleep disturbance, abnormal speech, stupor, torticollis. *CV:* Sustained increase in BP (hypertension), vasodilation, tachycardia, postural hypotension, angina pectoris, extrasystoles, hypotension, peripheral vascular disorder, syncope, thrombophlebitis, peripheral edema. *GI:* Anorexia, N&V, dry mouth, constipation, diarrhea, dyspepsia, flatulence, dysphagia, eructation, colitis, edema of tongue, esophagitis, gastroenteritis, gastritis, glossitis, gingivitis, hemorrhoids, ***rectal hemorrhage,*** melena, stomatitis, stomach ulcer, mouth ulceration. *Body as a whole:* Headache, asthenia, infection, chills, chest pain, trauma, yawn, weight loss, accidental injury, malaise, neck pain, enlarged abdomen, allergic reaction, cyst, facial edema, generalized edema, hangover effect, hernia, intentional injury, neck rigidity, moniliasis, substernal chest pain, pelvic pain, photosensitivity reaction. *Respiratory:* Bronchitis, dyspnea, asthma, chest congestion, epistaxis, hyperventilation, laryngismus, laryngitis, pneumonia, voice alteration. *Dermatologic:* Acne, alopecia, brittle nails, contact dermatitis, dry skin, herpes simplex, herpes zoster, maculopapular rash, urticaria. *Hematologic:* Ecchymosis, anemia, leukocytosis, leukopenia, lymphadenopathy, lymphocytosis, thrombocytopenia, thrombocythemia, abnormal WBCs. *Endocrine:* Hypothyroidism, hyperthyroidism, goiter. *Musculoskeletal:* Arthritis, arthrosis, bone pain, bone spurs, bursitis, joint disorder, myasthenia, tenosynovitis. *Ophthalmic:* Blurred vision, mydriasis, abnormal accommodation, abnormal vision, cataract, conjunctivitis, corneal lesion, diplopia, dry eyes, exophthalmos, eye pain, photophobia, subconjunctival hemorrhage, visual field defect. *GU:* Urinary retention, abnormal ejaculation, impotence, urinary frequency, impaired urination, disturbed orgasm, menstrual disorder, anorgasmia, dysuria, hematuria, metrorrhagia, vaginitis, amenorrhea, kidney calculus, cystitis, leukorrhea, menorrhagia, nocturia, bladder pain, breast pain, kidney pain, polyuria, prostatitis, pyelonephritis, pyuria, urinary incontinence, urinary urgency, enlarged uterine fibroids, ***uterine hemorrhage, vaginal hemorrhage,*** vaginal moniliasis. *Miscellaneous:* Sweating, tinnitus, taste perversion, thirst, diabetes mellitus, alcohol intolerance, gout, hypoglycemic reaction, hemochromatosis, ear pain, otitis media.

Withdrawal syndrome: Anxiety, agitation, tremors, vertigo, headache, nausea, tachycardia, tinnitus, akathisia.

Laboratory Test Considerations: ↑ Alkaline phosphatase, creatinine, AST, ALT. Glycosuria, hyperglycemia, hyperlipemia, bilirubinemia, hyperuricemia, hypercholesterolemia, hypoglycemia, hypokalemia, hyperkalemia, hyperphosphatemia, hyponatremia, hypophosphatemia, hypoproteinemia, uremia, albuminuria.

OD **Management of Overdose:** *Symptoms:* Extensions of side effects, especially somnolence. Other symptoms include prolongation of QTc, mild sinus tachycardia, and ***seizures.*** *Treatment:* General supportive measures; treat symptoms. Ensure an adequate airway, oxygenation, and ventilation. Monitor cardiac rhythm and VS. Activated charcoal, induction of emesis, or gastric lavage may be helpful.

Drug Interactions

Cimetidine / ↓ First-pass metabolism of venlafaxine

MAO inhibitors / Serious and possibly fatal reaction, including hyperthermia, rigidity, myoclonus, autonomic instability with rapid changes in VS, extreme agitation, coma

How Supplied: *Capsule, Extended-Release:* 37.5 mg, 75 mg, 150 mg; *Tablet:* 25 mg, 37.5 mg, 50 mg, 75 mg, 100 mg

V

Dosage

- **Tablets**

Depression.

Adults, initial: 75 mg/day given in two or three divided doses. Depending on the response, the dose can be increased to 150–225 mg/day in divided doses. Make dosage increments up to 75 mg/day at intervals of 4 or more days. Severely depressed clients may require 375 mg/day in divided doses. **Maintenance:** Sufficient studies have not been undertaken to determine length of treatment.

- **Capsules, Extended-Release**
  Depression.

Adults, initial: 75 mg once daily. Dose can be increased by up to 75 mg no more often than every 4 days, to a maximum of 225 mg/day.

HEALTH CARE CONSIDERATIONS

Administration/Storage

1. Take with food.
2. Reduce the dose by 50% with moderate hepatic impairment and by 25% with mild to moderate renal impairment.
3. When discontinuing venlafaxine, taper the dose over a 2– 4–week period to minimize the risk of withdrawal syndrome.
4. At least 14 days should elapse between discontinuation of a MAO inhibitor and initiation of venlafaxine therapy; at least 7 days should elapse after stopping venlafaxine before starting a MAO inhibitor.
5. Take the extended-release form in the morning.

Assessment

1. Record indications for therapy, onset, duration and characteristics of symptoms.
2. List other agents prescribed to ensure none interact unfavorably.
3. Monitor CBC, serum lipid levels, liver and renal function studies; reduce dose with hepatic or renal impairment.
4. Due to possible sustained hypertension, monitor HR and BP regularly.

Client/Family Teaching

1. Take only as directed; *do not* stop abruptly may cause withdrawal syndrome.
2. Do not perform activities that require mental alertness until drug effects realized; may cause dizziness or drowsiness.
3. Report any rash, hives, or other allergic manifestations immediately.
4. Drug may impair appetite and induce weight loss; report if excessive.
5. May experience anxiety, palpitations, headaches, and constipation; report if persistent or intolerable.
6. Avoid alcohol and any unprescribed or OTC preparations.
7. Use birth control. Notify provider if pregnant or intends to become pregnant while taking drug.
8. Any suicide ideations or abnormal behaviors should be reported. Due to the possibility of suicide, high-risk clients should be observed closely during initial therapy. Prescriptions should be written for the smallest quantity to reduce the risk of overdose. Have family supervise medication administration with severely depressed clients.

Outcome/Evaluate: Improvement in symptoms of depression

V

Verapamil

(ver-**AP**-ah-mil)

Pregnancy Category: C

Alti-Verapamil ✱, Apo-Verap ✱, Calan, Calan SR, Chronovera ✱, Covera HS, Gen-Verapamil SR ✱, Isoptin, Isoptin I.V. ✱, Isoptin SR, Novo-Veramil ✱, Novo-Veramil SR ✱, Nu-Verap ✱, Penta-Verapamil ✱, Taro-Verapamil ✱, Verelan **(Rx)**

Classification: Calcium channel blocking agent

See also *Calcium Channel Blocking Agents.*

Action/Kinetics: Slows AV conduction and prolongs effective refractory period. IV doses may slightly increase LV filling pressure. Moderately decreases myocardial contractility and peripheral vascular resistance. Worsening of heart failure may result if verapamil is given to clients with moderate to severe cardiac dysfunction. **Onset: PO,** 30 min; **IV,** 3–5 min. **Time to peak plasma levels (PO):** 1–2 hr (5–7 hr for extended-release). **t½, PO:** 4.5–12 hr with repetitive dosing; **IV, initial:** 4 min; **final:** 2–5 hr. **Therapeutic serum levels:** 0.08–0.3 mcg/mL. **Duration, PO:** 8–10 hr (24 hr for extended-release); **IV:** 10–20 min for hemodynamic effect and 2 hr for antiarrhythmic effect. Metabolized to norverapamil, which possesses 20% of the activity of verapamil.

NOTE: Covera HS is designed to deliver verapamil in concert with the 24-hr circadian variations in BP.

Uses: PO: Angina pectoris due to coronary artery spasm (Prinzmetal's variant), chronic stable angina including angina due to increased effort, unstable angina (preinfarction, crescendo). With digitalis to control rapid ventricular rate at rest and during stress in chronic atrial flutter or atrial fibrillation. Prophylaxis of repetitive paroxysmal supraventricular tachycardia. Essential hypertension. Sustained-release tablets are used to treat essential hypertension (Step I therapy). **IV:** Supraventricular tachyarrhythmias. Atrial flutter or fibrillation *Investigational:* PO for prophylaxis of migraine, manic depression (alternate therapy), exercise-induced asthma, recumbent nocturnal leg cramps, hypertrophic cardiomyopathy, cluster headaches.

Contraindications: Severe hypotension, second- or third-degree AV block, cardiogenic shock, severe CHF, sick sinus syndrome (unless client has artificial pacemaker), severe LV dysfunction. Cardiogenic shock and severe CHF unless secondary to SVT that can be treated with verapamil. Lactation. Use of verapamil, IV, with beta-adrenergic blocking agents (as both depress myocardial contractility and AV conduction). Ventricular tachycardia.

Special Concerns: Infants less than 6 months of age may not respond to verapamil. Use with caution in hypertrophic cardiomyopathy, impaired hepatic and renal function, and in the elderly.

Side Effects: *CV:* CHF, bradycardia, ***AV block, asystole,*** premature ventricular contractions and tachycardia (after IV use), peripheral and pulmonary edema, hypotension, syncope, palpitations, AV dissociation, ***MI, CVA.*** *GI:* Nausea, constipation, abdominal discomfort or cramps, dyspepsia, diarrhea, dry mouth. *CNS:* Dizziness, headache, sleep disturbances, depression, amnesia, paranoia, psychoses, hallucinations, jitteriness, confusion, drowsiness, vertigo. IV verapamil may increase intracranial pressure in clients with supratentorial tumors at the time of induction of anesthesia. *Dermatologic:* Rash, dermatitis, alopecia, urticaria, pruritus, erythema multiforme, ***Stevens-Johnson syndrome.*** *Respiratory:* Nasal or chest congestion, dyspnea, SOB, wheezing. *Musculoskeletal:* Paresthesia, asthenia, muscle cramps or inflammation, decreased neuromuscular transmission in Duchenne's muscular dystrophy. *Other:* Blurred vision, equilibrium disturbances, sexual difficulties, spotty menstruation, sweating, rotary nystagmus, flushing, gingival hyperplasia, polyuria, nocturia, gynecomastia, claudication, hyperkeratosis, purpura, petechiae, bruising, hematomas, tachyphylaxis.

Laboratory Test Considerations: ↑ Alkaline phosphatase, transaminase.

OD **Management of Overdose:** *Symptoms:* Extension of side effects. *Treatment:* Beta-adrenergics, IV calcium, vasopressors, pacing, and resuscitation.

Additional Drug Interactions

Antihypertensive agents / Additive hypotensive effects
Barbiturates / ↓ Bioavailability of verapamil
Calcium salts / ↓ Effect of verapamil
Carbamazepine / ↑ Effect of carbamazepine due to ↓ breakdown by liver
Cimetidine / ↑ Bioavailability of verapamil
Cyclosporine / ↑ Plasma levels of cyclosporine possibly leading to renal toxicity
Digoxin / ↑ Risk of digoxin toxicity due to ↑ plasma levels
Disopyramide / Additive depressant effects on myocardial contractility and AV conduction
Etomidate / Anesthetic effect of etomidate may be ↑ with prolonged respiratory depression and apnea
Lithium / ↓ Lithium plasma levels; lithium toxicity also observed
Muscle relaxants, nondepolarizing / ↑ Neuromuscular blockade due to effect of verapamil on calcium channels
Prazosin / Acute hypotensive effect
Quinidine / Possibility of bradycardia, hypotension, AV block, ventricular tachycardia, and pulmonary edema
Ranitidine / ↑ Bioavailability of verapamil
Rifampin / ↓ Effect of verapamil
Sulfinpyrazone / ↑ Clearance of verapamil
Theophyllines / ↑ Effect of theophyllines
Vitamin D / ↓ Effect of verapamil
Warfarin / Possible ↑ effect of either drug due to ↓ plasma protein binding

NOTE: Since verapamil is significantly bound to plasma proteins, interaction with other drugs bound to plasma proteins may occur.

How Supplied: *Capsule, extended release:* 240 mg; *Injection:* 2.5 mg/mL; *Tablet:* 40 mg, 80 mg, 120 mg; *Tablet, extended release:* 120 mg, 180 mg, 240 mg

Dosage

- **Tablets**

Angina at rest and chronic stable angina.

Individualized. Adults, initial: 80–120 mg t.i.d. (40 mg t.i.d. if client is sensitive to verapamil); **then,** increase dose to total of 240–480 mg/day. Covera HS is given once daily at bedtime in doses of either 180 or 240 mg.

Arrhythmias.

Dosage range in digitalized clients with chronic atrial fibrillation: 240–320 mg/day in divided doses t.i.d.–q.i.d. For prophylaxis of nondigitalized clients: 240–480 mg/day in divided doses t.i.d.–q.i.d. Maximum effects are seen within 48 hr.

Essential hypertension.

Initial, when used alone: 80 mg t.i.d. Doses up to 360 mg daily may be used. Effects are seen in the first week of therapy. In the elderly or in people of small stature, initial dose should be 40 mg t.i.d.

- **Extended-Release Capsules and Tablets**

Essential hypertension.

Initial: 240 mg/day in the a.m (120 mg/day in the elderly or people of small stature). If response is inadequate, increase dose to 240 mg in the a.m. and 120 mg in the evening and

V

then 240 mg q 12 hr. Covera HS is given once daily at bedtime in doses of either 180 or 240 mg.

- **IV, Slow**

Supraventricular tachyarrhythmias.

Adults, initial: 5–10 mg (0.075–0.15 mg/kg) given over 2 min (over 3 min in older clients); **then,** 10 mg (0.15 mg/kg) 30 min later if response is not adequate. **Infants, up to 1 year:** 0.1–0.2 mg/kg (0.75–2 mg) given as an IV bolus over 2 min; **1–15 years:** 0.1–0.3 mg/kg (2–5 mg, not to exceed 5 mg total dose) over 2 min. If response to initial dose is inadequate, it may be repeated after 30 min, but not more than a total of 10 mg should be given to clients from 1 to 15 years of age.

HEALTH CARE CONSIDERATIONS

See also *Health Care Considerations* for *Calcium Channel Blocking Agents.*

Administration/Storage

1. The SR tablets (120 mg) may be useful for small stature and elderly clients who require less medication.
2. Take the SR tablets with food.
3. Verelan pellet filled capsules may be carefully opened and the contents sprinkled on a spoonful of applesauce. Swallow the applesauce immediately without chewing and follow with a glass of cool water to ensure complete swallowing of the pellets. Subdividing the contents of a capsule is not recommended.

IV 4. Before administration, inspect ampules for particulate matter or discoloration.
5. Administer IV dosage under continuous ECG monitoring with resuscitation equipment readily available.
6. Give as a slow IV bolus (5–10 mg) over 2 min (3 min to elderly clients) to minimize toxic effects.
7. Store ampules at 15°C–30°C (59°F–86°F) and protect from light.
8. Do not give verapamil in an infusion line containing 0.45% NaCl with $NaHCO_3$ because a crystalline precipitate will form.
9. Do not give verapamil by IV push in the same line used for nafcillin infusion because a milky white precipitate will form.
10. Do not mix with albumin, amphotericin B, hydralazine, trimethoprim/sulfamethoxazole, or diluted with sodium lactate in PVC bags.
11. Verapamil will precipitate in any solution with a pH greater than 6.
12. Always individualize dose in the elderly because the pharmacologic effects are more pronounced and more prolonged.

Assessment

1. Record indications for therapy, onset and duration of symptoms. List agents trialed and outcome.
2. Review list of prescribed medications to ensure none interact.
3. Monitor ECG, CBC, liver and renal function studies; reduce dose with hepatic or renal impairment.

Interventions

1. Monitor VS; assess for bradycardia and hypotension, symptoms that may indicate overdosage. Verapamil may lower BP to dangerously low levels if BP already low.
2. *Do not* administer concurrently with IV beta-adrenergic blocking agents.
3. Unless treating verapamil overdosage, withhold any med that may elevate calcium levels.
4. Clients receiving concurrent digoxin therapy should be assessed for symptoms of toxicity and have digoxin levels checked periodically.
5. If disopyramide is to be used, do not administer for at least 48 hr before to 24 hr after verapamil dose.
6. Administer extended-release tablets with food to minimize fluctuations in serum levels.

Client/Family Teaching

1. Drug may cause dizziness and orthostatic effects; use caution.
2. Keep a log of BP and pulse for provider review.
3. Avoid alcohol, CNS depressants, and any OTC preparations without approval.
4. Continue life-style modifications (low-fat and low-salt diet, decreased alcohol consumption, no smoking, and regular exercise) in the overall goal of BP control.
5. Increase bulk and fiber in diet to prevent constipation. With higher doses constipation occurs more frequently. Report if bothersome or pronounced, as psyllium may be prescribed or, if severe, drug therapy may be changed.

Outcome/Evaluate

- ↓ Frequency/severity of anginal attacks
- Control of BP
- Restoration of stable rhythm
- Therapeutic drug levels (0.08–0.3 mcg/mL)

Vidarabine

(vye-**DAIR**-ah-been)
Pregnancy Category: C
Vira-A **(Rx)**
Classification: Antiviral

See also *Antiviral Agents* and *Anti-Infectives.*

Action/Kinetics: Phosphorylated in the cell to arabinosyl adenosine monophosphate (ara-AMP) or the triphosphate (ara-ATP). These compounds cause inhibition of viral DNA polymerase, inhibition of virus-induced ribonucleotide reductase. The drug may also incorporate into the viral DNA molecule leading to chain termination. Due to low solubility, systemic absorption is not expected to occur after ophthalmic use. Trace amounts seen in the aqueous humor only if there is a corneal epithelial defect.
Uses: Acute keratoconjunctivitis and recurrent epithelial keratitis caused by HSV types 1 and 2. Superficial keratitis caused by HSV that is resistant to idoxuridine or when toxic or hypersensitivity reactions have resulted from idoxuridine. It is more effective than idoxuridine for deep recurrent infections.
Contraindications: Hypersensitivity to drug. Concomitant use of corticosteroids usually contraindicated. Use in presence of sterile trophic ulcers.
Side Effects: Photophobia, lacrimation, conjunctival infection, foreign body sensation, temporal visual haze, burning, irritation, superficial punctate keratitis, pain, punctal occlusion, sensitivity to bright light.
Laboratory Test Considerations: ↑ Bilirubin, AST.
How Supplied: *Ophthalmic ointment:* 3%

Dosage

- **Ophthalmic Ointment, 3%**

½ in. applied to lower conjunctival sac 5 times/day at 3-hr intervals. Continue therapy for 7 days after complete reepithelialization but at reduced dosage (e.g., b.i.d.). If there are no signs of improvement after 7 days or if complete reepithelialization has not occurred within 21 days, consider other therapy.

HEALTH CARE CONSIDERATIONS

See also *General Health Considerations for All Anti-Infectives.*

Administration/Storage

1. To be effective, initiate as soon as possible, but no later than 72 hr after the appearance of vesicular lesions.
2. Topical corticosteroids or antibiotics may be used concomitantly with vidarabine, but benefits and risks must be assessed.
3. Wait 10 min before use of an additional topical ointment.
4. Ophthalmic use may result in sensitivity to bright light that can be minimized by wearing sunglasses.

Assessment: Record indications for therapy, onset, duration and clinical presentation. Must initiate within 72 hr of lesion appearance to be effective.

Client/Family Teaching

1. Take only as directed and do not share medications. Drug must be initiated within 72 hr of appearance of vesicular lesions to be effective.
2. Wash hands before and after applying ointment. If other agents prescribed, wait 10 min before application.
3. Ophthalmic ointment will cause a temporary haze after instillation. Avoid hazardous activities until vision clears.
4. Report any new, persistent, or bothersome side effects.
5. Wear sunglasses outside and avoid bright lights; may cause photophobic reactions.
6. Do not wear contact lenses until eye infection clears.
7. Remain under close ophthalmic supervision while receiving therapy for eye problem.

Outcome/Evaluate

- Healing of skin lesions
- Reepithelialization of herpetic eye lesions; healing in 1–3 weeks

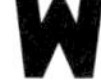
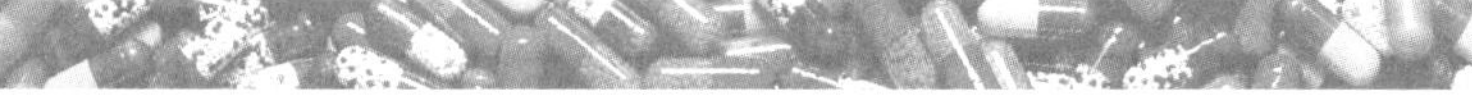

W

Warfarin sodium

(WAR-far-in)
Pregnancy Category: X
Coumadin, Warfilone ✱ **(Rx)**
Classification: Anticoagulant

See also *Anticoagulants.*
Action/Kinetics: Interferes with synthesis of vitamin K–dependent clotting factors resulting in depletion of clotting factors II, VII, IX, and X. Has no direct effect on an established thrombus although therapy may prevent further extension of a formed clot as well as secondary thromboembolic problems. Well absorbed from the GI tract although food affects the rate (but not the extent) of absorption. Suitable for parenteral administration. **Peak activity:** 1.5–3 days; **duration:** 2–5 days. **t½:** 1–2.5 days. Highly bound to plasma proteins. Metabolized in the

liver and inactive metabolites are excreted through the urine and feces.

Uses: Prophylaxis and treatment of venous thrombosis and its extension. Prophylaxis and treatment of atrial fibrillation with embolization. Prophylaxis and treatment of pulmonary embolism. Prophylaxis and treatment of thromboembolic complications associated with atrial fibrillation. *Investigational:* Adjunct to treat small cell carcinoma of the lung with chemotherapy and radiation. Prophylaxis of recurrent transient ischemic attacks and to reduce the risk of recurrent MI. In combination with aspirin to reduce risk of a second MI.

Additional Contraindications: Lactation. IM use. Use of a large loading dose (30 mg) is not recommended due to increased risk of hemorrhage and lack of more rapid protection.

Special Concerns: Geriatric clients may be more sensitive. Anticoagulant use in the following clients leads to increased risk: trauma, infection, renal insufficiency, sprue, vitamin K deficiency, severe to moderate hypertension, polycythemia vera, severe allergic disorders, vasculitis, indwelling catheters, severe diabetes, anaphylactic disorders, surgery or trauma resulting in large exposed raw surfaces. Use with caution in impaired hepatic and renal function. Safety and efficacy have not been determined in children less than 18 years of age. Careful monitoring and dosage regulation are required during dentistry and surgery.

Side Effects: *CV:* ***Hemorrhage*** is the main side effect and may occur from any tissue or organ. Symptoms of hemorrhage include headache, paralysis; pain in the joints, abdomen, or chest; difficulty in breathing or swallowing; SOB, unexplained swelling or shock. *GI:* N&V, diarrhea, sore mouth, mouth ulcers, anorexia, abdominal cramping, paralytic ileus, intestinal obstruction (due to intramural or submucosal hemorrhage). *Hepatic:* Hepatotoxicity, cholestatic jaundice. *Dermatologic:* Dermatitis, exfoliative dermatitis, urticaria, alopecia, necrosis or gangrene of the skin and other tissues (due to protein C deficiency). *Miscellaneous:* Pyrexia, red-orange urine, priapism, leukopenia, systemic cholesterol microembolization ("purple toes" syndrome), hypersensitivity reactions, compressive neuropathy secondary to hemorrhage adjacent to a nerve (rare).

Laboratory Test Considerations: False ↓ levels of serum theophylline determined by Schack and Waxler UV method (warfarin and dicumarol). Metabolites of indanedione derivatives may color alkaline urine red; color disappears upon acidification.

OD Management of Overdose: *Symptoms:* Early symptoms include melena, petechiae, microscopic hematuria, oozing from superficial injuries (e.g., nicks from shaving, excessive bruising, bleeding from gums after teeth brushing), excessive menstrual bleeding. *Treatment:* Discontinue therapy. Administer oral or parenteral phytonadione (e.g., 2.5–10 mg PO or 5–25 mg parenterally). In emergency situations, 200–250 mL fresh frozen plasma or commercial factor IX complex. Fresh whole blood may be needed in clients unresponsive to phytonadione.

Drug Interactions: Warfarin is responsible for more adverse drug interactions than any other group. Clients on anticoagulant therapy must be monitored carefully each time a drug is added or withdrawn. Monitoring usually involves determination of PT. In general, a lengthened PT means potentiation of the anticoagulant. Since potentiation may mean hemorrhages, a lengthened PT warrants **reduction of the dosage of the anticoagulant.** However, the anticoagulant dosage must again be increased when the second drug is discontinued. A shortened PT means inhibition of the anticoagulant and may require an increase in dosage.

Acetaminophen / ↑ Anticoagulant effect

Alcohol, ethyl / Chronic alcohol use ↓ effect of warfarin

Aminoglutethimide / ↓ Effect of warfarin due to ↑ breakdown by liver

Aminoglycoside antibiotics / ↑ Effect of warfarin due to interference with vitamin K

Amiodarone / ↑ Effect of warfarin due to ↓ breakdown by liver

Androgens / ↑ Effect of warfarin

Ascorbic acid / ↓ Effect of warfarin by unknown mechanism

Barbiturates / ↓ Effect of warfarin due to ↑ breakdown by liver

Beta-adrenergic blockers / ↑ Effect of wafarin

Carbamazepine / ↓ Effect of warfarin due to ↑ breakdown by liver

Cephalosporins / ↑ Effect of warfarin due to effects on platelet function

Chloral hydrate / ↑ Effect of warfarin due to ↓ binding to plasma proteins

Chloramphenicol / ↑ Effect of warfarin due to ↓ breakdown by liver

Cholestyramine / ↓ Anticoagulant effect due to binding in and ↓ absorption from GI tract

Cimetidine / ↑ Anticoagulant effect due to ↓ breakdown by liver

Clofibrate / ↑ Anticoagulant effect

Contraceptives, oral / ↓ Anticoagulant effect by ↑ activity of certain clotting factors (VII

and X); rarely, the opposite effect of ↑ risk of thromboembolism
Contrast media containing iodine / ↑ Effect of warfarin by ↑ PT
Corticosteroids / ↑ Effect of warfarin; also ↑ risk of GI bleeding due to ulcerogenic effect of steroids
Cyclophosphamide / ↑ Anticoagulant effect
Dextrothyroxine / ↑ Effect of warfarin
Dicloxacillin / ↓ Effect of warfarin
Diflunisal / ↑ Anticoagulant effect and ↑ risk of bleeding due to effect on platelet function and GI irritation
Disulfiram / ↑ Effect of warfarin
Erythromycin / ↑ Effect of warfarin
Estrogens / ↓ Anticoagulant response by ↑ activity of certain clotting factors; rarely, the opposite effect of ↑ risk of thromboembolism
Ethchlorvynol / ↓ Effect of warfarin
Etretinate / ↓ Effect of warfarin due to ↑ breakdown by liver
Fluconazole / ↑ Effect of warfarin
Gemfibrozil / ↑ Effect of warfarin
Glucagon / ↑ Effect of warfarin
Glutethimide / ↓ Effect of warfarin due to ↑ breakdown by liver
Griseofulvin / ↓ Effect of warfarin
Hydantoins / ↑ Effect of warfarin; also, ↑ hydantoin serum levels
Hypoglycemics, oral / ↑ Effect of warfarin due to ↓ plasma protein binding; also, ↑ effect of sulfonylureas
Ifosfamide / ↑ Effect of warfarin due to ↓ breakdown by liver and displacement from protein binding sites
Indomethacin / ↑ Effect of warfarin by an effect on platelet function; also, indomethacin is ulcerogenic cause GI hemorrhage
Isoniazid / ↑ Effect of warfarin
Ketoconazole / ↑ Effect of warfarin
Loop diuretics / ↑ Effect of warfarin by displacement from protein binding sites
Lovastatin / ↑ Effect of warfarin due to ↓ breakdown by liver
Metronidazole / ↑ Effect of warfarin due to ↓ breakdown by liver
Miconazole / ↑ Effect of warfarin
Mineral oil / ↑ Hypoprothrombinemia by ↓ absorption of vitamin K from GI tract; also mineral oil may ↓ absorption of warfarin from GI tract
Moricizine / ↑ Effect of warfarin
Nafcillin / ↓ Effect of warfarin
Nalidixic acid / ↑ Effect of warfarin due to displacement from protein binding sites
Nonsteroidal anti-inflammatory agents / ↑ Effect of warfarin and ↑ risk of bleeding due to effects on platelet function and GI irritation
Omeprazole / ↑ Effect of warfarin due to ↓ breakdown by liver
Penicillins / ↑ Effect of warfarin and ↑ risk of bleeding due to effects on platelet function
Phenylbutazone / ↑ Effect of warfarin due to ↓ breakdown by liver and ↑ displacement from protein binding sites
Propafenone / ↑ Effect of wafarin due to ↓ breakdown by liver
Propoxyphene / ↑ Effect of warfarin
Quinidine, quinine / ↑ Effect of warfarin due to ↓ breakdown by liver
Quinolones / ↑ Effect of warfarin
Rifampin / ↓ Anticoagulant effect due to ↑ breakdown by liver
Salicylates / ↑ Effect of warfarin and ↑ risk of bleeding due to effect on platelet function and GI irritation
Spironolactone / ↓ Effect of warfarin due to hemoconcentration of clotting factors due to diuresis
Streptokinase / ↑ Effect of warfarin
Sucralfate / ↓ Effect of warfarin
Sulfamethoxazole and Trimethoprim / ↑ Effect of warfarin due to ↓ breakdown by liver
Sulfinpyrazone / ↑ Anticoagulant effect due to ↓ breakdown by liver and inhibition of platelet aggregation
Sulfonamides / ↑ Effect of sulfonamides
Sulindac / ↑ Effect of warfarin
Tamoxifen / ↑ Effect of warfarin
Tetracyclines / ↑ Effect of warfarin due to interference with vitamin K
Thiazide diuretics / ↓ Effect of warfarin due to hemoconcentration of clotting factors
Thioamines / ↑ Effect of warfarin
Thiopurines / ↓ Effect of warfarin due to ↑ synthesis or activation of prothrombin
Thyroid hormones / ↑ Anticoagulant effect
Trazodone / ↓ Effect of warfarin
Thiazide diuretics / ↓ Effect of warfarin due to hemoconcentration of clotting factors due to diuresis
Troglitazone / Possible ↑ effect of warfarin due to ↓ breakdown by liver or displacement from plasma proteins
Urokinase / ↑ Effect of warfarin
Vitamin E / ↑ Effect of warfarin due to interference with vitamin K
Vitamin K / ↓ Effect of warfarin

How Supplied: *Powder for injection:* 5 mg; *Tablet:* 1 mg, 2 mg, 2.5 mg, 4 mg, 5 mg, 6 mg, 7.5 mg, 10 mg

Dosage

- **Tablets, IV**
  Induction.

W

Adults, initial: 5–10 mg/day for 2–4 days; **then,** adjust dose based on prothrombin or INR determinations. A lower dose should be used in geriatric or debilitated clients or clients with increased sensitivity. Dosage has not been established for children.

Maintenance.

Adults: 2–10 mg/day, based on prothrombin or INR.

Prevent blood clots with prosthetic heart valve replacement.

2–5 mg daily.

HEALTH CARE CONSIDERATIONS

See also *Health Care Considerations* for *Anticoagulants.*

Administration/Storage

1. Frequent monitoring of PT/INR is recommended during the first week of therapy, or during adjustment periods, and monthly thereafter.
2. Do not change brands; there may be differences in bioavailability.
3. To transfer from heparin therapy, give heparin and warfarin together from the first day (as there is a delayed onset of oral anticoagulant effects). Alternatively, warfarin may be started on the third to sixth day of heparin therapy.
4. Levels of anticoagulation that are recommended for specific indications by the American College of Chest Physicians and the National Heart, Lung, and Blood Institute should be followed.
5. Protect from light; store at controlled room temperature. Dispense in a tight, light-resistant container.
6. **IV** Give IV as a slow bolus injection over 1–2 min into a peripheral vein.
7. Reconstitute for IV use by adding 2.7 mL sterile water for injection. Inspect for particulate matter and discoloration.
8. After reconstitution, injection is stable for 4 hr at room temperature. There is no preservative; take care to assure sterility of prepared solution.
9. Do not use the vial for multiple use; discard unused solution.

W

Assessment

1. Record indications for therapy, onset and characteristics of symptoms.
2. List drugs currently prescribed to ensure that none interacts unfavorably by increasing or decreasing PT as a result of competition for protein binding at receptor sites.
3. Note any bleeding tendencies.
4. Determine if pregnant. May cause fetal malformations and neonatal hemorrhage.
5. Monitor ECG, CBC, PT/PTT, INR, liver and renal function studies.

Interventions

1. Request written parameters noting the desired range for PT or INR, once anticoagulated (orally). It usually takes 36–48 hr for drug to reach steady state; therefore allow time to equilibrate. The INR is the PT ratio (test/control) obtained from human brain thromboplastin and is universally considered most accurate to calculate dosage.
2. Drug inhibits production of factors II, VII, IX, and X; onset in response is delayed because of degradation of clotting factors that have already been synthesized.
3. Observe for "purple toes" syndrome related to inhibition of protein C and S.

Client/Family Teaching

1. Take oral warfarin as prescribed and at the same time each day.
2. This drug does not dissolve clots but decreases the clotting ability of the blood and helps to prevent the formation of harmful blood clots in the blood vessels and heart valves.
3. Avoid activities and contact sports that may cause injury or cuts and bruises. Use a soft toothbrush, electric razor to shave, wear shoes and use a night light to avoid falls at night.
4. Report immediately any unusual bruising or bleeding, dark brown or blood-tinged body secretions, injury or trauma, dizziness, abdominal pain or swelling, back pain, severe headaches, and joint swelling and pain.
5. May carry vitamin K for emergency use. (The usual dosage is 5–20 mg, to be used in the event of excessive bleeding.)
6. Avoid foods high in vitamin K: asparagus, broccoli, cabbage, brussels sprouts, spinach, turnips, milk, and cheese.
7. Use reliable birth control.
8. Menstruation may be prolonged and flow slightly increased. Report if excessive and unusual.
9. Skin eruptions may develop as an allergic reaction; report.
10. Do not change brands of drug unless approved; may alter response.
11. Wear identification and alert all providers of anticoagulant therapy.
12. Report as scheduled for labs to evaluate effectiveness of therapy and need for dosage changes.

Outcome/Evaluate

- Prevention/resolution of thrombus formation
- PT within desired range (1.5–2 times the control)
- INR within desired range (2.0–3.0 with standard therapy; 2.5–4.0 with high-dose therapy)

Z 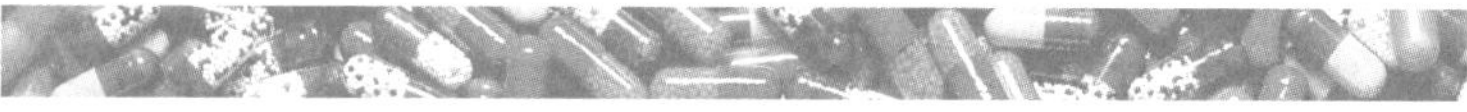

Zafirlukast

(zah-**FIR**-loo-kast)
Pregnancy Category: B
Accolate **(Rx)**
Classification: Antiasthmatic

Action/Kinetics: A selective and competitive antagonist of leukotriene receptors D_4 and E_4, which are components of slow-reacting substance of anaphylaxis. It is believed that cysteinyl leukotriene occupation of receptors causes asthma, including airway edema, smooth muscle constriction, and altered cellular activity associated with the inflammatory process. Zafirlukast inhibits bronchoconstriction caused by sulfur dioxide and cold air in clients with asthma. It also attenuates the early- and late-phase reaction in asthmatics caused by inhalation of antigens such as grass, cat dander, ragweed, and mixed antigens. Rapidly absorbed after PO use; bioavailabilty may be decreased when taken with food. **Peak plasma levels:** 3 hr. **t½, terminal:** About 10 hr. Over 99% bound to plasma proteins. Extensively metabolized in the liver, with about 90% excreted in the feces and 10% in the urine. Inhibits certain cytochrome P450 isoenzymes.

Uses: Prophylaxis and chronic treatment of asthma in adults and children 12 years of age and older.

Contraindications: Use to terminate an acute asthma attack, including status asthmaticus. Lactation.

Special Concerns: The clearance is reduced in clients 65 years of age and older. Safety and efficacy have not been determined in children less than 12 years of age.

Side Effects: *GI:* N&V, diarrhea, abdominal pain, dyspepsia. *CNS:* Headache, dizziness. *Hepatic:* Rarely, symptomatic hepatitis and hyperbilirubinemia. *Hypersensitivity reactions:* Urticaria, angioedema, rashes (with and without blistering). *Miscellaneous:* Infection, generalized pain, asthenia, accidental injury, myalgia, fever, back pain, systemic eosinophilia with vasculitis consistent with Churg-Strauss syndrome.

Laboratory Test Considerations: ↑ ALT.

Drug Interactions

Aspirin / ↑ Plasma levels of zafirlukast
Erythromycin / ↓ Plasma levels of zafirlukast
Terfenadine / ↓ Plasma levels of zafirlukast
Theophylline / ↓ Plasma levels of zafirlukast
Warfarin / Significant ↑ PT

How Supplied: *Tablet:* 20 mg

Dosage

- **Tablets**

Asthma.

Adults and children aged 12 and older: 20 mg b.i.d.

HEALTH CARE CONSIDERATIONS

Administration/Storage: Protect from light and moisture and store at controlled room temperatures of 20°C–25°C (68°F –77°F).

Assessment

1. Record indications for therapy, onset, duration, and characteristics of symptoms. List other agents trialed with the outcome.
2. Note cardiopulmonary assessment findings.
3. Monitor labs and PFTs.

Client/Family Teaching

1. Take 1 hr before or 2 hr after meals to prevent loss of bioavailability.
2. Take drug regularly during symptom-free periods. Do not increase or decrease dose without approval.
3. Drug is not appropriate for acute episodes of asthma. Continue all other antiasthma medications as prescribed.
4. Review peak flow meter use and set targets for intervention or additional therapy.
5. Avoid triggers, i.e., dust, chemicals, cigarette smoke, pollutants, pets, and perfumes.
6. Practice reliable birth control; do not breast feed during therapy.

Outcome/Evaluate: Inhibition of bronchoconstriction; improved breathing patterns

Zalcitabine (Dideoxycytidine, ddC)

(zal-**SIGH**-tah-been)
Pregnancy Category: C
Hivid **(Rx)**
Classification: Antiviral

See also *Antiviral Drugs,* and *Anti-Infectives.*

Action/Kinetics: Converted in cells to the active metabolite, dideoxycytidine 5'-triphosphate (ddCTP), by cellular enzymes. ddCTP serves as an alternative substrate to deoxycytidine triphosphate for HIV-reverse transcriptase, thereby inhibiting the in vitro rep-

Z

lication of HIV-1 and inhibiting viral DNA synthesis. The incorporation of ddCTP into the growing DNA chain leads to premature chain termination. ddCTP serves as a competitive inhibitor of the natural substrate for deoxycytidine triphosphate for the active site of the viral reverse transcriptase, which further inhibits viral DNA synthesis. Food reduces the rate of absorption. Does not appear to undergo significant metabolism by the liver. **Elimination t½:** 1–3 hr. Approximately 70% of a PO dose is excreted through the kidneys and 10% in the feces. Prolonged elimination (t½ up to 8.5 hr) is observed in clients with impaired renal function.

Uses: In combination with AZT in advanced HIV infections (CD_4 cell count of 300/mm³ or less and who have shown significant clinical or immunologic deterioration). Alone for HIV-infected adults with advanced disease who are intolerant to AZT or where the disease has progressed while taking AZT.

Contraindications: Hypersensitivity. Use in moderate or severe peripheral neuropathy or with drugs that have the potential to cause peripheral neuropathy (see *Drug Interactions*). Concomitant use with didanosine. Lactation.

Special Concerns: Use with extreme caution in clients with low CD_4 cell counts (< 50/mm³). Use with caution in clients with a history of pancreatitis or known risk factors for the development of pancreatitis. Clients with a C_{CR} less than 55 mL/min may be at a greater risk for toxicity due to decreased clearance. Clients may continue to develop opportunistic infections and other complications of HIV infection. Safety and efficacy have not been determined in HIV-infected children less than 13 years of age.

Side Effects: The incidence of certain side effects is dependent on the duration of use and the dose of the drug. *Neurologic:* Peripheral neuropathy (may be severe) characterized by numbness and burning dysesthesia involving the distal extremities; this may be followed by sharp shooting pains or severe continuous burning pain if the drug is not withdrawn. The neuropathy may progress to severe pain requiring narcotic analgesics and may be irreversible. *GI:* ***Fatal pancreatitis*** when given alone or with AZT. Esophageal ulcers, oral ulcers, nausea, dysphagia, anorexia, abdominal pain, vomiting, constipation, ulcerative stomatitis, aphthous stomatitis, diarrhea, dry mouth, dyspepsia, glossitis, ***rectal hemorrhage,*** hemorrhoids, enlarged abdomen, gum disorders, flatulence, anorexia, tongue ulceration, dysphagia, eructation, gastritis, ***GI hemorrhage,*** left quadrant pain, salivary gland enlargement, esophageal pain, esophagitis, rectal ulcers, melena, painful swallowing, mouth lesion, acute pharyngitis, abdominal bloating or cramps, anal/rectal pain, colitis, dental abscess, epigastric pain, gagging with pills, gingivitis, heartburn, ***hemorrhagic pancreatitis,*** increased salivation, odynophagia, painful sore gums, rectal mass, sore tongue, sore throat, tongue disorder, toothache, unformed/loose stools. *Dermatologic:* Rash (including erythematous, maculopapular, follicular), pruritus, night sweats, dermatitis, skin lesions, acne, alopecia, bullous eruptions, increased sweating, urticaria, hot flashes, lip blister or lesions, carbuncle/furuncle, cellulitis, dry skin, dry rash desquamation, exfoliative dermatitis, finger inflammation, impetigo, infection, itchy rash, moniliasis, mucocutaneous/skin disorder, nail disorder, photosensitivity, skin fissure, skin ulcer. *CNS:* Headache, dizziness, seizures, ataxia, abnormal coordination, Bell's palsy, dysphonia, hyperkinesia, hypokinesia, migraine, neuralgia, neuritis, stupor, aphasia, decreased neurologic function, disequilibrium, facial nerve palsy, focal motor seizures, memory loss, paralysis, speech disorder, ***status epilepticus,*** tremor, vertigo, hypertonia, hand tremor, twitching, confusion, impaired concentration, insomnia, agitation, depersonalization, hallucinations, emotional lability, nervousness, anxiety, depression, euphoria, manic reaction, dementia, amnesia, somnolence, abnormal thinking, crying, loss of memory, decreased concentration, acute psychotic disorder, acute stress reaction, decreased motivation, decreased sexual desire, mood swings, paranoid states, ***suicide attempt***. *Respiratory:* Coughing, dyspnea, respiratory distress, rales/rhonchi, nasal discharge, flu-like symptoms, cyanosis, acute nasopharyngitis, chest congestion, dry nasal mucosa, hemoptysis, sinus congestion, sinus pain, sinusitis, wheezing. *Musculoskeletal:* Myalgia, arthralgia, arthritis, arthropathy, cold extremities, leg cramps, myositis, joint pain or inflammation, weakness in leg muscle, generalized muscle weakness, back pain, backache, bone aches and pains, bursitis, pain in extremities, joint swelling, muscle disorder, muscle stiffness, muscle cramps, arthrosis, myopathy, neck pain, rib pain, stiff neck. *Hepatic:* Exacerbation of hepatic dysfunction, especially in those with preexisting liver disease or with a history of alcohol abuse. Abnormal hepatic function, hepatitis, jaundice, hepatocellular damage, hepatomegaly with steatosis, cholecystitis. *CV:* ***Cardiomyopathy,*** CHF, abnormal cardiac movement arrhythmia, atrial fibrillation, ***car-***

diac failure, cardiac dysrhythmias, heart racing, hypertension, palpitations, ***subarachnoid hemorrhage,*** syncope, tachycardia, ventricular ectopy, epistaxis. *Hematologic:* Anemia, leukopenia, thrombocytopenia, alteration of absolute neutrophil count, granulocytosis, eosinophilia, neutropenia, hemoglobinemia, neutrophilia, platelet alteration, purpura, thrombus, unspecified hematologic toxicity, alteration of WBCs. *Hypersensitivity:* Urticaria, ***anaphylaxis*** (rare). *Endocrine:* Diabetes mellitus, gout, hot flushes, hypoglycemia, hyperglycemia, hypocalcemia, hypophosphatemia, hypernatremia, hyponatremia, hypomagnesemia, hyperkalemia, hypokalemia, hyperlipidemia, polydipsia. *GU:* Dysuria, toxic nephropathy, polyuria, renal calculi, ***acute renal failure,*** hyperuricemia, increased frequency of micturition, abnormal renal function, renal cyst, albuminuria, bladder pain, genital lesion/ulcer, nocturia, painful/sore penis, penile edema, testicular swelling, urinary retention, vaginal itch/ulcer/pain, vaginal/cervix disorder. *Ophthalmologic:* Abnormal vision, burning or itching eyes, xerophthalmia, eye pain or abnormality, blurred or decreased vision, eye inflammation/irritation, eye redness/hemorrhage, increased tears, mucopurulent conjunctivitis, photophobia, dry eyes, unequal sized pupils, yellow sclera. *Otic:* Ear pain/blockage, fluid in ears, hearing loss, tinnitus. *Body as a whole:* Fatigue, fever, rigors, chest pain or tightness, weight decrease, pain, malaise, asthenia, generalized edema, general debilitation, chills, difficulty moving, facial pain or swelling, flank pain, flushing, pelvic/groin pain. *Miscellaneous:* Lymphadenopathy, taste perversion, decreased taste, parosmia, lactic acidosis.

Laboratory Test Considerations: ↑ ALT, AST, alkaline phosphatase, CPK, amylase, nonprotein nitrogen. Abnormal gamma-glutamyl transferase, GGT, LDH, lactate dehydrogenase, triglycerides, lipase. Bilirubinemia. ↓ Hematocrit.

Drug Interactions: The following drugs have the potential to cause peripheral neuropathy and should probably not be used concomitantly with zalcitabine: chloramphenicol, cisplatin, dapsone, disulfiram, ethionamide, glutethimide, gold, hydralazine, iodoquinol, isoniazid, metronidazole, nitrofurantoin, phenytoin, ribavirin, vincristine. Drugs such as amphotericin, foscarnet, and aminoglycosides may increase the risk of peripheral neuropathy by interfering with the renal clearance of zalcitabine, thus increasing plasma levels.

Antacids (Mg/Al-containing) / ↓ Absorption of zalcitabine
Cimetidine / ↓ Elimination of zalcitabine by ↓ renal tubular secretion
Pentamidine / ↑ Risk of fulminant pancreatitis
Probenecid / ↓ Elimination of zalcitabine by ↓ renal tubular secretion

How Supplied: *Tablet:* 0.375 mg, 0.75 mg

Dosage

- **Tablets**

In combination with AZT in advanced HIV infection.

Adults: 0.75 mg given at the same time with 200 mg AZT q 8 hr for a total daily dose of 2.25 mg zalcitabine and 600 mg AZT.

Alone in advanced HIV infection.

0.75 mg q 8 hr (2.25 mg/day).

HEALTH CARE CONSIDERATIONS

Administration/Storage

1. If C_{CR} is 10–40 mL/min, reduce the dose to 0.75 mg/12 hr; if C_{CR} is less than 10 mL/min, reduce the dose to 0.75 mg/24 hr.
2. Reduction of dosage is not required for client weights down to 30 kg.

Assessment

1. Clients with a history of pancreatitis or elevated serum amylase should be followed closely while on zalcitabine therapy.
2. Baseline serum amylase and triglyceride levels should be performed in clients with a history of pancreatitis, increased amylase, those on parenteral nutrition, or those with a history of drug abuse.
3. Frequent monitoring of hematologic indices is recommended to detect serious anemia or granulocytopenia. In clients manifesting hematologic toxicity, decreases in hemoglobin may occur as early as 2–4 weeks after beginning therapy, whereas granulocytopenia may be seen after 6–8 weeks of therapy.
4. Monitor CBC, CD_4 counts/viral loads, liver and renal function studies.
5. Assess for symptoms of peripheral neuropathy: pain, numbness, and tingling. If symptoms evident, the drug may be reintroduced at 50% of the initial dose (i.e., 0.375 mg/8 hr) once all symptoms related to the peripheral neuropathy have improved to mild symptoms. The drug should be permanently discontinued if severe discomfort due to peripheral neuropathy progresses for 1 week or longer.

Client/Family Teaching

1. Take only as directed on an empty stomach (with concurrently prescribed AZT) every 8 hr.

2. May continue to develop opportunistic infections and other complications of HIV infection; remain under close medical supervision.
3. Use reliable contraceptive and practice safe sex.
4. Drug is not a cure, but helps to alleviate and manage the symptoms of HIV infections.
5. Discontinue and report if symptoms of peripheral neuropathy occur, especially if the symptoms are bilateral and progress for more than 72 hr. Peripheral neuropathy may continue to worsen despite interruption of therapy. If the symptoms improve, then drug may be reintroduced at a lower dose.
6. Schedule retinal exams q 6 mo to assess for retinal depigmentation.
7. Identify local support groups that may assist client/family to understand and cope with this disease.

Outcome/Evaluate: Improved CD_4 cell counts, ↓ viral load, ↓ incidence of opportunistic infection, and improved survival rates in clients with advanced HIV infections

Zaleplon

(ZAL-leh-plon)
Pregnancy Category: C
Sonata **(Rx) (C-IV)**
Classification: Hypnotic

Action/Kinetics: Nonbenzodiazepine hypnotic. However, it interacts with the GABA-benzodiazepine receptor complex. It binds selectively to the brain omega-1 receptor located on the alpha subunit of $GABA_A$ receptor complex and potentiates t-butyl-bicyclophosphorothionate (TBPS) binding. Although it decreases the time to sleep, it does not increase total sleep time or decrease the number of awakenings. Rapidly and almost completely absorbed. **Peak plasma levels:** 1 hr. Undergoes significant first-pass metabolism. A high-fat or heavy meal prolongs absorption. Extensively metabolized to inactive metabolites which are excreted in the urine (70%) and feces (17%). **t½:** About 1 hr.
Uses: Short-term treatment of insomnia.
Contraindications: Use with alcohol, severe hepatic impairment, or during lactation.
Special Concerns: Use with caution in diseases or conditions that could affect metabolism or hemodynamic responses, in clients with compromised respiratory function, or in clients showing signs or symptoms of depression. Abuse potential is similar to benzodiazepine and benzodiazepine-like hypnotics. The products contain tartrazine (FD&C yellow #5) which may cause an allergic-type reaction, especially in those with aspirin hypersensitivity. May cause amnesia and dependence.
Side Effects: Listed are side effects with an incidence of 0.1% or greater. *CNS:* Dizziness, amnesia, somnolence, anxiety, paresthesia, depersonalization, hypesthesia, tremor, hallucinations, vertigo, depression, hypertonia, nervousness, abnormal thinking/concentration, abnormal gait, agitation, apathy, ataxia, circumoral paresthesia, confusion, emotional lability, euphoria, hyperesthesia, hyperkinesia, hypotonia, incoordination, insomnia, decreased libido, neuralgia, nystagmus. *GI:* Nausea, dyspepsia, anorexia, colitis, constipation, dry mouth, eructation, esophagitis, flatulence, gastritis, gastroenteritis, gingivitis, glossitis, increased appetite, melena, mouth ulceration, rectal hemorrhage, stomatitis. *CV:* Migraine, angina pectoris, bundle branch block, hypertension, hypotension, palpitation, syncope, tachycardia, vasodilation, ventricular extrasystoles. *Dermatologic:* Pruritus, rash, acne, alopecia, contact dermatitis, dry skin, eczema, maculopapular rash, skin hypertrophy, sweating, urticaria, vesiculobullous rash. *GU:* Bladder pain, breast pain, cystitis, decreased urine stream, dysuria, hematuria, impotence, kidney calculus, kidney pain, menorrhagia, metorrhagia, urinary frequency, urinary incontinence, urinary urgency, vaginitis, dysmenorrhea. *Respiratory:* Bronchitis, asthma, dyspnea, laryngitis, pneumonia, snoring, voice alteration. *Musculoskeletal:* Arthritis, arthrosis, bursitis, joint disorder (swelling, stiffness, pain), myasthenia, tenosynovitis. *Hematologic:* Anemia, ecchymosis, lymphadenopathy. *Metabolic:* Edema, gout, hypercholesterolemia, thirst, weight gain. *Ophthalmic:* Eye pain, abnormal vision, conjunctivitis, diplopia, dry eyes, photophobia, watery eyes. *Otic:* Ear pain, hyperacusis, tinnitus. *Body as a whole:* Headache, asthenia, myalgia, fever, malaise, chills, generalized edema. *Miscellaneous:* Abdominal pain, photosensitivity, peripheral edema, epistaxis, back pain, chest pain, substernal chest pain, face edema, hangover effect, neck rigidity, parosmia.

Drug Interactions

Cimetidine / Significantly ↑ zaleplon serum levels
CNS depressants (anticonvulsants, antihistamines, ethanol) / Additive CNS depression
Rifampin / Significantly ↓ zaleplon serum levels

How Supplied: *Capsules:* 5 mg, 10 mg

Dosage

• **Capsules**

Insomnia.

Adults, nonelderly: 10 mg for no more than 7–10 days. Consider 20 mg for the occasional client who does not benefit from the lower dose. Do not exceed a dose of 20 mg. **Mild to moderate hepatic impairment, elderly clients, or low-weight individuals:** 5 mg, not to exceed 10 mg..

HEALTH CARE CONSIDERATIONS

Assessment

1. Note characteristics of insomnia and assess for contributing factors.
2. Assess for depression, respiratory dysfunction, alcohol or drug dependence. Drug may cause dependence and amnesia.
3. Contains tartrazine (FD&C yellow #5); note any aspirin hypersensitivity.
4. Note drugs prescribed to ensure none interact; with cimetidine initially reduce zaleplon dose to 5 mg and assess response.
5. Monitor renal and LFTs; reduce dose with liver dysfunction.

Client/Family Teaching

1. Due to its rapid onset, ingest immediately prior to going to bed or after the client has gone to bed and experienced difficulty falling asleep.
2. Taking zaleplon with or immediately after a heavy, high-fat meal causes slower absorption leading to a reduced effect on sleep latency.
3. Do not engage in activities requiring mental alertness after ingesting drug and during the next day until drug effects realized.
4. Avoid alcohol and CNS depressants.
5. May experience amnesia. Obtain at least 4 hr sleep after ingestion and before activity.
6. If also taking cimetidine, take an initial lowered dose of 5 mg of zaleplon.
7. May experience withdrawal symptoms or worsening of insomnia with abrupt drug discontinuation especially with daily use for an extended period of time.
8. If behaviorial changes or unusual thinking occur involving aggressiveness, confusion, loss of personal identity, agitation, hallucinations, increased depression or suicide ideations, report.
9. Store out of the reach of children.

Outcome/Evaluate: Relief of insomnia

Zanamivir

(zah-**NAM**-ih-vir)

Pregnancy Category: B

Relenza **(Rx)**

Classification: Antiviral drug

Action/Kinetics: Selectively inhibits influenza virus neuraminidase. The enzyme allows virus release from infected cells, prevents virus aggregation, and possibly decreases virus inactivation by respiratory mucus. Zanamivir may alter virus particle aggregation and release. There is the possibility of emergence of resistance. About 4%–17% is absorbed systemically. **Peak serum levels:** 17–142 ng/mL within 1–2 hr after a 10-mg dose. Readily excreted as unchanged drug in the urine. **t½:** 2.5–5.1 hr after PO inhalation.

Uses: Treatment of uncomplicated acute illness due to influenza virus A and B (limited) in adults and adolescents (12 years and older) who have been symptomatic for 2 or less days. *Note:* There is no evidence that zanamivir is effective in any illness caused by agents other than influenza virus A and B.

Special Concerns: Use with caution during lactation. It is possible the elderly may be more sensitive to effects of the drug. Safety and efficacy have not been determined in children less than 12 years of age, in clients with underlying chronic pulmonary disease, for prophylactic use to prevent influenza (clients should still take annual flu vaccinations), or in those with high-risk underlying medical conditions.

Side Effects: *GI:* Diarrhea, N&V. *Respiratory:* Nasal signs and symptoms, bronchitis, cough, sinusitis, infections of the ear, nose, and throat. *Miscellaneous:* Dizziness, headache, malaise, fatigue, fever, abdominal pain, myalgia, arthralgia, urticaria.

Laboratory Test Considerations: ↑ Liver enzymes, CPK. Lymphopenia, neutropenia.

How Supplied: *Powder for Inhalation, Blisters:* 5 mg

Dosage

- **Powder for oral inhalation**

  Influenza treatment.

Adults and children over 12 years: 2 inhalations (one 5-mg blister per inhalation for a total dose of 10 mg) b.i.d. for 5 days. Two doses are taken on the first day of treatment whenever possible, provided there is 2 or more hr between doses. On subsequent days, doses are taken about 12 hr apart (i.e., morning and evening) at about the same time each day. Safety and efficacy of repeated treatment courses have not been studied.

HEALTH CARE CONSIDERATIONS

Administration/Storage: Store at 25°C (77°F).

Z

Assessment: Record indications for therapy, onset and characteristics of symptoms, and any other medical conditions and drug allergies known.

Client/Family Teaching

1. To be given by oral inhalation only, using the Diskhaler provided. Review/demonstrate use of the delivery system.
2. Do not puncture any Relenza Rotadisk blister until taking a dose using the Diskhaler.
3. Continue complete treatment despite feeling better. Take oral inhalations twice a day 12 hr apart at approximately the same time each day.
4. If client is to use an inhaled bronchodilator at the same time as zanamivir, use the bronchodilator before taking zanamivir.
5. Safety and efficacy of repeated treatment courses have not been evaluated.
6. Does not reduce the risk of transmisstion of flu to others.
7. Clients with COPD may experience bronchospasm with zanamivir; have a fast-acting inhaled bronchodilator available, stop zanamivir and contact provider immediately if experience worsening respiratory symptoms.

Outcome/Evaluate: Relief of influenza S&S

Zidovudine (Azidothymidine, AZT)

(zye-**DOH**-vyou-deen, ah-**zee**-doh-**THIGH**-mih-deen)

Pregnancy Category: C

Apo-Zidovudine ✱, Novo-AZT ✱, Retrovir **(Rx)**

Classification: Antiviral

See also *Antiviral Drugs* and *Anti-Infectives*.

Action/Kinetics: The active form of the drug is AZT triphosphate, which is derived from AZT by cellular enzymes. AZT triphosphate competes with thymidine triphosphate (the natural substrate) for incorporation into growing chains of viral DNA by retroviral reverse transcriptase. Once incorporated, AZT triphosphate causes premature termination of the growth of the DNA chain. Low concentrations of AZT also inhibit the activity of *Shigella, Klebsiella, Salmonella, Enterobacter, Escherichia coli,* and *Citrobacter,* although resistance develops rapidly. Rapidly absorbed from the GI tract and is distributed to both plasma and CSF. **Peak serum levels:** 0.1–1.5 hr. **t½:** approximately 1 hr. Metabolized rapidly by the liver and excreted through the urine.

Uses: PO: Initial treatment of HIV-infected adults who have a CD_4 cell count of 500/mm³ or less. Superior to either didanosine or zalcitabine monotherapy for initial treatment of HIV-infected clients who have not had previous antiretroviral therapy. To prevent HIV transmission from pregnant women to their fetuses. For HIV-infected children over 3 months of age who have HIV-related symptoms or are asymptomatic with abnormal laboratory values indicating significant immunosuppression. In combination with zalcitabine in selected clients with advanced HIV disease (CD_4 cell count of 300 cells/mm³ or less).

IV: Selected adults with symptomatic HIV infections who have a history of confirmed *Pneumocystis carinii* pneumonia or an absolute CD_4 (T_4 helper/inducer) lymphocyte count of less than 200 cells/mm³ in the peripheral blood prior to therapy.

Contraindications: Allergy to AZT or its components. Lactation.

Special Concerns: Use with caution in clients who have a hemoglobin level of less than 9.5 g/dL or a granulocyte count less than 1,000/mm³. AZT is not a cure for HIV; thus, clients may continue to acquire opportunistic infections and other illnesses associated with ARC or HIV. AZT has not been shown to reduce the risk of HIV transmission to others through sexual contact or blood contamination.

Side Effects: Adults. *Hematologic:* Anemia (severe), granulocytopenia. *Body as a whole:* Headache, asthenia, fever, diaphoresis, malaise, body odor, chills, edema of the lip, flu-like syndrome, hyperalgesia, abdominal/chest/back pain, lymphadenopathy. *GI:* Nausea, GI pain, diarrhea, anorexia, vomiting, dyspepsia, constipation, dysphagia, edema of the tongue, eructation, flatulence, bleeding gums, mouth ulcers, ***rectal hemorrhage.*** *CNS:* Somnolence, dizziness, paresthesia, insomnia, anxiety, confusion, emotional lability, depression, nervousness, vertigo, loss of mental acuity. *CV:* Vasodilation, syncope, vasculitis (rare). *Musculoskeletal:* Myalgia, myopathy, myositis, arthralgia, tremor, twitch, muscle spasm. *Respiratory:* Dyspnea, cough, epistaxis, rhinitis, pharyngitis, sinusitis, hoarseness. *Dermatologic:* Rash, pruritus, urticaria, acne, pigmentation changes of the skin and nails. *GU:* Dysuria, polyuria, urinary hesitancy or frequency. *Other:* Amblyopia, hearing loss, photophobia, ***severe hepatomegaly with steatosis,*** lactic acidosis, change in taste perception, hepatitis, pancreatitis, hypersensitivity reactions, including ***anaphylaxis,*** hyperbilirubinemia (rare), ***seizures.***

Children. The following side effects have

been observed in children, although any of the side effects reported for adults can also occur in children. *Body as a whole:* Granulocytopenia, anemia, fever, headache, phlebitis, bacteremia. *GI:* N&V, abdominal pain, diarrhea, weight loss. *CNS:* Decreased reflexes, nervousness, irritability, insomnia, ***seizures.*** *CV:* Abnormalities in ECG, left ventricular dilation, CHF, generalized edema, ***cardiomyopathy,*** S_3 gallop. *GU:* Hematuria, viral cystitis

OD **Management of Overdose:** *Symptoms:* N&V. Transient hematologic changes. Headache, dizziness, drowsiness, confusion, lethargy. *Treatment:* Treat symptoms. Hemodialysis will enhance the excretion of the primary metabolite of AZT.

Drug Interactions

Acetaminophen / ↑ Risk of granulocytopenia
Adriamycin / ↑ Risk of cytotoxicity, nephrotoxicity, or hematologic toxicity
Dapsone / ↑ Risk of cytotoxicity, nephrotoxicity, or hematologic toxicity
Flucytosine / ↑ Risk of cytotoxicity, nephrotoxicity, or hematologic toxicity
Fluconazole / ↑ Levels of AZT
Ganciclovir / ↑ Risk of hematologic toxicity
Interferon alfa / ↑ Risk of hematologic toxicity
Interferon beta-1b / ↑ Serum levels of AZT
Phenytoin / Levels of phenytoin may ↑, ↓, or remain unchanged; also, ↓ excretion of AZT
Probenecid / ↓ Biotransformation or renal excretion of AZT → flu-like symptoms, including myalgia, malaise or fever, and maculopapular rash
Rifampin / ↓ Levels of AZT
Trimethoprim / ↑ Serum levels of AZT
Vinblastine / ↑ Risk of cytotoxicity, nephrotoxicity, or hematologic toxicity
Vincristine / ↑ Risk of cytotoxicity, nephrotoxicity, or hematologic toxicity

How Supplied: *Capsule:* 100 mg; *Injection:* 10 mg/mL; *Syrup:* 50 mg/5 mL; *Tablet:* 300 mg

Dosage

- **Capsules, Syrup**

Symptomatic HIV infections.

Adults: 100 mg (one 100-mg capsule or 10 mL syrup) q 4 hr around the clock (i.e., total of 600 mg daily).

Asymptomatic HIV infections.

Adults: 100 mg q 4 hr while awake (500 mg/day); **Pediatric, 3 months–12 years, initial:** 180 mg/m² q 6 hr (720 mg/m²/day, not to exceed 200 mg q 6 hr).

Prevent transmission of HIV from mothers to their fetuses (after week 14 of pregnancy).

Maternal dosing: 100 mg 5 times a day until the start of labor. During labor and delivery, AZT IV at 2 mg/kg over 1 hr followed by continuous IV infusion of 1 mg/kg/hr until clamping of the umbilical cord. **Infant dosing:** 2 mg/kg PO q 6 hr beginning within 12 hr after birth and continuing through 6 weeks of age. Infants unable to take the drug PO may be given AZT IV at 1.5 mg/kg, infused over 30 min q 6 hr.

In combination with zalcitabine.

Zidovudine, 200 mg, with zalcitabine, 0.75 mg, q 8 hr.

- **IV**

1–2 mg/kg infused over 1 hr. The IV dose is given q 4 hr around the clock only until PO therapy can be instituted. Dosage adjustment may be necessary due to hematologic toxicity.

HEALTH CARE CONSIDERATIONS

See also *General Health Care Considerations for All Anti-Infectives.*

Administration/Storage

1. Protect capsules and syrup from light.
IV 2. Do not mix with blood products or protein solutions.
3. Remove dose from 20-mL vial and dilute in 5% dextrose injection to a concentration not to exceed 4 mg/mL. Administer calculated dose IV at a constant rate over 1 hr.
4. After dilution, the solution is stable at room temperature for 24 hr and if refrigerated (2°C–8°C, 35.6°F–46.4°F) for 48 hr. However, to ensure safety from microbial contamination, give within 8 hr if stored at room temperature and 24 hr if refrigerated.

Assessment

1. Record indications for therapy, onset, other therapies trialed and baseline CD_4 counts and viral load.
2. Initially monitor CBC at least q 2 weeks. If anemia or granulocytopenia severe, the dose must be adjusted or discontinued. Epoetin alfa recombinant may be administered with iron to stimulate RBC production. A blood transfusion may also be required.
3. Safety and effectiveness of chronic AZT therapy in adults are not known, especially in clients who have a less advanced form of disease.
4. When used to prevent maternal-fetal transmission of HIV, AZT should be initiated in pregnant women between 14 and 24 weeks of gestation; also, IV AZT should be given during labor up until the cord is clamped, and newborn infants should re-

Z

ceive AZT syrup. Mothers may not breast feed.

Client/Family Teaching

1. Take on an empty stomach q 4 hr ATC as ordered; sleep must be interrupted to take medication.
2. Report for all labs, especially CBC, because drug causes anemia, and additional medications or blood transfusions may be necessary.
3. Report early S&S of anemia, such as SOB, weakness, lightheadedness, or palpitations, and increased tiredness.
4. Consume 2–3 L/day fluids to ensure adequate hydration. Maintain a record of weights and I&O.
5. Report any symptoms of superinfections (e.g., furry tongue, mouth lesions, vaginal or rectal itching, thrush).
6. Avoid acetaminophen and any other unprescribed drugs that may exacerbate the toxicity of AZT.
7. Drug is not a cure but helps to alleviate and manage symptoms of HIV infections. May continue to develop opportunistic infections and other complications due to AIDS or ARC.
8. Do not share meds and do not exceed the recommended dose of AZT.
9. The risk of transmission of HIV to others through blood or sexual contact is not reduced in individuals on AZT therapy. Practice safe sex and do not share needles.
10. With pregnancy, AZT therapy should start after the 14-week gestation period to help prevent the transmission from mother to infant. Once delivered, do not nurse infant.
11. Identify local support groups that may assist client/family to understand and cope with this disease.

Outcome/Evaluate

- Control of symptoms of HIV, AIDS, or ARC
- ↑ CD_4 counts; ↓ viral load (HIV RNA)
- ↓ Maternal fetal HIV transmission

Zileuton

(zye-**LOO**-ton)

Pregnancy Category: C

Zyflo **(Rx)**

Classification: Antiasthmatic, leukotriene receptor inhibitor

Action/Kinetics: Specific inhibitor of 5-lipoxygenase; thus, inhibits the formation of leukotrienes. Leukotrienes are substances that induce various biological effects including aggregation of neutrophils and monocytes, leukocyte adhesion, increase of neutrophil and eosinophil migration, increased capillary permeability, and contraction of smooth muscle. These effects of leukotrienes contribute to edema, secretion of mucus, inflammation, and bronchoconstriction in asthmatic clients. By inhibiting leukotriene formation, zileuton reduces bronchoconstriction due to cold air challenge in asthmatics. Rapidly absorbed from the GI tract; **peak plasma levels:** 1.7 hr. Metabolized in liver and mainly excreted through the urine. **t½:** 2.5 hr.

Uses: Prophylaxis and chronic treatment of asthma in adults and children over 12 years of age.

Contraindications: Active liver disease or transaminase elevations greater than or equal to three times the upper limit of normal. Hypersenstivity. Treatment of bronchoconstriction in acute asthma attacks, including status asthmaticus. Lactation.

Special Concerns: Use with caution in clients who ingest large quantities of alcohol or who have a past history of liver disease. Safety and efficacy have not been determined in children less than 12 years of age.

Side Effects: *GI:* Dyspepsia, N&V constipation, flatulence. *CNS:* Headache, dizziness, insomnia, malaise, nervousness, somnolence. *Body as a whole:* Unspecified pain, abdominal pain, chest pain, asthenia, accidental injury, fever. *Musculoskeletal:* Myalgia, arthralgia, neck pain/rigidity. *GU:* UTI, vaginitis. *Miscellaneous:* Conjunctivitis, hypertonia, lymphadenopathy, pruritus.

Laboratory Test Considerations: ↑ LFTs. Low WBC count.

Drug Interactions

Propranolol / ↑ Effect of propranolol
Terfenadine / ↑ Effect of terfenadine due to ↓ clearance
Theophylline / Doubling of serum theophylline levels → ↑ effect
Warfarin / ↑ Prothrombin time

How Supplied: *Tablets:* 600 mg.

Dosage

- **Tablets**

Symptomatic treatment of asthma.

Adults and children over 12 years of age: 600 mg q.i.d.

HEALTH CARE CONSIDERATIONS

Administration/Storage

1. May be taken with meals and at bedtime.
2. Do not decrease the dose or stop taking any other antiasthmatics when taking zileuton.

Assessment

1. Record onset, characteristics, and severity of disease. Note triggers and list currently prescribed medications.

2. Monitor CBC, PFTs, and LFTs.
3. Screen for excessive alcohol use and any evidence of liver disease.

Client/Family Teaching

1. Take regularly as directed (may take with meals and at bedtime) and continue other antiasthmatic medications as prescribed.
2. Drug will not reverse bronchospasm during acute asthma attack; use bronchodilators and seek medical attention if symptoms are severe or peak flow readings indicate need.
3. Drug inhibits formation of those substances that cause bronchoconstrictive symptoms in asthmatics.
4. Use peak flow meter readings to monitor airway effectiveness, to increase medications, and to seek immediate medical attention.
5. Report immediately if experiencing RUQ pain, lethargy pruritus, jaundice, fatigue, or flu-like symptoms (S&S of liver toxicity).
6. Report for CBC, regularly scheduled LFTs and evaluation of pulmonary status. Bring record of peak flow readings.
7. Review triggers (i.e., smoke, cold air, and exercise) that may cause increased hyperresponsiveness which can last up to a week. If more than the usual or maximum number of inhalations of short-acting bronchodilator treatment in a 24-hr period are required, notify the provider.

Outcome/Evaluate: Asthma prophylaxis; improved airway exchange.

Zolmitriptan

(zohl-mih-**TRIP**-tin)
Pregnancy Category: C
Zomig **(Rx)**
Classification: Antimigraine drug

Action/Kinetics: Binds to serotonin 5-$HT_{1B/1D}$ receptors on intracranial blood vessels and in sensory nerves of trigeminal system. This results in cranial vessel constriction and inhibition of pro-inflammatory neuropeptide release. Well absorbed after PO use. **Peak plasma levels:** 2 hr. **t½, elimination:** 3 hr (for zolmitriptan and active metabolite). Excreted in feces and urine.

Uses: Treatment of acute migraine in adults with or without aura. Use only when there is clear diagnosis of migraine.

Contraindications: Prophylaxis of migraine or management of hemiplegic or basilar migraine. Use in angina pectoris, history of MI, documented or silent ischemia, ischemic heart disease, coronary artery vasospasm (including Prinzmetal's variant angina), other significant underlying CV disease. Also use in uncontrolled hypertension, within 24 hr of treatment with another serotonin HT_1 agonist or an ergotamine-containing or ergot-type drug (e.g., dihydroergotamine, methysergide). Concurrent use with MAO inhibitor or within 2 weeks of discontinuing MAO A inhibitor.

Special Concerns: Use with caution in liver disease and during lactation. A significant increase in BP may occur in those with moderate-to-severe hepatic impairment. Safety and efficacy have not been determined for cluster headache.

Side Effects: *GI:* Dry mouth, dyspepsia, dysphagia, nausea, increased appetite, tongue edema, esophagitis, gastroenteritis, abnormal liver function, thirst. *CV:* Palpitations, arrhythmias, hypertension, syncope. *Atypical sensations:* Hypesthesia, paresthesia, warm/cold sensation. *CNS:* Dizziness, somnolence, vertigo, agitation, anxiety, depression, emotional lability, insomnia. *Pain pressure sensations:* Chest pain, tightness, pressure and/or heaviness. Pain, tightness, or heaviness in the neck, throat, or jaw. Heaviness, pressure, tightness other than in the chest or neck. *Musculoskeletal:* Myalgia, myasthenia, back pain, leg cramps, tenosynovitis. *Respiratory:* Bronchitis, ***bronchospasm,*** epistaxis, hiccup, laryngitis, yawn. *Dermatologic:* Sweating, pruritus, rash, urticaria, ecchymosis, photosensitivity. *GU:* Hematuria, cystitis, polyuria, urinary frequency or urgency. *Body as a whole:* Asthenia, allergic reaction, chills, facial edema, edema, fever, malaise. *Miscellaneous:* Dry eye, eye pain, hyperacusis, ear pain, parosmia, tinnitus.

Drug Interactions

Cimetidine / Half life of zolmitriptan is doubled
Ergot-containing drugs / Prolonged vasospastic reactions
MAO Inhibitors / ↑ Levels of zolmitriptan
Oral contraceptives / ↑ Plasma levels of zolmitriptan
Selective serotonin reuptake inhibitors / Rarely, weakness, hyperreflexia, and incoordination

How Supplied: *Tablets:* 2.5 mg, 5 mg

Dosage

• **Tablets**

Migraine headaches.

Adults, initial: 2.5 mg or lower. Dose of 5 mg may be required. If headache returns, repeat dose after 2 hr, not to exceed 10 mg in 24-hr period.

Z

HEALTH CARE CONSIDERATIONS

Administration/Storage

1. Doses less than 2.5 mg may be obtained by manually breaking 2.5 mg tablet in half.
2. Safety of treating more than 3 headaches in 30 day period has not been established.
3. Use doses less than 2.5 mg in those with liver disease.

Assessment

1. Record frequency, duration, and characteristics of migraines. Note neurologist headache evaluation/diagnosis.
2. Note any evidence of history or cardiovascular disease as this precludes therapy.
3. List drugs prescribed to ensure none interact.
4. Determine if pregnant.
5. Monitor VS, ECG, liver, and renal function studies; reduce dose with dysfunction and monitor BP.

Client/Family Teaching

1. Take exactly as directed. Do not exceed dosage or dosing intervals of 2 hr apart and total of 10 mg/24 hr. Drug is strictly for migraine headaches.
2. Report if chest pain, SOB, chest tightness, or wheezing persists.
3. Do not perform activities that require mental alertness until drug effects realized.
4. Practice reliable contraception; report if pregnancy suspected.
5. Report any loss of effect, unusual, or adverse side effects.
6. Attempt to identify triggers.

Outcome/Evaluate: Relief of migraine headache

Zolpidem tartrate

(ZOL-pih-dem)

Pregnancy Category: B

Ambien **(Rx) (C-IV)**

Classification: Nonbarbiturate, nonbenzodiazepine sedative-hypnotic

Action/Kinetics: May act by subunit modulation of the GABA receptor chloride channel macromolecular complex resulting in sedative, anticonvulsant, anxiolytic, and myorelaxant properties. Although unrelated chemically to the benzodiazepines or barbiturates, it interacts with a GABA-benzodiazepine receptor complex and shares some of the pharmacologic effects of the benzodiazepines. Specifically, it binds the omega-1 receptor preferentially. No evidence of residual next-day effects or rebound insomnia at usual doses; little evidence for memory impairment. Sleep time spent in stage 3 to 4 (deep sleep) was comparable to placebo with only inconsistent, minor changes in REM sleep at recommended doses. Rapidly absorbed from the GI tract. **t½:** About 2.5 hr (increased in geriatric clients and those with impaired hepatic function). Bound significantly (92.5%) to plasma proteins. Food decreases the bioavailability of zolpidem. Metabolized in the liver; inactive metabolites are excreted primarily through the urine.

Uses: Short-term treatment of insomnia.

Contraindications: Lactation.

Special Concerns: Use with caution and at reduced dosage in clients with impaired hepatic function, in compromised respiratory function, in those with impaired renal function, and in clients with S&S of depression. Impaired motor or cognitive performance after repeated use or unusual sensitivity to hypnotic drugs may be noted in geriatric or debilitated clients. Closely observe individuals with a history of dependence on or abuse of drugs or alcohol. Safety and efficacy have not been determined in children less than 18 years of age.

Side Effects: *Symptoms of withdrawal:* Although there is no clear evidence of a withdrawal syndrome, the following symptoms were noted with zolpidem following placebo substitution: fatigue, nausea, flushing, lightheadedness, uncontrolled crying, emesis, stomach cramps, panic attack, nervousness, abdominal discomfort.

The most common side effects following use for up to 10 nights included drowsiness, dizziness, and diarrhea. The side effects listed in the following are for an incidence of 1% or greater. *CNS:* Headache, drowsiness, dizziness, lethargy, drugged feeling, lightheadedness, depression, abnormal dreams, amnesia, anxiety, nervousness, sleep disorder, ataxia, confusion, euphoria, insomnia, vertigo. *GI:* Nausea, diarrhea, dyspepsia, abdominal pain, constipation, anorexia, vomiting. *Musculoskeletal:* Myalgia, arthralgia. *Respiratory:* URI, sinusitis, pharyngitis, rhinitis. *Body as a whole:* Allergy, back pain, flu-like symptoms, chest pain, fatigue. *Ophthalmologic:* Diplopia, abnormal vision. *Miscellaneous:* Rash, UTI, palpitations, dry mouth, infection.

Laboratory Test Considerations: ↑ ALT, AST, BUN. Hyperglycemia, hypercholesterolemia, hyperlipidemia, abnormal hepatic function.

OD Management of Overdose: *Symptoms:* Symptoms ranging from somnolence to light coma. Rarely, CV and respiratory compromise. *Treatment:* Gastric lavage if appropriate. General symptomatic and supportive measures. IV fluids as needed. Flumaz-

Z

enil may be effective in reversing CNS depression. Monitor hypotension and CNS depression and treat appropriately. Sedative drugs should not be used, even if excitation occurs. Zolpidem is not dialyzable.
Drug Interactions: Additive CNS depressant effects are possible when combined with alcohol and other drugs with CNS depressant effects.
How Supplied: *Tablet:* 5 mg, 10 mg

Dosage

- **Tablets**
  Hypnotic.

Adults, individualized, usual: 10 mg just before bedtime. In hepatic insufficiency, use an initial dose of 5 mg.

HEALTH CARE CONSIDERATIONS

Administration/Storage

1. Limit therapy to 7–10 days. Reevaluate if the drug is required for more than 2–3 weeks.
2. Do not prescribe in quantities exceeding a 1-month supply.
3. Do not exceed 10 mg daily.

Assessment

1. Record indications for therapy, onset, duration, and characteristics of symptoms.
2. Record any respiratory dysfunction (sleep apnea).
3. Record any drug or alcohol dependence; assess for symptoms of depression.
4. Monitor LFTs.
5. Review sleep patterns and life-style. Identify underlying cause(s) of insomnia (i.e., napping during the daytime, lack of exercise, ↑ stress, depression).

Client/Family Teaching

1. Take only as directed, on an empty stomach at bedtime.
2. Do not perform any activities that require mental or physical alertness after ingesting medication. Evaluate response the following day to ensure that no residual depressant effects are evident.
3. Avoid alcohol and any unprescribed or OTC drugs.
4. Drug is only for short-term use; keep a log and identify factors that may be contributing to insomnia.
5. Review alternative methods for inducing sleep such as relaxation techniques, daily exercise, soft music, no daytime napping, guided imagery, white noise or special effects simulator.
6. Those with depression are at a higher risk for suicide or intentional overdose. Advise family that these clients warrant closer observation and limited prescriptions and to report any evidence of suicidal thoughts or aggressive behavior.
7. Keep out of reach of children and store in a safe place; drug has a high potential for abuse.

Outcome/Evaluate: Relief of insomnia

Zonisamide

(zoh-**NISS**-ah-myd)
Pregnancy Category: C
Zonegran **(Rx)**
Classification: Anticonvulsant, sulfonamide

See also *Anticonvulsants* and *Sulfonamides*
Action/Kinetics: Exact mechanism unknown. May stabilize neuronal membranes and suppress neuronal hypersynchronization through action at sodium and calcium channels. Does not affect GABA activity. **Metabolism:** hepatic. **t½:**63 hr. **Peak:** 2-6 hr.
Uses: Adjunct treatment of partial seizures in adults with epilepsy.
Contraindications: Hypersensitivity to sulfonamides or zonisamide.
Special Concerns: Rare, but potentially fatal sulfonamide reactions have occurred following the use of zonisamide. Reactions include Stevens-Johnson syndrome and toxic epidermal necrolysis, usually appearing within 2-16 weeks of starting the drug. Discontinue zonisamide if rash develops. Decreased sweating and hyperthemia requiring hospitalization have been reported in children. Safety and efficacy in children <16 years of age have not been established. Discontinue zonisamide in clients who develop acute renal failure or a significant sustained increase in creatinine/BUN concentration. Kidney stones have been reported. Use cautiously in clients with renal or hepatic dysfunction. Do not use if estimated C_{CR} <50 mL/minute. Significant CNS effects include psychiatric symptoms, psychomotor slowing, fatigue or somnolence. Abrupt withdrawal may precipitate seizures; discontinue or reduce doses gradually.
Side Effects: Adjunctive therapy, >10%: *CNS:* Somnolence, dizziness, headache. *GI:* Anorexia. **Adjunctive therapy, <10%:** *CNS:* Agitation/irritability, fatigue, tiredness, ataxia, confusion, decreased concentration, memory impairment, depression, insomnia, speech disorders, mental slowing, anxiety, nervousness, schizophrenic/schizophreniform behavior. *Dermatologic:* Rash, bruising. *GI:*

Z

Nausea, abdominal pain, diarrhea, dyspepsia, weight loss, constipation, dry mouth, taste perversion. *Neuromuscular/skeletal:* Paresthesia. *Ophthalmic:* Diplopia, nystagmus. *Respiratory:* Rhinitis. *Miscellaneous:* Flu-like syndrome.

Laboratory Test Considerations: Obtain LFTs and renal function studies prior to starting the drug.

OD **Management of Overdose:** *Treatment:* No specific antidotes available. Emesis or gastric lavage, with airway protection, should be done following a recent overdose. Supportive care and close observation are indicated. Renal dialysis may not be effective due to low protein binding (40%).

Drug Interactions: CYP3A4 enzyme substrate. Zonisamide does not appear to affect steady state levels of carbamazepine, phenytoin or valproate. Zonisamide half-life is decreased by carbamazepine, phenytoin, phenobarbital, and valproate. Other medications that induce or inhibit CYP3A4 would also be expected to affect serum levels of zonisamide. Avoid ETOH; may increase CNS depression.

How Supplied: *Capsule:* 100 mg

Dosage

- **Capsule**

Adjunctive treatment of partial seizures

Children >16 yrs. and adults, initial: 100 mg/day. Dose may be increased to 200 mg/day after 2 weeks. **Then,** dosage increases to 300 mg and 400 mg/day can be made with a minimum of 2 weeks between adjustments, in order to reach steady state at each dosage level. Doses of up to 600 mg/day have been studied. There is no evidence of increased response with doses above 400 mg/day. Slower titration and frequent monitoring are indicated in clients with renal or hepatic disease. Do **not** use if C_{CR} <50 mL/minute.

HEALTH CARE CONSIDERATIONS

See also *Health Care Considerations* for *Anticonvulsants* and *Sulfonamides*.

Administration/Storage: Store at controlled room temperature, 25°C (77°F). Protect from moisture and light.

Assessment

1. Record indications for therapy, onset and characteristics of seizures.
2. Monitor seizure frequency; monitor hepatic and renal function.
3. Ask client about drug allergies, especially sulfonamides.

Client/Family Teaching

1. Swallow capsule whole; do not chew, break, or crush capsule. Drink 6-8 glasses of water each day while using this medication.
2. May cause drowsiness, especially at higher doses. Do not drive a car or operate other complex machinery until effects can be determined.
3. Avoid alcohol use and other CNS depressants while taking this medication.
4. Contact provider immediately if seizures worsen or if any of the following symptoms occur: skin rash; sudden back pain, abdominal pain, blood in urine; fever, sore throat, oral ulcers or easy bruising.
5. Do not stop taking this or other seizure medications without talking with your healthcare provider first.

Outcome/Evaluate: Control of seizures.

APPENDIX 1

Controlled Substances in the United States and Canada

Controlled Substances Act—United States

The U.S. Federal Controlled Substances Act of 1970 placed drugs controlled by the Act into five categories or schedules based on their potential to cause psychologic and/or physical dependence as well as on their potential for abuse. The schedules are defined as follows:

Schedule (C-I): Includes substances for which there is a high abuse potential and no current approved medical use (e.g., heroin, marijuana, LSD, other hallucinogens, certain opiates and opium derivatives).

Schedule (C-II): Includes drugs that have a high abuse potential and a high ability to produce physical and/or psychologic dependence and for which there is a current approved or acceptable medical use.

Schedule (C-III): Includes drugs for which there is less potential for abuse than drugs in Schedule II and for which there is a current approved medical use. Certain drugs in this category are preparations containing limited quantities of codeine. Also, anabolic steroids are classified in Schedule III.

Schedule (C-IV): Includes drugs for which there is a relatively low abuse potential and for which there is a current approved medical use.

Schedule (C-V): Drugs in this category consist mainly of preparations containing limited amounts of certain narcotic drugs for use as antitussives and antidiarrheals. Federal law provides that limited quantities of these drugs (e.g., codeine) may be bought without a prescription by an individual at least 18 years of age. The product must be purchased from a pharmacist who must keep appropriate records. However, state laws vary, and in many states such products require a prescription.

Controlled Substances—Canada

In Canada, narcotics are governed by the Narcotics Control regulations and are designated by the letter N. Drugs that are considered subject to abuse, have an approved medical use, and are not narcotics are designated by the letter C.

Generally prescriptions for Schedule II (high-abuse-potential) drugs cannot be transmitted over the phone and they cannot be refilled. Prescriptions for Schedule III, IV, and V drugs may be refilled up to five times within 6 months. Schedule II drugs are not necessarily "stronger" than drugs in Schedules III, IV, or V; Schedule II drugs are classified as such due to their high abuse potential.

	Drug Schedule	
Drug	*United States*	*Canada*
Alfentanil	II	N
Alprazolam	IV	*
Amobarbital	II	C
Amphetamine	II	Not available
Aprobarbital	III	*
Benzphetamine	III	Not available
Buprenorphine	V	*
Butabarbital	III	C
Butorphanol	*	C
Chloral hydrate	IV	*
Chlordiazepoxide	IV	*
Clonazepam	IV	*
Clorazepate	IV	*
Codeine	II	N
Dextroamphetamine	II	C
Diazepam	IV	*
Diethylpropion	IV	C
Estazolam	IV	*
Ethchlorvynol	IV	*
Fenfluramine	IV	*
Fentanyl	II	N
Fluoxymesterone	III	*
Flurazepam	IV	*
Glutethimide	III	*
Halazepam	IV	Not available
Hydrocodone	Not available alone	N
Hydromorphone	II	N
Levomethadyl acetate HCl	II	Not available
Levorphanol	II	N
Lorazepam	IV	*
Mazindol	IV	*
Meperidine	II	N
Mephobarbital	IV	C
Meprobamate	IV	*
Methadone	II	N
Methamphetamine	II	Not available
Metharbital	III	C
Methylphenidate	II	C
Methyltestosteone	III	*
Methyprylon	III	*
Midazolam	IV	*
Morphine	II	N
Nalbuphine	*	C

* Not controlled

Nandrolone decanote	III	*
Nandrolone phenpropionate	III	*
Opium	II	N
Oxandrolone	III	*
Oxazepam	IV	*
Oxycodone	II	N
Oxymetholone	III	*
Oxymorphone	II	N
Paraldehyde	IV	*
Paregoric	III	N
Pemoline	IV	*
Pentazocine	IV	N
Pentobarbital		
PO, parenteral	II	C
Rectal	III	C
Phendimetrazine	III	Not available
Phenmetrazine	II	Not available
Phenobarbital	IV	C
Phentermine	IV	C
Prazepam	IV	Not available
Propoxyphene	IV	N
Remifentanil hydrochloride	II	-
Quazepam	IV	Not available
Secobarbital		
PO	II	C
Parenteral	II	*
Rectal	III	*
Stanozolol	III	*
Sufentanil	II	N
Talbutal	III	*
Temazepam	IV	*
Testosterone cypionate in oil	III	*
Testosterone enanthante in oil	III	*
Testosterone in aqueous suspension	III	*
Testosterone propionate in oil	III	*
Testosterone transdermal system	III	*
Triazolam	IV	*
Zaleplon	IV	-
Zolpidem tartrate	IV	*

*Not controlled

APPENDIX 2

Pregnancy Categories: FDA Assigned

The U.S. Food and Drug Administration's use-in-pregnancy rating system weighs the degree to which available information has ruled out risk to the fetus against the drug's potential benefit to the patient. The ratings, and their interpretation, are as follows:

Category	Interpretation
A	**CONTROLLED STUDIES SHOW NO RISK.** Adequate, well-controlled studies in pregnant women have failed to demonstrate a risk to the fetus in any trimester of pregnancy.
B	**NO EVIDENCE OF RISK IN HUMANS.** Adequate, well-controlled studies in pregnant women have not shown increased risk of fetal abnormalities despite adverse findings in animals, or, in the absence of adequate human studies, animal studies show no fetal risk. The chance of fetal harm is remote, but remains a possibility.
C	**RISK CANNOT BE RULED OUT.** Adequate, well-controlled human studies are lacking, and animal studies have shown a risk to the fetus or are lacking as well. There is a chance of fetal harm if the drug is administered during pregnancy; but the potential benefits may outweigh the potential risk.
D	**POSITIVE EVIDENCE OF RISK.** Studies in humans, or investigational or post-marketing data, have demonstrated fetal risk. Nevertheless, potential benefits from the use of the drug may outweigh the potential risk. For example, the drug may be acceptable if needed in a life-threatening situation or serious disease for which safer drugs cannot be used or are ineffective.
X	**CONTRAINDICATED IN PREGNANCY.** Studies in animals or humans, or investigational or post-marketing reports, have demonstrated positive evidence of fetal abnormalities or risk which clearly outweighs any possible benefit to the patient.

APPENDIX 3

Elements of a Prescription

In order to safely communicate the exact elements desired on a prescription, the following items should be addressed:

A. The prescriber: Name, address, phone number, and associated practice/speciality

B. The client: Name, age, address and social security number

C. The prescription itself: Name of the medication (generic or trade); quantity to be dispensed (e.g., tablets or capsules, 1 vial, 1 tube, volume of liquid); the strength of the medication (e.g., 125-mg tablets, 250 mg/5 mL, 80 mg/1 mL, 10%); and directions for use (e.g., 1 tablet po t.i.d.; 2 gtt to each eye q.i.d.; 1 teaspoonful po q 8 hr for 10 days; apply a thin film to lesions b.i.d. for 14 days)

D. Other elements: Date prescription is written, signature of the provider, number of refills; provider number: state license number and Drug Enforcement Agency (DEA) number (when applicable); and brand-product-only indication (when applicable)

A typical prescription is depicted as follows:

A. **Julia Bryan, MSN, RN, CPNP**
Pediatric Associates
1611 Kirkwood Highway
Wilmington, DE 19805
302-645-8261

Date: July 10, 2001

B. For: Kathryn Woods, Age 8
27 East Parkway
Lewes, DE 19958
123-555-1234

C. Rx Amoxicillin susp. 250 mg/5 mL
Disp. 150 mL
Sig: 1 teaspoon PO q 8 hr x 10 days

D. Refills: 0

Provider signature
Provider/State license number

Interpretation of prescription: The above prescription is written by Pediatric Nurse Practitioner Julia Bryan for Kathryn Woods and is for amoxicillin suspension. The concentration desired is 250 mg/5 mL. The directions for taking the medication are 1 teaspoon (i.e., 5 mL) by mouth every 8 hr for 10 days. The prescriber wants 150 mL dispensed and there are no refills allowed.

APPENDIX 4

Easy Formulas for IV Rate Calculation

In order to calculate the continuous drip rate for an IV infusion, the following information is necessary:

a. amount of solution to be infused
b. time for infusion to be administered
c. *drop factor (found in the tubing package)

$$\frac{\text{Total volume to be infused}}{\text{Total hours for infusion}} \times \frac{\text{*drop factor}}{\text{60 min/hr}} = \text{gtt/min}$$

*If drop factor is:
60 gtt/min, then use 1 in the formula
10 gtt/min, then use ⅙ in the formula
15 gtt/min, then use ¼ in the formula
20 gtt/min, then use ⅓ in the formula

This gives you $\frac{\text{gtt}}{\text{min}}$.

Example: Infuse 1,000 cc over 8 hr using tubing with a drop factor of 10 gtt/min.

$$\frac{\text{1,000 cc}}{\text{8 hr}} \times \frac{1}{6} = 20.8 \text{ or } 21 \ \frac{\text{gtt}}{\text{min}}$$

Complete equation is:

$$\frac{\text{1,000 cc}}{\text{8 hr}} \times \frac{\text{10 gtt/min}}{\text{60 min/1 hr}} = \frac{\text{1,000 cc}}{\text{8 hr}} \times \frac{\text{10 gtt}}{\text{cc}} \times \frac{\text{1hr}}{\text{60 min}} = 21 \ \frac{\text{gtt}}{\text{min}}$$

To get $\frac{\text{cc}}{\text{hr}}$ invert drop factor and multiply by $\frac{\text{gtt}}{\text{min}}$, or:

$$\frac{6}{1} \times 21 \ \frac{\text{gtt}}{\text{min}} = 126 \ \frac{\text{cc}}{\text{hr}}$$

When administering intermittent infusions, as with antibiotic therapy, use the following formula:

$$\text{Total volume to be infused} \div \frac{\text{minutes to administer}}{\text{60 min/hr}} = \frac{\text{mL}}{\text{hr}}$$

Example: Administer 3 g Zosyn in 100 cc of D5W over 45 min

$$100 \div \frac{45}{60} \text{ (invert to multiply)}$$

or

$$100 \times \frac{60}{45} = 133.3 \text{ or } 134 \ \frac{\text{mL}}{\text{hr}}$$

APPENDIX 5
Adult IVPB Medication Administration Guidelines and Riders

Adult IVPB Medication Guidelines

Medication	*Solutions(s)*	*Amount*	*Infuse Over*
Amikin (Amikacin)	D5W; NSS	250–500 mg/ 100 mL	30–60 min
Amphotericin B (Fungizone)	D5W	50 mg/500 mL	6 hr
Ampicillin (Polycillin-N)	NSS	1 g/50 mL	15–30 min
Ancef (Cefazolin Na)	D5W; NSS	1 g/50 mL	40 min
Azactam (Aztreonam)	D5W; NSS	1 g/50 mL	20–30 min
Bactrim (Septra/ Co-Trimoxazole)	D5W	Premixed, usually 5 mL/125 mL	60–90 min
Cefotan (Cefotetan disodium)	D5W; NSS	1–2 g/75 mL	30 min
Cipro (Ciprofloxacin)	D5W; NSS	400 mg/200 mL	60 min
Claforan (Cefotaxime)	D5W; NSS	1 g/50 mL	30 min
Cleocin (Clindamycin)	D5W; NSS	300–900 mg/ 100 mL	20–40 min
Decadron (Dexamethasone)	D5W; NSS	40 mg/50 mL	15–30 min
Doxycycline (Vibramycin)	D5W; NSS	100 mg/100 mL	1–2 hr
Erythromycin (Erythrocin)	NSS, RL	500 mg/100 mL	30–60 min
Famotidine (Pepcid)	D5W; NSS	20 mg/50–100 mL	15–30 min
Flagyl (Metronidazole)	Prepackaged	—	60 min
Foscavir (Foscarnet)	D5W	60–90 mg/kg q 8 hr	2 hr
Fortaz (Ceftazidime)	D5W; NSS	1–2 g/100 mL	30 min
Gentamycin (Garamycin)	D5W; NSS	80 mg/50 mL	30–60 min
Nafcillin (Nafcin)	D5W; NSS	1 g/50–100 mL	30–60 min
Penicillin G	D5W; NSS	5,000,000 U/ 100 mL	40 min
Primaxin (Imipenem-Cilastatin Na)	D5W; NSS	500 mg/100 mL	20–30 min
Rocephin (Ceftri-axone Na)	D5W; NSS	1–2 g/100 mL	30 min
Solumedrol (Methyl-prednisolone)	D5W; NSS	10–250 mg/50 mL	20 min

Tagamet (Cimetidine)	D5W; NSS	300 mg/50 mL	15–20 min
Tetracycline (Achromycin IV)	D5W; NSS	250–500 mg/100 mL	60 min
Tobramycin (Nebcin)	D5W; NSS	80 mg/100 mL	30 min
Vancomycin (Vancocin)	D5W; NSS	1 g/200 mL	60 min
Zantac (Ranitidine HCl)	D5W; NSS	50 mg/100 mL	15–20 min

Riders

When ordered for nonemergent IV infusion, the following guidelines may be used for administration:

- Calcium gluconate: 1 ampule Ca gluconate in 100 mL D5W given over 1 hr (each ampule contains approximately 940 mg Ca)

- Magnesium sulfate: 1 g in 100 mL D5W given over 1 hr

- Potassium chloride: 40 mEq in 150 mL D5W given over 4 hr or 60 mEq in 250 mL D5W given over 6 hr. With KCl, a good rule of thumb is not to infuse more than 10 mEq/hr.

- Potassium phosphate: 15 mM phosphate (contains 22 mEq K) in 100 mL D5W given over 2–3 hr

APPENDIX 6
Therapeutic Classification of Wounds and Dressings

A proliferation of products to enhance wound care management is available. Wounds heal best in a moist environment; thus moisture-retentive or occlusive dressings should be utilized. With a moist wound environment, granulation tissue formation and collagen synthesis are improved, cell migration and epithelial resurfacing occur faster, and crusts, scabs, and eschars do not form. Dressing categories will be listed with some sample product names, indications for therapy, action/kinetics, contraindications, adverse reactions, and evaluation/outcome criteria.

A careful wound assessment should be performed to determine the ulcer stage and any other factors contributing to the skin breakdown, such as infection or necrotic tissues. Wounds are staged by determining which tissue layers are involved:

WOUND STAGING

Stage I: Erythema of intact skin; nonblanchable

Stage II: Partial-thickness skin loss involving epidermis and/or dermis; appears as a shallow crater, blister, or abrasion. Includes partial or complete skin tear.

Stage III: Full-thickness skin loss of subcutaneous tissue involving damage or necrosis that may extend down to the fascia; appears as a deep crater.

Stage IV: Full-thickness skin loss with extensive necrosis, destruction, or damage to muscle, bone, or supporting structures; may also see sinus tracts or undermining with this stage.

Once the wound has been staged, an appropriate dressing choice may be made.

DRESSING CHOICE
by Wound Stage

Stage I: Wounds; management options:

Nonadherent dressing or
Barrier product
Moisture product or

Extra thin hydrocolloid or
Transparent dressing

Stage II: Wounds with

A: Scant or minimal drainage; management options:
Non-adherent gauze or
Transparent dressing or
Hydrogel or
Extra thin or Foam dressing

B: Moderate drainage; protect surrounding tissue and consider:
Hydrocolloid or
Continually moist saline soaked dressings or
Foam dressing

C: Extensive drainage, consider:
Absorption dressing or
Alginate (especially if drainage is sanguinous) or
Fibergel

Stage III: Wounds; protect surrounding tissue; check for undermining wound margins, as debridement of edges may be necessary

A. Scant or minimal drainage, consider:
Hydrogel or
Hydrocolloid paste with wafer or
Continually moist saline soaked dressing or
Foam dressing

B. Moderate drainage, consider:
Hydrocolloid paste with wafer or
Continually moist saline soaked packing or
Hypertonic saline gauze or
Fibergel or foam dressing
Alginate if drainage sanguinous

C. Excessive drainage, consider:
Absorption packing (hydrophillic) or
Continually moist saline soaked packing with hydrophillic sponge or
Fibergel or
Alginate (especially if sanguinous drainage)

Stage IV: Wounds, evaluate for surgical debridement and repair; with

A. Scant or minimal drainage, consider:
Hydrogel-soaked packing

B. Moderate drainage, consider:
Hypertonic saline gauze or
Fibergel or
Continually moist saline-soaked dressings

C. Excessive drainage, consider adding a:
Hydrophillic topper or packing or
Alginate dressing or
Fibergel

Dressing Category of
WOUND CARE PRODUCTS

I. Nonadherent Dressings—use on stage I and stage IIA with minimal drainage;

Nonimpregnated: Telfa, Release, Metalline, EXU-DRY, ETE-sterile Protective dressing

Impregnated: Adaptic, Scarlet Red, Vaseline Gauze, Xeroflo, Xeroform

USE/ACTION: useful for skin tears, skin grafts, and donor sites; occlusive, nontraumatic, nonadhesive. May require secondary dressing, such as gauze, to wrap area. Use an ATX ointment to keep wound bed moist and to prevent dressing adherence.

II. Transparent Films—use on stage I and stage IIA with minimal drainage

OpSite, Tegaderm, Transite, Bioclusive, Blister Film, Ensure-It, Omiderm, OpraFlex, Bioclusive, UniFlex, Varilmoist, Polyderm

USE/ACTION: adhesive elastomeric copolymer dressing; use with superficial wounds such as superficial burns, abrasions, wounds, donor sites; water resistant, permits easy wound visualization, nonbulky, comfortable, semipermeable, moisture retentive. Useful for autolytic debridement and does not require secondary dressing; minimally absorbent.

III. Hydrocolloids—use extra thin or transparent hydrocolloid on stage I and IIA; all others on Stage II and III wounds

DuoDERM, Restore, Hydrapad, Intact, IntraSite, 3M Tegasorb, ULTEC

USE/ACTION: adhesive wafers containing colloids and elastomers; may see wafer, powder or paste forms; water resistant, nonbulky, comfortable, occlusive or semipermeable, moisture retentive, excellent bacterial barrier, high tack (adhesive), useful for autolytic debridement and does not require secondary dressing.

IV. Gels/Hydrogels—use on stage IIA, IIIA, IVA wounds

Biolex, Carrington Dermal Wound Gel, Clear Site, Elasto-Gel, Gelicerm Wet/Granulate, Hydron Wound Dressing, IntraSite Gel, Nu-Gel, Second Skin, Spand-Gel, Vigilon.

USE/ACTION: single-polymer formulations; adhesive or nonadhesive; sheet or gel form; moisture retentive, lowers wound temperature resulting in decreased inflammation and pain, with cooling, soothing effects; autolysis of necrotic tissue; can be useful when infection is present; permits easy wound visualization, may use a transparent film or gauze dressing over gel forms to contain.

V. Exudate Absorbers—use on stage IIB, IIC, and IIIC wounds

Allevyn Cavity Wound Dressing, Bard Absorption dressing, Debrisan, Envisan Hydragran, Kaltostat, Mesalt hypertonic saline gauze, Sorosan, Algosteril, Aquacel

USE/ACTION: only for highly exudating wounds; can absorb several times their weight in exudate; materials such as starch, paste, beads, hypertonic saline gauze; moisture retentive, requires secondary dressing to contain. Nonadhesive, useful for autolytic debridement.

VI. Foams—nonadhesive, nonadhering polymeric dressings

Mitraflex, EPIGARD, Epi-Lock, LYOfoam, Allevyn

USE/ACTION: moisture retentive, comfortable, moderately absorptive, insulates the wound, nonadherent, compressible; very useful on leg ulcers.

VII: Cotton Mesh Gauzes—use cotton mesh gauze with large interstices, such as, Kerlix for debridement; use nonwoven gauze, such as Sof-Kling for secondary dressings, wrapping, or absorption

For heavy exudating wounds use absorbent toppers: Topper, ABD, Surgipad Combine dressing; or Hypertonic saline gauze (Mesalt) or wound pouches.

Use Montgomery straps to secure dressings or protect wound margins with a skin sealant.

USE/ACTION: wet to dry for debridement, packing of tunneling or undermining wounds, moderately absorptive, may be combined with NSS for granulation or antibiotic solutions for infections; dressings tend to be bulky and uncomfortable.

Moisture-Retentive Dressings

Side Effects:

Increased number of bacteria
Silent infections
Accumulation of exudates
Maceration of wound margins
Hypergranulation

Contraindications/Precautions:

Active cellulitis/vasculitis
Wound infection
Some are not appropriate for stage IV full-thickness wounds

Outcome/Evaluation:

Prevent further skin breakdown
Decreased infection
Promote healing of wound
Decreased pain
Enhancement of wound-healing process
Decreased size and depth of wound
Increased extremity mobility

Finally, dressing choice should change as the wound changes during the healing process. A good rule of thumb is to use wet-dry for debridement, and moisture-retentive for granulation, and always have someone experienced/trained in wound assessment and management evaluate your client.

APPENDIX 7

Commonly Accepted Therapeutic Drug Levels

Drug	Peak	Trough
	Aminoglycosides	
Amikacin	20–30 mcg/mL	1–5 mcg/mL
Gentamicin	5–10 mcg/mL	1–2 mcg/mL
Netilmicin	4–10 mcg/mL	1–2 mcg/mL
Streptomycin	25 mcg/mL	–
Tobramycin	4–10 mcg/mL	1–2 mcg/mL
Vancomycin	20–50 mcg/mL	1–5 mcg/mL

Drug	Therapeutic Range
Amiodarone	0.5–2.5 mcg/mL
Amitriptyline	50–200 ng/mL
Bepridil HCl	1–2 ng/mL
Carbamazepine	4–10 mcg/mL
Desipramine	50–200 ng/mL
Digoxin	0.5–2.2 ng/mL
Disopyramide	2–8 mcg/mL
Doxepin	50–200 ng/mL
Flecainide acetate	0.2–1.0 mcg/mL
Haloperidol	3–10 ng/mL
Heparin	1.5–3 times normal clotting time
Lidocaine	1.5–5 mcg/mL
Lithium	0.4–1.0 mEq/mL (maintenance)
Mezlocillin sodium	35–45 mcg/mL
Mexiletine HCl	0.5 mcg/mL
Milrinone	150–250 ng/mL
Nicardipine	0.028–0.05 mcg/mL
Nifedipine	0.025–0.1 mcg/mL
Phenobarbital	15–40 mcg/mL (as anticonvulsant)
Phenytoin	10–20 mcg/mL
Primidone	5–12 mcg/mL
Procainamide	4–8 mcg/mL

Drug	Therapeutic Range
Propafenone	0.5–3 mcg/mL
Propranolol	50–200 ng/mL
Quinidine	2–6 mcg/mL
Salicylic acid	150–300 mcg/mL (as anti-inflammatory)
Theophylline	10–20 mcg/mL (desired 7-12 mcg/mL)
Tocainide HCl	4–10 mcg/mL
Valproic acid	50–100 mcg/mL
Verapamil	0.08–0.3 mcg/mL

APPENDIX 8

Tables of Weights and Measures

Weights	Exact Equivalents	Approximate Equivalents
1 ounce (oz)	28.35 g	30 g
1 pound (lb)	453.6 g	454 g
1 gram (g)	0.0353 oz	0.035 oz
1 kilogram (kg)	2.205 lb	2.2 lb
Fluid Measures		
1 teaspoon (t)		5 mL
1 tablespoon (T)	3 tsp	15 mL (½ fl oz)
1 fluid ounce (fl oz)	29.57 mL	30 mL
1 pint (16 fl oz)	473.0 mL	473 mL
1 quart (32 fl oz)	946 mL	945 mL
1 gallon (128 fl oz)	3.785 L	3.8 L
1 milliliter (mL)	0.0352 fl oz (Imperial)	0.0345 fl oz
1 liter (L)	2.11 pt	2 pt
Lengths		
1 inch (in)	2.54 cm	2.5 cm
1 foot (ft)	30.48 cm	30.0 cm
1 yard (yd)	0.914 m	0.9 m
1 centimeter (cm)	0.3937 in	
1 meter (m)	39.4 in	

Approximate Conversions to Metric Measures

To Convert	To	Multiply By
Inches	Centimeters	2.54
Feet	Centimeters	30.48
Grains	Grams	0.065
Ounces	Grams	28.35
Pounds	Kilograms	0.45
Teaspoons, Medical	Milliliters	5.0
Tablespoons	Milliliters	15.0
Fluid ounces	Milliliters	29.57
Cups	Liters	0.24
Pints	Liters	0.47
Quarts	Liters	0.95
Gallons	Liters	3.8

Approximate Conversions to Metric Measures

To Convert	To	Multiply By
Millimeters	Inches	0.039
Centimeters	Inches	0.39
Grams	Grains	15.432
Kilograms	Pounds	2.2
Milliliters	Fluid ounces	0.034
Liters	Pints	2.1
Liters	Quarts	1.06
Liters	Gallons	0.26
Deg. Fahrenheit	Deg. Celsius	5/9 (after subtracting 32)
Deg. Celsius	Deg. Fahrenheit	9/5 (then add 32)

APPENDIX 9

Commonly Used Combination Drugs

NOTE: Please consult individual drugs for more extensive information.

NOTE: Table entries are alphabetized by generic name.

Accuretic (quinapril hydrochloride and hydrochlorothiazide)
Advair Diskus (fluticasone and salmeterol)
Aggrenox (aspirin and dipyridamole)
Aldactazide (spironolactone and hydrochlorothiazide)
Aldoril (methyldopa and hydrochlorothiazide)
Arthrotec (diclofenac sodium and misoprostol)
Atacand HCT (candesartan cilexetil and hydrochlorothiazide)
Axocet (butalbital and acetaminophen)
Brontex (codeine phosphate and guaifenesin)
Claritin-D (loratidine and pseudoephedrine)
Combivent (ipratropium bromide and albuterol sulfate)
Cosopt (dorzolamide hydrochloride and timolol maleate)
Darvocet-N50, Darvocet N-100 (acetaminophen and propoxyphene napsylate)
Darvon Compound 65 (aspirin, caffeine and propoxyphene hydrochloride)
Donnatal (atropine sulfate, hyoscyamine sulfate, scopolamine hydrobromide, and phenobarbital)
Dyazide, Maxzide, Maxide-25 MG, Apo-Triazide, Novo-Triamzide, Nu-Triazide, Protriazide (triamterene and hydrochlorothiazide)
Equagesic (aspirin and meprobamate)
Fiorinal (aspirin, butalbital and caffeine)
Fiorinal with codeine (aspirin, butalbital, caffeine, and codeine phosphate)
Glucovance (glyburide and metformin hydrochloride)
Hycodan (hydrocodone bitartrate and homatropine methylbromide)
Hyzaar (losartan potassium and hydrochlorothiazide)
Inderide, Inderide LA (propranolol hydrochloride and hydrochlorothiazide)
Kaletra (lopinavir and ritonavir)
Librax (chlordiazepoxide and clidinium bromide)
Lotrel (amlodipine and benazepril hydrochloride)
Malarone (atovaquone and proguanil hydrochloride)
Moduretic (amiloride and hydrochlorothiazide)
Pediazole (erythromycin ethylsuccinate and sulfisoxazole)
Prinzide, Zestoretic (lisinopril and hydrochlorothiazide)
Rifamate, Rimactane/INH (rifampin and isoniazid)
Rifater (rifampin, isoniazid and pyrazinamide)
Talwin NX (pentazocine hydrochloride and naloxone hydrochloride)
Triavil (amitriptyline hydrochloride and perphenazine)
Tylenol with codeine (acetaminophen and codeine phosphate)
Vaseretic (enalapril maleate and hydrochlorothiazide)
Vicoprofen (hydrocodone bitartrate and ibuprofen)
Ziac (bisoprolol fumarate and hydrochlorothiazide)

Generic Name (Content)	Trade Name	Use	Dose
Acetaminophen (300 mg/tablet or 120 mg/5mL), Codeine phosphate (15 mg–No. 2, 30 mg–No. 3, 60 mg–No. 4 tablets and 12 mg/5mL elixir).	Tylenol with Codeine (Rx, C-III: Tablets, C-V: Elixir).	Mild to moderate pain.	**Tablets. Adults, individualized, usual:** 1–2 No. 2 or No. 3 Tablets q 2–4 hr as needed for pain. Or, 1-No. 4 Tablet q 4 hr as needed. Maximum 24-hr dose: 360 mg codeine phosphate and 4,000 mg acetaminophen. **Elixir. Adults, individualized, usual:** 15 mL q 4 hr as needed; **pediatric, 7–12 years:** 10 mL t.i.d.–q.i.d.; **3–6 years:** 5 mL t.i.d.–q.i.d. Use cautiously with liver dysfunction.
Acetaminophen (325 or 650 mg), Propoxyphene napsylate (50 or 100 mg)	Darvocet-N 50, Darvocet-N 100 (Rx, C-IV)	Mild to moderate pain (may be used if fever is present)	2-Darvocet-N 50 tablets or 1-Darvocet-100 tablet q 4 hr, not to exceed 600 mg propoxyphene napsylate/day. Reduce dose in impaired renal/hepatic function.
Amiloride (5 mg), Hydrochlorothiazide (50mg)	Moduretic (Rx)	Hypertension or CHF, especially when hypokalemia occurs. May be used with other antihypertensives.	**Initial:** 1 tablet/day; **then**, can increase to 2 tablets/day.

Generic Name (Content)	Trade Name	Use	Dose
Amitriptyline HCl (10, 25, or 50 mg),Perphenazine (2 or 4 mg)	Triavil 2-10, 2-25, 4-10, 4-25, 4-50 (Rx)	Depression with moderate to severe anxiety and/or agitation (including those with chronic physical disease). Schizophrenia with symptoms of depression.	**Initial:** 1 Triavil 2-25 or 4-25 tablet t.i.d.–q.i.d. or 1 Triavil tablet 4-50 b.i.d. (for schizophrenia, use 2 Triavil 4-50 t.i.d. with a fourth dose at bedtime if needed). **Maintenance:** 1 Triavil 2-25 or 4-25 b.i.d.–q.i.d. or 1 Triavil 4-50 b.i.d.
Amlodipine (2.5 or 5 mg), Benazepril HCl (10 or 20 mg)	Lotrel 2.5/10, 5/10, or 5/20 (Rx)	Hypertension if control not achieved with either drug alone.	One 2.5/10, 5/10, or 5/20 capsule daily. For the small, elderly, frail, or hepatically impaired, initial amlodipine dose is 2.5 mg.
Aspirin (325 mg), Butalbital (50 mg), Caffeine (40 mg)	Fiorinal (Rx, C-III)	Tension headaches.	1–2 tablets or capsules q 4 hr, not to exceed 6 tablets or capsules/day.

Generic Name (Content)	Trade Name	Use	Dose
Aspirin (325 mg), Butalbital (50 mg), Caffeine (40 mg), Codeine phosphate (7.5 mg, 15 mg, or 30 mg)	Fiorinal with Codeine (Rx, C-III)	Analgesic for all types of pain.	**Initial:** 1–2 capsules; **then,** dose may be repeated, if necessary, up to maximum of 6 capsules/day.
Aspirin (389 mg), Caffeine (32.4 mg), Propoxyphene HCl (65 mg)	Darvon Compound 65 (Rx, C-IV)	Mild to moderate pain, with or without fever.	1-Capsule q 4 hr, not to exceed 390 mg propoxyphene HCl/day. Decrease total daily dose in impaired renal/hepatic function.
Aspirin (25 mg), Dipyridamole (200 mg)	Aggrenox (Rx)	Reduce risk of stroke in clients who have had transient ischemia of the brain or completed ischemic stroke due to thrombosis.	One capsule b.i.d., in the morning and evening. Swallow capsules whole without chewing.
Aspirin (325 mg), Meprobamate (200 mg)	Equagesic (Rx, C-IV)	Short-term treatment of pain due to musculoskeletal disease accompanied by anxiety and tension.	**Adults:** 1–2 tablets t.i.d.–q.i.d.

Generic Name (Content)	Trade Name	Use	Dose
Atovaquone (250 mg/tablet or 62.5 mg/pediatric tablet), Proguanil hydrochloride (100 mg/tablet or 25 mg/pediatric tablet)	Malarone	Prophylaxis of *Plasmodium falciparum* malaria including areas where chloroquine resistence seen. Treatment of acute, uncomplicated *P. falciparum,* even in areas where resistance to other drugs seen.	*Prophylaxis.* **Adults:** 1 adult tablet/day. **Children, 11-20 kg:** 1 pediatric tablet/day; **21-30 kg:** 2 pediatric tablets/day as a single dose; **31-40 kg:** 3 pediatric tablets/day as a single dose; **>40 kg:** 1 adult strength tablet/day. *Treatment.* **Adults:** 4 adult strength tablets/day as a single dose/day for 3 consecutive days. **Children, 11-20 kg:** 1 adult strength tablet/day for 3 consecutive days; **21-30 kg:** 2 adult strength tablets/day for 3 consecutive days; **31-40 kg:** 3 adult strength tablets/day for 3 consecutive days; **>40 kg:** Use adult dose. Take daily dose at same time each day with food or a milky drink.
Atropine sulfate (0.0194 mg), Hyoscyamine sulfate (0.1037 mg), Scopolamine HBr (0.0065 mg), Phenobarbital (16.2 mg) in each tablet, capsule, or 5 mL elixir	Donnatal (Rx)	Adjunct to treat irritable colon, spastic colon, mucous colitis, acute enterocolitis.	**Adults, usual:** 1–2 tablets or capsules t.i.d.–q.i.d. or 1-Extentab q 12 hr, or 5–10 mL elixir t.i.d.–q.i.d. **Pediatric:** Use elixir as follows: **4.5–9.0 kg:** 0.5 mL q 4 hr or 0.75 mL q 6 hr. **9.1–13.5 kg:** 1.0 mL q 4 hr or 1.5 mL q 6 hr; **13.6–22.6 kg:** 1.5 mL q 4 hr or 2.0 mL q 6 hr; **22.7–33.9 kg:** 2.5 mL q 4 hr or 3.75 mL q 6 hr; **34.0–45.3 kg:** 3.75 mL q 4 hr or 5 mL q 6 hr; **45.4 kg:** 5 mL q 4 hr or 7.5 mL q 6 hr.

Generic Name (Content)	Trade Name	Use	Dose
Bisoprolol fumarate (2.5, 5, or 10 mg), Hydrochlorothiazide (6.25 mg)	Ziac (Rx)	Mild to moderate hypertension (first-line therapy).	1 2.5/6.25 mg tablet once daily; dose may be increased q 14 days to a maximum of 2 10/6.25 tablets once daily.
Butalbital (50 mg), Acetaminophen (650 mg)	Axocet (Rx)	Tension headaches.	1 Capsule q 4 hr, not to exceed 6 capsules/day.
Candesartan cilexetil (16 mg or 32 mg), Hydrochlorothiazide (12.5 mg)	Atacand HCT 16-12.5 or Atacand HCT 32-12.5 (Rx)	Hypertension (not for initial treatment)	**Initial:** 1 tablet of Atacand HCT 16-12.5. Depending on response, can increase to Atacand 32-12.5
Chlordiazepoxide (5 mg), Clidinium Br (2.5 mg)	Librax (Rx)	Adjunct in the treatment of irritable colon, spastic colon, mucous colitis, and acute enterocolitis.	**Adults, individualized, usual:** 1–2 capsules t.i.d.–q.i.d before meals and at bedtime.
Codeine phosphate (10 mg/tablet or 20 mL), Guaifenesin (300 mg/tablet or 20 mL)	Brontex (Rx, C-III)	Relief of cough due to cold or inhaled irritants. Loosen mucus and thin bronchial secretions.	**Adults and children over 12 years:** 1 Tablet or 20 mL q 4 hr. **Children, 6–12 years:** 10 mL q 4 hr.

Generic Name (Content)	Trade Name	Use	Dose
Diclofenac sodium (50 or 75 mg), Misoprostol (200 mcg)	Arthrotec 50, Arthrotec 75 (Rx)	Osteoarthritis or rheumatoid arthritis in those at high risk of developing NSAID-induced gastric and duodenal ulcers.	*Osteoarthritis:* 1-Arthrotec 50 tablet with food t.i.d. If intolerance occurs, give Arthrotec 50 or Arthrotec 75 b.i.d., although this dose is less effective in preventing ulcers. *Rheumatoid arthritis:* 1-Arthrotec 50 tablet with food t.i.d. or q.i.d. If intolerance occurs, give Arthrotec 50 or Arthrotec 75 b.i.d., atlhough this dose is less effective in preventing ulcers.
Dorzolamide HCl (2%), Timolol maleate (0.5%)	Cosopt (Rx)	Reduce elevated IOP in open-angle glaucoma or ocular hypertension in those inadequately controlled with beta blockers.	**Adults:** 1 gtt in the affected eye(s) b.i.d.
Enalapril maleate (5 mg or 10 mg), Hydrochlorothiazide (12.5 or 25 mg)	Vaseretic (Rx)	Hypertenstion	**Adults:** 1-2 tablets once daily.
Erythromycin ethylsuccinate (200 mg) and Sulfisoxazole (600 mg) in 5 mL of oral suspension.	Pediazole (Rx)	Acute otitis media in children due to *Haemophilus influenzae.*	**Usual:** Equivalent of 50 mg/kg/day of erythromycin and 150 mg/kg/day of sulfisoxazole, up to a maximum of 6 g/day. **Over 45 kg:** 10 mL q 6 hr; **24 kg:** 7.5 mL q 6 hr; **16 kg:** 5 mL q 6 hr; **8 kg:** 2.5 mL q 6 hr; **less than 8 kg:** calculate dose according to body weight.

Generic Name (Content)	Trade Name	Use	Dose
Fluticasone (100 mcg), Salmetcrol (50 mcg)	Advair Diskus (Rx)	Maintenance treatment of asthma in clients 12 years and older.	One inhalation b.i.d. (morning and evening) approximately 12 hr apart.
Glyburide (1.25 mg, 2.5 mg, or 5 mg), Metformin hydrochloride (250 mg or 500 mg)	Glucovance (Rx)	Initial therapy, as an adjunct to diet and exercise, to treat type 2 diabetics whose hyperglycemia can not be treated by diet and exercise alone.	Individualize. **Initial:** 1.25 mg/250 mg once or twice daily with meals. **Use in previously treated clients (second-line therapy):** 2.5 mg/500 mg or 5 mg/500 mg b.i.d. with meals. Do not exceed 20 mg glyburide and 2000 mg metformin/day.
Hydrocodone bitartrate (5 mg), Homatropine methylbromide (1.5 mg) in each tablet or 5 mL	Hycodan (Rx, C-III)	Relief of symptoms of cough.	**Adults and children over 12 years:** 1 Tablet or 5 mL q 4–6 hr, not to exceed 6 tablets or 30 mL in 24 hr. **Children, 6–12 years:** ½ Tablet or 2.5 mL q 4–6 hr, as needed, not to exceed 3 tablets or 15 mL in 24 hr.

Generic Name (Content)	Trade Name	Use	Dose
Hydrocodone bitartrate (7.5 mg), Ibuprofen (200 mg)	Vicoprofen (Rx, C-III)	Short-term (less than 10 days) treatment of pain.	**Adults:** 1 tablet q 4 - 6 hr, as needed, not to exceed 5 tablets in a 24-hr period. Adjust dose/frequency of dosing to client needs.
Ipratropium bromide (18 mcg) and Albuterol sulfate (103 mcg) in each actuation of metered dose inhaler.	Combivent (Rx)	Treatment of COPD in those who are on regular aerosol bronchodilator therapy and who require a second bronchodilator.	2 Inhalations q 6 hr, not to exceed 12 inhalations/24 hr.
Lisinopril (20 mg), Hydrochlorothiazide (12.5 mg or 25 mg)	Prinzide 12.5 and 25, Zestoretic 20–12.5 and 20–25 (Rx)	Hypertension in clients where combination therapy is appropriate. Not for initial therapy.	**Individualized, usual:** 1 or 2 tablets daily of one of the products.
Lopinavir (133.3 mg/capsule, 80 mg/mL solution), Ritonavir (33.3 mg/capsule, 20 mg/mL solution)	Kaletra (Rx)	With other antiretroviral drugs to treat HIV infections.	3 Capsules or 5 mL b.i.d. with food.
Loratidine (5 mg), Pseudoephedrine (120 mg)	Claritin-D (Rx)	Relieve symptoms of seasonal allergic rhinitis, including asthma.	**Adults and children over 12 years:** 1 Tablet q 12 hr on an empty stomach. Give 1 tablet/day in those with a GFR less than 30 mL/min.

Generic Name (Content)	Trade Name	Use	Dose
Loratidine (10 mg), Pseudoephedrine (240 mg)	Claritin-D 24 Hour Extented Release (Rx)	Relieve symptoms of seasonal allergic rhinitis, including asthma.	**Adults:** 1 Tablet daily.
Losartan potassium (50 mg), Hydrochlorothiazide (12.5 mg)	Hyzaar (Rx)	Hypertension (not for initial treatment). Use when losartan alone is not effective or hydrochlorothiazide (25 mg) alone causes hypokalemia.	**Adults:** 1 Tablet daily. If BP not controlled after 3 weeks, can increase dose to a maximum of 2 tablets/day.
Methyldopa (250 or 500 mg), Hydrochlorothiazide (15, 25, 30, or 50 mg)	Aldoril 15, 25, D30, and D50 (Rx)	Hypertension (not for initial treatment).	**Adults:** 1 Tablet b.i.d.–t.i.d. for the first 48 hr; **then,** increase dose, depending on response, in intervals of not less than 2 days to a maximum daily dose of 3 g methyldopa and 100–200 mg hydrochlorothiazide.
Pentazocine HCl (50 mg), Naloxone HCl (0.5 mg)	Talwin NX (Rx, C-IV)	Moderate to severe pain.	**Adults:** 1 Tablet q 3–4 hr, up to 2 tablets q 3–4 hr. Daily dose should not exceed 600 mg pentazocine.

Generic Name (Content)	Trade Name	Use	Dose
Propranolol HCl (40, 80, 120, or 160 mg), Hydrochlorothiazide (25 or 50 mg)	Inderide 40/25, Inderide 80/25, Inderide LA 80/50, Inderide LA 120/50, Inderide LA 160/50 (Rx)	Hypertension (not for initial therapy).	*Inderide Tablets:* 1–2 tablets b.i.d., up to 320 mg propranolol/day. *Inderide LA Capsules:* 1 capsule per day.
Quinapril hydrochloride (10 mg or 20 mg), Hydrochlorothiazide (12.5 mg or 25 mg)	Accuretic (Rx)	Hypertension (not for initial treatment).	One 10/12.5 or 20/12.5 tablet/day if BP not controlled by quinapril alone. Also for those whose BP adequately controlled by 25 mg hydrochlorothiazide but have significant potassium loss. Those adequately treated with 20 mg quinapril and 25 mg hydrochlorothiazide may switch to 20/25 dosage form.
Rifampin (300 mg), Isoniazid (150 mg)	Rifamate, Rimactane/INH Dual Pack (Rx)	Pulmonary tuberculosis following completion of initial therapy. In malnourished clients, adolescents, or those predisposed to neuropathy, also treat with pyridoxine.	Two capsules once daily.

Generic Name (Content)	Trade Name	Use	Dose
Rifampin (120 mg), Isoniazid (50 mg), Pyrazinamide (300 mg)	Rifater (Rx)	nitial phase of the short-course (2 months) treatment of pulmonary tuberculosis. If resistance is high, add streptomycin or ethambutol. In malnourished clients, adolescents, or those predisposed to neuropathy, also treat with pyridoxine. Follow the 2-month course of treatment with Rifamate.	**Weight less than 44 kg:** 4 tablets/day given at the same time; **45–54 kg:** 5 tablets/day given at the same time; **Over 55 kg:** 6 tablets/day given at the same time.
Spironolactone (25 or 50 mg), Hydrochlorothiazide (25 or 50 mg)	Aldactazide 25 and 50 (Rx)	CHF, essential hypertension, nephrotic syndrome. Edema and/or ascites in cirrhosis of the liver.	*Edema*. **Adults, usual:** 100 mg of each drug daily (range 25–200 mg) given as single or divided doses. **Children, usual:** Equivalent to 1.65–3.3 mg/kg spironolactone. *Essential hypertension*. **Adults, usual:** 50–100 mg of each drug daily in single or divided doses.

Generic Name (Content)	Trade Name	Use	Dose
Triamterene (37.5 or 75 mg for capsules or tablets), Hydrochlorothiazide (25 mg for capsules, 25 or 50 mg for tablets)	Apo-Triazide, Dyazide, Maxzide, Maxide-25 MG, Novo-Triamzide, Nu-Triazide, Pro-Triazide (Rx)	Hypertension or edema in clients who manifest hypokalemia on hydrochlorothiazide alone. Not first line of therapy except in those in whom hypokalemia should be avoided	Triamterene/Hydrochlorothiazide: **37.5 mg/25 mg:** 1 or 2 capsules/tablets daily; **50 mg/25 mg:** 1 or 2 capsules b.i.d. after meals; **75 mg/50 mg:** 1 tablet daily.

APPENDIX 10
Drug/Food Interactions

A. DRUGS THAT SHOULD BE TAKEN WHILE FASTING

Ampicillin
AzoGantanol/Gantrisin
Bacampicillin
Bethanechol(may experience N&V)
Bisacodyl
Calcium carbonate
Captopril
Carbenicillin
Castor oil
Chloramphenicol
Cyclosporine gel caps only (do not take with fatty meals)
Demeclocycline (avoid high calcium foods/dairy products)
Dicloxacillin
Disopyramide
Digitalis preparations (not with high fiber foods)
Erythromycin base/estolate
Etidronate
Ferrous salts (not with tea, coffee, egg, cereals, fiber, or milk)
Flavoxate
Furosemide
Isoniazid
Isosorbide dinitrate
Ketoprofen (if GI distress occurs, may take with food)
Lansoprazole
Levodopa (not with high protein foods; meals delay absorption and peak plasma concentration; avoid caffeine)
Lisinopril
Lomustine (empty stomach will reduce nausea)
Methotrexate (milk, cream, or yogurt may decrease absorption)
Methyldopa (not with high protein foods; meals delay absorption and peak plasma concentration; avoid caffeine)
Nafcillin (inactivated by stomach acid; absorption variable with/without food)
Nalidixic acid
Naltrexone
Norfloxacin (milk, cream, or yogurt may decrease absorption)
Oxytetracycline (avoid dairy products and foods high in calcium)
Penicillamine (antacids, iron and food decreases absorption)
Penicillin
Phenytoin (if GI distress occurs, may take with food; food effect depends on preparation)
Propantheline
Rifampicin
Sotalol

Sulfamethoxazole
Tetracycline (avoid dairy products and foods high in calcium)
Theophylline (absorption of controlled release varies by preparation)
Thyroid hormone preparations (limit foods containing goitrogens)
Terbutaline sulfate
Trientine (antacids, iron, and food reduces absorption)
Trimethoprim

B. DRUGS THAT SHOULD BE TAKEN WITH FOOD

Buspirone
Carbamazepine (erratic absorption)
Chlorothiazide
Clofazimine
Gemfibrozil
Griseofulvin (high fat meals)
Isotretinoin
Labetatol
Lovastatin
Methenamine
Metoprolol
Nifedipine (grapefruit juice increases bioavailability)
Nitrofurantoin
Oxcarbazepine
Probucol (high fat meals)
Propranolol
Spironolactone
Trazodone
Verapamil SR (absorption varies by manufacturer; too rapid absorption may cause heart block)

C. CONSTIPATING AGENTS

Antacids
Anticholinergic drugs
  Antihistamines
  Anticholinergics
  Phenothiazines
  Tricyclic antidepressants
Corticosteroids
Clonidine
Ganglionic blocking agents
Iron supplements
Laxatives (when abused)
Lithium
MAO inhibitors
Muscle relaxants
Octreotide
Opioids
Prostaglandin synthesis inhibitors
  NSAIDS

D. DIARRHEAL AGENTS

Adrenergic neuron blockers: reserpine, guanethidine
Antibiotics (especially broad spectrum agents)
Cholinergic agonists and cholinesterase inhibitors
Erythromycin
Osmotic and stimulant laxatives
Metoclopramide
Quinidine

E. TYRAMINE CONTAINING FOODS

Moderate amounts of tyramine:

- Broad beans
- Raspberries
- Banana peel
- Cheese (all except cream cheese and cottage cheese)
- Imitation cheese
- Prepared meats (sausage, chopped liver, pate, salami, mortadella)
- Meat extracts
- Concentrated yeast extracts/Brewer's yeast
- Liquid and powdered protein supplements
- Fermented soy products: fermented bean curd, soya bean paste, miso soup
- Hydrolyzed protein extracts for sauces, soups, gravies
- Fermented cabbage products: sauerkraut, kimchee
- Chianti, vermouth
- Nonalcoholic beers
- Some non-United States brands of beer

Significant amounts of tyramine:

- Avocado
- Yogurt
- Cream from fresh pasteurized milk
- Soy sauce
- Peanuts
- Chocolate
- Red and white wines, port wines
- Distilled spirits

F. FOODS CONTAINING GOITROGENS

- Asparagus
- Brussels sprouts
- Cabbage
- Kale
- Lettuce
- Peas
- Soy beans
- Spinach
- Turnip greens
- Watercress
- Other leafy green vegetables

G. COUMARIN ANTICOAGULANTS AND DIETARY EFFECTS

Consumption of vitamin K enriched foods may counteract the effects of anticoagulants since the drugs act through antagonism of vitamin K. Advise the client on anticoagulants to maintain a steady, consistent intake of vitamin K containing foods. The drug monograph for warfarin clearly lists these foods. Additionally, certain herbal teas (Woodruff, tonka beans, melitot) contain natural coumarins that can potentiate the effects of Coumadin and should be avoided. Large amounts of avocado also potentiate the drug's effects. Brussels sprouts and other cruciferous vegetables increase the catabolism of warfarin thereby decreasing its anticoagulant activities.

H. GENERAL DRUG CLASS RECOMMENDATIONS

Antacids: take 1 hr after or between meals. Avoid dairy foods as the protein in them can increase stomach acid.

Antihistamines: take on an empty stomach to increase effectiveness.

Analgesic/Antipyretic: take on an empty stomach as food may slow the absorption.

NSAIDS: take with food or milk to prevent irritation of the stomach.

Corticosteroids: take with food to decrease stomach upset

Bronchodilators with theophylline: high-fat meals may increase bioavailability while high-carbohydrate meals may decrease it. Food increases absorption of Theo-24 and Uniphyl which may cause increased N&V, headache and irritability.

Diuretics: vary in interactions; some cause loss of potassium, calcium, and magnesium. Avoid salty food and natural black licorice as these increase K and Mg losses. Large doses of vitamin D can elevate blood pressure.

ACE inhibitors: take captopril and moexipril 1 hr before or 2 hrs after meals; food decreases absorption. Avoid high potassium foods as ACE increases K+.

HMG-CoA reductase inhibitors: take lovastatin with the evening meal to enhance absorption.

Anticoagulants: high vitamin K produces blood-clotting substance and may reduce drug effectiveness. Vitamin E >400 IU may prolong clotting time and increase bleeding risk.

Antibiotics: penicillin generally should be taken on an empty stomach; may take with food if GI upset occurs. Do not mix with acidic foods such as coffee, citrus fruits, and tomatoes as the acid interferes with absorption of penicillin, ampicillin, erythromycin and cloxacillin.

Quinolones: Take on an empty stomach 1 hr before or 2 hrs after meals. May take with food for GI upset but avoid calcium containing foods such as milk, yogurt, vitamins/minerals containing iron and antacids because they decrease drug concentrations. Caffeine containing products may lead to excitability and nervousness.

Cephalosporins: take on an empty stomach 1 hr before or 2 hrs after meals. May take with food if GI upset occurs.

Macrolides Take on an empty stomach 1 hr before or 2 hrs after meals. May take with food for GI upset.

Sulfonamides: take on an empty stomach 1 hr before or 2 hrs after meals. May take with food if GI upset occurs.

Tetracyclines: take on an empty stomach 1 hr before or 2 hrs after meals. May take with food but avoid dairy products, antacids, and vitamins containing iron with tetracycline.

Nitroimadazole (metronidazole): avoid alcohol or food prepared with alcohol for at least three days after finishing the medicine. Alcohol may cause nausea, abdominal cramps, vomiting, headaches, and flushing.

Laxatives: avoid dairy foods as calcium can decrease absorption.

MAO inhibitors: have many dietary restrictions, so follow dietary guidelines as prescribed. Foods or alcoholic beverages containing tyramine may cause a fatal increase in BP.

Anti-anxiety agents: caffeine may cause excitability, nervousness, and hyperactivity lessening the anti-anxiety drug effects.

Antidepressant drugs: may be taken with or without food.

Antifungals: avoid taking with dairy products; avoid alcohol.

H_2 blockers: may take with or without regard to food.

APPENDIX 11

Commonly Used Herbal Products

General Statement: Herbs are medicinal plants, also called botanicals or phytomedicines. Phytomedicines are medicinal products that contain plant material as their pharmacologically active component. They are often complex mixtures of compounds that generally do not exert a strong, immediate action. Consumers use herbal products as therapeutic agents for the treatment/cure of illness/disease symptoms and prophylactically to prevent disease and to maintain health and wellness. Consumer use of herbs and medicinal products over the past two decades has risen dramatically. These agents are found in retail pharmacies, grocery stores, health food shops, corner markets, and other large outlet stores as well as mail order and TV/Internet sales. Some major health insurance companies are including coverage for herbs under "alternative therapies" and many more are considering this coverage. Herbs are regulated as Dietary Supplements under the Dietary Supplement Health and Education Act of 1994 (DSHEA). Extracts are concentrated preparations of a liquid, powdered, or viscous consistency that are usually made from dried plant parts by maceration or percolation. Tincture is an alcoholic or hydroalcoholic solution prepared from botanicals. Plant juices are formed from the freshly harvested plant parts macerated in water and pressed. Herbal teas are potable infusions made from infusion (pour boiling water over the herb), decoction (cover herb with cold water and bring to a boil and simmer for 5-10 min), or cold maceration (place herb in tap water and let stand at room temperature for 6-8 hr). Always ask about herbs, vitamins, teas or other remedies that client may be using for a problem or to maintain health/wellness. Clients generally do not consider these as medicines and often fail to mention them during a drug history.

Commonly Used Herbal Products

The following table presents some of the commonly used herbal products. It is not intended to be an extensive listing of information for each product. Rather, the table contains important information regarding use(s), dose, side effects, and other information.

Name(s)	Use(s)	Dose	Contraindications	Side Effects	Other Information
Aloe gel, Aloe vera	Gel is used in cosmetics and topical products to heal wounds, burns, skin ulcers, frostbite, dry skin. Laxative.	Aloe vera powder, aqueous or aqueous-alcoholic extract in powder/liquid/tablets/capsule forms: 100–200 mg (internal use). Use smallest dose to maintain a soft stool.	Intestinal obstruction, Crohn's disease, ulcerative colitis, appendicitis, abdominal pain of unknown origin. Children under 12 years, pregnancy, lactation	GI cramps. Long term use/abuse: Potassium deficiency, albuminuria, hematuria.	Should not be used for longer than 1–2 weeks without medical advice. Potassium deficiency can be increased by simultaneous use of thiazides, corticosteroids, and licorice.
Bilberry fruit/leaf, blueberry	*Fruit:* Nonspecific, acute diarrhea. Mild inflammation of the mucous membranes of the mouth and throat. Improve night vision. *Leaf:* Arthritis, gout, dermatitis, hemorrhoids, CV problems, and prevention/treatment of GI, kidney, and GU symptoms and diseases.	**Fruit. External:** 10% decoction. **Internal:** 20–60 g/day of the fruit. **Leaf.** Used as a tea (1–2 teaspoons of the finely chopped leaf in 150 mL boiling water for 5–10 min.)	Chronic use of the leaf may cause anemia, jaundice, "wasting," excitation, and disturbances of muscle contraction.	Has an astringent effect. Consult a provider if diarrhea lasts for more than 3–4 days. Avoid prolonged use of the tea.	

Name(s)	Use(s)	Dose	Contraindications	Side Effects	Other Information
Cascara sagrada bark	Laxative.	**Capsules, fluid extract, syrup, tablets:** 20–30 mg hydroxyanthracene derivatives/day, calculated as cascaroside A. May be used as a tea (2 g finely chopped bark in 150 mL boiling water for 5–10 min). **Fluid extract:** 2–5 mL t.i.d. Use smallest dose to maintain a soft stool.	Intestinal obstruction, Crohn's disease, colitis, appendicitis, abdominal pain of unknown origin. Children under 12 years, pregnancy, lactation.	Abdominal cramps. Long term use/abuse: Potassium deficiency, albuminuria, hematuria, disturbed cardiac function.	Do not use for more than 1–2 weeks without medical advice. Potassium deficiency can be increased by concomitant use of thiazides, corticosteroids, and licorice root.
Cat's Claw	Diverticulitis, hemorrhoids, peptic ulcer disease, colitis, parasites, antihypertensive, hypocholesterolemic, AIDS (in combination with AZT)	**Capsules:** 300 mg t.i.d.; **Timed-release capsules:** 1000 mg once daily; **Liquid concentrate:** Diluted in water and taken 1–3 times/day; **Bark:** Used for tea (1 g root bark in 150 mL boiling water for 5–10 min).		Diarrhea (high doses), hypotension. May contribute to unusual bruising or bleeding gums.	Use with caution in those taking antihypertensives.

Name(s)	Use(s)	Dose	Contraindications	Side Effects	Other Information
Chamomile, German Chamomile	**Topical:** Inflammation of the mouth, skin, respiratory tract (inhalation). **Internal:** GI antispasmodic and anti-inflammatory. Allegedly has sedative, hypnotic, analgesic, and immunostimulant effects.	**PO. Dried flower heads:** 2–8 g t.i.d. or 1 cup of tea t.i.d.–q.i.d. **Liquid extract (1:1 in 45% alcohol):** 1–4 mL t.i.d. **Topical.** Prepared tea (use 4 tsp. of dried flower heads in 1.5 cups boiling water for 15 min; strain).		Anaphylaxis, dermatitis, other hypersensitivity reactions.	Cautious use in those allergic to ragweed, asters, chrysanthemums, or other members of the Asteraceae family. Do not confuse with Roman Chamomile.
Chondroitin Sulfate	Osteoarthritis, osteoporosis, ischemic heart disease, hyperlipidemia. Ophthalmic product (FDA-approved) for dry eyes, as a viscoelastic agent in cataract surgery, and to preserve corneas for transplantation.	**Osteoarthritis. PO:** 200–400 b.i.d.–t.i.d. or 1200 mg/day as a single dose.	Pregnancy, lactation.	Epigastric pain, nausea, allergic reactions.	Has also been used IM.

Name(s)	Use(s)	Dose	Contraindications	Side Effects	Other Information
Comfrey	**External:** Wound healing, ulcers, bruises/sprains. **Internal:** Stomach ulcers, "blood purifier," prevention of kidney stones, rheumatic/pulmonary disorders.	**Topical:** Ointments/other topical products containing 5–20% comfrey. **PO.** Do not exceed 100 mcg/day of pyrrolizidine alkaloids.	Pregnancy, lactation. Use on broken skin.	Hazardous to health due to hepatotoxic alkaloids; internal use not safe. Veno-occlusive disease.	Use for no more than 10 days; maximum use is 4–6 weeks/year.
Cranberry	Urinary tract infections, urinary deodorizer for incontient clients.	**PO. Juice:** 3 oz/day to prevent urinary infection and 12–32 oz/day to treat infection. **Capsules:** 6 capsules (equivalent to 3 oz juice)/day. Some recommend 300–400 mg of concentrated juice capsules b.i.d.		High doses can cause diarrhea and other GI symptoms.	Do not confuse with highbush cranberry.
Dong Quai	Menstrual cramps/irregularity, retarded flow, menopausal symptoms. Treatment of skin pigmentation and psoriasis.	**PO, women:** 3–4 g/day in divided doses with meals.	Pregnancy, lactation.	Severe photodermatitis and photosensitivity. Potentially carcinogenic and mutagenic.	May potentiate the effect of warfarin.

Name(s)	Use(s)	Dose	Contraindications	Side Effects	Other Information
Echinacea	**Topical:** Minor infections, snake/spider bites, poorly healing wounds, chronic ulcers. **Internal:** Viral, bacterial, and *Candida* infections, including colds, flu, urogenital, and upper respiratory tract infections. Immunostimulant.	**Topical:** Use cream or liquid t.i.d. **Internal:** 0.5–1 mL of the fluid extract (1:1 in 45% alcohol) t.i.d. or 300 mg of the solid extract (6.5:1) t.i.d.	Pregnancy. Use with immunosuppressants or in those with chronic progressive systemic diseases (e.g., tuberculosis, leucosis, multiple sclerosis, collagenosis).	N&V. Hypersensitivity reaction in those allergic to sunflower seeds/flowers. Tingling of the tongue; fever (due to the freshly pressed juice).	Use with caution in those with AIDS, rheumatoid arthritis, lupus, or leukemia.
Evening primrose oil	Breast disorders, premenstrual syndrome, hypercholesterolemia, eczema, psoriasis, multiple sclerosis, lupus erythematosus, antihypertensive.	**PO:** 4 g/day (maximum), equivalent to 300–360 mg gamma-linolenic acid.		Indigestion, nausea, soft stools, headache. Reduces platelet aggregation (monitor bleeding times and PT in those on antiplatelet drugs or warfarin).	If used with phenothiazines or TCAs, may worsen temporal lobe epilepsy or schizophrenia.

Name(s)	Use(s)	Dose	Contraindications	Side Effects	Other Information
Feverfew	Fever, arthritis. Prophylaxis for migraine headache.	**Dry powdered leaf capsules/tablets:** 300 mg 2–6 times/day. To prevent migraine, 50–100 mg of dried leaves/day have been used.	Pregnancy and in children less than 2 years.	Dizziness, lightheadedness, nausea, indigesion, bloating, gas, diarrhea or constipation, palpitations, heavy menstrual flow, contact dermatitis, rash. Aphthous ulcers due to chewing leaves. Rebound headache may occur if abruptly discontinued.	May take 4–6 months for beneficial effects. Reduces platelet aggregation (monitor bleeding times and PT in those on antiplatelet drugs or warfarin).
Garlic	Lower serum cholesterol and BP. Mild respiratory and GI tract infections. GI disturbances.	**PO:** 10 mg of allicin, a total of allicin potential of 4 mg/day, or 1 clove (4 g) of fresh garlic/day.	Topical use. Large doses in pregnancy and lactation.	Mouth and GI burning or irritation, heartburn, flatulence, N&V, diarrhea, changes in gut flora, allergic reactions, odor to skin/breath. May decrease blood sugar (monitor).	Reduces platelet aggregation (monitor bleeding times and PT in those on antiplatelet drugs or warfarin). May potentiate antihypertensives. To assure efficacy, monitor lipids for 3 months.

Name(s)	Use(s)	Dose	Contraindications	Side Effects	Other Information
Ginger, Jamaica Ginger, African Ginger, Cochin Ginger	Prevent morning sickness, motion sickness. Treat arthritis, muscle pain, migraine headache.	**Powdered ginger root:** Prevent motion sickness: 1 g 30 min before travel followed by 500 mg q.i.d. Prevent morning sickness: 250 mg q.i.d. Arthritis: 125–1,000 mg q.i.d., not to exceed 4 g/day.	With gallstones, use only after consultation with provider. Large doses during lactation.	High doses: GI discomfort if taken on an empty stomach; CNS depression, and cardiac arrhythmias.	Inhibits platelet aggregation (monitor bleeding times and PT in those on antiplatelet drugs or warfarin). May alter effect of calcium channel blockers.
Ginkgo biloba	Short-term memory loss, headache, vertigo, tinnitus due to vascular insufficiency. Depression. Intermittent claudication. Early Alzheimer's disease, senility. Diabetic retinopathy. Asthma.	100–300 mg/day, to provide 10 mg ginsenosides.	Pregnancy, lactation.	GI discomfort, headache, allergic skin reactions, contact dermatitis, severe allergic reactions, restlessness, diarrhea. Inhibits platelet aggregation (monitor bleeding time and PT in those taking anticoagulants).	May take up to 12 weeks for beneficial effect to be seen. Cross allergy in those allergic to poison ivy, poison oak, poison sumac, mango rind, and cashew shell oil.

Name(s)	Use(s)	Dose	Contraindications	Side Effects	Other Information
Ginseng root	Improve cognitive function/concentration, fatigue, stress, enhance immune function, menopausal symptoms, impotence/infertility, reduce cholesterol.	**PO:** 100–300 mg/day, to provide 10 mg ginsenosides.	Panax ginseng in newborns.	Breast tenderness, insomnia, diarrhea, skin eruptions, nervousness/excitation (decreases with use). Hypoglycemia (monitor diabetics). Decreased platelet adhesiveness (monitor bleeding times and PT in those taking anticoagulants).	May interfere with digoxin activity or monitoring.
Goldenseal	**External:** Treatment of trachoma. **Internal:** Diarrhea due to *E. coli*.	**Topical mouthwash:** Use t.i.d.–q.i.d. Prepare by steeping 6 g of dried herb in 150 mL boiling water for 5–10 min; strain and allow to cool. **Internal, dried root or rhizome:** 0.5–1 g t.i.d. **Use as a tea:** Prepare by simmering 0.5–1 g of dried root or rhizome in 150 mL boiling water for 5–10 min; strain. **Liquid extract (1:1, 60% ethanol):** 0.3–1 mL t.i.d. **Tincture (1:10, 60% ethanol):** 2–4 mL t.i.d.	Pregnancy (likely unsafe), lactation. Hypertension, infectious or inflammatory GI disease.	Chronic use: Digestive disorders, constipation, excitation, hallucinations, delirium, decrease in B vitamin absorption.	May interfere with antacids, sucralfate, H-2 antagonists, proton pump inhibitors, antihypertensives. Additive effects with CNS depressants.

Name(s)	Use(s)	Dose	Contraindications	Side Effects	Other Information
Grape Seed Extract, Muskat	Varicose veins, hypoxia secondary to atherosclerosis, myocardial or cerebral infarction.	**Capsules/Tablets, initial:** 75–300 mg/day for 3 weeks; **maintenance:** 40–80 mg/day. **Concentrate liquid:** 15 mLin one cup of hot or cold water.	In pregnancy/lactation, avoid amounts greater than in food.	None reported.	May increase the effect of warfarin.
Green Tea	Stomach disorders, vomiting, diarrhea, headaches, as a diuretic. Traditional use to promote health and prevent cancer (anti-oxidant effect). As a beverage.	No reliable information on safe and effective dose. As many as ten cups of tea/day are consumed by some.	Use in infants, lactation. Use in those with gastric/duodenal ulcers.	Hyperacidity, gastric irritation, decreased appetite, constipation, diarrhea, restlessness, irritability, insomnia, palpitations, vertigo.	Increased CNS stimulation when used with caffeine-containing products or ephedrine. Many possible drug interactions.
Hawthorn Flower, Fruit, Leaves	Heart failure, hypertension, arteriosclerosis, angina pectoris, Buerger's disease, paroxysmal tachycardia.	**Dried fruit:** 300–1,000 mg t.i.d. **Fruit fluid extract (1:1 in 25% alcohol):** 0.5–1 mL t.i.d. **Fruit tincture (1:5 in 45% alcohol):** 1–2 mL t.i.d.	Pregnancy, lactation. Use with cardiac glycoside-containing products.	Nausea, GI complaints, fatigue, hand rash, palpitations, headache, dizziness, sleeplessness, agitation, circulatory disturbances.	Additive effects when used with vasodilators or CNS depressants.

Name(s)	**Use(s)**	**Dose**	**Contraindications**	**Side Effects**	**Other Information**
Kava Kava	Stress, nervous anxiety, insomnia, restlessness.	**Anxiolytic:** 45–70 mg kavalactones t.i.d. **Sedative:** 180–210 mg kavalactones 1 hr before bedtime.	Alcohol use. Endogenous depression. Safety/efficacy not known in pregnancy/lactation.	GI discomfort, allergic skin reactions. Chronic use: Yellow discoloration of skin, hair, nails.	Additive effects with CNS depressants. May affect motor reflexes and judgment. May worsen Parkinson symptoms. Do not use more than 3 months without medical advice.
Licorice, Glycyrrhiza, Licorice Root	Upper respiratory tract mucous membrane inflammation. Gastric/duodenal ulcers.	**Root:** 5–15 g/day, equivalent to 200–600 mg glycyrrhizin.	Cholestatic liver disorders, liver cirrhosis, hypokalemia, hypertonia, severe kidney impairment, pregnancy.	Chronic use/high doses: Sodium and water retention, potassium loss, hypertension, edema, hypokalemia.	Use with thiazides increases potassium loss; may increase digitalis sensitivity. Do not use more than 4–6 weeks without medical advice.
Melatonin	Insomnia, especially to overcome jet lag or shift-work disorder.	**PO:** 0.3–5 mg at bedtime for sleep disturbances. For jet lag, 5 mg at bedtime for one week beginning three days before the flight.	Use in depression, children, pregnancy, lactation.	Headache, transient depression, daytime fatigue/drowsiness, dizziness, abdominal cramps, irritability, reduced alertness, tiredness.	Additive effects with CNS depressants. Use with caution if driving or operating hazardous machinery.

Name(s)	Use(s)	Dose	Contraindications	Side Effects	Other Information
Milk Thistle, Our Lady's Thistle	Liver cirrhosis, chronic hepatitis, gallstones, psoriasis, liver protectant from toxins (e.g., butyrophenones, phenothiazines, phenytoin, acetaminophen, alcohol, halothane).	**PO:** 200 mg t.i.d. standardized to provide at least 140 mg silymarin t.i.d. or 100–200 mg of phosphatidylcholine-bound silymarin b.i.d.		Loose stools (prevent by ingesting psyllium and oat bran), mild allergic reactions.	Possible cross allergy in those sensitive to ragweed, chrysanthemums, marigolds, daisies.
Saw Palmetto	Benign prostatic hypertrophy.	**PO:** 160 mg standardized fat-soluble extract b.i.d. (containing 85–95% fatty acids and sterols). Or, 0.5–1 g of the dried berry or one cup of tea t.i.d. Prepare tea by simmering 0.5–1 g dried berry in 150 mL boiling water for 5–10 min; strain.	Pregnancy, use in breast cancer.	Headache, mild abdominal pain, nausea, dizziness.	May require 4–6 weeks for effect to be seen. May interfere with oral contraceptive or hormone therapy. No significant effect on serum prostate-specific antigen levels. Due to lack of evidence, the FDA has banned all OTC medicines to treat BPH.

Name(s)	Use(s)	Dose	Contraindications	Side Effects	Other Information
Senna leaf	Laxative.	**PO:** 20–30 mg hydroxyanthracene derivatives/day calculated as sennoside B. Use lowest dose to maintain a soft stool.	Intestinal obstruction, Crohn's disease, colitis ulcerosa, appendicitis, abdominal pain of unknown origin. Children under 12 years. Pregnancy, lactation.	GI cramps, abdominal discomfort, colic. Chronic use/abuse: Potassium deficiency, albuminuria, hematuria, "sluggish" colon.	Loss of potassium may potentiate effect of cardiac glycosides, diuretics, and corticosteroids on heart function.
St. John's Wort	**External:** Herpes simplex I, minor wounds/burns. **Internal:** Mild to moderate depression, anxiety, antiviral (HIV, AIDS).	**External:** Apply oil or cream b.i.d.–t.i.d. **Internal:** 300 mg t.i.d., standardized to 0.3% hypericin extract.	Use with MAOIs, selective serotonin reuptake inhibitors, and other antidepressant drugs. Pregnancy, lactation.	Photosensitivity in fair-skinned clients. GI symptoms, fatigue, delayed hypersensitivity. Serotonin syndrome. Possible hypertensive crisis if taken with tyramine-containing foods.	To prevent GI upset, take with food.
Valerian	Insomnia, anxiety, stress.	**Insomnia:** 150–300 mg valerian extract (0.8% valeric acid) 30–45 min before bed. **Anxiety:** 150 mg q.i.d.	Pregnancy, lactation.	Morning drowsiness (rare), headache, excitability, cardiac disturbances, uneasy feeling.	Additive effect with CNS depressants. Do not confuse with Valium.

Name(s)	Use(s)	Dose	Contraindications	Side Effects	Other Information
Yohimbe Bark	Impotence, as an aphrodisiac. Exhaustion.	Available as a prescription drug with no FDA-approved uses.	Liver and kidney dysfunction. Pregnancy, lactation.	Nervous excitation, tremor, sleeplessness, anxiety, increased BP, tachycardia, N&V.	The FDA has determined the active compound (yohimbine) to be unsafe and ineffective for OTC use. Possibility of hypertensive crisis when taken with caffeine, tyramine-containing foods, or ephedrine. Additive therapeutic/toxic effects if taken with MAOIs. Interference with drugs to treat hypertension.

APPENDIX 12
Dosage Terminology

Initial dose – the first (starting) dose of the medication given

Maintenance dose – the amount of the drug given to keep bloodstream/tissue levels of a specific drug at therapeutic concentration

Maximum dose – the largest amount of a drug that can be given safely to humans (usually published in the product labeling information accompanying the drug)

Minimum dose – the smallest amount of a drug that will be effective

Therapeutic dose – the amount of a specific drug needed to cause the desired effect in a specific treatment regimen.

Divided dose – a fractional portion of the total dose given at specified intervals

Unit dose – an individually packed premeasured amount of medication for a one-time administration (one dose)

Lethal dose – the amount of medication that could kill a human (the amount varies with age and size, i.e., the amount of medication given to infants and children is usually much smaller that the amount given to adults)

Index

Valnac **(Betamethasone valerate)**, 202
Valproic acid (Depakene), **854**
Valsartan (Diovan), **856**
Valtrex **(Valacyclovir hydrochloride)**, 853
Vancenase AQ Forte **(Beclomethasone dipropionate)**, 197
Vancenase AQ Nasal **(Beclomethasone dipropionate)**, 197
Vancenase AQ 84 mcg Double Strength **(Beclomethasone dipropionate)**, 197
Vancenase Nasal Inhaler **(Beclomethasone dipropionate)**, 197
Vanceril **(Beclomethasone dipropionate)**, 197
Vanceril DS **(Beclomethasone dipropionate)**, 197
Vancocin **(Vancomycin hydrochloride)**, 857
Vancoled **(Vancomycin hydrochloride)**, 857
Vancomycin hydrochloride (Vancocin), **857**
Vantin **(Cefpodoxime proxetil)**, 245
Vaponefrin **(Epinephrine hydrochloride)**, 362
Vascor **(Bepridil hydrochloride)**, 201
Vaseretic (ENALAPRIL MALEATE AND HYDROCHLOROTHIAZIDE), 358
Vasotec **(Enalapril maleate)**, 356
Vasotec I.V. **(Enalapril maleate)**, 356
Vatronol Nose Drops **(Ephedrine sulfate)**, 361
Vectrin **(Minocycline hydrochloride)**, 583
Veetids '250' **(Penicillin V potassium)**, 666
Velosef **(Cephradine)**, 252
Velosulin Human BR **(Insulin injection)**, 462
Veltane **(Brompheniramine maleate)**, 215
Venlafaxine hydrochloride (Effexor), **858**
Ventodisk Disk/Diskhaler 🍁 **(Albuterol)**, 156
Ventolin **(Albuterol)**, 156
Ventolin Rotacaps **(Albuterol)**, 156
Verapamil (Calan, Isoptin), **860**
Verelan **(Verapamil)**, 860
Vermox **(Mebendazole)**, 542
Versed **(Midazolam hydrochloride)**, 579
Vesanoid **(Tretinoin)**, 837
Vexol **(Rimexolone)**, 750
Viagra **(Sildenafil citrate)**, 769
Vibramycin **(Doxycycline calcium)**, 349
Vibramycin **(Doxycycline hyclate)**, 349
Vibramycin **(Doxycycline monohydrate)**, 349
Vibramycin IV **(Doxycycline hyclate)**, 349
Vibra-Tabs **(Doxycycline hyclate)**, 349
Vibra-Tabs C-Pak 🍁 **(Doxycycline hyclate)**, 349
Vick's Formula 44 **(Dextromethorphan hydrobromide)**, 317
Vick's Formula 44 Pediatric Formula **(Dextromethorphan hydrobromide)**, 317
Vicks Sinex **(Phenylephrine hydrochloride)**, 679
Vicoprofen (HYDROCODONE BITARTRATE AND IBUPROFEN), 447
Vidarabine (Vira-A), **862**
Videx **(Didanosine)**, 323
Viokase **(Pancrelipase)**, 649
Viokase 🍁 **(Pancrelipase)**, 649
Vioxx **(Rofecoxib)**, 757
Vira-A **(Vidarabine)**, 862
Viracept **(Nelfinavir mesylate)**, 610
Viramune **(Nevirapine)**, 613
Visken **(Pindolol)**, 690
Vistacrom 🍁 **(Cromolyn sodium)**, 298
Vistaril **(Hydroxyzine hydrochloride)**, 452
Vistaril **(Hydroxyzine pamoate)**, 452
Vistazine 50 **(Hydroxyzine hydrochloride)**, 452
Vitamin A acid (Retin-A), **837**
Vitamin B_1 (Betaxin), **812**
Vitamin B_6 Nestrex, **727**
Vitamin B_{12} (Kaybovite-1000, Redisol), **299**
Vitamin K_1 (Aqua-Mephyton), **687**
Vitamins, 135
Vitinoin 🍁 **(Tretinoin)**, 837
Vitrasert **(Ganciclovir sodium)**, 415
Vivelle **(Estradiol transdermal system)**, 374
Vivol 🍁 **(Diazepam)**, 318
Vivox **(Doxycycline hyclate)**, 349
V-Lax **(Psyllium hydrophilic muciloid)**, 725
Volmax **(Albuterol)**, 156
Voltaren **(Diclofenac sodium)**, 320
Voltaren Ophthalmic **(Diclofenac sodium)**, 320
Voltaren Ophtha 🍁 **(Diclofenac sodium)**, 320
Voltaren Rapide 🍁 **(Diclofenac potassium)**, 320
Voltaren-XR **(Diclofenac sodium)**, 320

Warfarin sodium (Coumadin), **863**
Warfilone 🍁 **(Warfarin sodium)**, 863
Webber Calcium Carbonate 🍁 **(Calcium carbonate)**, 227
Wellbutrin **(Bupropion hydrochloride)**, 218
Wellbutrin SR **(Bupropion hydrochloride)**, 218
Wellcovorin **(Leucovorin calcium)**, 507
Wellferon **(Interferon alfa-n1 lymphoblastoid)**, 470
Westcort **(Hydrocortisone valerate)**, 448
Winpred 🍁 **(Prednisone)**, 707
Wycillin **(Penicillin G procaine, intramuscular)**, 665
Wymox **(Amoxicillin)**, 172
Wytensin **(Guanabenz acetate)**, 432

Xalatan **(Latanoprost)**, 504
Xanax **(Alprazolam)**, 161
Xanax TS 🍁 **(Alprazolam)**, 161
Xylocaine HCl IV for Cardiac Arrhythmias **(Lidocaine hydrochloride)**, 519
Xylocard 🍁 **(Lidocaine hydrochloride)**, 519

Zaditor **(Ketotifen fumarate)**, 497
Zafirlukast (Accolate), **867**
Zagam **(Sparfloxacin)**, 779
Zalcitabine (Hivid), **867**
Zaleplon (Sonata), **870**
Zanaflex **(Tizanidine hydrochloride)**, 821
Zanamivir (Relenza), **871**
Zantac **(Ranitidine hydrochloride)**, 739
Zantac-C 🍁 **(Ranitidine hydrochloride)**, 739
Zantac Efferdose **(Ranitidine hydrochloride)**, 739